Lung
Function

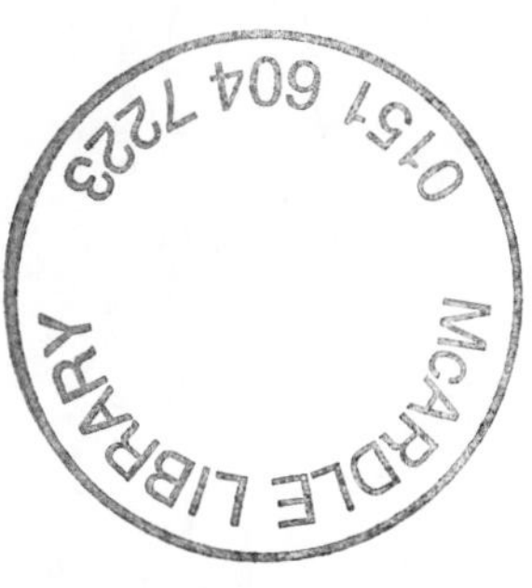

Lung Function

Physiology, Measurement and Application in Medicine

J. E. Cotes
DM, DSc (Oxon), FRCP, FFOM, Dhc, Warsaw
Visitor, University Department of Physiological Sciences
Formerly Reader in Respiratory Physiology,
External Scientific Staff of Medical Research Council, and
Honorary Consultant in Clinical Respiratory Physiology
Newcastle upon Tyne, UK

D. J. Chinn
BSc, PhD, MSc (Public Health)
Senior Research Fellow in Epidemiology,
Centre for Primary and Community Care,
University of Sunderland,
Sunderland, UK
(Present address: Senior Research Fellow,
School of Clinical Sciences and Community Health,
University of Edinburgh, UK)

M. R. Miller
BSc, MD, FRCP
Consultant Respiratory Physician
University Hospital Birmingham NHS Trust
Birmingham, UK

SIXTH EDITION

Blackwell
Publishing

© 1965, 1968, 1975, 1979, 1993, 2006 Blackwell Publishing Ltd
Blackwell Publishing, Inc., 350 Main Street, Malden, Massachusetts 02148-5020, USA
Blackwell Publishing Ltd, 9600 Garsington Road, Oxford OX4 2DQ, UK
Blackwell Publishing Asia Pty Ltd, 550 Swanston Street, Carlton, Victoria 3053, Australia

The right of the Author to be identified as the Author of this Work has been asserted in accordance with the Copyright, Designs and Patents Act 1988.

All rights reserved. No part of this publication may be reproduced, stored in a retrieval system, or transmitted, in any form or by any means, electronic, mechanical, photocopying, recording or otherwise, except as permitted by the UK Copyright, Designs and Patents Act 1988, without the prior permission of the publisher.

First published 1965
Second edition 1968
Third edition 1975
Fourth edition 1979
Fifth edition 1993
Polish edition 1969
Italian edition 1978
Sixth edition 2006

2 2006

Library of Congress Cataloging-in-Publication Data

Cotes, J. E.
Lung function : physiology, measurement and application in medicine / J.E. Cotes, D.J. Chinn, M.R. Miller.--6th ed.
p. ; cm.
Includes bibliographical references and index.
ISBN-13: 978-0-632-06493-9
ISBN-10: 0-632-06493-5
1. Pulmonary function tests. 2. Lungs--Physiology. 3. Respiration.
[DNLM: 1. Lung--Physiology. 2. Lung Diseases--physiopathology. 3. Respiratory Function Tests. 4. Respiratory Physiology. WF 600 C843L 2006] I. Chinn, D. J. (David J.) II. Miller, M. R. (Martin Raymond), 1949- III. Title.

RC734.P84C68 2006
616.2′40754--dc22

2005026837

ISBN-13: 978-0-6320-6493-9

A catalogue record for this title is available from the British Library

Set in 9.5/12pt Minion & ITC Stone Sans by TechBooks, New Delhi, India
Printed and bound in India by Replika Press PVT Ltd, Harayana, India

Commissioning Editor: Maria Khan
Editorial Assistant: Saskia Van der Linden
Development Editor: Rob Blundell
Production Controller: Kate Charman

For further information on Blackwell Publishing, visit our website:
http://www.blackwellpublishing.com

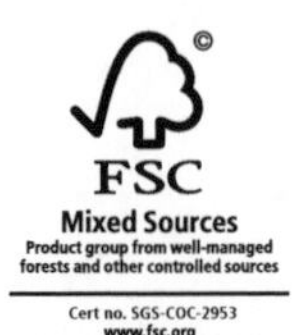

Contents

Part 5 Breathing During Sleep, 453

Part 6 Potentially Adverse Environments, 471

Part 7 Lung Function in Clinical Practice, 529

Foreword

It is not every day one of my icons asks for my opinion. This is that day and I am deeply honored to have been asked to write the Foreword to this edition of John Cotes' Lung Function. I have admired this book in its earlier incarnations and am happy to report this is perhaps the best of all.

For this 6th edition, Dr Cotes has been ably assisted by two other authorities in pulmonary medicine and lung physiology (Dr David Chinn and Dr Martin Miller) and obtained critiques by other experts for individual chapters. It is the most comprehensive and up-to-date book on lung function testing and pulmonary physiology available and has elements that will be of importance for everyone who works in the field. Moreover, it is a pleasure to read. The style is crisp, clean, and precise.

Early chapters cover the evolution of the earth's atmosphere, the early history of lung physiology and the developmental aspects of the respiratory system. They are followed by a chapter summarizing what you need to know to assess lung function including the equipment you need and measurement techniques. The discussion of numerical interpretation of lung function presents impressive illustrations showing how using numbers improperly can result in errors in interpreting physiologic variables. It was good to be reminded that errors can occur with as simple a process as how and when numbers are rounded and the discussion of why errors occur at the boundaries of the normal distributions was particularly insightful. Chapters on flow limitation and the forced volumes and flows provide clear information for both the expert and the novice.

There are sections on lung function physiology for the complete spectrum of human life (from birth to old age). Since I work mostly with adults, I was intrigued with the information on infant lung function. For older people, the mechanisms for the normal aging changes were particularly enlightening.

Reference values were covered in some detail, with emphasis on the issues that must be addressed to optimize the value of reference comparisons. The issues involved in choosing a set of reference values are addressed and there is an entire chapter on reference values in non-Caucasians.

There are chapters dedicated to special circumstances including high altitude, aviation physiology, exercise, near drowning, diving and hyperbaric oxygen therapy. Another chapter looks at respiratory hazards in home and occupational environments.

I found chapter 39 on Strategies for Assessment (of lung function) to be particularly informative. The reason airways resistance has not claimed a spot in routine pulmonary function testing is clarified. The chapter goes far beyond the primary tests offered in most laboratories and includes testing strategies for diseases. The comprehensive interpretative flow diagram is somewhat different from that included in the recently published American Thoracic Society (ATS)/European Respiratory Society (ERS) recommendations but is a good adjunct to it. The differences in the diagrams enhanced my understanding of the strategies in both.

Chapter 40 focuses on lung function in several lung disease categories that constitute the majority of all pulmonary patients, i.e. asthma, COPD, emphysema and lung fibrosis. This chapter in particular deepened my understanding of the physiology in each category. The descriptions of how other diseases affect the lungs was particularly illuminating. A large number of diseases are catalogued and the descriptions of lung effects are concise and helpful.

This is a book to read straight through and also to keep at the ready to address questions as they arise. Pulmonary technicians, laboratory directors, pulmonary physicians and pulmonary physiologists will all gain something here.

Robert O. Crapo
Professor of Medicine
University of Utah
Salt Lake City, Utah, USA

Preface

About the authors

John Cotes became interested in breathlessness as a result of taking part in athletics as a schoolboy. His subsequent career has spanned the development of modern lung function testing from its emergence out of aviation physiology at the end of World War II through to the present. The first edition of *Lung Function* in 1965 arose from this interest. It was a theoretical text and practical handbook, written to complement *The Lung* by Julius Comroe and colleagues [1], and the formula that he adopted worked well for five editions. The book has underpinned the subject for nearly half a century! For the present sixth edition new authors have been brought in and the text has been remodelled.

David Chinn is a clinical lung physiologist, teacher and research worker whose accuracy in clinical and longitudinal epidemiological studies of lung function has exceeded what many have thought possible. His authorship ensures that the new text is grounded on recent practical experience.

Martin Miller is a respiratory physician and clinical teacher who contributed materially to the Guidelines for the Measurement of Respiratory Function of the British Thoracic Society and Association for Respiratory Technology and Physiology [2]. He was a member of the European Respiratory Society Task Force on Peak Flow and the joint American Thoracic Society and European Respiratory Society Task Force on standardisation of lung function testing [3]. His authorship ensures that this book embraces current world thinking on symbols, methods and other aspects of standardisation and that it is clinically relevant.

Other significant contributors. The preparation of the manuscript entailed extensive consultations with other knowledgeable persons. Their contributions are indicated in the Acknowledgements section.

Aims and contents

The book gives a comprehensive account of lung function and its assessment in healthy persons and those with all types of respiratory disorder, against a background of respiratory, exercise and environmental physiology. It is a theoretical textbook and practical manual for respiratory physicians and surgeons, staff of lung function laboratories and others who have a professional interest in the function of the lungs at rest or on exercise and how it may be assessed. Physiologists, anthropologists, paediatricians, anaesthetists, occupational physicians, explorers, epidemiologists and respiratory nurses should also find the book useful.

The text incorporates the technical and methodological recommendations for lung function testing of the American Thoracic Society and European Respiratory Society up to the time of publication. The approach to measurement is through human anatomy, physiology and pathology, the basic sciences of maths, physics, chemistry and biology and applied clinical science (pathophysiology). Mathematical treatments are kept to a minimum and most can be skipped by readers not concerned with making measurements. However, the bottom-up approach has inevitably identified instances where current practice is at odds with basic theory. Such difficulties are discussed constructively and, where appropriate, alternative practices are suggested.

Comparison with previous editions

The text is based on that of the previous editions but is more clearly laid out with 44 chapters instead of 18, numbered sections and more concise writing. Amongst the new chapters are ones on respiratory surveys, respiratory muscles, neonatal assessment, exercise, sleep, high altitude, hyperbaria, the effects of cold and heat, respirable dusts, fumes and vapours, anaesthesia, surgery and respiratory rehabilitation. There is a compendium of lung function in selected individual diseases. The numbers of diagrams and illustrative cases have been increased materially. Unlike in previous editions most statements are attributed to original sources; these are given as numbered references at the end of chapters and the classification of references by topics has been abandoned. At the same time in the interests of brevity the number of authors for each citation has been reduced to the first three or four. Compared with the fifth edition the quantity of information in the book is greatly increased and is more accessible.

Using the book

This is a textbook of pure and applied respiratory physiology and the lung function component of respiratory medicine, including breathlessness. It is also a practical manual for assessing the function of the lungs and reporting on and interpreting the findings. Thus entry into the book can be at any of several levels.

The text progresses from basic science through lung mechanics, distribution of gas and blood in the lungs, gas exchange and respiratory control to more applied aspects, including exercise, sleep, unusual environments, breathing polluted air and changes in lung function in disease. Each topic is presented in a simple manner and can be explored separately. However, in life the topics interact, so what starts as a single structural or functional abnormality comes to embrace most aspects of function, including exercise. A common outcome is incapacitating breathlessness. In the book the primary features and methods of investigating each topic are described in appropriate detail, the implications are spelt out and cross-references are given to other sections in the book where there is additional information and/or practical examples. Inevitably, tracking the interactions through to their origins initially requires diligence, but this is likely to be rewarded by a clearer understanding of end results.

Feedback

As authors we have done our best to eliminate errors, but inevitably some will have evaded us. We invite readers to draw these lapses to our attention and also make other suggestions for improving any subsequent edition. Such material should be sent to LungFunction@Coterie.globalnet.co.uk

JE Cotes
DJ Chinn
MR Miller

References

1. Comroe JH, Forster RE, DuBois AB, Briscoe AW, Carlsen E. *The lung, clinical physiology and pulmonary function tests.* 2nd ed. Chicago, Year Book Medical Publishers, 1962.
2. Guidelines for the measurement of respiratory function; recommendations of the British Thoracic Society and the Association of Respiratory Technicians and Physiologists. *Respir Med* 1994; **88**: 165–194.
3. Miller MR, Hankinson J, Brusasco V et al. Standardisation of spirometry. In ATS/ERS Task Force: standarization of lung function testing. Brusasco V, Carpo R, Viegi G eds. *Eur Respir J.* 2005; **26**: 319–338.

Acknowledgements

In the preparation of the new text Martin Miller wrote the first drafts of the chapters in Parts 5 and 7. David Chinn drafted Chapter 8 and John Cotes supported by David Chinn drafted the remainder. David Chinn also prepared many new charts. All chapters were then revised and, where appropriate, the material was passed to independent referees. Considerable help in drafting the respective chapters was received from Professor Ole Pedersen (Chapter 13), Dr James (Jim) Reed (Chapter 23) and Professor Janet Stocks (Chapter 24). Dr Reed reviewed many of the physiological chapters and Dr Sarah Pearce the mainly clinical ones. Mr Kevin Hogben responded to many technical queries. Dr R.A.L. Brewis and Mr M.F. Clay kindly prepared the cartoons.

Comments and suggestions that led to improvements in individual chapters came from Dr Roger Carter, Dr Brendan Cooper, Dr Patricia Tweeddale and Professor Susan Hill (Chapter 2), Professor J.G. Widdicombe (Chapter 3), Professor Peter (PRM) Jones (Chapter 4), Professor Geoffrey Berry and Dr Charles Rossiter (Chapter 5), Dr Brendan Cooper (Chapter 7), Professor H. Ross Anderson (Chapter 8), Professor P.H. Quanjer and Dr Sarah Pearce (Chapter 15), Professor Michael (JMB) Hughes and Dr Alison Mackie (Chapter 18), Dr Colin Borland (Chapters 19 and 20), Professor Gareth Jones (Chapters 21 and 42), Professor Norman Jones (Chapter 22), Dr Derek Cramer, Dr James Martin, Dr Michael Rosenthal (Chapter 26), Dr Sally Singh (Chapter 29), Dr Ruth Cayton (Chapters 32 and 33), Dr James Milledge (Chapter 34), Dr Einer Thorsen (Chapter 35).

Members of staff at Blackwell Publishing prepared the manuscript for printing.

The authors are very appreciative of the help they received from so many people and apologise to any others whose names may have been left out (see Feedback above). The help came without commitment, and the authors corporately accept responsibility for the final product.

PART 1
Foundations

CHAPTER 1

Early Developments and Future Prospects

This chapter describes how the theory and practice of lung function testing have reached their present state of development and gives pointers to the future.

1.1 The gaseous environment

The basis of respiratory physiology is Claude Bernard's concept of a 'milieu interieur' that remains constant and stable despite changes in the environment. However, the two are not independent since life on earth has evolved symbiotically with changes in earth's atmosphere and this process is continuing. At first, the composition of the atmosphere was determined by physical processes, and then by the biological ones. Now changes in the composition of air are being driven by man's own actions. It remains to be seen how and to what extent the system will adapt.

Initially the atmosphere was mainly nitrogen. Then as the earth cooled, carbon dioxide was formed by chemical reactions beneath the earth's crust and released by volcanic activity. Some of the gas was taken up by combination with minerals and deposited as sediment at the bottom of the oceans. Oxygen was released, but immediately combined with iron and other elements, and so the atmospheric concentration was very low [1, 2]. Subsequently, the concentration of oxygen increased as a result of biological activity [3]. A hypothesis as to how this happened was proposed by Lovelock [4] whose concept of the living earth (Gaia) is on a par with evolution as one of the formative influences of our time.

Free oxygen first appeared some 3.5×10^9 years ago coincidentally with the development of organisms capable of photosynthesis. The organisms multiplied and their growth reduced significantly the atmospheric concentration of carbon dioxide. Some organisms (methanogens) developed an ability to form free methane gas. The methane was liberated into the atmosphere where it shielded the earth's surface from ultraviolet light. The shielding allowed ammonia gas to accumulate and this provided a substrate for the growth of photosynthesising organisms; as a result, at the beginning of the Proterozoic era some 2.3×10^9 years ago, the atmospheric concentration of oxygen began to rise. By geological standards the increase was rapid, from 0.1 to 1% over about one million years (Fig. 1.1).

When the ambient oxygen concentration reached 0.2%, aerobic organisms became abundant in the surface layers of lakes and oceans and at 2% life began to move onto the land. A concentration of 3% may have been attained some 1.99×10^9 years ago. At 10% photosynthesis was at its peak; this further raised the concentration of oxygen and lowered that of carbon dioxide. The changes reduced the available substrate (CO_2) and increased the formation of hydrogen peroxide, superoxide ions and atomic oxygen that were potentially lethal to cells. Photosynthesis was reduced in consequence. With other factors, the balance between promotion and inhibition of photosynthesis formed a feedback loop that stabilised the atmospheric concentration of oxygen at its present level (21.93%, $F_{I,O_2} = 0.2193$).

The concentration of oxygen stabilised at the start of the Phanerozoic era some 6×10^8 years ago. It led to the evolution of animals with skeletons. Thereafter, the concentrations of carbon dioxide, and to some extent oxygen, appear to have oscillated in response to secondary factors. These included fluctuations in the balance between the relative dominance of plants and animals. Some 5×10^8 years ago the species that were net consumers of oxygen (e.g. bacteria, fungi and insects) were in the ascendancy and CO_2 levels were relatively high. Then, plants that fix CO_2 as lignin appeared and the levels fell. The plants

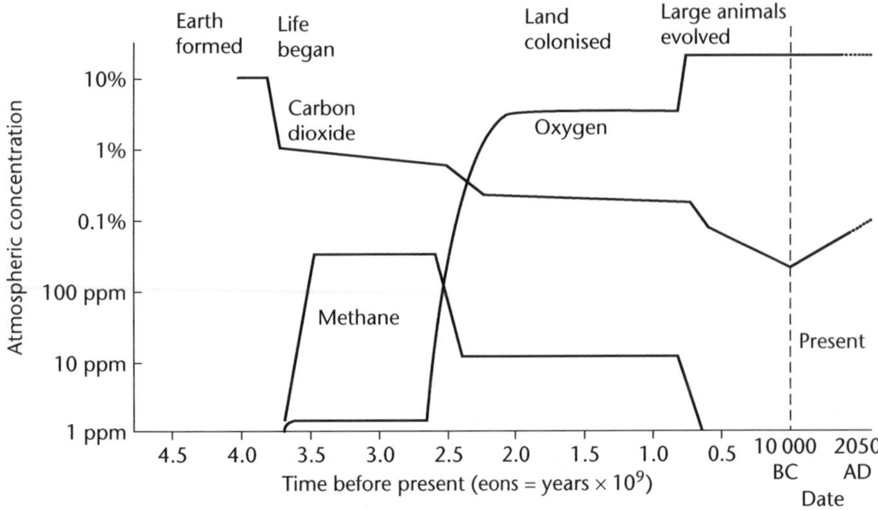

Fig. 1.1 Approximate timescale for the evolution of the gaseous environment. Source: After [4].

led to the evolution of dinosaurs and other animals that could feed off and digest the cellulose. The species flourished and the cycle was reversed. From time to time the sequence was unsettled by dust clouds from meteors and volcanic eruptions. The dust interfered with photosynthesis by obscuring the sun, but up to the present the equilibrium has always been restored.

Currently, the atmosphere is under threat from human activity. Clearance of forests and the replacement of grassland by buildings and roads are reducing the earth's capacity for photosynthesis. Hence, the amount of carbon dioxide removed from air is falling. Concurrently, the quantity released is increasing because of massive combustion of fossil fuels. As a result, the earth's temperature is rising and this is increasing the formation of methane gas that could raise the temperature further. However it also has other effects, and so the long-term outcome is unpredictable. In the short term any change in gaseous equilibrium is likely to occur slowly.

In summary, living organisms first appeared in an anaerobic environment that they helped to convert to an aerobic one. Hence they were adapting to the new conditions as they were creating them. On this account, the capacity to tolerate conditions of hypoxia and hypercapnia are part of man's heritage. How this is achieved is described in subsequent chapters. The evolutionary history also indicates the importance of natural protection against oxygen radicals. However, there is only limited evidence for Berken and Marshall's suggestion [1] that the relevant mechanisms emerged during periods of what we would now regard as hyperoxia.

1.2 Functional evolution of the lung

Aerobic organisms developed in an aqueous medium where the amount of oxygen is determined by its partial pressure and by the solubility; this is such that the concentration in water is only about one fortieth of that in air (Table 1.1). By contrast carbon dioxide is highly soluble, so at physiological partial pressures the concentration in water is nearly as great as in air. The differences in solubility have consequences for gas exchange [5].

Table 1.1 Atmospheric concentrations and solubility in water of oxygen and carbon dioxide.

	Units	Oxygen	Carbon dioxide
Atmospheric concentration	vol./vol.	0.2093	0.003
Solubility in water at 1 atm:			
Temperature 20°C*	vol. of gas(STPD) / vol. of water	0.031	0.88
Temperature 37°C*	vol. of gas(STPD) / vol. of water	0.024	0.55

*Solubility in blood plasma is approximately 10% less.

For the fish the problem of obtaining sufficient oxygen was solved by the evolution of the gill system. This organ is perfused by a large volume of water from which almost all the oxygen is extracted; the blood leaving the bronchial clefts contains oxygen in a concentration equal to that in blood leaving the lung in man. However, the water perfusing the gill takes with it the carbon dioxide in solution and this lowers the CO_2 tension in the blood to less than 0.7 kPa (5 mm Hg). Mainly on this account the blood pH is relatively high (approximately 8.0 pH units at a temperature of 20°C). At higher water temperatures the pH falls to approach that in the blood of man. Concurrently, the solubility of oxygen in water delivered to the gill clefts is reduced.

In hot climates a high ambient temperature might cause streams to dry up, leaving any fish stranded. To meet this hazard some fish developed lung-like pouches in the back of the pharynx; they also developed primitive limbs with which to crawl along streambeds in search of water. For this type of existence a gill for the exchange of carbon dioxide and a primitive lung for exchanging oxygen formed a life-saving combination. The lung was further developed in the reptiles. In birds the pouches were adapted as reservoirs from which air was pumped through parabronchi; these supplied air to the diffusive zones where the whole of the surface was lined with capillaries. This arrangement resulted in a very compact lung with a high capacity to transfer gas. The amphibians developed in a different way by shedding their scales to leave a soft vascular skin; this replaced the gill as a means of exchanging carbon dioxide with the surrounding water. Somewhere between these diverging species emerged the primitive mammals and eventually man.

1.3 Early studies of lung function

Erasistratus (c. 280 BC) and Galen (129–201) demonstrated the role of the diaphragm as a muscle of respiration, the origin and function of the phrenic nerve and the function of the intercostal and accessory muscles. The function of the diaphragm was further explored by da Vinci (1452–1519) who observed that during inspiration the lung expanded in all directions following the movement of the thoracic cage. The lung collapse that followed puncture of the pleura was described by Vesalius (1514–1564).

The need for fresh air was recognised by Galen who believed it reacted with the blood in the left heart and arteries to produce the 'vital spirit'. The absence of a visible communication between the pulmonary artery and the pulmonary vein led him to suggest that blood passed through invisible pores between the two sides of the heart; thus, he failed to comprehend the function of the lung. This was surmised by Ibn-al-Nafis (c. 1210–1289) and by Servetus (1511–1553) who separately recognised the impermeability of the interventricular septum and proposed that blood passed from the pulmonary artery through the lung to the pulmonary vein. Harvey (1578–1657) demonstrated that blood circulated through the lung and Malpighi (1628–1694) showed that the blood capillaries were in close proximity to the smallest air spaces. These observations prepared the way for a correct understanding of lung function.

The role of ventilation in maintaining life was demonstrated by Vesalius who was able to restore the activity of the heart in an apnoeic dog by insufflating air into the trachea through a reed. Hooke (1635–1703) subsequently showed that the essential factor was a supply of fresh air. Boyle (1627–1691) and, to a lesser extent Mayow (1643–1679), demonstrated that the constituent of air that supported combustion also supported life. Lower (1631–1691) further showed that the uptake of air in the lung caused the blood to change colour. These discoveries laid the foundations for subsequent studies of gas exchange but their importance was not immediately apparent. The confusion was such that on 22 January 1666, after a meeting of the Royal Society on the subject of respiration, Samuel Pepys wrote in his diary: 'it is not to this day known, or concluded on among physicians how the action is managed by nature, or for what use it is'.

1.4 The past 350 years

The information about the lung that was necessary for the birth of respiratory physiology was available by about the year 1667. Thereafter aspects of the subject developed at different rates, reflecting their immediate interest and the techniques that were available for their investigation.

1.4.1 Lung volumes

The volume of air that a man can inhale during a single deep breath was first measured by Borelli (1679). Subsequent work established that this quantity in an average adult is about 200–300 in^3 (3.3–4.9 l) at ambient temperature. The need for a temperature correction was pointed out by Goodwyn (1788). In 1831 Thackrah showed the volume of air to be less in women than in men and to be reduced amongst workers in flax and other occupations due to the inhalation of dust [6]. The measurement of vital capacity was put on a quantitative basis by Hutchinson in 1846 [7]. Hutchinson defined it as 'the greatest voluntary expiration following the deepest inspiration' and designed a spirometer for its estimation. He showed that the vital capacity is related to the height such that 'for every inch of height (from 5 to 6 ft) eight additional cu. inches of air at 60°F are given out by forced expiration'. The equivalent parameter in metric units is 5.8 l m^{-1}, which is similar to values used today (Section 26.5). He further showed that the vital capacity decreased with age and was reduced by excess weight and by disease of the lung. The measurement of residual volume by a gas dilution method was first performed by Davy (1800). The method using whole body plethysmography was developed by DuBois and colleagues (1956).

1.4.2 Lung mechanics

The role of the elastic recoil of the lung in causing expiration was demonstrated by Donders (1853) who was the first to measure the retractive force. This work was extended by Dixon and Brodie (1903) and by Cloetta (1913). Concurrently, Rohrer (1915) was applying the concepts of Newtonian mechanics to explain the relationship between the force exerted by the respiratory muscles and the rate of airflow. This approach was extended by his successors Neergaard and Wirz (1927) who used the pneumotachograph of Fleisch (1925). Neergaard also demonstrated the role of surface forces in the lung by comparing the relationship of the lung volume to the retractive force when the air in the lung was replaced by water. This work was repeated independently by Radford (1954) who, with Pattle (1955) Clements (1956) and Avery and Mead (1959), established the physiological and chemical significance of lung surfactant. Knowledge of the viscoelastic properties of the lung was extended by Bayliss and Robertson (1939), Dean and Visscher (1941), Rahn, Otis, Chadwick and Fenn (1946), Mead and Whittenberger (1953), and their many collaborators; a seminal review was prepared by Mead [8]. The role of antitrypsin in protecting the lung from proteolytic enzymes was discovered by Eriksson [9].

1.4.3 Ventilatory capacity

The relationship of breathlessness on exertion to vital capacity was considered by Peabody (1915). He also compared the ventilation during exercise with that during breathing carbon dioxide. The use of the forced vital capacity was introduced by Strohl (1919). The role of changes in lung distensibility in causing breathlessness was explored by Christie (1934). The maximal breathing capacity was introduced as a dynamic test of lung function by Jansen, Knipping and Stromberger (1932) who calculated it from the forced vital capacity. The maximal voluntary ventilation was first measured by Hermannsen (1933). The use of the proportion of the vital capacity that could be expired in one second as a guide to airways obstruction was introduced by Tiffeneau (1948). The measurement was facilitated through the addition of a timing device to the spirometer by Gaensler (1951) and subsequently by McDermott and colleagues (1960). A convenient and reasonably accurate peak flowmeter was developed by Wright (1959) and other instruments followed.

1.4.4 Blood chemistry and gas exchange in the lung

During the eighteenth century, the lung's role as an organ of gas exchange was obscured by the belief of Lavoisier (1777) and others that it was the site of combustion. This was disproved by Magnus (1837) who used an extraction technique to analyse the gases in arterial and venous bloods. The use of such data for the calculation of cardiac output was proposed by Fick (1870), whilst the true site of oxidation was demonstrated by Pflüger (1872). The techniques for analysing gases were improved by Haldane and described in *Methods of Air Analysis* (1899); an improved method for determining the concentrations in the blood was described by Haldane and Barcroft (1902). The tonometer methods for measuring the blood gas tensions were developed by Bohr (1890) and Krogh (1910); other technical advances were reported by Peters and Van Slyke in *Quantitative Clinical Chemistry* (1932). The application of these and other techniques to human arterial blood was made possible through the introduction by Hurter (1912) of the procedure of arterial puncture.

The relationship of the pressure to the content of oxygen in the blood was explored by Paul Bert and described in *La Pression Barometrique* (1878); in this he showed that the pressure and not the concentration of gases in the atmosphere is of physiological significance. The oxygen dissociation curve was described by Bohr (1904). With Hasselbalch and Krogh (1904), Bohr showed that its shape is greatly influenced by the coexisting tension of carbon dioxide. Further advances were made by Barcroft and summarised in *The Respiratory Function of the Blood* (1914). The dissociation curve for carbon dioxide was described by Christiansen, Douglas and Haldane (1914) and the chemical reactions were further explored by Hasselbalch, Hastings, Roughton, Sendroy, Stadie and others. Some of this work is described by L.J. Henderson in *Blood: A Study in General Physiology* (1928).

The exchange of gas across the alveolar capillary membrane was considered by Bohr (1891). He found that the tension of oxygen was sometimes higher in the arterial blood than in the alveolar gas and concluded that oxygen was secreted by the alveolar cells. The measurements were in error, but the hypothesis was supported by Haldane and Smith (1896–1898); these workers inhaled gas containing carbon monoxide (CO), and observed differences between the observed and expected CO tensions in blood. This could best be explained by secretion of oxygen. Their view was opposed by the Kroghs (1910) and by Barcroft, who believed correctly that the transfer of oxygen took place solely by diffusion. The controversy led Bohr (1909) to develop his integration method for determining the mean tension of oxygen in the pulmonary capillaries and to calculate the diffusing capacity of the lung for carbon monoxide. It also stimulated physiological expeditions to high altitudes, including to Pikes Peak, described by Douglas, Haldane, Y. Henderson and Schneider (1913), and to Cerro de Pasco, described by Barcroft in the second edition of *The Respiratory Function of the Blood.* Studies of conditions at high altitude were also undertaken by Dill, Christensen and Edwards (1936), and by Houston and Riley (1947). Subsequently, interest shifted to the Himalayas where the physiological adaptations necessary for the ascent of Mount Everest were investigated by Pugh (1964) and West (1983), amongst others. Meanwhile, the transfer of oxygen from alveolar gas to pulmonary capillary blood was explored by Lilienthal and Riley (1946) and Piiper (1961). Understanding of the transfer of carbon monoxide was advanced by Roughton and Forster (1957). The single breath method for the measurement of transfer factor (diffusing capacity) for carbon monoxide was developed by Marie Krogh (1915) and improved under Comroe's guidance by Forster, Fowler and colleagues (1954). The anatomical basis of gas exchange was described in quantitative terms by Weibel (1963).

The distribution of gas in the lung was considered by Zuntz (1882) who introduced the concept of dead space; this was first measured at post-mortem by Loewy (1894). The dead space for carbon dioxide was measured during life by Bohr (1891) as well as by Haldane and others who used the method of sampling the alveolar gas devised by Haldane and Priestley (1905). By this method Douglas and Haldane (1912) showed that the dead space increased with the depth of inspiration, but the magnitude of the increase was disputed by Krogh and Lindhard (1913–1914) who sampled the end tidal gas. Part of the increase was believed by Haldane to represent ventilation of the alveolar ducts and atria where the ventilation per unit of perfusion (i.e. the ventilation–perfusion ratio) was higher than in the alveoli. Haldane, Meakins and Priestley (1918–1919) explored the effects of uneven lung function upon the composition of alveolar gas and arterial blood. The application of these concepts to patients with lung disease was described by Meakins and Davies in *Respiratory Function in Disease* (1925).

The role of the pulmonary circulation was clarified through the application of the newly discovered technique of cardiac catheterisation by Cournand (1942) and by McMichael and

Sharpey-Schafer (1944). However, there was disagreement as to whether or not it was ethical to apply the technique to healthy people. The mechanisms underlying uneven lung function were further illuminated by the development of bronchospirometry by Jacobaeus (1932), the concept of regional inhomegeneity by Rauwerda (1945), the respiratory mass spectrometer by Fowler (1957), the oxygen electrode by Clark (1953) and radioisotope assay methods by Knipping (1955). These techniques were used to good effect by Rahn and Fenn (1955), Gilson and colleagues (1955) and West (1969) who, with Wagner (1974), developed the multiple inert gas elimination technique for describing ventilation–perfusion inequality.

1.4.5 Control of respiration

Knowledge of the central nervous regulation of respiration stems from the observations of Legallois (1812) and Flourens (1824) that a lesion in a small area of the medulla oblongata caused breathing to cease. The location of the respiratory region was defined with increasing precision by many workers, including Lumsden (1923) and Pitts, Magoun and Ranson (1939). At an early stage, Hering and Breuer (1868) separately showed that the region received, via the vagi, sensory information on the distension of the lung. This provided the basis for a mechanism of self-regulation whereby the inflation of the lung tended to terminate inspiration and to initiate expiration whilst deflation of the lung had the opposite effect.

Activity in single vagal fibres was recorded by Adrian (1933) and others. Their work paved the way for dramatic advances in understanding the role of pulmonary receptors. Subsequent contributors included Whitteridge (1950) and his pupils Paintal, Widdicombe and Guz. Sears (1963) showed that the muscle spindles in the respiratory muscles played a part in regulation, whilst Campbell and Howell (1963) explored the role they might play in the sensation of dyspnoea. The Hering–Breuer centenary symposium provided a seminal review [10]; it also introduced respiratory physiologists to some psychological techniques for the quantification of breathlessness.

The stimulant effects upon respiration of both a relative deficiency of oxygen and a moderate excess of carbon dioxide were known to Pflüger (1868) who believed the former to be the more important factor. In this he was in agreement with Rosenthal (1862). Evidence for the role of carbon dioxide was provided by Miescher-Rusch (1885), whilst Geppert and Zuntz (1888) demonstrated the stimulant action of other products of metabolism. The action of carbon dioxide in man was investigated quantitatively by Haldane and Priestley (1905) who, over a wide range of barometric pressures, demonstrated that the ventilation was adjusted to maintain the alveolar carbon dioxide tension at a constant level.

J.S. Haldane's great contribution is summarised in *Respiration* (1922). It was republished jointly with Priestley in 1935. The role of the blood hydrogen ion concentration in controlling breathing was suggested by Winterstein (1911) and elaborated, amongst others, by Yandell Henderson in *Adventures in Respiration* (1938). Gesell (1923) believed the response of the respiratory region of the brain to be affected by the metabolism of chemosensitive cells. The role of hypoxaemia was advanced through the identification by Heymans (1926) and De Castro (1930) of the chemoreceptors in the carotid and aortic bodies; their function was further studied by Comroe and Schmidt (1938). The interdependence of the responses of ventilation to hypercapnia and hypoxaemia was demonstrated by Nielsen and Smith (1951), whilst the effects of inhalation of oxygen were studied by Leonard Hill and Flack (1910), A.V. Hill, Long and Lupton (1924), Asmussen and Nielsen (1946), Comroe and Dripps (1950), Dejours (1966) and others. The combined effects on respiration of these and other factors were synthesised into a multiple theory of respiratory regulation by Gray in *Pulmonary Ventilation and its Physiological Regulation* (1950).

1.4.6 Energy expenditure during exercise

The rates of exchange of oxygen and carbon dioxide in the lung were measured by Lavoisier (1784) who showed that they varied with the level of activity. The relationship of resting metabolism to body surface area was demonstrated by Robiquet and Thillaye (1839). The underlying biochemical processes were investigated by Liebig (1842), Voit (1857), Rubner (1883) and others. One important landmark was the demonstration by Fletcher and Hopkins (1907) that lactic acid was produced in muscles during anaerobic contractions.

The measurement of human metabolism by indirect calorimetry was facilitated by Zuntz (1891) when he developed a portable apparatus. The method was validated by Atwater and Rosa (1897) using a human calorimeter. Other equipment was introduced by Tissot (1904), Douglas (1911), Benedict and Roth (1922), Kofranyi and Michaelis (1940), Müller and Franz (1952) and Wolff (1958). The need to relate the results to the body mass of the subjects was recognised by Frentzel and Reach (1901). The energy expenditure during activity was measured by many workers, including Benedict (1915), whilst the relationship to the speed of locomotion was analysed in detail by Magne (1920), A.V. Hill and his colleagues, including Lupton (1922), Atzler and Herbst (1927), Fenn (1930), Margaria (1939) and others.

1.5 Practical assessment of lung function

Most of the physiological concepts described in this chapter were applied to the assessment of patients with respiratory disease, starting with the vital capacity in the early nineteenth century [7]. In the 1930s, Knipping's laboratory in Hamburg was setting the trend, using a wide range of tests, all of which have their counterparts today (Table 1.2).

In 1950, when Comroe reviewed the subject, the scope of the tests had broadened to include aspects of lung mechanics. However, the forced expiratory volume was scarcely known outside France and no test had reached its current form. This mainly

Table 1.2 Tests of respiratory efficiency in Knipping's laboratory.

Aspect	Test	Normal level
Anatomical	Vital capacity	>70% pred.
Physiological	Ventilation equivalent for O_2	<3 1/100 ml
	Ventilating power	Not defined
	Respiratory style (t_{exp}/t_{insp})	<1.4
	Composition of arterial blood	
Epiratory force	Mercury U-tube (Flak) test	40 mm Hg > 40 s
Symptoms	Dyspnoea ratio	
	(VE recovery/VE rest)	Average 1.64

Source: [11].

happened during the next 12 years (Table 1.3); the developments were aided by a transfer of technical expertise from wartime aviation medicine [35]. Photographs of some of those who contributed are given in Fig. 1.2.

Since the 1960s, the means for calibration have been improved, the convenience of the tests increased and the subtlety of interpretation extended. New tests have mainly emerged in the related fields of medical physics and anthropometry. Some of them are included in the present account.

The changes have led to the loss of many procedures from the days when laboratory equipment comprised beautiful glassware and 'bits and pieces' held together by 'string and sealing wax'. The methods were often very practical (Fig. 1.3 and Table 1.4) and the routine analysis of expired gas was usually performed with greater accuracy than is the case today (Table 1.3, [34]).

1.6 The position today

Modern lung function testing is based on detailed understanding of the underlying physiology. This has been reviewed extensively in many publications. The most comprehensive is *The Lung, Scientific Foundations*, edited by Crystal and colleagues [38]. Other reviews are listed in the appropriate chapters of the present account.

1.7 Future prospects

The mechanisms that underlie the respiratory function of the lung are now quite well understood. The practical assessment

Table 1.3 Some developments in the post-war period 1945–1965.

Aspect	Authors	Year	Reference
Obstruction index	Tiffeneau	1948	[12]
Closed circuit spirometry	Gilson and Hugh-Jones	1949	[13]
Symbols	Pappenheimer et al.	1950	[14]
Dynamic spirometry	Gaensler	1951	[15]
Bronchial provocation	Tiffeneau and Drutel	1951	[16]
Exchange of inert gases	Kety	1951	[17]
Gas exchange			
O_2	Riley and Cournand	1951	[18]
CO_2	Roughton	1954	[19]
O_2 and CO_2	Rahn and Fenn	1955	[5]
Blood PO_2 electrode	Clark et al.	1953	[20]
Lung mechanics	Mead and Whittenberger	1953	[21]
First Entretiens de Nancy*	Sadoul	1954	[22]
Body plethysmography	DuBois et al.	1956	[23]
Distribution of gas	Otis et al.	1956	[24]
The Lung	Comroe et al.	1955	[25]
Single breath Dl_{CO}	Forster et al.	1954	[26]
	Jones and Mead	1961	[27]
Terminology			
FEV_1	Gandevia and Hugh-Jones	1957	[28]
Tl	Cotes	1963	[29]
Respir. Mass spectrometry	Fowler and Hugh-Jones	1957	[30]
Peak flow meter	Wright and McKerrow	1959	[31]
Flow–volume curve	Fry and Hyatt	1960	[32]
Progressive cycling test	Borg and Dahlstrom	1962	[33]
Quality control – gas analysis	Cotes and Woolmer	1962	[34]

*Led to formation of Societas Europea Physiologiae Clinicae Respiratoriae (SEPCR), forerunner of European Respiratory Society.

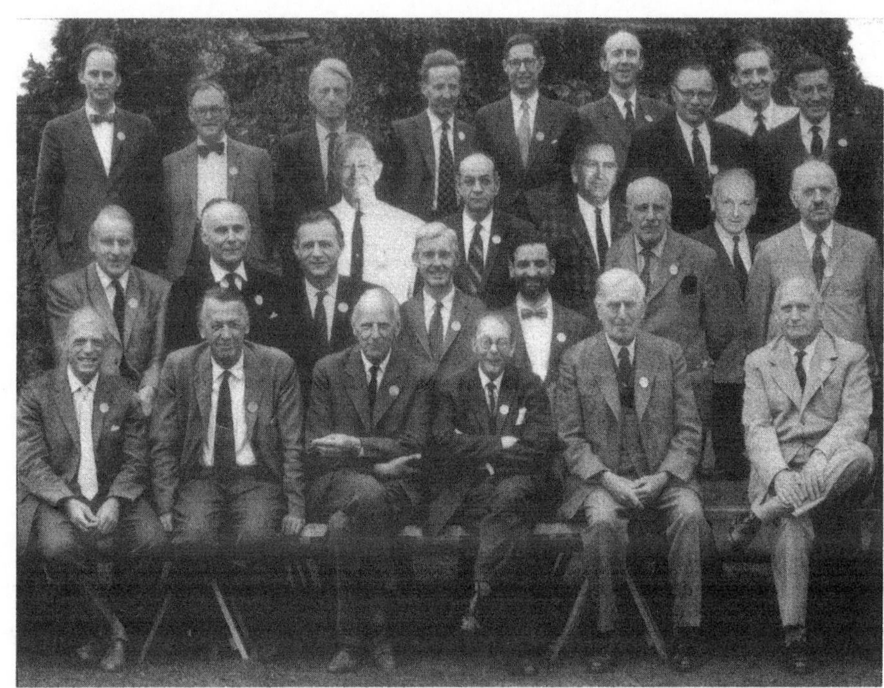

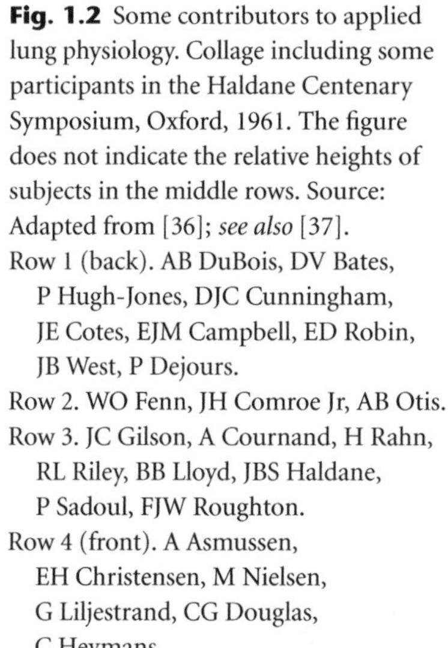

Fig. 1.2 Some contributors to applied lung physiology. Collage including some participants in the Haldane Centenary Symposium, Oxford, 1961. The figure does not indicate the relative heights of subjects in the middle rows. Source: Adapted from [36]; *see also* [37].
Row 1 (back). AB DuBois, DV Bates, P Hugh-Jones, DJC Cunningham, JE Cotes, EJM Campbell, ED Robin, JB West, P Dejours.
Row 2. WO Fenn, JH Comroe Jr, AB Otis.
Row 3. JC Gilson, A Cournand, H Rahn, RL Riley, BB Lloyd, JBS Haldane, P Sadoul, FJW Roughton.
Row 4 (front). A Asmussen, EH Christensen, M Nielsen, G Liljestrand, CG Douglas, C Heymans.

of lung function is an accepted part of clinical medicine, occupational medicine and epidemiology. The techniques for assessment have been standardised between workers in different countries and computerised equipment has become available in bewildering variety; thus the subject has matured.

Forthcoming challenges are to hold onto what we now know in the face of competition from other disciplines, exploit emerging technologies and discover how to benefit from recent developments in pharmacology and molecular and cell biology, including the mapping of the human genome (Table 1.5).

The immediate benefits are likely to be considerable and in the longer term they could be immense. But they will only be realised if high standards are maintained; this might be done by building on the techniques and underlying physiology that are described in this book.

Table 1.4 Reagents for use with the chemical absorption methods of gas analysis at or above 20°C.

Acid rinse		Glycerol	21 ml
		H_2SO_4 (concentrated)	1 ml
		Na_2SO_4 (anhydrous)	66.4 g
		H_2O	400 ml
40 mg of pulverised $K_2Cr_2O_7$ is added to 50 ml of this solution immediately before use.			
Absorber for CO_2		KOH	8.86 g
		$K_2Cr_2O_7$	40 mg
		H_2O	100 ml
Absorber for O_2	A	KOH	5 g
		H_2O	100 ml
	B	$Na_2SO_4 \cdot 2H_2O$	24 g
		Anthraquinone	0.1 g
The oxygen reagent is made up by dissolving 1.3 g of B in 10 ml of A. In this form it will only keep for a few days but the components will keep indefinitely.			

Table 1.5 Future directions of research.

Topic	Aspect	Location
Emerging technologies [39]	Exercise flow–volume loops	Section 28.8.1
	Negative pressure assisted flows	Section 12.5.1
	Forced oscillations for measuring resistance	Section 14.4.4
Understanding human respiration [40]	All	This book
Environmental contaminants	Determinants of chronic respiratory disorders	Chapters 38 and 39
Molecular biology [41–43]	Genetic basis for normal respiratory function	Chapter 27
	Diagnosing and evaluating treatments for genetic respiratory disorders	Chapter 39
Lung function	Better use of exercise tests	Part 4

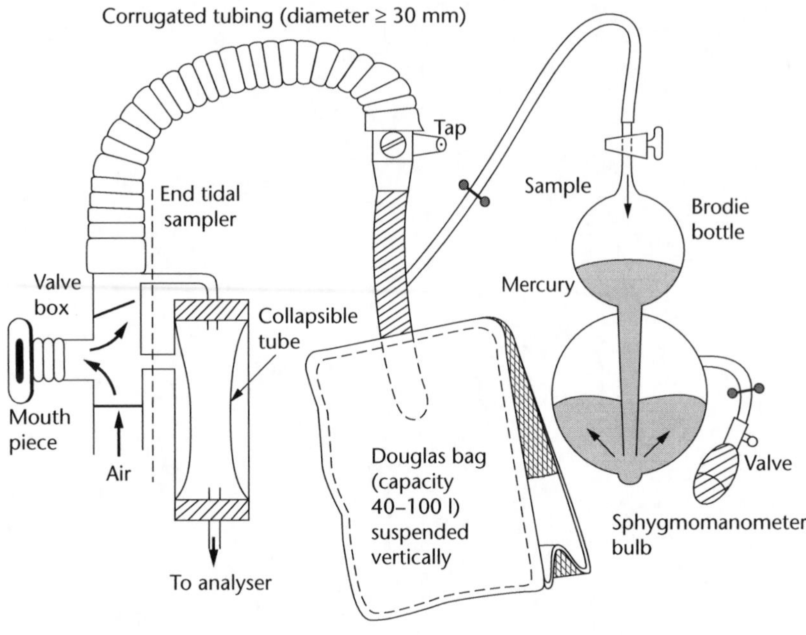

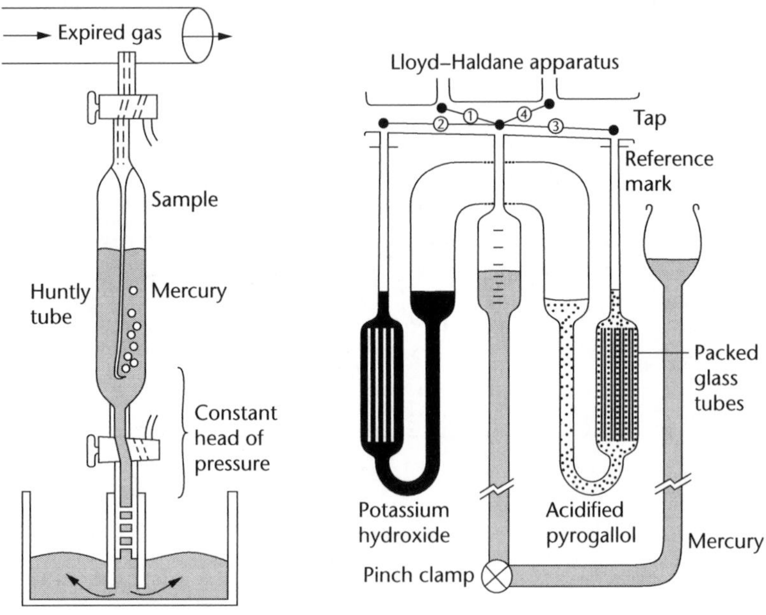

Fig. 1.3 Traditional equipment for collecting and sampling expired gas. The Douglas bag is suspended vertically. Prior to use, its dead space is flushed with expired gas. After collection, the gas is mixed by pummelling the bag and a small amount is passed through the side arm. A sample is then transferred to a Brodie bottle (capacity 50 ml) or direct into a chemical gas analyser (e.g. Lloyd-Haldane, lower right; also Table 1.4). Gas volume is measured by using a wet gas meter and constant flow pump that cuts out at a predetermined negative pressure. Alternatively a Tissot spirometer (capacity 100 l) is used. The sampler for end tidal gas (top left) is operated by the pressure changes in the valve box. The sample collects in the collapsible tube and is sucked off at a flow of 50–200 ml min^{-1} into a Huntly tube or other apparatus. The Huntly tube (capacity 50 ml, lower left) provides a means of collecting a representative sample of mixed gas over a period of 1 or 2 min.

1.8 References

1. Berken LV, Marshall LC. Limitation on oxygen concentration in a primitive planetary atmosphere. *J Atmos Sci* 1966; **23**: 133–143.
2. Pearce F. The kingdom of Gaia. *New Scientist* 2001; **2295**: 30–33.
3. Thomas L. The world's biggest membrane. *New Engl J Med* 1973; **289**: 576–577.
4. Lovelock J. *The ages of Gaia.* Oxford: Oxford University Press, 1988.
5. Rahn H, Fenn WO. *A graphical analysis of the respiratory gas exchange.* Washington, DC: American Physiological Society, 1955.
6. Thackrah CT. The effects of art, trades and professions on health and longevity. In: Meiklejohn A, ed. *The life, work and times of Charles Turner Thackrah.* Edinburgh: E&S Livingstone, 1831/1957.
7. Hutchinson J. On the capacity of the lungs, and on the respiratory functions, with a view of establishing a precise and easy method of detecting disease by the spirometer. *Med Chir Trans (Lond)* 1846; **29**: 137–252.
8. Mead J. Mechanical properties of lungs. *Physiol Rev* 1961; **41**: 281–330.
9. Eriksson S. Studies in α-antitrypsin deficiency. *Acta Med Scand* 1965: **177** (Suppl 432): 1–85.
10. Porter R., ed. *Breathing: Hering–Breuer Centenary Symposium.* London: Churchill, 1970: 59–71.
11. Moncrieff A. *Tests for respiratory efficiency.* Medical Research Council, Special Reports Series No. 198. London: HMSO, 1934.

12. Yernault JC. The birth and development of the forced expiratory manoeuvre: a tribute to Robert Tiffeneau (1910–1961). *Eur Respir J* 1997; **10**: 2704–2710, see also Chapter 12, ref. 30 (page 141).
13. Gilson JC, Hugh-Jones P. The measurement of the total lung volume and breathing capacity. *Clin Sci* 1949; **7**: 185–216.
14. Pappenheimer JR, Comroe JH, Cournand A et al. Standardization of definitions and symbols in respiratory physiology. *Fed Proc* 1950; **9**: 602–605.
15. Gaensler EA. Analysis of the ventilatory defect by timed vital capacity measurements. *Am Rev Tuberc* 1951; **64**: 256–278.
16. Tiffeneau R, Drutel P. Étude des facteurs alvéolaires et bronchiques de la ventilation pulmonaire. *J Fr Med Chir Thorac* 1951; **5**: 209–232, 316–334.
17. Kety SS. The theory and application of the exchange of inert gas at the lungs and tissues. *Pharmacol Rev* 1951; **3**: 1–41.
18. Riley RL, Cournand A. Analysis of factors affecting partial pressures of oxygen and carbon dioxide in gas and blood of lungs: theory. *J Appl Physiol* 1951; **4**: 77–101.
19. Roughton RJW. Respiratory function of blood. In: Booth WM, ed. *Respiratory physiology in aviation.* Texas: School of Aviation Medicine. 1954; USAF project 21-2301-0003.
20. Clark LC Jr, Wolf R, Granger D, Taylor Z. Continuous recording of blood oxygen tension by polarography. *J Appl Physiol* 1953; **6**: 189–193.
21. Mead J, Whittenberger JL. Physical properties of human lungs measured during spontaneous respiration. *J Appl Physiol* 1953; **5**: 779–796.
22. Faculté de Médicine de Nancy. Entretiens sur la physio-pathologie Respiratoire. *Rev Med Nancy* 1954; **79**: 625–804.
23. DuBois AB, Botelho SY, Bedell GN et al. A rapid plethysmographic method for measuring thoracic gas volume: a comparison with a nitrogen washout method for measuring functional residual capacity in normal subjects. *J Clin Invest* 1956; **35**: 322–326.
24. Otis AB, McKerrow CB, Bartlett RA et al. Mechanical factors in distribution of pulmonary ventilation. *J Appl Physiol* 1956; **8**: 427–443.
25. Comroe JH Jr, Forster RE, DuBois AB, Briscoe WA, Carlsen E. *The lung, clinical physiology and pulmonary function tests.* Chicago: Year Book Medical Publishing Inc., 1955.
26. Forster RE, Fowler WS, Bates DV, Van Lingen B. The absorption of carbon monoxide by the lungs during breath holding. *J Clin Invest* 1954; **33**: 1135–1145.
27. Jones RS, Mead F. A theoretical and experimental analysis of anomalies in the estimation of pulmonary diffusing capacity by the single breath method. *Q J Exp Physiol* 1961; **46**: 131–143.
28. Gandevia B, Hugh-Jones P. Terminology for measurements of ventilatory capacity. *Thorax* 1957; **12**: 290–293.
29. Cotes JE. Term for exchange of gas in the lungs. *Lancet* 1963; **2**: 843, see also Chapter 20, ref. 1 (page 255).
30. Fowler KT, Hugh-Jones P. Mass spectrometry applied to clinical practice and research. *Br Med J* 1957; **1**: 1205–1211.
31. Wright BM, McKerrow CB. Maximum forced expiratory flow rate as a measure of ventilatory capacity. *Br Med J* 1959; **2**: 1041–1047.
32. Fry DL, Hyatt RE. Pulmonary mechanics. A unified analysis of the relationship between pressure, volume and gas flow in the lungs of normal and diseased human subjects. *Am J Med* 1960; **29**: 672–689.
33. Borg GAV, Dahlstrom H. The reliability and validity of a physical work test. *Acta Physiol Scand* 1962; **55**: 353–361.
34. Cotes JE, Woolmer RF. A comparison between twentyseven laboratories of the results of analysis of an expired gas sample. *J Physiol (Lond)* 1962; **163**: 36P–37P.
35. Otis AB, Rahn H. Development of concepts in Rochester, New York, in the 1940s. *Pulm Gas Exch* 1980; **1**: 33–66.
36. Cunningham DJC, Lloyd BB, eds. The regulation of human respiration. In: *Proceedings of JS Haldane Centenary Symposium.* Oxford: Blackwell Scientific Publications, 1963.
37. West JB, ed. *Respiratory physiology: people and ideas.* New York: Oxford University Press, 1996.
38. Crystal RG, West JB, Weibel ER, Barnes PJ, eds. *The lung, scientific foundations,* vols 1 and 2, 2nd ed. Philadelphia: Lippincott-Raven, 1997.
39. Johnson BD, Beck KC, Zeballos RJ, Weisman IM. Advances in pulmonary laboratory testing. *Chest* 1999; **116**: 1377–1387.
40. American Thoracic Society. Updates: future directions for research on diseases of the lungs. *Am J Respir Crit Care Med* 1998; **158**: 320–334.
41. Barnes PJ. The fate of respiratory physiology. *Eur Respir J* 1994; **7**: 635–636.
42. Barnes PJ. Genetics and pulmonary medicine, 9: Molecular genetics of chronic obstructive pulmonary disease. *Thorax* 1999; **54**: 245–252.
43. Wilk JB, Djousse L, Arnett DK et al. Evidence for major genes influencing pulmonary function in the NHLBI Family Heart Study. *Genet Epidemiol* 2000; **19**: 81–94.

Further reading

Christie RV. The elastic properties of the emphysematous lung and their clinical significance. *J Clin Invest* 1934; **13**: 295–321.

Comroe JH Jr, ed. *Pulmonary and respiratory physiology, Parts 1 and 2.* Benchmark papers in human physiology/5 & 6. Stroudsburg, PA: Dowden, Hutchinson & Ross, 1976.

Comroe JH. *Retrospectoscope. Insights into medical discovery.* Menlo Park, CA: Von Gehr, 1977.

Cunningham DJC, Lloyd BB. The regulation of human respiration. In: *Proc. JS Haldane Centenary Symposium.* Oxford: Blackwell Scientific Publications, 1963.

Derenne J-Ph, Debru A, Grassino AE, Whitlaw WA. History of diaphragm physiology: the achievements of Galen. *Eur Resp J* 1995; **8**: 154–160.

Fishman AP, Dickinson DW, eds. *Circulation of the blood: men and ideas.* New York: Oxford University Press, 1982.

Gilson JC, Hugh-Jones P, Oldham PD, Meade F. Lung function in coal workers' pneumoconiosis. *Spec Rep Med Res Coun (Lond)* 1955; **290**.

Hughes JM, Bates DV. Historical review: the carbon monoxide diffusing capacity (DLCO) and its membrane (DM) and red cell (Theta, Vc) components. *Respir Physiol Neurobiol* 2003; **138**: 115–142.

Macklem PT. A century of the mechanics of breathing. *Am J Respir Crit Care Med* 2004; **170**: 10–15.

Meneely GR, Kaltreider NL. Use of helium for determination of pulmonary capacity. *Proc Soc Exper Biol Med.* 1941; **46**: 266–269.

Milic-Emili J. Regional distribution of gas in the lung. *Canad Respir J* 2000; **7**: 71–76.

Otis AB. History of respiratory mechanics. In: Macklem PT, Mead J, eds. *Handbook of physiology, Vol. 3: Mechanisms of breathing* (Section 3). Bethesda, MD: American Physiological Society, 1986: 1–12.

Sadoul P. Exploration de la fonction pulmonaire dans les pneumoconioses. In: *Proc 27th Congrès Internat. de Medécine du Travail*, Strasbourg, 1954, Cahors, Coueslant.

Sprigge JS. Historical note. Sir Humphry Davy; his researches in respiratory physiology and his debt to Antoine Lavoisier. *Anaesthesia* 2002; **57**: 357–364.

West JB, ed. *High altitude physiology*. Benchmark papers in human physiology/15. Stroudsburg, PA: Hutchinson & Ross, 1981.

Yernault JC, Pride N, Laszlo G. How the measurement of residual volume developed after Davy (1800). *Eur Respir J* 2000; **16**: 561–564.

CHAPTER 2

Getting Started

The chapter summarises the basic information needed to enter the subject of lung function testing, discover what is entailed in setting up a laboratory and start using this book.

2.1 Brief description of the lungs and their function

The gas exchanger. The lung is a sophisticated conglomerate of alveolar air sacs that has several functions. The principal one is as the body's organ of gas exchange. It also provides air for phonation and buoyancy during immersion in water. The latter function was important during man's evolution. The lung is at risk of being traumatised if the barometric pressure changes abruptly.

Connection to atmosphere. The alveoli are connected with the atmospheric air via branching tubes (bronchioles, bronchi and trachea). The atmosphere is a source of oxygen for metabolism and a sump for carbon dioxide, which is the principal waste product. The airways are also a portal of entry for potentially noxious gases, particles, respirable fibres and micro-organisms. Much of this material is removed in the nose and airways. The remainder is either exhaled or ingested and to some extent inactivated by phagocytic cells.

Respiratory muscles. The lungs are ventilated through the actions of respiratory muscles. The principal muscle is the diaphragm; this functions as a piston within the thoracic cage formed by the ribs and vertebral column. The ribs are stabilised and moved by intercostal muscles. Their functions can be supplemented by the actions of skeletal muscles that are attached to the thoracic cage; some of the muscles form the anterior abdominal wall.

Lung volumes and ventilatory capacity. The lung volume at the equilibrium position of the thoracic cage is functional residual capacity (FRC). Inspiration to total lung capacity (TLC) is effected by the respiratory muscles stretching the elastic tissue of the lungs. Expiration to residual volume (RV) is effected by the elastic tissue squeezing air from the lungs. The exhalation is accompanied by inward movement of the thoracic cage.

Vital capacity (VC) is the maximal tidal excursion from TLC to RV, or vice versa. When the full expiratory manoeuvre is performed with maximal effort the volume of air expired in the first second reflects the maximal ventilatory capacity of the lung. This forced expiratory volume in 1 s (FEV_1) is a widely used index of lung function.

The lungs grow during childhood; subsequently they deteriorate as a result of ageing and intercurrent illnesses. Smoking causes additional damage.

The normal levels of lung volume and other indices of function (reference values) are defined in terms of age and stature (height) for the two sexes separately. For optimal accuracy, allowance should also be made for ethnic group and body composition.

Blood supply. The output of the right ventricle of the heart flows into the pulmonary artery and thence into capillaries present in the walls of alveoli. Here the blood is conditioned by exchange of oxygen and carbon dioxide with alveolar gas.

Control of respiration. Ventilation of the lungs is controlled by respiratory centres in the brain. These have an intrinsic rhythmicity. Their function is modulated by information from other parts of the brain including its contained blood, the carotid bodies (which monitor the oxygen and carbon dioxide in arterial blood), the lungs via the vagus nerves and the skeletal muscles. Drive to ventilation is increased in many circumstances, including exercise and when the partial pressure of oxygen in inspired air is reduced by ascent to high altitude. The drive is reduced when the function of the respiratory centres is depressed.

Matching of lung ventilation and perfusion. Ventilation and perfusion of individual lung units are influenced by anatomical factors and gravitational force. In the absence of control mechanisms these factors would lead to imperfect gas exchange from imbalance between ventilation ($\dot{V}$) and perfusion ($\dot{Q}$). The difficulty is overcome by adjustments to the calibres of individual small airways and blood vessels.

Gas exchange. Ventilation of the lungs renews the contained gas down to the level of the respiratory bronchioles. From there to the surface of the alveoli – a distance of approximately 1 mm – the movement of gases is by diffusion. The subsequent stages for oxygen uptake include solution in the fluid of the alveolar lining, diffusion from that point across the alveolar wall into plasma in the alveolar capillary and chemical combination with haemoglobin present in red blood cells. The capacity of these processes can be represented by the transfer factor (Tl); this is the amount of gas that transfers from alveolar gas to capillary blood per minute per unit partial pressure gradient across the alveolar capillary membrane. The transfer factor is usually measured using carbon monoxide as the indicator gas.

2.2 Deviations from average normal lung function

Overall function. Lung function and capacity for exercise are correlated. However, the scope for improving the function by training is rather limited. The size of the lungs is reduced by obesity.

Airways. The commonest abnormality in lung function arises from narrowing of airways. This can be episodic or persistent and may or may not be ameliorated by therapy. Causes include recurrent episodes of bronchitis, smoking and bronchial hyperresponsiveness, which can be associated with asthma. The presenting symptom is often wheeze or breathlessness on exertion. The FRC is usually increased and the FEV_1 reduced but the latter can often be restored towards normal by inhalation of a bronchodilator drug.

Parenchyma. The parenchymal tissue of the lung is attenuated in patients with emphysema. The elasticity of the tissue that remains is then reduced and the TLC is often increased. Conversely, in alveolitis and interstitial fibrosis the amount of tissue and the elasticity are increased, whilst the TLC is reduced. Both types of disease of the lung parenchyma are associated with a reduced transfer factor and a fall in the blood oxygen level during exercise (hypoxaemia). Restriction to lung expansion is also a feature of abnormalities of the pleura, chest wall and respiratory muscles.

Cardiac overload. Overload of the right ventricle can result from pulmonary vasoconstriction secondary to persistent narrowing of airways or from obliteration of blood vessels by fibrous tissue or other cause. These changes can lead on to congestive cardiac failure.

A rise in left atrial pressure from any cause (for example, mitral stenosis or failure of the left ventricle) leads to pulmonary congestion; this may progress to oedema. The consequences include rapid, shallow breathing from stimulation of pulmonary J-receptors and changes in gas exchange.

Respiratory control. Excessive ventilation (hyperventilation) occurs during pregnancy, in some disorders that affect the lung parenchyma, diabetic acidosis, anxiety, malingering and other conditions. Hypoventilation can result from depression of the respiratory centres in the brain (for example by drugs or by severe hypoxaemia, or hypercapnia), and some abnormalities of the chest wall or respiratory muscles. The condition may lead on to stopping of breathing (apnoea), either intermittently or altogether. Apnoea during sleep can occur as a result of obstruction of the upper airways.

2.3 Uses of lung function tests

Respiratory medicine and surgery. Measurements of FEV_1 and VC before and often after inhalation of a bronchodilator aerosol are necessary for diagnosis and day-to-day management of many respiratory patients, both adults and children. Information on lung volumes, transfer factor and the physiological responses to progressive exercise contribute to diagnosis and assessment of patients with abnormalities of the lung parenchyma, including patients who may go on to lung surgery and transplantation of the lungs or heart. Exercise tests are an essential adjunct to programmes of respiratory rehabilitation, including portable oxygen therapy. Dedicated procedures are used for diagnosis of sleep apnoea and for monitoring treatment.

General surgery. Lung function is one consideration in determining suitability for general anaesthesia.

Occupational medicine. Knowledge of lung function is necessary for the diagnosis and management of most occupational disorders of the lung, including the pneumoconioses, extrinsic allergic alveolitis and occupational asthma. Diagnosis of the latter condition can depend on the response to inhalation challenge undertaken in the lung function laboratory.

Lung function and the response to exercise are essential components of assessment of disability and fitness for work. They also contribute to the pre-employment assessment, to routine surveillance throughout employment, and to appraisals for medicolegal purposes.

Screening at work and in epidemiology. The FEV_1, VC and peak expiratory flow have been used in community surveys to provide evidence on overall respiratory health and life expectancy. In occupational surveys the mean levels in a work force can identify respiratory hazards at an early stage. Individual results can identify persons in need of medical treatment. Screening of targeted groups within a general population can sometimes be helpful but non-selective screening for evidence of respiratory disease is seldom cost-effective.

Human biology. The size of the lungs relative to the size of the person varies depending on ethnic group and a host of environmental factors. These are still being documented.

Physically active pursuits. Lung function and capacity for exercise contribute to performance in athletics, mountaineering, competitive sports, fire fighting and rescue work and other high-level activities. The tests can identify the need for and response to physical training.

Abnormal environments. Exposure to high or low barometric pressures exerts both acute and long-term effects upon the lungs. Inappropriately rapid changes in pressure also have significant effects. Hence, most codes of practice for aircrew and for professional underwater divers require the long-term monitoring of personnel. Patients and members of the general public may need individual, specialist assessment prior to exposure.

2.4 Assessment of lung function

Guidelines. These have been prepared by respiratory learned societies and are comprehensive ([1–6], also references in individual chapters). However, the recommendations are not always concordant, some are compromises and some have not been fully validated. Thus, there is need for an independent viewpoint.

Criteria for tests. Over the past 50 years many lung function tests have been introduced and many have been abandoned. The choice has been mainly empirical. However, a set of criteria for selecting tests was proposed early in the evolution of the subject [7] and the current version has a wide measure of support (Table 2.1). The criteria are relevant for evaluating any new test that may emerge in future.

Which measurements? Four domains where lung function tests are undertaken are shown in Table 2.2, together with tests that are appropriate for each location and purpose. All assessments should include accurate measurement of stature and a record of age, smoking status, gender, ethnic group and respiratory symptoms. Body mass or composition is usually also necessary. A fuller list of procedures is in Table 2.3.

2.5 Setting up a laboratory

Location. Some patients will be disabled, and so the laboratory should be accessible to the car park, chest clinic, ward and toilets. However, observing the patient take a short walk can assist in diagnosis and be of therapeutic value, and so close proximity is not essential. Laboratories may also conduct cardiac evaluations for which similar considerations apply. Proximity to the radiographic and physiotherapy departments can be advantageous.

Table 2.1 Criteria for tests.

Aspect	Criterion	Presentation
Acceptability	Safe, simple and not unpleasant for subject	Arbitrary
Objectivity	Result not too much under subject's control	
Repeatability	Closeness of agreement over a short space of time with same method, observer, instrument, location and conditions of use	Differences between replicates
Reproducibility	As above but with a change in one or more of the conditions	
Accuracy	Results do not deviate systematically from the correct values	Amount or percentage
Validity	Test should be relevant and discriminatory in the relevant circumstances	
Sensitivity	A high proportion of affected persons should be identified as abnormal	Percentage
Specificity	A high proportion of unaffected persons should be identified as normal	Percentage
False positives	Relatively few normal persons should be wrongly identified as having the condition	Percentage or likelihood ratio (LR)*
False negatives	Relatively few persons with the condition should escape detection	Percentage or likelihood ratio (LR)†
Technical considerations	Test should be of short duration, require compact equipment that is convenient to use, calibrate and service and for which intermediate results can be displayed for purposes of quality control	Arbitrary

$$\text{* LR of a positive test} = \frac{\text{probability of obtaining an abnormal test result in diseased subjects}}{\text{probability of obtaining an abnormal test result in disease-free subjects}}$$

This can be represented as Sensitivity/(100 – Specificity).

$$\text{† LR of a negative test} = \frac{\text{probability of obtaining a normal test result in diseased subjects}}{\text{probability of obtaining a normal test result in disease-free subjects}}$$

This can be represented as (100 – Sensitivity)/Specificity.

Table 2.2 Tests for use in different circumstances.

	Time (min)*
Basic screening.	
Stature. Questionnaire	10
Forced expiration test for measurement of FEV_1, FVC and/or peak expiratory flow. Other tests have also been recommended	15
Primary care/Consulting room	
Stature. Measurement of VC, FEV_1 and related indices before and after inhalation of bronchodilator aerosol	20–70†
Secondary care/District hospital	
Essential measurements	
Stature and body mass	5
VC and FEV_1 before and after inhalation of bronchodilator aerosol	20–70†
Transfer factor for carbon monoxide	20
Arterial blood gas tensions (unless measured elsewhere)	10–20
Chest radiology	
Recommended measurements	
Total lung capacity and subdivisions	20
Physiological response to exercise (preferably on a treadmill, Section 29.4.1)	20–40
Body fat and fat-free body mass	10
Simple monitoring of respiratory muscle strength	10
Simple monitoring for sleep apnoea	12h
Specialist centre. All the above with appropriate additions, e.g.	
Airway resistance by whole body plethysmography	15
Compliance of the lung by oesophageal intubation	20
Assessment of function of respiratory muscles	10–20
Full assessment for sleep apnoea (polysomnography)	12h
Challenge tests for bronchial hyperresponsiveness and extrinsic asthma	30–60
Skin allergy tests if not done previously	20
CT and other scans	

* Timings are a rough guide and will depend on the patient's condition, cooperation and safety.
† The time depends on which drug is being used (Section 15.7.2).

Staff qualifications and training. The presence of two clinical respiratory physiologists is a working minimum (see Footnote 2.1). Both should have received four years of basic training leading to a diploma in physiological measurement or hold an appropriate higher qualification. One member should be trained in health and safety issues and all staff should be competent in cardiopulmonary resuscitation. Medical cover should be available in the building. Staff should be capable of adopting an unassuming and friendly but firm approach (e.g. see Section 30.4.3) and not mind performing the tests on themselves. This can be necessary both to supplement verbal instructions to new patients and to check on instrument calibrations.

Footnote 2.1. 'Clinical respiratory physiologist' is used here to describe any person judged competent under his or her national accreditation arrangements to conduct lung function assessments in a clinical setting. The term covers, for example, clinical scientist, medical technical officer, respiratory therapist, respiratory technologist, lung function technician and respiratory nurse.

The formal training of staff is a responsibility of the head of department [8]. It should include regular attendance at departmental meetings where lung function is integrated with other aspects of individual cases. Participation in continual professional development courses and scientific meetings along with clinical respiratory physiologists from other centres is also necessary. Such gatherings are arranged by national and international respiratory societies (Table 2.4). Clinical respiratory physiologists should be members of whichever of their national, professional societies hold meetings for those working in lung function laboratories.

Equipment. The equipment should preferably be compact, robust and easy to calibrate, clean and service adequately. Arrangements should be made for long-term servicing and details of it recorded in an equipment logbook. The measurements should be in a form that meets the specification of the user. This includes both physical characteristics (e.g. Table 2.5) and conventions for selecting and processing the measurements. The technical specification provided by the manufacturer should be scrutinised,

Table 2.3 Checklist of respiratory laboratory procedures.

Lung mechanics
- Peak expiratory flow
- Spirometry
- Flow–volume curves (maximal and partial)
- Lung volumes (gas dilution, body plethysmography, radiography)
- Chest wall mechanics • Lung compliance
- Respiratory muscle function
- Resistance (oscillometry, plethysmography, oesophageal manometry, airflow interruption)

Gas exchange (rest and exercise)
- Blood sampling (ear lobe and arterial)
- Blood analysis (gases, pH, haemoglobin, pulse oximetry, transcutaneous measurements)
- Gas analysis (O_2 uptake, CO_2 output)
- Transfer factor and components
- Distributions of blood flow and ventilation ($\dot{V}_A/\dot{Q}$)
- Physiological and anatomical shunts

Ventilatory control at rest
- Tidal breathing, pattern and minute ventilation
- Hyperventilation responses, hypoxic and hypercapnic challenge, pressure output
- Response to mechanical loading
- Flight (altitude) simulation
- Diving simulation

Sleep studies
- Simple screening (oximetry, actigraphy, snore detection)
- Limited multichannel studies (oxygen saturation, cardiac frequency, airflow, chest wall movement)
- Full polysomnography, incorporating electrophysiology
- Assessment of interventions (mechanical, pharmacological, etc.)

Physique
- Body mass and composition, stature

Physiological responses to exercise
- 6/12 min walk tests, shuttle walk tests, step tests, exercise-induced asthma Cardiorespiratory exercise testing
- Gas exchange, ventilation and work rate
- Blood gases
- Respiratory and other symptoms
- Cardiac responses (cardiac frequency, 12 lead ECG, blood pressure, cardiac output)
- Maximal exercise, disability assessment

Responses to therapeutic interventions

Pharmacological interventions
- Supplemental oxygen (rest and exercise), bronchodilators, corticosteroids, antibiotics, etc.
- Non-pharmacological interventions
- Non-invasive ventilatory support
- Pulmonary rehabilitation including exercise retraining, inspiratory muscle training

Impact of respiratory disease
- Symptoms (indirect and direct methods)
- Health status (generic and disease-specific questionnaires)

Systemic and airway responsiveness
- Bronchodilator response
- Skin allergen testing
- Bronchial challenge testing
- Exercise-induced asthma
- Cough reflex

Acute and domiciliary services and support
- Planning assessments, interpreting results, surveying patients

Source: S Hill, personal communication, 2004.

Table 2.4 Websites for some respiratory societies.

Country/continent	Society	Address*
United Kingdom	Association for Respiratory Technology and Physiology(ARTP)	www.artp.org.uk
United Kingdom	British Thoracic Society	www.brit-thoracic.org.uk
Europe	European Respiratory Society (ERS)	www.ersnet.org
Europe	International Union Against Tuberculosis and Lung Diseases	www.iuatld.org
North America	American Thoracic Society (ATS)	www.thoracic.org
Canada	Canadian Thoracic Society	www.lung.ca/cts
Latin America	Latin American Thoracic Association	www.alat.brz.net
Australasia	Australia & New Zealand Society of Respiratory Science (ANZSRS)	www.anzsrs.org.au
Australasia	Thoracic Society of Australia & New Zealand	www.thoracic.org.au
Middle East	Arab Respiratory Society	www.imhotep.net/ars.html
Japan	Japanese Respiratory Society	www.jrs.or.jp
South Africa	South African Thoracic Society	www.pulmonology.co.za

* Sites include hyperlinks to other web addresses.

Table 2.5 Qualitative appraisal of assessment procedures for the study of lung mechanics.

Aspects of lung function and method or apparatus	Technical aspects*						Use	Location (Chapter or Section)
	Simplicity	Reproducibility	Ease of calibration	Portability	Capital cost	Cheap to run		
Lung volumes								10.3
Closed circuit spirometry	B	A–B	A–B	C	C	C	Routine	
Forced rebreathing	B	B	B	A	B	A	Surveys	
Plethysmography	C	A–B	B	D	D	B	Specialist centre	
Radiography	C	A–B	C	D	D	C	Research	
Ventilatory capacity								12.3 to 12.6
Peak flowmeter	A	A	B	A	A	A	Clinic	
Bellows spirometer	A	A	A–C	A	A	A	Clinic	
Rolling seal spirometer	B	A	B	B–C	C	B	L.F. Lab	
Pneumotachography	B	A	B	B	D	A	L.F. Lab	
Resistance to flow								Ch 14
Airway interruptor	B	B	C	A	B	A	Surveys	
Forced oscillation	C	C	C	C	B	B	L.F. Lab	
Plethysmography	C	A–B	B	D	D	B	Specialist centre	
Oesophageal balloon, etc.	C	C	C	C	C	C	Research	
Lung elasticity								11.8
Oesophageal balloon, etc.	C	C	C	C	C	C	Specialist centre	

* Scale A–D: A indicates simple test, yielding reproducible results from equipment that is easily calibrated, cheap to buy and run. D indicates complex test, yielding non-reproducible results from equipment that is not easily calibrated, not portable, expensive to buy and run.

including the algorithms in any software for calculating intermediate results. Alternative non-standard procedures are usually best avoided. If in doubt, expert advice should be sought from experienced colleagues; these are sometimes only to be found in other institutions.

The need for advice is greatest with multi-purpose equipment. Such equipment is often economical and can be satisfactory, but may not meet the technical specifications for all the intended applications. The stepwise acquisition of dedicated quality instruments can be a better policy.

Bringing a test into use. Before applying a new test the clinical respiratory physiologist should receive appropriate training. The manufacturer sometimes provides this. The equipment should be calibrated under the conditions in which it is to be used (Section 7.15) and the result recorded in a book kept for this purpose. The clinical respiratory physiologists should then try out the test on themselves and on volunteer visitors and patients.

The reproducibility and accuracy of the equipment and operator together should next be determined (Section 7.15). The accuracy should not be in doubt if the calibration is satisfactory and the correct procedure followed. Despite this, systematic errors can occur. They are usually due to neglect of some apparently trivial aspect of the procedure or a defect in the equipment that is not readily amenable to calibration. The operator performing a biological calibration can detect such errors. This entails applying the test to a group of subjects with apparently normal lungs. The results should be comparable with those published in the literature (Chapter 26). To ensure that this level of performance is maintained, a routine should be established for the regular repetition of the calibration. Only at this stage is the equipment ready for use.

2.6 Conduct of assessments

The appointment, arrangements and underlying considerations. Arrangements for the appointment should lead to the appropriate measurements being made including those needed for interpretation. This is best achieved by including in the form completed by the referring doctor both a clear statement as to why the patient has been referred and the option that the choice of tests be delegated to the laboratory (Fig. 2.1).

For the patient the notification should usually include an indication of the likely duration of the procedures. Patients should be asked to bring their reading glasses and wear loose clothing. It is advisable that they do not smoke or consume alcohol on the day of the test or attend soon after undertaking heavy exercise or eating a big meal. Any medication should be taken at the normal times; the clinical respiratory physiologist should record the times. However, where the response to bronchodilator is of interest, the patient may be asked not to use any bronchodilator drug or inhaler during the four hours prior to the appointment. Exposure to cold air should be avoided.

RESPIRATORY FUNCTION SERVICE REQUEST FORM		
Patient details:		How will patient come to lab?
Surname:	DOB:	Walking ☐
Forenames:	Hosp Number:	Chair ☐
Address:	Hospital/ward/clinic for report	Ambulance:
	Consultant:	One man ☐
		Two man ☐
Give Clinical Details		

Indicate both the "PROBLEM TO BE INVESTIGATED" and "TESTS" required			
PROBLEM TO BE INVESTIGATED		**TESTS TICK EITHER A or B**	
Airflow obstruction present?	☐	A Lab to decide	☐
reversibility?	☐	B Please undertake:	☐
induced by exercise?	☐	Spirometry – focus on:	
extra-thoracic?	☐	FEV_1 and Vital capacity	☐
baseline for therapy	☐	Response to bronchodilator	☐
inhaler technique suspect?	☐	State drug type..........................	
Transfer defect present?	☐	Therapeutic dose	☐
exercise desaturation?	☐	High dose (nebulised)	☐
Restrictive disorder?	☐	Test patient's technique with their inhaler	☐
Breathlessness – cause? (state haemoglobin)	☐	Assess inhaler device patient uses best	☐
Respiratory muscle weakness?	☐	Maximal flow volume curves	☐
Pre-operative assessment	☐	Lung volumes (Helium dilution)	☐
Factors limiting exercise?	☐	Gas transfer test (Tlco) State haemogloblin.................	☐
Other (please state):	☐	Maximal mouth pressures	☐
		Airways resistance (body box)	☐
OTHER CLINICAL PROBLEMS:		Exercise test: with oximetry	☐
		with respiratory data	☐
		Walking test (6 mins)	☐
		Shuttle test	☐
		Exercise-induced asthma: Detection	☐
MO's signature..		Protection against	☐
Print name...		Challenge test: Histamine	☐
Bleep / extension....................Date............		Metacholine	☐

Fig. 2.1 Example of a request form for lung function tests. Source: P. Tweeddale, personal communication, 2001.

Most appointments are likely to be during normal working hours. Very disabled patients are best seen in the middle of the day. Immunocompromised patients should be seen at the beginning of the day and patients with a high risk of infection should be left to the end of the day. Serial measurements should preferably be made in a post-absorptive state at a specific time of day and season of the year. The air temperature in the laboratory should be within the range 16–25°C (60–77°F).

Consent and other preliminaries to assessment. Prior to the patient being seen, the request form and other relevant material, for example the clinical notes and chest radiograph or radiologist's report, should be used to decide which measurements are needed. The chest radiograph can also provide an independent estimate of TLC (Section 10.3.4).

On attendance the subject, or in the case of young children the parent, is given a simple factual description of why lung function is to be measured and what is entailed. Tests for research purposes should have had ethics approval. Questions should be encouraged and answered, and explicit consent for the procedure should be obtained. A check should be made for any contraindications to the tests being considered.

The next step may be to supplement the clinical information, possibly by asking the questions contained in the British Medical Research Council Questionnaire of respiratory symptoms (Fig. 8.2, page 88). The questionnaire is available in most languages. If an adult patient is to be exercised, the blood pressure should be recorded and the electrocardiogram (ECG) inspected for abnormalities.

Quality control. At the beginning and end of the measurement session the necessary calibrations should be undertaken and the result noted (Section 7.16). A record must be kept of the procedures undertaken by each patient, the times when the measurements were made and any untoward effects. This should be recorded in the laboratory logbook.

Order of testing. At initial assessment stature, body mass and, for some applications, body composition should be measured. At subsequent assessments the latter measurements may need to be repeated (Section 4.7). The first lung function measurements are of FEV_1 and FVC by dynamic spirometry. Next, if the patient is in the habit of using a bronchodilator aerosol, this should be inhaled. The FEV_1 is then repeated after an appropriate interval and the remaining measurements undertaken, ending with exercise. Unless it is proposed to assess bronchial lability it is not helpful to give the bronchodilator late in the assessment.

Afterwards. After the measurements have been completed the subject should be thanked for participating and supplied with precise information as to when the results will be available, to whom they will be sent and how he or she can have access to them. It is advisable to confirm if the measurements were technically satisfactory. The practice of commenting on the results as they come up on the printer can be helpful if they lead to the subject improving his or her performance but may cause misapprehensions that are difficult to correct subsequently.

Reporting the results. An assessment of lung function is not complete until the result has been compiled and reported on. A report generated by an automated measurement system can be used but for a comprehensive assessment an individual report is preferable (Fig. 2.2). It should be based on all the relevant information. To achieve this the report form should include personal details about the subject, anthropometric measurements, the results, the reference values, any previous result that may be relevant and spaces for a comment and clinical, biochemical and radiographic information. These items should be to hand when the comment is prepared.

The anthropometric measurements and the clinical information will usually be obtained at the time of assessment and the chest radiograph and biochemical results (if available) coded at the time of preparing the comment. Reference values appropriate for most circumstances are given in Chapter 26.

The results and the reference values may be inserted into the report sheet by the clinical respiratory physiologist who made the measurements; alternatively, the data can be processed and printed automatically. In this event the report should be checked and initialled by the clinical respiratory physiologist as evidence for its accuracy.

Someone who was familiar with the patient's condition would traditionally have prepared the report. Now, independently prepared or automated reports are widely used; these can be of limited usefulness or even misleading on account of not considering all the relevant information. A report prepared from within the laboratory is preferable. It can be typed or written by hand and then photocopied.

The reporters base their comments on the list of results and they must be able to rely on their accuracy. Their trust should be founded on familiarity with the equipment, an adequate laboratory routine and a procedure for finding faults involving both the clinical respiratory physiologist who made the measurements and the reporter (Section 7.16). Direct discussion between the parties improves the quality control. It can also contribute to clinical management, since the patient sometimes shares information with technical staff that he or she does not tell the physician!

The interpretation of the measurements should be based on all the individual findings. Each of these will be compared with the reference value, normally either a previous result for that subject or one obtained from tables. For the principal indices the result under scrutiny can conveniently be allocated to one of four categories: normal, or slightly, moderately or grossly abnormal (e.g. Section 26.8).

If abnormality is suspected or established, the next step is to discover its nature. This will entail recognition of a characteristic pattern of abnormality such as one of the syndromes of abnormal function described in Chapter 38 or of physiological

LUNG FUNCTION REPORT		Result	Ref value	SD units
Name:	Date	/ /	-	-
Address:	FEV_1 Pre-br (l)			
	drug:................ Post-br (l)		-	
	time(min): Diff (l or %)		-	-
Hospital number:	FVC Pre-br (l)			
Consultant:	Post-br (l)		-	
Date: / / DOB: / /	Diff (l or %)		-	-
Age: Sex:	FEV% (%)			
Occupation:	PEF Pre-br ($l.s^{-1}$)			
Ethnicity:	Post-br ($l.s^{-1}$)		-	
Clinical diagnosis:	Diff ($l.s^{-1}$ or %)		-	-
	$FEF_{50\%FVC}$ ($l.s^{-1}$)			
ECG:	$FEF_{75\%FVC}$ ($l.s^{-1}$)			
BP (systemic):	AWR on insp ($kPa.l.^{-1}.s$)			
Bronchitis [a]:	At lung volume (l)		-	-
Wheeze [a]:	TLC Helium dil (l)			
Breathlessness grade [a]:	VC (l)			
Smoking:	FRC (l)			
X-ray:	RV (l)			
	RV% (%)			
Height (m): Weight (kg):	Cstat insp ($l.kPa^{-1}$)[b]			
BMI ($kg.m^{-2}$):	Cstat exp ($l.kPa^{-1}$)[b]			
FFM (kg): Fat %:	Recoil pr (max) (kPa)[b]			
Hb ($g.dl^{-1}$):	*P*static (TLC-20%VC) (kPa)[b]			
COMMENT:	MEP (TLC) (kPa)[b]			
	MIP (FRC) (kPa)[b]			
	MIP (RV) (kPa)[b]			
	*Tl*co ($mmol.min^{-1}. kPa^{-1}$)[c]			
	*Tl*co (adj for VA)			
	kco (*Tl*/VA)			
	Mixing index (VA'/VA)			

EXERCISE RESULTS				
Treadmill / Bike		Submax	Ref Submax / max	Max result
O_2 uptake	(mmol or $l. min^{-1}$)		/	
$\dot{V}_{E, air}$	($l. min^{-1}$)		/	
R			/	
$\dot{V}_{E, O_2}$	($l. min^{-1}$)		/	
Vt_{30}	(l)		/ -	-
*f*C	(min^{-1})		/	
ΔSa_{O_2}	(%)		/	
Pa,O_2	(kPa)[b]		/	
Pa,CO_2	(kPa)[b]		/	
Vd/*Vt*	(%)		/	
$\dot{Q}va / \dot{Q}t$	(%)		/	
$\dot{Q}t$	($l.min^{-1}$)		/	
SV (max)	(l)			

Report prepared by:

[a] from MRC questionnaire on respiratory symptoms

[b] In traditional units pressure is in cmH_2O or mm Hg.

[c] In traditional units $ml.min^{-1}.mmHg^{-1}$

Fig. 2.2 Example of a lung function report form.

adaptation described in Parts 3 to 6. For the report to be conclusive the pattern should be consistent with all the physiological results, the clinical features, the appearance of the chest radiograph and other information about the person being assessed. Inconsistencies within or between any of these classes of information should lead to reappraisal of the findings with a view to achieving a comprehensive interpretation or deciding how the inconsistency should be resolved. Strategies for assessment are in Chapter 39.

2.7 References

1. Miller MR, Hankinson J, Brusasco V et al. ATS/ERS Task Force: standardisation of spirometry. *Eur Respir J.* 2005; **26**: 319–338.
2. Quanjer PhH, ed. Standardized lung function testing. *Bull Eur Physiopathol Respir* 1983; **19** (Suppl 5): 1–95.
3. American Thoracic Society. Lung function testing; selection of reference values and interpretative strategies. *Am Rev Respir Dis* 1991; **144**: 1202–1218.
4. Quanjer PhH, Tammeling GJ, Cotes JE et al. Standardized lung function testing: lung volumes and forced ventilatory flows: 1993 update. *Eur Respir J* 1993; **6** (Suppl 16): 4–40.
5. Guidelines for the measurement of respiratory function; recommendations of the British Thoracic Society and the Association of Respiratory Technicians and Physiologists. *Respir Med* 1994; **88**: 165–194.
6. Stocks J, Sly P, Morris MG, Frey U. Standards for infant respiratory function testing: what(ever) next? *Eur Respir J* 2000; **16**: 581–584. [This article makes extensive reference to best practices.]
7. Gilson JC, Hugh-Jones P, Oldham PD, Meade F. Lung function in coal workers' pneumoconiosis. *Spec Rep Med Res Coun (Lond)* 1955; **290**: 114–124, 150–201.
8. Gardner RM, Clausen JL, Epler GR et al. (on behalf of the ATS). Pulmonary function laboratory personnel qualifications. *Am Rev Respir Dis* 1986; **134**: 623–624.

Further reading

Brewis RAL, Gibson GJ, Geddes DM, eds. *Respiratory medicine,* 2nd ed. London: Baillière Tindall, 1995.

Chang HK, Paiva M, eds. *Lung biology in health and disease, Vol. 40: Respiratory physiology – an analytical approach.* New York: Marcel Dekker, 1989.

Crystal RG, Barnes PJ, West JB, Weibel ER, eds. *The lung: scientific foundations,* vols 1 and 2, 2nd ed. Philadelphia: Lippincott-Raven, 1997.

Hughes JMB, Pride NB, eds. *Lung function tests: physiological principles and clinical applications.* London: Saunders, 1999.

Murray JF, Nadel JA, Mason RJ, Boushey HA. *Textbook of respiratory medicine,* 3rd ed. London: WB Saunders, 2000.

Lumb A. *Nunn's applied respiratory physiology,* 5th ed. London: Butterworths, 2000.

West JB, ed. *Lung biology in health and disease, Vol. 3: Bioengineering aspects of the lung.* New York: Marcel Dekker, 1977.

CHAPTER 3

Development and Functional Anatomy of the Respiratory System

The structure of the respiratory system is the key to its function. This chapter describes the main features.

3.1 Introduction

Access to the lungs is through the upper airways; these are described below. The lungs occupy the thoracic cavity, which is a space bounded by the chest wall and the diaphragm. The space is lubricated by fluid present in the pleura. The cavity is subdivided by the mediastinum and by the heart extending out into the left thoracic space. On this account the left lung is somewhat smaller than the right lung, with respective weights in healthy young adult males of approximately 500 and 600 g. The shape is nearly pyramidal with a height of approximately 20 cm and a density when fully inflated of about 0.2 kg dm^{-3}. The lungs connect with the internal environment via the pulmonary artery, pulmonary vein, lymphatics and vagus nerves.

The lungs can be visualised by chest radiography, bronchography, computer-assisted tomography (CT scans), magnetic resonance imaging (MRI) and use of radio-tagged particles and gases. The movements can be observed, inspected by X-ray screening and listened to with a stethoscope. Endoscopic techniques can be used to inspect and take samples from the airways, the pleural space and the mediastinum. Hence, the lungs are very accessible to observation during life as well as subsequently.

3.2 Functional anatomy of the upper airways

The upper airways comprise the nose, the nasopharynx and the oropharynx. Their relative positions are indicated in Fig. 3.1.

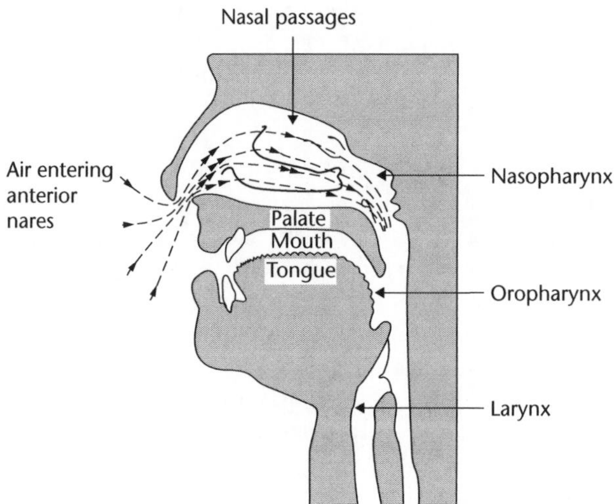

Fig. 3.1 Functional anatomy of the nose. The small cross-sectional area of the anterior nares results in a high linear velocity (indicated by arrows). This leads to the larger particles impacting on the anterior tip of the turbinate bones. Source: Adapted from [1].

The air passages are lined by ciliated cubical or columnar epithelium interspersed with goblet cells and receptors or free nerve endings supplied by the trigeminal and glossopharyngeal nerves (Section 3.3.10).

The main function of the upper airways is to condition the air that is inspired. In addition, the pharynx and epiglottis are adapted to compensate for the defect in design that led to the conduits to the lungs and stomach crossing over in the pharynx instead of being separate. The crossing is a consequence of the lungs budding off the ventral surface of the primitive endodermal tube. In retrospect an origin from the lateral or dorsal surfaces might have been better!

Conditioning the incoming gas. During nasal breathing the incoming air is warmed and humidified by passing over the richly vascular ciliated epithelium of the nasopharynx. Close contact over a wide area is ensured by the presence of the turbinate bones. These lead to the pathway being circuitous, the passages narrow (width approximately 2 mm) and the area of epithelium relatively large (approximately 50 cm^2). As a result, except under conditions of extreme cold (Section 36.2), air enters the trachea at near to body temperature and almost fully saturated with water vapour. The process of equilibration with the internal environment is completed in the lungs. It is reversed during exhalation when some of the heat and moisture in the gas leaving the lungs is returned to the nasal epithelium.

Purifying the incoming gas. Atmospheric air is seldom completely free of contaminants. It almost always contains some particles and may contain foreign gases, for example ammonia, sulphur dioxide or hydrogen sulphide. Depending on its solubility a proportion of any contaminant gas is taken up or modified in the nose and upper airways. However, the protection that is provided to the lungs is incomplete. The nasal apparatus is more successful in removing particulate material, though here, unlike in rodents, the lung airways also contribute to the protection of the alveoli (Section 37.2.2).

Control of air movement in the oropharynx. The oropharynx is normally open for the flow of air as a consequence of tonic contractions of the respective abductor muscles. These include the genioglossus, tensor palati and medial pterygoid muscles. The tone is greater on inspiration than on expiration. The resulting slight obstruction to flow of gas is a component of total pulmonary resistance (Section 14.3.2). The tone in the muscles is reduced during sleep and minimal during snoring. It is absent in some types of obstructive sleep apnoea (Section 32.4.1).

3.3 The lungs

3.3.1 Early stages in development

The laryngotracheal groove forms in the endodermal tube when the embryo is approximately 26 days of age. The lung bud forms almost immediately and divides progressively, so that in normal circumstances the bronchial structure of the lung is complete by the sixteenth week [2]. If development is retarded before this time the number of airway generations can be reduced. The bronchi are lined by columnar epithelium and are closely packed together to give the lung a *pseudoglandular* appearance. The bronchi are separated by mesenchymal tissue, which at this stage already contains blood vessels. During the following two months (weeks 16–24) the mesenchyme differentiates further with extensive growth of capillaries. By birth the branching network of pulmonary arteries and veins is complete.

At about the twenty-first week the epithelium of some peripheral airways becomes flattened; this is associated with the airways becoming more conspicuous, and hence the designation *canalicular stage* of foetal development. Alveolar type I and type II cells are now recognisable, the latter containing osmiophilic bodies, indicating the appearance of surface-active material. This has the property of lowering the surface tension at the air to tissue interface (Section 11.3). The lung is now capable of normal expansion and of supporting life.

By about the twenty-eighth week the first true alveoli appear in the walls of some peripheral airways, indicating the appearance of respiratory bronchioles. Growing out from them are short channels, designated *transitional ducts,* which in turn produce peripheral saccules, and hence the *saccular stage of development.* The saccules are present at birth. The interstitium now contains the capillary network and numerous cells; some of these lay down elastic material where the future alveoli are to be formed. Subsequently, the transitional ducts and saccules develop into alveolar ducts, atria and alveoli [3]. The latter continue to increase during the first 4 years of extrauterine life. During this period the double layer of capillaries between alveoli merge to form a single layer. At this point the formation of new alveoli normally ceases. The process of fusion reduces the quantity of interalveolar tissue. It is associated with holes appearing in some interalveolar septa; these are the pores of Kohn (Section 3.3.5). The lungs continue to grow up to or beyond puberty (Section 25.3). During this time the increase in lung volume is achieved by enlargement of all structures, not by proliferation of alveoli. The increases in size are not uniform; for example the diameters of peripheral airways increase relatively more than those of the proximal airways. As a result the airflow resistance falls [4].

The anatomical development of the lung has been described by Thurlbeck [5] and Zeltner and Burri [6] amongst others. The changes at birth are in Section 24.2.

The lung develops from both epidermal and mesodermal cells. They grow by proliferation, migration, differentiation and adhesion and these processes involve interactions with extracellular matrix, platelets and other bodies. The substances in the matrix include fibronectin, laminin, collagen and elastin.

Development is initiated and regulated by a host of factors. In the case of the pulmonary vascular bed, they include growth factors from fibroblasts, platelets, endothelial cells, heparin-binding growth factor, platelet endothelial cell adhesion molecules and other components. The outcomes are both strategic in the branching morphology and local in the detailed structure of the lung. The stimuli arise from the interactions that have been mentioned, supplemented by environmental factors. The latter includes the prevailing tension of oxygen, the amount of blood flow through the lungs and the extent of lung movement. The movements are associated with local stresses that lead to the deposition of elastic tissue. The processes are easily deranged, for example, by too much or too little oxygen or exposure to some herbicides. Oligohydramnios or other abnormality that impairs foetal breathing can cause congenital pulmonary hypoplasia. Growth hormones contribute to the overall size of the lung. Glucocorticoid action promotes the maturation of preformed alveolar epithelium and the synthesis of surfactant compounds, and so their use can be therapeutic (Section 24.3.2). However, at an earlier stage of development corticosteroid drugs can suppress the formation of new alveoli [7]. The subject has been reviewed by Gaultier and colleagues [8].

3.3.2 Bronchopulmonary anatomy

The right lung is subdivided into upper, middle and lower lobes; each connects with a branch of the right main bronchus. The bronchus to the right lower lobe is a nearly linear continuation of the trachea. The left lung is subdivided into the upper and lower lobes and the lingula; the latter is supplied by the lingular or lower division of the left upper lobe bronchus and is analogous to the middle lobe of the right lung. The lobes are divided into segments; these are listed in Table 3.1.

Within each segment the bronchus subdivides and gives off between 10 and 25 branches, of which the diameters in adults range from about 1 cm downwards; the path length from the carina is in the range 8–23 cm.

The *pattern of branching* is described in terms of models of which two are in common use. In Weibel's model [9] the right and left main bronchi constitute generation one and the generation number is increased at each dichotomy. This is useful for describing the larger airways, for example in relation to bronchoscopy. The model breaks down when describing the peripheral airways because these are allocated to different generations depending on their distance from the carina; this obscures the relationship of branch number to diameter. In addition, if a common path length is assumed, the model overestimates the number of terminal units and predicts incorrectly that the total cross-sectional area of the respiratory tract increases progressively, with distance from the carina resembling the contour of a trumpet. These errors are avoided by ordering the airways from the periphery as is done in the procedure of Horsfield and Cumming [10] (Fig. 3.2). Their model correctly describes the distribution of airway cross-sectional area as onion-shaped, with a maximum some 12 cm from the carina. The average numbers and dimensions of airways in the different orders are given in Fig. 3.3.

Table 3.1 Nomenclature of bronchopulmonary anatomy.

Right lung		Left lung	
Bronchi	Segments	Bronchi	Segments
Upper lobe	Apical (1)	Upper lobe	Apical (1)
	Posterior (2)		Apicoposterior (1)
	Anterior (3)		Anterior (2)
Middle lobe	Lateral (4)		Superior (3) (lingula)
	Medial (5)		Inferior (4) (lingula)
Lower lobe	Apical (6)	Lower lobe	Apical (5)
	Medial basal (7)		Medial basal (6)
	Anterior basal (8)		Anterior basal (7)
	Lateral basal (9)		Lateral basal (8)
	Posterior basal (10)		Posterior basal (9)

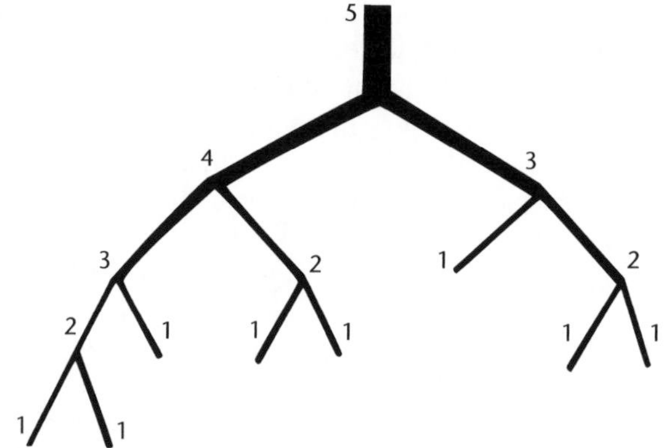

Fig. 3.2 Model of the bronchial tree showing asymmetrical branching. The ordering starts at the periphery. Where two branches meet the parent branch is one order higher than the higher ordered daughter branch. Source: [10].

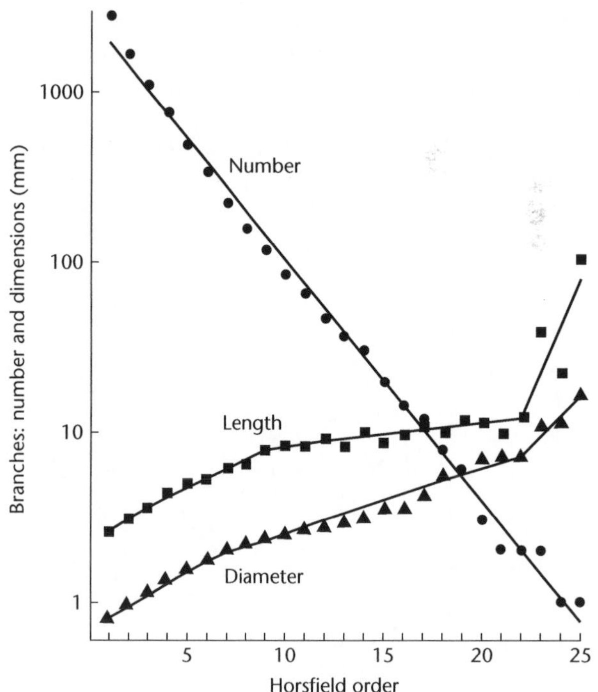

Fig. 3.3 Number, mean diameter and mean length of branches in each Horsfield order of a cast of the human bronchial tree. Straight lines represent the regression equations. The ordering starts three bifurcations up from the terminal bronchioles ($n \approx 25{,}000$). Source: [11].

The two-dimensional model of Weibel and that of Horsfield and Cumming do not allow for the spatial arrangement of airway structure. Kitaoka and colleagues developed a three-dimensional model of the human airway tree down to the level of the terminal bronchiole [12]. The model predicts 54,611 branches, with 27,306 terminal bronchioles with an average diameter of 0.48 mm (SD 0.06 mm). The lung volume is 6388 ml, and the total airway volume is 174 ml. It differs from that of Horsfield by predicting more terminal bronchioles with a wider distribution of generation numbers. The model agrees well with morphometric characteristics from casts of the bronchial tree and may have benefits over the Horsfield model in, for example, CT analysis.

3.3.3 Intrapulmonary airways

The intrapulmonary airways are of endothelial origin and are fully differentiated by the sixteenth week of gestation. The proximal airways (i.e. bronchi) have cartilage in their walls, mucous glands beneath the basement membrane and columnar epithelium. The distal subdivisions are bronchioles and differ from the bronchi in having no cartilage or mucous glands and being lined by cubical rather than columnar epithelium. Both types of cell are ciliated and are interspersed with goblet cells (Fig. 3.4). The cilia provide the driving force for the mucociliary escalator that clears debris from the surface of airways (Section 37.2.2). To this end the motion of cilia is normally forwards and backwards in the line of flow. The beat frequency in young persons is of the order of 12 Hz. It declines slightly with age [14]. The function of cilia is deranged in primary ciliary dyskinesia and as a consequence of exposure to cold, infection, smoking, harmful gases and other insults (Section 36.3 and Chapter 37).

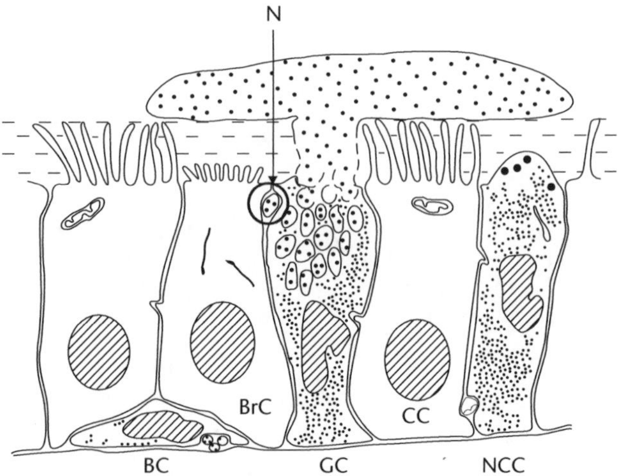

Fig. 3.4 Human bronchial epithelium traced from an electron micrograph. BrC, brush cell; GC, goblet cell; CC, ciliated cell; NCC, non-ciliated cell; BC, basement cell; N, nerve cell with irritant receptor. Source: Courtesy of P.K. Jeffery [13].

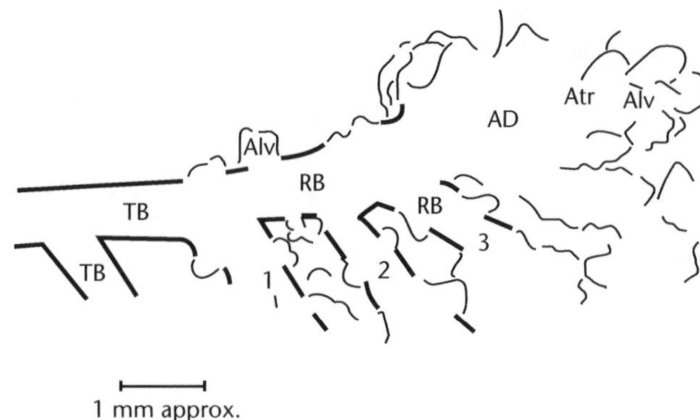

Fig. 3.5 The normal anatomy of the air-containing structures of the acinus (the respiratory portion of the bronchiolar tree). The figure shows terminal bronchioles (TB), three orders of respiratory bronchioles (RB1, 2 and 3), an alveolar duct (AD), atrium (Atr) and alveoli (Alv). The acinus is approximately spherical and of average diameter 6 mm. Source: [16].

The average densities of surface mucus cells and submucosal gland ducts in human trachea have been estimated respectively at 6000–7000 cells and 10 ducts per mm^2 of surface epithelium [15]. Goblet cells make up about 15% of the columnar cells.

The goblet cells end distally at the level of the terminal bronchiole; these airways are the most distal bronchioles to have a continuous layer of smooth muscle, and hence no alveoli opening off their walls. The terminal bronchioles have an internal diameter in the range 0.3–1.0 mm; their total number in the two lungs is of the order of 25,000. Clusters of between 3 and 5 terminal bronchioles constitute the secondary lobules. Some of these units are surrounded by fibrous septa that render them visible to the naked eye. The portion of lung distal to one terminal brochiole is called an *acinus* (Fig. 3.5).

3.3.4 Acinus

The structure of the acinus has been investigated quantitatively amongst others by Weibel, who made measurements on sections using random samples [9], and by Horsfield and Hansen and their respective colleagues, who attempted three-dimensional reconstructions [17, 18].

A typical acinus contains some 14 respiratory bronchioles; these are bronchioles that have alveoli opening from their walls. Each of them has shallow alveoli in its wall and communicates with approximately 100 alveolar ducts and air sacs. Between these structures the epithelium comprises ciliated cubical cells and Clara cells; these resemble the alveolar type II cells and, like them, have a secretory function (Section 11.3). A small pulmonary artery usually adjoins the first-order respiratory bronchiole, and so the distribution of air spaces is not symmetrical.

More air spaces are present on the second- and third-order respiratory bronchioles. The largest spaces are alveolar ducts of which there are up to eight orders; the diameter is in the range 0.6–2 mm. Air sacs are smaller and have few distinctive features.

Each *alveolar duct* is lined by flattened epithelial cells and is supported by a spring-like spiral fibre of collagen, elastin and smooth muscle cells. The alveoli emerge from between the turns of the spiral, usually 5–8 per turn; they are roughly hexagonal in shape except for the terminal alveolus, which is spherical. There are between 10 and 30 alveoli per duct and this unit constitutes a primary lobule. The vessels run between the alveolar duct systems and surround the alveoli.

3.3.5 Collateral channels

The alveoli communicate with each other through the pores of Kohn, which are discrete holes in the walls between alveoli, often with a cuboidal type II alveolar cell forming part of the aperture (Section 11.3). The pores probably form during the process of thinning of alveolar septa that occurs after birth (Section 3.3.1) and then expand as the alveoli enlarge during the first few years of life. Their absence in infancy is a factor in young children being relatively susceptible to atelectasis. Accessory communications between some bronchioles and their adjacent alveoli have been described by Lambert [19] and there are also communications between alveolar ducts and between respiratory bronchioles; their diameter is up to 200 μm. These communications permit collateral ventilation between adjacent portions of lung tissue. Larger communications occur in the lungs of some other mammals, for example dogs, in which there is less interlobular connective tissue than in man.

3.3.6 Alveoli

Most alveoli are formed in the first 2 years of extrauterine life. Their size increases throughout the period of growth. Hence there is an approximately 20-fold increase in surface area between birth and adulthood. The number of alveoli in the two lungs together varies directly with the final lung volume and is usually in the range (200–600) $\times$ 10^6[20]. The average diameter is 0.25 mm; it is independent of the size of the lungs [21]. The total surface area estimated by light microscopy is approximately 70–80 m^2. Using electron microscopy the estimate is doubled [22]. The alveoli are lined by type I alveolar cells (epithelial cells) whose thickness away from the nuclei is in the range 0.04–0.07 μm. The cells lie on a basement membrane (Fig. 3.6). For 2 alveoli that are adjacent the basement membranes enclose the components of the interalveolar septum, including reticulin fibres, elastic fibres, the histiocytes (macrophages) and capillaries with their lining of endothelial cells. The total thickness of the alveolar capillary membrane is normally in the range 0.15–0.5 μm. The alveoli are lined with a film of lipopolysaccharide (surfactant) that is secreted by the alveolar type II cells (Section 11.3).

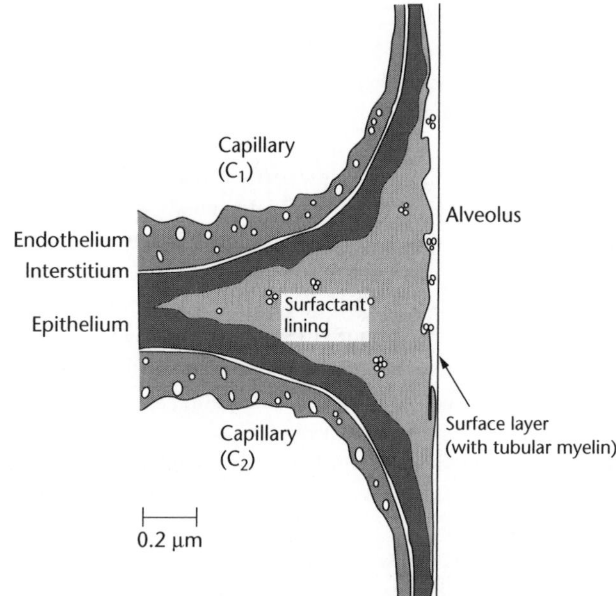

Fig. 3.6 Line drawing of a photomicrograph showing the surfactant lining of part of an alveolus at the junction between two alveolar capillaries (C_1 and C_2). The lining layer contains tubular myelin and is indicated by an arrow; the lining bridges over amorphous fluid (hypophase) in the trough between the capillaries. The alveolar capillary membrane comprising endothelium, interstitium, epithelium and surface layer is thickened in consequence (scale 0.2 μm). Source: [23].

The epithelial cells (type I) are in close apposition and have minimal gaps between them; the mean pore size is 0.5 nm. As a result, alveolar oedema is rare in healthy persons. It has been described during maximal exercise. The condition is commoner in racehorses when it is associated with very high transmural capillary pressures (up to 40 mm Hg) [24]. By contrast to the epithelial cells, the endothelial cells that line alveolar capillaries are separated by clefts and by pores of diameter 12–15 nm. The pores open when the capillary is distended; in this circumstance a filtrate of plasma-containing albumen will pass into the interstitial space. On this account interstitial oedema will occur if the capillary intravascular pressure is increased or the plasma osmotic pressure is reduced.

3.3.7 Pulmonary circulation

The pulmonary artery is developed from the artery to the left sixth branchial arch and is the main source of blood for the lung. It conveys most of the cardiac output from the right ventricle to the alveolar capillaries. The pulmonary artery divides into right and left pulmonary arteries and these in turn subdivide to provide up to eight generations of elastic-walled vessels of diameter more than 2 mm. Distal branches of diameters 2 mm down to 0.3 mm are small muscular pulmonary arteries; they run beside the airways that supply the parenchyma of the lung. Other vessels enter the periphery of the lung units where they provide a collateral circulation. The arteries end as terminal arterioles that supply the individual acini; these vessels have thin walls, a diameter of less than 150 μm, and a surrounding perivascular space. Accumulation of fluid in the space can interfere with blood flow (Sections 17.1.3 and 18.4.4). The arterioles deliver blood to capillary networks that lie in the septa between the alveoli; the networks drain into pulmonary venules in the periphery of the lobules. The venules unite to form veins that run in the septa and join to form the main pulmonary veins that end in the left atrium of the heart.

Pulmonary arterioles do not anastomose with each other but they may communicate with the pulmonary veins through anastomotic channels bypassing the alveolar capillaries; the significance of the channels is not known. Blood that has not traversed the alveolar capillaries may flow directly into the pulmonary veins or left atrium from the bronchial arteries and veins and the lower oesophageal veins. Entry can also occur if there is anomalous drainage from the coronary sinus or azygos veins.

Blood from the coronary circulation can enter the left ventricle through the thebesian veins; however, the amount is normally less than 0.4% of cardiac output and the total quantity of blood that bypasses the alveolar capillaries is usually small (see Fig. 18.1, page 211). This physiological shunt can be increased in a number of diseases including pulmonary fibrosis, bronchiectasis, bronchial carcinoma and portal hypertension.

The physiology of the pulmonary circulation is considered in Chapter 17.

3.3.8 Bronchial arteries

These structures arise from the thoracic aorta. Their related arterioles provide nutrients to the visceral pleura, pulmonary arteries and conducting airways down to and including the respiratory bronchioles. Structures distal to the bronchioles, including the primary lobules, are supplied by branches of the pulmonary artery. The bronchial veins anastomose with the pulmonary veins. The bronchial arterioles communicate with the pulmonary arterioles in newborn infants but not in later life except when the pulmonary arteriolar flow is reduced by lung disease. In this circumstance, oxygenated bronchiolar blood can enter the pulmonary circulation.

3.3.9 Pulmonary lymphatics

The lymphatics drain the connective tissue spaces of the lung down to the level of the primary lobules including the interlobular, subpleural, peribronchial and perivascular spaces. They run proximally from the level of the alveolar ducts into lymph nodes that adjoin the respiratory bronchioles. From here the drainage is into nodes, which lie along the course of the bronchi and at the hilum of the lung. The latter drain into the cervical, para-aortic, subdiaphragmatic and anterior mediastinal nodes. Flow of lymph also occurs into plexuses of lymphatics that lie beneath the pleura and into channels that accompany the pulmonary veins. Flow is directional because of the presence of valves. Lymphatics have not been observed in the walls of atria or alveoli. The final lymphatic outflow for the left lung is into the thoracic duct and for the right lung the right lymphatic duct; these vessels enter systemic veins at the junctions of the subclavian and internal jugular veins.

3.3.10 Innervation

The autonomic nerve supply to the lung is from the vagi and the fibres of the cervical and the upper six thoracic ganglia of the sympathetic nervous system. The postganglionic sympathetic fibres enter the pulmonary plexus; this forms a sheath round the bronchi and the bronchioles in which are embedded the parasympathetic ganglia. The ganglia provide a parasympathetic cholinergic motor innervation to the bronchial smooth muscle, the secretory epithelium and the bronchial glands. The plexus provides a sympathetic adrenergic motor innervation; this supplies the bronchial and pulmonary blood vessels and submucosal glands but not the bronchial smooth muscle. The latter deficiency is compensated for by a high density of adrenoceptors, especially β_2 receptors (Section 15.7.1). An additional autonomic nerve supply to the lung is provided by the peptidergic or non-adrenergic, non-cholinergic system (NANC). The mediators for NANC include vasoactive intestinal peptide and substance P, which respectively relax and constrict bronchial smooth muscle. The role of the system has been investigated by Richardson [25] amongst others.

3.3.11 Pulmonary receptors

The sensory nerves arise from receptors in the upper respiratory tract, the lung and the pulmonary vascular bed; some are listed in Table 3.2.

The role of the receptors in the upper airways is mainly protective. The pulmonary receptors contribute to the pattern of breathing in a wide range of circumstances of which some are discussed subsequently. In addition, nodes of epithelioid cells resembling those in the carotid body (Section 23.5) occur in the glomus pulmonale; this is located near the bifurcation of the pulmonary artery. Other types of receptors have also been described; many have still to be investigated in detail.

Table 3.2 Features of some respiratory receptors.

Site/name	Location	Nerve/type	Stimuli	Responses
Nose	Epithelium/mucosa	Trigeminal myelinated /C-fibre	Dusts Vapours Irritants Cold Mediators Touch	Sneeze Apnoea Bronchodilatation/ constriction Hypotension Bradycardia
Nasopharynx	Epithelium/mucosa	Glossopharyngeal myelinated	Pressure/touch	Sniff/aspiration reflex Hypertension Bronchodilatation
Oropharynx/epiglottis	Epithelium/mucosa	Glossopharyngeal myelinated	Pressure/touch	Swallow
Larynx	Epithelium/mucosa/muscle	Laryngeal, superior/ recurrent myelinated/ C-fibre	Pressure Cold/flow Irritants Muscle contraction Mediators	Cough Apnoea Expiration Laryngo- and bronchoconstriction Mucus secretion Hypertension Change in fC
Airways: rapidly adapting receptors (RARs)	Epithelium/mucosa	Vagus/small myelinated	Dusts Irritants Mediators Touch Deep breaths Bronchoconstriction Airway diseases	Cough Deep breaths Hyperpnoea Laryngo and bronchoconstriction Mucus secretion
Airways: slowly adapting receptors (SARs)	Smooth muscle	Vagus/large myelinated	Inflation Smooth muscle contraction Hypocarbia	Inhibit inspiration Prolong expiration Bronchodilatation
Airways: C-fibre receptors (formerly J receptors, also in acinus)	Epithelium	Vagus/non-myelinated	Irritants Mediators Airway diseases	Apnoea Tachypnoea Laryngo- and bronchoconstriction Hypotension Bradycardia Mucus secretion
Acinus: C-fibre receptors	Alveolar wall	Vagus/non-myelinated	As for bronchial C-fibre receptors	As for bronchial C-fibre receptors
Neuroepithelial bodies	Airway epithelium	Vagus/spinal non-myelinated	Hypoxia, irritants	Uncertain ? local reflexes

Source: [26].

3.4 References

1. Swift DL, Proctor DF. Access of air to the respiratory tract. In: Brain JD, Proctor DF, Reid LM, eds. *Respiratory defence mechanisms, Part 1: Lung biology in health and disease*, Vol. 1. New York: Marcel Dekker, 1997: 63–93.
2. Bucher U, Reid L. Development of the intrasegmental bronchial tree: the pattern of branching and development of cartilage at various stages of intrauterine life. *Thorax* 1961; **16**: 207–218.
3. Hislop A, Reid L. Development of the acinus in the human lung. *Thorax* 1974; **29**: 90–94.

4. Hogg JC, Williams J, Richardson JB et al. Age as a factor in the distribution of lower airway conductance and in the pathologic anatomy of obstructive lung disease. *N Engl J Med* 1970; **111**: 1283–1287.
5. Thurlbeck WM. Postnatal growth and development of the lung. *Am Rev Respir Dis* 1975; **111**: 803–844.
6. Zeltner TB, Burri PH. The postnatal development and growth of the human lung, II: Morphology. *Respir Physiol* 1987; **67**: 269–282.
7. Massaro GD, Massaro D. Formation of pulmonary alveoli and gas-exchange surface area: quantitation and regulation. *Ann Rev Physiol* 1996; **58**: 73–92.
8. Gaultier C, Bourbon JR, Post M, eds. *Lung development.* New York: Oxford University Press, 1999.
9. Weibel ER. *Morphometry of the human lung.* Berlin: Springer, 1963.
10. Horsfield K, Cumming G. Morphology of the bronchial tree in man. *J Appl Physiol* 1968; **24**: 373–383.
11. Horsfield K. *Handbook of physiology. The respiratory system*, Vol. III. Bethesda, MD: American Physiological Society, 1986: 75–86.
12. Kitaoka H, Takaki R, Suki B. A three-dimensional model of the human airway tree. *J Appl Physiol* 1999; **87**: 2207–2217.
13. Jeffery PK, Reid LM. Ultrastructure of normal large bronchi. *Les Bronches* 1973; **23**: 368–380.
14. Chilvers MA, Rutman A, O'Callaghan C. Functional analysis of cilia and ciliated epithelial ultrastructure in healthy children and young adults. *Thorax* 2003; **58**: 333–338.
15. Ellefsen P, Tos M. Goblet cells in the human trachea: quantitative studies of a pathological biopsy material. *Arch Otolaryngol* 1972; **95**: 547–555.
16. Reid L. The secondary lobule in the adult human lung, with special reference to its appearance in bronchograms. *Thorax* 1958; **13**: 110–115.
17. Horsfield K, Relea FG, Cumming G. Diameter, length and branching ratios in the bronchial tree. *Respir Physiol* 1976; **26**: 351–356.
18. Hansen JE, Ampaya EP, Bryant GH, Gavin JJ. Branching pattern of airways and air spaces of a single human terminal bronchiole. *J Appl Physiol* 1975; **38**: 983–989.
19. Lambert MW. Accessory bronchiole-alveolar communications. *J Pathol Bacteriol* 1955; **70**: 311–314.
20. Angus GE, Thurlbeck WM. Number of alveoli in the human lung. *J Appl Physiol* 1972; **32**: 483–485.
21. Ochs M, Nyengaard JR, Jung A et al. The number of alveoli in the human lung. *Am J Respir Crit Care Med* 2004; **169**: 120–124.
22. Gehr P, Bachofen M, Weibel ER. The normal human lung: ultrastructure and morphometric estimation of diffusing capacity. *Resp Physiol* 1978; **32**: 121–140.
23. Weibel ER. *Handbook of physiology. The respiratory system*, Vol. III. Bethesda, MD: American Physiological Society, 1986: 100.
24. West JB. Cellular responses to mechanical stress: pulmonary capillary stress failure. *J Appl Physiol* 2000; **89**: 2483–2489.
25. Richardson JB. State of art. Nerve supply to the lungs. *Am Rev Respir Dis* 1979; **119**: 785–802.
26. Widdicombe JG. Airway receptors. *Resp Physiol* 2001; **125**: 3–15.

Further reading

Fillenz M, Widdicombe JG. Receptors of the lungs and airways. In: Neil E, ed. *Enteroceptors, Vol. 3/1: Handbook of sensory physiology.* Berlin: Springer-Verlag, 1972: 81–112.

Fung YC. A model of the lung structure and its validation. *J Appl Physiol* 1988; **64**: 2132–2141.

Hafeli-Bleuer B, Weibel ER. Morphometry of the human pulmonary acinus. *Anal Rec* 1988; **220**: 401–414.

Helms PJ. Lung growth: implications for the development of disease. *Thorax* 1994; **49**: 440–441.

Hislop A, Reid L. Pulmonary arterial development during childhood: branching, pattern and structure. *Thorax* 1973; **28**: 129–135.

Jeffrey PK. Airway mucosa: secretory cells, mucus and mucin genes. *Eur Respir J* 1997, **10**: 1655–1662.

Lauweryns JM. The juxta-alveolar lymphatics in the human adult lung. *Am Rev Respir Dis* 1970; **102**: 877–885.

Lee LY, Pisarri TE. Afferent properties and reflex functions of bronchopulmonary C-fibers. *Respir Physiol* 2001; **125**: 47–65.

Meyrick B, Reid L. The alveolar wall. *Br J Dis Chest* 1970; **64**: 121–140.

Miserocchi G, Mortola J, Sant 'Ambrogio G. Localization of pulmonary stretch receptors in the airways of the dog. *J Physiol (Lond)* 1973; **235**: 775–782.

Parker H, Horsfield K, Cumming G. Morphology of distal airways in the human lung. *J Appl Physiol* 1971; **31**: 386–391.

Raskin SP, Herman PG. Interacinar pathways in the human lung. *Am Rev Respir Dis* 1975; **111**: 489–495.

Ravin MB, Epstein RM, Malm JR. Contribution of thebesian veins to the physiologic shunt in anaesthetized man. *J Appl Physiol* 1965; **20**: 1148–1152.

Thurlbeck WM, Haines JR. Bronchial dimensions and stature. *Am Rev Respir Dis* 1975; **112**: 142–145.

Whimster WF. The microanatomy of the alveolar duct system. *Thorax* 1970; **25**: 141–149.

Widdicombe JG. Overview of neural pathways in allergy and asthma. *Pul Pharmacol Ther* 2003; **16**: 23–30.

Widdicombe JH, Bastacky SJ, Wu DX, Lee CY. Regulation of depth and composition of airway surface liquid. *Eur Respir J* 1997; **10**: 2892–2897.

Wilson TA, Bachofen H. A model for mechanical structure of the alveolar duct. *J Appl Physiol* 1982; **52**: 1064–1070.

CHAPTER 4

Body size and anthropometric measurements

This chapter indicates why anthropometric features should be included in any comprehensive assessment of lung function and describes some appropriate measurements.

4.1 Bodily components are matched for size

The several stages in the transfer of oxygen from the atmosphere to blood in alveolar capillaries are summarised in Chapter 2. The capacities of the different stages are in proportion [1] and related to body size and composition. Compared with a small person or one with much fat and little muscle, a larger, leaner or more athletic person is likely to have a larger total lung capacity, transfer factor, cardiac stroke volume and quantity of skeletal muscle (Fig. 4.1). Cardiac frequency is lower in consequence. Some associations with body composition in persons of European descent are summarised in Table 4.1. For other ethnic groups the findings are similar (Chapter 27). These observations indicate that reference values for functional indices in individuals should take account of body size and composition. Allowance is made by including in the reference equations one or more terms for anthropometric features. The most commonly used feature is stature, but for maximal accuracy other features should be included as well. The form of the equations is described in Section 5.6.1 and the equations themselves in Chapter 26.

The principal indices of human body size and composition and information about their measurement are summarised in Table 4.2. The subject is currently evolving. There is an extensive literature, including some that is particularly relevant to lung function [7–10]. Sources of equipment for measuring body composition are given in Footnote 4.1.

4.2 Growth and ageing

Growth begins in the uterus and is reflected in the mass and body length at birth. These features influence future growth and susceptibility to illness [11]. However, the dimensions are poor predictors of adult physique. Subsequent to birth, the relative growth in stature is maximal in infancy when it affects the head, neck and trunk more than the legs. There is a second peak at adolescence that affects mainly the legs. This adolescent growth spurt begins at approximately age 12 years in girls and age 14 in boys. The growth spurt is terminated through the attainment of adult stature, by which time the epiphyses of long bones have become closed. In most girls this occurs at about age 15 years, but in Western societies there is anecdotal evidence that some girls are now maturing later. The cessation of growth is often followed by a period during which the quantity of body fat increases. The

Footnote 4.1. In the UK, anthropometric equipment (including Holtain skinfold calipers) can be obtained from Holtain Ltd., Crosswell, Crymmych, Dyfed. SA41 3UF. Harpenden skinfold calipers are supplied by British Indicators Ltd., Quality House, 46-56 Dumfries St, Luton, Beds. LU1 5BP. For North America, see [9].

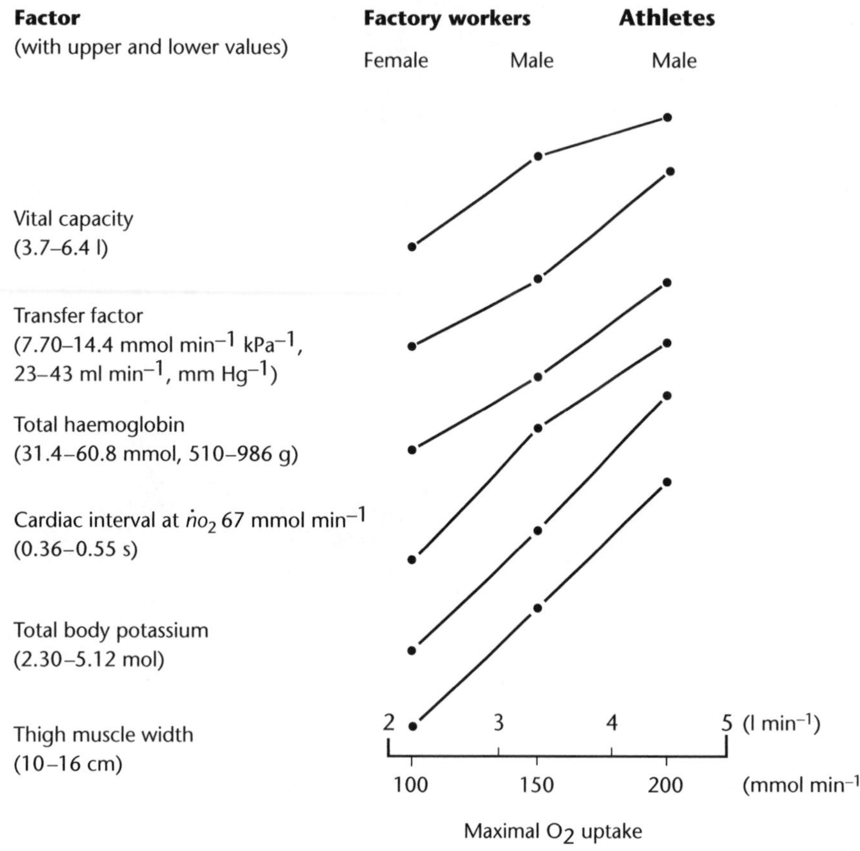

Fig. 4.1 Concordance between variables that relate to the maximal oxygen uptake. Source: [2].

Table 4.1 Contributions of Fat% and FFMI‡ to descriptions of physiological function.

Index	Contribution* Fat%	Contribution* FFMI	Effect on gender difference†	Effect on coefficient on age
Total lung capacity	–	+	Eliminated	Becomes positive in men
Vital capacity	–	+	Eliminated	Becomes less negative
Inspiratory capacity	ns	+	Eliminated	Term not significant anyway
Expiratory reserve volume	–	–	None anyway	Becomes less negative
Residual volume	–	ns	No change	No change
Transfer factor	ns	+	No change	No change
Exercise cardiac frequency ($f$csub-max)	ns	–	Eliminated	Not known
Maximal O_2 uptake ($\dot{V}O_2$max)	ns	+	Eliminated	Not known

*When significant (– or +) the confidence limits of the reference value are narrowed. ns: not significant.
†After allowing for age, stature and, in case of exercise indices, the level of habitual activity.
‡Fat free mass · stature^{-2}.
Source: [3–6].

Table 4.2 Anthropometric dimensions, indices and measurement techniques.*

Dimensions	Indices	Measurement techniques
Lengths	Stature (St) = sitting height + leg length†	Stadiometer
	Sitting height = trunk length + head and neck lengths	
	Ulna or other long bone	Anthropometer
Mass	Body mass (BM) [hence body mass index (BM St^{-2})]	Scales
	Fat-free mass (FFM) [=BM(1 – Fat%/100)]	See below
Breadths	Biacromial and bi-iliac diameters (shoulder and hip widths)	Anthropometer
	Mid-thoracic width	
	Epicondylar diameter of humerus (hence frame size)	Calipers
Girth	Waist and hip girths (hence waist/hip ratio)	Spring loaded tape
Bone mass	Site to be specified	Computerised tomography (CT)
		Magnetic resonance imaging (MRI)
		Dual X-ray absorptiometry (also for Fat%)
Body fat	Fat as percentage body mass (Fat%)	Underwater weighing (densitometry)
		Skinfold calipers and nomogram
		Ultrasonic probe
		Derived from body cell mass or total body water
		Excess mass adjusted for frame size
Abdominal fat	Waist circumference	Measuring tape
	Anterior abdominal skinfold thickness	Skinfold calipers
Muscle	Thigh muscle width and total leg muscle volume	CT, MRI or other method
	Fat-free mass (FFM), hence FFM Index (FFM St^{-2})	As for Fat%
	Body cell mass (BCM)	Total body potassium, measured as K^{40}
	Total body water (TBW)	Dilution of deuterium
		Bioelectrical impedance
Haemoglobin	Total body haemoglobin (THb)	Carbon monoxide uptake

*For details see text.

†Leg length can be obtained from this relationship or measured as distance from greater trochanter to floor with subject standing.

'puppy fat' usually disappears in early adult life (Section 25.3.2). Boys on average attain their adult stature at age 19 years, but a minority continues to grow in stature up to age 25 years. During this time thoracic width increases as well (Section 4.4, *also* [12]). This affects the lung function (Section 25.3.3).

The process of growth is controlled by growth hormone that enters the blood from the anterior pituitary gland. The release occurs mainly during sleep and is reduced if sleep is disturbed by nocturnal asthma. Treatment of the asthma by daily administration of steroid drugs can also suppress the production of the hormone sufficient to retard growth, but administration on alternate days seldom has this effect. Production of growth hormone is also reduced by malnutrition, intercurrent infection and other causes of suboptimal health. If the reason for the slowing is corrected, the period of growth is extended, but despite this, the final stature is usually below the expected level. Growth is promoted by a recumbent posture, appropriate nutrition and absence of infections. It is stimulated by increased exposure to growth hormone. The source of the additional hormone is endogenous in acromegaly or when production of growth hormone is increased by prolonged exercise. The source is exogenous if hormone is administered deliberately.

Once adult stature has been attained the skeletal dimensions normally remain relatively constant. However in later life, stature declines on account of thinning and compression of intervertebral discs. This occurs particularly in some women at and beyond the menopause. The decline in stature can be accentuated if the loss of bone mineral that occurs with age [13] causes collapse of vertebrae. An increase in curvature or twisting of the spine can also occur from other causes. In this circumstance the stature used for predicting the normal lung function should be estimated from the arm span (see below).

4.3 Stature (body length)

4.3.1 Overview

During the course of evolution the adult stature of primates increased up to a peak of approximately 2 m in Neanderthal man. *Homo sapiens* was initially shorter, but his stature has also increased. Some ethnic groups are taller than others. Recently there has been a further increase, particularly in the Netherlands (Holland) where a stature of 2 m is now relatively common. Equipment for measurement of stature should accommodate this development.

Stature (standing height) can be represented as the sum of leg length and sitting height. As a result, stature and sitting height are correlated. Both are also correlated with all the primary indices of lung function. The correlations are higher for stature than for sitting height, probably because the inclusion of leg length leads to a better representation of body size. On this account, stature is the principal reference variable for describing indices of lung function.

Errors in the measurement of stature can seriously affect reference values. For example, based on population data for men and women [3] the mean errors associated with a 2 cm (1.2%) error in measured stature were for total lung capacity (3%), forced vital capacity (2.7%), forced expiratory volume (2.4%) and transfer factor (1.7%). Such errors could distort medical decisions. Hence, accuracy in measurement is as important for stature as for indices of lung function. Where stature is difficult to measure or the outcome is not representative a surrogate can often be used instead (see below).

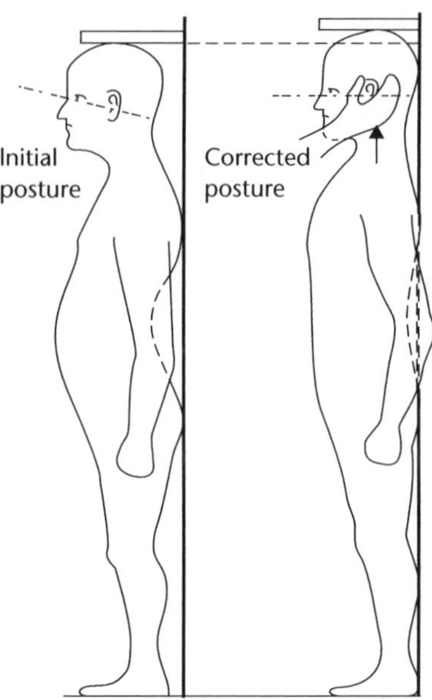

Fig. 4.2 Procedure for measurement of stature showing the effects of moving the head into the Frankfort plane (dotted and dashed line horizontal) and then applying traction. For details see text.

4.3.2 Measurement of stature and sitting height

Measurement of stature. The measurement is made using a stadiometer (e.g. Harpenden), as this leaves the observer with both hands free to position the subject. The heels should be together and the subject as tall as possible with the heels, calf, buttocks and back preferably touching the stadiometer. When this position is achieved the observer cups the angles of the mandible in both hands, tilts the subject's face so that the lower orbital margin is level with the external auditory meatus and applies gentle upward traction to the head. Compared with subjects who are standing erect but unsupported this procedure can increase the apparent height by up to 5 cm (Fig. 4.2). It can also eliminate diurnal variation and improve the reproducibility, which is then less than 2 mm. The accuracy is similar, provided the stadiometer is reading correctly. Calibration is with standard rods (Section 7.15.1).

Measurement of sitting height. The procedure is as for stature, but with the subject seated on a high stool. The stool should have a level firm top. The muscles of the buttock should be relaxed. Relaxation can be helped by arranging that the feet are supported on an adjustable footrest (e.g. Holtain sitting height stool).

Estimating stature from span. If the spine is deformed, or one leg shorter than the other, the measured stature is less than the biological stature. In this circumstance, the span from fingertip to fingertip with arms and fingers stretched out laterally can be used instead. In most children, but not Negro or Aboriginal children, the two dimensions are interchangeable. In adults the relationship between stature and span is linear and declines with age in men, but not apparently in women (Table 4.3). However, depending on the objective, an allowance for age in excess of that at peak lung function (which occurs at age 20–25 yr) may or may not be appropriate. If the measured span is also likely to be unrepresentative, the length of one of the long bones can be considered instead (Table 4.2).

The span is obtained from the demi-span; this is the length from the tip of the longest finger to the centre of the sternal notch or vertebral spine. The subject stands with the left arm fully extended and abducted in the transverse plane of the body. Some subjects have difficulty in achieving this posture without assistance, for example by facing a wall and pressing against it. The span is twice the demi-span, as measured with a tape.

Table 4.3 Regression equations for estimating stature from span in adults (ages 20–88 years).*

Gender	Ethnic group	*a*	*b*	*c*	SE
Males	Caucasian	0.63	0.10	68.7	4.12
	Black	0.65	0.083	60.1	3.04
Females	Caucasian	0.79	–	33.1	3.09
	Black	0.61	–	59.1	3.69

*The equations have the form Stature (cm) = *a* (span, cm) – *b* (age, year) + *c* ± SE.
Source: [14].

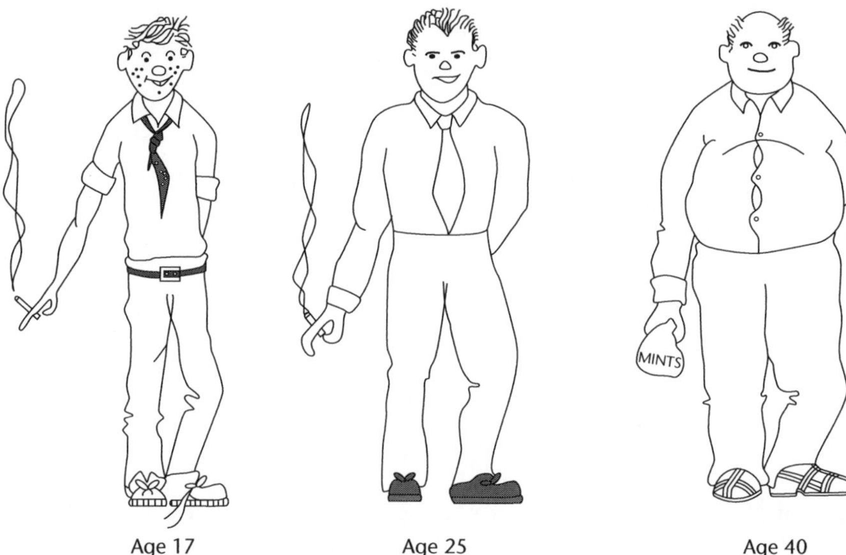

Fig. 4.3 Evolution of physique in a fairly typical sedentary male. The first step change is mainly skeletal. The second can be accentuated by, for example, discontinuing smoking.

4.4 Body width

Growth in body width continues for a few years after growth in stature has ceased (Fig. 4.3). As a result, an allowance for width can contribute to the prediction of lung function in adolescent boys (Section 25.3.3). Bi-epicondylar width of the humerus is correlated with body width and can also be used. Its measurement is described under body mass below.

Measurement. Body widths are measured at the levels of the acromial processes of the scapula, the mid-thorax and the iliac crests. The measurer stands behind the subject and uses an anthropometer (large callipers). The calliper blades are applied fairly firmly so as to compress the soft tissues. For the biacromial diameter the shoulders should be relaxed and pulled slightly forwards; the outer edges of the acromial processes are located by palpation. Thoracic width is at the junction between the third and fourth sternebrae. Bi-iliac diameter is across the iliac crests at their maximal diameter.

4.5 Body depth and girth

The depth of the thorax and abdomen is usually expressed in terms of girth (circumference). Chest depth is seldom used. *Mid sternal girth* is chest circumference. Its main use is for measurement of chest expansion, which is the increase in chest girth from complete expiration to full inspiration. The expansion decreases with age. It was formerly used as a guide to physical fitness.

Waist and hip circumferences. These indices reflect both the size of the trunk and the quantity of fat. The latter increases with age, but fat distribution varies with age (Fig. 4.3) and on average differs between the sexes (Fig. 4.4). In middle-aged men the additional fat is mainly intra-abdominal (for example a 'beer

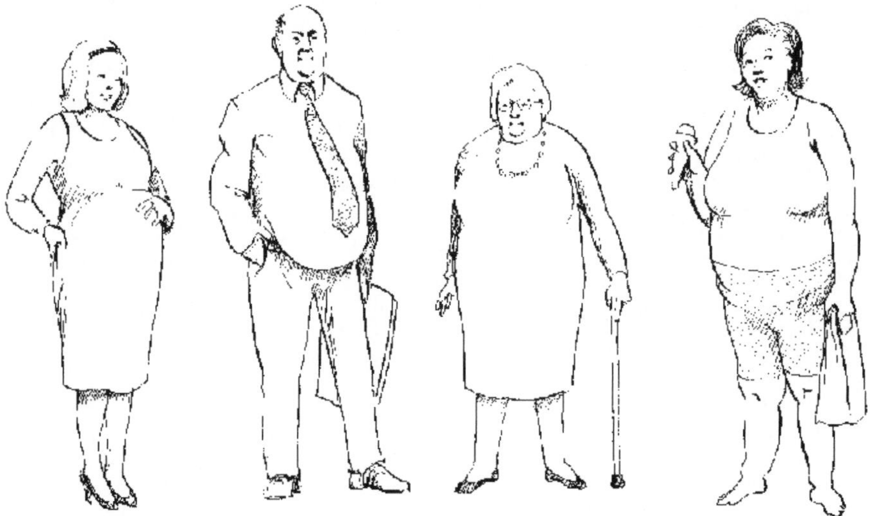

Fig. 4.4 Body shapes that affect the lungs. A full abdomen raises the diaphragm, a big bosom encourages shallow breathing and intrathoracic fat leaves less space for air. Fat on the hips is of no consequence.

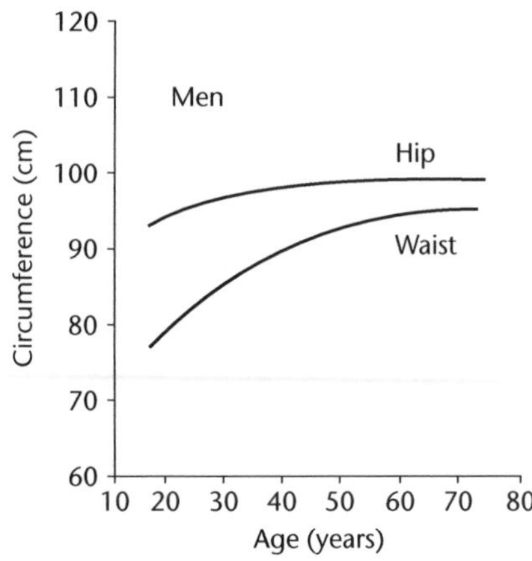

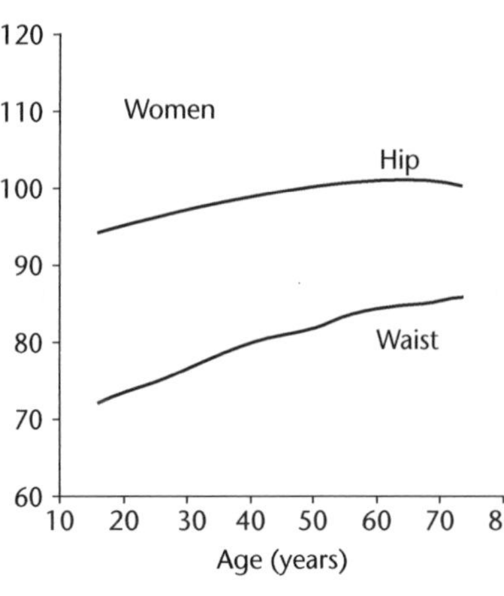

Fig. 4.5 Relationship of hip and waist circumferences (cm) on age in men and women. Source: [15].

belly' or paunch). It results in a marked increase in waist circumference (Fig. 4.5). In pregnant women the increasing size of the gravid uterus (Section 25.8.2) similarly raises the diaphragm and reduces the residual and expiratory reserve volumes; indices that include these volumes (e.g. TLC, FRC, VC) are also reduced. In middle-aged women the extra fat is usually around the hips, where it has little effect upon the lungs.

The waist circumference in centimetres or as a ratio to hip circumference or stature can indicate the extent to which abdominal fat (or other cause of abdominal distension) contributes to the position of the diaphragm [16, 17]. The association of the indices with lung function is stronger in men than women [18]. The waist/hip ratio is normally less than 0.9. The waist circumference is also used in general medicine and in cardiology, where a high value (>1 m) is associated with increased risk of cardiovascular disease. In one such study the subjects were drivers and conductors employed by London Transport and the circumferences were obtained from the company records of the sizes of employees' trousers [19].

Measurement of girth. Girth is measured using a non-stretchable steel tape with spring-loaded handles so that the tension applied to the skin can be constant. The tape should be horizontal, flat against the skin and not twisted. For trunk girths, the subject is partially undressed and stands symmetrically. Except for maximal chest expansion, measurements are made during tidal breathing. Thoracic girth is at the junction of the third and fourth sternebrae. Waist girth is the circumference at the mid-point between the lowest rib and the iliac crest. Hip girth is the maximal pelvic circumference at the level of the greater trochanters.

4.6 Body mass and body mass index

During childhood and adolescence the mass of the body increases in parallel with skeletal growth. In adults through into middle age the mass often continues to increase but at a slower rate. Adults who put on weight usually accumulate fat. However, in persons who undertake physical training, a gain in weight is due to an increased quantity of muscle and mineralisation of bone. The quantity of fat may then be relatively small. In later life the body mass often stabilises, and then declines. The reductions affect all bodily compartments, including fat, muscle, fluid and bone (e.g. Fig. 4.6). These changes influence the lung function and capacity

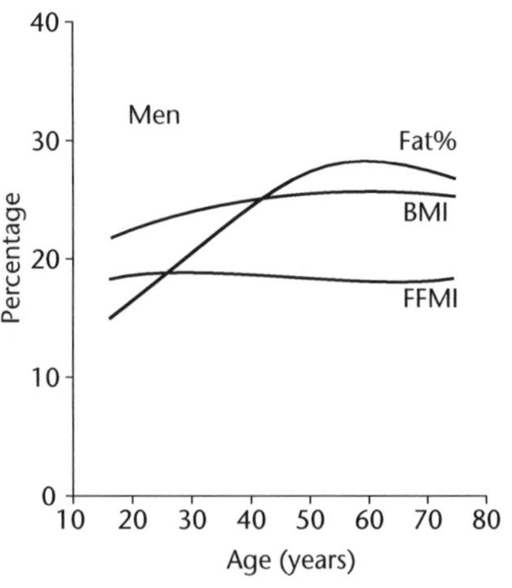

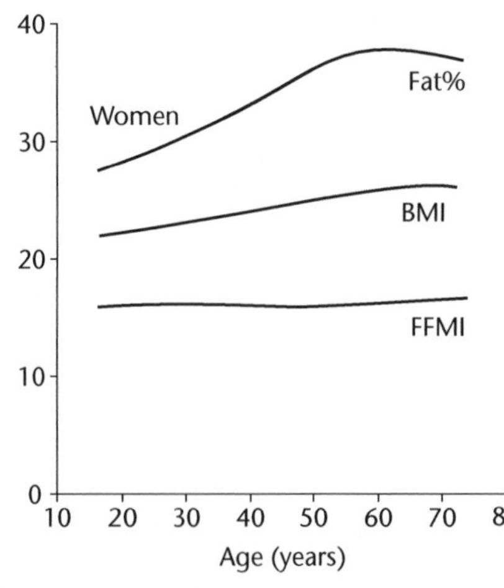

Fig. 4.6 Relationship of Fat%, BMI ($kg\ m^{-2}$) and FFMI ($kg\ m^{-2}$) on age in men and women. Source: [15].

for exercise and are best described in terms of simple indices of body fat and muscle.

In most men, and to a lesser extent in women, a *change* in fat is the largest single cause for a *change* in lung function [20]. It is also the commonest cause for a change in body mass. Hence, for interpreting longitudinal measurements of lung function *the body mass should be measured as part of the assessment.*

The component of body mass that is attributable to stature can be allowed for arithmetically (Section 5.3). In adults the outcome is body mass index [21], also called Quetelet's index after the Belgian mathematician who described it in 1835 [22]:

$$\text{Body mass index (BMI)} = \text{body mass} \times \text{stature}^{-2} \qquad (4.1)$$

In adults, but not in children, BMI is nearly independent of stature. For youngsters, body mass $\times$ stature^{-3} more nearly achieves this goal [23], but BMI is more widely used. In the absence of extra muscle, the range for healthy adults of all ages and both sexes is 18.5–25 kg m^{-2}; a BMI in excess of 30 kg m^{-2} is evidence for obesity [24].

BMI has the important limitation of not distinguishing between body fat and muscle (Table 4.4). Both compartments can affect the lungs, and so interpretation is difficult when their effects have opposite signs (Table 4.1).

Relative weight. Standardisation of mass for frame size can be achieved by using the correlation that exists between bone mass and elbow width. The association is the basis of the classification of the Metropolitan Life Assurance Company of New York [26]. Their relative weights are body mass standardised for age, height and frame size, expressed as elbow width. The width, i.e. the bi-epicondylar diameter of the humerus, is measured on the left side using calipers. The usefulness of this index as a reference variable for lung function has still to be explored.

Measurement of body mass. The measurement has a high accuracy (<0.01 kg) provided the weighing machine is calibrated. This is done using a set of 20 kg weights to check linearity as well as accuracy (Section 7.15). An allowance is made for the weight of the clothing. To this end the measurement is made after the subject has removed outer clothing and shoes; an assumed value for the remaining garments (usually 2 kg) is then subtracted from the observed weight.

Table 4.4 An example of BMI being a poor guide to its constituents; data from fire brigades men before and after physical training.

Index	Before	After	Difference
Maximal O_2 uptake (mmol min^{-1})	133	151	18.2*
Fat%	19.6	16.0	−3.58*
Fat-free mass (kg)	61.7	64.4	2.79*
Body mass index (kg m^{-2})	24.4	23.9	ns

* $P < 0.01$; ns: not significant.
Source: [25].

4.7 Body composition

4.7.1 Fat% and fat-free mass

The body mass is divisible into compartments; these overlap because of the ways in which they are defined (Table 4.2). The simplest subdivision is into a fat compartment and a remainder, of which approximately 40% is muscle. The fat compartment is expressed as percentage of body mass (Fat%) and the remainder as fat-free mass (FFM, kg).

Fat% is independent of stature, and so the effects of these two attributes can be considered concurrently without error from co-linearity (Section 5.6.2). FFM resembles body mass in being correlated with stature. The association is reduced or eliminated by expressing FFM as fat-free mass index (FFMI). This is given by:

$$\text{FFMI} = \text{FFM} \times \text{stature}^{-2} \qquad (4.2)$$

The fat and muscle compartments have different associations with age (Fig. 4.6). They also make different contributions to lung function and the responses to exercise; in general the fat component reduces performance, except in swimming where it increases buoyancy, whilst muscle enhances it. For some indices of function either Fat% or FFMI is informative whilst the other is not. For other indices, the contributions of Fat% and FFMI are synergistic or operate in opposition. Making allowance for body composition increases the precision of reference values, reduces or eliminates gender differences in function and modifies the apparent deterioration in function with age (Table 4.1). Hence compared with using body mass, making even approximate allowances for the separate contributions of body fat and muscle can be informative.

4.7.2 Measurement of Fat% and FFM

In early attempts to measure Fat%, the density of the body was obtained from measurements of body mass with the subjects in air and during submersion in water at 35°C. Allowance was made for air present in the lungs. The density was used to partition the mass into a fat compartment (density 0.9, i.e. 900 kg m^{-3}) and an FFM compartment for which the density was on average 1.1 [27]. This estimate was based on compositional analysis of five cadavers [28]. No allowance was made for differences between individuals in the volume and density of bone or the quantity of body water. In practice, the contributions of these variables to body density varies with physique. The bone density also exhibits ethnic variation with values for adult Negroes exceeding those for Caucasians. On this account, traditional underwater weighing underestimated the fat mass of Negroes by approximately 3 kg.

A valid correction is now possible [29]. The main use of the procedure is for calibrating the simpler methods [30]. In a lung function laboratory underwater weighing can be replaced by measurement of body volume by plethysmography and the result used to calculate body density. The reliability of the method is uncertain [31, 32].

According to the two-compartment model, if body mass and either Fat% or FFM are measured or estimated, the other can be obtained by difference:

$$\text{FFM (kg)} = \text{body mass} \times (100 - \text{Fat\%})/100 \qquad (4.3)$$

The respective merits of the different ways of deriving and using the two-compartment model have been reviewed [7]. A four-compartment model (fat, intra- and extracellular water and bone mineral [33, 34]) should be better, but present methods for identifying the components are not appropriate for a routine lung function laboratory.

Methods that estimate Fat%

Skinfold method. The subcutaneous fat is expressed as skinfold thickness measured with calipers. The method requires only simple equipment and can provide a result in all subjects. The reproducibility is 4% when applied by trained observers (Reed JW, Chinn DJ, unpublished work, 1980). It is recommended for routine use. The method is described below.

The depth of subcutaneous adipose tissue (SCAT). SCAT can be estimated by near-infrared interactance (NIRA) or dual energy X-ray absorptiometry (DEXA). NIRA is based on the relative absorption when skin over the biceps muscle is irradiated using two or more infrared sources. DEXA uses a paired photon source, and hence entails exposure to ionising radiation. However, the dosage is low and the time taken is relatively short. The method appears to have great potential in centres with appropriate expertise. However, the existence of several versions of the equipment, with different software and calibration procedures, has led to results from different centres that are not always comparable [7].

Methods that estimate FFM

Total body potassium. The measurable quantity that most nearly approximates to FFM is the active cell mass of the body. This can be obtained as total body potassium, since the potassium is mainly intracellular. The method entails measuring the emission of pairs of γ particles from disintegration of the naturally occurring isotope K^{40} [35]. The particles are identified by coincidence counting in a whole body counter. The results can be used interchangeably with those by the skinfold method for describing physiological variables [5]. However, whole body counters are available only in a few centres.

Total body water (TBW). For a subject who is in fluid balance the TBW provides a reasonable estimate of body muscle and hence FFM and Fat%. The standard method entails the intravenous injection of a bolus of deuterium and is not suitable for routine use. The TBW can also be estimated in terms of its content of electrolytes, from measurement of the electrical impedance of the body. The latter procedure is quick, simple and acceptable for the subject and is accurate when circumstances are favourable. However, the method has inherent limitations that are described below.

Estimation of TBW by bioelectrical impedance analysis. The impedance is measured from the transmission of electrical signals between electrodes applied to the hands and feet. A range of frequencies is used to partition the body water into extra- and intracellular compartments. Electrical theory requires that the compartments are each of uniform conductivity, fixed cross-sectional area and uniform current density [36]. Since these conditions are not met the signals are interpreted empirically. The method requires that good electrical contact is made through the skin, and hence degreasing is important, especially where body oils have been applied. The electrodes should be at least 5 cm apart and located precisely in accordance with the instructions of the manufacturer. The interpretation of the signals assumes that the subject is in fluid balance, and hence in a thermally neutral environment, a post-absorptive state and with an empty bladder. When these conditions are met the impedance method can be very precise for subjects that resemble those on whom the method was calibrated. For other subjects, especially those of a different ethnic group, the method is unreliable, as it also is in small children. In addition, the method appears not to be satisfactory for longitudinal measurements. Some of these difficulties may be resolved, but until they are the skinfold methods are more reliable [37].

Details of skinfold method for estimating Fat% and FFM

The thickness of the skin-plus-subcutaneous tissues at specified sites on the left side of the body is measured with skin calipers (e.g. Holtain). In the Durnin, Womersley version of the method [38], four sites are used over the biceps and triceps muscles, below the angle of the scapula in the line of the muscle, and above the anterior superior iliac spine; here the line is that of the external oblique muscle. The sites are marked with a skin pencil. For the upper arm, the olecranon process is marked with the elbow flexed, and then the arm is allowed to hang free. The measurements are made at a level midway between this point and the acromion process. The anterior and posterior skinfolds should be in the long axis of the limb (Fig. 4.7). They should be picked up between thumb and index finger of the left hand, without pinching or including muscle. The calipers are applied without delay and the reading is taken after 2 s. In the hands of trained observers the resulting estimate of body density agrees well with that by underwater weighing (coefficient of variation 4% [7]). The density is converted to FFM using Siri's equation [27]:

$$\text{Fat\%} = [1 - (4.95/D - 4.5)] \times 100 \qquad (4.4)$$

where D is body density.

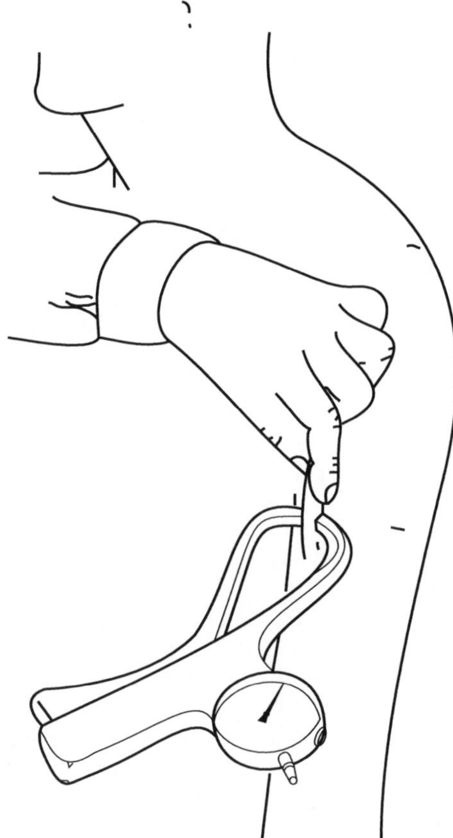

Fig. 4.7 Measurement of skinfold thickness.

Other skinfolds can also be used. For example, in the method of Jackson and colleagues the primary sites for women are the triceps, supra-iliac and anterior mid-thigh, but other sites can be used as well [39, 40].

Table 4.5 Equations relating Fat% (y) to the sum of the triceps and subscapular skinfold thickness (x) in children and adolescents (age range 8–17 years).*

	Regression coefficients			
	a	b	Constant c	SE
Males				
$x < 35$ mm	1.21	−0.008	See below	3.6%
$x > 35$ mm	0.783	–	1.6	
Females				
$x < 35$ mm	1.33	−0.013	−2.5	3.9%
$x > 35$ mm	0.546	–	9.7	

Constant term for males in relation to stage of puberty and ethnic group ($x < 35$ mm)

Ethnic group	Before	At	After puberty
Caucasian	−1.7	−3.4	−5.5
Negro	−3.5	−5.2	−6.8

*The equations have the form $y = ax + bx^2 + c$.
Source: [41].

The percentage of body mass that is fat is calculated from the sum of two or more skinfold thicknesses using empirical relationships that also include age. For children and adolescents the relationships of Slaughter and colleagues are recommended (Table 4.5) and for adults the equations of Durnin and Womersley (Table 4.6 and Fig. 4.8).

The thickness of subcutaneous fat at specified sites also has a local relevance. The subscapular skinfold thickness reflects the central thoracic fat [18], whilst the thigh fat can be used

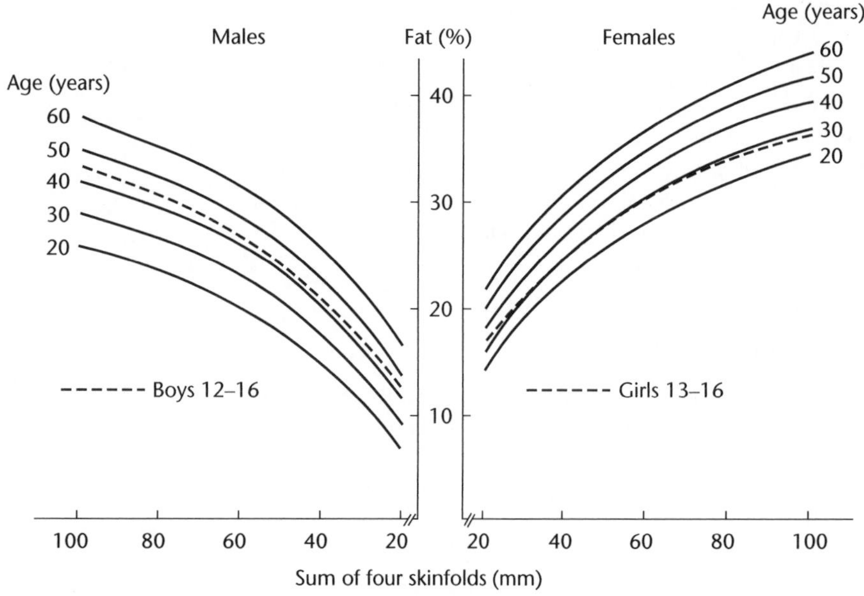

Fig. 4.8 Graphical representation of the equations of Durnin and Womersley relating the sum of four skinfold thicknesses to percentage of body mass which is fat. The coefficient of variation of the estimate is of the order of 6%. For details see text. Source: [38].

Table 4.6 Equations of Durnin and Womersley for estimating body density (D, kg m^{-3}) in adult Caucasians from the sum (x) of four skinfolds (biceps, triceps, subscapula and supra-illiac)*

Age group (Years)	Men		Women	
	a	b	a	b
17–19	1162.0	63.0	1154.9	67.8
20–29	1163.1	63.2	1159.9	71.7
30–39	1142.2	54.4	1142.3	63.2
40–49	1162.0	70.0	1133.3	61.2
50–70	1171.5	77.9	1133.9	64.5

*Equation: $D = a - b \operatorname{Log}_{10} x$.
Source: [38].

in conjunction with thigh circumference to obtain thigh muscle plus bone width [4].

4.8 Distributions of fat and muscle: a forward look

Lung function is influenced by the amounts of body fat and muscle and the extent to which these compartments impinge upon the thorax. In the case of muscle, the primary and accessory muscles of respiration make a direct contribution to lung function (Section 25.5.1). A convenient surrogate for strength is FFMI, but there are alternatives (Table 4.2), some of which are appropriate for respiratory surveys. The same indices can also be a guide to stroke volume, and hence to cardiac frequency during submaximal exercise and maximal oxygen uptake (Sections 28.5.2 and 28.8.4).

Indices of body fat similarly relate to the lung function. Their contribution is particularly relevant now that in some communities people are becoming leaner on account of food shortages whilst in others there are changes in eating patterns leading to an epidemic of obesity.

On scientific grounds there is an overwhelming case for anthropometric indices being part of the repertoire of the lung function laboratory. The missing ingredient is the imagination to take the measurements seriously. Their acquisition would lead to improved reference values for lung function and exercise, and hence an enhanced contribution by lung function laboratories to their parent discipline.

4.9 Conclusion

Anthropometric indices should be measured with the same attention to detail as the physiological ones. Stature and body mass should be reported routinely. The partitioning of body mass into fat and fat-free compartments should form part of any physiological assessment that includes measurement of lung volumes or performance of an exercise test. Simple indices that reflect body fat and muscle should be obtained on respiratory surveys.

4.10 References

1. Holmgren A, Åstrand P-O. DL and the dimensions and functional capacities of the O_2transport system in humans. *J Appl Physiol* 1966; **21**: 1463–1470.
2. Cotes JE, Davies CTM. Factors underlying the capacity for exercise: a study in physiological anthropometry. *Proc R Soc Med* 1969; **62**: 620–624.
3. Cotes JE, Chinn DJ, Reed JW. Body mass, fat% and fat-free mass as reference variables for lung function: effects on terms for age and gender. *Thorax* 2001; **56**: 839–844
4. Cotes JE, Berry G, Burkinshaw L et al. Cardiac frequency during submaximal exercise in young adults; relation to lean body mass, total body potassium and amount of leg muscle. *Q J Exp Physiol* 1973; **58**: 239–250.
5. von Dobeln W. Human standard and maximal metabolic rate in relation to fat free body mass. *Acta Physiol Scand* 1956; **37** (Suppl 126): 1–79.
6. Weller JJ, El-Gamal FM, Parker L et al. Indirect estimation of maximal oxygen uptake for study of working populations. *Br J Ind Med* 1988; **45**: 532–537.
7. Jones PRM, Norgan NG. Anthropometry and the assessment of body composition. In: Harries M, Williams C, Stanish WD, Micheli LJ, eds. *Oxford textbook of sports medicine*, 2nd ed. Oxford: Oxford University Press, 1998: 207–221.
8. Davies PSW, Cole TJ, eds. *Body composition techniques in health and disease.* Society for the study of human biology symposium series, Vol. 36. Cambridge: Cambridge University Press, 1995.
9. Lohman TG, Roche AF, Martorell R, eds. *Anthropometric standardisation reference manual.* Champaign, IL: Human Kinetics Books, 1988.
10. Gauld LM, Kappers J, Carlin JB, Robertson CF. Prediction of childhood pulmonary function using ulna length. *Am J Respir Crit Care Med* 2003; **168**: 804–809.
11. Barker DJP. *Mothers, babies and health in later life.* Edinburgh; Churchill Livingstone, 1998.
12. DeGroodt EG, van Pelt W, Borsboom GJJM et al. Growth of lung and thorax dimensions during the pubertal growth spurt. *Eur Respir J* 1988; **1**: 102–108.
13. Heaney RP, Abrams S, Dawson-Hughes B et al. Peak bone mass. *Osteoporos Int.* 2000; **11**: 985–1009.
14. Parker JM, Dillard TA, Phillips YY. Arm span–height relationships in patients referred for spirometry. *Am J Respir Crit Care Med* 1996; **154**: 533–536.
15. Allied Dunbar National Fitness Survey: main findings. Northampton, UK: The Sports Council and the Health Education Authority, 1992.
16. Jones PRM, Hunt JM, Brown TP, Norgan NG. Waist–hip circumference ratio and its relation to age and overweight in British men. *Hum Nutr Clin Nutr* 1986; **40C**: 239–247.
17. Ashwell M, Cole TJ, Dixon AK. Ratio of waist circumference to height is strong predictor of intra-abdominal fat. *Br Med J* 1996; **313**: 559–560.
18. Lazarus R, Gore CJ, Booth M et al. Effects of body composition and fat distribution on ventilatory function in adults. *Am J Clin Nutr* 1998; **68**: 35–41.
19. Morris JN, Kagan A, Pattison DC et al. Incidence and prediction of ischaemic heart disease in London busmen. *Lancet* 1966; **2**: 555–559.

20. Chinn DJ, Cotes JE, Reed JW. Changes in body mass can affect interpretation of longitudinal measurements of ventilatory capacity (FEV_1 & FVC). *Thorax* 1996; **51**: 699–704.
21. Keys A, Fidanza F, Karvonen MJ et al. Indices of relative weight and obesity. *J Chronic Dis* 1972; **25**: 329–343.
22. Quetelet A. *Sur l'homme et le developpement de ses facultés, ou essai de physique sociale.* Paris: Bachelier, 1835.
23. Cole TJ. The influence of height on the decline in ventilatory function. *Int J Epidemiol* 1974; **3**: 145–152.
24. World Health Organisation. Obesity: preventing and managing the global epidemic. Report of a WHO Consultation, Geneva, 3–5 June 1997 (WHO /NUT/98.1). Geneva: WHO, 1998.
25. Brown A, Cotes, Mortimore IL, Reed JW. An exercise training programme for firemen. *Ergonomics* 1982; **25**: 793–800.
26. Metropolitan Life Insurance Companies. Metropolitan height and weight tables. *Stat Bull Metropo Life Insur Co* 1983; **64**: 1–9.
27. Siri WE. The gross composition of the body. *Adv Biol Med Phys* 1956; **4**: 239–280.
28. Brozek J, Grande F, Anderson JT, Keys A. Densitometric analysis of body composition: revision of some quantitative assumptions. *Ann N Y Acad Sci* 1963; **110**: 113–140.
29. Wagner DR, Heyward VH. Validity of two-compartment models for estimating body fat in black men. *J Appl Physiol* 2001; **90**: 649–656.
30. Lohman TG. Assessment of body composition in children. *Pediatr Exerc Sci* 1989; **1**: 19–30.
31. Wagner DR, Heyward VH, Gibson AL. Validation of air displacement plethysmography for assessing body composition. *Med Sci Sports Exerc* 2000; **32**: 1339–1344.
32. Parker L, Reilly JJ, Slater C et al. Validity of six field and laboratory methods for measurement of body composition in boys. *Obes Res* 2003; **11**: 852–858.
33. Clasey JL, Kanaley JA, Wideman L et al. Validity of methods of body composition assessment in young and older men and women. *J Appl Physiol* 1999; **86**: 1728–1738.
34. Fields DA, Goran MI. Body composition techniques and the four-compartment model in children. *J Appl Physiol* 2000; **89**: 613–620.
35. Burkinshaw L. Measurement of body composition in vivo. In: Orton CG, ed. *Progress in medical radiation physics,* Vol. 2. New York: Plenum Press, 1985: 113–137.
36. Baumgartner RN, Chumlea WC, Roche AF. Bioelectric impedance for body composition. *Exerc Sport Sci Rev* 1990; **18**: 193–224.
37. Norgan NG. The assessment of body composition of populations. In: Davies PSW, Cole TJ, eds. *Body composition techniques in health and disease.* Society for the study of human biology symposium series, Vol. 36. Cambridge: Cambridge University Press, 1995: 195–221.
38. Durnin JVGA, Womersley J. Body fat assessed from total body density and its estimation from skinfold thickness: measurements on 481 men and women aged from 16 to 72 years. *Br J Nutr* 1974; **32**: 77–97.
39. Jackson AS, Pollock ML. Generalized equations for predicting body density of men. *Br J Nutr* 1978; **40**: 497–504.
40. Jackson AS, Pollock ML, Ward A. Generalized equations for predicting body density of women. *Med Sci Ex Sport* 1980; **12**: 175–182.
41. Slaughter MH, Lohman TG, Boileau RA et al. Skinfold equations for estimation of body fatness in children and youth. *Hum Biol* 1988; **60**: 709–723.

Further reading

Chumlea WC, Guo SS, Steinbaugh ML. Prediction of stature from knee height for black and white adults and children with application to mobility-impaired or handicapped persons. *J Am Diet Assoc* 1994; **94**: 1385–1388.

Cole TJ, Henson GL, Tremble JM, Colley NV. Birthweight for length: ponderal index, body mass index or Benn index? *Ann Hum Biol* 1997; **24**: 289–298.

Dempster P, Aitkens S. A new air displacement method for the determination of human body composition. *Med Sci Sports Exerc* 1995; **27**: 1692–1697.

Dewit O, Fuller NJ, Fewtrell MS et al. Whole body air displacement plethysmography compared with hydrodensitometry for body composition analysis. *Arch Dis Child* 2000; **82**: 159–164.

CHAPTER 5

Numerical Interpretation of Physiological Variables

The way numbers are used can make or mar the derivation and interpretation of physiological indices. This chapter identifies some good practices.

5.1 Introduction

Microprocessors and computers have revolutionised the manipulation of numbers. Results can be calculated and displayed almost instantaneously. Sophisticated allowances can be made for nuisance and confounding variables. Statistical analyses can be performed and graphs produced at the touch of a key. Now the difficulties are to ensure that indices do not proliferate unnecessarily, are appropriate for their purpose and are calculated and interpreted correctly. This is not always the case at present; however, there are accessible texts that contain the relevant information [e.g. 1–3].

Many indices in current use are conceptually unsound and some are calculated using equations that do not reflect the realities of the measurement or the underlying physiology. Decision trees used for interpretation may not allow for some critical indices being determined by more than one factor. Statistical analyses may not take account of co-linearity between variables. To avoid these and other pitfalls, operators need some knowledge, a sceptical outlook and much attention to detail. They should understand the algorithms that underlie numerical results produced by equipment in their laboratory and the decision tree used for interpretation. This high level of awareness should extend to persons who confirm the reports and write any papers that may arise from the measurements (see also Chapter 2).

5.2 Simple arithmetic

5.2.1 Manipulating numbers

Rounding off. Indices that are calculated electronically often contain more digits than are appropriate, considering that the accuracy of measurement is seldom better than 1%. Hence, primary results should be rounded off to three meaningful digits. The only valid convention is to round off downwards all terminal digits of five or less and to round upwards the terminal digits six to nine. For example if the number 10.45 is rounded off downwards to 10.4 and then to 10, it is still a good estimate of the original. However, if the rounding off is upwards, 10.45 becomes 10.5 and then 11, which is a less good estimate of what was first reported.

Rounding off should not extend to the intermediate calculations of statistical analyses; these depend for their accuracy on using all the digits that are available.

Performing calculations. Equations that include brackets and terms for addition/subtraction and multiplication/division should be processed in the right order. The wrong order will lead to error (e.g. eqn. 10.2, page 114). The convention should be followed that any exponent is processed first. Within a bracket any multiplication and/or division should precede any addition or subtraction. An example is given below.

5.2.2 Averaging ratios

Some lung function results are expressed as ratios or percentages having the form y/x or $100 \times y/x(\%)$. In circumstances where this format is appropriate, there may be a need to calculate the average ratio. This should be the average of the individual ratios (y_1/x_1, etc.) and not the ratio of the average values for y and x. For example, if there are two values each for x and y, the average of their ratios is $0.5(y_1/x_1 + y_2/x_2)$. It is not $0.5(y_1 + y_2)/0.5(x_1 + x_2)$.

5.2.3 Decimal age

Age is commonly expressed in years rounded off to the nearest whole number. This may not be sufficiently precise for children or for longitudinal studies involving measurements made annually or after an interval of a few years. The requisite precision is obtained by expressing the age at assessment or the interval between assessments in decimal years. Age is obtained by subtracting the decimal date at birth from that at the assessment. The interval is obtained in a similar fashion. Decimal dates for each day of the year can be read off a list (Table 5.1) or computed using an equation based on that for the Julian date (Table 5.2), courtesy of CE Rossiter.

5.3 Relationship of one variable to another

Very frequently there is a need to standardise one variable for another that is dependent on it (Table 5.3). For the standardisation to be accurate the relationship between the variables should be known. The relationship can be complex, but usually it is quite

Table 5.1 Date expressed as decimal years.

	Month (name and number)											
Day	Jan 1	Feb 2	Mar 3	Apr 4	May 5	Jun 6	Jul 7	Aug 8	Sep 9	Oct 10	Nov 11	Dec 12
1	000	085	162	247	329	414	496	581	666	748	833	915
2	003	088	164	249	332	416	499	584	668	751	836	918
3	005	090	167	252	334	419	501	586	671	753	838	921
4	008	093	170	255	337	422	504	589	674	756	841	923
5	011	096	173	258	340	425	507	592	677	759	844	926
6	014	099	175	260	342	427	510	595	679	762	847	929
7	016	101	178	263	345	430	512	597	682	764	849	932
8	019	104	181	266	348	433	515	600	685	767	852	934
9	022	107	184	268	351	436	518	603	688	770	855	937
10	025	110	186	271	353	438	521	605	690	773	858	940
11	027	112	189	274	356	441	523	608	693	775	860	942
12	030	115	192	277	359	444	526	611	696	778	863	945
13	033	118	195	279	362	447	529	614	699	781	866	948
14	036	121	197	282	364	449	532	616	701	784	868	951
15	038	123	200	285	367	452	534	619	704	786	871	953
16	041	126	203	288	370	455	537	622	707	789	874	956
17	044	129	205	290	373	458	540	625	710	792	877	959
18	047	132	208	293	375	460	542	627	712	795	879	962
19	049	134	211	296	378	463	545	630	715	797	882	964
20	052	137	214	299	381	466	548	633	718	800	885	967
21	055	140	216	301	384	468	551	636	721	803	888	970
22	058	142	219	304	386	471	553	638	723	805	890	973
23	060	145	222	307	389	474	556	641	726	808	893	975
24	063	148	225	310	392	477	559	644	729	811	896	978
25	066	151	227	312	395	479	562	647	731	814	899	981
26	068	153	230	315	397	482	564	649	734	816	901	984
27	071	156	233	318	400	485	567	652	737	819	904	986
28	074	159	236	321	403	488	570	655	740	822	907	989
29	077	159	238	323	405	490	573	658	742	825	910	992
30	079	–	241	326	408	493	575	660	745	827	912	995
31	082	–	244	–	411	–	578	663	–	830	–	997

Example: 16 August 2001 is 2001.622.

Table 5.2 Calculation of decimal age.*

No. of days since 1/1/1900 = *Integer*(365.25 × *Y*) + *Integer*(30.6001 × (*M* + 1)) + *D* − 694037

Integer is that part of a number that precedes the decimal point, e.g. Integer(12.6) = 12

Y = Year (4 digits)

M = Month (up to 12)

D = Days (up to 31)

Then, Age = {(No. of days from 1/1/1900 to assessment) − (No. of days to birthday)}/365.25

Example: To calculate age on 6 July 2001 if born on 24 February 1924:
For 24 February 1924:
No. of days from 1900 to birthday
= *Integer*(365.25 × 1924) + *Integer*(30.6001 × 3) + 24 − 694037
= 702741 + 91 + 24 − 694037 = 8819
Similarly for 6 July 2001: Number of days from 1900 = 37078
Hence: Age = (37078 − 8819)/365.25 = 77.369 years

* The number of days from 1 January 1900 to any specified date can be calculated exactly from the relationship shown in the table based on the full calculation of the Julian date.

Table 5.3 Uses of relationships of *y* on *x*.

1 Making allowance for *x* prior to interpreting *y* (e.g. in a report)
2 Identifying a value for *y* at a given value of *x* (e.g. a reference value)
3 Linearising data prior to statistical analysis
In the case of an exponential relationship, this is done by using natural logarithms
4 Describing a physiological or biochemical process (modelling)
5 Demonstrating a property of biological organisms (allometry)

simple. This is the case in Fig. 5.1 where the relationship of *y* to *x* is a curve going through the origin (in this case an exponential relationship). Over a limited range the relationship of *y* to *x* can be represented by a straight line (linear model). The other simple alternative is a straight line through the origin (proportional model), but such a model is not appropriate here. Indeed, few biological relationships are of this form.

5.3.1 Proportional relationships

The relationships have the form $y = mx$. Hence:

$$y/x = m \qquad (5.1)$$

Proportionality can be expressed as a percentage. The equation states in mathematical notation that expressing *y* in the form y/x renders it independent of *x*. Few relationships are of this form. A rare example is FEV_1/FVC. In most circumstances this index is independent of FVC. Hence it can be used as a guide to airway calibre without regard to the size of the lungs. Unfortunately this property holds only for relationships that are truly proportional. It does not hold for the data illustrated in Fig. 5.1. In the orig-

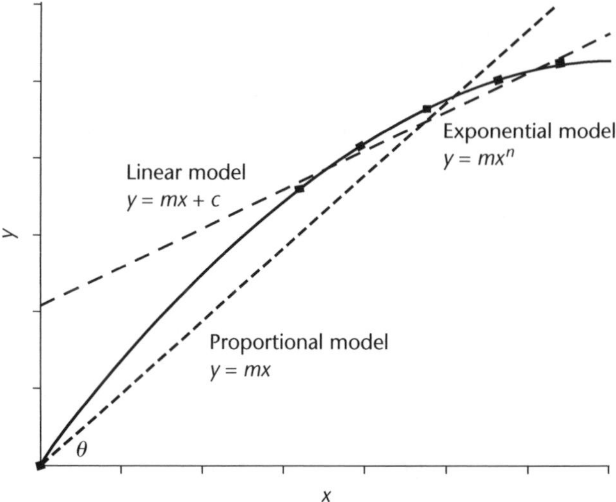

Fig. 5.1 Data points that are described accurately by an exponential relationship, approximately by a linear relationship and not at all by a proportional relationship. The data are for transfer factor in a subject who performed the measurement at several lung volumes. See also Fig. 20.7, page 251.

inal version of Fig. 20.7, *y* is transfer factor for the lungs (*T*l) and *x* is alveolar volume (*V*a). y/x is *K*co; this index is often wrongly interpreted as *T*l standardised for *V*a. In fact the angle θ (the angle defining the proportional relationship) and hence *K*co varies inversely with *V*a, and so at any level of gas transfer, subjects with small lungs have higher values for *K*co than those with larger lungs. Errors in diagnosis can follow from this misunderstanding (Section 20.9.2). Similar errors can occur with other indices (Table 5.4).

5.3.2 Linear relationships

These have the form:

$$y = mx + c \qquad (5.2)$$

The relationships are often empirical and valid only over a limited range of values of *x*. Provided this is recognised the relationships can be most useful. Examples abound throughout the book (e.g. Fig. 5.1).

5.3.3 Simple curves through the origin

The curves are often exponential, in which case they become linear when converted to natural logarithms, i.e.:

$$y = e^c x^m \qquad (5.3)$$

where *e* (the base of natural logarithms) has the approximate value 2.71828...
Hence:

$$\ln y = m \ln x + c \qquad (5.4)$$

Table 5.4 Examples of ratio indices that are mathematically unsound because they are correlated with their denominators.

Original form	Valid alternative	Location
Body mass/stature	Body mass/(stature)^{x*}	[4]
FEV_1/stature	FEV_1/(stature)^{x*}	[5, 6]
Ventilation equivalent ($\dot{V}E/\dot{V}O_2$)	Use linear regression or $\dot{V}_{E45}$†	Section 28.4.3
Oxygen pulse ($\dot{V}O_2/fC$)	Use linear regression or fC_{45}†	Section 28.6.1
Aerobic power ($\dot{V}O_2$/body mass)	$\dot{V}O_2$ max/(body mass)$^{0.67}$	[7]
KCO ($T1/V$A)	$T1$ with or without standardisation for VA‡	Section 20.9.1

* x is usually between 2 and 3 depending on circumstances.
† See Fig. 29.1, page 418.

A relationship of this form is used to describe variation of lung function with stature in children studied cross-sectionally (Table 26.5, page 336). The model has the useful feature that, if, as in this example, the value for m is effectively constant between subjects then the result for each subject is defined by the parameter c. The proportional difference between two subjects or groups of subjects is then expressed by:

$$100(c_1 - c_2)\% \tag{5.5}$$

An example is the difference in lung function between boys and girls (Table 25.4, page 320).

5.4 Interpreting a possible change in an index

Comparison of two results before and after an illness, an intervention, or the passage of time is an every day occurrence in chest medicine. The commonest instance is when looking for a possible improvement in FEV_1 following inhalation of a test dose of bronchodilator aerosol. Such comparisons are subject to error from a number of sources (Table 5.5).

Table 5.5 Errors when looking for change in an index.

1. Methods on two occasions not comparable (need for quality controls; Section 7.16).
2. Random errors conceal a real change only detectable with more subjects. Minimal numbers (sample size) for a specified level of certainty can be calculated (eqn. 5.6).
3. Bias in the initial measurement is magnified in the difference. Hence allow for regression to the mean (Section 5.4.2).
4. Model used to interpret the changes may not be appropriate. This is particularly the case for proportional relationships (Table 5.4).
5. Interpretation invalid because not all factors have been controlled. Error can affect comparisons within the subjects (e.g. Section 15.7.2) or between subjects (selection bias or measurement bias; Table 8.7, page 94).

5.4.1 Sample size required to detect a meaningful difference

The minimal sample size needed to measure a difference that would be considered relevant in the circumstances can be calculated in terms of the standard deviation (SD) of the measurement, the degree of certainty that is required and the meaningful difference. Then:

$$n = \frac{2[(Z_\alpha + Z_\beta) \times \text{sd between individuals}]^2}{(y_1 - y_2)^2} \tag{5.6}$$

where the denominator is the meaningful difference, Z_α and Z_β are standard normal deviates corresponding to the level of statistical significance (α) and the chance of not detecting a difference of $y_1 - y_2$ units (β). Then, in the case of FEV (SD between individuals $\sim$ 0.5 l), if the meaningful difference is 0.25 l, and α is taken as 0.05 ($Z_\alpha = 1.96$) and β 0.1 ($Z_\beta = 1.64$) then the number of subjects (n) is 104 [1]. Determination of sample size is also considered in Section 8.2.3.

Equation 5.6 can be used in other circumstances, for example, to determine what would be a meaningful change in FEV_1 following inhalation of a bronchodilator. Thus, if $n = 3$ blows, $\alpha = 0.05$, $\beta = 0.1$ and the within-blows SD $= 0.05$ l (see Table 8.5, page 86), the meaningful change ($y_1 - y_2$) is 0.147 l. The assumptions are that the three readings at each test session are independent and approximately normally distributed with about equal standard deviations. When the within-blows variability is greater, as may occur with patients or with other indices the meaningful difference will be larger [8].

5.4.2 Regression to the mean

Where x_1 and x_2 are the initial and final values, the difference term ($x_1 - x_2$) is inevitably correlated with the initial level (x_1). This may lead to error in the interpretation of such data ([9, 10], *also* Fig. 5.2). The error is avoided when the change is related to the mean level (eqn. 5.7) or the result is expressed in natural logarithms (eqn. 5.8).

$$\begin{aligned}\text{Change} &= (x_1 - x_2)/0.5(x_1 + x_2) \\ &= \Delta x/\bar{x} \text{ or } 100 \times \Delta x/\bar{x}\ \%\end{aligned} \tag{5.7}$$

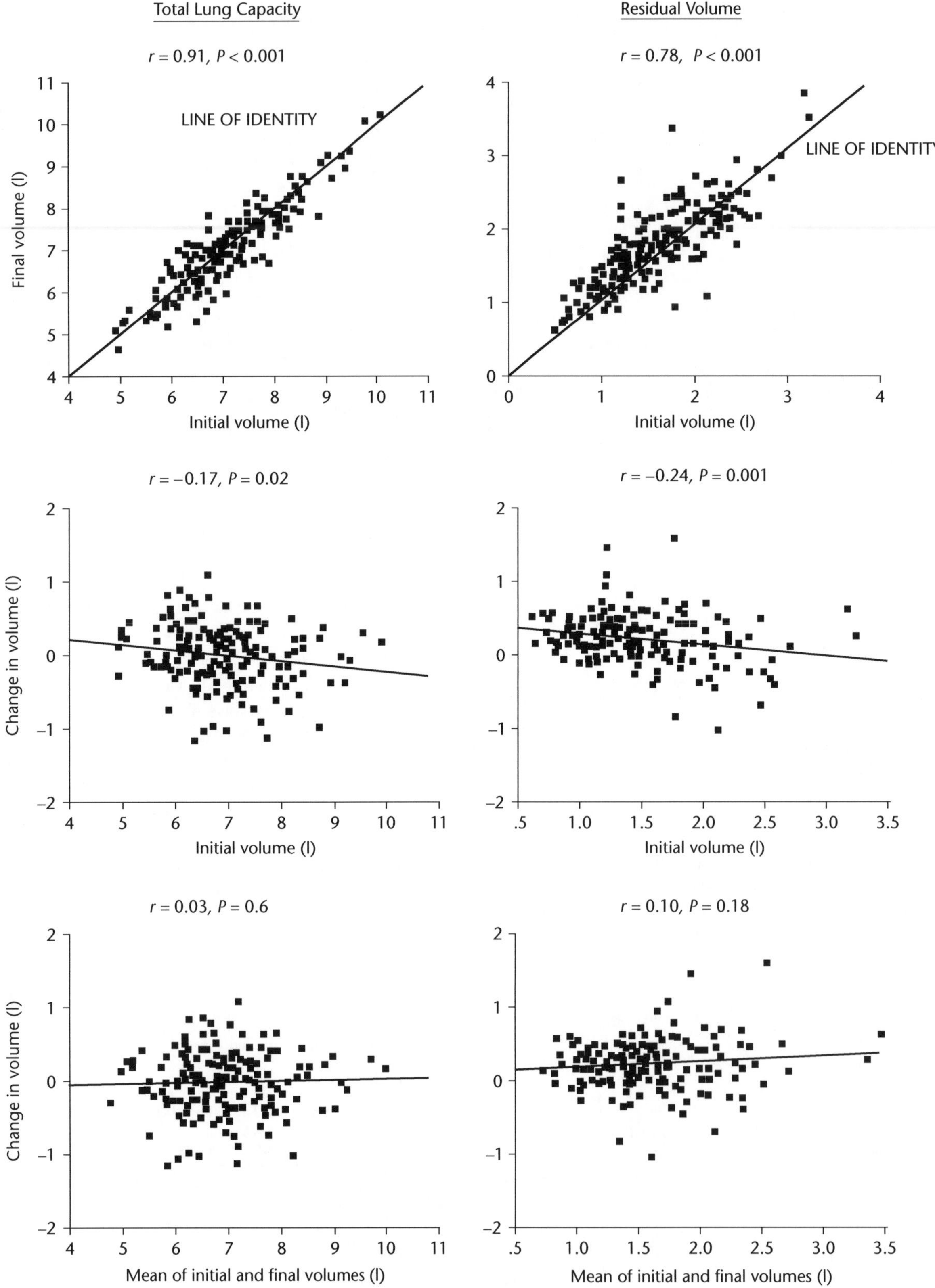

Fig. 5.2 Relationships of changes in lung function over 6 years to the initial and mean levels amongst 175 men. The graphs show the errors that can arise from neglecting regression to the mean, c.f. [9]. For details see text.

This equation should be used to report the short-term change in an index following a challenge test. In a cohort study conducted over months or years the $\Delta x/\bar{x}$ term should be divided by the interval between measurements to obtain the *annual* change.

When the rate of change of a variable is proportional to its magnitude, then $dx/dt = kx$, where k is the constant of proportionality and is the proper measure of the proportional changes. Integrating gives $\ln x = \ln x_0 + kt$, where x_0 is the value of x at time zero and ln indicates the natural logarithm. With observations x_1 at time t_1 and x_2 at time t_2:

$$\ln x_1 = \ln x_0 + k\,t_1 \quad \text{and} \quad \ln x_2 = \ln x_0 + k\,t_2$$

so that:

$$k\% = (\ln x_1 - \ln x_2)/(t_1 - t_2) \tag{5.8}$$

The *numerator* in eqn. 5.8 and the $\Delta x/\bar{x}$ in eqn. 5.7 differ to an extent that for practical purposes is negligible [11].

5.4.3 Choice of model for paired observations

Interpretation of any observations entails making allowances for biological variability and technical factors in the measurements. Interpretation of paired observations also entails using a model that avoids error from regression to the mean, as described above. The simplest procedure is to relate the individual differences to their respective mean levels. Graphical representations of such data are shown in Fig. 5.2. The data relate to change in TLC and RV over 6 years in 175 men. The initial and final values are highly correlated (upper graphs). The difference between occasions was negatively correlated with the initial value (middle graphs) but independent of the mean level of function (lower graphs). The figure illustrates the error in analysis that can arise from neglect of regression to the mean. The interpretation of change between years was very different when a valid procedure was used.

The model $(\Delta x/\bar{x})$ has been applied extensively in medical research and is known as the Oldham transformation or Bland–Altman plot [11, 12]. It should also be used in a clinical context, for example to assess the response to a bronchodilator drug (Section 15.7.2).

Serial observations. Paired observations are the simplest form of serial observations, e.g. when assessing bronchodilation (Chapter 15).

5.5 Normal and skewed distributions

A variable that has been measured on a group of subjects can be described by a mean value with its standard deviation. The latter indicates the spread of values about the mean and the calculation requires that the distribution is symmetrical; when this is the case the distribution is said to be Gaussian or 'normal' (Fig. 5.3).

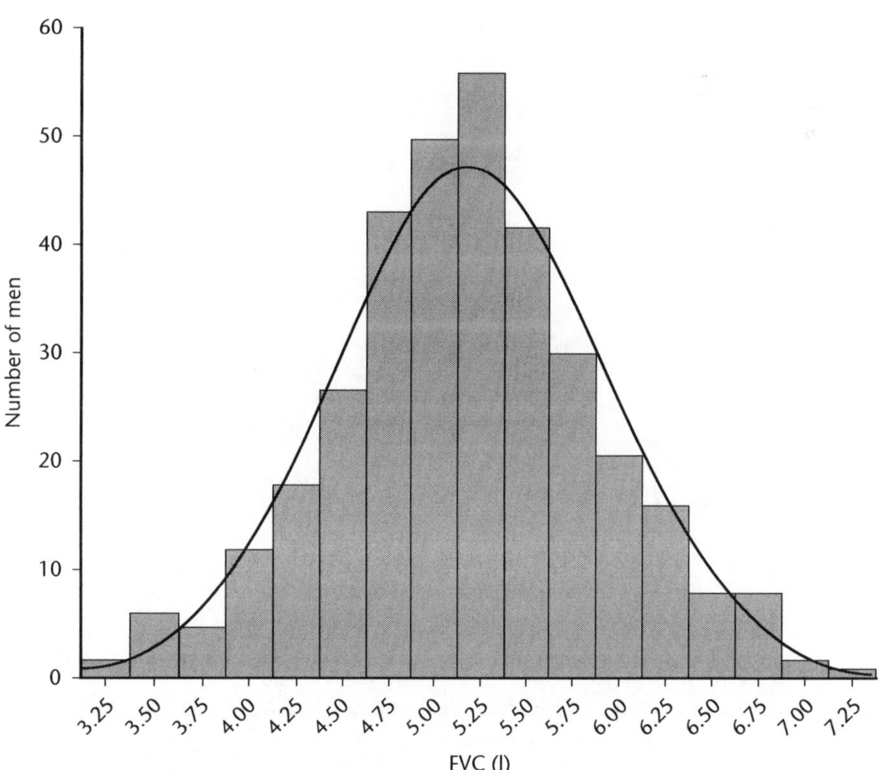

Fig. 5.3 Example of a variable that fits a Gaussian distribution: FVC in 346 men (mean = 5.18, SD 0.73 litres).

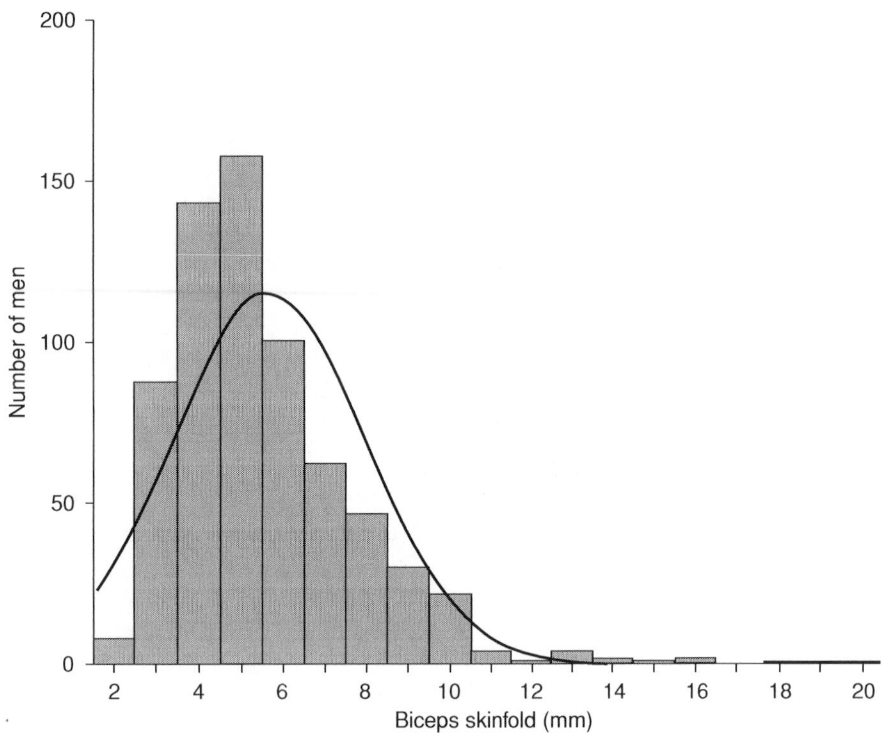

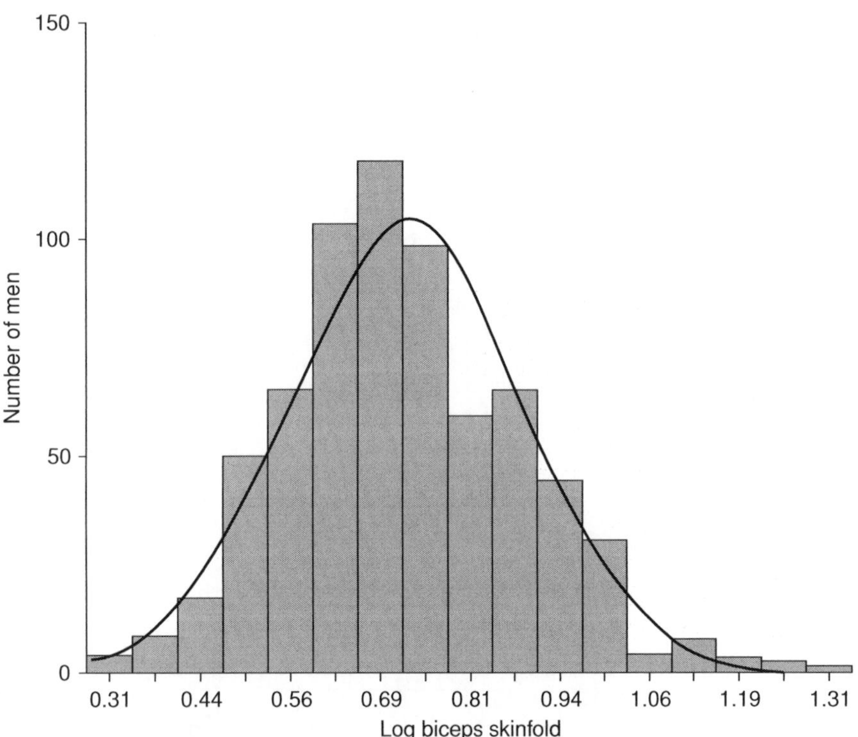

Fig. 5.4 Example of a variable with a positively skewed distribution and its log transformation:Biceps skinfold 678 men (mean 6.0 mm, SD 2.34 mm).

Where the distribution is asymmetrical and skewed it must be transformed into a normal one prior to statistical analysis using parametric procedures such as the Student *t*-test. Normalisation entails transforming the original numbers, for example by taking logarithms (Fig. 5.4), using the squares or cubes of the numbers or taking their reciprocals. A quadratic or cubic transformation arises from a logarithmic one, as in eqns. 5.3 and 5.4. In the former equation the coefficient of proportionality m is sometimes called the allometric constant (Table 5.3).

5.6 Relationship of one variable to several others

5.6.1 Multiple regression

A multiple regression equation is used to describe a variable that is dependent on several others. For example, FEV_1 in adults is often described in terms of age and stature (eqn. 5.12, below). FEV_1 is the dependent variable. The distribution of the independent variables (stature and age) is usually normal. If this is not the case the data are transformed prior to analysis by applying one of the transformations described in the preceding paragraph. Then:

$$y = mx + m'z + c \qquad (5.9)$$

where y is FEV_1, x is stature in metres, z is age in years and m and m' are the partial regression coefficients on stature and age, respectively. The model implies that the increment of lung function per unit of stature is the same for short and tall people; this appears to be the case. The model also implies that the decline in lung function that occurs from one year to the next is the same at all ages and is independent of stature. This is only approximately correct. A way of allowing for the interaction is described below.

The relationship of y on x and z can be simplified if either x or z can be expressed in the form of a proportionality. Thus in the above example, Cole [5] has shown that, in adults, a proportionality exists between FEV_1 and the square of the stature (x^2). On this account, FEV_1 can be related to age independent of stature, using the form:

$$y/x^2 = m'z + c' \qquad (5.10)$$

The proportionality can also be used to standardise FEV_1 or other index to a common stature, which for men might be 1.72 m. The standardised value (FEV_1 std) is then given by:

$$FEV_1\ \text{std} = FEV_1\ \text{observed} \times (1.72)^2/\text{measured stature}^2 \qquad (5.11)$$

In addition to age and stature the dependent variable (y) can often be related to other characteristics of the subject. The characteristics might be expressed numerically as a continuous variable or as belonging to one or other group of subjects (a categorical variable). In the case of FEV_1 the additional continuous variables might be Fat% and fat-free mass index (Section 25.5.1). The categorical variables could be gender, ethnic group, occupational exposure and whether or not the subject was a smoker. The contributions of these independent variables can be analysed by introducing appropriate terms into the multiple regression equation. The continuous variables are treated as in eqn. 5.9. The categorical or dummy variables are allocated the value 1 if they are present and 0 if they are absent for the subject in question.

The effect of smoking increases with age; this interaction is allowed for by including the term age × smoking. Hence, for men of one ethnic group:

$$\begin{aligned} FEV_1 = a &+ b(\text{stature}) + c(\text{age}) + d(\text{smoking}) \\ &+ e(\text{age} \times \text{smoking}) \\ &+ f(\text{occupational exposure}) + \text{etc.} \end{aligned} \qquad (5.12)$$

The smoking variable is defined here as 1 for smokers and 0 for non-smokers, so the regression coefficient of FEV_1 on age is c for non-smokers and $c + e$ for smokers. The effect of being a former smoker can be allowed for by including another categorical term for ex-smoking.

An equation of this type is often used to describe the FEV_1 of subjects participating in an occupational respiratory survey (Chapter 8). The values of the coefficient terms are obtained by multiple regression analysis using an appropriate computer software package (e.g. Statistical Package for Social Sciences, SPSS). However, prior to the analysis the independent variables should be scrutinised to establish that they are truly independent and not inter-correlated (co-linear), as this will affect the reliability of the result.

5.6.2 Co-linearity

Two variables are co-linear when they are to some extent interrelated (correlated). The relationship can take one of the forms described for simple relationships above. The extent of the association is described by the correlation coefficient, which is in the range from 0, when the variables are truly independent, to 1.0, when they are perfectly related and effectively synonymous. The level of co-linearity that can be tolerated in a multiple regression analysis varies with circumstances; the partial correlation coefficient should probably not exceed 0.4 [9]. Higher correlations between independent (predictor) variables in the same equation make the model unstable. The commonest form of co-linearity is with respect to age.

5.6.3 Allowing for effects of age

Relation to calendar age and to initial level. In adults the deterioration in lung function with age is usually represented as linear (eqn. 5.12). This is a first approximation to a more subtle relationship, because deterioration is to some extent progressive and increases with age. The progression can be included by having in the model an additional term age^n, where the exponent n is usually 2 or 3. [13]. The term can apply either to all ages included in the analysis or to subjects of greater than a certain age. The latter procedure is known as splining [14]. The need for one or more exponential terms can be assessed by comparing the observed values for the dependent variable (e.g. FEV_1) with the

Table 5.6 Some statistical terms.

Mean	Average value; measure of location
Median	Middle value when data ordered; measure of location for skewed data
Standard deviation, SD $= [\sum(x_i - \bar{x})^2/(n-1)]^{0.5}$	Describes spread of data
Standard error, SE $=$ SD$/n^{0.5}$ or $(n-1)^{0.5}$	Indicates precision of an estimated mean value (e.g. that for data from a population study)
Residual standard deviation (RSD)	SD about regression line
Standard error of the estimate (SEE)	As for RSD
Correlation coefficient (r)	Extent to which two variables provide the same information (range 0–1)
Coefficient of variation, ($\bar{x}$/SD) %	Measure of repeatability of a test result
Variance (R^2), $s^2 = \sum(x_i-\bar{x})^2/(n-1)$	Measure of variability (spread) in data
R^2 (square of the correlation coefficient)	In regression analysis describes the proportion of total variance in dependent variable that is explained by the predictor variables
95% confidence interval (of an estimated mean)	Range within which the true mean is likely to lie (with 95% confidence)
Type I error	Incorrect rejection of null hypothesis (false positive result)*
Type II error	Failure to detect a real difference (false negative result)*

* The probability of the error occurring can be calculated.

values predicted by the multiple regression equation. The difference should be independent of age. Such a comparison is known as analysis of residuals. Complex models can also be developed, but are subject to the law of diminishing returns [15, 16]. Improving the specificity of the variables can be more informative [17].

The decline with age is usually related to the level of lung function and hence to body size. This association can be accommodated by including in the model a term for initial level of lung function for the index under consideration. The term eliminates the weak interaction whereby tall persons (who tend to have large lungs) have larger age regression coefficients than short persons.

Age as a surrogate for another variable. A term for age is to some extent a surrogate for other terms whose effects vary with age. For example, the amount of body fat varies with age, and hence the partial regression coefficient on age (m' in eqn. 5.9) is altered if a term for Fat% is included in the equation [17].

Contrived co-linearity. Error can be introduced into the term for age if another variable that includes age is added to the model. The commonest of these is the amount smoked expressed in pack-years (number of packs of 20 cigarettes smoked per day multiplied by duration of smoking in years). Another is cumulative dust exposure, expressed over a lifetime spent in a dusty industry. Both these indices are co-linear with age; their inclusion in a multiple regression model that also contains a term for age can lead to the contribution of age being misinterpreted.

5.6.4 Variation about the regression equation

The variation is expressed as a residual standard deviation (RSD); this describes the scatter about the equation, which is the same along its length. However, the accuracy of estimates of lung function obtained using the equation varies according to how far the explanatory variables are from their mean values. Predictions for extreme values may not be reliable. RSD and some other statistical terms are given in Table 5.6.

The properties of the standard deviation are such that the mean ±1 SD embrace 68% of the observations. Of the remainder, 16% exceed the mean by more than 1 SD and 16% are less than the mean by at least a similar amount. The corresponding figures for 1.64 SD and for 1.96 SD are 5 and 2.5% (Table 5.7).

A result that deviates from the expected value by more than 1 SD merits scrutiny if the deviation is in the direction of abnormal lung function. One that deviates by more than 1.64 SD is usually taken to indicate that the function is abnormal. This will be true in 95% of such cases but in 5% the result will be an outlier in a person with healthy lungs. Thus using this criterion, there is a 5%

Table 5.7 Values for the standardised deviate (Z) associated with different cumulative frequencies (percentiles) in a normal (Gaussian) distribution.

	Percentile (%)	
Z value*	Z negative	Z positive
1.960	2.5	97.5
1.645	5	95
1.282	10	90
1.036	15	85
0.842	20	80
0.674	25	75
0.524	30	70
0.385	35	65
0.253	40	60
0.126	45	55
0.000	50	50

*Z = (observed value − expected value)/RSD.

risk of achieving a false positive result (type I error). The statistical approach assumes that subjects for investigation are selected at random from the reference population. This condition can be met in respiratory surveys. In other circumstances selection for investigation is often biased towards those at the abnormal end of the Gaussian distribution; such persons are more likely to develop symptoms and be referred for assessment compared with others whose lung function was initially above average. Thus, the false positive rate of 5% is an underestimate. The border line group is likely to contain a disproportionate number of heavy smokers, the obese, persons who take little exercise, the anxious, and women whose lung function may have been underestimated on account of their foundation garments (Section 12.6.2).

5.6.5 Logistic regression analysis

This form of multiple regression analysis is used to describe a dichotomous categorical variable, i.e. one which is present or absent, for example whether or not the subject is a current smoker or has the features that characterise chronic bronchitis (Fig. 8.2, page 88). Again, the independent variables should not exhibit co-linearity. Some computer software packages for logistic regression analysis have limitations and so should not be used uncritically. Thus, at this stage if not earlier, a statistician should be consulted.

5.6.6 Principal components analysis (PCA)

PCA is a multivariate method of reducing a large set of measurements into a smaller number of independent principal components each one of which is a linear combination of the original measurements. Because the components are independent of one another they may be used as predictor variables together in multiple regression analyses. For example, in a study exploring the relationship between lung size in adolescents and body dimensions (e.g. shoulder width, chest width, chest depth, sternum length and hip width) PCA may be used to condense the five body dimensions into two principal components that can be regressed against total lung capacity standardised for stature.

The main advantages of PCA are first that an unwieldy number of related variables can be condensed into a usable form, and second, the resulting factors can sometimes be recognised as having biological relevance [e.g. 18, 19]. However, in many instances their only significance is statistical. The factors should be obtained and interpreted under the guidance of a statistician.

5.7 References

1. Armitage P, Berry G, Matthews JNS. *Statistical methods in medical research*, 4th ed. Oxford: Blackwell Scientific Publications, 2001.
2. Altman DG. *Practical statistics for medical research*, 2nd ed. London: Chapman & Hall, 1999.
3. Cambpell MJ, Machin D. *Medical statistics, a common sense approach.* Chichester: John Wiley & Sons, 1993.
4. Tanner JM. Fallacy of per-weight and per-surface area standards, and their relation to spurious correlation. *J Appl Physiol* 1949; **2**: 1–15.
5. Cole TJ. Linear and proportional regression models in the prediction of ventilatory function. *J Roy Stat Soc A*, 1975; **138**: 297–328.
6. Fletcher C, Peto R, Tinker C, Speizer FE. *The natural history of chronic bronchitis and emphysema.* Oxford: Oxford University Press, 1976.
7. Åstrand P-O, Rodahl K. *Textbook of work physiology*, 3rd ed. London: McGraw-Hill, 1986.
8. Whitaker CJ, Chinn DJ, Lee WR. The statistical reliability of indices derived from the closing volume and flow volume traces. *Bull Eur Physiopathol Respir* 1978; **14**: 237–247.
9. Oldham PD. *Measurement in medicine. The interpretation of numerical data.* London: English University Press, 1968.
10. Rossiter C. Contribution to discussion. *Scand J Respir Dis* 1976; **57**: 315–316.
11. Oldham PD. A note on the analysis of repeated measurements of the same subjects. *J Chronic Dis* 1962; **15**: 969–977.
12. Bland JM, Altman DG. Statistical methods for assessing agreement between two methods of clinical measurement. *Lancet* 1986; **i**: 307–310.
13. Burrows B, Lebowitz MD, Camilli AE, Knudson RJ. Longitudinal changes in forced expiratory volume in one second in adults: methodologic considerations and findings in healthy nonsmokers. *Am Rev Respir Dis* 1986; **133**: 974–980.
14. Sherrill DL, Lebowitz MD, Knudson RJ, Burrows B. Smoking and symptom effects on the curves of lung function growth and decline. *Am Rev Resp Dis* 1991; **144**: 17–22.
15. Rosen MJ, Sorkin JD, Goldberg AP et al. Predictors of age-related decline in maximal aerobic capacity; a comparison of four statistical models. *J Appl Physiol* 1998; **84**: 2163–2170.
16. Nevill AM, Holder RL. Scaling, normalizing and 'per ratio' standards; an allometric modeling approach. *J Appl Physiol* 1995; **79**: 1027–1031.
17. JE Cotes, DJ Chinn, JW Reed. Body mass, fat% and fat-free mass as reference variables for lung function: effects on terms for age and gender. *Thorax* 2001; **56**: 839–844.
18. Gilson JC, Hugh-Jones P, Oldham PD, Meade F. Lung function in coal workers' pneumoconiosis. Gas-distribution and transfer. *Spec Rep Med Res Coun (Lond)* 1955; **290**: 114–124, 150–201.
19. Cowie H, Lloyd MH, Soutar CA. Study of lung function data by principal components analysis. *Thorax* 1985; **40**: 438–443.

CHAPTER 6

Basic Terminology and Gas Laws

This chapter reports symbols and abbreviations that are used in respiratory physiology and clinical lung function testing, together with the units of measurement and the physical gas laws that underlie them.

6.1 Glossary of terms

The terms used in respiratory physiology are defined in the text and listed in the index. Some general terms not specific to respiratory physiology are defined in Table 6.1.

6.2 Abbreviations and primary symbols

Some lung function indices are designated by abbreviations and others by symbols. The former are made up of the initial letters of the words that describe the measurements. Examples are given in Table 6.2, together with the section numbers in the text where the indices are defined. Abbreviations used when describing anthropometry are given in Table 6.3.

The symbols come mainly from biochemistry and biophysics; their use in respiratory physiology was codified in 1950 by Pappenheimer and colleagues [2] and a major revision was made in 1980 by the Commission of Respiratory Physiology of the International Union of Physiological Sciences [3]. Refinements have been introduced by the American Physiological Society [4] and by a working group of the European Community for Coal and Steel [5]. The latter has also provided translations of terms in major European languages. Recommendations exist for standardisation of terms used in paediatric pulmonary function testing [6]. Symbols are printed in italics (Table 6.4).

Derivatives with respect to time are portrayed in a traditional manner. Volume per unit of time (i.e. $V \div t$) is $\dot{V}$ in the gas phase and $\dot{Q}$ in the blood phase; the units are $l\ min^{-1}$. The rate of change of volume with time, i.e dV/dt, is represented by $\dot{v}$ in the units $l\ s^{-1}$. This usage is adopted for the present account. Alternatively, a mathematical notation may be used as in Table 6.4, which lists the primary symbols and, where appropriate, their mathematical equivalents.

6.3 Suffixes

A primary symbol is usually qualified by suffixes that define the anatomical site or substance to which the measurement refers, as well as other information that clarifies the meaning of the symbol in the context in which it is used. Suffixes are printed in roman type. The anatomical site is usually represented by the first letter of its name; this is usually written in lower case except when the measurement refers to the gas phase. The mean or average value at a particular site is represented by a bar over the corresponding suffix. Thus, the partial pressure of oxygen in alveolar gas is P_{A,O_2}; in mixed venous blood the oxygen tension is $P_{\bar{v},O_2}$, and in systemic arterial blood it is P_{a,O_2}. Other suffixes are listed in Table 6.5. The concepts *partial pressure* and *gas tension* are considered below.

6.4 Units

The units used in respiratory physiology have evolved in line with scientific practice. However, the rate of change has been uneven and this has led to the present unsatisfactory situation in which many countries including all European countries have adopted standard international (SI) units for most indices whilst others including the United States have continued to use more traditional units. The two conventions have in common the litre as

Table 6.1 General terms used in respiratory physiology.

Term	Description*
Acidaemia	A relative excess of hydrogen ions in blood (*vs alkalaemia*)
Airways obstruction	Narrowing or occlusion of airways (often inferred from airflow *limitation* which is then the correct usage)
Anoxia	Absence of oxygen
Apnoea	Cessation of breathing
Asphyxia	Hypoxia and hypercapnia due to severe diminution in ventilation
Bradypnoea	Decreased frequency of breathing (*vs tachypnoea*)
Bronchoconstriction	Airways obstruction due to increased tone of bronchial smooth muscle (*vs bronchodilatation*)
Cyanosis	A bluish discoloration of lips or buccal mucous membrane
Dyspnoea	A consciousness of difficulty in breathing
Hypercapnia	A relatively high tension of carbon dioxide in blood (*vs hypocapnia*)
Hyperinflation	An increase in functional residual capacity (measured or inferred)
Hyperpnoea	An increase in ventilation relative to the metabolic rate (*vs hypopnoea*)
Hyperventilation	An increase in ventilation sufficient to cause hypocapnia (*vs hypoventilation*)
Hypoxaemia	A relative deficiency of oxygen in blood
Hypoxia	A relatively low tension of oxygen at a specified site
Lactacidaemia	Acidaemia due to a raised concentration of lactic acid
Metabolic acidosis	An increase in blood non-volatile acids or reduction in basic substances; if compensated, the blood HCO_3 is reduced and the pH normal (*vs metabolic alkalosis*)
Orthopnoea	Dyspnoea on lying flat
Reference values	Values with which the results under consideration may be compared
Respiratory acidosis	An increase in blood carbon dioxide tension; if compensated, the blood HCO_3^- is increased and the pH normal (*vs respiratory alkalosis*)
Steady state	The condition of equilibrium for a particular variable

* In these descriptions the term 'relative' is used with respect to that for a healthy person breathing air at sea level. The blood concentrations relate to the systemic arterial circulation.

Table 6.2 Abbreviations used to indicate some respiratory indices.*

Abbreviation	Index	Units†	Section no.
Lung volume‡			
CC	Closing capacity	l (or % TLC)	16.1.8
CV	Closing volume	l (or % VC)	16.1.8
ERV	Expiratory reserve volume	l	10.1
EVC	Expiratory vital capacity	l	10.1
FRC	Functional residual capacity	l	10.1
IC	Inspiratory capacity	l	10.1
IRV	Inspiratory reserve volume	l	10.1
IVC	Inspiratory vital capacity	l	10.1
RV	Residual volume (symbol V_R)	l	10.1
RV%	100 × RV/TLC	%	10.1
TGV	Thoracic gas volume	l	10.1
TLC	Total lung capacity	l	10.1
Ventilatory capacity‡			
FEF	Forced expiratory flow	$l\ s^{-1}$	12.5.1
FET	Forced expiratory time	s	12.4.2
FEV_t	Forced expiratory volume	l	12.4.1
FEV_t%	Percentage expired‡ (i.e. 100 × FEV_t/FVC)	%	12.4.1
FIF	Forced inspiratory flow	$l\ s^{-1}$	12.4.1
FIV	Forced inspiratory volume	l	12.4.1
FMF	Forced mid-expiratory flow ($FEF_{25-75\%}$)	$l\ s^{-1}$	12.4.1

Continued

Table 6.2 *(Continued)*

Abbreviation	Index	Units†	Section no.
FVC	Forced vital capacity	l	12.4.1
IMBC	Indirect maximal breathing capacity (estimated from FEV_1)	l min^{-1}	12.2.2
IVPF	Isovolume pressure–flow curve		13.2
MBC	Maximal breathing capacity	l min^{-1}	12.2
MEF	Maximal expiratory flow (now FEF)	l s^{-1}	12.4.1
MEFV	Maximal expiratory flow–volume curve		12.5
MMF	Maximal mid-expiratory flow (now $FEF_{25-75\%}$)	l s^{-1}	12.4.1
MR	Moment ratio		12.4.2
MTT	Mean transit time	s	12.4.2
MVV	Maximal voluntary ventilation§	l min^{-1}	12.2
PEF	Peak expiratory flow	l s^{-1}	12.3
PEFV	Partial expiratory flow–volume curve		12.5
PIF	Peak inspiratory flow	l s^{-1}	–
SDTT	Standard deviation of transit times	s	12.4.2
TVC	Timed vital capacity (now replaced by FEV_t)	l	
VC	Vital capacity	l	10.1
Lung mechanics			
AWR	Airway resistance (alt. *R*aw)	kPa (or cm H_2O) $l^{-1}s$	14.3.4
EPP	Equal pressure point		13.3
Gas exchange			
A-a, d	Alveolar–arterial tension difference (for O_2 or CO_2)	kPa or mm Hg	21.5.2
RER	Respiratory exchange ratio		7.8.2
RQ	Respiratory quotient		7.8.2
TF	Transfer factor (*T*l preferred)	mmol min^{-1} kPa^{-1} or ml min^{-1} mm Hg^{-1}	19.3.5
Response to exercise			
AT	Anaerobic threshold**	mmol O_2 (or l STPD) min^{-1}	28.4.6
EEV	Excess exercise ventilation	l min^{-1}	28.4.2
PFI	Physical fitness index		28.12
SV	Stroke volume	ml	28.6.1
VE	Ventilation equivalent††		28.4.3
Other			
CAO	Chronic airways obstruction		40.3
COHb	Carboxyhaemoglobin	%	19.4.2
COPD	Chronic obstructive pulmonary disease		40.3
MEP	Maximal expiratory pressure (also *P*E, mo, max)	kPa or cm H_2O	9.9.3
MIP‡‡	Maximal inspiratory pressure (also *P*E, mo, max)	kPa or cm H_2O	9.9.3
PEEP	Positive end-expiratory pressure		42.5.1
Sniff Pdi	Sniff transdiaphragmatic pressure	kPa or cm H_2O	9.9.3
Sniff na	Sniff nasal pressure	kPa or cm H_2O	9.9.3
Sniff oes	Sniff oesophageal pressure	kPa or cm H_2O	9.9.3

* The indices are commonly reported in Standard International (SI) units except in the United States where traditional units are used (Section 6.4).

† Volumes are in l BTPS (Section 6.4). The SI unit of time is seconds but minutes is permitted and is often more appropriate. Other units are in Table 6.6.

‡ The time in seconds or the segment of the forced expiratory spirogram should be indicated, e.g. FEV_1, $FEF_{25-75\%FVC}$, $FEF_{75-85\%FVC}$, $FEF_{200-1200}$. Flows generated by forced expiratory effort and measured after expiration from TLC of specified volumes of gas (expressed as % of FVC) are designated $FEF_{x\%FVC}$ (where x = TLC − x% FVC, e.g. $FEF_{75\%FVC}$). Where the volume of gas is that remaining in the lung this should be indicated. The alternative usage (MEF, MMF) is no longer recommended [1].

§ The frequency of breathing should be indicated, e.g. MVV_F, if uncontrolled, and MVV_{40}, if controlled at 40 min^{-1}.

** Owles' point or inflection point is preferable (Section 28.4.6).

†† Also called ventilatory equivalent of oxygen.

‡‡ The lung volume at which the pressure is measured (usually RV or FRC) should be specified.

Table 6.3 Abbreviations used to indicate some anthropometric indices.

Abbreviation	Index	Units	Section no.
BM	Body mass	Kg	4.6
BMI	Body mass index (BM St^{-2})	kg m^{-2}	4.6
BSA	Body surface area	m^2	–
ChD	Chest depth	cm	4.5
ChW	Chest width	cm	4.4
Fat%	Percentage of body mass that is fat	%	4.7
FFM	Fat-free mass	kg	4.7
FFMI	Fat-free mass index (FFM St^{-2})	kg m^{-2}	4.7
SH	Sitting height	m	4.3
ShW	Shoulder width (biacromial width)	cm	4.4
St	Stature (standing height)	m	4.3

Table 6.4 Primary symbols used in respiratory physiology.

C	Concentration in blood, *also* compliance
sC	Specific compliance
D	Diffusing capacity*
E	Elastance
F	Fractional concentration in dry gas
f	Frequency
G	Conductance
sG	Specific conductance
K	*Tl*/*V*A = *K* CO, after Krogh†
k	Coefficient of lung distensibility
$\dot{n}$ (*n′*)	Amount of substance per unit time
P	Pressure
Q	Volume of blood
$\dot{Q}$ (*Q′*)	Volume of blood per unit time
R	Respiratory exchange rate, *also* resistance
S	Saturation, *also* ventilatory response to CO_2
T	Transfer factor*
t	Time
V	Volume of gas
$\dot{V}$ (*V′*)	Volume of gas per unit time
$\dot{v}$ (*V″*)	Instantaneous flow rate of gas

* *D* symbolises the rate constant for movement of substances by diffusion, e.g. across the alveolar capillary membrane. It can represent the rate constant for transfer of substances by multiple processes that include both diffusion and chemical reaction, e.g. transfer from alveolar gas to red cells in alveolar capillaries, but for this application the term transfer factor (symbol *T*) is more appropriate (Section 19.3.5).
† Related to Krogh's factor (*k*), which is in absolute units (Section 20.9.1).

Table 6.5 Some suffixes used in respiratory physiology.

A	Alveolar (e.g. *V*A)
a	Arterial (e.g. *Pa*,O_2)
an	Anatomical (e.g. *V*an,ds)
aw	Airway (e.g. *R*aw)
B	Barometric (e.g. *P*B)
C	Cardiac (e.g. *f*C)
c	Capillary (e.g. *P*c,O_2)
c′	End capillary (e.g. *P*c′,CO_2)
di	Diaphragm (e.g. *P*di)
d	Dead space (e.g. *V*d)
dyn	Dynamic (e.g. *C*dyn)
E	Expired (e.g. $\dot{V}_E$)
el	Elastic (e.g. *P*el)*
ex	Exercise (e.g. $\dot{V}_E$ ex)
I (or insp)	Inspired (e.g. *t*I)
int	Interrupter (e.g. *R*tot th,int)
iso-$\dot{v}$	Isoflow (e.g. *V* iso-$\dot{v}$)
l	Lung (e.g. *T*l)
m	Alveolar capillary membrane (e.g. *D*m)
mb	Multibreath (e.g. RV,mb)
max	Maximal (e.g. $\dot{V}$E, max ex)
oes	Oesophageal (e.g. *P*oes)
PA	Pulmonary artery (e.g. *P*PA)
pl	Pleural (e.g. *P*pl)
R	Respiration (e.g. *f*R)
rb	Rebreathing (e.g. *S*CO_2,rb)
s	Shunt (e.g. $\dot{Q}$s)
sb	Single breath (e.g. *T*l,CO.sb)
ss	Steady state (e.g. *T*l,CO.ss)
st	Static (e.g. *C*st)
t	Tidal (e.g. *V*t)
th	Thoracic (e.g. *R*th)
ti	Tissue (e.g. *R*ti)
tm	Transmural (e.g. *P*tm)
tot	Total (e.g. *t*tot)
$\bar{v}$	Mixed venous (e.g. *P*$\bar{v}$,CO_2)
va	Venous admixture (e.g. $\dot{Q}$va)

* Elastic recoil pressure is preferable (Section 11.3).

the unit of volume, degrees Celsius for temperature and seconds or minutes as units of time. Blood pressure is in kilopascals or millimetres of mercury. For some other applications within the traditional system of units the mm Hg has been replaced by the Torr (after the Italian physicist Torricelli). The SI system differs from the traditional in using metric units for length, mass and their derivatives, including pressure (where the appropriate unit is the kilopascal), energy (joules) and power (watts). The amount of a chemical substance is in molar units, usually millimoles. SI units are used in the present account together with some commonly used traditional equivalents. Of these the mm Hg has been retained as a unit of pressure or gas tension in preference to the Torr, which, whilst familiar to respiratory physiologists, appears not to be widely known in medicine. The conversion factors between SI and traditional units are given in Table 6.6.

6.5 Partial pressure and gas tension (use of Dalton's law)

Partial pressure is the subject of Dalton's law. This states that in any mixture of gases in a container each gas exerts the same pressure it would if it were present alone. For example, gas present in

Table 6.6 Derivation of SI from traditional units.

Category	SI unit	Conversion factor
Temperature	Degrees Celsius (°C, i.e. °K − 273)	(°F − 32) × 5/9
Pressure	Kilopascal (kPa, i.e. kilonewton per square metre)	mm Hg* × 0.1333 (or ÷ 7.50)
		cm H_2O × 0.0981 (or ÷ 10.2)
		atm × 101.3 (or bar × 100)
Length	Centimetre (10^{-2}m)	in. × 2.54 (or ÷ 0.394)
	Metre (m)	in. ÷ 39.37 (or × 0.0254)
	Kilometre (1000 m)	miles × 8/5 (or × 1.609, or ÷ 0.621)
Mass	Gram (10^{-3}kg)	oz × 28.3
	Kilogram (kg)	lb ÷ 2.2 (or × 0.4536)
Volume	Litre (dm^3)	ft^3 × 28.316
Velocity	Metre per second	mph ÷ 2.24
	Metre per minute	ft s^{-1} ÷ 3.28 (or × 0.3048)
		mph × 26.8
Energy	Joule (J, i.e. kg m^2s^{-2})†	cal × 4.184
Power	Watt (W, i.e. J s^{-1})†	kp m min^{-1} × 0.163‡
		(or ÷ 6.12)
		hp × 745.7, or for metric hp × 745.5
Frequency	Hertz (Hz, i.e. s^{-1})	
Amount of substance in gaseous form	Milllimole (mmol)§	For most gases ml STPD ÷ 22.4 but for CO_2 ÷ 22.26
Compliance	l kPa^{-1}	l cm H_2O^{-1} × 10.2 (or ÷ 0.098)
Resistance	kPa l^{-1}s	cm H_2O l^{-1}s × 0.098 (or ÷ 10.2)
Conductance	l $s^{-1}$$kPa^{-1}$	l s^{-1}cm H_2O^{-1} × 10.2 (or ÷ 0.098)
Ventilatory response to CO_2	l min^{-1} kPa^{-1}	l min^{-1} mm Hg^{-1} × 7.5
Transfer factor	$mmol^{-1}$ min^{-1} kPa^{-1}	ml min^{-1}mm Hg^{-1} × 0.335 (or ÷ 2.986)

* 1 mm Hg is approximately 1 Torr (Section 6.4).
† See also Section 29.4.3.
‡ kp is kilopond (Section 29.3.2).
§ Molar concentration (mol l^{-1}) = *P*(atm)/*RT*(°K), where *R* (gas constant) = 0.0821 l atm °$K^{-1}mol^{-1}$.

the lungs (alveolar gas) comprises oxygen (O_2), carbon dioxide (CO_2), inert gases which are mainly nitrogen, and hence designated N_2, and water vapour (H_2O). Except when the airways are obstructed the sum of the partial pressures is equal to the barometric pressure. Thus:

$$P_B = P_{A,O_2} + P_{A,CO_2} + P_{A,N_2} + P_{A,H_2O} \quad (6.1)$$

The partial pressure of water vapour (P_{A,H_2O}) is that for gas at body temperature, saturated with water vapour. When body temperature is 37°C, the aqueous vapour pressure is 6.3 kPa (47 mm Hg or Torr). The pressure of dry gas is obtained by subtracting the water vapour pressure from the barometric pressure. Hence from eqn. 6.1:

$$P_B - P_{H_2O}(37) = P_{A,O_2} + P_{A,CO_2} + P_{A,N_2} \quad (6.2)$$

When a gaseous substance is in solution in a liquid, for example blood, the effective partial pressure or tension is that which the substance would exert in gas in equilibrium with the liquid in question. This is irrespective of whether or not a stable gaseous phase is present. In its absence, the sum of the tensions of all gases present in the liquid need not add up to the barometric pressure. For example, in the mixed venous blood the tensions of oxygen, carbon dioxide and nitrogen are on average, 5, 6 and 77 kPa (40, 46 and 574 mm Hg) respectively. The sum of these tensions is 88 kPa (660 mm Hg), which is less than the average pressure of dry gas in the lungs at sea level, i.e. 101.3 − 6.3 = 95 kPa (760 − 47 = 713 mm Hg). This means that if a small bubble of air is introduced into a vein (e.g. in relation to venipuncture or decompression sickness), it will come to have this relative composition and will be reabsorbed.

6.6 Standardisation of volumes for temperature and pressure (use of Boyle's and Charles' laws)

Measurements of gas volume are made at the temperature and pressure of the recording equipment where the gas molecules are at ambient temperature and pressure (ATP); expired gas is usually also saturated with water vapour and in these circumstances its condition is designated ATPS. Ambient conditions vary and so the volumes need to be converted to a standard condition, which for most purposes is that obtaining in the lung; here the gas is at body temperature and pressure and saturated with water vapour (BTPS). In the traditional system of units the *quantity* of a gas is reported as a volume under standard conditions of temperature ($t = 0°C$), at one atmosphere of pressure [$P = 101.3$ kPa or 760 mm Hg (Torr)] and dry as a result of elimination of water vapour. A volume in these units is said to be at STPD (standard temperature and pressure dry). In the SI system the quantity of a gas is reported in millimoles.

The relationship of gas volume to pressure is described by Boyle's law, which states that at a constant temperature a gas volume is inversely related to its pressure. Hence, $P \propto 1/V$ and $PV=$ a constant, k. The relationship of volume to ambient temperature is the subject of Charles' law, which states that at a constant pressure a gas volume is proportional to its absolute temperature in Kelvin (T). Hence, $V = k'T$; this can be rewritten as $V = k'(273 + t)$, where t is temperature in degrees Celsius. The two equations are combined in the general gas equation; this represents that for a given mass of gas under two sets of conditions, $P_1V_1/T_1 = P_2V_2/T_2$. The equation is used to convert gas volumes to BTPS or STPD from measurements made at ATP. For this purpose:

$$V_{BTPS} = V_{ATP} \times \frac{273+37}{273+t} \times \frac{P_B - P_{H_2O}(t)}{P_B - P_{H_2O}(37)} \quad (6.3)$$

$$V_{STPD} = V_{ATP} \times \frac{273}{273+t} \times \frac{P_B - P_{H_2O}(t)}{P_{B,Standard}} \quad (6.4)$$

where V is gas volume under the conditions specified, t is ambient temperature and 37 is body temperature (both in degrees Celsius), P_B is barometric pressure and P_{H_2O} is aqueous vapour pressure at the temperature indicated. Water vapour pressures for saturated gas at different temperatures are listed in Table 6.7, together with factors for converting gas volumes from ATPS to BTPS and STPD. They have been calculated for standard barometric pressure and may be used when the actual pressure deviates by less than 2.5%. In other circumstances conversion should be made using the equations. When this is done on a computer the aqueous vapour pressure over the range 10–40°C (kPa or mm Hg) may be represented by the following equation due to Berry:

$$P_{H_2O,t} = 0.1333(9.993 - 0.3952t + 0.03775t^2) \text{ kPa} \quad (6.5)$$

where 0.1333 converts from mm Hg (Torr) to kilopascals and t is as defined above. The error in P_{H_2O} derived in this way is less than 0.09 kPa (0.7 mm Hg).

Table 6.7 Factors for conversion of volumes from ATPS to STPD and BTPS.

Ambient temperature (°C)	Aqueous vapour pressure		Factor to convert to	
	KPa	mm Hg	STPD	BTPS
10	1.23	9.2	0.952	1.153
11	1.31	9.8	0.949	1.148
12	1.40	10.5	0.945	1.143
13	1.49	11.2	0.940	1.138
14	1.60	12.0	0.936	1.133
15	1.71	12.8	0.932	1.128
16	1.81	13.6	0.928	1.123
17	1.93	14.5	0.924	1.118
18	2.07	15.5	0.920	1.113
19	2.20	16.5	0.916	1.108
20	2.33	17.5	0.911	1.102
21	2.49	18.7	0.906	1.096
22	2.64	19.8	0.902	1.091
23	2.81	21.1	0.897	1.085
24	2.99	22.4	0.893	1.080
25	3.17	23.8	0.888	1.075
26	3.36	25.2	0.883	1.069
27	3.56	26.7	0.878	1.063
28	3.77	28.3	0.874	1.057
29	4.00	30.0	0.869	1.051
30	4.24	31.8	0.864	1.045
31	4.47	33.7	0.859	1.039
32	4.76	35.7	0.853	1.032
33	5.03	37.7	0.848	1.026
34	5.32	39.9	0.843	1.020
35	5.62	42.2	0.838	1.014
36	5.95	44.6	0.832	1.007
37	6.28	47.1	0.826	1.000
38*	6.63	49.7	0.821	0.994
39*	6.99	52.4	0.816	0.987
40*	7.37	55.3	0.810	0.980

* At above body temperature gas in a bellows or other waterless spirometer is not fully saturated with water vapour. The appropriate factor is then midway between the value quoted and that for body temperature.

6.7 Graham's law of diffusion

The relationship between the molecular size of a gas and its rate of diffusion is described by Graham's law, which states that for a given temperature and pressure the diffusion rate is inversely proportional to the square root of the molecular weight. Hence, small molecules diffuse faster than large ones.

$$\text{Diffusion rate} \propto 1/\sqrt{\text{MW}} \quad (6.6)$$

The application of Graham's law in describing diffusion in the gas phase is in Section 19.2.3.

6.8 Henry's law

The relationship between the pressure of a gas and the quantity in solution under equilibrium conditions is described by Henry's law. This states that the amount of gas dissolved in a liquid is proportional to the partial pressure of the gas in contact with the liquid, provided no chemical reaction takes place. The amount varies with the temperature and so this should be specified.

Henry's law is used to describe the consequences of exposure to changes in barometric pressure such as occurs in divers or when working at high altitude (Sections 35.3 and 34.1).

6.9 Terminology for lung imaging

Computed tomography and magnetic resonance imaging provide information that can complement the assessment of lung function. The techniques have generated their own terminology [7, 8].

6.10 References

1. Miller MR, Hankinson J, Brusasco V et al. Standardization of spirometry. Official statement of the American Thoracic Society and the European Respiratory Society. *Eur Respir J*, 2005; **26**: 319–338.
2. Pappenheimer JR, Comroe JH, Cournand A et al.Standardization of definitions and symbols in respiratory physiology. *Fed Proc* 1950; **9**: 602–605.
3. Commission of Respiratory Physiology of the International Union of Physiological Sciences. Geneva: UNESCO, 1980.
4. Pulmonary terms and symbols: a report of the ACCP-ATS Joint Committee on Pulmonary Nomenclature. *Chest* 1975; **67**: 583–593.
5. Quanjer PhH, Tammeling GJ, Cotes JE et al. Symbols, abbreviations and units. Working party on standardisation of lung function tests, European Community for Steel and Coal. *Eur Respir J* 1993; **6** (Suppl 16): 85–100.
6. Quanjer PhH, Sly PD, Stocks J. Uniform symbols, abbreviations and units in pediatric pulmonary function testing. *Pediatr Pulmonol* 1997; **24**: 2–11.
7. Webb WR, Muller NL, Naidich DP. Standardised terms for high-resolution computed tomography of the lung: a proposed glossary. *J Thorac Imaging* 1993; **8**: 167–175.
8. Austin JH, Muller NL, Friedman PJ et al. Glossary of terms for CT of the lungs: recommendations of the Nomenclature Committee of the Fleischner Society. *Radiology* 1996; **200**: 327–331.

Further reading

Cooper JD, Billingham M, Egan T et al. A working formulation for the standardisation of nomenclature and for clinical staging of chronic dysfunction in lung allografts. International Society for Heart and Lung Transplantation. *J Heart Lung Transplant* 1993; **12**: 713–716.

Cotes JE. SI units in respiratory medicine. *Am Rev Respir Dis* 1975; **112**: 753–755.

Daves ML. The language of the lungs. *Am J Roentgenol* 1994; **162**: 21–22.

Kendrick AH. Historical development of the gas laws. *Breath* 1990; **39**: 3–10.

Snider GL. What is in a name? Names, definitions, descriptions and diagnostic criteria of diseases, with emphasis on chronic obstructive pulmonary disease. *Respiration* 1995; **62**: 297–301.

CHAPTER 7

Basic Equipment and Measurement Techniques

This chapter describes some aspects of equipment and techniques used to investigate lung function.

7.1 Introduction

For assessing lung function the basic measurements are the volume, flow, pressure and chemical composition of respired gas, in a variety of circumstances. The measurements are usually made using transducers sensitive to linear displacement, or physical gas analysers. In modern equipment the sensors are incorporated in semi or fully automated devices that are often relatively simple to use and yield fully processed results online or with only minimal delay. Traditional methods usually measured the required attributes directly but were slower and often required manipulative skill. However, they could yield accurate results when set up by dedicated, trained personnel. In the case of gas sampling and analysis, traditional procedures often entailed exposure to mercury vapour and corrosive chemicals. In many countries the requirements of health and safety regulations have led to the procedures being discontinued.

7.2 Computers

The introduction of computers into the lung function laboratory has revolutionised the tasks of technical personnel [1]. The advantages outweigh the disadvantages (Table 7.1), but the changes in working practices have altered the skills required of technicians. In addition, the responsibility for obtaining accurate results is now shared between the operator and the manufacturer of the equipment; hence the manufacturer's instructions on setting up and calibration need to be followed meticulously. But, the operator should have checked and accepted as valid the conventions adopted in the computer program for calculation of intermediate results and reference values. These should be supplied by the manufacturer and not left concealed within a 'black box'.

7.3 Measurement of gas volumes and flows

A volume of gas is usually best measured with a spirometer and a flow with a flow-measuring device. However, flow can also be obtained from volume by differentiation with respect to time and volume from flow by integration in a similar manner. Thus the distinction between volume- and flow-measuring devices has been reduced, but not eliminated. The various instruments

Table 7.1 Some advantages and disadvantages of using automated equipment.

Advantages	Disadvantages
Throughput is increased	Initial cost can be high
Measurement errors are less common	Servicing and upgrades can be costly
Complex calculations are performed accurately	System failure can be a disaster
Running costs are lower	Back-up facilities are essential
Quality assurance can be automated	Test routines become inflexible
Inter-lab differences can be reduced	Reference values cannot readily be altered
Data can be stored and retrieved readily	Technicians lose practical skills
Reports, audits and invoices can be generated automatically	Atypical circumstances may be overlooked

Source: Adapted from [1].

inevitably differ in their physical characteristics and these should be appropriate for the intended application.

The instrument chosen should meet or exceed the standards of accuracy for volume and dynamic characteristics published in the joint recommendations of the American Thoracic Society (ATS) and European Respiratory Society (ERS) [2]. This document draws together previous standards set by each authoritative body separately [3, 4]. Recommendations of the European Coal and Steel Community (on behalf of the ERS) not covered in the joint recommendations are retained in the present account (Table 7.2).

Table 7.2 Minimal standards for equipment used for measurement of gas volumes and dynamic flow rates: recommendations of the European Coal and Steel Community (ECSC) and joint working parties of the American Thoracic Society (ATS) and European Respiratory Society (ERS).

	ECSC	Joint ATS/ERS
Volume range	0–8 l	0.5–8 l
Volume accuracy	±3% or ±50 ml*	±3% or ±50 ml*
Volume resolution†	25 ml	Not stated
Driving pressure	<0.03 kPa	Not stated
Paper speed, slow	0.03 m min^{-1}	Not stated
Paper speed, fast	0.02 m s^{-1}	At least 0.02 m s^{-1}
Recording time	15 s accurate to ±1%	At least 15 s
Flow range	0–15 l s^{-1}	±14 l s^{-1}
Flow accuracy	±3.5% or ±0.07 l s^{-1}*	±5% or ±0.2 l s^{-1}*
Dynamic resistance	<0.05 kPa l^{-1} s	<0.15 kPa (1.5 cm H_2O) l^{-1} s‡
Inertia	<0.001 kPa l^{-1} s^2	Not stated
Maximal mouth pressure	<0.6 kPa	Not stated
Dynamic response	3–20 Hz§	Flat (±5%) up to 15 Hz (for PEF)

* Whichever is greater.
† Minimal detectable change in volume.
‡ At a flow of 14 l s^{-1}.
§ The response should be flat (within 5%) at 3 Hz for FEV_1, $FEF_{25-75\%}$ and $FEF_{75\%FVC}$, 5 Hz for $FEF_{50\%FVC}$, and 20 Hz for PEF and $FEF_{25\%FVC}$.
Source: [2, 3].

7.3.1 Volume-measuring devices

Spirometer. Gas volume is usually measured in a spirometer. This can take the form of a cylinder, piston, wedge or bellows of known dimensions (Table 7.3). A spirometer used for studying adults should have a volume displacement of at least 8 l. The container is sealed by a trough of water, an expansile bellows or a rolling seal. Where water is used the level should be maintained constant by regular checking. In a rolling seal spirometer the piston is made of thin-walled stainless steel and mounted horizontally or vertically on low-friction bearings. These features are intended to minimise respectively the inertia and resistance to movement of the system. The piston is connected to the inside wall of the housing by a silicon rubber seal that rolls over itself.

The displacement of the spirometer should be linear with volume and the equipment should comply with the standards (Table 7.2). Procedures for calibration are in Section 7.15 below.

The pressure of gas in both lungs and spirometer is atmospheric, and so the correction of volume for pressure is straightforward (Section 6.6). Correction for temperature is more of a problem as air leaving the lungs has a temperature of about 33–35°C [5, 6] whereas that in the spirometer is usually at

Table 7.3 Some types of volume displacement spirometers.

Type	Shape	Seal	Common features	Applications
Benedict, Roth	Long cylinder (diameter ≈ 20 cm)	Water	Water oscillation, low dead-space	Closed circuit
Tissot	Large cylinder	Water	High inertia	Storing gas
Mendel, Bernstein	Wide	Water	Small displacement	Dynamic volumes
Krogh	Wedge	Water	Small displacement	Dynamic volumes
Vitalograph	Wedge	Bellows	High inertia	FEV_1 and FVC
McDermott	Cube	Bellows	Low resistance and inertia	Dynamic volumes and flow rates
Rolling seal	Wide piston	Rolling seal	Low resistance and inertia	All

ambient temperature. Hence the exhaled gas gives up heat to the spirometer. If the materials used for the spirometer conduct heat and have a high thermal capacity, the exhaled gas rapidly achieves thermal equilibrium and this is also the case if the exhalation is slow. However, equilibrium may not be achieved following a rapid exhalation into a spirometer made of components having a low thermal conductivity; in this event, an error in the measured volume of up to 5–6% can occur [7].

Spirometers are used for measurement of vital capacity, dynamic lung volumes and flows and for measurement of total lung capacity and its subdivisions. The latter application is described in Section 10.3.1, which also details how the spirometer should be tested for leaks.

In some spirometers the volume signal is differentiated to yield flow. In this event the spirometer should have a frequency response of at least 15 Hz [2], the output should be linear and the differentiator should be accurate to 1% of the signal. Alternatively, the signal from the spirometer can be expressed as volume per 10 ms; in this event, each increment is a flow. Volume is obtained by summation [8]. Methods of calibration are in Section 7.15 below.

Gas meters. Traditional wet gas meters measure gas volume by means of a bladed paddle-wheel that dips in a trough of water. The axle should be level and the gas delivered at a steady rate. The meters are still used in conjunction with Douglas bags for calibrating modern automated equipment (Figs 1.3, page 10 and Section 29.5.3).

A dry gas meter comprises two interconnected bellows that fill alternately. Volume is measured by displacement and 1% accuracy can be achieved over complete cycles of the mechanism. Over segments of the cycle the calibration is alinear. These devices have largely been replaced by pneumotachographs with integrators.

Impedance plethysmograph. In this instrument [9], the sensor is an expansile wire coil round the torso. The coil acts as the inductive element in an oscillatory circuit. Changes in torso diameter with respiration alter the inductance and hence the frequency of the oscillator and this is detected as a direct current (DC) signal. In the commercial model (Respitrace) two sensors are used respectively to monitor expansion of the upper chest and abdomen and the signals are summed after calibration to ensure that they are comparable. Then:

$$\Delta V_m = a\Delta_{RC} + b\Delta_{Abd} \tag{7.1}$$

where ΔV_m is volume change at the mouth, Δ_{RC} and Δ_{Abd} are the changes in the signals respectively from the rib cage and the abdominal transducers, *a* and *b* are calibration factors, also called volume-motion coefficients [10]. This two-compartment model is adequate for tidal breathing but not for vital capacity manoeuvres. Calibration is done by one of several methods including voluntarily altering the position of rib cage and diaphragm during breath holding (isovolume method) and fractionating the tidal breaths into segments. The variability under favourable conditions is approximately 6% but is more during deep breathing. Recalibration is advisable following body movement. The instrument is used for monitoring ventilation during sleep and when the nose and mouth are involved with other activity, for example phonation or assisted ventilation.

7.3.2 Flow-measuring devices

Respiratory flow can vary from 0.5 ml s^{-1} in a premature infant during tidal breathing to about 16 l s^{-1} in a large adult performing a forced expiratory manoeuvre. Hence a range of instruments is needed to meet all circumstances. Flow-measuring devices should have a stable baseline, be sensitive to small changes in flow and meet the technical specifications. These are defined separately for adults (Table 7.2) and for infants [11]. The specification for children is that for adults.

Pneumotachograph. A pneumotachograph records airflow in terms of the reduction in pressure that occurs across a suitable resistance (Fig. 7.1).

The pressure drop, *P*, between two arbitrary points in a flow stream can be approximated from the Navier–Stokes equation:

$$P = Pa + Pc + Pf \tag{7.2}$$

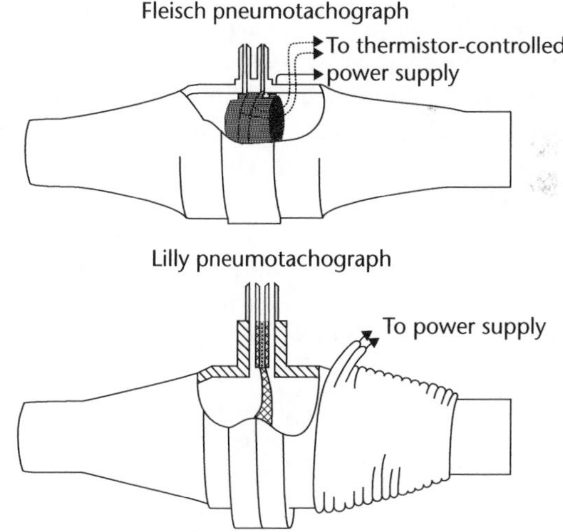

Fig. 7.1 Fleisch- and Lilly-type pneumotachographs each fitted with thermostat and heater. The Fleisch device has a series of capillary tubes or tightly packed corrugated channels. The approaching gas should have a square front. Flow becomes laminar in the middle section of the capillaries where the pressure drop is measured [12]. The tubes connecting the resistance to the transducer should be of equal length and diameter. The Lilly device has a mesh perpendicular to flow. The flow should be laminar [13]. The pressure drop across the resistance is monitored using a differential manometer. The voltage signal is used to provide flow and, by integration, volume.

where Pa is the pressure increment or decrement due to linear acceleration or deceleration between the two points, Pc is the pressure change due to convective acceleration between the two points, and Pf is the pressure change due to frictional losses. In a pneumotachograph, Pa is minimised by placing the pressure ports close together, and Pc is minimised by ensuring that the inlet and outlet diameters of the pneumotachograph are the same. In this way the pressure drop can be simplified to $P = Pf$, and in fully developed laminar flow using the Hagen–Poiseuille equation P can be given by:

$$P = Pf = 8\mu LQ/(\pi r^4) \tag{7.3}$$

where μ is the gas viscosity, r is the radius of the tube, L is the length of the tube and Q is the flow. Thus the pressure drop is linearly related to flow and is dependent on gas viscosity. A Fleisch pneumotachograph has small capillaries with a suitable entry length before the pressure ports so that laminar flow is achieved. It is critical that the flow profile upstream to the Fleisch head is a square front and not laminar (facilitated by using an upstream mesh inside the pneumotachograph) so that the flow in the peripheral capillaries is representative of the total flow. If the flow in the capillaries is not laminar then:

$$P = Pf \propto \mu Q^2/\rho \tag{7.4}$$

where ρ is the gas density. Thus, in turbulent flow the pressure drop is no longer linearly related to flow and is now also density dependent.

The pneumotachograph head should be dry and its temperature should preferably be that of expired gas leaving the mouth (approximately 33–35°C). This reduces condensation of water vapour that otherwise alters the viscous resistance offered by the capillaries and it also minimises fluctuations in gas temperature which would affect gas viscosity.

The Fleisch pneumotachograph is compact because the capillary tubes used to eliminate turbulence in the air stream can be relatively short. In the Lilly type the tendency for turbulence is limited by using a tapered tube, but this device is not as linear as the Fleisch. In practice, the accuracy and acceptability of a pneumotachograph and hence the range of flows over which it can be used depends on the sensitivity of the pressure transducer and the physical characteristics of the resistance. The model that is used should be appropriate for the application.

Aspects of calibration. Calibration of flow meters was historically carried out using rotameters, but these require their own independent calibration and are not simple to use. An alternative method is to integrate the flow to derive volume and compare this with the discharged known volume from a calibrated 1-l or preferably 3-l syringe. The discharge is made several times using a range of flows and a calibration factor derived from the average of the volumes recorded. As pneumotachographs are never perfectly linear this means the calibration factor is not biased towards one end of the flow range. A pump system can be used to deliver accurate, constant flows to check the linearity of the flow meter. A calibration curve that is alinear but apparently stable can be linearised by electronic means; both the linearity and the stability should be checked. Drift in analogue integrators can be a problem that can be reduced by automatic re-zeroing. Modern transducers are generally very stable and so numerical integration by computer after analogue to digital conversion is the preferred method.

A calibration curve will be in error if the gas viscosity alters over a period of measurement, for example during an exhalation following inhalation of a single breath of 80% helium in oxygen. This source of error can be avoided by interposing a bag-in-box between the mouthpiece and the pneumotachograph (Fig. 16.5, page 187). Alternatively, the flow can be measured using a spirometer and differentiator. The spirometer is calibrated volumetrically and the differentiator is calibrated by comparing its output (flow) with the spirometer trace recorded during a series of 1- or 3-l syringe volumes each delivered at constant flow over different time intervals.

Turbine. The principal feature is a vane mounted centrally in a tube. Air flowing down the tube rotates the vane at a speed that is proportional to the flow. An optical sensor detects the rotations and the signal is fed to a microprocessor to calculate flow and volume. The device is not normally affected by the composition of the gas flowing through it and so can be used for measuring inspiratory and expiratory flows consecutively. Errors can arise from secretions affecting the rotor and at low flows from the gas not actuating the mechanism. Gas may then pass unregistered, in which case the forced vital capacity will be underestimated, particularly in patients with flow limitation.

Anemometers. In the hot wire anemometer the airflow cools the wire, which results in a change in its electrical resistance. Compared with a pressure device, the instrument is usually linear over a smaller range of flow rates.

In the *Wright anemometer* a rotor in a tube is driven by air that enters through oblique slots cut in the wall. The shape and size of the slots determine the flow characteristics. The instrument is very compact but the calibration curve can be alinear and some air can pass the vane before it starts to rotate. These difficulties have now largely been overcome, for example, by programming a microprocessor to construct a calibration curve. The calibration can be checked using a standard volume of gas delivered from a syringe with different amounts of force. In one version of the instrument, the signal from the anemometer is used to drive a trigger device for sampling the respired gas; this instrument (Miser) is suitable for field studies of energy expenditure.

In constant pressure, variable orifice anemometers (e.g. *Wright peak flow meter*) a slot aperture in communication with a mouthpiece is initially covered by a moveable vane or piston restrained by a constant tension spring. Forcible exhalation into the instrument uncovers the aperture to the extent needed to maintain a constant pressure in the mouthpiece. The maximal enlargement of the slot and associated excursion of the vane reflect the peak expiratory flow. The meter should be linear over the range 0–14 $l\,s^{-1}$ and the frequency response should be flat up to a frequency of 15 Hz [2], though 20 Hz may be preferable [3].

The initial calibration of the Wright peak flow meter (original version) was performed biologically using subjects whose peak flow was also registered using a pneumotachograph. The relationship of this calibration to that obtained using steady flows from a rotameter is given by eqn. 7.5:

$$\mathrm{PEF}(\mathrm{l\,s^{-1}}) = 0.017[0.95\dot{V}\,(\mathrm{l\,min^{-1}}) + 47] \quad (7.5)$$

where PEF is the corrected peak flow reading, $\dot{V}$ is the rotameter reading and 0.017 converts from $l\,min^{-1}$ to $l\,s^{-1}$. Other versions of the meter can be calibrated against the original (held by the manufacturer) or another pneumotachograph using volunteer subjects whose PEF values cover the range of the instrument under test. The pneumotachograph should be dried between blows using a fan.

With some anemometers calibration can be performed with a computer-controlled pump; this requires that the resistance of the instrument does not affect the pump. Use of the procedure has demonstrated alinearity and inappropriate damping in some peak flow meters [14]. The errors can invalidate comparisons of flows before and after inhalation of a bronchodilator aerosol (Section 15.7). One strategy to reduce the alinearity and associated clinical problems is to use an adjusted scale based on a single, internationally agreed standard [15]. Technical aspects of registering peak expiratory flow have been reviewed [2, 16]. The measurement is in Section 12.3.2.

Ultrasound. In an ultrasound airflow meter sound pulses are transmitted diagonally across a tube through which gas is flowing [17]. Two transducers on either side of the tube emit and receive the pulses. Flow is derived from the difference in the transit time of the upstream and downstream sound pulses. The device has no moving parts and the signal is uninfluenced by changes in gas composition, temperature or pressure. It has been used in ventilated and spontaneously breathing children for measurements of functional residual capacity using sulphur hexaflouride wash-in and washout [18].

7.4 Measurement of respiratory pressure

Simple manometer. A pressure that is steady or changing only very slowly can be measured directly with a U tube manometer containing a liquid of known density, for example water (density 1 $g\,ml^{-1}$) or mercury (density 13.6 $g\,ml^{-1}$). The pressure is equal to the product of the density and the height of the column of the liquid that the unknown pressure will support. Manometers still have a role in calibration of pressure-measuring devices and for measuring the resistance characteristics of physiological equipment. The method is illustrated in Fig. 7.2.

Table 7.4 Pressures likely to be encountered in different circumstances.

Circumstances	Pressure
Maximal respiratory pressure	±30 kPa (≈ 300 cm H_2O)
Sniff nasal pressure	−20 kPa (≈ 200 cm H_2O)
Oesophageal pressure	±3 kPa (≈ 30 cm H_2O)
Body plethysmography	
Mouth pressure	±2 kPa
Box pressure*	$\pm 2 \times 10^{-2}$ kPa

* The two signals should be *in phase* up to 10 Hz [3].

Electric manometers. Pressure transducers convert a change in pressure into an electrical signal. The pressure is applied to one side of a diaphragm, crystal, or other device of which the opposite side is at atmospheric pressure. The measured pressure is then with respect to atmospheric pressure. An example is the measurement of respiratory pressure at the mouth. In a differential pressure transducer, such as is used with a pneumotachograph, the pressure at the second site is applied to the other side of the diaphragm. Details of the connections are given in the caption to Fig. 7.1.

The movement of the diaphragm or the distortion of the crystal lattice is detected as a change in electrical resistance, capacitance or inductance. For measurement of the pressure drop across a pneumotachograph, use is made of a low-pressure differential transducer, whilst for the pressure at the tip of a long catheter there is need for a high-pressure, low-volume displacement transducer.

Where two or more pressure transducers are used concurrently, as occurs in the whole body plethysmograph, they should preferably be of the same type in order that their outputs can be synchronised.

The electromanometers used for recording pressure should have an accuracy and resolution of less than 2% of the maximal pressure that it is proposed to measure (Table 7.4). The time required for 95% response should be of the order of 0.01 s.

With appropriate damping and suitable recording equipment most manometers can be used to follow cyclical fluctuations in pressure occurring with a frequency of up to about 40 Hz; this is adequate for most purposes (e.g. Table 7.2). Manometers that meet more stringent specifications are also available.

7.5 Other electronic apparatus

Amplifiers. The output from the transducer is coupled to an amplifier; this should have characteristics to match both the transducer and the recorder that it is proposed to use. Semiconductor integrated circuit amplifiers are widely used as they combine a high gain (amplification) with a high input resistance and operate at a low DC voltage and current, and hence are electrically safe. This class of amplifiers includes integrated circuit

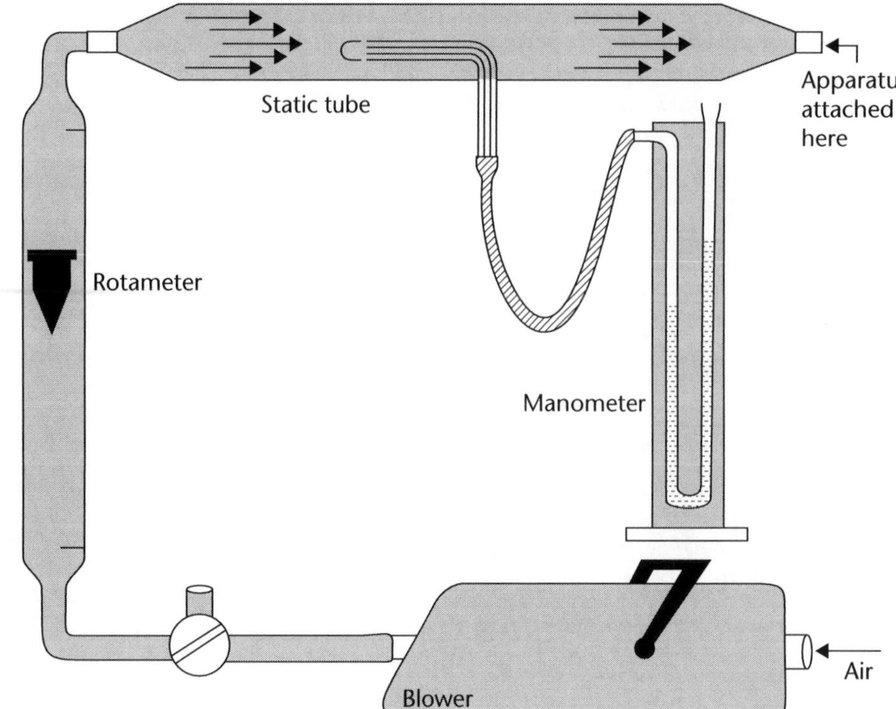

Fig. 7.2 Static tube and other equipment for determining the resistance to air flow imposed by items of physiological apparatus. The outer tube has an internal diameter of 5 cm and the angle of the cones is 7°. The inner tube is of diameter 8 mm and length 10.5 cm; it is perforated by seven holes (diameter 0.97 mm) located 3.2 cm downstream from the hemispherical head. The outer tube should ideally extend for 1 m on either side of the static tube. The pressure is recorded at selected flow rates before and after connection of the apparatus to be tested; the resistance at these flow rates is then obtained by difference. The method is satisfactory when, as is usually the case, the back pressure is less than 0.2 kPa (2.0 cm H_2O). For higher pressures the reading on the rotameter should be adjusted for the change in the density of the gas according to the following relationship:

$$\dot{V} = \dot{V}_0 \sqrt{\frac{(P_B + P)}{P_B}}$$

where $\dot{V}_0$ and $\dot{V}$ are the initial and corrected readings on the rotameter, P_B is barometric pressure and P is the pressure difference registered by the manometer.

operational amplifiers; they can be used with glass electrodes for the measurement of pH and P_{CO_2} where an input resistance in excess of $10^{11}\,\Omega$ is required.

Direct writing Y/t or X/Y chart recorder. In modern applications computers are widely used for data acquisition, processing and display. However, direct-writing Y/t and X/Y recorders are still used when an instantaneous printed record of events is required, for example an electrocardiogram. Twin coordinate (X/Y) chart recorders in which two variables are recorded simultaneously along two axes at right angles are seldom used because, except with servo-assistance that is expensive, the frequency response is low (approximately 1 Hz). This limitation can be overcome by the use of microcircuits to store the incoming signals that are then replayed at a slower rate. In this way signals with respect to time can be recorded over a deflection of 250 mm with an accuracy of 0.2%, and a frequency response of up to 20 kHz. For X/Y displays similar advantages can be obtained.

Analogue to digital converters. Data acquisition by computer is done through an analogue to digital (A/D) converter that transforms an analogue output DC voltage from a spirometer, gas analyser or other device into a digital value. A key feature of an A/D converter is the number of binary digits (bits) into which the voltage range is divided. This determines the resolution of the monitoring device. For example, a 10-bit converter can express a voltage range in 1024 (2^{10}) parts. Hence, for an 8-l spirometer, with a voltage output of 0–5 V full-scale deflection, the resolution would be 5 V/1024 or 4.8 mV per bit (equivalent to 7.8 ml volume displacement per bit). In modern equipment 12-bit converters are commonplace and in some circumstances are recommended to achieve even better resolution [4].

The signal should be sampled at a rate at least twice that of the highest frequency contained in the signal [4]. This should be at least 15 Hz [2] and probably 20 Hz [3] for recording peak flow but sampling rates of 100 Hz are commonly employed in automated equipment.

7.6 Connecting the subject to the equipment

Most respiratory procedures entail making measurements on respired gas via a mouthpiece. The nasopharynx is sealed off either reflexly, as when exhaling forcibly through the mouth, or by use of a nose clip. The mouthpiece is a round or nearly oval rigid tube of cross-sectional area at least 5 cm^2, equivalent to a tube of diameter 2.5 cm. Subjects unable to tolerate a mouthpiece can use a well-fitting oronasal mask. The fit is achieved by selecting one from a number of semi-rigid face pieces or by using a face piece with a soft inflatable edge and fastening it using a relatively tight harness. The fit can be assessed by closing the outlet and having the subject sniff. Any valve box should have a small dead-space [19] and low flow resistance. Volume- or flow-measuring devices can be attached and the expired gas can be channelled past a sampling point or a mixing chamber if a representative sample is required (Fig. 29.6, page 424).

The respiratory equipment should not itself hinder the flow of gas into or out of the lungs and on this account should have an acceptably low flow resistance (Table 7.5). However, despite this precaution the use of a mouthpiece or oronasal mask can alter the pattern of breathing. Under resting conditions the principal change in normal supine subjects is an increase in tidal volume of approximately 15% with a mouthpiece and nose clip and 30% with a mask [21, 22]. The distortion can be avoided by replacing the mouthpiece with a ventilated canopy (bias flow spirometry) or by recording the respiratory excursion of the thorax and abdomen by a suitable means. This might be by photography, light sensors, plethysmography or by magnetometers, strain gauges or other sensors applied to the torso. Such methods are suitable only for a few applications; for the majority a mouthpiece is used and any interaction with breathing is ignored.

Table 7.5 Inspiratory flow resistances that do not themselves reduce the ventilation minute volume ($\dot{V}_E$).*

	Suction	
$\dot{V}_E$ (l min^{-1})	kPa	cm H_2O
<10	0.5	5.0
10–30	0.25	2.5
30–100	0.10	1.0
>100	0.07	0.7

Note: Expiratory flow resistances should not exceed twice these levels. For protective respirators in order to avoid undue discomfort (but not hypoventilation) Bentley and others [20] recommend that maximal peak pressure does not exceed 1.7 kPa (17 cm H_2O).

* Resistance is expressed as suction needed to generate a flow of 85 l min^{-1} (3 ft^3 min^{-1}).

7.7 Analysis of gases

In a lung function laboratory, gas analysis is commonly undertaken by exploiting a physical property of the gas. Chemical methods have mostly been abandoned, but have a role for calibration (e.g. Table 1.4, page 9). For the physiological gases oxygen, carbon dioxide and carbon monoxide, their physical properties determined how they might be analyzed. For other gases both the physical property and the ability to quantify it have influenced decisions on use. In most instances the property is not unique to one gas and so the presence of other gases must be allowed for (Table 7.6).

Table 7.6 Physical methods for analysis of gases.

Physical attributes	Gases for which appropriate	Other gases which interfere
Chemiluminescence	NO	H_2O, CO_2, Ethane
Differential absorption (gas chromatography)	All	–
Flame conductivity	C_2H_2 and other hydrocarbons	O_2, CO_2
Gamma emission	^{85}Kr, $^{15}O_2$, $^{17}O_2$, ^{133}Xe	–
Infrared absorption	CO_2, CO, N_2O, C_2H_2, CH_4, SF_6	H_2O*
Kinematic viscosity	He, H_2, SF_6	†
Mass	All	See text
Paramagnetic properties	O_2, NO	–
pH in solution	CO_2	†
Photoionisation	O_2	†
Polarographic potential	O_2	†
Refraction index	He	–
Sound transmission	He, H_2	O_2, CO_2, H_2O
Thermal conductivity	He, CO_2, N_2O, H_2	O_2, H_2O
Ultraviolet emission	N_2	CO_2, H_2O, SF_6

* Other gases including oxygen can give rise to collision broadening of the absorption bands for the gas to be analysed; the broadening alters the calibration.

† Variable depending on conditions.

The most universal attribute is mass, which for most purposes is equal to the gram molecular weight; this is the basis for resolution in respiratory mass spectrometers such as that originally developed by Fowler [23]. Most instruments are able to analyse simultaneously up to four gases having molecular weights in the range 1–200. The response time is about 0.1 s. The resolution is normally to one mass unit. This constrains the analysis of some gas mixtures, for example those that contain carbon monoxide and nitrogen, since both gases have molecular weights of about 28. The difficulty can extend to the analysis of nitrogen in the presence of carbon dioxide, because up to 0.6% of the CO_2 can be reduced to carbon monoxide during passage through the instrument. Carbon monoxide can be analysed as an isotope, for example $C^{18}O$. Nitrous oxide overlaps with carbon dioxide (mass of approximately 44), but the former gas is oxidised to nitric oxide that can be detected separately. In addition, the concentration of water vapour may be in error if the vapour condenses to form water droplets in the sampling tube. This and other errors can usually be allowed for by computation.

7.8 Measurement of oxygen consumption and respiratory exchange ratio

7.8.1 Oxygen consumption

The consumption of oxygen by a subject can be measured by closed circuit spirometry (Section 10.3.1) but more often is calculated from the volume and composition of the respired gas. Gas may first be dried and then analysed using a paramagnetic analyser for oxygen and infrared analyser for carbon dioxide. The remainder is then nitrogen plus the rare gases (98.9 and 1.1% respectively). Alternatively, a mass spectrometer can be used. The consumption of oxygen per minute is the difference between the amounts of oxygen that enter and leave the lung. Thus:

$$\dot{n}O_2 = 1000/22.4(\dot{V}\text{I} \times F\text{I},_{O_2} - \dot{V}\text{E} \times F\text{E},_{O_2})\ \text{mmol min}^{-1} \quad (7.6)$$

where $\dot{n}O_2$ is the consumption of oxygen in mmol min^{-1}, $\dot{V}\text{I}$ and $\dot{V}\text{E}$ are the volumes of gas that are respectively inspired and expired per minute in l STPD; the other symbols are defined in Table 7.7. The ratio (1000/22.4) converts the term within the bracket from l min^{-1} to mmol min^{-1}. It should be omitted when traditional units are used (Table 6.6, page 56). Application of eqn. 7.6 entails measuring the volumes of both the inspired and expired gas since the two differ on account of the oxygen that is absorbed seldom being replaced by an exactly equal volume of carbon dioxide. However, under steady-state conditions breathing air the difference does not extend to nitrogen. This gas with or without the rare gases can therefore be used to correct for the change in volume. To this end the volume of nitrogen entering and leaving the lung per minute is represented as follows:

$$\dot{V}\text{I} \times F\text{I},_{N_2} = \dot{V}\text{E} \times F\text{E},_{N_2} \quad (7.7)$$

This relationship is then restated:

The volume of gas inspired per litre of gas expired = $\dot{V}\text{I}/\dot{V}\text{E} = F\text{E},_{N_2}/F\text{I},_{N_2}$

The volume of O_2 inspired per litre of gas expired = $F\text{I},_{O_2} \times F\text{E},_{N_2}/F\text{I},_{N_2} = 0.2648 \times F\text{E},_{N_2}$ (including rare gases)

The volume of O_2 absorbed per litre of gas expired = $0.2648 \times F\text{E},_{N_2} - F\text{E},_{O_2}$

Hence in SI units O_2 consumption per minute

$$= (1000/22.4)\,\dot{V}\text{E} \times (0.2648 \times F\text{E},_{N_2} - F\text{E},_{O_2})\ \text{mmol min}^{-1} \quad (7.8)$$

For $\dot{V}o_2$ in l min^{-1} the term (1000/22.4) is omitted.

When, instead of the expired minute volume, the inspired minute volume is recorded it may be converted into the corresponding expired minute volume via eqn. 7.7. Thus:

$$\dot{V}\text{E} = \dot{V}\text{I} \times F\text{I},_{N_2}/F\text{E},_{N_2} \quad (7.9)$$

If it is convenient to analyse only one gas, the concentration of oxygen should be obtained and used in an empirical equation such as proposed by Musgrove and Doré [24]. Alternatively, the analysis may be performed before and after the absorption of carbon dioxide.

Table 7.7 Symbols for quantities used in the calculation of consumption of oxygen (from Chapter 6).

	Inspired concentration*	Expired concentration
Oxygen	$F\text{I},O_2$ (0.2093)*	$F\text{E},O_2$
Carbon dioxide	$F\text{I},CO_2$ (0.0003)	$F\text{E},CO_2$
Nitrogen (including rare gases)	$F\text{I},N_2$ (0.7904)	$F\text{E},N_2$

* These fractional concentrations are for breathing air.

7.8.2 Respiratory exchange ratio

The respiratory exchange ratio is the ratio of the rate at which carbon dioxide leaves the lungs in expired gas to the rate of consumption of oxygen. Under steady-state conditions the ratio is representative of the metabolism of the subject and is called the *respiratory quotient*. It is calculated in the following manner:

$$R = CO_2 \text{ output} \div O_2 \text{ uptake} = F\text{E},_{CO_2}/(0.2648\,F\text{E},_{N_2} - F\text{E},_{O_2}) \quad (7.10)$$

where R is the respiratory exchange ratio.

7.9 Collection and storage of blood

Collection. Arterialised capillary blood is easier to obtain than an arterial sample and is often used as a substitute for it [25–27]. The capillary samples are analysed by methods that collectively require only a small quantity of blood (<0.1 ml). The measurements include capillary blood pH, the tensions of carbon dioxide and oxygen, the concentration of sodium bicarbonate, the saturation of haemoglobin with oxygen or carbon monoxide and the concentration of lactic acid. The preferred sites for blood collection are the skin of the heel in an infant, or the ear lobe or pulp of a finger in a child or adult.

The part is rendered hyperaemic by local heat and application of a rubefacient cream (see Footnote 7.1).

The skin is cleaned by the evaporation of alcohol and a stab incision is made with a surgical needle or spring-loaded small blade. In the case of the ear the stab is 3 mm above the lower border of the ear lobe through to a sterile rubber bung or cork placed behind the ear. Free flow of blood is essential. The blood is sampled by capillary attraction into a heparin-coated glass capillary tube (100 μl).

Despite good correlations between ear lobe and arterial samples taken simultaneously in the same patient the limits of agreement for $P\text{O}_2$ can be wide both at rest [28] and on exercise [29]. In these studies the $P\text{O}_2$ of blood from the ear lobe was lower, on average, than that from the artery and differences were larger in the normal range of $P\text{O}_2$. The difference arose because of a significant venous admixture in blood sampled from the ear lobe. By comparison, the errors and limits of agreement for $P\text{CO}_2$ were smaller. However, if accurate or repeated estimates of $P\text{O}_2$ are required, the arterial blood should be sampled directly [27]. The arterial sites, in order of preference, are the radial, brachial, dorsalis pedis and femoral arteries. In neonates an umbilical artery catheter can be used. With practice, the radial artery is satisfactory in most patients, usually has good collateral circulation, and produces the lowest incidence of complications. Training in the procedure is essential.

Storage. The leakage of oxygen from blood is greater when the sample is stored in plastic compared with glass syringes [30] and the relative losses are greater when the partial pressure of oxygen is high [31, 32]. Even in glass syringes the gaseous composition of freshly drawn arterial blood begins to change within 5 min at room temperature (22°C). This is due to metabolic activity principally by white blood cells, which, over the first 10 min, reduces $P\text{O}_2$ by about 0.5 kPa min^{-1}. The corresponding rise in $P\text{CO}_2$ is trivial as CO_2 is buffered in the blood [31, 32]. Storage of the sample on ice reduces the change in $P\text{O}_2$ by a factor of 4. Accordingly, if routine blood gas analysis is likely to be delayed the sample should be collected in a glass syringe, stored on ice at 0°C and the analyses of $P\text{O}_2$ and $P\text{CO}_2$ performed within an hour.

Samples for lactate or pyruvate analysis should be delivered immediately into trichloroacetic acid at 0°C, centrifuged and stored at −10°C, after which they can be analysed at leisure.

Footnote 7.1. Examples of rubefacient creams are Transvasin (Reckitt & Colman), Ralgex (Beecham Proprietaries) and Algipan (Wyeth Laboratories, Maidenhead).

Safe handling. Blood samples represent a biohazard; hence all persons who are involved in taking blood or who come into contact with samples must be trained in appropriate safe procedures. These include avoidance of stick injuries, disposal of samples, hyperdermic needles and swabs and cleaning up of spillages. All samples should be treated as potentially infectious and staff should wear protective clothing, including disposable gloves. Any skin abrasions or cuts should be covered appropriately [25].

7.10 Analysis of blood for oxygen

The amount of oxygen in the blood is usually reported in one of three ways: The *content* is the volume in ml STPD per 100 ml of blood. The *saturation* is the content as a percentage of the capacity when the blood is exposed to a high tension of oxygen. The *tension or partial pressure* of oxygen is that in air in equilibrium with the blood (Section 6.5). The saturation can be deduced from the tension by reference to the blood dissociation curve (e.g. Fig. 21.1, page 260); conversely, the tension of oxygen can be deduced from the saturation over the range where there is a linear relationship between these variables. Outside this range the tension of oxygen can only be determined by a direct method.

7.10.1 Content of oxygen and saturation of haemoglobin

Volumetric method. Oxygen saturation is the ratio of oxygen content to the oxygen-binding capacity of either all the haemoglobin or the available haemoglobin present in the blood sample. These quantities are respectively fractional saturation and functional saturation. The difference between them is usually about 2%.

Oxygen saturation is calculated as follows:

$$\text{Saturation } (Sa, \text{O}_2) = \frac{\text{Content of oxygen}}{\text{Capacity of oxygen}} \times 100\% \qquad (7.11)$$

The content of oxygen was formerly determined from the volume that is liberated when potassium ferricyanide solution is added to a measured amount of blood in a closed container. The volume is estimated either from the change in pressure at constant volume by the method of Van Slyke, or from the change in volume at constant pressure by the method of Haldane. The capacity is determined by similar analysis of blood that has been saturated with oxygen; an allowance is then made for the volume of oxygen that is dissolved in the plasma. At a tension of oxygen of 13.3 kPa (100 Torr) it is 0.13 mmol l^{-1} (0.3 ml per 100 ml) whilst at a tension of 93 kPa (700 Torr) it is 0.9 mmol l^{-1} (2.0 ml per 100 ml).

Spectrophotometric methods. In a spectrophotometer the saturation is obtained from the proportion of haemoglobin that is present in a reduced form. This is ascertained by passing a ray of light through haemoglobin in solution and measuring the absorption at two wavelengths. These are (i) an isobestic point where the absorption is the same for the oxygenated and the reduced haemoglobin, e.g. 805 nm (8050 Å); (ii) a wavelength where the absorption is very different for the two haemoglobins, e.g. 650 nm (6500 Å). Other combinations of wavelengths can also be used. The blood should be haemolysed before analysis as otherwise the light beam is partly scattered by the red cells. This type of spectrophotometer is also known as a co-oximeter.

Error can occur from the presence of carboxyhaemoglobin but this can be minimised by use of appropriate wavelengths, filters and computations.

The capacity of haemoglobin for oxygen is a simple function of the amount of haemoglobin present (Section 21.2). The amount can be determined after its conversion to cyanmethaemoglobin by the method of Drabkin [33]. This technique is adequate for most purposes. However, it also detects methaemoglobin where this is present in the blood, for example in patients with polycythaemia. In this event the oxygen capacity can be overestimated.

Pulse oximetry. Oximetry is the adaptation of the spectrophotographic method for use *in vivo* by application of a sensor to the earlobe, finger, heel or other site. In pulse oximetry the contribution from tissues other than blood is minimised by confining the measurements to the time when the vessels are distended by the pulse wave [34]. The sensor contains light emitting diodes producing wavelengths in the red zone (e.g. 650 nm) and infrared zone (e.g. 940 nm). The absorption spectra vary according to the form of haemoglobin (Fig. 7.3). The measurements are subject to errors on account of the presence of carboxyhaemoglobin (oxygen saturation overestimated) and methaemoglobin (oxygen saturation underestimated) and the variation in the degree of dilatation of blood vessels affecting the amount of blood in the light path. The latter is reduced by timing the measurements with respect to the pulse wave and securing maximal vasodilatation (see above 'Collection and storage of blood'). Error can also arise if the sensor is applied over the site of piercing of the ear or over nail polish or stain applied to the skin. Pigmentation of the skin can also absorb light, resulting in problems of signal quality in persons with particularly dark skin [36]. Where the sensors function correctly the error in readings of Sa,o_2 due to skin colour appear not to be of clinical significance [25, 36]. Skin discolouration may occur from metabolites of drugs and from use of indicator dyes [25]. Pulse oximeter readings should be interpreted with caution and considered only a guide to blood oxygenation.

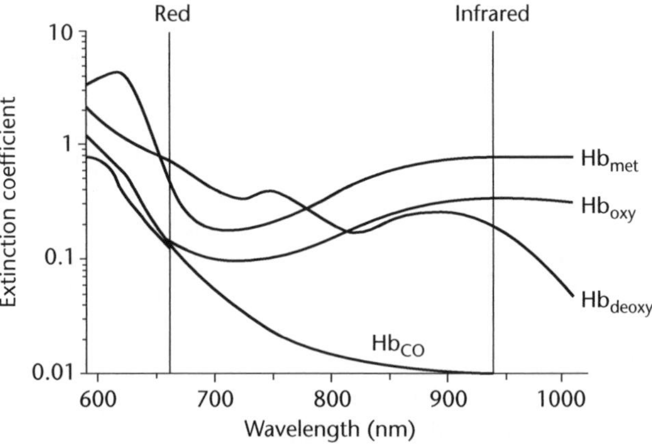

Fig. 7.3 The absorption spectra of different states of haemoglobin across wavelengths of light in the red and infrared range. Source: Adapted from [35].

Pulse oximeters under-read Sa,o_2 in patients with pulsatile veins. Conditions in which this can occur include tricuspid incompetence with regurgitation, arteriovenous fistulae and right heart block [37].

Pulse oximetry at the ear is recommended for exercise studies and at the finger or heel for critical care monitoring, anaesthesia, sleep studies and measurements in infants. When in use, the device should be protected from extraneous light, maintained at a constant temperature and attached securely. The practice of setting the instrument at 100% after the subject has breathed oxygen for 10 min is not now considered necessary.

The accuracy is usually better than ±3% except when the saturation is much reduced (<70%); in this range some instruments perform better than others [38, 39]. *In vitro* calibration devices have been described and used to compare oximeters [40, 41].

Polarographic method. The quantity of oxygen in a measured volume of blood can be deduced from the change in oxygen tension that occurs when the oxygen is liberated from combination with haemoglobin by potassium ferricyanide or carbon monoxide in solution. The tension is measured by polarography (see below), which can also be used to construct the haemoglobin dissociation curve. For this purpose oxygenated blood and blood previously equilibrated with 100% nitrogen are mixed in known proportions; the concentration of red cells should be the same in both and the reservoirs in which the bloods are contained should be agitated before the blood is withdrawn. Alternatively, the content of oxygen may be increased progressively by electrolysis [42].

7.10.2 Tension of oxygen in blood

The tension of oxygen in the blood may be determined in several ways, each of which, in skilled hands, has a standard deviation of approximately 0.25 kPa (2 Torr).

Dissociation curve method. Over the range 2.5–9 kPa (20–70 Torr) the tension of oxygen can be determined from the saturation of haemoglobin by means of the blood dissociation curve for oxygen (Fig. 21.1, page 260); a correction should be made if the body temperature departs to a material extent from 37°C or the pH of the blood is other than 7.4.

Riley bubble method. When the tension of oxygen does not exceed about 13 kPa (100 Torr) it can be determined by a volumetric

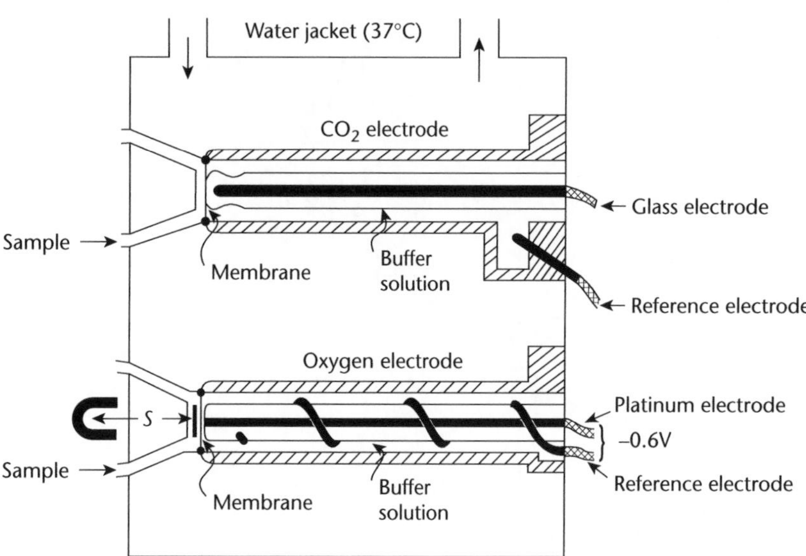

Fig. 7.4 Electrode analysers for the measurement of blood–gas tensions. The gas to be analysed diffuses through the semipermeable membrane of polyethylene or other material into the buffer solution which bathes the electrode. For carbon dioxide, the change in pH is measured with a glass electrode. The electrode is calibrated with gas or water containing carbon dioxide at a known tension. For oxygen, the current which flows between the platinum and reference electrodes is passed into an electrometer amplifier coupled to a recorder of the potentiometer type. When the diameter of the platinum electrode exceeds about 0.025 mm the blood is agitated by rotating the magnetically coupled stirring bar (*S*) at about 25 Hz. Calibration is usually carried out with gas or with blood equilibrated with oxygen at known tensions.

equilibrium method such as that evolved by Riley [43] from the earlier method of Krogh. Success with the method depends upon the correct manipulation of a Roughton–Scholander syringe and requires a delicate touch. This is best learnt in a laboratory where the method is used. The method takes 20–25 min per sample, employs inexpensive apparatus that is simple to maintain and also yields the tension of carbon dioxide. It is suitable for field laboratories or when the electrical supply is variable.

Polarography. For most applications the tension of oxygen is best determined by polarography. By this method the oxygen in a sample of gas or in solution in blood at 37°C is brought into contact with a platinum electrode to which a potential difference of −0.6 V is applied (Fig. 7.4). The current that flows is then a function of the rate of reduction of oxygen at the tip of the electrode; the rate depends upon the diameter of the electrode and the tension of oxygen in the solution. An electrode of diameter 0.025 mm is commonly used because measurements can then be made on unstirred capillary blood. The electrode is protected from protein deposits by a membrane made of polyethylene or polytetrafluoroethylene (PTFE) (thickness 0.025 mm) [44]. This also permits the access of molecules of oxygen and carbon dioxide but not those of other substances whose presence could interfere with the response. Routine calibration is carried out using humidified gases at 37°C containing oxygen at known tensions. The gases are conditioned by bubbling through water. For greater accuracy and when setting up the equipment calibration should also be performed using blood. This is conditioned in a swirling or a rotating-disc tonometer or by bubbling, using an antifoam agent and a vessel coated with silicone. To avoid cooling of the blood during bubbling, the rate of flow of the gas should be relatively slow (<100 ml min^{-1}) and to avoid a rise in the tension of oxygen due to surface forces in the bubbles their diameters should be relatively large (2–7 mm). The calibration of the polarograph is linear for both water and blood, the coefficient of proportionality varying between 0.93 and 1.0, depending on the electrode.

The method is suitable for gaseous oxygen as well as for oxygen in blood or other fluid. Alternative electrode systems include one based on a silver–lead galvanic cell (fuel cell). The cell has a typical response time of about 30 s and is used for *in vitro* measurements, for example, in portable oxygen analysers used at the bedside. In the zirconium oxygen analyser the response time is less than 200 ms, making it suitable for breath-by-breath measurements in exercise tests.

The polarograph electrode can be incorporated in a syringe or arterial catheter or applied to the skin for measurement of transcutaneous oxygen tension. The skin locally is heated to 43–45°C to promote vasodilatation when the skin and capillary oxygen tensions approximate that in arterial blood. When used for continuous monitoring the electrodes should be re-sited 4 hourly to avoid skin burns [25]. The transcutaneous method is suitable for neonates and most patients in intensive care. It can also be used for respiratory patients amongst whom Hutchinson and colleagues [45] observed the following relationship of transcutaneous to arterial oxygen tension:

$$Pa,o_2 = 1.14(Ptc,o_2 - 0.66) \tag{7.12}$$

where Pa,o_2 and Ptc,o_2 are respectively arterial and transcutaneous oxygen tension (kPa). The accuracy of the method can be increased if, concurrent with one of the measurements, a sample of arterial blood is drawn and then analysed in the laboratory.

When the temperature of the equipment (usually 37°C) differs from that of the blood at the time of collection the measured tensions also differ from those which obtain in the body. A correction for this effect of the difference in temperature can be made by use of the factors given in Fig. 7.5.

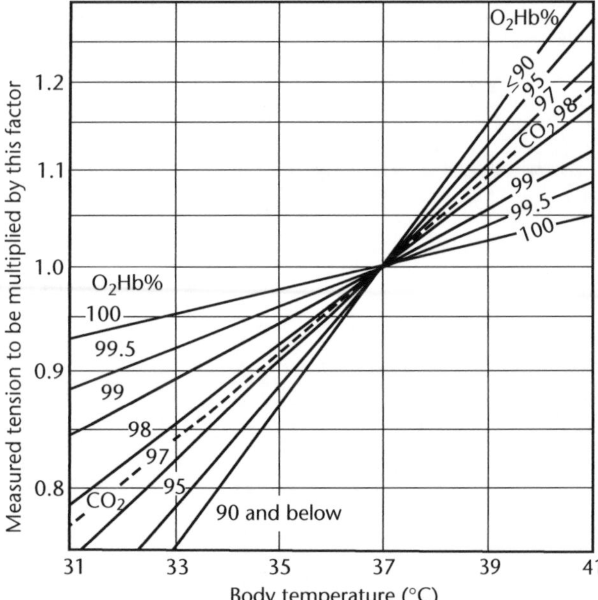

Fig. 7.5 Nomogram showing the factors by which the blood–gas tensions obtained by measurement at 37°C should be multiplied in order to obtain the correct tensions at body temperature; the factors for oxygen are a function of the saturation of haemoglobin. Source: [46].

7.11 Analysis of blood for carbon dioxide

7.11.1 Direct methods

The tension and the content of carbon dioxide and the concentration of hydrogen ions in the blood plasma are related approximately through the Henderson–Hasselbalch equation, which is derived by application of the law of mass action to carbonic acid (H_2CO_3). The relationship is of the form:

$$CO_2 + H_2O \rightleftharpoons H_2CO_3 \rightleftharpoons H^+ + HCO_3^- \quad (7.13)$$

Hence by the law of mass action:

$$[H_2CO_3] = K[H^+][HCO_3^-] \quad (7.14)$$

or, on rearrangement:

$$\frac{1}{H^+} = \frac{K[HCO_3^-]}{[H_2CO_3]} \quad (7.15)$$

Then, taking logs on both sides:

$$\text{pH} = \text{pK} + \log_{10}\frac{[HCO_3^-]}{[H_2CO_3]} \quad (7.16)$$

where $[HCO_3^-]$ is the concentration of bicarbonate and pH is the log of the reciprocal of the concentration of hydrogen ions in mol l^{-1}. $[H_2CO_3]$ is the concentration of carbonic acid: it is a function of the tension and the solubility of the carbon dioxide in human plasma, such that:

$$[H_2CO_3] = S \times P\text{CO}_2 \text{ mol l}^{-1} \quad (7.17)$$

where S is a modified Bunsen absorption coefficient, which, for plasma at 37°C, is in SI units 0.231 and in traditional units 0.0306, and pK is the dissociation exponent and is usually assumed to have a constant value of 6.10. The assumption is adequate in normal circumstances but very different values for pH have been obtained in subjects in whom the acid–base balance was disturbed. The variation has been explained as being due to the presence in plasma of the ionic species $H_2CO_3 \cdot HCO_3^-$ that is not represented in the equation [47]. Neglect of this substance effectively invalidates the equation in abnormal circumstances (see Section 22.3.2).

For describing the *in vitro* relationship between the tension of carbon dioxide in blood and the plasma pH, allowances should be made for the concentrations of haemoglobin and titratable non-carbonic acid (base); the latter is called base excess. It may be subdivided into two components, one reflecting endogenous metabolic processes including the production and oxidation of lactic acid (Section 28.9.2) and the other associated with the transport, storage and control activities of the kidneys, the gastrointestinal tract and the skeleton. The resulting Van Slyke equation has been arranged in a form suitable for a programmable calculator by Siggaard-Anderson [48]:

$$[HCO_3^-] - 24.4 = -(2.3[\text{Hb}] + 7.7) \times (\text{pH} - 7.40) + \frac{\text{BE}}{1 - 0.023[\text{Hb}]} \quad (7.18)$$

where [Hb] is blood concentration of haemoglobin in mmol l^{-1} and BE is base excess in the same units; the other terms are as defined above.

When some of the variables in eqns. 7.16 and 7.18 are known, the remainder may be obtained by calculation or by use of the equivalent nomogram (Fig. 7.6). Usually the pH is measured with a glass electrode and the tension of carbon dioxide with a CO_2 electrode (see below). The method then yields the plasma bicarbonate concentration, the base excess and the total CO_2 content of plasma. Other approaches are also used (Section 22.3.2).

Henderson–Hasselbalch equation. Measured values for pH and concentration of bicarbonate are substituted in eqn. 7.16.

Interpolation: Astrup technique. For this purpose three measurements of pH at 37°C are made on the sample of blood to be analysed, first without modification and then after equilibration with saturated gas containing, respectively, lower and higher tensions of carbon dioxide than the unknown sample. Gas mixtures containing carbon dioxide in the fractional concentrations 0.04 and 0.08 with the remainder in air or oxygen are usually appropriate. The pH values of the latter two blood samples are plotted

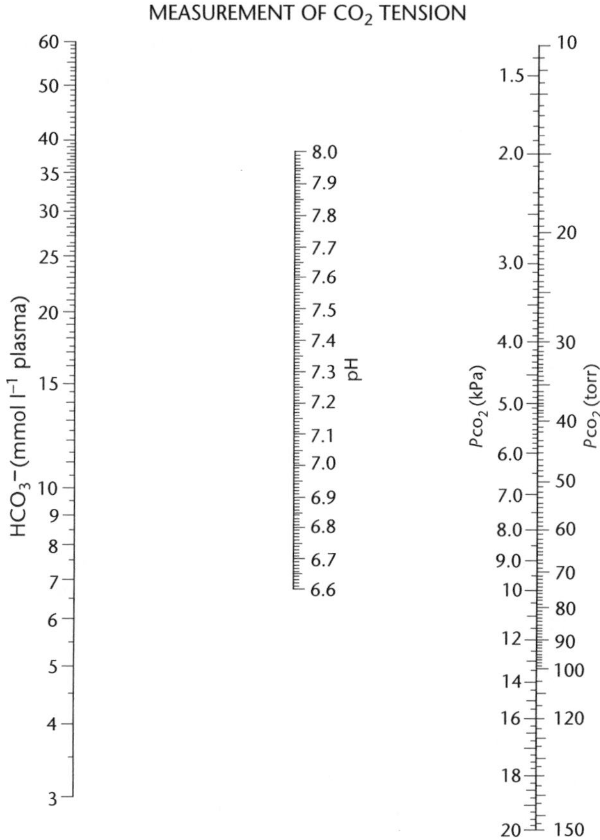

Fig. 7.6 Graphical solution of the Henderson–Hasselbalch equation for blood at 38°C. Source: [49]

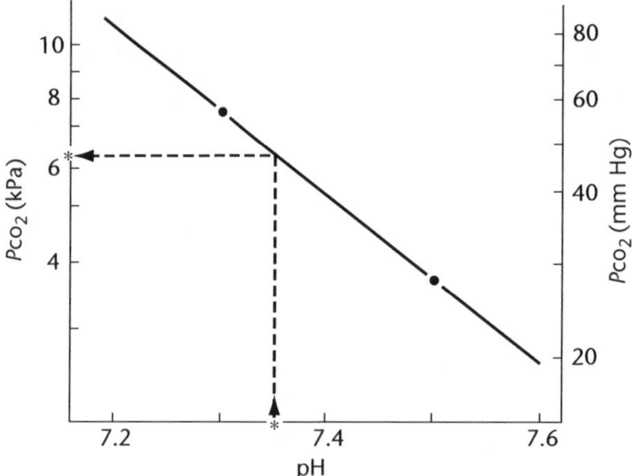

Fig. 7.7 Interpolation method for estimating the tension of carbon dioxide in blood. The pH, log Pco_2 relationship for the unknown sample is constructed from measurements of the pH of 2 aliquots of blood equilibrated respectively with appropriate mixtures of carbon dioxide in air (e.g. Fco_2 0.04 and 0.08, closed circles). X is the pH of the unknown sample before equilibration. For oxygenated blood asterisk indicates the corresponding Pco_2.

on semi-log paper against values for the corresponding tensions of carbon dioxide; when the blood is equilibrated at sea level with the above gas mixtures these tensions are respectively 3.8 and 7.6 kPa (28.5 and 57 Torr) (Fig. 7.7). The line joining the points describes the relationship between the pH and the $P\text{co}_2$ for fully oxygenated blood under the condition of study. Provided that the unknown sample is at least 90% saturated, the Pco_2 that corresponds to the pH of the unknown sample is then obtained by interpolation. If the saturation is less than 90%, this value should be corrected by a small amount. The method may be applied to 0.1 ml of blood when, during normoxia, the standard deviation of a single estimate of Pco_2 is approximately 0.25 kPa (2.0 Torr). In the presence of hypoxaemia, due to the operation of the Haldane effect (Section 21.2), the method leads to an underestimation of the tension of carbon dioxide; this may be allowed for in the manner described by Siggaard-Andersen [50].

CO_2 *electrode.* The instrument (Fig. 7.4) consists of a glass electrode for the measurement of pH [51]. The electrode is bathed in a thin film of bicarbonate buffer solution and contained by a PTFE membrane that separates it from the blood. By this arrangement a constant concentration of bicarbonate is maintained in the buffer solution that surrounds the electrode. The pH is then a simple function of the tension of carbon dioxide in the solution, which, as a result of diffusion across the membrane, is equal to that in the unknown sample. The electrode is calibrated with either humidified gas containing a known partial pressure of carbon dioxide or water with which the gas has been equilibrated. The method is now standard in most laboratories.

Correction factors for use when the temperature of the blood at the time of the analysis differs from that at which it is collected are shown in Fig. 7.5. The corresponding factors for blood pH are listed in Table 7.8.

Table 7.8 Factors for correcting the blood pH to the temperature of the body (t_b°C) when the measurements are made at 38°C (pH_{38}).*

pH_{38}	Factor
7.00–7.15	0.0127
7.16–7.30	0.0136
7.31–7.45	0.0142
7.46–7.60	0.0149

* They are derived for a CO_2 content in plasma of 25 mmol l^{-1} and are used in the form $pH_b = pH_{38} - \text{factor}\,(t_b - 38)$. Source: [52].

Riley equilibration method. By this method the tensions of carbon dioxide and oxygen in blood are determined concurrently (see above Riley bubble method).

7.11.2 Indirect methods

The tension of carbon dioxide in the mixed venous blood is similar to that in the tissues and, at rest, exceeds the tension in the arterial blood by approximately 0.8 kPa (6 Torr). The tension can be obtained by a rebreathing method in which the lung is used as a tonometer [53]. The method can be used at rest or on exercise (Section 17.3.2). It requires a three-way tap that is fitted between a bag of capacity approximately 2 l and a mask or mouthpiece. The bag has a small-bore side connection from which a sample of gas can be drawn off for analysis. The bag initially contains 1.0 or 1.5 l of oxygen. To make the measurement the subject first rebreathes from the bag for a period of 1.5 min or until the ventilation begins to rise. This manoeuvre raises the tension of carbon dioxide in the lung-bag system to near the level of the mixed venous blood. It also leads to some carbon dioxide being retained in the body. This may be eliminated by allowing the subject to breathe air for a period of 3 min. The rebreathing is then repeated for 20 s or five breaths; this manoeuvre raises the tension of carbon dioxide in the bag to the level of oxygenated mixed venous blood. A gas sample from the bag is now analysed for carbon dioxide to an absolute accuracy of 0.1% in an infrared or simple chemical analyser. Subsequently, the rebreathing is repeated to confirm that equilibrium has in fact been achieved. The tension of carbon dioxide is calculated as follows:

$$P\bar{v}{,}\mathrm{CO_2}(\text{indirect}) = F\mathrm{A{,}CO_2} \times (P\mathrm{B} - P\mathrm{H_2O}) \tag{7.19}$$

where $P\bar{v}$, $\mathrm{CO_2}$ is the tension of carbon dioxide in the oxygenated mixed venous blood, $F\mathrm{A{,}CO_2}$ is the fractional concentration of carbon dioxide in the bag and ($P\mathrm{B} - P\mathrm{H_2O}$) is the pressure of dry gas in the lungs at 37°C. The tension of carbon dioxide in arterial blood is less than that in the mixed venous blood by, on average, 0.8 kPa (6 Torr).

Success with the method depends on the volume of oxygen in the bag being no larger than is needed for the rebreathing manoeuvre. The connection between the bag and the subject should be gas-tight and the tap should only be turned in the intervals after the subject has completed an expiration and before the start of the next inspiration. The method is useful for the study of subjects with normal lungs, for the screening of outpatients and for hospital inpatients who have been fitted with a tracheotomy tube. In other acutely ill patients spuriously low values are sometimes obtained, especially when the tidal volume is small or the subject is restless or semi-conscious. In such circumstances the $P\mathrm{a{,}CO_2}$ should be measured directly.

7.12 Use of isotopes (including radioisotopes) to study lung function

Many stable atoms have companion isotopes of different atomic number that are to some extent unstable. Over time, this leads to their disintegrating with the release of radiation. Isotopes can contribute to understanding of lung function in several ways. The differences in mass are used to extend the range of substances that can be analysed concurrently in a respiratory mass spectrometer (Table 7.9).

Table 7.9 Examples where an alternative mass for a substance has extended the scope of respiratory mass spectrometry.

Difficulty	Solution
Carbon monoxide has the same atomic number as nitrogen	Use CO made with an isotope of oxygen or carbon
Newly inhaled O_2 or CO_2 cannot be identified separate from the resident gas	Use an appropriate isotope for the gas to be inspired
Pairs of stable soluble and insoluble tracer gases of comparable density are scarce	Use argon (atomic number 18) and freon-22 (e.g. Fig. 18.8, page 221).

Measurement of the radiation emitted during the disintegration of an isotope is an alternative to assessment of thermal conductivity or other physical or chemical attribute. This approach has permitted the use of a very small bolus of gas for investigation of lung gas distribution (Section 16.2.5). A radioisotope can also be used for its convenience as in some indicator-dilution methods for cardiac output (Section 17.3.2). The dose of radiation is tiny, but such methods are now seldom recommended.

High-energy gamma (γ) radiation has the valuable property of being able to penetrate the chest wall. This allows the assessment of the distribution and persistence in the lung of labelled gas or aerosol particles delivered by inhalation or intravenous infusion. The applications include assessment of regional ventilation and perfusion, visualisation of bronchial dilatation or stenosis and investigation of deposition and clearance of inhaled particles. Some of these functions are now undertaken using high-resolution computer-assisted tomography (HRCT); alternative methods that do not involve ionising radiation are in process of development [e.g. 54, 55]. Currently, methods based on scanning the chest are used to investigate the matching of ventilation to perfusion and to measure regional lung volume, ventilation and perfusion (Figs 7.8 and 7.9). The particular application dictates the physical and chemical characteristics of the test substance, of which some are given in Tables 7.10 and 7.11. Measurement aspects of the methods are given here. Applications are in Section 18.6.

The radiation is detected by luminescent crystals that light up on impact. Currently, the number of impacts is usually counted by a gamma camera of which the main element is a battery of photomultiplier tubes (Fig. 7.9). Radioactive decay is a random phenomenon and so the number of counts per second is reported as the mean with its standard deviation; for acceptable accuracy an adequate number of counts should be recorded (see Fig. 7.9).

Detection is broadly confined to one energy level; this is achieved using a pulse height analyser whose 'window' is set to reject all γ-energies except the principal energy of the radioisotope in question. The width of the window is usually ±20% of the peak energy. The diameter of the camera is equal to that of the lungs and a 40.6 cm (16 in.) crystal is used. The crystal is protected from low-energy background and scattered radiation by

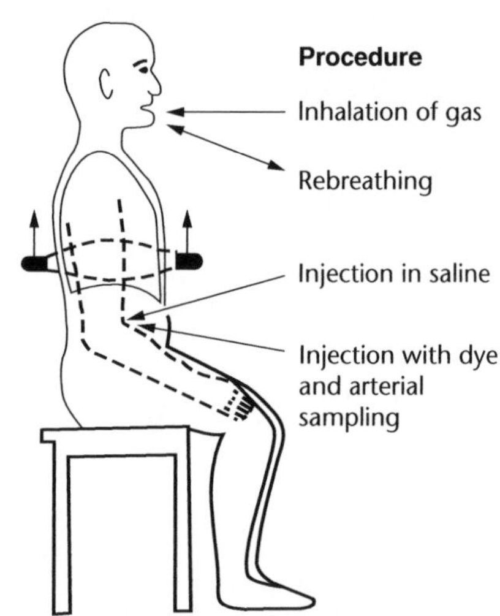

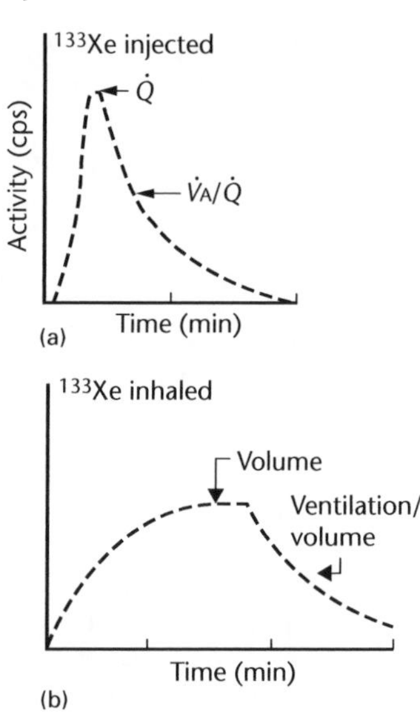

Fig. 7.8 Assessment of regional lung function using ^{133}Xe. To maximise the yield the counters are placed on both sides of the chest. (a) After injection the initial peak reflects the regional blood flow ($\dot{Q}$); the isotope then passes into the gas phase where the clearance during normal breathing reflects the ventilation of lung tissue which is perfused. A slow washout indicates a low ventilation–perfusion ratio ($\dot{V}/\dot{Q}$). (b) During rebreathing the plateau count rate when mixing is complete, reflects the volume of lung gas in the field of counting. The slopes of the wash-in and washout curves indicate the ventilation per unit volume. Source: After [55].

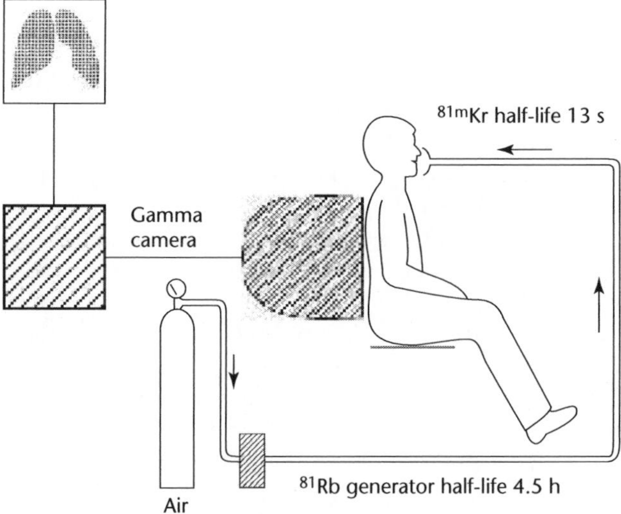

Fig. 7.9 Gamma camera being used for a ventilation scan following normal tidal breathing of gas containing ^{81m}Kr (half-life 13 s; Table 7.10). The output from the camera can be colour coded to highlight regions of contrasting activity. Counting is continued until a predetermined number of counts has been accumulated; the number might be 300,000, which during tidal breathing could occupy 12 respiratory cycles. Under the conditions indicated, the alveolar concentration would be less than inspired concentration and reflect the ventilation per unit of lung volume. A different relationship would obtain during voluntary hyperventilation. A perfusion scan can be obtained nearly concurrently. Source: After [56].

a lead shield of which the thickness is determined by the energy of the relevant radiation.

In the thorax some radiation is absorbed by the tissue of the chest wall and to a lesser extent the lung. The amount varies inversely with the γ-emission energy (Table 7.10). For a low-energy isotope (e.g. ^{133}Xe), the activity that is recorded is mainly from the lung tissue immediately beneath the detectors. The amount of lung tissue and the thickness of the chest wall vary down the lung and so counts made at apex and base cannot be compared directly. However, this geometric factor is eliminated when the ratios of two counts are compared. For the ratio to be meaningful the tissue absorption should be the same for both signals. When this condition is met, valid regional comparisons can be made for ventilation/perfusion, ventilation/volume and perfusion/volume. Error due to tissue absorption is increased if isotopes of different energy are used.

Error can also arise from isotope leaving the lungs and entering the chest wall via the systemic circulation. This is likely to occur with soluble and partially soluble isotopes (e.g. ^{133}Xe) but not with insoluble isotopes or those having a very short half-life (e.g. ^{81m}Kr). Correction for the chest wall activity can be made in some circumstances. Recirculation of isotope can also occur into the lung.

Activity in the depth of the lungs can be detected using counters on both sides of the chest (Fig. 7.8), but for low-energy isotopes the sensitivity is poor. It can be increased by using high-energy isotopes, particularly those that emit pairs of positrons; these are discharged in opposite directions and are detected by coincidence counting using banks of detectors on both sides of the chest. Coincidence counting provides a high signal-to-noise ratio and permits three-dimensional tomography with a spatial resolution of approximately 0.7 cm. Positron-emitting isotopes other than ^{18}F are produced in a cyclotron and have a short half-life (Table 7.10), and so can only be used on site.

Radiation dose. The radiation exposure from most pulmonary isotopic procedures is low and mainly confined to the lungs. A typical ^{81m}Kr scan gives 0.2 mSv and a ^{133}Xe or ^{99m}Tc study 0.4–2 mSv effective dose. The average background radiation

Table 7.10 Properties of some radioisotope gases used for studying the lung; the absorption is for a 2.5-cm-thick layer of soft tissue.

Isotope	Source	Half-life	γ–Energy (keV)	Absorption (%)	Example of use
Inert gas					
^{133}Xe	Nuclear reactor	5.3 days	80	45	Ventilation/perfusion scan*
^{81m}Kr	^{81}Rb†	13 s	190	38	Ventilation scan and regional tomography‡
^{18}F	Cyclotron	120 min	511	28	Glucose metabolism
Reactive gas					
^{11}CO¶	Cyclotron	20 min	511	28	Lung haemoglobin
Technetium					
^{99m}Tc	^{99}Mo‖	6 h	140	40	See Table 7.11
^{99m}Tc-DTPA**					Lung clearance
^{99m}Tc-MAA††					Perfusion studies*

* For assessment of perfusion the isotope is administered dissolved in saline.
† In United Kingdom available from MRC Cyclotron Unit, Hammersmith Hospital, London.
‡ Single photon emission computed tomography (SPECT).
¶ Positron emitter.
‖ Molybdenum from nuclear reactor.
** Diethylenetriamine pentacetate, administered as an aerosol.
†† Albumin macroaggregates.

Table 7.11 Some radioisotope substances used to investigate the lung.*

Perfusion distribution	^{99m}Tc-HMPAO† (lipophilic aerosol)
	^{99m}Tc-albumin macroaggregates diameter 30–50 μm‡
Ventilation distribution	^{99m}Tc-albumin (aerosol) diameter 1–2 μm
Pulmonary embolism	^{111}In-P256 binds to fibrinogen receptors (or albumin microspheres)
	^{99m}Tc-albumin macroaggregates
Alveolar capillary permeability	
Endothelium	^{113m}In-transferrin
Epithelium	^{99m}Tc-DTPA¶ (aerosol)
Trapped haemoglobin	^{11}CO (gas)‖
Lung metabolism	^{18}F deoxyglucose‖ (combines with glucose-6-phosphate)

* The substances are administered intravenously except where indicated.
† Hexamethylene propyleneamine oxime.
‡ Combined with renal scans can assess A-V shunts.
¶ Diethylenetriamine pentacetate.
‖ Detected by positron emission tomography (PET).

absorbed by a person in the United Kingdom is approximately 2.5 mSv per annum.

7.13 Sterilisation and disinfection of equipment

The equipment used for assessment of lung function should be free from respiratory hazards including accumulated secretions and potentially harmful bacteria or fungi. Patients should be protected from the equipment, and the equipment and technicians from the patients. Reports of cross-infection are rare and bacteria that deposit on the inside surfaces of spirometry tubing are unlikely to be re-aerosolised [57]. Despite these considerations the disinfection of equipment should be part of the laboratory's daily routine [2–4, 58, 59].

Disinfection inactivates pathogenic micro-organisms whereas sterilisation destroys all microbial life and spores. After each test the mouthpiece, mask and rubber breathing valves should be either discarded or washed in antiseptic detergent in water above 70°C, rinsed, soaked for 30 min in antiseptic solution and then air dried. The connecting tubes, valve box and rebreathing bags should be disinfected, rinsed and drained. The other components should be dismantled for cleaning at weekly or monthly intervals depending on the frequency of use. Nose clips and the external surfaces of equipment need attention, particularly if they have been exposed to potentially infective secretions. Nose clips with rubber rather than sponge mounts are preferable as they are easier to clean and last longer [58].

Special care is needed in relation to high-risk patients including those who may have infective hepatitis, multidrug resistant organisms (e.g. tubercle bacilli or *Staphylococcus aureus*) or whose immunological defence mechanisms are impaired. A simple procedure is to interpose a disposable bag-in-box assembly between patient and apparatus [60]. Alternatively, a disposable, in-line filter can be used, though this will not guarantee entrapment of all micro-organisms [61, 62]. Filters provide limited protection in proportion to the added respiratory resistance, but at the cost of impairing the lung function. For example, use of a filter has been associated with statistically significant but clinically small differences in FEV_1, airway resistance and specific conductance [63]. The resistance of the filter should be <0.15 kPa l^{-1} s (<1.5 cm H_2O l^{-1} s) and an allowance should be made for the added dead-space [64]. The use of single-patient, in-line filters does not eliminate the need for periodic decontamination of respiratory circuits [58, 59].

Testing a high-risk patient may best be left to the end of the day [58, 59]. After the test the closed breathing circuits should be sterilised. However, except for equipment that has been designed with the needs of sterilisation in mind, methods currently available are seldom completely effective. Thus, the ease with which any new equipment can be sterilised should be noted prior to purchase and the recommendations of the manufacturer and of any local infection control policy should be adhered to.

Disinfectant materials can be corrosive to equipment and may pose a health risk to staff who should wear gloves and take other precautions as necessary [25, 58].

7.14 Care of gas cylinders

The presence of high-pressure gas cylinders in a laboratory represents a significant hazard to staff and visitors. All connectors and gas flow regulators should be kept clean. No oil or grease should ever be applied. The gas cylinders are tested at high pressure before they are supplied; they should be retested at intervals to detect any deterioration with use. They should also be treated with respect; for example, all cylinders should be labelled with contents and date, and when in an upright position they should be clamped to the wall or otherwise supported. Cylinders should only be moved using approved trolleys; they should never be dropped or exposed to high temperature. Leakage of gas should be looked for using soap solution or the sampling probe of an appropriate gas analyser. A leak that cannot be controlled by tightening a retaining nut or screwing a valve finger tight should be referred for specialist scrutiny.

All gas mixtures used for lung function tests should have a certificate of analysis and be approved for medical use.

7.15 Calibration of equipment

On two occasions, 18 years apart, standard gas mixtures were circulated to a number of lung function laboratories; on both occasions the results of the analysis varied by up to 10%, yet the instruments were capable of a 1% accuracy (Table 7.12). Similarly, for patients examined in several laboratories the variability between the laboratories greatly exceeds that when the measurements are repeated in the same laboratory [66–69]. Such studies have amply demonstrated the importance of all aspects of calibration yet the subject continues to have a low priority and to be an important cause of discrepant results.

Faults in equipment can arise during manufacture or transit; they can also occur from the ageing of the components, or their interaction with other equipment. In addition, the performance may be affected by the temperature, humidity or electromagnetic field in the laboratory as well as by the manner of use, which will also vary. The effect of these factors upon the performance of the instrument should be established by accurate calibration, which should be carried out both when the equipment is received and at appropriate intervals thereafter. The calibration should be performed in circumstances that simulate as closely as possible the actual conditions of use. The properties to be checked should include repeatability, reproducibility, accuracy (linearity) and response time [59]. The results should be compared with earlier ones, based on records in a book kept for the purpose.

Repeatability reflects the extent to which a result varies when it is repeated within a session using the same equipment and same observer.

Reproducibility reflects the extent to which a result varies when it is repeated with changed conditions, for example, using a different observer or instrument, or repeating measurements over a longer period of time such as following administration of a bronchodilator.

Variability that is independent of the mean level is described by the standard error of the mean. Alternatively, where the error is a proportional one, the coefficient of variation (standard deviation × 100/mean) is used. For physical measurements the latter is normally less than 0.5%. Biological measurements are rather less reproducible with coefficients of variation of the order of 2% for stature and forced expiratory volume, 5% for transfer factor and 15% for compliance. The variability of biological measurements is greater between sessions and from day to day (reproducibility) compared with measurements made at a single session (repeatability). A high level of reproducibility is of particular importance when serial measurements of lung function are used to assess the changes over time; this is usually done

Table 7.12 Variability in gas analysis between 57 lung function laboratories in the United Kingdom.

Gas	Concentrations (%)	Reproducibility* (%)	Percentage of samples accurate to 1%	Main faults in instrument calibration
Oxygen	11–18	1.8–5.3	48	Zero error
Carbon dioxide	3.8	8.9	28†	Curvilinearirty
Carbon monoxide	0.1–0.3	3.2–4.9	14	Curvilinearirty
Helium	8–14	3.0–3.2	37†	

* Based on analysis of gas in small cylinders; the gas concentration as assessed in the reference laboratory varied by less than 0.6%.
† The resulting errors in the calculated respiratory exchange ratio and transfer factor exceeded 5% in respectively 28 and 20% of instances.
Source: [65].

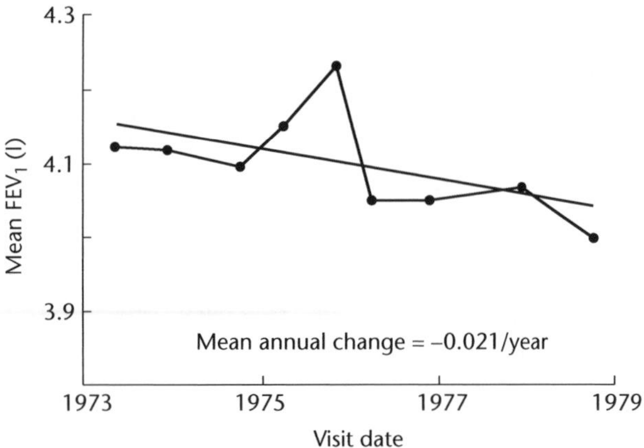

Fig. 7.10 Mean levels of FEV_1 for 33 subjects assessed on nine occasions between April 1973 and October 1978. The downward trend was interrupted by one anomalous result; the mechanism is unclear. Source: [70].

using groups of subjects (e.g. Fig. 7.10). The repeatability and reproducibility will normally be assessed when a new measurement is introduced into the laboratory and as part of the training program for new staff.

Accuracy reflects the extent to which a result deviates from an absolute standard. The standard will normally be defined in terms of length, mass and time from which can be derived volume, concentration, flow rate, resistance (or conductance) and elastance. Examples of laboratory standards are given in Table 7.13. They include a gas syringe, flow–volume simulator and calibration gas mixtures; the latter can be purchased or prepared in the laboratory (Fig. 7.11). The tolerance on the standard should be established. For physical measurements the accuracy should normally be better than 1%. The minimal standards for equipment used for measurements of gas volume and flow are given in Table 7.2. A procedure for calibrating a spirometer is illustrated in Fig. 7.12.

The standard is used to construct a calibration graph in which the correct result on the *y*-axis is related to the observed result on the *x*-axis. The relationship should lie on the line of identity, which for equal scales on the two axes is a straight line at an angle of 45° to both axes and passing through the origin. Alternatively, there may be a proportional or zero error or the relationship may be alinear (Fig. 7.13 on page 78).

Causes for some of these deviations are indicated in Table 7.12; they can be detected when calibration is performed at a minimum of three points but not when two or even one point is used as in some physical gas analysers. The calibration will normally be undertaken at the beginning and end of each measurement session but for instruments that are subject to drift an appropriate check should be performed for each patient. Very stable instruments can be calibrated once a month (e.g. most helium katharometers).

Response time. This is the sum of the *delay time* between application of the signal and the start of the response and the *rise time* to 95% of the final response. In the case of a gas analyser both the delay and the rise time vary over a wide range, reflecting the method of sampling the gas and the type of analyser. For pressure transducers and pneumotachographs the two times should be short and there should be no overshoot; this aspect should

Table 7.13 Calibration of laboratory equipment.

Feature	Equipment	Standard
Permeability	Douglas bag	Calibration gas
Linearity	Volume recorders	Gas syringe (1 or 3 l)
	Flow recorders	Calibrated rotameters
		Flow–volume simulator
	Peak flow meter	Flow generating pump
	Pressure transducer	Mercury or water manometer
	Gas analyser	Calibration gas
	Stadiometer	Calibration rod
	Scales	Standard weights
Resistance	Volume- and flow-measuring devices	Static tube (Fig. 7.2)
Paper speed	Chart recorder	Stop watch
Response time	Flow and pressure recorders	Square wave impulse*
Frequency response	Flow and pressure recorders	Sinusoidal wave impulse†

* A square wave can be generated by the abrupt release of gas previously stored in a drum or a balloon at a known pressure. When the gas is released manually or by bursting the balloon with a pin the rise time is of the order of 0.01 s. The volume which is released is closer to that which is calculated from the adiabatic than from the isothermal relationship for gases, i.e. $PVg = RT$, where g is the ratio of the specific heats of a gas at constant pressure and constant volume (Cp and Cv respectively). Thus $g = Cp/Cv = 1.4$ for air.

† A sinusoidal wave form can be generated by a piston-type pump. A wave form that more nearly resembles normal breathing may be produced using an appropriate cam.

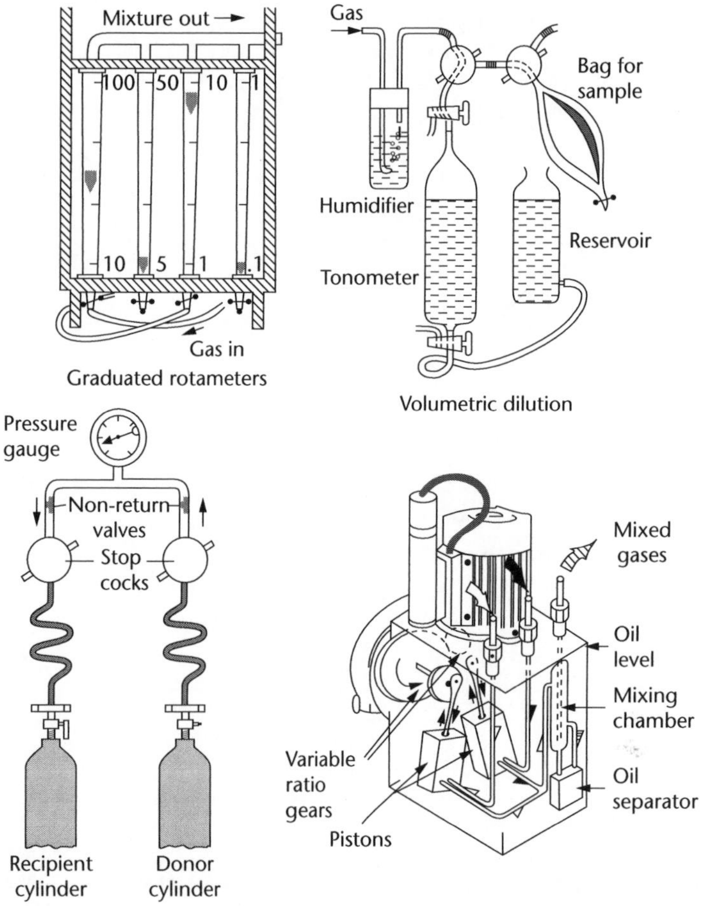

Fig. 7.11 Equipment for making up gas mixtures. *Upper right.* Preparation by volumetric dilution when only a small quantity is required. The bag should be evacuated initially, and then the dead-space of the apparatus should be flushed before each gas is added. *Upper left.* Graduated rotameters may be used to prepare gas mixtures for immediate use. The range of flow rates should reflect the intended gas concentrations in the final mixture; ranges for air of 0.1–1.0 l min^{-1}, 1.0–10.0 l min^{-1} and 10.0–100 l min^{-1}, with additional calibration charts for oxygen, nitrogen and carbon dioxide are adequate. *Lower left.* Gas mixtures prepared in high-pressure cylinders. The pressure gauge should be of high quality and for convenience have a dial of diameter at least 12.5 cm (5 in.). The cylinders and copper tubing should be sound and the gases transferred slowly; they should subsequently be mixed by laying the cylinder horizontal. The procedure should be undertaken with due care, by trained personnel working in a dedicated building. *Lower right.* The Wösthoff pump mixes two gases in predetermined proportions using two pistons of fixed volume driven by variable ratio gears.

form part of the calibration. For other instruments the response time will normally be assessed when the equipment is set up or if there is reason to believe that it may be faulty. Response times for instruments that are used concurrently should be synchronised either physically or electronically.

7.15.1 Anthropometry equipment

Calibration procedures should extend to equipment used to measure the anthropometric indices as these are used to derive reference values. For example, a stadiometer should be checked daily with a rod of known length. The accuracy and linearity of weighing scales should be checked using calibration weights (for example, at least 4× 20 kg). The frequency of calibration will depend on the type of scales (balance, spring-loaded or electronic), their age and the amount of use. Skinfold calipers and impedance devices used to measure body composition should be calibrated periodically by the manufacturer.

7.15.2 Linearity of gas analysers

A linear gas analyser is one in which the response to a given change in gas concentration is the same at all levels of concentration over the range of the instrument. The linearity may be a property of the detection system or achieved by electronic means. In most circumstances it is assessed by analysing a minimum of three gas mixtures of known composition and plotting the result (Fig. 7.13). The method depends critically on knowing precisely the concentrations of the calibration gases.

A simpler and more accurate alternative is available to laboratories where lung volumes are measured by closed circuit spirometry with helium, analysed with a katharometer, used as the indicator gas. The method entails establishing the linearity of the katharometer and the dead-space of the spirometer by a serial dilution method and then using the equipment to check the linearity of other analysers.

Helium analyser. The linearity of a helium analyser may be assessed by serial dilution of a mixture of helium in air contained in a closed circuit spirometer. The procedure also yields the volume of the instrument dead-space. This is the minimal volume of the system when the water level and/or the quantity of soda lime are set correctly. To make the assessment the analyser is zeroed on room air and the spirometer set up in a closed circuit, with a concentration of helium close to full-scale deflection on the katharometer. The mouthpiece tap is opened, the spirometer

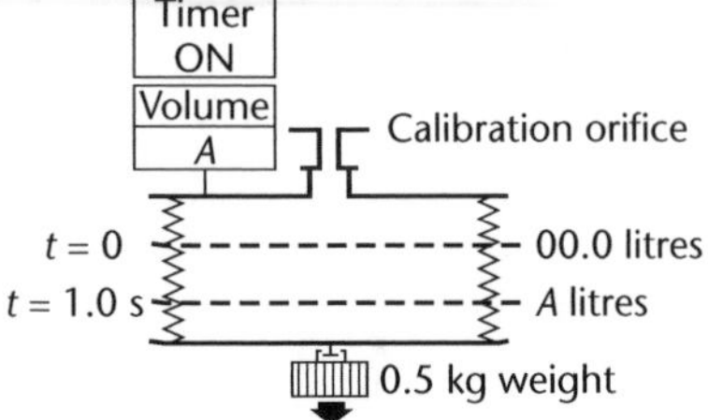

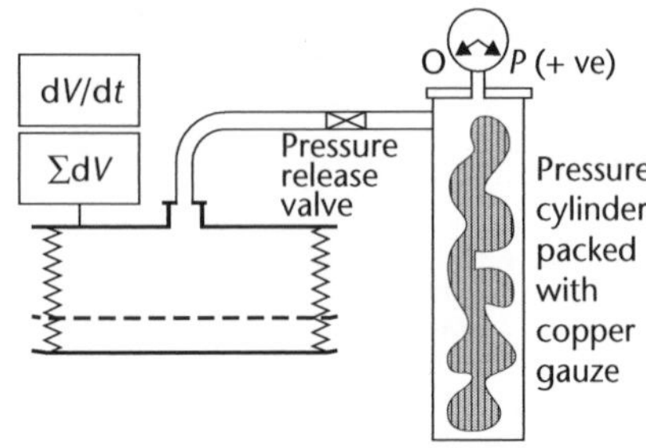

Fig. 7.12 Calibration of a spirometer with a vertically fitted bellows showing the use of a calibrated syringe, a standard orifice and weight and a flow–volume simulator.

emptied, the tap closed and the initial helium noted. Gas from a cylinder of medical air is run into the spirometer in 0.5- to 1-l steps, each time noting the new helium concentration. The reciprocal of the helium concentration is plotted against the volume added (Fig. 7.14). A curved line is evidence that the helium analyser is alinear. If, as is usually the case, the relationship is linear the intercept on the volume axis is the instrument's dead-space (3.08 l in the example).

Carbon monoxide and carbon dioxide analysers. The linearity of an infrared carbon monoxide analyser may be checked against a linear helium analyser. The CO analyser is zeroed on room air and a large bag filled with the gas mixture used for the measurement of transfer factor. The initial concentration is recorded and then the mixture is diluted with air from a syringe or cylinder of medical air. The mixture is reanalysed and the concentrations of helium and carbon monoxide are expressed as a ratio of their respective initial values. The dilution is repeated serially and the ratios tabulated and plotted against one another. Equivalent ratios indicate that the CO analyser is linear. If the ratios differ, the plot may be used to correct the observed alveolar CO concentrations (see Fig. 20.2, page 240). However, alinearity in excess of 0.5% of full scale is evidence that the analyser is in need of urgent attention [71]. The linearity of the CO analyser should be checked weekly.

The linearity of an infrared carbon dioxide analyser may be checked in a similar manner using a suitable mixture of helium and carbon dioxide made up in air, oxygen or nitrogen, depending on the application. The choice of background gas influences the calibration. For example, an infrared CO_2 analyser calibrated in a N_2/CO_2 mixture will under-read by about 8% in an oxygen-rich mixture. Accordingly, the N_2/O_2 ratio of the calibrating mixture should be appropriate for the intended application [72].

Oxygen analyser. The linearity of an oxygen analyser can be checked against a linear helium analyser. Prior to this the zero of the oxygen analyser should have been checked with "white-spot" nitrogen or, if unavailable, with 100% helium, when true zero reads 0.3% because of helium's paramagnetic properties. The span is then fixed using air from outside the building or from a cylinder. Finally, the linearity is checked by serial dilution of a large bag of transfer test gas mixture using white-spot nitrogen as the diluent. The helium meter is slightly sensitive to oxygen, and so the reading may need to be corrected using an electric compensator, if fitted. The ratios of subsequent to initial helium concentration are compared with the corresponding oxygen ratios. Similarly, the accuracy of any oxygen compensator circuit can be checked by serial dilution of the transfer test gas mixture

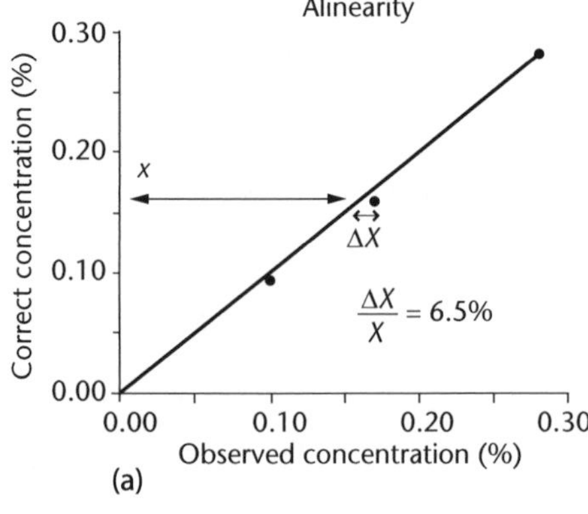

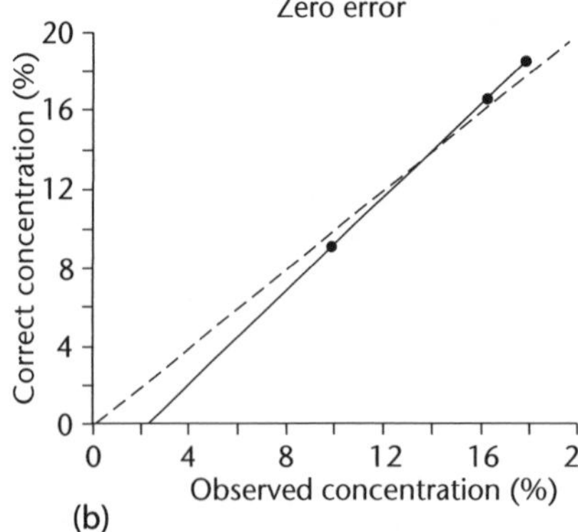

Fig. 7.13 Examples of faulty calibration. (a) Alinearity, which in this example is 6.5%. (b) Zero error; in this case more than 2% absolute concentration. Source: [65].

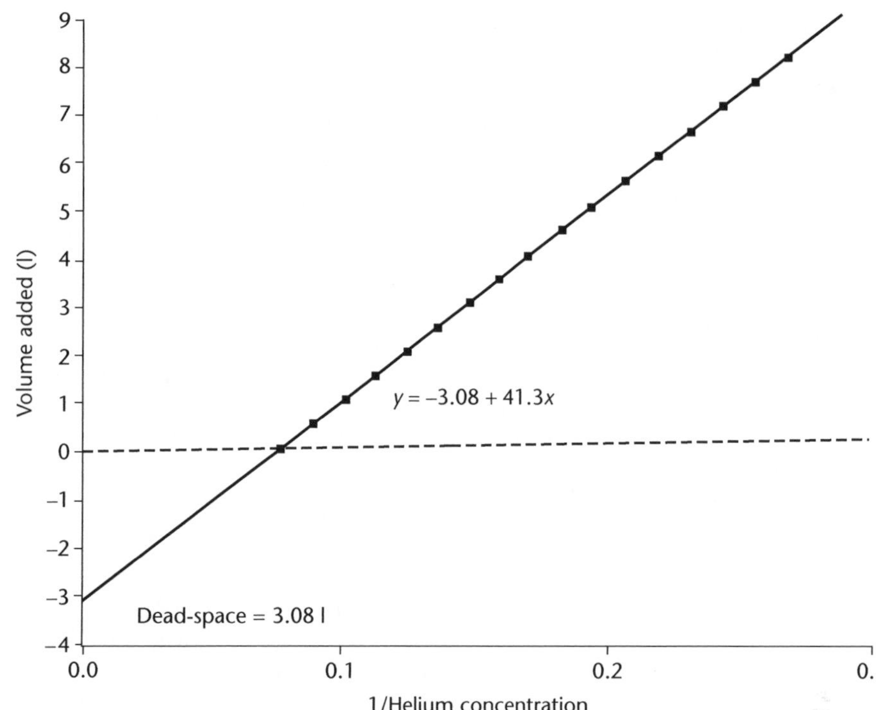

Fig. 7.14 Procedure for testing the linearity of a helium meter. For details see text.

made up in oxygen (as used for estimation of *D*m and *V*c), again using nitrogen as diluent.

7.16 Quality control

Achieving and maintaining high standards of measurement and service is not easy. The processes can be helped by the laboratory having a quality assurance program [2, 73]. This should be based on a written protocol outlining all aspects of the work, including details of equipment, measurement procedures, reference values with age ranges and staff training. The protocol should indicate the nature, frequency and recording of all ongoing checks on equipment and the performance of individual practitioners. The physical checks on equipment should be supplemented by 'biological' calibrations made by recording regularly the test results of key personnel [74, 75]. The mean and standard deviation (σ) of the day-to-day variation in lung function measures should be established for each key person. The routinely collected data should be plotted on a control chart marked with the statistical limits expected [76]. A convenient rule is to consider a deviation beyond 3σ, whether below or above that expected, as evidence that the system is 'out of control'. Biological calibrations can identify equipment faults not detected by computer-driven automated calibration procedures [77].

Test results from individual practitioners should be scrutinised at regular intervals by other members of laboratory staff or by an independent arbiter to ensure quality standards are being maintained. This is necessary in order to identify any short cuts or other substandard practices that may otherwise creep into the measurement techniques of individual staff (Section 2.5).

7.17 Manufacturers

A list of companies can be found on the European Respiratory Society website under the Buyer's guide (http://www.ersnet.org).

7.18 References

1. Gardner RM, Clausen JL, Cotton, DJ et al (on behalf of the ATS). Computer guidelines for pulmonary laboratories. *Am Rev Respir Dis* 1986; **134**: 628–629.
2. Miller MR, Hankinson J, Brusasco V et al. Standardization of spirometry. Official statement of the American Thoracic Society and the European Respiratory Society. *Eur Respir J*, 2005; **26**: 319–338.
3. Quanjer Ph H, Tammeling GJ, Cotes JE et al. Standardized Lung Function Testing (Lung volumes and forced ventilatory flows 1993 update). *Eur Respir J* 1993; **6** (Suppl 16): 5–40
4. ATS. Standardization of spirometry, 1994 update. *Am J Respir Crit Care Med* 1995; **152**: 1107–1136.
5. Cole P. Recordings of respiratory air temperature. *J Laryngol* 1954; **68**: 295–307.
6. Madan I, Bright P, Miller MR. Expired air temperature at the mouth during a maximal forced expiratory manoeuvre. *Eur Respir J* 1993; **6**: 1556–1562.
7. Pincock AC, Miller MR. The effect of temperature on recording spirograms *Am Rev Respir Dis* 1983; **128**: 894–898.
8. McDermott M, McDermott TJ. Digital incremental techniques applied to spirometry. *Proc Roy Soc Med* 1977; **70**: 169–171.
9. Milledge JS, Stott FD. Inductive plethysmography – a new respiratory transducer. *J Physiol (Lond)* 1977; **267**: 4P–5P.
10. Konno K, Mead J. Static volume–pressure characteristics of the rib cage and abdomen. *J Appl Physiol* 1968; **24**: 544–548.

11. Frey U, Stocks J, Coates A et al (on behalf of the ERS/ATS taskforce). Specifications for equipment used for infant pulmonary function testing. *Eur Respir J* 2000; **16**: 731–740.
12. Fleisch A. Der Pneumotachograph: ein Apparat zur Beischwindigkeitregstrierung der Atemluft. *Arch Ges Physiol* 1925; **209**: 713–722.
13. Lilly JC. Flow meter for recording respiratory flow of human subject. In: Comroe JH, ed. *Methods in medical research*, Vol. 2. Chicago: Year Book, 1950: 113–121.
14. Miller MR, Dickinson SA, Hitchings DJ. The accuracy of portable peak flow meters. *Thorax* 1992; **47**: 904–909.
15. Miller MR, Quanjer PH. Peak flow meters: a problem of scale. *BMJ* 1994; **308**: 548–549.
16. Quanjer PH, Lebowitz MD, Gregg I et al. Peak expiratory flow: conclusions and recommendations of a Working Party of the European Respiratory Society. *Eur Respir J* 1997; **10** (Suppl 24): 2S–8S.
17. Buess C, Pietsch P, Guggenbuhl W, Koller EA. A pulsed diagonal-beam ultrasonic airflow meter. *J Appl Physiol* 1986; **61**: 1195–1199.
18. Schibler A, Henning R. Measurement of functional residual capacity in rabbits and children using an ultrasonic flow meter. *Pediatr Res* 2001; **49**: 581–588.
19. Cormack RS. A technique for evaluating expired air mixing devices. *Br J Anaesth* 1972; **44**: 8–18.
20. Bentley RA, Griffin OG, Love RG et al. Acceptable levels for breathing resistance of respiratory apparatus. *Arch Environ Health* 1973; **27**: 273–280.
21. Askanazi J, Silverberg PA, Foster RJ et al. Effects of respiratory apparatus on breathing pattern. *J Appl Physiol* 1980; **48**: 577–580.
22. Perez W, Tobin MJ. Separation of factors responsible for change in breathing pattern induced by instrumentation. *J Appl Physiol* 1985; **59**: 1515–1520.
23. Fowler KT, Hugh-Jones P. Mass spectrometry applied to clinical practice and research. *Br Med J* 1957; **1**: 1205–1211.
24. Musgrove J, Doré C. A nomogram for the calculation of oxygen uptake. *J Appl Physiol* 1974; **36**: 606–607.
25. Guidelines for the measurement of respiratory function; recommendations of the British Thoracic Society and the Association of Respiratory Technicians and Physiologists. *Respir Med* 1994; **88**: 165–194.
26. Pitkin AD, Roberts CM, Wedzicha JA. Arterialised earlobe blood gas analysis: an underused technique. *Thorax* 1994; **49**: 364–366.
27. Williams AJ. ABC of oxygen. Assessing and interpreting arterial blood gases and acid–base balance. *BMJ* 1998; **317**: 1213–1216.
28. Sauty A, Uldry C, Debetaz LF et al. Differences in Po_2 and Pco_2 between arterial and arterialised earlobe samples. *Eur Respir J* 1996; **9**: 186–189.
29. Fajac I, Texereau J, Rivoal V et al Blood gas measurement during exercise: a comparative study between arterialised earlobe sampling and direct arterial puncture in adults. *Eur Respir J* 1998; **11**: 712–715.
30. Scott PV, Horton JN, Mapleson WW. Leakage of oxygen from blood and water samples stored in plastic and glass syringes. *BMJ* 1971; **3**: 512–516
31. Pretto JJ, Rochford PD. Effects of sample storage time, temperature and syringe type on blood gas tensions in samples with high oxygen partial pressures. *Thorax* 1994; **49**: 610–612.
32. Smeenk FWJM, Janssen JDJ, Arends BJ et al. Effects of four different methods of sampling arterial blood and storage time on gas tensions and shunt calculation in the 100% oxygen test. *Eur Respir J* 1997; **10**: 910–913.
33. Fish RG, Lee MR. Technical and experimental errors in the spectroscopic determination of oxygen saturation. *J Clin Pathol* 1963; **16**: 476–478.
34. Polange JA. Pulse oximetry: technical aspects of machine design. *Int Anesthesiol Clin* 1987; **25**: 137–153.
35. Barker SJ, Tremper KK. Pulse oximetry: applications and limitations. *Int Anesthesiol Clin* 1987; **25**: 155–175.
36. Ries AL, Prewitt LM, Johnson JJ. Skin color and ear oximetry. *Chest* 1989; **96**: 287–290.
37. Moyle JTB, Hahn CEW, Adams AP. *Pulse oximetry*, revised ed. London: BMJ Books, 1998.
38. Severinghaus JW, Naifeh KH, Koh SO. Errors in 14 pulse oximeters during profound hypoxia. *J Clin Monit* 1989; **5**: 72–81.
39. Hannhart B, Haberer J-P, Saunier C, Laxenaire M-C. Accuracy and precision of fourteen pulse oximeters. *Eur Respir J* 1991; **4**: 115–119.
40. Volgyesi GA, Kolesar R, Lerman J. An in vitro model for evaluating the accuracy of pulse oximeters. *Can J Anaesth* 1990; **37** (Suppl): S88.
41. Reynolds KJ, Moyle JTB, Sykes MK, Hahn CEW. Response of 10 pulse oximeters to an in vitro test system. *Br J Anaesth* 1992; **68**: 365–369.
42. Longmuir IS, Chow J. Rapid method for determining effect of agents on oxyhaemoglobin dissociation curves. *J Appl Physiol* 1970; **28**: 343–345.
43. Riley RL, Campbell EJM, Shephard RH. A bubble method for estimation of Pco_2 and Po_2 in whole blood. *J Appl Physiol* 1957; **11**: 245–249.
44. Clark LC Jr, Wolf R, Granger D, Taylor Z. Continuous recording of blood oxygen tension by polarography. *J Appl Physiol* 1953; **6**: 189–193.
45. Hutchinson DCS, Rocca G, Honeybourne D. Estimation of arterial oxygen tension in adult subjects using a transcutaneous electrode. *Thorax* 1981; **36**: 473–477.
46. Kelman GR, Nunn JF. Nomograms for correction of blood Po_2, Pco_2, pH and base excess for time and temperature. *J Appl Physiol* 1966; **21**: 1484–1490.
47. Flear CTG, Roberts SW, Hayes S et al. $PK_1{'}$ and bicarbonate concentration in plasma. *Clin Chem* 1987; **33**: 13–20.
48. Siggaard-Anderson O. The Van Slyke equation. *Scand J Clin Lab Invest* 1977; **37** (Suppl 146): 15–19.
49. Siggaard-Anderson O. Blood acid–base alignment nomogram. *Scand J Clin Lab Invest* 1963; **15**: 211–217.
50. Siggard-Anderson O. The acid–base status of the blood. *Scand J Clin Lab Invest* 1963; **15** (Suppl 70): 1–134.
51. Severinghaus JW, Bradley AF. Electrodes for blood Po_2 and Pco_2 determination. *J Appl Physiol* 1958; **13**: 515–520.
52. Adamson K Jr, Daniel SS, Gandy D, James LS. Influence of temperature on blood pH of the human adult and newborn. *J Appl Physiol* 1964; **19**: 897–900.
53. Campbell EJM, Howell JBL. Rebreathing method for measurement of mixed venous Pco_2. *BMJ* 1962; **2**: 630–633.
54. Kauczor HU, Hanke A, van Beek EJ. Assessment of lung ventilation by MR imaging: current status and future perspectives. *Eur Radiol* 2002; **12**: 1962–1970.
55. Brand P, Letzel S, Buchta M et al. Can aerosol derived airway morphometry detect early, asymptomatical lung emphysema? *J Aerosol Med* 2003; **16**: 143–151.

56. West JB. Distribution of pulmonary blood flow and ventilation measured with radioactive gases. *Scand J Respir Dis* 1966; **62** (Suppl): 9–13.
57. Hiebert T, Miles J, Okelson GC. Contaminated aerosol recovery from pulmonary function testing equipment. *Am J Respir Crit Care Med* 1999; **159**: 610–612.
58. Kendrick AH, Johns DP, Leeming JP. Infection control of lung function equipment: a practical approach. *Resp Med* 2003; **97**: 1163–1179.
59. Miller MR, Crapo R, Hankinson J. General considerations for lung function testing. The official statement of the American Thoracic Society and the European Respiratory Society. *Eur Respir J*, 2005; **26**: 153–161.
60. Denison DM, Cramer DS, Hanson PJV. Lung function testing and AIDS. *Resp Med* 1989; **83**: 133–138.
61. Leeming JP, Pryce-Roberts DM, Kendrick AH, Smith EC. The efficacy of filters used in respiratory function apparatus. *J Hosp Infect* 1995; **31**: 205–210.
62. Castel O, Planchon C, Denjean A. Assessment of three filters for respiratory function tests. *Rev Mal Respir* 1998; **15**: 759–764.
63. Fuso L, Accardo D, Bevignani G et al. Effects of a filter at the mouth on pulmonary function tests. *Eur Respir J* 1995; **8**: 314–317.
64. Clausen JL. Lung volume equipment and infection control. *Eur Respir J* 1997; **10**: 1928–1932.
65. Chinn DJ, Naruse Y, Cotes JE. Accuracy of gas analysis in lung function laboratories. *Thorax* 1986; **41**: 133–137.
66. Saunders KB. Current practice in 6 London lung function laboratories. *Proc R Soc Med* 1977; **70**: 162–163.
67. Mushtaq M, Hayton R, Watts T et al. An audit of pulmonary function laboratories in the West Midlands. *Resp Med* 1995; **89**: 263–270.
68. Dowson LJ, Mushtaq M, Watts T et al. A re-audit of pulmonary function laboratories in the West Midlands. *Resp Med* 1998; **92**: 1155–1162.
69. Viegi G, Simoni M, Pistelli F et al Inter-laboratory comparison of flow–volume curve measurements as quality control procedure in the framework of an international epidemiological study (PEACE project). *Resp Med* 2000; **94**: 194–203.
70. Diem JE, Jones RN, Hendrick DJ et al. Five-year longitudinal study of workers employed in a new toluene di-isocyanate manufacturing plant. *Am Rev Respir Dis* 1982; **126**: 420–428.
71. MacIntyre NR, Crapo RO, Viegi G et al. Standardization of the single breath determination of carbon monoxide uptake in the lung. The official statement of the American Thoracic Society and the European Respiratory Society. *Eur Respir J* 2005; **26**: in press.
72. Arieli R, Ertracht O, Daskalovic Y. Infrared CO_2 analyzer error: an effect of background gas (N_2 and O_2). *J Appl Physiol* 1999; **86**: 647–650.
73. Gardner RM, Clausen JL, Crapo RO et al (on behalf of the ATS). Quality assurance in pulmonary function laboratories. *Am Rev Respir Dis* 1986; **134**: 625–627.
74. Kangalee KM, Abboud RT. Interlaboratory and intralaboratory variability in pulmonary function testing – a 13-year study using a normal biologic control. *Chest* 1992; **101**: 88–92.
75. Van den Boom G, van der Star LM, Folgering H et al. Volume calibration alone may be misleading. *Resp Med* 1999; **93**: 643–647.
76. International Organisation for Standardisation. *Shewhart control charts: statistical methods for quality control*, ISO 8258. Geneva: ISO, 1991.
77. Revill SM, Morgan MDL. Biological quality control for exercise testing. *Thorax* 2000; **55**: 63–66.

Further reading

Becquemin MH, Camus F, Lucet JC et al. Recommandations sur le bienfondé et l'efficacité des filtres en exploration fonctionnelle respiratoire. Texte intégral d'un rapport d'experts sollicité et validé par le CLIN-central le 28 Avril 1997. *Rev Mal Respir* 1999; **16**: 585–588.

Bushman JA, Calvert JR, Stockwell J. A new method for the calibration of peak flow meters. *Med Eng Phys* 1997; **19**: 359–365.

Child F, Clayton S, Davies S et al. How should airways resistance be measured in young children: mask or mouthpiece? *Eur Respir J* 2001; **17**: 1244–1249.

Hankinson JL, Crapo RO. Standard flow-time waveforms for testing of PEF meters. *Am J Resp Crit Care Med* 1995; **152**: 696–701.

Health and Safety Commission. *Safe working and the prevention of infection in clinical laboratories.* London: HMSO, 1991.

Holland WP, Boender W, Bos JA, Huygen PE. A simple handheld pushbutton device for in situ calibration of pneumotachographs. *J Appl Physiol* 1994; **77**: 2042–2047.

Hughes JMB. Short life radionucleotides and regional lung function. *Br J Radiol* 1979; **52**: 353–370.

Kharitonov S, Alving K, Barnes PJ. ERS Task Force Report. Exhaled and nasal nitric oxide measurements: recommendations. *Eur Respir J* 1997; **10**: 1683–1693.

Rhodes CG, Hughes JMB. Pulmonary studies using positron emission tomography. *Eur Resp Dis* 1995; **8**: 1001–1017.

van der Mark ThW, Kort E, Meijer RJ et al. Water vapour and carbon dioxide decrease nitric oxide readings. *Eur Respir J* 1997; **10**: 2120–2123.

Wimberley PD, Burnett RW, Covington AK et al International Federation of Clinical Chemistry (IFCC). Scientific Division. Committee on pH, blood gases and electrolytes. Guidelines for transcutaneous P_{O_2} and P_{CO_2} measurement. *Ann Biol Clin (Paris)* 1990; **48**: 39–43.

CHAPTER 8
Respiratory Surveys

Respiratory surveys that include measurement of lung function can provide invaluable information on the respiratory health of communities. This chapter describes how the survey should be conducted.

8.1 Indications

Respiratory surveys are used to establish the prevalence of respiratory disorders (e.g. asthma), identify causes of respiratory symptoms in communities or occupational groups, confirm the effectiveness of protective strategies and establish levels of pulmonary function amongst healthy people (reference values). Sometimes a survey will be directed towards more than one objective, but the principal objective should have priority.

8.2 Planning the survey

The survey is likely to be expensive of time and resources and so the exact need for it should be established in detailed discussion. The participants should have the relevant background information and be informed about the recent literature. Depending on the objective the planning team might include a medical practitioner, a project worker (who might be a respiratory physiologist or research nurse), an administrator, a statistician and, perhaps, an epidemiologist. One or more representatives from the target population, which might be from a factory, hospital or community, should also be consulted.

The aim of the preliminary discussion is to decide on the research question to be answered. For example, the question might be 'what is the prevalence of childhood asthma and does it vary with environmental pollution?' The survey can also entail an intervention. For it to be successful the question should be simple and answerable.

Success also depends on forward planning and this should include deciding on the data that are required, the subjects on whom they will be obtained, the instruments to be used and membership of the investigating team. Consideration must also be given to data processing, handling and analysis. The steps are outlined in Table 8.1.

8.2.1 Writing objectives

Objectives are explicit and realistic statements about the intended *outcome* of the survey process. They arise from but are narrower than the aims of the study. For example, if the aim is to derive reference equations for lung size in adolescents, one objective might be to measure the TLC and its subdivisions by closed circuit helium dilution in 100 males aged 16–19 years.

8.2.2 Choice of design for a descriptive survey

A survey is usually either cross-sectional in time, or longitudinal if it follows a cohort of subjects over time. Alternatively, features of cases may be compared with those of control subjects in a retrospective (case-control) study. Each type has its strengths and weaknesses (Tables 8.2 to 8.4) and the choice depends on the research question being asked. For example, a study seeking to

Table 8.1 Checklist for planning a respiratory survey.

Step	Task
1	Formulate the question
2	Write the objectives
3	Choose study design
4	Determine the sample size
5	Identify the target population
6	Select the study population
7	Choose the survey instruments
8	Write the study protocol
9	Estimate costs
10	Secure ethics approval and funding
11	Recruit and train staff
12	Prepare the timetable for: Fieldwork Preparing data for analysis Statistical analysis Report writing

estimate the prevalence of a symptom or disease in a population would use a cross-sectional design. The investigation of causal association between a disease and a putative risk factor would require a cohort, or longitudinal design. Finally, a case-control design would be appropriate for a study to identify factors associated with development of a rare disease.

Cross-sectional surveys. In a cross-sectional study each participant is examined once. This allows an investigator to estimate the prevalence of a disease, symptom or risk factor at a single point or period in time and to explore associations between disease frequency and potential causative factors. The associations may not be considered confirmatory because the investigator cannot be certain which came first, the disease or the risk factor. Cross-sectional studies are useful in formulating hypotheses about possible causal associations that may be tested in a cohort study.

Table 8.2 Strengths and weaknesses of the cross-sectional study design.

Strengths:
- One point in time
- Can generate hypotheses by determining associations
- Often cheap to set up
- Results can be obtained quickly
- Can be repeated in different settings

Weaknesses:
- Not good for assessment of cause and effect (temporality)
- Because it is made at one point in time it deals only with 'survivors'
- Not good for rare conditions
- Cannot predict future health outcomes

Table 8.3 Strengths and weaknesses of a cohort (longitudinal) study design.

Strengths:
- Can illuminate time sequences (which came first, the exposure or the disease)
- Good for studies of causation
- Can quantify risk of developing an abnormality
- Can quantify attributable risk and, therefore, the likely impact on health status from eliminating the causative factor
- Less prone to observer bias in data collection at the start of the study (investigators will not know which participant is likely to develop the abnormality)
- Can assess multiple outcomes in the same study

Weaknesses:
- Requires commitment to maintain standards
- Can be expensive in time and resources
- Results may not be available for years, during which time exposure conditions may have changed
- Prone to bias from selective loss from the cohort
- No control over extraneous factors that might affect the outcome, e.g. change in tobacco taxation
- Not useful for rare diseases

A cross-sectional design is appropriate for studies of reference values. Healthy individuals of different ages and body size are identified from a target population and information obtained on them is analysed to provide prediction equations. Some model equations are given in Section 5.6 and criteria for choosing subjects for different applications (for example when it is appropriate to include asymptomatic smokers) in Section 26.1.

Cohort study. Cohort studies are also known as follow-up or longitudinal studies. The follow-up may be prospective as in a study of growth, or retrospective, as in some studies of occupational cancer. The cohort may be divided into two or more subgroups

Table 8.4 Strengths and weaknesses of a case-control study.

Strengths:
- Good for rare conditions
- Cases should be easily identifiable (and presumably available)
- Relatively cheap
- Relatively quick
- Can be done from hospital setting
- Needs relatively fewer subjects (cf. cross-sectional study)
- Can explore several potentially causative factors

Weaknesses:
- Suitable controls can be difficult to identify
- Matching for confounders (e.g. age, gender) may not be adequate
- Results can only support, not prove, causal associations (temporality)
- Subject to reporting bias, e.g. from patient's memory or notes
- Cases recruited from hospital may not be 'representative' of all cases with the condition (selective survival)

according to the exposure to a risk factor; the exposure is then a categorical variable (Section 5.6). Cohort studies may progress over many years and involve more than one repeat examination. The interval between observations may be several years or a few months, as in surveys of occupational asthma or growth in children.

Cohort studies suffer from selective loss to follow-up. For example, persons with inferior lung function or respiratory symptoms may not re-attend for testing and their absence from the follow-up data set can bias the outcome. Accordingly, detailed efforts are required to maintain contacts with participants. The studies are also technically demanding in that the observations must be comparable throughout the period of follow-up. The comparability is with respect to equipment, conditions of measurement, quality of all observations and details of interpretation of individual features. It is greatly helped if the same equipment and observers can be retained throughout. There may also be need to capture additional information, for example data on exposure of participants during intervals between attendances.

When investigating a new hazard, a prospective cohort study sometimes grows out of a cross-sectional one. Ideally this should only happen if the cohort is suitable for both purposes, which is not always the case. However, where it is a possibility, the participants should be alerted at their initial examination. This will minimise anxiety that may arise from an unexpected recall at a later date.

Case-control study. A case-control or case-referent study is used to identify factors that contribute to a disease process, usually one that has a low prevalence in the community. To this end, individuals with the disease are identified and aspects of their lifestyle and exposures are compared with those of suitable control subjects. The choice of controls can critically influence the result.

8.2.3 Sample size calculations

The sample size is a compromise between that needed for statistical reliability and that which is realistically possible given the resources available. It is an important aspect of study design but is frequently overlooked. Studies with too few observations in relation to their intended accuracy and the question being asked have a low statistical power, and hence are unethical and waste resources. Procedures for determining sample size are summarised here. Details are given elsewhere [1–4].

Disease prevalence. The accuracy of an estimate of disease prevalence in a target population is determined by the actual prevalence and by the number of subjects studied. Then, for a disease prevalence expressed as the proportion (P), the standard error (SE) of P is given by:

$$\mathrm{SE}(P) = \sqrt{P(1-P)/n} \qquad (8.1)$$

where n is the size of the sample. When planning a survey this equation may be used to determine the sample size needed assuming a 'best guess' for the true prevalence and what would be considered an acceptable SE. Thus:

$$n = P(1-P)/[\mathrm{SE}(P)]^2 \qquad (8.2)$$

Example: If the prevalence of asthma in school children was thought to be about 15% ($P = 0.15$) and the investigator wanted to estimate it with an SE of 0.03, then from eqn. 8.2 the survey would need to examine 142 children.

It is common practice to report a prevalence and the confidence interval associated with it. The confidence interval (CI) for P is a range of values within which the 'true' population prevalence is likely to lie, with a given level of confidence, for example 95%. The 95% CI is calculated as:

$$P \pm 1.96 \times \mathrm{SE}(P) \qquad (8.3)$$

where 1.96 is the two-sided 95th percentile interval from the normal distribution that encompasses 95% of observations. In the example above, if $P = 0.15$ and $n = 142$, the $\mathrm{SE}(P) = 0.03$ and the 95% CI will be:

Lower limit $= 0.15 - (1.96 \times 0.03) = 0.09$

Upper limit $= 0.15 + (1.96 \times 0.03) = 0.21$

So, the investigator may be 95% confident that the true proportion lies between 0.09 and 0.21. If a more precise estimate is required, the study will require a larger sample. The relationship between P, $\mathrm{SE}(P)$ and n is given in Fig. 8.1.

Comparison between groups. In any study comparing, for example, the lung function of two matched groups of persons there is likely to be a difference between them. The question is whether the observed difference could have occurred by chance or reflects a true difference between the two groups. In this example a 'null hypothesis' is proposed that there is no difference in lung function between the two groups. Then, four items of information are required to determine a sample size necessary to ensure a robust chance of detecting a difference between the two groups if such a difference truly exists. These are:

1 The acceptable level of risk that the two results will be considered different when in reality they are the same. This is a false positive result and constitutes a type I error [1, 2]. The associated error rate (α) is the probability of the comparison rejecting the null hypothesis when it is true. This is the P value in a significance test and is arbitrarily set at 5% for which the standard normal deviate $Z_\alpha = 1.96$ (two-sided 95th percentile; Table 5.7, page 50).

2 The acceptable level of risk that a real difference will be missed. This is a false negative result and constitutes a type II error. The associated error rate (β) is normally set at less than 20% for which the standard normal deviate $Z_\beta = 1.28$ (one-sided 90th percentile, for 90% power) or 0.84 (one-sided 80th percentile, for 80% power). Here the power of the test is $1 - \beta$, which is

the probability of the test correctly rejecting the null hypothesis when it is false.

3 The variability of the measurement. This can be determined experimentally or taken from the literature. An example is given in Table 8.5.

4 The size of whatever difference between the groups is considered meaningful or clinically important (also called the *effect size*). This quantity depends on the judgement of the principal investigators and is usually a 'best guess'.

Example: How many subjects would be needed to detect a mean difference (effect size) of 0.2 l in a comparison of FEV_1 between two matched groups of men (gp1 and gp2)?

Effect size $(\Delta) = 0.2$ l

Standard deviation (SD) gp1 = 0.5 l

Standard deviation (SD) gp2 = 0.5 l

$Z_\alpha = 1.96$

$Z_\beta = 0.84$ (80% power)

Then, minimum n for *each* group $= (Z_\alpha + Z_\beta)^2[(\text{SD, gp1})^2 + (\text{SD, gp2})^2]/(\Delta^2) = (1.96 + 0.84)^2(0.5^2 + 0.5^2)/(0.2^2) = 98$, *per group*

For 90% power, 131 subjects would be required for each group.

When determining sample size the investigator should allow for non-attendance and failure to perform the respiratory function tests properly. The latter depends on the respiratory health and cognitive ability of the subjects and the complexity of the test. With forced expiratory manoeuvres the failure rate is small [5]. By contrast the failure rate for the single breath nitrogen test has been reported as in the range 16–58% [6–8]. The lower figure should be achieved if a valid result is to be obtained. When planning cohort studies the investigator must adjust the desired sample size for the estimated dropout rate during follow-up. When this is done, the sample size should be estimated with a 90% power; then, if the loss of subjects is greater than originally estimated the study may still retain enough subjects to provide an analysis with at least 80% power, which should be the minimum requirement.

8.2.4 Identify the target population and select the study sample

In order to obtain a result that is representative of a particular population all the members should be identified. For a factory population this will involve personnel records and may include past employees. Electoral records may be used for community studies of adults eligible to vote. Alternatively, in the United Kingdom, all members of a community, including children, may be identified from Health Authority lists of persons registered with a general practitioner. No source should be used uncritically as records may be out of date. For example, O'Mahony and colleagues [9] noted that in a UK survey of 2000 randomly selected persons aged 45 and above, registered addresses were inaccurate in 11% of cases. Furthermore, 2.1% of registered persons were dead. The error rate was relatively greater in elderly compared with younger persons.

If the population is too large to be studied in full then a sample should be used. Sampling is best done using randomisation

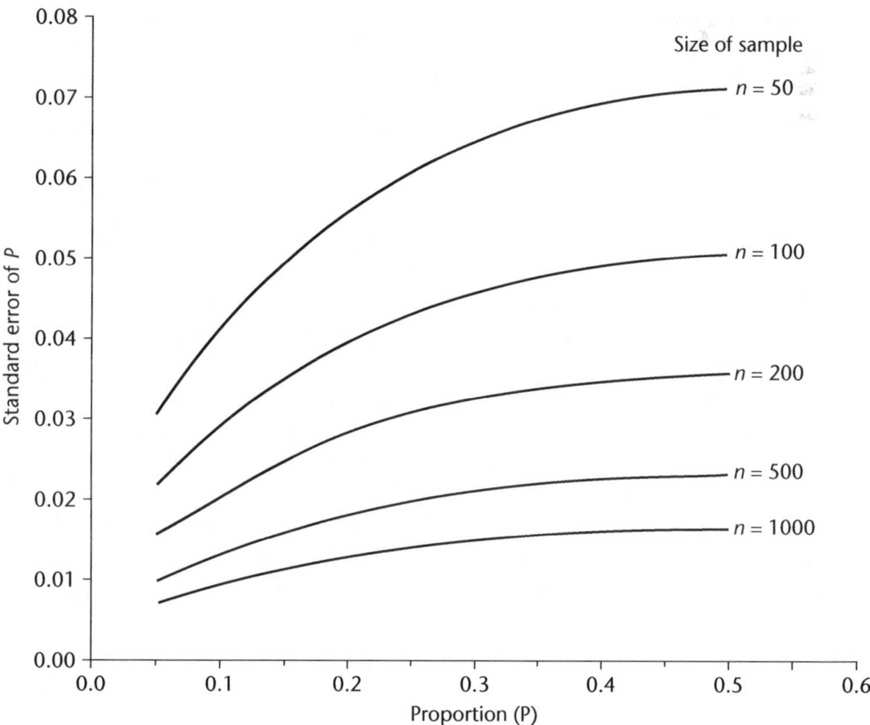

Fig. 8.1 The relationship between sample size and accuracy of the estimate (standard error) for a proportion P.

Table 8.5 Sample size required in relation to length of follow-up and frequency of measurements to detect a difference in annual change of FEV_1 of 0.03 l $year^{-1}$ between two groups, with a significance level (type I error) of 0.05.

	Interval between measurements									Equivalent number needed for a cross-sectional study∗	
	6 months			1 year			Beginning and end only				
Length of follow-up (years)	SD† (l $year^{-1}$)	Power 80%	Power 90%	SD† (l $year^{-1}$)	Power 80%	Power 90%	SD† (l $year^{-1}$)	Power 80%	Power 90%	Power 80%	Power 90%
1	0.174	528	707	0.174	528	707	0.174	528	707	4361	5837
2	0.086	129	173	0.094	154	206	0.094	154	206	1090	1459
3	0.060	63	84	0.067	78	105	0.069	83	111	485	649
4	0.051	45	61	0.055	53	71	0.058	59	79	273	365
5	0.046	37	49	0.049	42	56	0.052	47	63	174	233
6	0.044	34	45	0.046	37	49	0.049	42	56	121	162
7	0.042	31	41	0.044	34	45	0.047	39	52	89	119
8	0.042	31	41	0.043	32	43	0.045	35	47	68	91
9	0.041	29	39	0.042	31	41	0.044	34	45	54	72
10	0.041	29	39	0.042	31	41	0.043	32	43	44	58

Note: For a cohort study the accuracy of the estimation of change in lung function will be related to the length of follow-up and the frequency of repeated measures. Berry [3] estimated the three sources of error associated with change in the FEV_1 by using published data. These are the measurement error on a single occasion (standard deviation of mean of three blows, about 0.05 l), the between-occasion standard deviation (about 0.12 l) and the variability between individuals of the linear decline in FEV_1, which is related to the frequency of measurements and length of follow-up. These latter figures were used to calculate sample size required to detect a difference in annual FEV_1 of 0.03 l per year between two matched groups of individuals. The table also shows the number of subjects required in an equivalent cross-sectional study of individuals exposed for the follow-up period. For example, a cross-sectional study of persons exposed to an occupational hazard for 4 years would require 273 in each group (80% power) to detect, at 5% significance in a two-sided test, a difference of 0.12 l (difference in annual change of 0.03 l per year for 4 years). A cohort study based on 4 years annual follow-up (5 measurements in total) would require 53 persons in each group to detect an equivalent effect (80% power) and 59 persons in each group if the FEV_1 was measured at the beginning and end of the 4-year period.

∗ Individuals exposed for length of follow-up and assuming a standard deviation between individuals of 0.5 l.

† Estimated standard deviation of linear decline in FEV_1.

Source: Modified from Berry [3].

tables, whereby each member of the target population has an *equal* chance of being chosen for the sample.

In a stratified sample the entire population is subdivided into component groups on the basis of age or other variable. A random selection is then made from within each subgroup to satisfy a predetermined sampling strategy. For example, if the refusal rate is likely to be greater in one subgroup than another then 'over-sampling' in the 'hard to engage' group may be justifiable. However, it is no substitute for determined canvassing to bring as many as possible of the sample into the study. A response rate of 90% or more should be the target. A lower response rate may compromise the results if the participants are not representative of the target population. For example, in a postal survey of 7000 randomly selected persons the prevalence of asthma-related symptoms was significantly greater in early responders compared with that in late responders who were sent a second questionnaire and non-responders who were interviewed by telephone [10]. The responders were more likely to be symptomatic and the influence of non-response was to overestimate true prevalence of symptoms in the community.

8.2.5 Survey instruments for testing lung function

Respiratory epidemiology was developed around the measurement of ventilatory capacity (forced expiratory volume and vital capacity; Chapter 12) and this procedure is still the most widely used. Other aspects of function can be measured in the field including gas transfer, lung volumes, bronchial lability and exercise capacity. The criteria for selecting tests are reviewed elsewhere (Table 2.1, page 15). In summary, the tests should be acceptable to the population under study and relate to the aspect of lung function under scrutiny. The instruments should be robust and easily calibrated under field conditions. They should conform to international standards (Section 7.3). As a general rule, instruments used for diagnostic purposes should be selected over those used for monitoring (for example, mini Wright peak flowmeters) as they will be more accurate and have better performance characteristics. Instruments used for monitoring may, in some circumstances, be judged suitable for follow-up surveys of, for example, cross-shift changes in occupational studies.

The quality of measurements needs to be high, and if this cannot be guaranteed, the survey should normally be delayed until circumstances can be improved.

The operators should be fully trained and all equipment calibrated before and after each measurement session. These prerequisites apply as much to the measurement of stature (Section 4.3) as of lung function. Several surveys have been invalidated by neglect of this precaution! In all respects the standards for a survey should not fall below those expected for a good lung function laboratory, including the quality control processes.

8.2.6 Questionnaires

Questionnaires are used to collect items of information that will complement and assist in the interpretation of the lung function measurements. The items can include respiratory and cardiac symptoms, occupational exposures, aspects of lifestyle (e.g. smoking history and habitual activity) and quality of life. Many questionnaires exist and, in general, it is preferable to chose a validated questionnaire rather than devise a new one. However, caution may be needed when adopting a questionnaire for use in a population for which it was not designed. This is because questionnaires generally reflect the cultural norms of the society in which they were developed. Some items may not translate well and there may even be confusion in the interpretation of English as used in countries worldwide.

If there is no previously validated, published questionnaire fit for the purpose then the investigator will need to develop a specific tool. The design of a questionnaire is a complex and lengthy process that can become onerous and should not be undertaken lightly. There are many stages involved in the process, including defining the scope of the questionnaire, deciding the wording and ordering of questions, checking for ambiguities, developing the scales and piloting it [11].

Questionnaires may be administered by interviewer or self-administered. Interviews should be undertaken in quiet surroundings, not overheard by others, by appropriately trained staff using a consistent interview style within and between observers. The interview should not be rushed and the interviewer should adopt a quiet manner using the exact wording on the questionnaire whilst maintaining eye-to-eye contact with the interviewee. Clear instructions must be given on responding to the questions.

Self-administered questionnaires require very precise wording with clear instructions on what is required. The size of the print should accommodate those with poor vision. Questionnaires may be distributed by post or through a workplace, with a view to their being completed prior to attendance for lung function testing. Alternatively, the texts may be handed out on attendance, to be completed prior to the tests or whilst the subject is waiting between tests. Whichever method is adopted the replies should be checked with the respondent before the end of the test session.

Respiratory symptom questionnaires. Many respiratory questionnaires are based on the British Medical Research Council (BMRC) questionnaire on respiratory symptoms. This was designed for investigating chronic bronchitis and is commonly used in conjunction with measurements of ventilatory capacity [12, 13]. The 1976 version is recommended (Fig. 8.2). The questionnaire can be extended with additional questions on wheeze, angina and occupation. It has the advantages of having been properly validated, and so minimises bias in data collection, and of translation into over 100 languages so that comparisons can be made between different populations [e.g. 14–16]. The questionnaire has been modified on numerous occasions and some of the changes have been detrimental [17] and so the choice of version is important. In addition, for an untested population the meanings of words and even the concepts may not be appropriate. Thus the question 'do you ever produce phlegm from your chest' may elicit negative responses if the local cultural practice prohibits expectoration in favour of swallowing the phlegm. Similarly, the information conveyed by the question 'do you usually bring up phlegm from your chest first thing in the morning in the winter?' is subtly different when asked of a person working night shifts compared with one who rises from bed in the morning.

Additional respiratory symptom questionnaires are referenced in Table 8.6. They differ in many important respects and so the choice of which to use should be made carefully. Any new questionnaire enquiring into respiratory symptoms should be calibrated against the BMRC questionnaire [25].

Cough score. The questions on cough in the MRC questionnaire do not indicate its intensity. This can be assessed using a semi-quantitative scoring technique developed by Field [24]. The method is directed to persons with mild symptoms who do not cough on most days for as much as 3 months in the year and can relate to any time interval to suit the investigator, for example, over the past 4 weeks (Fig. 8.3).

Health-related quality of life. Respiratory questionnaires identify symptoms in respiratory patients that influence their quality of life, which is designated health-related quality of life (HRQoL). It is greatly influenced by the reaction of the subject to the symptoms and by the extent to which the reaction is modified by environmental factors. For example, depending on the other factors, dyspnoea on exertion can be overcome, tolerated, or lead to avoidance of exercise, increased dependency, loss of self-esteem, anxiety and depression. Hence, HRQoL provides a broader view of the overall impact of a respiratory illness than the loss of lung function and reduced response to exercise. These three aspects are designated respectively handicap, respiratory impairment and respiratory disability (Section 30.1).

Quantitative measures of the quality of life are not always easy to interpret, for example:

1 Some patients with severe disability still rate their quality of life as good. This has been described as a 'disability paradox' [26].

Use the actual wording of each question. Enter in the boxes 1 = Yes, 2 = No, or other codes as appropriate. When in doubt record as no.

Preamble
I am going to ask you some questions, mainly about your chest. I should like you to answer **Yes** or **No** whenever possible.

Cough
1. Do you **usually** cough first thing in the morning in the winter? ☐

2. Do you **usually** cough during the day – or at night – in the winter? ☐

If Yes to 1 or 2
3. Do you cough like this on most days for as much as three months each year? ☐

Phlegm
4. Do you **usually** bring up any phlegm from your chest first thing in the morning in the winter? ☐

5. Do you **usually** bring up any phlegm from your chest during the day – or at night – in the winter? ☐

If Yes to 4 or 5

6. Do you bring up phlegm like this on most days for as much as three months each year? ☐

Periods of cough and phlegm

7a. In the past three years have you had a period of (increased) cough and phlegm lasting for three weeks or more? ☐

If Yes
7b. Have you had more than one such period? ☐

Breathlessness

If the subject is disabled from walking by any condition other than heart or lung disease, omit question 8 and enter 1 here. ☐

8a. Are you troubled by shortness of breath when hurrying on level ground or walking up a slight hill? ☐

If Yes
8b. Do you get short of breath walking with other people of your own age on level ground? ☐

If Yes
8c. Do you have to stop for breath when walking at your own pace on level ground? ☐

Wheezing

9a. Does your chest ever sound wheezing or whistling? ☐

If Yes
9b. Do you get this on most days – or nights? ☐

10a. Have you ever had attacks of shortness of breath with wheezing? ☐

If yes
10b. Is/was your breathing absolutely normal between attacks? ☐

Chest illness

11a. During the past three years have you had any chest illness which has kept you from your usual activities for as much as a week? ☐

If Yes
11b. Did you bring up more phlegm than usual in any of these illnesses? ☐

If Yes
11c. Have you had more than one illness like this in the past three years? ☐

Past illnesses
Have you ever had:

12a. An injury or operation affecting the chest ☐

12b. Heart trouble ☐

12c. Bronchitis ☐

12d. Pneumonia ☐

12e. Pleurisy ☐

12f. Pulmonary tuberculosis ☐

12g. Bronchial asthma ☐

12h. Other chest trouble ☐

12i. Hay fever ☐

Fig. 8.2 The MRC questionnaire on respiratory symptoms (1976 version).

Tobacco smoking **1 = Yes, 2 = No**

13a. Do you smoke? ☐

If No
13b. Have you ever smoked as much as one cigarette a day (or one cigar a week or an ounce of tobacco a month) for as long as a year? ☐

If No to both parts of question 13, omit remaining questions on smoking

14a. Do (did) you inhale the smoke ? ☐

If Yes
14b. Would you say you inhaled the smoke slightly = 1, moderately = 2 or deeply = 3 ☐

15. How old were you when you started smoking regularly? ☐☐

16a. Do (did) you smoke manufactured cigarettes? ☐

If Yes
16b. How many do (did) you usually smoke per day on weekdays? ☐☐

16c. How many per day at weekends? ☐☐

16d. Do (did) you usually smoke plain [=1] or filter tip [=2] cigarettes? ☐

16e. What brands do (did) you usually smoke? ☐☐☐
....

17a. Do (did) you smoke hand-rolled cigarettes? ☐

If Yes
17b. How much tobacco do (did) you usually smoke per week in this way? ☐☐☐

17c. Do (did) you put filters in these cigarettes? ☐

18a. Do (did) you smoke a pipe? ☐

If Yes
18b. How much pipe tobacco do (did) you usually smoke per week? ☐☐☐

19a. Do (did) you smoke small cigars? ☐

If Yes
19b. How many of these do (did) you usually smoke per day? ☐☐

20a. Do (did) you smoke other cigars? ☐

If Yes
20b. How many of these do (did) you usually smoke per week? ☐☐

For present smokers
21a. Have you been cutting down your smoking over the past year? ☐

For ex-smokers
21b. When did you last give up smoking? Month: ☐☐ Year: ☐☐

Additional observations

Instructions for using the questionnaire are available from the authors (*see* Feedback on page x).

Fig. 8.2 *Continued*

Table 8.6 Respiratory symptom questionnaires for use in surveys.

Questionnaire	Reference	Comment*
Medical Research Council (MRC)	[12, 13]	IA. Widely used. Revised 1966, 1976 and 1986. 1976 version grades wheeze into 'occasional' and 'regular'
American Thoracic Society, Division of Lung Diseases (ATS-DLD-78)	[18]	SA or IA. Recommended for age 13 and above. Includes family history of chest disease
International Union Against Tuberculosis and Lung Disease (IUATLD)	[19]	SA. Designed to compare the prevalence of asthma in international studies
European Community for Coal and Steel (ECSC) 1987 update.†	[20]	IA. Includes questions to diagnose asthma and passive smoking. Wheeze not graded
European Community Respiratory Health Survey (ECRHS)	[21]	SA and IA. Developed from standardised questionnaires used in multinational studies and designed to estimate the prevalence of asthma and asthma-like symptoms in adults aged 20–44 years. Includes SA screening questions for asthma
International Study of Asthma and Allergies in Childhood (ISAAC)	[22]	PA and/or SA. Designed to estimate the prevalence of asthma and allergic disease, including eczema and rhinitis in children aged 6–7 and 13–14 years. Video questionnaire available for older children
Infants and preschool children	[23]	PA. Relates to preceding 3 months. Measures impact of symptoms on child and family
'Cough' score	[24]	IA. Uses 10-point scale. Method can be adapted for other symptoms

* Questionnaire self-administered (SA) or administered by interviewer (IA) or parent (PA).

† Versions in many languages available from ECSC Division of Employment and Social Affairs, Luxembourg.

Card number	Order (1 or 2)	Statement
1	1	I cough occasionally
	2	I rarely ever cough
2	1	I rarely ever cough
	2	I cough a little on most days
3	1	I cough a little on most days
	2	I cough occasionally
4	1	I cough occasionally
	2	I cough a little every day
5	1	I cough a little every day
	2	I cough a little on most days
6	1	I cough a little on most days
	2	I cough a lot every day
7	1	I cough a lot every day
	2	I cough a little every day
8	1	I cough a little every day
	2	I cough all the time
9	1	I cough all the time
	2	I cough a lot every day

Scoring sheet:

	Card number								
	1	2	3	4	5	6	7	8	9
Statement number	2	1	2	~~1~~	~~2~~	~~1~~	~~2~~	~~1~~	~~2~~
	~~1~~	~~2~~	~~1~~	2	1	2	1	2	1

Fig. 8.3 Cough frequency statements and their order on the nine cards. Source: After Field [24].
The test equipment comprises 9 cards, each containing two questions out of a list of six. The cards are shuffled and presented to the subject who is asked to compare the statements and select the one that is nearer to the truth. Neither may be true but one statement will be closer to the truth than the other. For each card the statement nominated by the subject is marked and the cross-over point from the lower to upper line indicates the cough score (4 in this example). The procedure takes about five minutes. The success of the test depends on the subject being able to mentally rank the pairs of questions consistently. With suitable wording the technique can be adapted for other respiratory symptoms.

2 Impaired quality of life in respiratory patients can be due in part to other conditions. Hence, HRQoL can vary independent of the respiratory status [27].
3 Cultural and ethnic differences need to be taken into account.
4 The distribution of scores is sometimes skewed with a few subjects showing atypical features and this is not always taken into account in the statistical analysis (Section 5.5).
5 The HRQoL score is the sum of components that reflect different attributes of living. Their relative importance differs with circumstances and may vary with time. As a result no one questionnaire is appropriate for all applications.

The scores can relate to individual domains (e.g. dyspnoea) and are usually combined in a single, global score. Changes in the global measure at follow-up can mislead if an improvement in one domain is offset by deterioration in another.

Many questionnaires for assessing HRQoL have been proposed, but few of them have been properly validated [28–30]. Some that are widely used for respiratory patients are described below. A list of suitable questionnaires is available on the ATS website (http://www.thoracic.org).

Chronic Respiratory Questionnaire (CRQ) of Guyatt and colleagues. [31]. The CRQ assesses four dimensions: fatigue, dyspnoea, emotional functioning and mastery over the patient's disease. There are 19 questions (20 items), and the questionnaire is administered by a trained interviewer and takes 15–25 min to complete. The questionnaire has been validated and its repeatability and sensitivity to change established. The CRQ is not fully standardised as each patient is asked to identify the five most important activities that have induced dyspnoea in the previous 2 weeks. Thus, it is tailored to each patient, and so a standard score cannot be calculated and used for inter-patient comparisons. However, the CRQ is used widely and has contributed to cohort studies evaluating rehabilitation programs and therapeutic trials. The minimally important clinical difference in CRQ score is 0.5 (on a 7-point scale).

Self-reported versions of the questionnaire are available [32, 33]. One at least was as sensitive as the interviewer-administered version in a study of patients undergoing respiratory rehabilitation [34].

St George's Respiratory Questionnaire (SGRQ) of Jones and colleagues. [27, 35]. The SGRQ was developed for persons with diseases of the airways that result in airways obstruction, including asthma. It addresses (1) symptoms, (2) activities that relate to breathlessness and (3) disturbance to daily life. The latter includes the psychological impact but not scores for anxiety or depression. There are 76 items, weighted according to the distress that is associated with each aspect. The questionnaire is self-administered and takes about 10 min to complete. This is best done in a quiet room away from interference from carers or other patients but in the presence of the investigator who should answer any queries. The three topics are each scored 0–100, with a high score indicating poor quality of life. A global score can be calculated. The minimally important clinical difference was determined as 4% by the authors.

The weightings were determined from studies of 140 adult asthmatics in six countries; the weights were concordant between five of them (England, Finland, Italy, United States and Thailand) but higher by, on average, 19% in the Netherlands.

Asthma Quality of Life Questionnaire (AQLQ) of Juniper and colleagues. [36]. The questionnaire contains 32 items covering four domains: activity limitation, symptoms, emotional function and environmental stimuli. It is administered by an interviewer and takes about 10 min to complete. Average scores are derived, without weightings, to reflect the four domains and the overall quality of life. The average scores range from 1 to 7, with a low score indicating a poor quality of life. Summary scores are reproducible when the clinical condition is stable and are sensitive to small within-patient changes. A difference of 0.5 units is meaningful. The within-subject standard deviation of change is reported as 0.64, and so the sample size needed for a two-sided test with type I and type II errors of 0.05 and 0.1, respectively, is 35 per group [37].

An individualised and standardised version of the scale has been developed as well as a mini-version, which contains 15 items and is self-administered [38]. In a study of 40 patients it compared favourably with the original 32-item questionnaire but was less precise with larger within-subject standard deviations. Accordingly, the sample sizes required for cross-sectional and longitudinal surveys will be greater.

The 32-item and mini-AQLQ questionnaires are reported in appendices to their respective publications [37, 38]. Detailed instructions on use of the questionnaires are available from the authors. Both versions of the AQLQ have been translated into other languages.

A quality of life questionnaire has been developed for use in children [39] and parents of children [40].

8.2.7 Write the study protocol

A written protocol is obligatory. It establishes the ground rules and dictates to the team what information is required and how it should be obtained. The protocol also assists the team make decisions regarding the inevitable protocol violations that will occur during the course of the study. All relevant details should be noted in the protocol including definitions of, for example, an ex-smoker, and the procedure for handling 'test failures' [5]. The coding frame for the data should be specified including the rules for handling test failures and registering missing data; blank entries are unacceptable. A protocol informs the analysis and provides a basis for the final report, particularly when this is left to a team member not familiar with the day-to-day running of the survey. The protocol should provide all the information necessary for another investigator to repeat the study elsewhere.

The protocol should specify a procedure for persons with abnormal findings. The procedure should be included in any information leaflet given to the subject prior to obtaining informed consent for their participation in the survey. It may be a requirement in the application for ethics approval.

8.2.8 Secure ethics approval and funding

Ethics permission is necessary and takes time, particularly if the study is multicentred and requires consideration by more than one ethics committee. The application should include the question, objectives, protocol and details of funding.

The funding should cover the cost of training and retaining staff for the duration of the project. In longitudinal studies delays are common and so the estimate of time should not be parsimonious. Other costs are likely to include hire charges, rent, the costs of servicing equipment, purchasing consumable stores, travel by staff and possibly by subjects, data analysis, preparation of reports and overheads. With so many items the overall cost is likely to be high; it must be seen to be value for money.

8.2.9 Recruit and train staff

Surveys are team ventures to which newly recruited members make essential contributions. Desirable qualities include enthusiasm to surmount the inevitable difficulties, a sensitive personality to engage the subjects and drive to encourage subjects to give of their best. Specialist training in lung function testing is essential (Section 2.5). It is also necessary that staff follow the protocol without deviation. This can be difficult. For example, experienced laboratory staff may need to modify their practices and nurses to take more than their customary care when measuring stature.

The team approach extends to each member possessing and being familiar with the protocol, participating in regular discussions, reviews and progress meetings and taking and sharing responsibility for solving difficulties, not passing them on. The outcome can be very satisfying – and often great fun!

8.3 Conducting the survey

Prior to launching the survey it is imperative to undertake a pilot of the full survey methodology, including the preparation of the data for inputting onto the database. Faults in the process will be exposed and the lessons learned will contribute to eventual success. Without a pilot, and the lessons from it, the study may fall apart and not be salvageable.

8.3.1 Collecting the data

Working in the field remote from the familiarity of the host laboratory can pose many difficulties. Suitable premises are essential. They should be accessible, have sufficient space in at least two rooms that are quiet, appropriately heated and ventilated, supplied with water, electricity, a telephone and have a toilet nearby. A reception area is usually necessary. Premises should meet health and safety regulations. In addition, a personal assessment and security check will be necessary where staff are working alone.

The accommodation might be in a factory, school, community centre, health centre, prison or other establishment. A purpose built mobile laboratory is ideal, provided space and access to facilities can be arranged. The laboratory should be secure but remain operational when not in use so that the temperature can be maintained and electronic equipment left on.

Working hours should fit in with the availability of subjects (for example, shift workers) and, if in a factory, with the production schedules. Timetabling should be generous to allow for latecomers. Posting reminder notices can reduce the proportion that needs to be 'chased up'. The notices can also reinforce the request not to smoke on the day of the tests.

The procedure usually begins with collection of personal information and questionnaires, followed by anthropometry and physiological assessment. The order of tests should make use of time that might otherwise be spent whilst residual test gases are cleared from the lungs (Table 2.2, page 16). If the response to bronchodilators is part of the assessment, the schedule should allow sufficient time for administering the drug to naïve subjects as well as the obligatory time to achieve its full effect.

The results of each day's work should be stored off the site, preferably in the host laboratory. The requirements of data protection legislation must be adhered to.

Special arrangements, including chaperoning, are necessary for home visits when the observer may experience additional hazards of, for example, high-rise buildings, unsavoury surroundings, background distractions, dogs, inquisitive children and partners who overhear and challenge the participant's replies to questions.

8.3.2 Preparing the data for analysis

Errors can arise at any time from the period of data collection through to the subsequent processing. Transcription errors can arise when recording the prime measurements, inputting values into the computer or calculator, writing down intermediate results and manipulating the database. Confusion can arise when reading characters written by other observers and so a neat, orderly writing style is desirable.

During the data collection an ongoing check should be made to maintain standards. The checks should detect measurement 'drift' and lapses by individual observers (Fig. 8.4). Such deficiencies are difficult to rectify if data processing is delayed until all the information has been collected.

Data should be added to the database during the course of the survey, as the opportunity arises. This allows early identification of inconsistencies with the coding scheme and enables the team leaders to monitor progress and check intermediate results. Entries should be made for the observers, the equipment (if more than one instrument), the temperature and time of day.

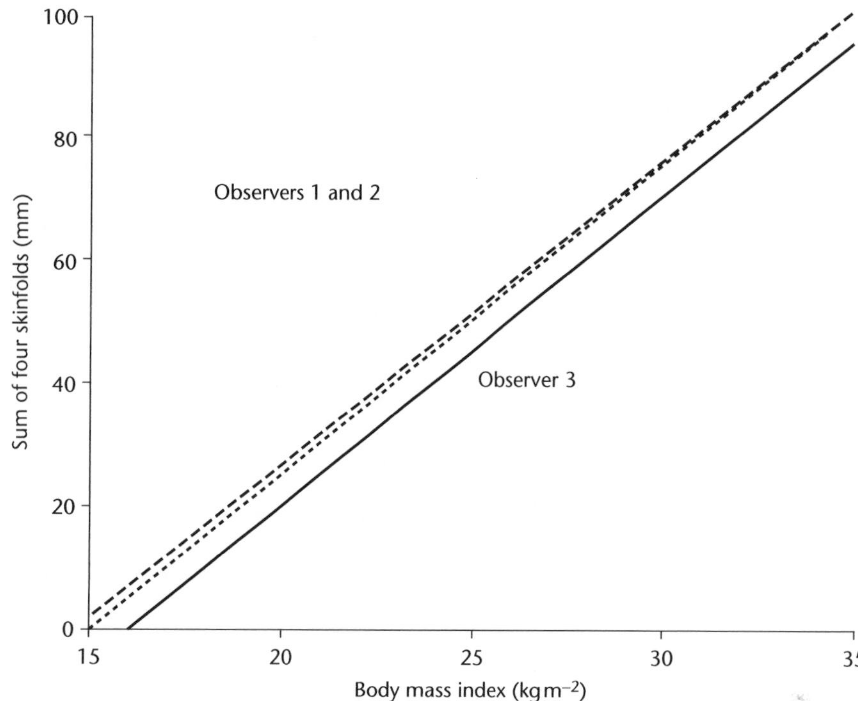

Fig. 8.4 Observer variation in measurement of skinfolds showing the linear regression lines of the sum of four skinfolds on body mass index. Observer 3 recorded consistently less than observers 1 and 2.
Note: In an occupational survey three observers were recording skinfold thicknesses at four sites to estimate the percent body fat. Before the survey the observers trained together and their results on the same group of 12 volunteer subjects had been equivalent. After 8 weeks on-site a plot of the sum of skinfolds against body mass index showed that the first two observers were making comparable measurements but the third observer was recording consistently lower skinfolds. This was traced to an underestimation in the measurement of the subscapula skinfold. The technique was reviewed, the aberrant observer was retrained and the subjects seen by that observer re-examined.

In addition, if more than one person is updating the database, he or she should be coded as well. Backup copies of the database should be updated daily.

Information should be collected at an appropriate level of accuracy. For example, age in children and intervals between examinations during a longitudinal study should be to the nearest day not year. This can be done by recording the actual dates or calculating age in decimal years (Table 5.2, page 44).

Prior to the final analysis the data should be checked rigorously. Ideally this should be done against all the original records, which should not be discarded. If this is not possible, use of a 10–20% random sample is usually sufficient. If the error rate is judged too high, the remaining records should be checked as well. The data should then be 'cleaned'. Obvious errors include that numbers are of the wrong order of magnitude or are internally inconsistent; for example, FVC is not greater than the TLC or less than FEV_1. Exercise tidal volume might be recorded as exceeding FVC, or V_A the TLC. Outliers may be recognised by scrutinising the minimum and maximum values for each variable and generating simple plots of indices of lung function against appropriate reference variables such as age and stature. Other plots suitable for identifying rogue results are body mass against stature, Fat% against body mass index (body mass $\times$ stature^{-2}) and stature against age (particularly in children).

8.3.3 Statistical analysis and storage of data

The statistician on the planning team should undertake the analysis. Where this is not practicable the investigator has the options of informing and working with another or undertaking the analysis in-house. Training in data analysis and familiarity with the statistical package is essential (see Footnote 8.1).

The first steps in statistical analysis include checking the distribution of the individual variables in a frequency histogram, transforming skewed data where this is desirable and exploring interrelationships between variables using simple correlations. Lung function indices usually are analysed by simple *t*-tests, analysis of variance, analysis of covariance, simple and multiple regression analysis. Analysis of dichotomous variables (for example, respiratory symptoms coded as present or absent) is undertaken with simple or multiple logistic regression (Section 5.6).

Survey data that are appropriately anonymised are a valuable resource. Thus, once the analysis has been completed and the paper published the data should be stored for future use. To this end the data should be treated to conform to the requirements of data protection regulations. Storage can be with the parent institution or a repository (see Footnote 8.2). Backup copies should be maintained and it is advisable to store the study protocol alongside the raw data.

Footnote 8.1. One package in the public domain is Epi Info 2000©. The software and its manual are available free over the Internet from the Centers for Disease Control and Prevention, Atlanta (www.cdc.gov/epiinfo). The software is used widely in epidemiological investigations, and the manual is available in many languages.

Footnote 8.2. In the United Kingdom, data from population surveys may be deposited in the Data Archive kept by the Economic and Social Research Council at the University of Essex (www.data-archive.ac.uk). Access to the data and the study protocol is either on request or via the depositors.

Table 8.7 Principal sources of bias in respiratory surveys.

Source	Comment
Design	Bias arising from any aspect of study design, e.g. failure to account for confounding, faulty randomisation, temporal differences in examination of subgroups. Unequal allocation of subjects with similar characteristics to different observers
Ascertainment	Variation in definitions used between or within studies (e.g. criteria to define an ex-smoker, or an asthmatic)
Selection	Failure to ensure that all members of the target population have an equal chance of selection. For example, when subjects with poor reading skills or visual impairment are approached by letter
Response	Systematic error from differences in characteristics between those who accept and those who decline an invitation to participate
Follow-up	Error in cohort studies arising from differences in characteristics between those who return for reassessment and those who drop out, for whatever reason
Measurement	Systematic error from faulty calibration, use of inaccurate standards, inaccurate measurement, differences between instruments used to collect data from different subgroups, data handling procedures by different observers, digit preference
Interviewer	Systematic error from the observers' conscious or subconscious collection of selective information
Recall	Selective memory in recall of events
Reporting	Respondents may perceive and/or report the same information in different ways depending on their personal circumstances
Observer	Differences in technique between and within observers. Should be minimised by training but can never be eliminated fully
Measurement decay	Error from a change in the measurement process over time. Can occur due to change in instrument performance or from change in technique by observers
Lead time	Failure to initiate follow-up of two or more comparison groups at a comparable time
Analysis	Inappropriate use of statistical methods and inferences drawn from them. Failure to treat outliers identically in all subgroup analyses. Differences in procedures for handling data from test failures. Neglect of confounding factors

8.4 Interpretation of the findings

The most exciting part of a survey is making sense of the data, the process whereby the numbers are turned into information. Answers to the original research question should emerge and other questions may emanate that will lead to further studies. The process is iterative and all team members should contribute to the discussions. Presentation before other colleagues and at professional meetings can prove invaluable and give depth to the report.

8.5 Writing the report

The study is only completed by the publication of a full account in a scientific journal. This should focus on the research question, including the extent to which it has been answered, the statement of objectives and the implications for further work. Any limitations should be mentioned, including places where bias or error might have been introduced (Table 8.7). The investigators should draft the report as soon as practicable after the analysis has been completed. At this stage it can be submitted to the funding body or commissioner of the work and used when applying for another grant. Release of the findings and submission for publication should be delayed until colleagues and others working in the field have subjected the work to comment. The process inevitably takes time though, in practice, there is often great urgency as the topic may attract much public interest or the investigator's career or the viability of the parent institution may depend on it. In this event, strong coffee, cold towels and burning midnight oil may be the only way ahead!

8.6 References

1. Altman DG. *Practical statistics for medical research*, 2nd ed. London: Chapman & Hall, 1999.
2. Kirkwood BR. *Essentials of medical statistics*, 2nd ed. Oxford: Blackwell Science, 1997.
3. Berry G. Longitudinal observations, their usefulness and limitations with special reference to the forced expiratory volume. *Bull Physiopathol Respir* 1974; **10**: 643–655.
4. Hofstra WB, Sont JK, Sterk PJ et al. Sample size estimation in studies monitoring exercise-induced bronchoconstriction in asthmatic children. *Thorax* 1997; **52**: 739–741.
5. Becklake M. Epidemiology of spirometric test failure. *Br J Ind Med* 1990; **47**: 73–74.

6. El-Gamal FMH. *Welding fumes as a cause of impaired lung function in shipyard workers.* PhD thesis, University of Newcastle-upon-Tyne, 1986.
7. Viegi G, Paoletti P, Di Pede F et al. Single breath nitrogen test in an epidemiologic survey in North Italy. Reliability, reference values and relationships with symptoms. *Chest* 1988; **93**: 1213–1220.
8. Teculescu DB, Damel M-C, Costantino E et al. Computerized single-breath nitrogen washout: predicted values in a rural French community. *Lung* 1996; **174**: 43–55.
9. O'Mahony PG, Thomson RG, Rodgers H et al. Accuracy of the family health services authority register in Newcastle upon Tyne, UK as a sampling frame for population studies. *J Epidemiol Commun Health* 1997; **51**: 206–207.
10. de Marco R, Verlato G, Zanolin E et al. Nonresponse bias in EC Respiratory Health Survey in Italy. *Eur Respir J* 1994; **7**: 2139–2145.
11. Stone DH. Design a questionnaire. *BMJ* 1993; **307**: 1264–1266.
12. Medical Research Council on the Aetiology of Chronic Bronchitis. Standardised questionnaire on respiratory symptoms. *BMJ* 1960; **ii**: 1665.
13. Medical Research Council. Definition and classification of chronic bronchitis for clinical and epidemiological purposes. *Lancet* 1965; **i**: 775–779.
14. Olsen HC, Gilson JC. Respiratory symptoms, bronchitis and ventilatory capacity in men. *BMJ* 1960; **i**: 450–456.
15. Wilhelmsen L. Effects on bronchopulmonary symptoms, ventilation and lung mechanics of abstinence from tobacco smoking. *Scand J Resp Dis* 1967; **48**: 407–414.
16. Malik MA, Moss E, Lee WR. Prediction values for the ventilatory capacity in male West Pakistani workers in the United Kingdom. *Thorax* 1972; **27**: 611–619.
17. Cotes JE. Medical Research Council Questionnaire on respiratory symptoms (1986). Correspondence. *Lancet* 1987; **2**: 1028.
18. American Thoracic Society Epidemiological Standardisation Project. Recommended respiratory disease questionnaires for use with adults and children in epidemiological research. *Am Rev Respir Dis* 1978; **118**: 7–53.
19. Burney P, Chinn S. Developing a new questionnaire for measuring the prevalence and distribution of asthma. *Chest* 1987; **91** (Suppl): 79S–83S.
20. Minette. A. Questionnaire of the European Community for Coal and Steel (ECSC) on respiratory symptoms. 1987 updating of the 1962 and 1967 questionnaires for studying chronic bronchitis and emphysema. *Eur Respir J* 1989; **2**: 165–177.
21. Burney PGJ, Luczynska C, Chinn S, Jarvis D. The European Community Respiratory Health Survey. *Eur Respir J.* 1994; **7**: 954–960.
22. Asher MI, Keil U, Anderson HR et al. International study of asthma and allergies in childhood (ISAAC): rationale and methods. *Eur Respir J.* 1995; **8**: 483–491.
23. Powell CVE, McNamara P, Solis A, Shaw NJ. A parent completed questionnaire to describe the patterns of wheezing and other respiratory symptoms in infants and preschool children. *Arch Dis Child* 2002; **87**: 376–379.
24. Field GB. The application of a quantitative estimate of cough frequency to epidemiological surveys. *Int J Epidemiol* 1974; **3**: 135–143.
25. Samet JM. A historical and epidemiologic perspective on respiratory symptoms questionnaires. *Am J Epidemiol* 1978; **108**: 435–446.
26. Carr AJ, Higginson IJ. Are quality of life measures patient centred? *BMJ* 2001; **322**: 1357–1360.
27. Jones PW. Quality of life measurement for patients with diseases of the airways. *Thorax* 1991; **46**: 676–682.
28. Bowling A. *Measuring disease. A review of disease-specific quality of life measurement scales*, 2nd ed. Milton Keynes, UK: Open University Press, 2001.
29. Lareau SC, Breslin EH, Meek PM. Functional status instruments: outcome measure in the evaluation of patients with chronic obstructive pulmonary disease. *Heart Lung.* 1996; **25**: 212–224.
30. Curtis JR, Martin DP, Martin TR. Patient-assessed health outcomes in chronic lung disease. *Am J Respir Crit Care Med* 1997; **156**: 1032–1039.
31. Guyatt GH, Berman LB, Townsend M et al. A measure of quality of life for clinical trials in chronic lung disease. *Thorax* 1987; **42**: 773–778.
32. Williams JEA, Singh SJ, Sewell L et al.Development of a self-reported Chronic Respiratory Questionnaire (CRQ-SR). *Thorax* 2001; **56**: 954–959.
33. Rutten-van Molken M, Roos B, Van Noord JA. An empirical comparison of the St George's Respiratory Questionnaire (SGRQ) and the Chronic Respiratory Disease Questionnaire (CRQ) in a clinical trial setting. *Thorax* 1999; **54**: 995–1003.
34. Williams JEA, Singh SJ, Sewell L, Morgan MDL. Health status measurement: sensitivity of the self-reported Chronic Respiratory Questionnaire (CRQ-SR) in pulmonary rehabilitation. *Thorax* 2003; **58**: 515–518.
35. Jones, PW, Quirk FH, Bayeystock CM et al. A self-complete measure of health status for chronic airflow limitation. The St George's Respiratory Questionnaire. *Am Rev Respir Dis* 1992; **145**: 1321–1327.
36. Juniper EF, Guyatt GH, Epstein RS et al. Evaluation of impairment of health related quality of life in asthma: development of a questionnaire for use in clinical trials. *Thorax* 1992; **47**: 76–83.
37. Juniper EF, Guyatt GH, Ferrie PJ, Griffith LE. Measuring quality of life in asthma. *Am Rev Resp Dis* 1993; **147**: 832–838.
38. Juniper EF, Guyatt GH, Cox FM et al. Development and validation of the Mini Asthma Quality of Life Questionnaire. *Eur Respir J* 1999; **14**: 32–38.
39. Juniper EF. Guyatt DH, Feeny D et al. Measuring quality of life in children with asthma. *Qual Life Res* 1996a; **5**: 35–46.
40. Juniper EF. Guyatt DH, Feeny D et al. Measuring quality of life in the parents of children with asthma. *Qual Life Res* 1996b; **5**: 27–34.

Further reading

Coggon D, Rose G, Barker DJP. *Epidemiology for the uninitiated*, 4th ed. London: BMJ, 1997.

Florey C. *Methods for cohort studies of chronic airflow limitation.* Copenhagen: WHO Regional Office for Europe, 1982.

Helsing KJ, Comstock GW, Speizer FE et al. Comparison of three standardized questionnaires on respiratory symptoms. *Am Rev Respir Dis* 1979; **120**: 1221–1231.

Hunt SM. The problem of quality of life. *Qual Life Res* 1997; **6**: 205–212.
Sackett DL. Bias in analytic research. *J Chron Dis* 1979; **32**: 51–63.
Silman AJ, Macfarlane GJ. *Epidemiological studies. A practical guide*, 2nd ed. Cambridge, UK: Cambridge University Press, 2002.
Toelle BG, Peat JK, Salome CM et al. Toward a definition of asthma for epidemiology. *Am Rev Respir Dis* 1992; **146**: 633–637.
Usherwood T. *Introduction to project management in health research. A guide for new researchers.* Buckingham: Open University Press, 1996.

PART 2

Physiology and Measurement of Lung Function

CHAPTER 9

Thoracic Cage and Respiratory Muscles

The thoracic cage and associated muscles enclose and provide the power for moving the lungs. This chapter describes the main features and how they can be assessed.

9.1 Introduction

Inspiration. Expansion of the chest cage takes place as a result of upward and outward movement of the ribs and downward movement of the diaphragm; it is achieved by contraction of the intercostal muscles and the muscle of the diaphragm. The expansion of the thoracic cavity lowers the pressure at the pleural surface of the lung relative to that in the surrounding atmosphere; air then enters and expands the lung. The expansion is not uniform throughout the lung. In an upright posture when inspiration begins from functional residual capacity the expansion is predominantly at the lung bases but, when inspiration follows a full expiration, the expansion is initially greater at the apex than at the base. The movement is effected by the operation of gravitational force and elastic, resistive and inertial forces in the lung; these factors are discussed in subsequent pages.

Expiration. During the expiratory phase of the respiratory cycle, the inspiratory muscles relax and the intrapleural pressure becomes less negative with respect to atmospheric pressure. The elastic recoil of the lung tissue then compresses the alveolar gas and raises its pressure above that at the mouth. This change reverses the direction of gas flow. The process occurs passively without much assistance from the respiratory or accessory muscles of respiration but, even during quiet expiration, some intercostal muscles contract to a small extent. During vigorous breathing expiration is assisted by contraction of the abdominal muscles that raises the intra-abdominal pressure forcing the diaphragm upwards. Compression by the thorax can contribute when expiration begins from near total lung capacity or when the elbows are used to reduce the size of the rib cage. These changes increase the intrapleural pressure, which rises towards the atmospheric pressure and then exceeds it. High intrapleural pressure initially increases the rate of expiration but its continuation may hinder expiration by compressing the airways (Section 12.5.1).

Overall function. The thoracic cage functions as a unit that moves air with greater efficiency than might be predicted from the behaviour of the component structures [1–3]. Hence the findings from classical studies that consider each structure in isolation provide an incomplete picture of what occurs *in vivo.* Whole body studies and models are also needed [4, 5].

9.2 Ribs

Overview. Posteriorly the ribs articulate with the thoracic vertebrae. Anteriorly the upper six ribs articulate with the sternum, whilst the 7th to 10th ribs are joined to the costal cartilages; the 11th and 12th ribs have no anterior connections other than the soft tissue in the wall of the abdomen. The first ribs on both sides of the body move together about a transverse axis through the costovertebral joints; rotation about this axis increases the antero-posterior diameter of the thoracic inlet and raises the sternum. This movement is effected by the contraction of the scaleni and the sterno-cleido-mastoid muscles.

Ribs 2–6. The 2nd–6th ribs move about two axes that lie, respectively, in the transverse and antero-posterior planes of the body. However, a single axis of rotation can describe both movements. The axis is common to both sides of the thorax and passes through the necks of the ribs; movement about this axis increases the antero-posterior diameter of the thorax and raises the sternum. It has been likened to the movement of the handle of a farmyard pump. In females, due to greater mobility of the upper ribs, this movement is relatively larger than in males. The second axis of rotation of the ribs is separate for each side of the thorax and is through the angles of the ribs and the costosternal joints. Rotation about this axis causes an outward and upward movement of the middle part of the ribs and an increase in the transverse diameter of the thorax. This movement has been likened to that of the handle of a bucket.

Ribs 7–10. The 7th–10th ribs exhibit the bucket-handle motion since rotation about their antero-posterior axes causes widening of the thorax. However, they do not exhibit the pump-handle movement. Instead, a rotatory movement in the transverse plane depresses the sternum and reduces the antero-posterior diameter of the chest.

9.3 Intercostal muscles

The internal and external intercostal muscles form two incomplete layers between each rib and the one below. The function of the muscles during respiration has been deduced with the aid of electrodes placed either on the surface of the thorax or in the muscle. Bipolar needle electrodes are commonly used because the recordings are not affected by extraneous electrical activity from other tissues.

External intercostals. Most fibres of the external intercostal muscles (*intercostales externi*) are in the posterior regions of the intercostal spaces. At the back of the thorax the fibres pass obliquely downwards and laterally, and at the side of the thorax downwards, forwards and medially from each rib to the one below. They contract during inspiration and relax during expiration. During quiet breathing the time of relaxation coincides with the start of expiration but during vigorous breathing the time of relaxation is delayed; this has the effect of smoothing the transition between inspiration and expiration.

Internal intercostals. Most of the fibres of the internal intercostal muscles (*intercostales interna*) are in the anterior regions of the intercostal spaces where they pass obliquely downwards and backwards. The function of the fibres is determined by the incline of the structures to which they are attached. The interchondral or *parasternal intercostals* lie between the costal cartilages. Their fibres slope upwards, resembling those of the external intercostal muscles. Like them, they contract during inspiration and have an inspiratory function. The associated electrical activity (EMG) can be used to monitor inspiration. The interosseous fibres lie between the ribs where they slope downwards and forwards. When the lungs are moderately inflated these fibres contract during expiration and have an expiratory function. They also contract during speech.

Paralysis of the intercostal muscles reduces both the rigidity of the chest wall and the lateral bucket-handle movement of the ribs. The intercostal spaces are then flaccid, and exhibit paradoxical movement, inwards during the inspiratory phase and outwards during the expiratory phase of the respiratory cycle.

9.4 Muscles acting on the upper rib cage

The *scaleni* arise from the transverse processes of the lower five cervical vertebrae and are inserted into the first and second ribs. Those fibres that arise from the tips of the transverse processes constitute the *levator costae* muscles. Both sets of muscles are active during normal inspiration, to which they contribute by moving the sternum towards the head.

During vigorous breathing or as a prelude to expiratory manoeuvres such as sneezing, the inspiratory action of the diaphragm, scalene and intercostal muscles is supplemented by that of accessory muscles. The sterno-cleido-mastoid muscles arise from the mastoid processes and are inserted into the manubrium sterni and medial third of the clavicle. They become hypertrophied in patients with high tetraplegia. The *pectoralis major and minor* and the upper fibres of the *latissimus dorsi* can also have an inspiratory function. All these muscles act upon the chest cage from other parts of the skeleton and their effects are additive. Their effectiveness appears to be enhanced when the shoulder girdle is braced by the subject gripping a fixed object. For this reason a breathless patient may stand gripping a window sill or a banister on stairs. However, bracing also reduces ribcage stability and the subject merits further investigation [6]. The suction developed at the airway opening ($P\text{ao}$) by an accessory muscle is related to the mass of the muscle and its fractional change in length during passive inflation [7]. Hence,

$$P\text{ao} = m\delta[\Delta L/(L\Delta V\text{L})]_{\text{Rel}} \tag{9.1}$$

where m is the muscle mass, δ is the maximal muscle tension per unit cross-sectional area, $\Delta L/L$ is the fractional change in muscle length per unit volume increase of the relaxed chest wall $(\Delta V\text{L})_{\text{Rel}}$. Furthermore, where two muscles are active the effect on $P\text{ao}$ is essentially additive [7] though the relationship is not perfect as the length of the muscle depends on the configuration of the chest wall which, in turn, is influenced by the force developed by other muscles.

The triangularis sterni muscles connect the inner surfaces of the ribs to the sternum; they have an expiratory function during exercise or manoeuvres that entail expiration (for example sneezing).

9.5 Diaphragm

Functional anatomy. The muscles of the diaphragm arise from around the floor of the thoracic cavity, including the arcuate ligaments and crura, lower six ribs and the xyphoid process of the sternum. Medial and lateral arcuate ligaments bridge over the psoas major and quadratus lumborum muscles from insertions, respectively, over the body and transverse process of the first lumbar vertebra and the twelfth rib. A median arcuate ligament bridges over the aorta. From its origins the muscle fibres of the diaphragm pass upwards to converge on the central tendon, which mostly lies beneath and is attached to the pericardium. The inferior vena cava passes through the central tendon of the diaphragm whereas the oesophagus passes through the muscular portion. In this position the muscle acts as a sphincter and can prevent regurgitation of gastric contents [8].

The costal and crural fibres of the diaphragm receive their innervation via the phrenic nerve from, respectively, the upper and lower cervical segments of the spinal cord. When all the fibres of the diaphragm contract together the central tendon is pulled downwards. The movement resembles that of a piston with a rolling seal. It leads to an increase in depth of the thoracic cavity and an increase in pressure in the abdomen including that part which is enclosed within the lower ribs. The increased abdominal pressure acts on the visceral surface of the ribs to displace them outwards. Upward and outward movement of the ribs and eversion of the lower margin of the thorax also follows contraction of the costal fibres of the diaphragm in isolation. This movement is a consequence of the position that the fibres normally occupy and does not occur when the fibres are horizontal; it therefore does not occur when the diaphragm is flat, as in some cases of emphysema. In these circumstances a contraction of the muscle of the diaphragm reduces the transverse and possibly the posterior–anterior diameters of the lower margin of the thorax. In supine obese subjects a similar response occurs. Isolated contraction of the posterior crural fibres of the diaphragm is believed to displace the rib cage downwards but not to influence the thoracic diameter ([9], also Fig. 9.1).

The diaphragm contracts during inspiration and is relaxed throughout the greater part of expiration. During quiet breathing it is the principal muscle of inspiration; then its tidal excursion in adults is on average 1.5 cm. During deep breathing Wade [11] has shown that the excursion relative to the insertion of the diaphragm can be as much as 10 cm. This movement is responsible for about 75% of the volume of gas that is inhaled; the remaining 25% is attributable to movement of the ribs. Thus, total paralysis of the diaphragm greatly reduces the ability to ventilate the lungs but respiration can be maintained without it. Unilateral paralysis in subjects with normal lungs causes a reduction in the ventilatory capacity of about 20%; the decline is greater when the work of breathing is increased by disease of the lungs, pleura or thoracic cage. The paralysed half of the diaphragm moves paradoxically by rising in the thorax during inspiration and falling during expiration; the movement reflects the differences in pressure between the thorax and the abdomen during the two phases of the respiratory cycle. Unilateral paralysis of the diaphragm may be diagnosed by asking the subject to sniff during X-ray screening of the chest or during ultrasonography of the diaphragm.

The maximal pressure that can be developed by the diaphragm varies with lung volume; that during inspiration against a closed airway is greatest when the inspiratory manoeuvre is performed from near to residual volume (Fig. 9.2).

In the absence of muscular contraction the position of the diaphragm is determined by the pressure difference between the peritoneum and pleura and, hence, that between stomach and the thoracic oesophagus; the latter is designated ΔPdi. It is usually measured in the oesophagus with respect to atmospheric pressure (Section 9.9.3) and can be achieved by sniffing. The measurement can contribute to investigation of diaphragmatic weakness (Section 39.3.3).

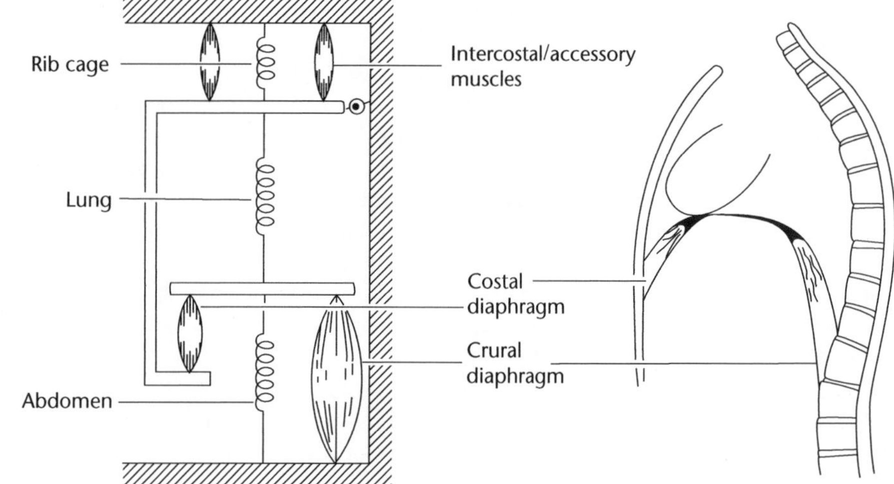

Fig. 9.1 Diagram that illustrates the respective actions of the costal and crural fibres of the diaphragm. The hatched area represents the vertebral column, the inverted L-shaped bar the rib cage, and the transverse bar the diaphragm; this is assumed to remain horizontal. The springs represent the elastic recoil of rib cage, lungs and diaphragm. Both parts of the muscle of the diaphragm depress the central tendon. The costal fibres elevate the rib cage and evert the lower costal margin. The crural fibres depress the rib cage through the mediation of lung elasticity. Source: Adapted from [10].

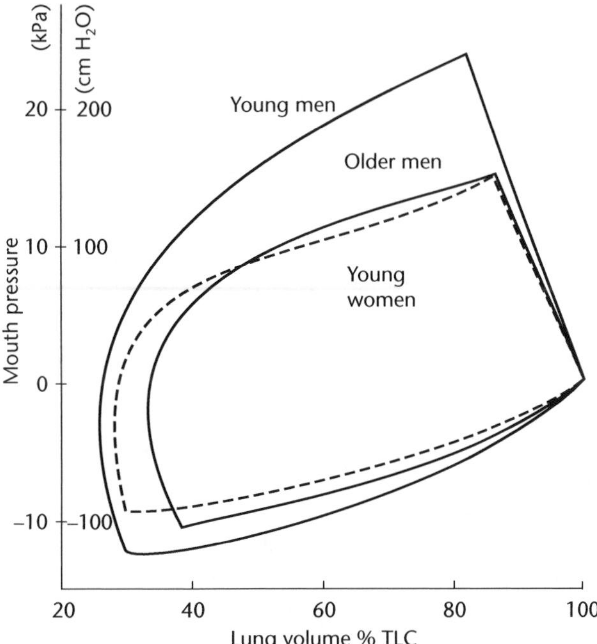

Fig. 9.2 Maximal volume–pressure loops showing the forces which can be developed by the respiratory muscles, including the accessory muscles, at different lung volumes. The data were for groups of subjects breathing with maximal effort into and out of air-tight containers of capacity 1.5–200 l. Source: [12].

Diaphragmatic fibre type and function. The diaphragm is a skeletal muscle that is adapted for both sustained and intense activities as are required during heavy exercise and during coughing and sneezing. As a result a relatively high proportion of the muscle fibres have an above average resistance to fatigue. The proportion has been estimated as 80%, comprising 55% type 1 and 25% type 2a fibres (described in Section 28.9.1) compared with approximately 40% in limb muscles [13]. This distribution results in relatively high mitochondrial density and associated maximal blood flow and capillary density. The oxidative capacity is relatively high in consequence [14]. Nevertheless, when it is over loaded, for example by maximal breathing for 2 min, the diaphragm is susceptible to fatigue [15]. This can be demonstrated by serial measurements of ΔPdi, max and by electromyography that shows a shift in the EMG frequency spectrum towards lower frequencies. In such studies the lung volume should be controlled [16]. The features of diaphragmatic weakness and a strategy and procedures for assessing diaphragmatic function are in Sections 9.9 and 41.8.

The proportions of the different fibre types is responsive to environmental factors. Ageing and malnutrition result in atrophy of type 1 fibres, leading to reduced endurance, and of type 2 fibres leading to reduced strength. Some chronic lung diseases, for example COPD, are associated with an increased work of breathing. This can cause work hypertrophy of the diaphragm and other respiratory muscles. However, the disease process can also cause hyperinflation that leads to the muscle fibres operating at below their optimum length. These two sets of changes are in opposition to each other and, depending on circumstances one or other will be dominant [17, 18].

Muscle training for strength and endurance can improve the function of the diaphragm and other respiratory muscles [19]; however, the optimal response is usually obtained only when breathing exercises are combined with other forms of training ([20, 21], Section 44.4).

9.6 Abdominal muscles

The abdominal muscles support and protect the abdominal contents and contribute to movement of the trunk. In appropriate circumstances they can contribute to all phases of respiration.

Expiratory function. This has two components. Firstly, contraction of fibres that arise from or are inserted into the lower ribs or costal cartilages reduces the anterio-posterior and transverse diameters of the thorax. Secondly, a rise in intra-abdominal pressure displaces the central tendon of the diaphragm in a cranial direction. These functions are apparent when breathing is increased by exercise or forced expiration. In adults once the minute volume exceeds approximately 40 l min^{-1} contraction of these muscles occurs towards the end of expiration. During maximal breathing it occurs throughout expiration. The muscles are also active during the expiratory efforts that are associated with phonation, coughing and sneezing.

The principal expiratory muscle is transversus abdominis [4, 22], with assistance from the internal oblique and rectus abdominus muscles. The latter occupies the medial half of the anterior abdominal wall and contributes to sitting up from a supine position. The external oblique muscle contributes to rotational movements but does not contribute to respiration in man.

Stabilising the chest wall. As well as causing expiration the abdominal muscles appear to have a subsidiary role of stabilising the rib cage or even causing some degree of chest expansion. Thus in the dog, De Troyer found that isolated stimulation of the external oblique muscle expanded the lower ribs. Stimulation of the internal oblique and transversus abdominus muscles did not influence the position of the ribs. In man, on account of the different configuration of the thorax, the abdominal muscles have two actions that are to some extent in opposition. The main action is to promote expiration by pulling down and deflating the lower part of the rib cage, but at the same time the rise in intra-abdominal pressure passively stretches the diaphragm and this tends to expand the lower part of the chest wall [23].

Contribution to inspiration. During inspiration the abdominal muscles contribute to the function of the diaphragm by raising the intra-abdominal pressure. This causes cranial displacement of the central tendon which, in turn, lengthens the muscle fibres of the diaphragm and increases their force of contraction. The additional contraction has the effect of everting the lower costal margin. This synergistic action of the abdominal muscles has been demonstrated on changing from a supine to an upright posture, during exercise, voluntary hyperventilation and when the chemical drive to ventilation is increased [24].

9.7 Pulmonary energetics

9.7.1 Mechanical work done in breathing (work of breathing)

The mechanical work done in ventilating the lungs is expressed over a whole breathing cycle comprising inspiration and expiration. It has three components associated, respectively, with expanding the lungs with its enclosing structures and overcoming the inertia and resistance to movement of the lungs, chest wall and abdomen (see Chapter 14). The work done in overcoming the elastic recoil of the lungs and chest wall operates only during inspiration (Section 11.2). The recoil varies with lung volume and the associated component of the overall pressure can be separated from the resistive and inertial components by considering the pressure across the relevant structures when the lungs are stationary and the muscles relaxed. (Fig. 11.3, page 120). The resulting work can be represented by a similar diagram for a whole breathing cycle (Fig. 9.3).

Over a small range of volumes above functional residual capacity the static compliance of the lungs is represented by the slope of the diagonal ABC. Also shown is the corresponding static recoil relationship for the chest wall, which at functional residual capacity, is of equal magnitude but of opposite sign to that for the lung. The two relationships intersect at FRC, which is indicated by the point A. During inspiration the work that is done by the inspiratory muscles in overcoming the elastic recoil of the lungs and chest wall is represented by the triangle ACD; it includes a component from the chest wall which assists lung expansion at small lung volumes but opposes it at larger volume. These are represented by the areas AE0 and EGD. The energy is stored in the stretched tissues. Additional inspiratory work is done in overcoming the resistance and inertia of the lung and thorax. The resistive components are illustrated in the diagram. During expiration the energy that is stored in the distended lung is used in part to overcome the forces that resist expiration, including the resistance of the airways and lung tissue. This work is represented by the area C Exp.AC. Some of the stored energy is also used to overcome the resistance of the chest wall and the remainder is dissipated as heat.

The total work done on the lungs by the inspiratory muscles is represented by the area A Insp.CZA. This quantity has been found to be a linear function of the hypercapnoeic drive to respiration [26]. However, the total work, i.e. that represented by the area A Insp CDFA, cannot easily be measured except when the force is applied externally to a subject in whom the respiratory muscles are paralysed; the results do not then apply to spontaneous breathing. The limiting condition within which the Campbell diagram operates is the maximal volume–pressure curve for the lung (Fig. 9.2). The method provides a reasonably accurate estimate of the work of breathing at rest, but during exercise on account of distortion of the chest wall the work may be underestimated by up to 25% [27].

9.7.2 Physiological cost of breathing

Circulatory cost. The fuel for respiratory work is delivered to the muscles by the circulation. Most of the delivery is to the diaphragm except when expiration is obstructed and then more blood flow goes to the expiratory muscles. The diaphragmatic blood flow varies with the rate of respiratory work and is normally in the range 0.08–0.33 ml g^{-1} min^{-1}. Higher flows are

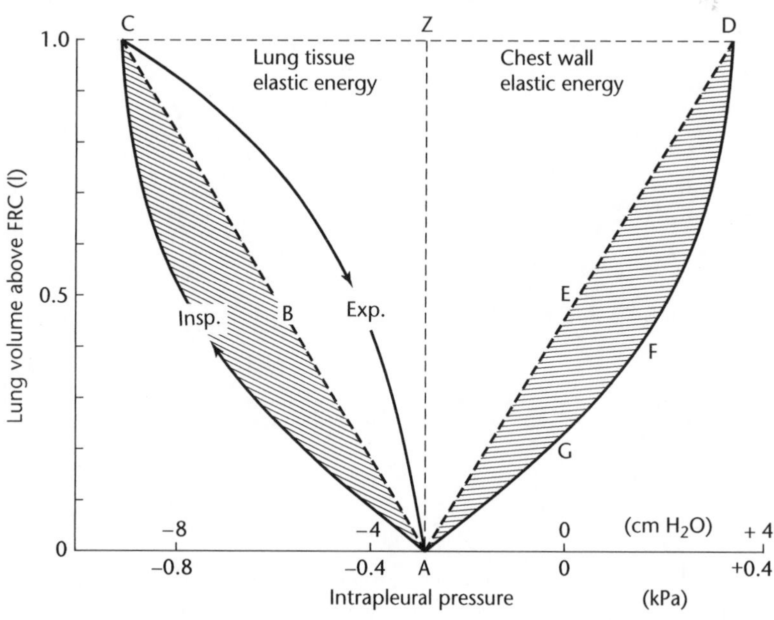

Fig. 9.3 Diagram (after Campbell) illustrating the relationship of the lung volume above functional residual capacity to the intrapleural pressure during quiet breathing. The slopes of the lines AC and AD represent the static compliance, respectively, of the lung and of the chest wall. These data may be obtained in the manner indicated in the caption to Fig. 11.3 (page 120). The hatched areas represent work done during inspiration in overcoming resistance of the airways (oblique hatching) and chest wall (horizontal hatching). The use of the diagram to calculate the total work done by the inspiratory muscles is described in the text. Source: [25].

observed if inspiration is obstructed. The diaphragmatic blood flow is well preserved during conditions of low cardiac output including shock when the flow may exceed 20% of cardiac output. The blood flow sustains the aerobic oxidation of carbohydrate and free fatty acids. Rapid glycolysis seldom occurs except when the diaphragm is driven by external phrenic nerve stimulation.

Oxygen cost. The oxygen consumed by the respiratory muscles is normally only a small proportion of total oxygen consumption so it is difficult to measure accurately in man. One method applied in ventilated patients has been to measure the drop in oxygen uptake as a result of intermittent positive pressure ventilation being switched on. Another has been to measure the increase in oxygen consumption above resting that occurs when the ventilation is increased, for example by voluntary hyperventilation, use of an external dead space, or by adding carbon dioxide to the inspired gas. The method is described in Section 7.8.1. In normal subjects under quiet resting conditions the oxygen cost of breathing is approximately 5–10 ml min^{-1} (0.25–0.5 mmol min^{-1}) and the cost per litre of ventilation is proportionately less. The quantity represents about 2% of total oxygen consumption (1–3% of the total). The cost is doubled at a ventilation minute volume of 40 l min^{-1} and is materially higher during strenuous exercise (Fig. 9.4). In patients with lung diseases requiring artificial ventilation the average has been reported as 75 ml min^{-1} (range 8–286) accounting for 24% of total oxygen consumption [28, 29].

A situation can then arise when a further increase in ventilation requires the consumption of more additional oxygen than enters the pulmonary capillary blood as a result of the extra ventilation. This can occur during maximal exercise or at rest if the work of breathing is greatly increased by obstruction to the airways. The energy cost of breathing is also high in patients with pulmonary fibrosis and in obese subjects in whom there is increased resistance to movement of the thoracic cage and abdomen and/or increased inertia. In all these circumstances an increase in the work of breathing can limit exercise and precipitate respiratory failure [30, 31].

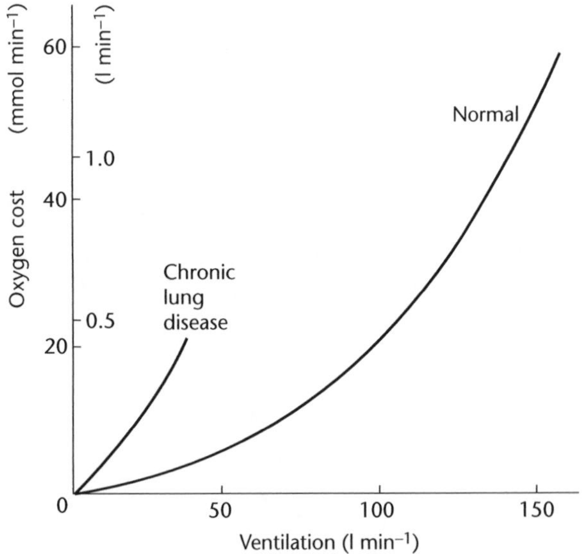

Fig. 9.4 The approximate oxygen cost of breathing in a healthy man and in a patient with severe lung disease Source: [28].

9.8 Constraints on contraction of respiratory muscles

In health. In an upright posture the responses of the chest wall and lungs to contraction of the respiratory muscles are normally symmetrical and unconstrained. In a prone or supine posture the lung volume at functional residual capacity is reduced on account of the mass of the thorax opposing the normal elasticity of the chest cage. The effect on the respiratory muscles is small for static contraction and the inspiratory capacity is increased by a nearly proportional amount (Section 10.2). Gas exchange is, if anything, improved in a prone position (and to a lesser extent a supine position) because in this posture the vertical gradient of gravitational force down the lungs is relatively small (Section 17.1.3). However, the posture may affect the dynamic force that the muscles can exert.

In a lateral decubitus position the expansion of the lower hemithorax is diminished. However, the blood flow is redistributed to the dependent lung and, on account of compensatory mechanisms (Section 18.1.1), the ventilation tends to follow the blood flow. As a result the effect on gas exchange is relatively small [32].

Differential expansion of the upper and lower parts of the chest wall can also be achieved voluntarily by adopting an upper thoracic or abdominal style of breathing. These differences are transmitted to the lung [33].

In disease. The respiratory muscles respond to a reduction in the distensibility of the lungs with a corresponding reduction in lung expansion. The changes may be local as with extensive localised apical tuberculosis or pleural disease, or generalised where there is diffuse airways obstruction [34] or interstitial fibrosis. In all these circumstances the function of the muscles is preserved. By contrast, when the bases of the lungs are inflated by air trapping or emphysema the diaphragm becomes flattened and its mechanical function is impaired. Respiration is then more dependent on the intercostal and accessory muscles of inspiration. The diaphragm adapts by shortening through losing sarcomeres and this goes some way to preserving its ability to generate force [35]. In addition, expiration becomes an active process to which the abdominal muscles make a material contribution [35, 36].

In anklyosing spondylitis the costo-vertebral joints become inflamed and calcified. This reduces the mobility of the chest wall (Section 41.7). However, except when there is kyphoscoliosis the diaphragm performs normally and the functional defect is confined to mild restriction to expansion of the lungs [37]. With kyphoscoloisis the inspiratory function of the respiratory

Table 9.1 Procedures that can throw light on the function of respiratory muscles.

Aspect	Principal techniques	Comment
Overall respiratory function	Lung function and exercise tests	Results need to be looked at from this point of view
Respiratory muscle strength	Measurement of maximal pressure including after sniff and phrenic nerve stimulation	Practicable in most lung function laboratories
Electromyography and related tests	Graphic and audible recording from respiratory muscles	Requires special training. Can assess muscle function
Respiratory muscle endurance	Incremental ventilation and loading tests	More data are needed
Respiratory muscle fatigue	Ability to generate pressure after successive periods of stimulation	Can be used to monitor therapy
Function of chest wall	Relationships between movement of chest wall and changes in volume and pressure	Mainly basic physiology. Few applications so far
Muscle imaging	Visual and ultrasound images of diaphragm and accessory muscles of respiration	Used in research
Control mechanisms	See Chapter 23	

Source: Adapted from [45].

muscles is impaired and the work of breathing is increased [38, 39]. This combination predisposes to ventilatory failure [40] (also Section 41.7). In Parkinson's disease the skeletal muscles become rigid and patients experience difficulty in performing repetitive tasks such as walking and breathing [41]. The strength and endurance of the respiratory muscles are impaired. There can also be obstruction to the upper airways. The changes can cause breathlessness on exertion [31, 42]. The condition is ameliorated by treatment (Section 41.8.5).

9.9 Impaired function of respiratory muscles

9.9.1 Weakness of respiratory muscles

Causes. Weakness of respiratory muscles can occur on account of mechanical derangement (as in kyphoscoliosis or hyperinflation), in association with a critical or chronic illness (the latter leading to muscle wasting and disuse atrophy) and as a result of a neurological or muscular disorder (Footnote 9.1)

Consequences. Weakness of inspiratory muscles reduces the inspiratory capacity and weakness of expiratory muscles can reduce the expiratory reserve volume. Hence, on both accounts the vital capacity and total lung capacity are reduced. The reduction in TLC has the incidental consequence of reducing the transfer factor and hence increasing the transfer factor per litre of lung volume (Tl/V_A also called K_{CO}) [43]. Consideration of K_{CO} as an index of gas exchange should take account of the loss of lung volume (Section 20.9.1). The diminution in vital capacity on moving from an upright to supine posture is enhanced [44]. In addition the ventilatory capacity is reduced; this affects the capacity for exercise (Section 28.8.1). By the time the reduction has reached 30% the patient is likely to have sought medical advice. There is progressive hypoxaemia and aggravation of any tendency to sleep apnoea. If the reduction in vital capacity exceeds 50% then hypoventilation is likely with hypercapnia and a poor prognosis.

Depending on circumstances weakness of respiratory muscles may respond to physical training, including strength and endurance training and general exercises. The need for training can be assessed by testing respiratory muscle function and some of the same procedures are also used to monitor progress. In view of the prospect of making a material difference to the quality of life of some respiratory patients the procedures are currently being used to an increasing extent in pulmonary function laboratories (Section 44.4).

9.9.2 Identification of abnormal function of respiratory muscles

The principal attributes for investigation are loss of muscle strength, impaired endurance and fatigue. Their relevance for an individual patient arises from the symptoms and clinical features, and the decision to look for abnormality in this branch of respiratory function requires a high level of clinical suspicion. The process is best undertaken in stages (Table 9.1).

Footnote 9.1. Some neurological and muscular causes of weakness of respiratory muscles: cerebral causes (e.g. hemiplegia), spinal cord lesions (e.g. multiple sclerosis), damage to anterior horn cells (e.g. motor neurone disease), phrenic nerve lesion (e.g. polyneuritis), blocked neuro-muscular junction (curare, myasthenia gravis), impaired muscle function (e.g. metabolic or electrolyte disorder). Additional causes are given in Chapter 41, especially Section 41.8 and Sections 41.20 to 41.26.

Some options, e.g. assessment of the components of overall lung function and the response to exercise, may have been explored prior to attention becoming focused on the respiratory muscles. The others, with the possible exception of electrophysiological and imaging techniques, are within the scope of most lung function laboratories.

9.9.3 Assessment of loss of muscle strength

Measurement of pressure. The force generated by contraction of respiratory muscles is applied to the lungs and thoracic cage where it generates both pressure and movement in variable proportions. The proportions depend on the local geometry, the elasticity of the lungs and chest wall, and the inertia and resistance to movement of the structures that are moved. The force cannot be measured directly and the closest surrogate is to measure pressure across a relevant structure under defined conditions. Thus, the structures must be stationary, so there is no resistive or inertial component to the measurement and the volume should be specified as this goes some way towards standardising the effective length of the muscle. It also standardises for lung and chest wall elasticity.

The sites of pressure measurement include the nose, mouth (hence alveolar pressure), oesophagus (hence pleural pressure) and stomach (subdiaphragmatic pressure). The methods for deriving alveolar pressure and oesophageal pressure, including the features and use of an oesophageal balloon are discussed in Sections 14.4 and 11.8.1. The mouth is also the site for measurement of maximal inspiratory and expiratory pressure for the respiratory muscles acting together. All these pressures are with respect to atmospheric pressure so inspiratory pressures are negative. As a result, weakness of inspiratory muscles *raises* the maximal inspiratory pressure (i.e. it becomes less negative), but the maximal suction is reduced. Thus, there is scope for confusion that is apparent in some publications. In the case of pressure change across the diaphragm between gastric and oesophageal pressures (Pdi) the response to contraction of the muscle is considered to be positive [45].

Pressure is measured using a transducer (Section 7.4). For the present applications it should have a resolution of 0.5 cm H_2O and a range of ± 200 cm H_2O, or their equivalents in SI units (0.05 and ± 20 kPa). The frequency response should exceed 10 Hz. For measurement of differential pressures (e.g. Pdi) a differential manometer can be used, but it is preferable to have a separate transducer for each site so the quality of the information can be assessed [45].

Maximal pressures can be generated by voluntary effort (as for maximal inspiratory or expiratory pressure), by maximal sniffing and by stimulation of one or both phrenic nerves when the contraction is nearly specific to the diaphragm.

Maximal inspiratory and expiratory pressures at the mouth. The subject should be seated and wear a nose clip. Connection with the equipment is via a mouthpiece with a flange that is inserted between the gum and the cheek. The mouthpiece leads into a short tube that is closed at the end. There is a side arm for connection to the pressure transducer and there should be a small leak (e.g. a tube of internal diameter 2 mm and length 25 mm) that allows movement of air into and out of the mouthpiece. The leak prevents the subject from closing the glottis on inspiration and relying on the muscles of the cheeks during expiration. Maximal expiratory pressure (PE,mo,max, MEP or PE,max) is measured during maximal expiratory effort from or near total lung capacity, whilst maximal inspiratory pressure (PI,mo,max, MIP or PI,max) is from residual volume or functional residual capacity. One or more training sessions should be provided [46]. The training might lead to the subject using one or both hands to secure a good fit about the mouthpiece and avoiding using the muscles of the cheeks. The maximal effort should be for approximately 1.5 s. Maximal encouragement should be given (cf. Fig. 12.5, page 138). The measurement is the maximal sustained pressure over 1 s and the result is the maximal value from 3 determinations that agree to within 20% [45]. The result is compared with reference values that can take into account age, stature, sex and body mass (Section 26.2). Fat-free mass can also be used where it is available (Section 4.7.1).

In clinical practice a value for PI,mo,max that does not reach -80 cm H_2O (-8 kPa) is likely to be abnormal. If the PE,mo,max is normal this suggests isolated diaphragmatic weakness. In other circumstances an apparently abnormal result may reflect a flat diaphragm from any cause (Section 9.8) or be an indication for further investigations. In the case of serial measurements for differences to be meaningful they should exceed 20% ([45], also Section 15.7.2).

The PE, mo, max is mainly due to active contraction of the transversus abdominis muscle. This can be elicited by voluntary effort or by coughing. The resulting rise in abdominal pressure can be monitored by measurement of intragastric pressure (see below). In addition, features of the contraction can be explored by electromyography using surface electrodes.

Measurement of mouth pressure has the limitations that not all subjects can exert a maximal effort. In this circumstance a sniff or stimulation of one or both phrenic nerves may be appropriate [47]. When this is done the mouth pressure may not be a reliable guide to the resulting twitch pressure [48].

Weakness of the diaphragm. The diaphragm is a relatively accessible muscle to study on account of contracting in response to a sniff or to stimulation of one or both phrenic nerves in the neck. In addition, its force of contraction can be monitored by measurement of Pdi. This is the difference between two measurements of pressure made simultaneously below and above the diaphragm. The techniques can also be used to assess loss of endurance and fatigue (Sections 9.9.4 and 9.9.5).

Pressure below the diaphragm is measured as intragastric pressure. This is monitored by a pressure transducer connected to a catheter that is passed into the stomach from the nose (Section 11.8.1). The same techniques and equipment are used for intraoesophageal pressure. However, recent advances in instrumentation have led to replacement of conventional transducers with miniaturised versions placed in the tips of the catheters [49]. The properties of the two transducers should be identical. The *P*di is best obtained by electronic subtraction (see above).

Maximal contraction of the diaphragm is obtained by performing a maximal sniff manoeuvre or by *phrenic nerve stimulation* (PNS). In some circumstances the intranasal pressure during the sniff (*P*nas,sn) can also be used as a surrogate for oesophageal pressure [50]; this is particularly the case for studies on healthy subjects.

The sniff pressure (*P*nas,sn) is obtained after lodging a catheter connected to a transducer into one of the two nares; both nares should be patent. A reasonably airtight seal should be made in whatever manner seems appropriate. The pressure should be monitored from a side hole below the catheter tip. The subject will usually sit and perform the sniffs starting from the end of a normal expiration. In normal circumstances a series of some 5–10 maximal sniffs will be undertaken by which time the resulting pressures will usually have reached a plateau. The method is dependent on the cooperation of the subject and can yield submaximal values in COPD due to airway narrowing. In this event the pressure can be measured in the oesophagus (*P*oes,sn). Where the conditions are met a suction <70 cm H_2O (7.0 kPa) is usually evidence for diaphragmatic weakness. However, the diagnosis is more secure when the procedure is combined with PNS (see below) [51].

PNS is used to achieve controlled supra-maximal contraction of one or both diaphragms. The stimulus can be an electric current or a magnetic stimulus that creates an electric field in the vicinity of the nerve; the abbreviation PNS is usually reserved for the electric current. It is applied to the neck via small electrodes. Where the electrodes are monopolar, one is applied to the skin below the clavicle. The other is applied to the phrenic nerve where it lies below the posterior border of the sternocleidomastoid muscle at the level of the cricoid cartilage. With bipolar electrodes both are applied at this site. The resulting contraction is then confined to the diaphragm but finding the correct location can be more difficult. For maximal contraction the shock is in the range 30–50 mA and the duration 0.1 ms. Specific contra-indication to all forms of PNS include the presence of metal objects anywhere in the body, and the wearing of a cardiac pacemaker. Ear protectors can be used.

An alternative stimulus for PNS is cervical magnetic stimulation (CMS). The subject is usually seated, but a recumbent position can be used [52]. Depending on the posture, the active site is in the vicinity of the 7th cervical vertebra or at the side of the neck. The procedure is relatively painless but less specific to the diaphragm than with electrical stimulation; this can lead to the resulting twitch contraction being stronger [53]. When the twitch pressure is measured at the mouth (*P*mo,tw) a suction of less than 10 cm H_2O, especially when combined with an abnormal *P*nas,sn, is highly suggestive of impaired diaphragmatic function (reference [54] reviews the subject). The procedure can be combined with intra-oesophageal electromyography; this gives a better signal compared with using surface electrodes [55]. However, any electromyogram record (EMG) should be obtained using equipment that is tolerant of the procedure. In addition, information stored by electromagnetic means should be kept out of the magnetic field.

Some features of respiratory muscle weakness are summarised in Table 9.2.

9.9.4 Assessment of respiratory muscle endurance

Maximal sustained or incremental ventilation. The maximal ability of the respiratory muscles to deliver output over time varies inversely with the load. This is a feature common to all skeletal muscles. The rate at which the performance declines provides a measure of the endurance. It is most easily assessed in terms of ability to sustain maximal ventilation. The base line is the maximal voluntary ventilation (MVV). The index is measured

Table 9.2 Summary of principal features of respiratory muscle weakness.

Measurement	Technique	Abnormal result
Symptoms, physical signs and related investigations	Clinical	Abnormal features
Vital capacity	Spirometry	>30% reduction from sitting to supine
Maximal inspiratory pressure at mouth (P_{I}.mo,max)	Suction against shutter	<–8 kPa (–80 cm H_2O)
Nasopharyngeal pressure (P_I,nas,sn)	Nasal probe	<–6 kPa (–60 cm H_2O)
Oesophageal pressure (P_I,oes,sn)	Oesophageal catheter	
Transdiaphragmatic pressure (*P*di,sn) (*P*di,tw)	Gastric and either nasal or oesophageal catheters Cervical magnetic stimulation	Men <1.0 kPa (10 cm H_2O) Women <0.7 kPa (7 cm H_2O)*
Phrenic nerve conduction time	EMG	>9.5 ms

*Pressures with respect to that above diaphram (see text).

over 12 s and expressed in l min^{-1} (Section 12.2). The simplest procedure is to measure the decline that occurs when maximal breathing is sustained for 4 min (4 min MVV). The procedure can be standardised by measuring the time for which the subject can maintain a ventilation equal to 80% of the 12 s MVV [56, 57]. However, the acceptability is low. It can be improved by measuring the time for progressively increasing levels of ventilation starting at 20% of MVV, then increasing the ventilation by 10% every third minute [58]. The method has the advantages of simplicity and assessing expiration as well as inspiration, but the result is influenced by the mechanical properties of the lungs and chest wall as well as by the endurance [45].

Other tests. In a research context, procedures for assessing endurance can be based on output variables other than ventilation (e.g. respiratory work) and on tasks other than ventilation. The output variables can include the ability to sustain a given pressure or flow pattern in a variety of circumstances [59]. The tasks can include breathing against a partially obstructed external airway, for example a narrow tube (resistance), an elastic hindrance such as breathing from a closed container, or a threshold load comprising a valve with finite opening pressure.

9.9.5 Assessment of respiratory muscle fatigue

Fatigue is usually considered to be present when the performance of a muscle declines as a consequence of a task being repeated a number of times during a session and then recovers afterwards. This definition does not allow for the possible existence of chronic fatigue. Central fatigue is due to a reduction in respiratory drive, alternatively there is some degree of central inhibition to breathing. Peripheral fatigue reflects loss of function at or peripheral to the neuromuscular junctions and can be of a high or low frequency type. In high frequency fatigue there is a reduction in the force generated in response to high frequency stimulation of the muscle (frequencies in the range 50–100 Hz). The commonest immediate cause is a reduction in transmission of signals across neuromuscular junctions. High frequency fatigue induced by stimulation of a phrenic nerve has been observed to recover rapidly [60]. Low frequency fatigue is loss of force generation in response to stimulation at a low frequency, in the range 1–20 Hz. It reflects a diminution in the contractile process in the muscle, such as that which occurs as a result of sustained maximal voluntary ventilation [15]. Unlike central and peripheral high frequency fatigue the recovery from low frequency fatigue takes a finite time (minutes or hours rather than seconds). The condition is usually associated with a rather shallow, rapid pattern of breathing and a variable distribution of inspiration as between its thoracic and abdominal components. These features can be observed in patients but are not diagnostic.

Fatigue can be represented as occurring as a consequence of repeated application of a load above a threshold load that can be applied repeatedly without fatigue. The threshold varies inversely with the time for which the load is applied. This has led to the concept of a pressure–time index that can be for the rib cage muscles (rc) or the diaphragm (di). The corresponding pressures are pleural pressure (Ppl) and trans-diaphragmatic pressure (Pdi), where the pressure is obtained as described above (Section 9.9.3). Then, for the diaphragm:

$$\text{Pressure–time index } (P\text{tdi}) = (P\text{di}/P\text{di,max})(\text{T}_\text{I}/\text{T}_\text{TOT})$$

where the right-hand term is time of inspiration as a fraction of breath duration. The corresponding index for rib cage muscles is obtained by substitution. The threshold for fatigue varies with the muscle group and is normally in the range 0.15–0.3 [61]. The threshold in patients appears not to have been established.

Fatigue can be assessed in terms of the ability to repeatedly generate a pressure. To do this voluntarily requires a high level of participation by the subject that may not be a realistic expectation. The pressure can also be generated by muscle stimulation but repeated stimulations can be disagreeable.

Fatigued muscles relax relatively slowly, so comparison of the inspiratory muscle relaxation rate before and after induction of fatigue can provide useful information. The relaxation rate is the decline in pressure following a sniff or other form of muscle contraction. The rate can be with respect to the pressure fall in 10 ms or be expressed as a time constant (Section 20.9.1). The rate is slowed in COPD [62]. However, interpretation of the test is not straightforward. In a research setting a more certain result can be obtained from measurement of the pressures generated in response to electrical or magnetic stimulation of the muscle (e.g. [16] and [45]). The subject has been reviewed [45].

9.10 References

1. De Troyer A, Cappello M, Meurant N, Scillia P. Synergism between the canine left and right hemidiaphragms. *J Appl Physiol* 2003; **94**: 1757–1765.
2. De Troyer A. Interaction between the canine diaphragm and intercostal muscles in lung expansion. *J Appl Physiol* 2005; **98**: 795–803.
3. Cappello M, De Troyer A. Role of rib cage elastance in the coupling between the abdominal muscles and the lung. *J Appl Physiol* 2004; **97**: 85–90.
4. Misuri G, Colagrande S, Gorini M et al. *In vivo* ultrasound assessment of respiratory function of abdominal muscles in normal subjects. *Eur J Physiol* 1997; **10**: 2861–2867.
5. Wilson TA, De Troyer A. The two mechanisms of intercostal muscle action on the lung. *J Appl Physiol* 2004; **96**: 463–468.
6. Prandi E, CoutureJ, Bellemare F. In normal subjects bracing impairs the function of the inspiratory muscles. *Eur Respir J* 1999; **13**: 1078–1085.
7. Legrand A, Wilson TA, De Troyer A. Rib cage muscle interaction in airway pressure generation. *J Appl Physiol* 1998; **85**: 198–203.
8. Pickering M, Jones JF. The diaphragm: two physiological muscles in one. *J Anat* 2002; **201**: 305–312.
9. De Troyer A, Estenne M. Functional anatomy of the respiratory muscles. *Clin Chest Med* 1988; **9**: 175–193.
10. Macklem PT, Macklem DM, De Troyer A. A model of inspiratory muscle mechanics. *J Appl Physiol* 1983; **55**: 547–557.

11. Wade OL. Movements of thoracic cage and diaphragm in respiration. *J Physiol (Lond)* 1954; **124**: 193–212.
12. Cook CD, Mead J, Orzalesi MM. Static volume–pressure characteristics of the respiratory system during maximal efforts. *J Appl Physiol* 1964; **19**: 1016–1022.
13. Rochester DF. The diaphragm: contractile properties and fatigue. *J Clin Invest* 1985; **75**: 1397–1402.
14. Edwards RHT, Faulkner JA. Structure and function of the respiratory muscles. In: Roussos C, Macklem PT, eds. *The Thorax*, Part A. New York: Marcel Dekker, 1986: 297–326.
15. Hamnegard CH, Wragg S, Kyroussis D et al. Diaphragm fatigue following maximal ventilation in man. *Eur Respir J* 1996; **9**: 241–247.
16. Polkey MI, Kyroussis D, Hamnegard C-H et al. Paired phrenic nerve stimuli for the detection of diaphragm fatigue in humans. *Eur Respir J* 1997; **10**: 1859–1864.
17. Similowski T, Yan S, Gauthier AP et al. Contractile properties of the human diaphragm during chronic hyperinflation. *N Engl J Med* 1991; **325**: 917–923.
18. De Troyer A. Effect of hyperinflation on the diaphragm. *Eur Respir J* 1997; **10**: 708–713.
19. Leith DE, Bradley M. Ventilatory muscle strength and endurance training. *J Appl Physiol* 1976; **41**: 508–516.
20. Smith K, Cook D, Guyatt GH et al. Respiratory muscle training in chronic airflow limitation: a meta analysis. *Am Rev Respir Dis* 1992; **145**: 533–539.
21. Salman GF, Mosier MC, Beasley BW, Calkins DR. Rehabilitation for patients with chronic obstructive pulmonry disease: meta-analysis of randomised control trials. *J Gen Intern Med* 2003; **18**: 213–221.
22. De Troyer A, Estenne M, Ninane V et al. Transversus abdominis muscle function in humans. *J Appl Physiol* 1990; **68**: 1010–1016.
23. De Troyer A, Sampson M, Sigirst S et al. How the abdominal muscles act on the rib cage. *J Appl Physiol* 1983; **54**: 465–469.
24. Martin J, De Troyer A. The behaviour of the abdominal muscles during inspiratory mechanical loading. *Respir Physiol* 1982; **50**: 63–73.
25. Campbell EJM, Agostini E, Newsom Davis J. *The respiratory muscles: mechanics and neural control.* London: Lloyd_Luke, 1970.
26. Milic-Emili J, Tyler JM. Relation between work output of respiratory muscles and end-tidal CO_2 tension. *J Appl Physiol* 1963; **18**: 497–504.
27. Goldman MD, Grimby G, Mead J. Mechanical work of breathing derived from rib cage and abdominal V-P partitioning. *J Appl Physiol* 1976; **41**: 752–763.
28. Cournand A, Richards DW, Bader RA et al. The oxygen cost of breathing. *Trans Assoc Am Physicians* 1954; **67**: 162–173.
29. Field S, Kelly SM, Macklem PT. The oxygen cost of breathing in patients with cardiorespiratory disease. *Am Rev Respir Dis* 1982; **126**: 9–13.
30. Roussos C, Campbell EJM. Respiratory muscle energetics. In: Macklem PT, Mead J, eds. *Handbook of physiology, Vol. 3: The respiratory system*, Part 1. Bethesda, MD: American Physiological Society, 1986: 481–509.
31. Aliverti A, Macklem PT. How and why is exercise limited in COPD? *Respiration* 2001; **68**: 229–239.
32. Bhuyan U, Peters AM, Gordon I et al. Effects of posture on the distribution of pulmonary ventilation and perfusion in children and adults. *Thorax* 1989; **44**: 480–484.
33. McCool FD, Loring SH, Mead J. Rib cage distortion during voluntary and involuntary breathing. *J Appl Physiol* 1985; **58**: 1703–1712.
34. Ringel ER, Loring SH, McFadden ER Jr, Ingram RH Jr. Chest wall configuration changes before and during acute obstructive episodes in asthma. *Am Rev Respir Dis* 1983; **128**: 607–610.
35. De Troyer A. Effect of hyperinflation on the diaphragm. *Eur Respir J* 1997; **10**: 708–713.
36. De Troyer A, Peche R, Yernault JC, Estenne M. Neck muscle activity in patients with severe chronic obstructive pulmonary disease. *Am J Respir Crit Care Med* 1994; **150**: 41–47.
37. Haslock I. Ankylosing spondylitis. *Baillieres Clin Rheumatol* 1993; **7**: 99–115.
38. Lisboa C, Morento R, Fava M et al. Inspiratory muscle function in patients with severe kyphoscoliosis. *Am Rev Respir Dis* 1985; **132**: 48–52.
39. Estenne M, Derom E, De Troyer A. Neck and abdominal muscle activity in patients with severe thoracic scoliosis. *Am J Respir Crit Care Med* 1998; **158**: 452–457.
40. Rochester DF. Respiratory muscles and ventilatory failure: 1993 perspective. *Am J Med Sci* 1993; **305**: 394–402.
41. Tzlepis GE, McCool FD, Friedman JH, Hoppin FG Jr. Respiratory muscle dysfunction in Parkinson's diseases. *Am Rev Respir Dis* 1988; **138**: 266–271.
42. Weiner P, Inzelberg R, Davidovich A et al. Respiratory muscle performance and the perception of dyspnoea in Parkinson's disease. *Can J Neurol Sci* 2002; **29**: 68–72.
43. Hart N, Cramer D, Ward SP et al. Effect of pattern and severity of respiratory muscle weakness on carbon monoxide gas transfer and lung volumes. *Eur Respir J* 2002; **20**: 996–1002.
44. Allen SM, Hunt B, Green M. Fall in vital capacity with posture. *Br J Dis Chest* 1985; **79**: 267–271.
45. American Thoracic Society and European Respiratory Society. ATS/ERS statement on respiratory muscle testing. *Am J Respir Crit Care Med* 2002; **166**: 518–624.
46. Smeltzer SC, Lavietes MH. Reliability of maximal respiratory pressures in multiple sclerosis. *Chest* 1999; **115**: 1546–1552.
47. Chaudri MB, Liu C, Watson L et al. Sniff nasal respiratory pressure as a marker of respiratory function in motor neurone disease. *Eur Respir J* 2000; **15**: 539–542.
48. Laghi F, Tobin MJ. Relationship between transdiaphragmatic and mouth twitch pressures at functional residual capacity. *Eur Respir J* 1997; **10**: 530–536.
49. Evans SA, Watson L, Cowley AJ et al. Normal range for transdiaphragmatic pressures during sniffs with catheter mounted transducers. *Thorax* 1993; **48**: 750–753.
50. Heritier F, Rahm F, Pasche P, Fitting JW. Sniff nasal inspiratory pressure. A noninvasive assessment of inspiratory muscle strength. *Am J Respir Crit Care Med* 1994; **150**: 1678–1683.
51. Hughes PD, Polkey MI, Kyroussis D et al. Measurement of sniff nasal and diaphragm twitch mouth pressure in patients. *Thorax* 1998; **53**: 96–100.
52. Polkey MI, Duguet A, Luo Y et al. Anterior magnetic phrenic nerve stimulation: laboratory and clinical evaluation. *Intensive Care Med* 2000; **26**: 1065–1075.
53. Mills GH, Kyroussis D, Hamnegard CH et al. Cervical magnetic stimulation of the phrenic nerves in bilateral diaphragm paralysis. *Am J Respir Crit Care Med* 1997; **155**: 1565–1569.

54. Man WD-C, Moxham J, Polkey MI. Magnetic stimulation for the measurement of respiratory and skeletal muscle function. *Eur Respir J* 2004; **24**: 846–860.
55. Luo YM, Harris ML, Lyall RA et al. Assessment of diaphragm paralysis with oesophageal electromyography and unilateral magnetic phrenic nerve stimulation. *Eur Respir J* 2000; **15**: 596–599.
56. Keens TG, Krastins IRB, Wannamaker EM et al. Ventilatory muscle endurance training in normal subjects and patients with cystic fibrosis. *Am Rev Respir Dis* 1977; **116**: 853–860.
57. Belman MJ, Mittman C. Ventilatory muscle training improves exercise capacity in chronic obstructive lung disease patients. *Am Rev Respir Dis* 1980; **121**: 273–280.
58. Mancini DM, Henson D, LaManca J, Levine S. Evidence of reduced respiratory muscle endurance in patients with heart failure . *J Am Coll Cardiol* 1994; **24**: 972–981.
59. Nickerson BG, Keens TG. Measuring ventilatory muscle endurance in humans as sustainable inspiratory pressure. *J Appl Physiol* 1982; **52**: 768–772.
60. Aubier M, Farkas G, De Troyer A et al. Detection of respiratory fatigue in man by phrenic stimulation. *J Appl Physiol* 1981; **50**: 538–544.
61. Zocchi L, Fitting JW, Majani U et al. Effect of pressure and timing of contraction on human rib cage muscle fatigue. *Am Rev Respir Dis* 1993; **147**: 857–864.
62. Kyroussis D, Polkey MI, Keilty SEJ et al. Exhaustive exercise slows inspiratory muscle relaxation rate in chronic obstructive pulmonary disease. *Am J Respir Crit Care Med* 1996; **153**: 787–793.

Further reading

Otis AB. The work of breathing. *Physiol Rev* 1954; **34**: 449–458.

Roussos Ch, ed. *The Thorax*, 2nd ed. New York: Marcel Dekker, 1995: 1405–1461.

CHAPTER 10

Lung Volumes

The size of the lung is conveniently described by the amounts of gas it contains at the end of a full inspiration, a normal expiration and a complete expiration. Measurement of these volumes was the first lung function test. This chapter describes present day procedures.

10.1 Definitions

The amounts of gas in the lungs at different levels of inflation are represented as volumes when they are single components and capacities when they comprise two or more components. They are normally defined for a subject seated in an upright posture wearing loose clothes so that the movement of the lungs is not restrained. The volumes can be represented on a spirogram (Fig. 10.1).

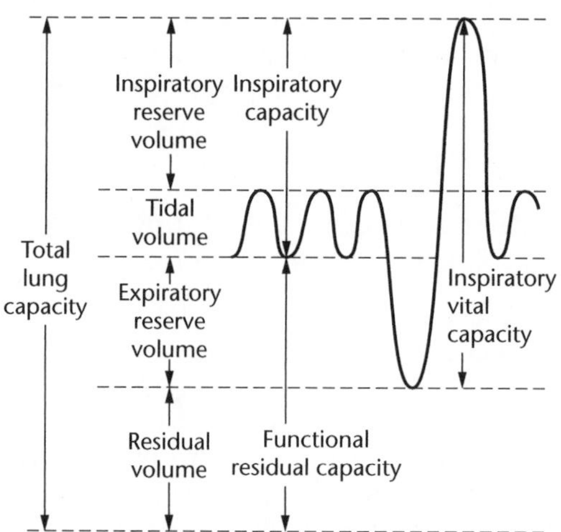

Fig. 10.1 Spirogram labelled to show the subdivisions of total lung capacity. Vital capacity is displayed as inspiratory vital capacity. Expiratory and two-stage vital capacity are defined in Section 10.1.2. The volumes are expressed in l BTPS (Section 6.5).

10.1.1 Total lung capacity and its subdivisions

Total lung capacity (TLC) is the maximal volume of air contained in the lungs at the end of a full inspiration. It has three principal and several subsidiary components; these are defined in terms of their relationships to normal tidal breathing and to full expiration.

Functional residual capacity (FRC) is the volume of air contained in the lungs at the end of a normal quiet expiration. It has two components: ERV and RV.

Expiratory reserve volume (ERV) is the volume of air that can be exhaled by a full expiration starting from FRC.

Residual volume (RV) is the volume of air remaining in the lungs at the end of a full expiration.

Inspiratory capacity (IC) is the maximal volume of air that can be inhaled from FRC. IC is the sum of *tidal volume* (Vt), where Vt is the volume inhaled and exhaled in each breath, and *inspiratory reserve volume* (IRV), where IRV is the maximal additional volume that can be inhaled prior to the subject attaining TLC.

10.1.2 Vital capacity and variants thereof

Vital capacity (VC) is the maximal volume of air that can be inhaled from RV (hence IVC) or exhaled from TLC (hence EVC). For the latter procedure, expiration is usually slow and relaxed (hence *relaxed* EVC). It may also be forced with maximal effort (hence *forced vital capacity*, FVC). In addition, the VC can be represented as the sum of IC and ERV obtained during separate inspiratory and expiratory manoeuvres from FRC; this estimate is designated as *two-stage vital capacity*.

In persons with healthy lungs the various procedures yield similar estimates of VC. However, in airway disease, on account of dynamic compression (Section 12.5.1), the FVC can be reduced compared with the other estimates.

10.1.3 Other volumes

Thoracic gas volume (TGV) is the volume of gas in the lungs under specified conditions. It is usually measured by whole body plethysmography, when it includes gas in any non-ventilated parts of the lung and that present in the abdomen.

Alveolar volume (V_A) is the total volume of gas available for exchanges with blood under the prevailing circumstances. It is expressed as lung volume less the volume of the conducting airways (anatomical dead space; Section 16.1.3). In practice, V_A usually refers to the volume at the end of a full inspiration and is measured as part of the determination of transfer factor by the single breath carbon monoxide method (Section 20.4).

Variants of FRC: These are described below.

10.2 Features of lung volumes

Orders of magnitude. Reasonable estimates for total lung capacity are 90 ml at birth, 1.5 l at age 7 years and 5.5–6.5 l in adult women and men, independent of age. There is wide variation depending on body size, ethnic group and other factors. Residual volume is approximately 25% of TLC in children and young adults, increasing to approximately 40% in old age; vital capacity decreases with age an amount in proportion to the rise in RV (Chapters 25, 26 and 27).

Some determinants: TLC. A position of full inspiration is reached when the maximal force developed by inspiratory muscles no longer exceeds the combined elastic recoil of the lungs and thoracic cage. The force is determined by anatomical factors (Sections 9.2 to 9.6), nutrition, and the extent to which the muscles are used (Section 28.12). The elastic recoil is reviewed in Chapter 11. The end-point of inspiration is influenced by the tension within the lung and is partly under reflex control.

FRC. The measurement is normally made with the subject seated and the respiratory muscles relaxed. The position of the chest wall is then the resting respiratory level at which the respiratory muscles are relaxed and the elastic recoil of the lungs and thoracic cage (including the diaphragm) are equal and opposite. This volume is sometimes called the *relaxation volume* (V_r) to distinguish it from when the respiratory muscles are not relaxed, for example during exercise or if there is material bronchial obstruction or obstruction to extra-thoracic airways. V_r is reduced during sleep (Section 32.4.4). The term *end-expiratory lung volume* (EELV) is also used [1]. EELV is reduced during exercise and increased when the subject is bronchoconstricted. Thus, the circumstances should be specified.

RV. The volume of gas at the end of a full expiration reflects a balance between the strength of the accessory muscles of expiration, the inherent compressibility of the rib cage and closure of airways; the last reflects insufficient traction by the stroma of the lung to keep the airways open (Section 11.4). In children and young adults the traction (elastic recoil) is high, and so expiration is limited by the extent to which the respiratory muscles can deform the chest wall [2]. The airways do not close (cf. Section 11.5.1). With increasing age the limiting factor becomes a diminution in elastic recoil; this leads to narrowing and eventually closure of some airways. As a result, RV increases with age.

Some external factors. Adoption of a supine posture reduces FRC by about 25% and increases IC by a nearly similar amount. The changes are due to elevation of the diaphragm by pressure from the lower ribs and abdominal contents, together with constraint on movement of the ribs. Additional displacement occurs in pregnancy (Section 25.8.2) and when abdominal fat is increased (Section 4.5, also Fig. 4.3, page 35). Posture has relatively little effect on TLC and RV. However, the posture influences the volume of blood in alveolar capillaries (V_c) via its effect on the distribution of blood as between the lungs, abdomen and lower limbs. The act of lying down materially increases V_c and reduces vital capacity by approximately 7% on this account. The change can be reversed by reducing the vascular pressure in the lungs relative to that in the legs through applying negative *g* in a human centrifuge.

Training of the muscles of the shoulder girdle increases IC and TLC whilst accumulation of body fat and muscle reduce ERV and hence FRC (see above, *also* [3]).

Diseases of the lung, including asthma, chronic obstructive pulmonary disease (COPD), emphysema and diffuse interstitial fibrosis, can profoundly affect the lung volumes (Table 10.1, *also* Chapter 40 and [4]).

10.3 Measurement of TLC and its subdivisions

Measurement of the lung volumes starts with spirometry. This gives vital capacity and the subdivisions IC and ERV but not residual volume or TLC. The second stage is the measurement of functional residual capacity from which residual volume can be obtained by subtraction of expiratory reserve volume. The FRC is measured by a closed or open circuit gas dilution method or by whole body plethysmography. Alternatively, TLC can be estimated using three-dimensional chest radiography.

The present methods are updated versions of those listed in Table 1.3 (page 8). They have been reviewed and revised on numerous occasions [5–11].

Table 10.1 Typical effects of mild generalised chronic lung diseases on lung volumes and forced expiratory flows.

	Underlying changes				Consequences		
	Elastic recoil	Respiratory muscles*	Airway smooth muscle	Epithelium	TLC	RV	Expiratory flow
Asthma	N or ↓†	Variable	Hypertrophy	Inflammation	N or ↑	↑	↓
COPD	N	Normal	Normal or +	Thickening‡	N	↑	↓
Emphysema	↓	Reduced	Normal	Normal	↑	↑↑	↓
Fibrosis	↑	§	Normal	§	↓	N or ↓	N or ↓

* Mechanical advantage under which respiratory muscles operate.
† Arrows indicate directions of deviations from normal (N).
‡ Compare Fig. 3.4 (page 26).
§ Variable depending on aetiology or circumstances.

10.3.1 Closed circuit gas dilution method

This method is recommended for routine measurement of lung volumes in patients other than those with communicable diseases. It has the additional merit of providing the laboratory with an accurate, self-contained method for calibrating gas analysers (Section 7.15).

Principle. The subject rebreathes from a closed circuit spirometer containing some helium or other indicator gas made up in 21% oxygen with the remainder gas nitrogen. During rebreathing the indicator mixes with the alveolar gas. The spirometer concentration falls, whilst the alveolar concentration rises until the two are equal. The dilution of the indicator reflects the ratio of the volume of the spirometer to that of the spirometer plus alveolar gas; if the spirometer volume is known, the alveolar volume can be calculated. Helium is commonly used as the indicator because the appropriate analyser (katharometer) is accurate, robust and cheap. The overall accuracy of the method is approximately 2% except in subjects with grossly impaired lung mixing. For such individuals the residual volume is likely to be underestimated compared with the plethysmographic method or by radiography; the error can be minimised in the manner described below.

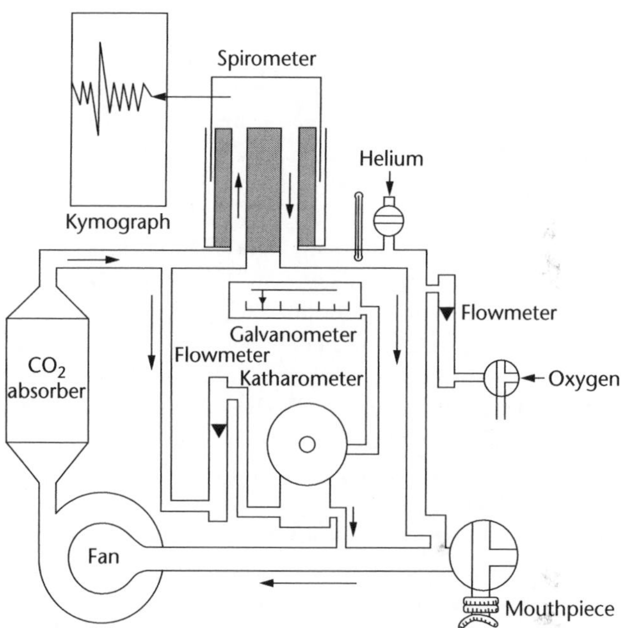

Fig. 10.2 Traditional closed-circuit apparatus for the measurement of total lung capacity and its subdivisions. The apparatus may be combined with that for measurement of transfer factor by the single breath (breath holding) method (Section 20.4.1).

Equipment. The method requires a katharometer or other appropriate analyser (see Table 7.6, page 65) and a spirometer of at least 8 l volume displacement [5]. This should record on a kymograph (paper speed 5 cm/min) or electronic recorder. The recording system should have a resolution of 25 ml. The breathing circuit is fitted with a soda lime canister for absorbing carbon dioxide. The canister should be mounted vertically to ensure uniform distribution of the granules and changed after every 20 determinations or when the CO_2 concentration in the circuit rises above 0.5%. A fan with an output of not less than 180 l min^{-1} (Fig. 10.2) secures both the mixing of the gases and a steady flow through the katharometer; the pressure in the mouthpiece should be atmospheric when the fan is running. This can be checked by having the mouthpiece open to air whilst the pump is running; the volume of gas in the circuit should remain constant. The temperature of the circulating gas should be recorded.

Testing for leaks. When setting up the apparatus the circuit should be tested for leaks. In the case of a water spirometer this is done by running the kymograph for 10 min, with the pump switched on, the mouthpiece occluded and a 2-kg weight placed on the bell. For a rolling seal spirometer a leak test may be undertaken in the closed system by placing sustained manual pressure on the recording arm on the kymograph and watching for a change in volume. For other systems, the stability of the helium concentration in the circuit is a good guide. To this end the mouthpiece should be closed, helium added to the circuit and the pump left running for 10 min. If there is outward leakage of gas, the source should be traced by application of soap solution to all joints and seals, including, if appropriate, the shaft of the pump, the rim of the soda lime canister and joins in the tubing. The fabric of the bell and tubing should be inspected and repaired or replaced if necessary.

Calibration. The checks should embrace the spirometer, the helium analyser and the dead space of the apparatus. Details are in Section 7.15.

Procedure. To measure functional residual capacity, the circuit is flushed with air and the spirometer bell set at an appropriate level, usually 2 l. Gas containing 80% helium and 20% oxygen is then added to raise the concentration of helium to near full-scale deflection on the katharometer. Meanwhile, the subject applies a nose clip, sits beside the apparatus and breathes air through the mouthpiece. At the end of a normal expiration, he or she is connected into the spirometer and rebreathes from the circuit. During rebreathing, oxygen is added at a rate that is adjusted to keep the volume at the end of expiration at a constant level; in some apparatus this is done automatically. The rate should be equal to the oxygen consumption of the subject, normally 0.2–0.25 l min^{-1}. The final adjustment should normally be made within the first minute of rebreathing. Any subsequent alteration will detract from the gaseous equilibrium within the spirometer–lung system. It may also conceal a change in end-expiratory level due to leakage at the mouth. During rebreathing the concentration of helium in the circuit falls at a steady but diminishing rate; this reflects gas mixing in the lung and a small loss of helium by solution in body fluid and passage into the stomach. Gas mixing is considered to have been achieved when the concentration does not change materially over 30 s. The acceptable fluctuations about the plateau value depend on the initial helium concentration. When this is 14% the plateau should be ±0.02%. This point is reached within 5 min in healthy subjects and up to 20 min in patients with emphysema.

Once equilibrium has been reached, the subject is asked to make a relaxed but full expiration to residual volume, and then return to normal tidal breathing. The manoeuvre is repeated twice. At this stage additional air may need to be introduced into the spirometer to ensure that the subject will be able to inspire fully from it. Three inspiratory vital capacity manoeuvres can then be made. For each of them the operator urges the subject to maximal expiratory and inspiratory effort. The resulting kymograph records, together with the initial and final helium concentrations, spirometer temperature, barometric pressure and apparatus dead space, provide the information for obtaining all the subdivisions of total lung capacity (Fig. 10.1). Except when automated equipment is used, the next stage is to measure the tracings.

In outline, functional residual capacity is given by:

$$\mathrm{FRC} = V(\mathrm{He}_1 - \mathrm{He}_2)/\mathrm{He}_2 \text{ l BTPS} \qquad (10.1)$$

where FRC is functional residual capacity, V is volume of gas in the circuit (both in l BTPS) and He_1 and He_2 are initial and final concentrations of helium. The latter is the concentration at the end of rebreathing except when no plateau has been reached. If this is due to an inadequate oxygen flow rate, the correct concentration can sometimes be estimated from the graph relating helium concentration to time by backward extrapolation of the curve to zero time. However, the procedure is not always reliable. Equation 10.1 neglects any displacement of the volume axis that may arise from the subject being switched into the breathing circuit at a volume other than FRC or from a change in resting respiratory level during rebreathing. The displacement can readily be allowed for (eqn. 10.2). In addition, a correction is needed because the gas in the spirometer is at ambient temperature and pressure (ATPS). For a spirometer temperature of t°C, a barometric pressure of P_B and a water vapour pressure at t°C of $P_{H_2O}(t)$, the functional residual capacity (l BTPS) may be calculated as follows:

$$\mathrm{FRC} = \left[\frac{[\mathrm{He}_1(V_1 + V\mathrm{ds})]}{[\mathrm{He}_2]} - (V_2 + V\mathrm{ds})\right] \times \frac{310}{(273 + t)} \times \frac{[P_B - P_{H_2O}(t)]}{[P_B - P_{H_2O}(37)]} \qquad (10.2)$$

where V_1 and V_2 are the volume of gas in the spirometer at switch in and at equilibrium and Vds is the dead space of the closed circuit apparatus. This and subsequent equations should be applied using the convention that within brackets, the procedures of multiplication and division precede those of addition and subtraction (Section 5.2.1).

A single measurement of FRC that is technically satisfactory is likely to have 95% confidence limits of ±0.4 l. The accuracy can be improved by repeating the measurement. In adults duplicates should agree to within 0.2 l [5, 6, 12].

Once FRC has been measured, the total lung capacity and its other subdivisions are obtained in the manner shown in Fig. 10.1. The largest technically acceptable value for IVC should be used. In the case of ERV there is ambivalence as to whether the largest [5] or the mean [6, 11] of several efforts should be used. The choice is important, as it will inevitably affect the estimate of RV and TLC. The most important estimate of ERV is likely to be the first one made after helium equilibrium (He_2) is reached. Then, other estimates should be judged against it and the resting end-expiratory position to determine their acceptability. Where the end-expiratory position moves markedly between manoeuvres, subsequent estimates of ERV should be discarded. There may then be a case for obtaining RV as TLC minus IVC [11].

Air trapping. As well as yielding the lung volumes, closed circuit spirometry can provide visual evidence for air trapping. This is present when, after a full inspiration, the resting respiratory level remains elevated for several breaths instead of returning immediately to its previous level (Fig. 10.3). The phenomenon is due to the trapping of gas behind small airways that became patent

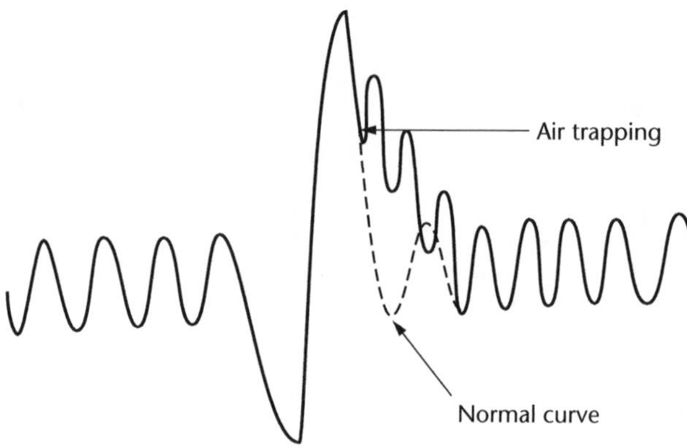

Fig. 10.3 Spirogram illustrating air trapping during measurement of the total lung capacity by the closed circuit method. After a full inspiration the spirogram returns gradually over a series of breaths to its previous level. In this it differs from the spirogram for a healthy subject where the return is immediate. Trace reads from left to right with inspiration upwards.

during the forced inspiration and closed prematurely during the subsequent expiration. The closure can be due to diminished elastic recoil by the lung tissue or to surface forces acting on the airways. Its presence should be noted on the lung function report.

10.3.2 Alternative closed circuit methods

During respiratory surveys there may be insufficient time or laboratory space for the closed circuit measurement of lung volume. If the subjects have relatively normal lungs, the lung volumes can be estimated using single breath or forced rebreathing techniques.

Single breath methods. The single breath measurement is usually made in conjunction with either a single breath test of lung mixing, for example the single breath nitrogen test (Section 16.2.2), or the single breath measurement of transfer factor (Section 20.4). These methods underestimate the lung volume in subjects with airflow limitation. The underestimation is less in the case of the transfer factor measurement, which entails breath holding, than in the mixing test, which does not. The underestimation can be allowed for empirically [13, 14] but the correction is inevitably approximate. Greater accuracy can be secured by the forced rebreathing technique.

Forced rebreathing technique. In the version of Wilmore [15] as modified by Sterk and colleagues [16], the subject exhales to residual volume and is then connected to a bag-in-bottle system, which is completely filled with 6–8 l of 100% oxygen. The subject inhales slowly to total lung capacity, exhales slowly to residual volume and then takes eight deep breaths each of duration 2 s. During rebreathing the flow is monitored with a heated pneumotachograph, and volume is measured with a spirometer and nitrogen concentration at the mouth using a nitrogen analyser or respiratory mass spectrometer. The residual volume is calculated per breath for the last three breaths and the value at breath number 7.5 obtained by interpolation. Residual volume is given by:

$$\mathrm{RV}n = V\mathrm{B} \times F\mathrm{B,N_2}/[(F\mathrm{A,N_2} - F\mathrm{B,N_2}) + V\mathrm{I} - V\mathrm{Cmax}] \quad (10.3)$$

where RVn is residual volume at breath n, and $F\mathrm{B,N_2}$ and $F\mathrm{A,N_2}$ are fractional concentrations of nitrogen respectively in the bag (measured during inspiration) and alveolar gas when breathing air. $V\mathrm{B}$, $V\mathrm{I}$ and VCmax are respectively the volume of oxygen in the bag, inspired volume and vital capacity, all at body temperature saturated with water vapour. $F\mathrm{A,N_2}$ is obtained from mean expired nitrogen concentration (area under the expired concentration–volume curve divided by expired volume) corrected for anatomical dead space [i.e. $F\mathrm{E,N_2} \times V\mathrm{t}/(V\mathrm{t} - V\mathrm{ad})$, where $F\mathrm{E,N_2}$ is mean expired nitrogen concentration, Vt is tidal volume and Vad is anatomical dead space.] The within-subject standard deviation is reported as 7.7%. The method requires practice. It is suitable for healthy subjects and for use in respiratory surveys but not for patients with impaired lung mixing.

10.3.3 Open circuit gas dilution method

Principle. The nitrogen present in the alveolar gas is flushed out of the lung by the subject breathing oxygen; the expired gas is collected and the quantity of nitrogen is determined by analysis. The change in alveolar nitrogen concentration over the period of washout is also measured and these two quantities are used to calculate the lung volume at the start of washout. Allowance is made for nitrogen that enters the lung from the pulmonary capillary blood and lung tissue as soon as the concentration in the alveolar gas becomes less than that in the body [7]. This technique has the advantage of also providing information on the effectiveness of gas mixing in the lung (Section 16.2.4); it has the disadvantages of requiring both very accurate gas analysis and an allowance for the volume of nitrogen that leaves the blood during the test. The assumed volume is an average and may not be appropriate for an individual subject. The method is not recommended for routine measurements except where lung-gas mixing is of special interest.

Practical details. The subject should wear a nose clip and breathe through a mouthpiece and valve box. A seated upright posture is recommended. The inspiratory port of the valve box should connect to a demand system supplying oxygen that is nitrogen-free. The expired port will usually connect to a Douglas bag (Fig. 1.3, page 10) or Tissot spirometer. Expired volume can also be obtained using a pneumotachograph and integrator, but allowance should then be made for any effect on the instrument calibration of the gas composition changing during the procedure. Gas density and thermal conductivity are amongst the variables to be considered (Table 7.6, page 65).

To start the procedure, the subject makes a full expiration and a sample of alveolar gas is collected (Fig. 1.3, page 10). Then at the end of a normal expiration, he or she is connected to the oxygen supply. Breathing oxygen is continued for 7 min or until the alveolar nitrogen level has fallen to a fractional concentration of 0.02. At this point a second alveolar sample is obtained. Both samples are analysed for nitrogen; this can be done directly using a nitrogen meter or respiratory mass spectrometer (cf. Table 7.6). Alternatively, the concentration can be obtained by difference following analysis of the gas for oxygen and carbon dioxide. The required accuracy is of the order of 0.01%, which for an FRC of 3 l will result in a measurement error of ±60 ml (±2%). The FRC is calculated as follows:

$$\mathrm{FRC} = \frac{(V\mathrm{E} + V\mathrm{ds})(F\mathrm{E,N_2} - F\mathrm{I,N_2})}{F\mathrm{A_1,N_2} - F\mathrm{A_2,N_2}} - 0.275\ \mathrm{l\ BTPS} \qquad (10.4)$$

where VE and Vds in l BTPS are the volumes of the gas expired during the period of breathing oxygen and the dead space of the collecting system, $F\mathrm{I,N_2}$ and $F\mathrm{E,N_2}$ are the fractional concentrations of nitrogen in the oxygen and in the mixed expired gas and $F\mathrm{A_1,N_2}$ and $F\mathrm{A_2,N_2}$ refer to the concentrations in the alveolar gas before and at the end of the period of breathing oxygen. The volume of 0.275 l is a correction expressed in terms of alveolar gas during breathing air, for the nitrogen that entered the alveoli from the blood during the period of breathing oxygen.

10.3.4 Radiographic method

Principle. The thoracic cavity is subdivided into a number of transverse slices whose width and depth are obtained by measurement of posteroanterior and left lateral chest radiography or by computer-assisted tomography (CT scanning). The radiographs are taken at full inspiration. The volume of each slice is calculated from the thickness of the slice and the appropriate width and depth measurements; the latter are corrected for magnification due to the film being a finite distance from the centre of the thorax. The slice volumes are summed to give a total cavity volume from which lung volume is obtained by subtracting the volume of the heart and other structures [8].

Practical details. The usual method is that of Barnhard and colleagues and is performed manually [17]. The slices are considered to be elliptical cylinders for which the volume is given by:

$$\text{slice volume} = 0.25\pi \times \text{width} \times \text{depth} \times \text{thickness} \qquad (10.5)$$

Five slices are used and their limits are given in Fig. 10.4. The heart is considered as a whole ellipsoid; the appropriate dimensions and the equation for calculating its volume are given in Section 17.4. The space beneath the dome of each half of

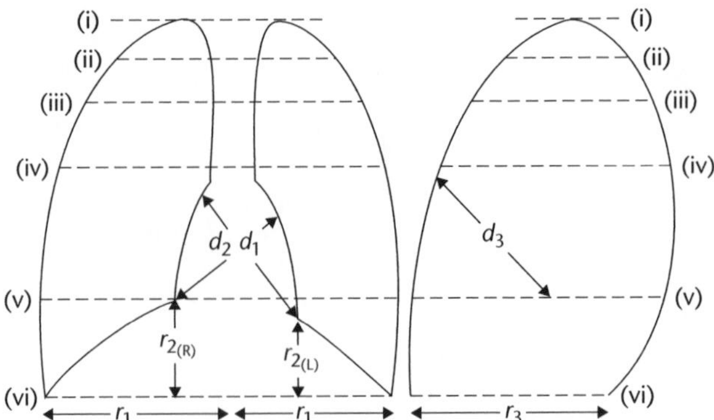

Fig. 10.4 Measurements used for calculation of radiographic lung volume by the method of Barnhard. The distances (i)–(ii) and (ii)–(iii) are each 2.5 cm. (v) is at the upper border of diaphragm and (vi) between the two costophrenic angles. (iv) is midway between (iii) and (v). d_2 and d_3 are respectively at right angles to and parallel with d_1, which terminates at the junction of the right atrium with the left border of the heart; within these constraints all three are maximal intracardiac dimensions. Source: [18]

the diaphragm (Vsd) is treated as one eighth of an ellipsoid. Its volume is given by:

$$V\mathrm{sd} = 0.13\pi \times \text{width} \times \text{depth} \times \text{height} \qquad (10.6)$$

where the width and depth are taken from line (vi) in the figure (i.e. r_1 and r_3) and the height is the vertical distance from the line to the appropriate cardiophrenic angle, i.e. $r_{2(R)}$ and $r_{2(L)}$.

In more sophisticated versions of the method the radiographs are marked by hand then scanned and the coordinates of successive points fed into a computer. The improved method of Pierce and colleagues uses 200 slices and has been reported as having an overall accuracy of ±0.2 l [19]. An increase in the number of slices, as can be obtained by modern CT technology, does not further increase the accuracy [20]. However, the technique allows for the selective exclusion of the great vessels and other structures [21] and this might be an advantage.

10.3.5 Plethysmographic methods

TGV is usually measured by *whole body plethysmography* as part of another procedure; this can be measurement of specific airway conductance (TGV/airway resistance; Section 14.3.4). The method is also used to delineate both partial and maximal flow–volume curves without the compression artefact that occurs when the curves are obtained by spirometry (Section 12.5.1). The plethysmographic method of measuring lung volume has been standardised [5, 9] and is described in Section 14.6.2.

Changes in lung volume can be monitored in terms of the associated changes in thoracic volume observed using sensors on the walls of the chest and abdomen. The sensors can generate electronic signals directly, as in *inductive plethysmography* in which the trunk is enveloped in a garment (e.g. Respitrace [22]) or markers whose positions are determined optically. The latter procedure has been described as *optoelectronic plethysmography* [23]. Both methods are subject to movement artefacts, require careful calibration [24] and depend on modelling the respective contributions to a change in volume of its thoracic and abdominal components. Inductive plethysmography is used extensively, including for recumbent subjects (e.g. Section 32.3.3). The optical method has also been applied to respiratory patients during cycle ergometry to assess the presence and extent of dynamic hyperinflation (Section 13.6).

10.4 References

1. Leith DE, Brown R. Human lung volumes and the mechanisms that set them. *Eur Respir J* 1999; **13**: 468–472.
2. Leith DE, Mead J. Mechanisms determining residual volume of the lungs in normal subjects. *J Appl Physiol* 1967; **23**: 221–227.
3. Gaultier C, Crapo R. Effects of nutrition, growth hormone disturbances, training, altitude and sleep on lung volumes. *Eur Respir J* 1997; **10**: 2913–2919.
4. Bancalari E, Clausen J. Pathophysiology of changes in absolute lung volumes. *Eur Respir J* 1998; **12**: 248–258.
5. Quanjer PH, Tammelling GJ, Cotes JE et al. Standardization of lung function tests. *Eur Respir J* 1993; **6** (Suppl 16): 5–40.
6. Brown R, Leith DE, Enright PL. Multiple breath helium dilution measurements of lung volumes in adults. *Eur Respir J* 1998; **11**: 246–255.
7. Newth CJL, Enright P, Johnson RL. Multiple-breath nitrogen washout techniques: including measurements with patients on ventilators. *Eur Respir J* 1997; **10**: 2174–2185.
8. Clausen J. Measurement of absolute lung volumes by imaging techniques. *Eur Respir J* 1997; **10**: 2427–2431.
9. Coates AL, Peslin R, Rodenstein D, Stocks J. Measurement of lung volume by plethysmography. *Eur Respir J* 1997; **10**: 1415–1427.
10. Stocks J, Sly PD, Tepper RS, Morgan WJ, eds. *Infant respiratory function testing.* New York: John Wiley & Sons, Inc., 1996.
11. Wanger J, Clausen JL, Coates A et al. Standardization of the measurement of lung volume. Official statement of the American Thoracic Society and the European Respiratory Society. *Eur Respir J* 2005; **26**: 211–222.
12. Hankinson JL, Stocks J, Peslin R. Reproducibility of lung volume measurements. *Eur Respir J* 1998; **11**: 1787–1790.
13. Van Ganse W, Comhaire F, Van der Straeten M. Alveolar volume and transfer factor determined by single breath dilution of a test gas at various apnoea times. *Scand J Resp Dis* 1970; **51**: 82–92.
14. Punjabi NM, Shade D, Wise RA. Correction of single-breath helium lung volumes in patients with airflow obstruction. *Chest* 1998; **114**: 907–918.
15. Wilmore JH. A simplified method for determination of residual lung volumes. *J Appl Physiol* 1969; **27**: 96–100.
16. Sterk PJ, Quanjer PhH, van der Maas LLJ et al. The validity of the single-breath nitrogen determination of residual volume. *Bull Eur Physiopathol Respir* 1980; **16**: 195–213.
17. Barnhard HJ, Pierce JA, Joyce JW, Bates JH. Roentgenographic determination of total lung capacity: a new method evaluated in health, emphysema and congestive heart failure. *Am J Med* 1960; **28**: 51–60.
18. O'Shea J, Lapp NL, Russakoff AD et al. Determination of lung volumes from chest films. *Thorax* 1970; **25**: 544–549.
19. Pierce RJ, Brown DJ, Denison DM. Radiographic, scintigraphic and gas-dilution estimates of individual lung and lobar volumes in man. *Thorax* 1980; **35**: 773–780.
20. Schlesinger AE, White DK, Mallory GB et al. Estimation of total lung capacity from chest radiography and chest CT in children: comparison with body plethysmography. *Am J Roentgenol* 1995; **165**: 151–154.
21. Walter D, De Man B, Iatrou M, Edic PM. Future generation CT imaging. *Thorac Surg Clin* 2004; **14**: 135–149.
22. Leino K, Nunes S, Valta P, Takala J. Validation of a new respiratory inductive plethysmograph. *Acta Anaesthesiol Scand* 2001; **45**: 104–111.
23. Dellaca RL, Aliverti A, Pelosi P et al. Estimation of end-expiratory lung volume variations by optoelectronic plethysmography. *Crit Care Med* 2001; **29**:1807–1811.
24. Banzett RB, Mahan ST, Garner DM et al. A simple and reliable method to calibrate respiratory magnetometers and Respitrace. *J Appl Physiol* 1995; **79**: 2169–2176; correspondence *J Appl Physiol* 1996; **81**: 516–517.

Further reading

Birath G, Swenson EW. A correction factor for helium absorption in lung volume determinations. *Scand J Clin Lab Invest* 1956; **8**: 155–158.

Clausen JL. Lung volume equipment and infection control. *Eur Respir J* 1997; **10**: 1928–1932.

Darling RC, Cournand A, Richards DW Jr. Studies on the intrapulmonary mixture of gases, III: Open circuit method for measuring residual air. *J Clin Invest* 1940; **19**: 609–618.

Demedts M, van de Woestijne KP. Which technique for total lung capacity measurement? *Bull Eur Physiopathol Respir* 1980; **16**: 705–709.

Fairshter RD. Effect of a deep inspiration on expiratory flow in normals and patients with chronic obstructive pulmonary disease. *Bull Eur Physiopathol Respir* 1986; **22**: 119–125.

Gollogly S, Smith JT, White SK et al. The volume of lung parenchyma as a function of age: a review of 1050 normal CT scans of the chest with three-dimensional volumetric reconstruction of the pulmonary system. *Spine* 2004; **29**: 2061–2066.

Jones HA, Davies EE, Hughes JMB. A rapid rebreathing method for measurement of pulmonary gas volume in humans. *J Appl Physiol* 1986; **60**: 311–316.

Loiseau A, Loiseau P, Saumon G. A simple method for correcting single breath total lung capacity for underestimation. *Thorax* 1990; **45**: 873–877.

Pichurko BM, Ingram RH Jr. Effects of airway tone and volume history on maximal expiratory flow in asthma. *J Appl Physiol* 1987; **62**: 1133–1140.

Wheatley JR, Pare PD, Engel LA. Reversibility of induced bronchoconstriction by deep inspiration in asthmatic and normal subjects. *Eur Respir J* 1989; **2**: 331–339.

CHAPTER 11

Lung and Chest Wall Elasticity

The elasticity of the respiratory system preserves the patency of airways and is the main driving force for expiration. This chapter describes its features and how it is assessed. The roles of superimposed dynamic forces are considered elsewhere, particularly in Chapter 13.

11.1 Functional anatomy

When a normal subject inhales maximally after a forced expiration the volume of gas in the lung increases approximately fourfold. For the expansion to be uniform this would require an increase in linear dimensions of the lung by a factor of $4^{1/3}$ or 1.6 which nearly happens in practice. However, regional differences in expansion occur on account of the pyramidal shape of the lung, the confining role of the visceral pleura and the operation of gravitational force (Fig. 11.1). Most expansion takes place in the alveolar ducts and alveoli. These structures enlarge to a similar extent [2]. By doing so they maintain constant branching angles between airways. This isotropic expansion is made possible by the structure of the lung tissue and the surface-tension properties of the material that lines the alveoli.

The framework of the lungs is made up of bundles of elastic and collagen fibres that extend from the large airways down to the alveoli and across to the pleura and blood vessels. The two types of fibre are frequently in apposition and together they form the scaffolding of the lung. Weibel has described this as resembling crumpled wire netting [3]. The constituent fibres are relatively indistensible but they can move in relation to each other so the bundles of fibres lengthen and uncurl and alter their relative positions like the threads of a nylon stocking when it is put on. Expansion of the lungs affects all its parts, but mainly the lung parenchyma. Here, during an inspiration that starts from residual volume, the coils of the spiral fibres of the alveolar ducts expand longitudinally; this enlarges the mouths of the alveoli that lie between the coils. The accordion-like expansion is associated with stretching of the alveolar septa, smoothing of undulations in alveolar walls (also called crumpling), opening up of pleats in the septa and recruitment of previously collapsed alveoli. The changes increase the area of alveolar surface and, by doing so facilitate the exchange of gas across the alveolar capillary membrane. The expansion also enlarges the minority of alveolar capillaries that lie near the junctions of septa but flatten the remainder. Overall, an increase in lung volume reduces the volume of alveolar capillary blood that is available for exchange of gas (Fig. 11.2).

During normal expiration the changes in shape and dimensions are reversed. Deflation of the lungs can also occur from contraction of muscle fibres present in the bundles that support the alveolar ducts and related structures. This pneumoconstriction does not necessarily affect the larger airways.

In the absence of constriction the network of fibres confer stability on the lungs because a local change in volume causes lengthening and/or shortening of elastic and collagen fibres in

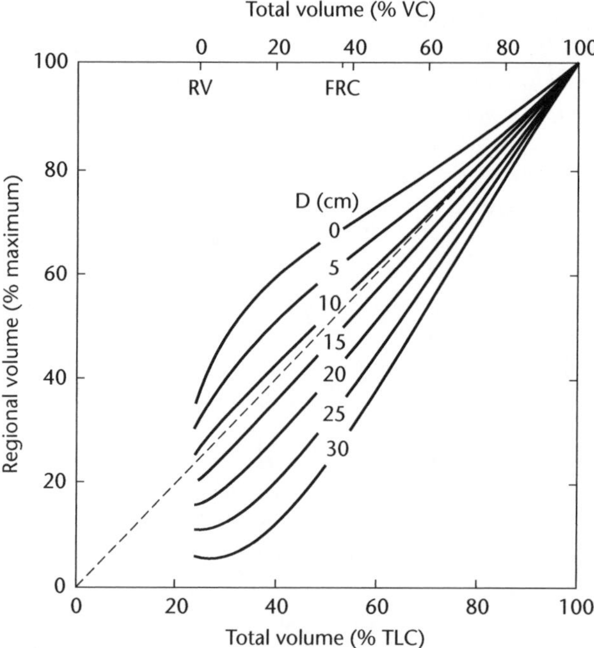

Fig. 11.1 Milic's onion. Diagram quantifying the influence of gravitational force on regional lung volumes. The ordinate is regional lung volume and the abscissa overall lung volume both as percentages of maximum. The lines are for regions of lung defined by vertical distance from the apex (in cm). At all degrees of expansion below the maximum the upper regions are relatively more expanded than the lower ones. Source: [1].

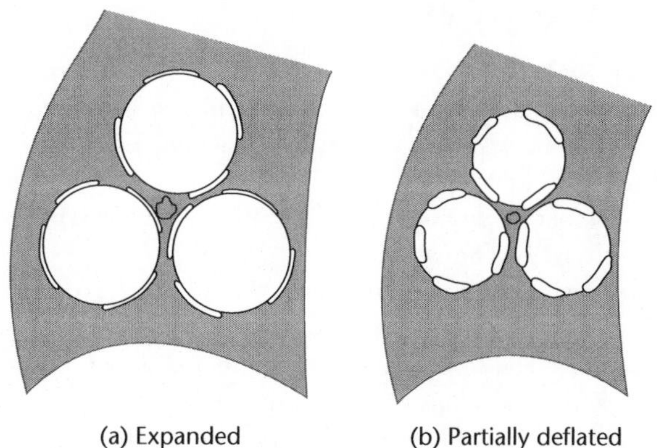

Fig. 11.2 Diagram illustrating the effect of lung expansion upon the size of the alveolar capillaries. When the lungs are expanded (left) the capillaries in the alveolar walls are attenuated and the volume of blood which they contain is less than when the lung is partially deflated (right); by contrast the alveolar corner vessels and the extra-alveolar vessels in the interstitial spaces are increased in size due to traction from the surrounding structures. Source: [4].

the immediate vicinity. It also deforms some alveoli and hence alters the local surface tension. This mechanism operates to reduce uneven lung function. It has been described as interdependence [5].

Stress and strain. Interdependence ameliorates the effects of local stresses; these are forces that act on surfaces throughout the lungs. They give rise to strains (i.e. the resulting deformations). Stresses have many causes. They include differences in compliance of structures within the lungs, constraints imposed by the shape of the lungs, gravitational force that causes a vertical gradient of pressure down the lungs [6] and the effects of adjacent structures. Stress can also be caused by trauma. The consequences are both structural and functional. They include reinforcement of or weakness in the collagen net (e.g. emphysema, Section 40.3) and uneven expansion and perfusion of the lungs (Chapters 16 and 17). The stresses can be analysed mechanically [7].

11.2 Elastic recoil

During inspiration, contraction of respiratory muscles stretches the elastic and collagen tissues network of the lungs and pleura; it also overcomes the surface tension that is present at the interfaces between the air in alveoli and the fluid that lines alveolar walls. These features constitute an elastic hindrance to inspiration. At most lung volumes the hindrance is mainly due to surface tension, but if the lungs are nearly fully distended the recoil of the elastic and collagen fibres contributes as well.

The work that is done in stretching the lung is not dissipated as heat; instead the energy is stored in the structures, which have been stretched, then expended to drive the subsequent expiration. This entails shrinking the lungs back to their previous volume. Hence, normal expiration is a passive process, which is effected by the elastic recoil of the lung tissue. The process becomes unstable at near to full expiration (Section 16.1.8).

The magnitude of the elastic recoil (static recoil pressure) is only apparent when the lungs are completely stationary, since in this circumstance no energy is expended in moving air against the resistance offered by the airways (cf. pendelluft phenomenon, Section 16.1.9). The static recoil pressure varies with lung volume (Fig. 11.3).

The slope of the relationship between pressure (*P*st) and volume (V) describes the distensibility of the lungs. The slope at functional residual capacity is called the *compliance of the lungs* (Section 11.6); it is a chord measurement to a curvilinear function that can be described by a sigmoidal equation [9] and has a different slope when measured on inspiration and on expiration. This is because, when the lungs are ventilated, the change in volume lags behind the change in pressure; the phenomenon is an example of hysteresis. It leads to the graph relating volume to pressure (V/P curve) taking the form of an ellipse (Fig. 11.4, left-hand curve).

11.3 Lung surface tension

The right hand curve in Fig. 11.4 is for the same lung filled with saline. The saline inactivates the force of surface tension acting at the gas-to-tissue interface. In this circumstance the recoil

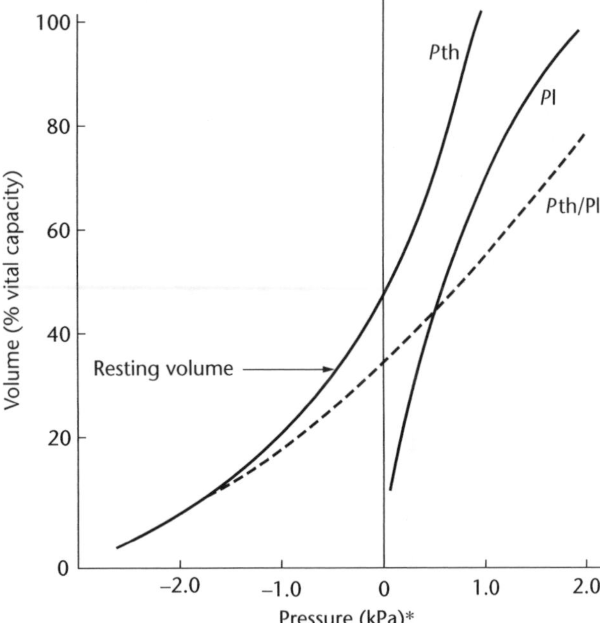

Fig. 11.3 Static volume–pressure curves for the thoracic cage (Pth) and the lung (Pl) separately and in combination. They were obtained from measurements of pressure in the pharynx and in the oesophagus during relaxation against a closed mouthpiece after inspiration from a spirometer. The relationship can also be obtained in other ways, e.g., during relaxation whilst breathing from a pressurised container.
*For pressure in cm H_2O multiply these numbers by 10.
Source: [8]

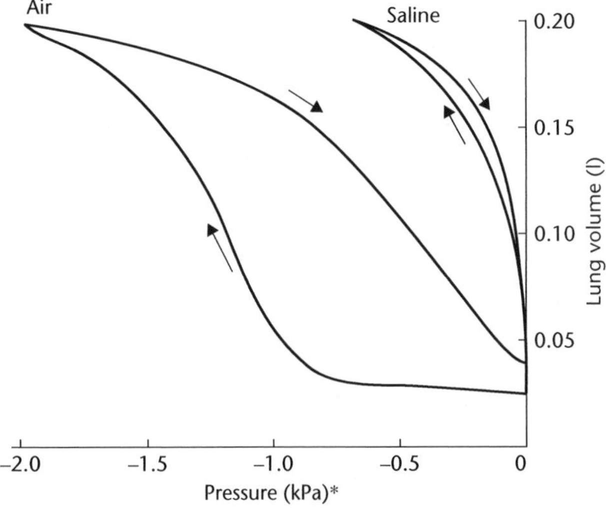

Fig. 11.4 Pressure–volume curves for an isolated cat lung suspended in air. On the left the lung is filled with air and the curve exhibits hysteresis. On the right the lung is filled with saline; this eliminates the surface forces and hence the hysteresis. As a result the compliance of the lung (i.e. the slope of the V/P curve at mid-capacity) is increased. The directions of the arrows indicate inflation and deflation.
*For pressure in cm H_2O multiply these numbers by 10.
Source: [10].

pressure is reduced and the area of the ellipse (i.e. the extent of hysteresis) is less. The reduction was evidence for the elastic recoil being mainly due to the operation of surface forces and not to stretching of the fibrous stroma in the lungs.

The association of elastic recoil with surface tension was reported by Neergaard in 1929 and subsequently independently by Radford [10, 11]. At about the same time Pattle demonstrated that fluid expelled from lung tissue had an extremely low surface tension [12]. Clements and his colleagues further found that the surface tension of a film of extract was less when the material was condensed into a small area than when it was expanded [13]. This important property of the surface layer has the effect of stabilising the lungs during expiration (Section 11.5.1).

The action of the surface film is due to the presence of a lipopolysaccharide, dipalmitoyl lecithin called surfactant; this is formed in the mitochondria of cuboidal granular pneumonocytes (type II alveolar cells) present in the alveolar walls. An important component is surfactant protein B [14]. The surfactant is stored as lamellar bodies prior to being secreted onto the epithelium of the alveoli and alveolar ducts where it forms a monomolecular layer. The layer extends into the respiratory bronchioles. It is relatively smooth due to it bridging over irregularities in the epithelial surface which are filled with liquid hypophase (see Fig. 3.6, page 27); this contains apoproteins, alveolar macrophages and tubular myelin, comprising concertina-like packets of dipalmitoyl lecithin: the latter is in a form which can be reinserted into the surface layer.

11.4 Patency of airways

For the lungs to function effectively the alveolar gas must be in communication with the environment, hence all classes of airways should be open. Four structural factors contribute to the patency of airways.

1 *Scaffolding.* The architecture of the lungs is supported by cartilage in the walls of bronchi and by the erectile action of distended blood vessels in the lung parenchyma. These features contribute to the lungs containing air.

2 *Guy lines.* The smaller airways are supported by bundles of elastic and other fibres that are inserted into and exert traction on the walls of airways (Section 11.1). The guy lines transfer much of the pressure gradient between the outside air and the pleural space to the immediate vicinity of small airways. This has the effect of holding the airways open. The action resembles that of guy lines that hold out the walls of a tent. The traction exerted by the guy lines varies with lung volume.

3 *Safety net.* The bundles of fibres, including collagen fibres, that permeate the lungs act as a safety net to limit over-expansion and prevent the lungs from rupturing.

4 *Surface tension.* The surface tension of the fluid lining the alveoli exerts a force that tends to shrink or even close these structures, hence to expand others, including small airways.

The effect of surface tension on the diameter of a small structure was first described by Young and expressed mathematically by Laplace [15]. Young observed that the pressure in a bubble was related directly to the surface tension and inversely to the radius of curvature. Hence, the law of Young and Laplace:

$$P = 2T/r \tag{11.1}$$

where P is the pressure within an air bubble surrounded by liquid, r is the radius of the bubble and T is the surface tension at the air to liquid interface. For a cylindrical air space the coefficient term is reduced from two to one whilst for a soap bubble, which has two surfaces, it is doubled to four. Within the lung not all the air spaces are of the same size. Hence, according to eqn. 11.1 the smaller ones should empty into the larger. In addition, during expiration, all air spaces should be at risk of collapse on account of their volume diminishing. In practice these undesirable events are prevented because the force of surface tension is reduced by surfactant.

11.5 Closure of air-filled structures

11.5.1 Closure of airways

During normal breathing the elastic recoil of lung tissue operates in the manner described above to keep the alveoli in communication with the environment. As part of this process the intrapleural pressure is below atmospheric pressure. At full expiration, in all but relatively young subjects, the intrapleural pressure becomes positive. Yet the lungs still contain air. This situation can only arise because air is trapped behind blockages somewhere between the large airways and the alveoli. The air remains trapped after intubation of a bronchus and this led Hughes and colleagues to suggest that the site of closure is in the terminal bronchi [16].

The distribution of the trapped gas is determined in part by the lungs being subject to gravitational force. During expiration, this leads to airways at the base of the lungs closing first (Section 16.1.8). At the point of maximal closure the volume of gas remaining in the lungs is the *residual volume* (Section 10.1.1), and the lung volume above residual at which closure is first detectable is the *closing volume* (Section 16.2.5). Premature closure increases the residual volume; the commonest cause is the loss of lung elasticity (increase of compliance), which occurs with increasing age (Section 25.9.1) and with emphysema (Section 40.3). Premature generalised closure can also occur as a consequence of narrowing of airways from other causes, including contraction of bronchial muscles and thickening of airway walls (e.g. Section 37.3). Localised closure can be due to a foreign body or a space-occupying lesion, for example a bronchial carcinoma or aortic aneurysm. The consequent atelectasis is considered below.

Retardation of the process of airway closure prolongs the expiration and reduces the residual volume. This occurs when the quantity of collagen in lung tissue is increased secondary to diffuse interstitial fibrosis or one of its antecedent conditions (Section 40.4).

When an airway is closed, its walls are in apposition and surface tension forces tend to hold them together. Such an airway reopens during a subsequent inspiration. In man, the suction needed to effect reopening is approximately 0.4 kPa; this critical opening pressure is achieved by over-expansion of regions of lungs not subject to closure, so the elastic recoil that these regions exert is increased. The process is an example of interdependence [5]. The lung volume at reopening is usually below that at the end of a normal expiration [17].

The manner of reopening was investigated by Macklem, who suggested that it began from the central end [18]. At bronchial bifurcations this could lead to one branch opening before the other or to the formation of a bubble or meniscus of fluid, which might then move up and down an airway causing a variable obstruction.

The closure of airways is the main cause for the inspiratory and expiratory limbs of the static pressure–volume curve forming a loop instead of being superimposed (Fig. 11.4). This situation is described as hysteresis (asynchrony) and reflects that the change in lung volume lags behind the driving force, which is the change in pleural pressure. For the cat lung shown in the figure the critical opening pressure was approximately 0.8 kPa. The inspiratory and expiratory curves converged on a maximal volume (volume asymptote) slightly in excess of 0.2 l. This volume was determined by the collagenous stroma of the lung and pleura because the organ was not restrained by the chest wall.

11.5.2 Closure of alveoli

Peripheral air spaces begin to develop early in foetal life but they are effectively indistensible until the lungs start to produce surfactant at about the 24th week of gestation. This process is delayed in babies with hyaline membrane disease of the lung (Section 24.3.2). The presence of surfactant enables the airspaces to fill with air during the first few breaths after birth. Subsequently, they do not collapse unless either the production of surfactant is reduced or conditions predisposing to collapse supervene. Production of surfactant is interfered with if the lung parenchyma is damaged by breathing oxygen-enriched air (Section 35.7.2), by severe shock and by diversion of pulmonary blood flow through an extracorporeal circulation (see 'acute lung injury', Section 41.12).

In the presence of surfactant, collapse of alveoli is due to absorption of gas distal to an obstructed airway. The obstruction can be a direct consequence of a local phenomenon (e.g. space occupying lesion or foreign body). Alternatively, the process can be facilitated by any manoeuvre that promotes airway closure, for example sustained coughing, ventilation of the lung at near to residual volume and, in air-force pilots, exposure to centrifugal force (high "g"). The gas is more likely to be absorbed completely if it is very soluble (see below), or if the effective alveolar diameter is reduced by interstitial or alveolar oedema.

11.5.3 Consequences of airway closure

Distal to an obstruction the alveolar gases very quickly come into equilibrium with the gases in the blood. Here, the sum of the tensions of the oxygen, carbon dioxide, nitrogen and water vapour is less than atmospheric pressure, so the gas is gradually absorbed. If the constituent gas is 100% oxygen, as can be the case for pilots in some aircraft or patients receiving some forms of oxygen therapy, or if the subject is breathing a soluble anaesthetic gas the rate of gas uptake is greatly increased. In this circumstance a brief closure, which would normally be transient, can progress to total collapse (atelectasis) on account of all the gas having been absorbed. In an isolated lung, atelectasis can also result from degassing *in vacuo*.

Reexpansion of an atelectatic volume of lung is achieved if the subject maximises the lung retractive force through making a full inspiration. The reexpansion of collapsed alveoli occurs haphazardly and not in a regular sequence. This instability is due to interaction between the surface tension of the fluid lining of the alveoli and the force exerted by the stroma of the lung. A theoretical model that accounts for this feature was developed by Mead (Fig. 11.5).

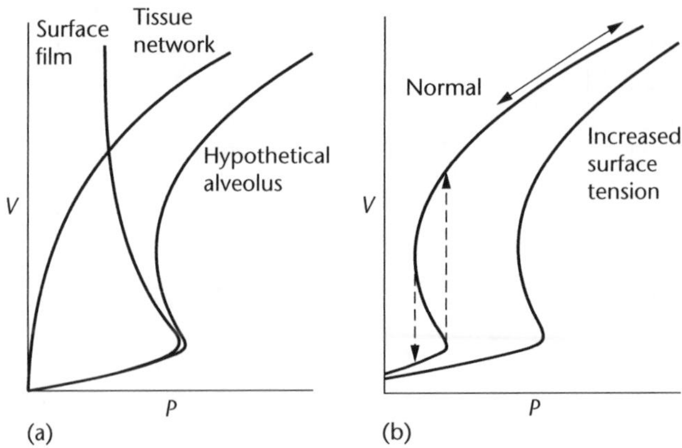

Fig. 11.5 Diagram illustrating the volume–pressure characteristic of a hypothetical alveolus. It is the sum of two components due, respectively, to the tissue network of the lungs and to the surface film (left-hand diagram). For the tissue network and for the surface film when the alveolus is not expanded beyond a hemisphere, the volume is directly related to the pressure; for the surface film at larger alveolar volumes (i.e. beyond the inflection in the curve) the volume increases abruptly unless the pressure is greatly reduced or the film is supported.

When the curves are combined to yield the alveolar curve (right-hand diagram) the kinked portion between the interrupted lines represents a region of instability. The alveolus during its initial inflation will follow the curve up to the point of inflection when the volume will increase abruptly to the new level indicated by the right-hand vertical arrow. During deflation it will follow the curve down to the left-hand vertical arrow when the volume will suddenly decrease. During normal tidal breathing the alveolus will move within the limits indicated by the double-headed arrow where the relationship is stable.

When the surface tension is increased a higher pressure is required in order to expand the alveolus; in addition the alveolus is now unstable over the range of pressures to which it is normally exposed. For both these reasons a rise in the surface tension is likely to be associated with atelectasis. Source [19]

11.6 Compliance of the lungs

The elasticity of the lungs is essential for its proper function; it is depicted by the static volume–pressure curve (Fig. 11.3); it is the sum of components for individual lung units [20] and can be described mathematically. The most convenient model is a mono-exponential equation. This has been shown by Colebatch to fit the upper half of the expiratory curves of normal subjects and most patients [21] and has the form:

$$V = A - Be^{-kP\text{st}} \qquad (11.2)$$

where *P*st is static transpulmonary pressure, *A* is the derived asymptote on the volume axis in excess of total lung capacity and *B* is the volume decrement below *A* at which transpulmonary pressure is zero (Section 11.8.3 and Fig. 11.7 below). The exponent *k* is a shape factor which, in conjunction with the lung volume, describes the slope of the volume–pressure curve per litre of volume, (i.e. $k = dV/dP\text{st}\,(A–V)^{-1}$),and is analogous to the specific compliance (see below). The derivation neglects the quantity of tissue present in the lung. In healthy adults *k* is of the order of 12 ± 1.5 Pa^{-1} (0.12 ± 0.015 cm H_2O^{-1}); it is increased with emphysema and reduced with stiff lungs.

The volume–pressure curve can also be described by the static recoil pressure at total lung capacity and by the static compliance, where the latter is the slope of the central linear part of the curve. The slope may be approximated by a straight line:

$$Cl,\text{st} = \Delta V/\Delta P\text{st} \qquad (11.3)$$

where *C*l,st is static lung compliance, *V* is volume (litres BTPS) and *P*st is static recoil pressure (kPa). On account of hysteresis the slope is influenced by whether the volume–pressure curve is obtained starting from full inspiration or from residual volume (Section 11.8.2). The former expiratory curve is more consistent so it is the compliance on expiration that is usually reported.

Static compliance of the lung. This is the change in lung volume per unit change in the transpulmonary pressure (i.e. the pressure difference between the interior of the alveoli and the pleural surface of the lungs). It is a measure of distensibility, and in normal adults has a mean value of 2.4 (SD 1.4) l kPa^{-1} (0.24 l cm H_2O^{-1}) (Table 26.16, page 347). Lower values are obtained in children and in women compared with men on account of their lungs being smaller (Chapters 25 and 26). A lung of high compliance expands to a greater extent than one of low compliance when both are exposed to the same increase in transpulmonary pressure.

In lungs of normal structure, the size influences the compliance since it determines the proportional expansion when the

Table 11.1 Factors that affect static lung compliance.

Aspect	Compliance low	Compliance high
Lung of normal structure*	Small person	Large person
	Feeble respiratory muscles	Some athletes
	Airway closure	Some asthmatics (asymptomatic)
Lung surfactant	Respiratory distress syndrome	
	Surfactant protein B deficiency	
Fibrous stroma	Disorders of lung parenchyma†	Age, Emphysema (especially with smoking and deficiency of α_1 anti-trypsin).
		Semicarbazide (breaks cross-linkages)
Visceral pleural	Thickened secondary to TB, asbestos exposure, haemothorax	
Tone in muscle of alveolar ducts	Histamine	Bronchodilator drugs
	Serotonin	
	Hypoxia	
Pulmonary blood volume	Mitral stenosis	Isocapnoeic hypoxia
	Left ventricular failure	Pulmonary stenosis
	Polycythaemia (?)	Haemorrhage (?)

* Specific lung compliance usually normal; the principal exception is airway closure with alveolar volume measured by plethysmography.
† Tidal volume is reduced, especially on exercise.

volume of the lungs is increased by a fixed amount. For example, an increase in lung size of 1 l represents a larger proportional expansion for the lungs of a child than for that of an adult; the increase in recoil pressure is correspondingly greater and the compliance is less in consequence. However, when the lung volume is expressed in dimensionless units (e.g. as a fraction of the total lung capacity) the relationship of recoil pressure to lung volume is found to be independent of lung size. This has the effect that the compliance per litre of lung volume, which is the *specific compliance*, is effectively constant. The specific compliance (sC) is usually reported for expiration at functional residual capacity; it then has a value in normal subjects of 0.8 (range 0.3 to 1.4) kPa^{-1} (0.08, range 0.03 to 0.14 cm H_2O^{-1}).

Some factors that influence the static lung compliance are listed in Table 11.1.

A patient seldom detects a change in *stiffness* of the lungs, despite its functional importance. However, the associated rapid shallow breathing can be conspicuous to all. In addition, if the patient requires assisted ventilation, for example in relation to anaesthesia for a surgical operation or respiratory distress syndrome, the anaesthetist may notice that the force required to inflate the lung is increased. Information on the lower and upper inflection points of the volume–pressure curve can then contribute to safe and effective ventilation [22]. This application of the V–P curve can be particularly helpful in infants.

Dynamic compliance. The lung compliance is normally measured as static compliance when the lungs are stationary (Section 11.8.2). The distensibility can also be estimated during normal tidal breathing from measurements of lung volume and oesophageal pressure made at the ends of inspiration and expiration when the lungs are *apparently* stationary. The index so obtained is called the *dynamic compliance* (Cdyn). In subjects with healthy lungs the two measurements yield similar results. However, in the presence of narrowing of small airways the dynamic compliance is reduced. The reduction is due to movement of gas *within the lungs* influencing the transpulmonary pressure (Section 16.1.9). In this circumstance the relationship of the dynamic compliance to the respiratory frequency is an index of airflow resistance (see frequency dependence of compliance in Section 11.8.4).

11.7 Compliance of the chest wall

The relationship of the pressure change across the chest wall to thoracic volume is illustrated in Fig. 11.3. Its shape is the mirror image of that of lung tissue, but the slopes of the middle halves of both curves are similar so, in normal circumstances, the compliance of the chest wall resembles that of the lungs. The curve itself is displaced to the left and the static pressure gradient across the thoracic cage is zero when the volume is approximately 45% of the vital capacity. Hence, at smaller volumes the elastic recoil of the thoracic cage exerts an inspiratory effect; this tends to expand the lung. The effect can be demonstrated if the thorax is opened (as at autopsy or during thoracic surgery) or if the pleural pressure is raised to atmospheric pressure by admission of air into

Table 11.2 Some causes of a reduced chest wall compliance.

Impaired mobility	Increasing age Disease of chondro-vertebral joints, e.g. ankylosing spondylitis Damage to thoracic vertebrae
Changes in soft tissues	Scarring of the skin of the chest e.g. by burns, radiotherapy or skin disease Central obesity Large bosom from any cause

the pleural space (pneumothorax). Under these circumstances, whilst the lungs collapse, the rib cage expands.

At near to total lung capacity the elasticity of the chest wall summates with that of the lungs, so muscular action is needed to achieve further expansion. Conversely, in young subjects at near to residual volume, force must be applied to compress the rib cage further.

In normal subjects the chest wall compliance is on average 2.3 (SD 1.3) l kPa^{-1} (0.23 (SD 0.13) l cm H_2O^{-1}), but many factors may reduce it (Table 11.2).

Posture exerts a profound influence on thoracic compliance through affecting the position and mobility of the ribs and the position of the diaphragm, including the upward force exerted by the muscles and contents of the abdomen (Section 9.8).

11.8 Measurement techniques

The measurement entails constructing a static volume–pressure curve (Figs 11.3 and 11.4 left). For this purpose it is necessary to measure the pressure gradient from alveoli to pleura. The alveolar pressure can be measured at the mouth under conditions of zero flow. Pleural pressure cannot readily be measured directly. It is usually obtained indirectly from measurement of pressure in the oesophagus.

11.8.1 Measurement of pleural and oesophageal pressure

Pleural pressure. The lungs have a finite density of approximately 0.2 g ml^{-1} and consequently the pressure in the pleural space is less negative at the base of the lungs than at the apex. When the subject is seated the pressure gradient between these points is approximately 0.5 kPa (5 cm H_2O). An average pressure may be obtained by inducing a small artificial pneumothorax and then measuring the pressure directly. However, the induction may itself affect the pressure and on ethical grounds it is only justifiable if the pleura is to be cannulated for medical reasons.

Oesophageal pressure. The pleural pressure is transmitted to the oesophagus so in favourable circumstances oesophageal pressure can substitute for pleural pressure. Furthermore, for measurement of compliance the measurement of interest is the *change* in pleural pressure, which is adequately recorded in the oesophagus. Ideally the site should be at the level of the middle of the lungs. Difficulty arises if the tone of the oesophageal wall is increased, if there is peristalsis, or if the oesophagus is compressed by the heart or affected by cardiac pulsations. Peristalsis occurs during swallowing and in anticipation of meals, whilst the cardiac artefact is increased by a supine posture. Accordingly, a time remote from meals and an upright posture are recommended.

Oesophageal catheter and balloon. Oesophageal pressure relative to mouth pressure is measured using a differential pressure transducer of small internal volume (Section 7.4). The transducer is connected to an air-filled polyethylene tube of internal diameter 1–1.5 mm, which is passed through the nose or mouth into the oesophagus. To obtain a representative pressure in the oesophagus, the end of the tube is surrounded by a thin-walled latex rubber balloon; its optimal dimensions are: length 10 cm, diameter 1 cm, and wall thickness 0.06 mm. The balloon should be tapered at its upper end to fit closely round the tube, which should be perforated in several places at near to the point of attachment. After injecting 6 ml of air down the tube with a syringe there should be no measurable pressure within the balloon. The air is then withdrawn and 0.4 ml reinjected. The recorded pressure is that in the air bubble at the upper end of the balloon [23].

As an alternative to a balloon, the tube can be filled with water. The system then has a more rapid frequency response but is liable to error due to hydrostatic forces and to the pressure being measured at only a single point. In addition, the presence of water in the oesophagus may provoke peristalsis.

Inserting the balloon. The operator establishes which of the subject's nostrils is widest by asking him or her to sniff through each in turn. In the few cases where a local anaesthetic is necessary, inquiry is made into previous drug sensitivity. The dose is 1 ml of 3% lignocaine hydrochloride solution (xylocaine) administered through a spray fitted with a long nozzle; the spray is directed to both the front and back of the nasopharynx and 5 min are allowed for anaesthesia to develop.

To make the insertion the operator faces the subject who sits with the neck slightly flexed. The operator lubricates the balloon with a tasteless lubricant (e.g. K-Y, Johnson and Johnson), and passes it gently into the nose whilst the subject makes a series of swallowing manoeuvres. Swallowing is assisted by having the subject suck up water from a glass through a flexible drinking straw held between the lips. The tube should now descend into the oesophagus. This should be checked by seeing that the tube has passed over the back of the tongue and is not coiled in the nasopharynx as sometimes occurs if the tube is very flexible. Swallowing is continued until the balloon enters the stomach. In this position sniffing should cause a rise in the pressure in the tube. After this has been confirmed, the tube is withdrawn 10 cm or more into the oesophagus where sniffing should now cause a fall rather than a rise in the pressure. The balloon is too high if the recorded pressure is affected by the subject performing a forced expiratory or inspiratory manoeuvre against a closed mouthpiece, or by moving the neck or by the observer pressing on the supra-sternal notch. Placement is satisfactory when a respiratory rhythm is obtained that is not obscured by pressure fluctuations transmitted from the heart. The main source of error is tonic contraction of the oesophageal muscle. This is particularly liable to occur at near to total lung capacity and is best overcome by waiting. Peristaltic contractions have duration of 2 s–5 s and occur especially in the lower part of the oesophagus; monitoring the pressure on an oscilloscope may identify them. Contractions due to the procedure usually disappear within a few minutes. Those due to hunger may be alleviated by a cup of tea.

11.8.2 Measurement of static lung compliance

The static compliance of the lungs is measured during breath holding at different volumes or during a very slow expiration. Volume is measured with a spirometer or by integration of the output from a pneumotachograph. Pleural pressure is measured indirectly from the oesophagus (see above). The alternative of using the supra-sternal notch as a null-point indicator is not satisfactory.

Outline. Consecutive measurements of oesophageal pressure and mouth pressure are made at a number of lung volumes throughout inspiration and expiration, starting from residual volume. The test breath is preceded by one or two full inspirations to total lung capacity; these prevent closure of some airways that might otherwise influence the result. The volume steps are made by closing the airways with a shutter for periods of about 1 s at steps of approximately 500 ml. During interruption the subject should not breathe but relax against the shutter. Provided that the glottis is open when the flow of gas is interrupted, equalisation of pressure occurs between the alveoli and the mouth. Equalisation is usually complete within 0.4 s, but at near to total lung capacity a time of 2 or 3 s may be required for the elastic recoil of the lung to accommodate to the change of volume.

Practical details. Pressure and volume are plotted in the form of a volume–pressure diagram such as that illustrated in Fig. 11.3. The compliance is the slope of the middle linear part of the tracing; it is usually measured over 1l starting from functional residual capacity. The pressure difference across the lungs is obtained by using a differential manometer to subtract mouth pressure from oesophageal pressure. The conditions are static so the recording equipment can have a relatively slow response time, for example a water manometer of small bore and recording spirometer. The procedure is simplified by using a differential electromanometer and a twin co-ordinate chart recorder in which the volume and the pressure are displayed on 2 axes at right angles. The record can be analysed directly provided there are no artefacts due to cardiac systole. These are best avoided by synchronising the periods of recording to follow the *R* wave of the ECG. Alternatively, the pressure fluctuations due to cardiac systole can be identified by the oesophageal pressure being recorded against time during periods when the airway is occluded by the shutter (see Fig. 11.6).

Compliance (slope) is measured for inspiration and expiration separately but the latter is usually reported because it is not as affected by hysteresis (Fig. 11.4). The pressure–volume diagram is also used to obtain the elastic recoil of the lung. This can be reported for inspiration and expiration separately at a lung volume 1 l or 20% below total lung capacity; alternatively the lung volume can be reported at a standard transpulmonary pressure, for example 0.5 kPa. The maximal recoil pressure at total lung capacity is also reported; it has the disadvantage of being rather variable, except when measured with the subject relaxing against the closed shutter. During the procedure the additional measurement of the rate of airflow immediately prior to interruption permits the calculation of pulmonary resistance and hence the relationship of pulmonary conductance to lung recoil pressure (Section 14.3.6).

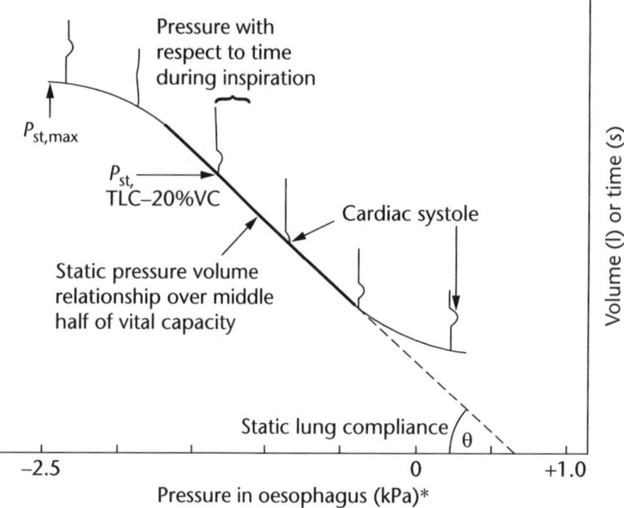

Fig. 11.6 Method for measuring static lung compliance using an interrupter and *X–Y* recorder [24]. The shutter interrupts the subject's airflow during slow inspiration or expiration; it is actuated for alternate periods of 1 s. After each interruption there is an interval of 0.4 s before the pen makes contact with the recorder paper. During the next 0.6 s pressure is recorded on the *X* axis. On the *Y* axis volume is recorded at the instant when the pen touches the paper; the time is recorded for the remainder of each interruption. The static lung compliance is the slope of the line joining the starting points of the tracings, except when these are deflected by pressure fluctuations due to cardiac systole. The fluctuations are apparent on the record so can be allowed for. *P*st is the elastic recoil pressure of the lung.
*For pressure in cm H_2O multiply these numbers by 10.

Comment. Static lung compliance is the most fundamental of all indices of lung function, but for practical assessment has largely been superseded by other tests (also see Section 11.10).

11.8.3 Exponential coefficient of lung distensibility (*k*)

Outline. The index (*k*) is the exponent in the equation used to describe the shape of the upper part of the static volume–pressure curve (eqn. 11.2). The volume is expressed as percentage of total lung capacity and is obtained using a volume displacement

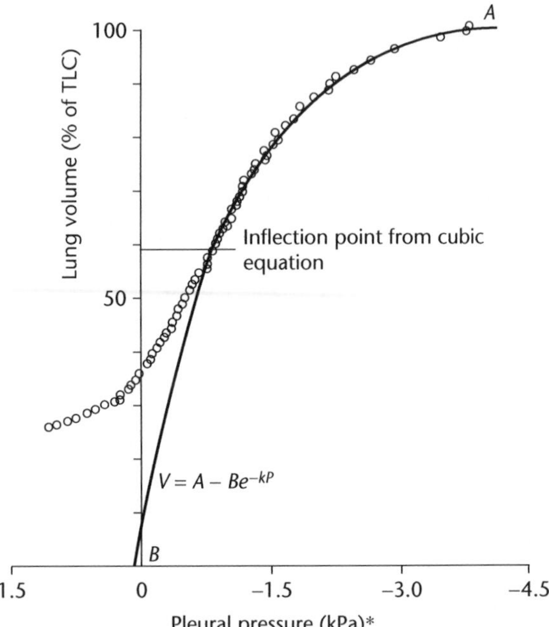

Fig. 11.7 Quasi-static P–V curve from a normal subject in the units % TLC and kPa. The continuous line is an exponential curve fitted to the data above the inflection point. $k = 0.120$ cm H_2O^{-1}.
*To obtain pressure in cm H_2O multiply these numbers by 10. Source [25]

plethysmograph. Pressure is obtained following oesophageal intubation as for static lung compliance.

Practical details. The method requires 30–40 pairs of observations between total lung capacity and where the curve ceases to be exponential. The subject performs the test expiration very slowly (flow rate $< 0.2\,\mathrm{l\,s^{-1}}$) without interruptions and the data points are obtained every quarter of a second [25], but to reduce variability the points can be running averages over the previous 0.5 s. The curves should be of good quality and free from artefacts due to oesophageal contractions, swallowing or closure of the glottis. The cutoff point is near to functional residual capacity. It can be identified as the point of inflection of a cubic equation fitted to the whole curve (Fig. 11.7). Subsequently, a mono-exponential equation is fitted to the data from this point up to total lung capacity. The residual variance about the curve expressed as a percentage of the total variance for volume over the range used should not exceed 10%.

Comment. The procedure for measuring k is technically demanding and low values are obtained if airways close during the test expiration. Hence, except in expert hands, the measurement of choice is that of static compliance.

11.8.4 Measurement of dynamic compliance

Outline. Dynamic compliance is measured during tidal breathing when the relationship between lung volume and pressure is not linear as in Fig. 11.3 but takes the form of an ellipse (see Fig. 9.3, page 103). This is formed by two arcs that join points of zero flow at the mouth just prior to the commencement of inspiration and expiration (A and C in the figure). Then, subject to the assumption indicated below the dynamic compliance is the slope of the straight line joining the two points. The method depends on the oesophageal pressure at these points being representative of the static recoil pressure of the lungs. This is the case in normal circumstances but not when the pressure is augmented by a resistive component from internal movement of air within the lungs (Section 16.1.9).

Practical details. Pressure is measured by a transducer selected to have a high frequency response and a range of 0–2.0 kPa (0–20 cm H_2O). Volume is measured with either a spirometer, which is modified by the connection of a potentiometer to the axle of the pulley wheel, or a pneumotachograph fitted with electronic integration, or a plethysmograph. The pressure and volume channels should be in phase and the dynamic responses of the pneumotachograph and pressure transducer should be similar. The pressure and volume are displayed synchronously on an x–y recorder or via a computer program. For convenience of measurement a mark is made on the pressure trace to indicate times when the flow is zero. The slope of the line through the points of zero flow on the diagram is estimated manually using a protractor or by computation. For greater accuracy the component of pressure that is applied to overcome the lung resistance is eliminated by electronic means. During very quiet breathing (i.e. in the absence of turbulence) this is done using the proportional relationship that exists between the velocity of airflow and the resistive pressure. The pressure record is backed off by an amount proportional to the velocity of airflow, which, in turn, is obtained from the output of the pneumotachograph before integration. In this way the short axis of the volume–pressure ellipse (Inspn-B-Expn. in Fig. 9.3, page 103) is narrowed down to a straight line. Alternatively, the dynamic compliance can be obtained during the measurement of the pulmonary resistance by the pressure–flow method ([26], also Section 14.4.5).

The measurement of dynamic compliance is normally made during slow quiet breathing when the resistive component of the pressure swing is minimal. The resistive component can be increased by performing the measurement at imposed breathing frequencies up to 60 per min. In the presence of airway obstruction the dynamic compliance falls as the frequency is increased. This *frequency dependence of compliance* can provide evidence for narrowing of small lung airways [27]. To avoid technical artifacts the tidal volume and the resting respiratory level must be kept constant. To obtain the change with frequency the dynamic compliance at each frequency is expressed as a percentage of the static compliance.

Comment. Dynamic compliance is used for studying the function of small lung airways and its measurement can provide an additional dimension to bronchodilatation (Fig. 15.1, page 168). It is seldom used for routine assessment of patients.

11.8.5 Total thoracic compliance

The total compliance of the respiratory system is the resultant compliances of the lungs and chest wall; these two attributes are in series so can be summed in terms of their elastances. Hence,

$$1/C\text{th} = 1/C\text{l} + 1/C\text{cw} \tag{11.4}$$

where C is compliance and th, l and cw refer respectively to the thorax, lungs and chest wall. The relationship can be used to derive chest wall compliance from separate static measurements of total thoracic and lung compliance. The principal requirement for the former measurement is that the respiratory muscles should be relaxed. This can often be achieved voluntarily (e.g. Fig. 11.3). It can also be obtained during anaesthesia. In infants reflex relaxation can often be achieved by gentle manual ventilation in conjunction with sedation. Alternatively, relaxation can be induced by occluding the airway (Section 24.4.5). The absence of muscle contractions should be confirmed by electromyography (Table 9.1, page 105).

A dynamic estimate of total thoracic compliance can be obtained during measurement of total respiratory resistance by the forced oscillation method (Section 14.4.4).

Comment. In premature infants the chest wall is relatively compliant, so thoracic compliance provides a good estimate of lung compliance. Subsequently, chest wall compliance decreases progressively with age. In most adults it is of nearly equal magnitude to lung compliance. The thoracic compliance is then mainly a nuisance variable.

Measurement in the Intensive Therapy Unit (ITU). In patients who are apnoeic and ventilated via a cuffed endotracheal tube the information needed to construct a static volume–pressure curve for the lungs and thorax is readily available. Pressure is monitored at the open end of the endotracheal tube (designated pressure at airway opening, Pao). It is recorded before and after tidal inflations with predetermined volumes from the ventilator or injection of air in 100 ml increments from a syringe. The Pao at end-inspiration is usually stable, but in some patients it declines exponentially to an equilibrium value. The decline reflects movement of air within the lungs and occurs when airways resistance is increased. The pressure before the decline can be used to calculate dynamic compliance. However, for constructing a static $V-P$ curve the pressure should be that after a steady level has been established; this may take up to 2 s. The subsequent plateau should persist for 300 ms. The drop in pressure is also informative since, in conjunction with the airflow immediately prior to the cessation of inspiration it can be used to calculate airways resistance. The resistance can be used to monitor the response to bronchodilator aerosol administered during ventilation.

Essential precautions with the method are that the cuff of the endotracheal tube should not allow leakage of air, the patient should not be making spontaneous respiratory efforts and the ventilator tubing should be indistensible. Alternatively, if it is distensible an allowance should be made for its compliance.

Comment. In ITU the static pressure–volume curve of the lungs can indicate optimal settings for ventilator therapy, contribute to diagnosis and be a means for monitoring the patient's progress. The curve can be separated from that for the thoracic cage if the oesophageal pressure is measured concurrently. However, the value so obtained can be in error when the subject is supine (Section 11.8.1).

11.9 Distensibility of conducting airways

The conducting airways are distensible structures, though in the larger airways this property is limited by the presence of cartilage and in all of them it can be overridden by contraction of bronchial smooth muscle. To measure the distensibility the muscle should be relaxed. *In vitro* the measurement can be of compliance ($\Delta V/\Delta P$) or a related attribute [28]. *In vivo* neither the volume nor the distending pressure of any single class of airway can be identified. Instead the volume can be that of trachea, bronchi and bronchioles together when it is anatomical deadspace (Section 16.1.3). Alternatively, in the case of an airway identified by a scanning technique, the diameter or length can be used instead. For airways that are extrapulmonary the distending pressure is pleural pressure. For intrapulmonary airways the pleural pressure is modified by being transmitted to the airway walls via the fibrous and elastic stroma of the lungs (Section 11.1). The transmission is further modified by disease processes that involve the lung parenchyma, including emphysema and interstitial fibrosis. The modifications are reflected in pleural pressure, so strictly this quantity should be used as the denominator. Alternatively, if the lung parenchyma is normal the lung volume can be used instead.

Measurement of the relationship of anatomical dead space to lung volume has been found to be an acceptable and rapid procedure. It has been used to show that the airway distensibility is reduced by thickening of the bronchial subepithelial tissue in patients with mild asthma [29]. Serial observations should be informative.

Practical details. The index ΔVd is the slope of the relationship of anatomical dead space to lung volume. The volume is varied by expiration from total lung capacity measured by a standard method (Section 10.3). The anatomical dead space is obtained by the method of Fowler. This can be applied as several lung volumes using nitrogen as the indicator gas (Section 16.2.3). Alternatively the indicator can be carbon dioxide, in which case the successive volumes can be obtained in the course of a single respiratory manoeuvre performed during closed circuit spirometry (Figs 11.8a, b).

In the method of Johns and colleagues [30], the subject adopts an upright-seated posture with the head erect. He or she breathes at a frequency of 25 min^{-1}. The first tidal breath is from total

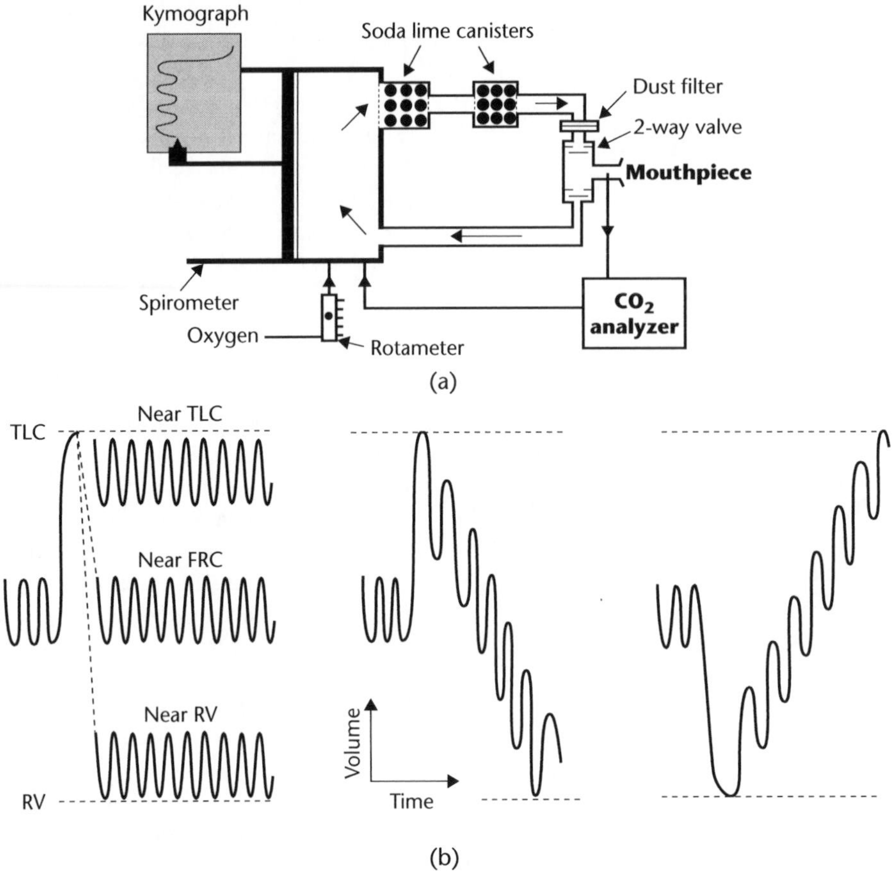

Fig. 11.8 (a) Schematic diagram of the apparatus used to measure ΔVd. (b) Spirogram illustrating the respiratory manoeuvre. Source: [30]

lung capacity and the subsequent breaths are from progressively decreasing volumes (Fig. 11.8b). Preliminary instruction is necessary. To obtain sufficient data points the manoeuvre is performed in triplicate. The dead space of each breath is calculated in the standard way; this can be done using a computer programme obtainable from the authors. The reproducibility of the index is reported as 9%.

11.10 Concluding remarks

The elasticity of lung tissue drives expiration and contributes to the stability of lung tissue. Deviations outside the normal range occur in many circumstances in association with material symptoms, impaired lung function and a risk of premature death. Hence, the static compliance is a fundamental dimension of lung function. Its magnitude is of great theoretical interest and practical importance and its measurement has contributed immensely to understanding how respiration is conducted.

Unfortunately the procedure for measuring static lung compliance has a poor acceptability and is technically demanding. The reproducibility is less than for most other indices. In addition, much of the relevant clinical information can now be inferred from scanning techniques that visualise deviations from normal lung structure. For these reasons static lung compliance is seldom measured on a routine basis. However, the procedure can resolve doubt as to the respective contributions to lung function of emphysema and fibrosis in cases where both are present [31] and the measurement is a necessary aid to understanding how respiration occurs. The case for measuring the underlying pressure–volume relationship is particularly strong in relation to assisted ventilation [32, 33]. The measurement of compliance should form part of the resources and teaching repertoire of every comprehensive lung function and academic respiratory laboratory.

11.11 References

1. Milic-Emili J, Henderson JA, Dolovich MB et al. Regional distribution of inspired gas in the lung. *J Appl Physiol* 1966; **21**: 749–759.
2. Storey WS, Staub NC. Ventilation of terminal air units. *J Appl Physiol* 1962; **17**: 391–397.
3. Weibel ER. *Morphometry of the human lung*. Berlin: Springer, 1963.
4. Howell JBL. Permutt S, Proctor DF, Riley RL. Effect of inflation of the lung on different parts of the vascular bed. *J Appl Physiol* 1961; **16**: 71–76.

5. Mead J, Takishima T, Leith D. Stress distribution in lungs: a model of pulmonary elasticity. *J Appl Physiol* 1970; **28**: 596–608.
6. Vawter DL, Matthew SFL, West JB. Effect of shape and size of lung and chest wall on stresses in the lung. *J Appl Physiol* 1975; **39**: 9–17.
7. Lai-Fook SJ. Stress distribution in the lung. In: Crystal RG, West JB, Weibel ER, Barnes P, eds. *The lung: scientific foundations.* 2nd ed. Philadelphia: Lippincott-Raven, 1997: 1177–1186.
8. Knowles JH, Hong SK, Rahn H. Possible errors using esophageal balloon in determination of pressure–volume characteristics of the lung and thoracic cage. *J Appl Physiol* 1959; **14**: 525–530.
9. Venegas JG, Harris RS, Simon BA. A comprehensive equation for the pulmonary pressure–volume curve. *J Appl Physiol* 1998; **84**: 389–395.
10. Radford EP Jr. Recent studies of mechanical properties of mammalian lungs. In: Remington JW, ed. *Tissue elasticity.* Bethesda, MD: American Physiological Society, 1957: 177–190.
11. Clements JA. Lung surface tension and surfactant: the early years. In: West JB, ed. *Respiratory physiology: people and ideas.* Oxford: Oxford University Press 1995; 208–229.
12. Pattle RE. Properties, function and origin of the alveolar lining layer. *Nature* 1955; **175**: 1125–1126.
13. Clements JA, Hustead RF, Johnson RP, Gribetz I. Pulmonary surface tension and alveolar stability. *J Appl Physiol* 1961; **16**: 444–450.
14. Whitsett JA, Nogee LM, Weaver TE, Horowitz AD. Human surfactant protein B: structure, function, regulation and genetic disease. *Physiol Rev* 1995; **75**: 749–757.
15. Tenney SDM. A tangled web: Young, Laplace and the surface tension law. *NIPS* 1993; **8**: 179–183.
16. Hughes JM. Site of airway closure in dog lungs. *Bull Physiopathol Respir* 1970; **6**: 877–879.
17. Craig DB, Wahba WM, Don HF et al. 'Closing volume' and its relationship to gas exchange in seated and supine positions. *J Appl Physiol* 1971: **31**: 717–721.
18. Macklem PT, Wilson NJ. Measurement of intrabronchial pressure in man. *J Appl Physiol* 1965; **20**: 653–663.
19. Mead J. Mechanical properties of lungs. *Physiol Rev.* 1961; **41**: 281–330.
20. Jonson B, Svantesson C. Elastic pressure–volume curves: what information do they convey? *Thorax* 1999; **54**: 82–87.
21. Colebatch HJH, Greaves IA, Ng CKY. Exponential analysis of elastic recoil and ageing in healthy males and females. *J Appl Physiol* 1979; **47**: 683–691.
22. Amato MB, Barbas CS, Medeiros DM et al. Effect of a protective-ventilation strategy on mortality in the acute respiratory distress syndrome. *N Engl J Med* 1998; **338**: 347–354.
23. Baydur A, Cha E-J, Sassoon CSH. Validation of esophageal balloon technique at different lung volumes and postures. *J Appl Physiol* 1987; **62**: 315–321.
24. Hart A, McKerrow CB, Reynolds JA. A method of using an X-Y recorder in measuring the lung compliance. *J Physiol (Lond)* 1966; **184**: 50P–52P.
25. Gugger M, Wraith PK, Sudlow MF. A new method of analysing pulmonary quasi-static pressure–volume curves in normal subjects and in patients with chronic airflow obstruction. *Clin Sci* 1990; **78**: 365–369.
26. Officer TM, Pellegrino R, Brusasco V, Rodarte JR. Measurement of pulmonary resistance and dynamic compliance with airway obstruction. *J Appl Physiol* 1988; **85**: 1982–1988.
27. Hoz RE, Berger KI, Klugh TT et al. Frequency dependence of compliance in the evaluation of patients with unexplained respiratory symptoms. *Respir Med* 2000; **94**: 221–227.
28. Hughes JMB, Hoppin FG, Mead J. Effect of lung inflation on bronchial length and diameter in excised lungs. *J Appl Physiol* 1972; **32**: 25–35.
29. Ward C, Johns DP, Bish R et al. Reduced airway distensibility, fixed airflow limitation and airway wall remodelling in asthma. *Am J Respir Crit Care Med* 2001; **164**: 1718–1721.
30. Johns DP, Wilson J, Harding R, Walters EH. Airway distensibility in healthy and asthmatic subjects: effect of lung volume history. *J Appl Physiol* 2000; **88**: 1413–1420.
31. Osborne S, Hogg JC, Wright JL et al. Exponential analysis of the pressure–volume curve. *Am Rev Respir Dis* 1988;**137**: 1083–1088.
32. Maggiore SM, Brochard L. Pressure–volume curve: methods and meaning. *Minerva Anestesiol* 2001; **67**: 228–237.
33. Antonaglia V, Peratoner A, De Simoni L et al. Bedside assessment of respiratory viscoelastic properties in ventilated patients. *Eur Respir J* 2000; **16**: 302–308.

Further reading (see also Section 1.8)

Bachofen H, Schurch S, Urbinelli M, Weibel ER. Relations among alveolar surface tension, surface area, volume, and recoil pressure. *J Appl Physiol* 1987; **62**: 1878–1887.

Bayliss LE, Robertson GW. The visco-elastic properties of the lungs. *Q J Exp Physiol* 1939; **29**: 27–47.

Budiansky B, Kimmel E. Elastic moduli of lungs. *J Appl Mech* 1990; **54**: 351–358.

Carson J. On the elasticity of the lungs. *Philos Trans R Soc Lond* 1820; **110**: 29–44.

Gibson GJ, Pride NB, Davis J, Schroter RC. Exponential description of the static pressure–volume curve of normal and diseased lungs. *Am Rev Respir Dis* 1979; **120**: 799–811.

Milic-Emili J, Mead J, Turner JM. Topography of esophageal pressure as a function of posture in man. *J Appl Physiol* 1964; **19**: 212–216.

Niewoehner DE, Kleinerman J. Morphometric study of elastic fibers in normal and emphysematous human lungs. *Am Rev Resp Dis* 1977; **115**: 15–21.

Rahn H, Otis AB, Chadwich LE, Fenn WO. The pressure–volume diagram of the thorax and lung. *Am J Physiol* l946; **146**: 161–178.

Smith JC, Stamenovic D. Surface forces in lungs. 1. Alveolar surface tension-lung volume relationships. *J Appl Physiol* 1986; **60**: 1341–1350.

Stamenovic D, Wilson TA. A strain energy function for lung parenchyma. *J Biomech Eng* 1985; **107**: 81–86.

Trop D, Peeters R, van de Woestijne KP. Localization of recording site in the esophagus by means of cardiac artifacts. *J Appl Physiol* 1970; **29**: 283–287.

Van Golde LMG, Batenburg JJ, Robertson B. The pulmonary surfactant system: biochemical aspects and functional significance. *Physiol Rev* 1988; **68**: 374–455.

CHAPTER 12

Forced Ventilatory Volumes and Flows (Ventilatory Capacity)

This chapter describes indices of ventilatory capacity and how they are measured. The measurements are the 'bread and butter' of lung function testing.

12.1 Introduction

Ventilatory capacity is the term used to describe the maximal ability to move gas rapidly in and out of the lung. It includes both maximal breathing and single forced inspirations and expirations. Ventilatory capacity integrates the characteristics of the whole respiratory apparatus, including the lungs, thoracic cage and respiratory muscles with their control mechanisms. The capacity is one of the factors that determine maximal exercise ability (Section 28.8). A reduced capacity secondary to narrowing of airways is the commonest cause of undue breathlessness on exertion. Tests of ventilatory capacity constitute the first and sometimes the only stage in the physiological assessment of respiratory symptoms in patients of all ages. The tests are used for clinical management, in respiratory surveys and for assessing respiratory impairment (Table 12.1). They can be performed satisfactorily by most subjects from age 5 year upwards, but failure to do so can itself provide useful information [1, 2]. The procedures have been subject to international scrutiny and the resulting protocols [3–5] should be adhered to in most circumstances.

12.2 Maximal breathing

12.2.1 Definitions

Maximal breathing capacity (MBC) is the maximal volume of air that a subject can breathe per min; the circumstances should be defined. When the manoeuvre is performed by voluntary effort, the index is called *maximal voluntary ventilation* (MVV); it is usually measured over 15 s. For a longer period, e.g. 4 min, the term *sustained* MVV or *sustained* MBC is used [6]. *Maximal ventilation during rebreathing carbon dioxide* and *maximal exercise ventilation* are also reported. The performance of maximal ventilation replicates a single breath of appropriate size and duration. This is the basis for *Indirect* MBC (Table 12.2). The index is the sum of 40 forced expirations from total lung capacity each of 0.75 s duration [8]. It provides a guide to the maximal exercise ventilation of respiratory patients, but other arithmetic models fit the data better [12].

Table 12.1 Some indices of ventilatory capacity.

Index	Comment	Reproducibility*
Individual tests		
Maximal voluntary ventilation (MVV)	overall test, effort dependent, can assess endurance	≈ 4–6%
Peak expiratory flow (PEF)	reflects large airway calibre, used to monitor bronchial lability	
Indices from volume–time curves		
Forced expiratory volume		
in 0.5 s or 0.75 s ($FEV_{0.5}$, $FEV_{0.75}$)	can be used in children	
in first second (FEV_1)	overall test, first choice in most circumstances	≈ 2–3%
in 6 s (FEV_6)	surrogate for FVC	
Forced vital capacity (FVC)	component of FEV% and other indices	≈ 2–3%
Forced expiratory time (FET)	clinical guide to expiratory narrowing of airways	> 8%
Inspiratory vital capacity (IVC)	used in Tiffeneau index (FEV_1/IVC)	≈ 2–3%
Forced mid-expiratory flow (FMF or $FEF_{25-75\%}$), formerly MMEF or MMF	detects mild airflow limitation (respiratory surveys)	≈ 4–6%
Transit time (mean, SD etc)	usefulness unproven	≈ 4–6%
Indices from flow–volume loop†		
$FEF_{25\%FVC}$	PEF is probably more useful	≈ 4–6%
$FEF_{50\%FVC}$	$FEF_{25-75\%}$ is more useful	≈ 4–6%
$FEF_{75\%FVC}$	may reflect small airway calibre. [$FEF_{75-85\%}$ is also used]	>8%
$FEF_{40\%TLC}$, pleth	is independent of dynamic compression	≈ 4–6%
$FIF_{50\%FVC}$	reduced by upper airway obstruction and respiratory muscle weakness. Is effort dependent. Has low acceptability.	>8%
Density dependence	mainly of research interest	no information

* Reference values are given in Chapter 26.
† Flow after the stated percentage has been expired or inspired.

Table 12.2 Interrelations between indices of ventilatory capacity.

Variable to be predicted	Predictor	Relationship*†	Source
Maximal voluntary ventilation	FEV_1	$MVV = 34.7\ FEV_1^{0.985}$ (simplifies to $35 \times FEV_1$) (C of V 18%, R^2 0.73)	[7]
Indirect maximal breathing capacity	$FEV_{0.75}$	$IMBC = 40 \times FEV_{0.75}$	[8]
$FEV_{0.75}$	FEV_1	$FEV_{0.75} = 0.92\ FEV_1 - 0.07$ (95% limits ± 8%)	[9]
Maximal exercise ventilation in respiratory patients	FEV_1	$\dot{V}_E$ max ex = 35 FEV_1	[10]
		$\dot{V}_E$ max ex = 18.9 FEV_1 + 19.7 ($R^2 = 0.67$)	[11]
		$\dot{V}_E$ max ex = 33.1 $FEV_1^{0.73}$ (C of V 18%)	[12]
Maximal exercise tidal volume	VC	V_t max ex = 0.65 VC – 0.64 (SD 0.21)	[13]

* Volumes are expressed in litres and ventilation in $l\ min^{-1}$.
† C of V = coefficient of variation (Section 7.15).

12.2.2 Background

The MBC reflects mainly the calibre of large airways, the respiratory effort and the condition of the thoracic cage. The procedure requires a high level of motivation and can be disagreeable so it is not suitable for routine use. It has been superseded by single breath tests, except sometimes as a guide to maximal ventilation during exercise (Section 28.8) and for assessing training of respiratory muscles.

12.2.3 Measurement

MVV is measured over 15 s using a rolling seal spirometer or pneumotachograph with an acceptably low flow resistance (Section 7.3.2). Alternatively, use can be made of a bellows spirometer or a water spirometer with large cross sectional area [14]; any valves and the absorber for carbon dioxide should have been removed. During rebreathing, CO_2 accumulates in the apparatus so there is no risk of hypocapnia. When a pneumotachograph is used in open circuit the CO_2 is lost to atmosphere. It should preferable be replaced by addition of CO_2 to the inspired gas [$F_{I,CO_2} = 0.05$], but this is not essential.

The general conditions for respiratory measurements should be adhered to (Sections 2.6 and 12.6.2). A nose clip should be used. During the test the observer urges the subject to achieve the greatest possible depth and frequency of breathing. The frequency should preferably exceed 80 min^{-1} and should be reported (Sections 6.2 and 6.3). A record of the ventilation should also be retained if one is available. The result is usually the average of two technically satisfactory measurements.

The outcome of the test is influenced by the rapport that develops between observer and subject and both can find the procedure tiring. Partly for this reason the measurement is made infrequently.

12.3 Peak expiratory flow

12.3.1 Background

Peak expiratory flow (PEF) is the maximal flow achieved during a forced expiration following a full inspiration. The peak obtained in this way can be exceeded involuntarily during coughing. The flow reflects the strength of the expiratory muscles, the mechanical properties of the lungs and airways and the inertia, resistance and sensitivity of the recording equipment. PEF is particularly susceptible to dynamic compression of extrapulmonary airways because whilst such airways are subject to pleural pressure, their walls are not supported by traction from lung tissue. The determinants of maximal flow are given in Chapter 13. The subject has been reviewed [15].

The bronchi and larger bronchioles are subject to reflex bronchoconstriction as in extrinsic asthma; hence, PEF is recommended for monitoring persons who may have occupational asthma (Sections 15.8.5 and 37.7.6). The index is also widely used by health professionals and by patients for detection and management of variable airflow limitation. PEF is unsuitable for patients with COPD or emphysema, on account of the disease processes involving small airways as well as the larger ones (Chapter 40). The ventilatory impairment assessed using PEF may then be underestimated compared with using FEV_1, which is the preferred index for assessment of such patients [16]. In addition, because PEF is dependent on expiratory effort it is unsuitable for debilitated patients or those who are acutely ill; again, the use of FEV_1 is preferable.

In most circumstances these limitations of using PEF outweigh the benefits from the equipment being readily portable, the procedure rapid and the manoeuvre not difficult to perform. For most applications FEV_1 should be used instead.

12.3.2 Measurement

In the laboratory the PEF can be obtained during the course of measurement of FEV_1 and FVC. It is then used to check that expiration was maximal (Section 12.4.1). For this purpose the equipment should be capable of measuring flow, for example a pneumotachograph, turbine or servo-spirometer. With a turbine spirometer the PEF derived from a short, sharp exhalation can be systematically higher by 3–5% than that obtained from a full expiration [17]; in that study, although the overall difference was small the limits of agreement were wide (–58 to +38 l min^{-1}).

In the clinic or for respiratory surveys PEF may be measured using a portable peak flow meter. This method may underestimate PEF compared with that obtained using a low resistance pneumotachograph [18]. Before use the meter should be inspected to establish that nothing is loose, the ratchet does not slip and the filter, if fitted, is clean. The procedure for calibration is described in Section 7.3.2 and involves use of a flow generating pump (Section 7.15). Where a pump is not available the calibration checks should be against secondary standards or biological controls [15].

The choice of model is important as portable peak flow meters vary in performance characteristics, including their frequency response [19, 20], accuracy and linearity [21–24]. Some models are seriously alinear and this can affect the interpretation of serial measurements, for example in community studies of air pollution [25] and clinical studies of patients with asthma [26]. To overcome the difficulty, models that meet the European standard EN 13826 are available for purchase. In addition, meters can be tested using standard waveforms [27]. Calibration factors are available for unmodified Wright peak flow meters purchased prior to September 2004 (Table 12.3).

The measurement of PEF is best performed seated without a nose clip. The flow should represent an appreciable movement of gas generated from the chest and not a pulse wave as can come from puffing or from blowing out and then contracting the muscles of the cheeks. If the last is a problem the cheeks can be held flat with the hand. The correct procedure should be demonstrated.

During the measurement the neck should be in a natural position and not flexed, the prior inspiration should be complete and the forced expiration should follow without delay. A pause or breath hold for as short a time as 2 s reduces the elastic properties of the central airways and can decrease the PEF by up to 10% [28]. Coughing is also unacceptable. Once the peak flow has been registered the subject should discontinue the expiration.

When a portable instrument is used the result is reported as litres BTPS min^{-1}; in other circumstances the flow is in l s^{-1}. Usual practice is to record the highest value from a set of three

Table 12.3 Calibration factors for Wright peak flow meters purchased in the UK prior to September 1st 2004.

Device	Calibration factor	RSD ($l\ min^{-1}$)
Large meter (round dial)	PEFcorrected = 53.2 + 0.585 PEFobs + 0.00075 $(PEFobs)^2$	6
Mini-Wright meter	PEFcorrected = 47.4 + 0.373 PEFobs + 0.00090 $(PEFobs)^2$	7

Source: [21]

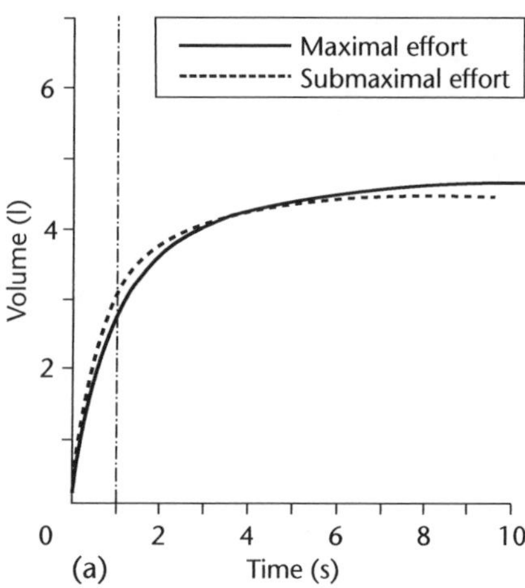

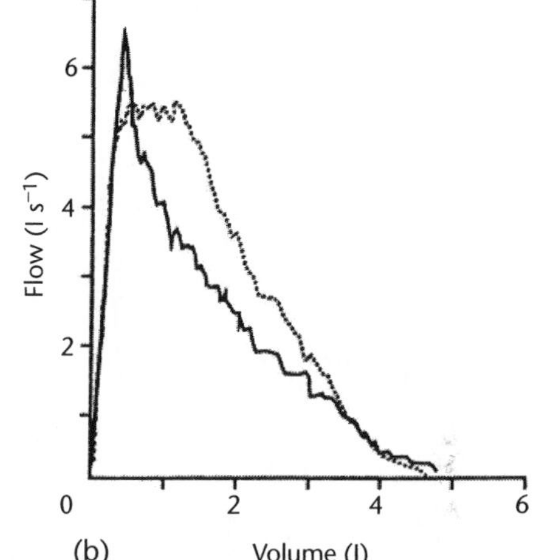

Fig. 12.1 Expiratory volume–time curves recorded by a healthy person who expired with maximal and submaximal effort after a full inspiration. Right. The flow–volume curves that relate to the same expirations. Features of the two curves are discussed in the text.

acceptable blows; of these the best two should not differ by more than $40\ l\ min^{-1}$. With care, a change in PEF of 6% to 8% in adults and 9% to 10% in youths can be statistically significant [29].

12.4 Indices from single breath volume – time curves (see also Footnote 12.1)

12.4.1 Indices based on volume

For these indices the *volume* of gas expired or inspired during one full respiratory manoeuvre made with maximal effort is related to time from the start of the manoeuvre (e.g. Fig. 12.1 (left)). The procedure has the merit that the equipment can be relatively unsophisticated. However, to make allowance for inertia and the biological and instrumental response times the start time is defined by back extrapolation as described below.

Forced expiratory volume and related indices. The forced expiratory volume in one second (FEV_1) is the volume of gas expired during the first second of a forced expiration following a full inspiration [10]. The index was pioneered by Tiffeneau and Pinelli [30] and by Gaensler [31]. It is very reproducible and is recommended for most applications in respiratory, clinical, occupational and paediatric medicine, including for assessing the response to a bronchodilator or constrictor aerosol (Section 15.7.2) and in respiratory surveys. Other time intervals, for example $FEV_{0.5}$ or $FEV_{0.75}$, can also be used. In adults and most children the volumes obtained using these time intervals are highly correlated (e.g. Table 12.2). The test is performed with maximal effort, so the result includes the effect of any retardation of flow caused by dynamic compression of airways during the expiration (Section 13.2). Where this occurs the flow is greater if the expiratory effort is submaximal [32, 33]. The phenomenon has been described as inverse effort dependence [34]. The associated index is the *relaxed expiratory flow* over the relevant time interval (Fig. 12.1). The use of this index is not recommended.

Forced inspiratory volume in 1 s (FIV_1) is the inspiratory equivalent of the FEV_1. FIV is effort dependent and not particularly easy or agreeable to perform. It can shed light on suspected obstruction to extrathoracic airways, but better discrimination is obtained by using $FIF_{50\%FVC}$ (Section 12.5.2).

Forced vital capacity (FVC) is the volume of gas expired when the forced expiratory manoeuvre is continued to full expiration. In most healthy persons this point is reached within 6 s (hence FEV_6), but in the presence of airflow limitation from narrow or unduly collapsible airways the expiration can continue for much longer (up to 15 s). In this circumstance the FEV_6 is a poor guide to FVC. In addition, due to dynamic compression the FVC is then less than some other estimates of vital capacity,

Footnote 12.1. This Section describes the indices. The procedures for measurement are in Section 12.6.

including inspiratory vital capacity (IVC) and two-stage vital capacity (Sections 10.1.2 and 13.2).

FVC is measured concurrent with FEV_1 and its main application is to standardize forced expiratory volume (FEV_1) for lung size using the relationship:

$$FEV_1\% = (FEV_1/FVC) \times 100 \qquad (12.1)$$

The relationship is a component of most lung function reports. However, to avoid an effect from dynamic compression, the denominator should preferably be IVC, two-stage vital capacity [35], or relaxed expiratory vital capacity (EVC) if one of these indices is available. The convention that is used should be reported.

FVC enters into the derivation by spirometry of indices of forced expiratory flow, including forced mid-expiratory flow ($FEF_{25-75\%}$), flows after a specified proportion of FVC has been expired (e.g. $FEF_{50\%FVC}$ and $FEF_{75\%FVC}$) and the volume of isoflow (Section 12.7). It provides an acceptable measure of vital capacity in occupational and epidemiological respiratory surveys. Whether or not this is also the case for FEV_6 depends on the objectives of the study.

Forced expired volume as percentage of forced vital capacity. $FEV_1\%$ is used as a guide to airway calibre (Section 38.3.1) and has the merit that, unlike FEV_1 it is nearly independent of lung size, body size and stature. $FEV_1\%$ may be misinterpreted if vital capacity is affected by increased strength or weakness of the accessory muscles of respiration (Section 25.5) or by dynamic compression, or if residual volume varies semi-independently. Thus, a reduced $FEV_1\%$ should not be interpreted as evidence for airflow limitation unless FEV_1 is itself reduced.

Bronchodilator and constrictor aerosols affect the denominator as well as the numerator of $FEV_1\%$. As a result the ratio is an insensitive guide to bronchial lability or responsiveness to a bronchodilator drug (e.g. Fig. 15.2, page 168 and Table 15.2, page 168). A similar consideration applies to the use of $FEF_{25\%-75\%}$, $FEF_{50\%FVC}$ and $FEF_{75\%FVC}$. Usually FEV_1 will be used instead.

Forced mid-expiratory flow (FMF) was formerly maximal mid-expiratory flow (MMEF). Now the recommended usage is *forced expiratory flow* ($FEF_{25-75\%FVC}$) [5]. The index is the average flow over the middle half of the forced vital capacity during maximally forced expiration [36]. It is used for detecting the early stages of airflow limitation, but not for clinical management of patients.

Other volume-based indices of forced expiratory flow. The *maximal expiratory flow* ($FEF_{200-1200}$) is the average flow over the first litre of expiration starting after 200 ml has been expired. This index has been superceded by PEF.

The *forced late expiratory flow* is the average flow between 75% and 85% of the expired vital capacity ($FEF_{75-85\%FVC}$). The index can be measured using equipment that does not meet the technical specification for instantaneous flows (e.g. Vitalograph recording to 12 s). It is believed to reflect the calibre of small airways. Similar information can be obtained more directly by using $FEF_{75\%FVC}$ (formerly $MEF_{25\%FVC}$, Section 12.5.1). The reproducibility of the index is poor.

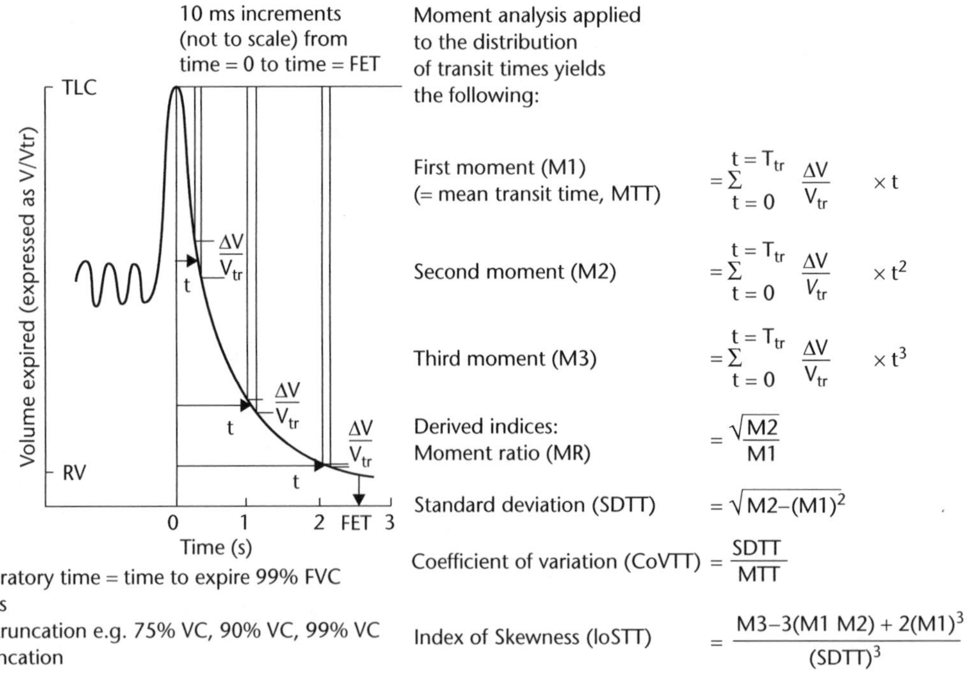

Fig. 12.2 Derivation of transit time indices. Source: [37]

12.4.2 Indices expressed as times

Forced expiratory time (FET). This index is the time taken to expire a specified portion of the forced vital capacity e.g. 99% (hence $FET_{99\%}$). It has a poor reproducibility. If spirometry is not available $FET_{100\%}$ can be measured using a stopwatch. A time in excess of 4 s is evidence for some degree of airflow limitation.

Mean transit time and derivatives. The *mean transit time* (MTT) is the mean time taken for gas molecules to leave the lung during the forced exhalation of either the full forced vital capacity (i.e. 100%) or a designated proportion of it (e.g. 90%). The volume associated with each time is expressed as a fraction of whatever proportion is chosen (Fig. 12.2). This process normalises the spirogram with respect to the volume. The MTT is calculated by moment analysis applied to the normalised spirogram and is equal to the first moment about the origin. For the full spirogram the volume expired in successive time intervals (e.g. 10 ms) is expressed as a proportion of the FVC (ΔV/FVC) and is multiplied by the time from the start of the breath (t) determined by back-extrapolation, as for measurement of the FEV_1. The MTT is the sum of the products, $\Sigma(\Delta V/\text{FVC} \times t)$, and is effectively the area under the normalised spirogram. The second and third moments about the origin are calculated using t^2 and t^3, respectively. The three moments are used to calculate dispersion indices including the *standard deviation of transit times* (SDTT), the *coefficient of variation* (CofVTT [i.e. SDTT $\times$ 100/MTT%]), an *index of skewness* (IOS) and various *moment ratios.* The use of t^2 and t^3 result in the calculated indices being influenced markedly by late events in the spirogram, thus they should be sensitive to prolongation of the expiration as occurs in airflow limitation. However, the variability between breaths can be large and this reduces the sensitivity of the test. Much of the variability is towards the end of expiration and can be avoided by omitting this part of the breath. Initially truncation was with respect to time at 6 s [38] but this process is unsound [39] and, instead, the spirogram should be truncated with respect to volume at, e.g. 90% (range 75%–99%). In practice three acceptable volume–time curves are recorded (Section 12.6.3). The measurements are either derived from the averaged moments [40] or taken from the curve that has the shortest MTT [37] or largest FVC. However, the methodology is not yet fully standardised.

Transit time indices differ from the forced expiratory flows in being derived from all or most of the forced expiration, being relatively independent of vital capacity and body size and focussing attention on lung units that empty late in expiration. In addition, airway disease results in a reduction in forced expiratory flows but an increase in transit time indices. This eliminates some of the difficulties experienced when interpreting changes in expiratory flows when expressed as standardised residuals from reference values. An important advantage favouring transit time analysis is that errors in calibration of volume between instruments should not influence the measurements, provided that the volume recording is linear and the timing is accurate. This facilitates comparisons between different studies. The indices were proposed for detecting minor degrees of airway narrowing, particularly in persons in whom FEV_1 and $FEF_{50\%FVC}$ were still relatively normal [41]. The MTT is highly correlated with $FEV_1\%$, which has the advantage of being more easily measured. However, for a comprehensive assessment the MTT should be reported with at least one of its indices of dispersion, of which the moment ratio is probably the measure of choice [39]. Despite these apparent advantages the practical usefulness of the indices has still to be established.

12.5 Indices from the relationship of flow to volume

The flow–volume curve depicts the relationship of respiratory flow to lung volume [42]. The curve can be for expiration alone or for expiration and inspiration (flow–volume loop). The flow can be spontaneous, as during exercise, or made with maximal effort and the volume excursion can be maximal or submaximal; in the latter instance it starts from the end of a normal inspiration and is called a partial expiratory flow–volume curve. The relevant circumstances should be recorded. For an expiratory curve obtained after a full inspiration and performed with maximal effort the volume axis is forced vital capacity.

Flow–volume curves illustrate the relationship of flow to lung volume at the instant of measurement (Figs 12.3 and 12.4). Hence, at any point on the curve the physiologically relevant volume is thoracic gas volume (TGV) as measured using whole body plethysmography (Section 14.6). However, on account of its convenience, the volume of gas measured at the mouth is often used instead when the volume is taken as that expired from total lung capacity down to the point where the flow is recorded. The gas remaining in the lung is then TLC less volume expired. This is nearly correct when airway calibre is normal. But when the airways are narrow the expiratory effort compresses the thoracic gas, so the TGV associated with the observed flow is overestimated. As a result, when flow–volume spirometry is performed in the presence of dynamic compression the volume signal is out of phase with flow. In this circumstance precise interpretation of the flow index is not possible [43].

12.5.1 Expiratory flow–volume curve

Expiratory flow–volume ($\dot{v}$–V) curves (Fig. 12.3) can be considered as having three parts. Of these, the initial rapidly rising limb and the inflection are dependent on the expiratory force that is applied. The inflection provides an index of peak expiratory flow and can indicate whether or not expiration has been performed with maximal effort (Section 12.6.2). The descending limb, after the volume has reduced to approximately 70% of total lung capacity, is nearly independent of expiratory effort and is effectively linear (Section 13.2). The linearity is lost and the limb becomes concave in the presence of obstruction to intrathoracic

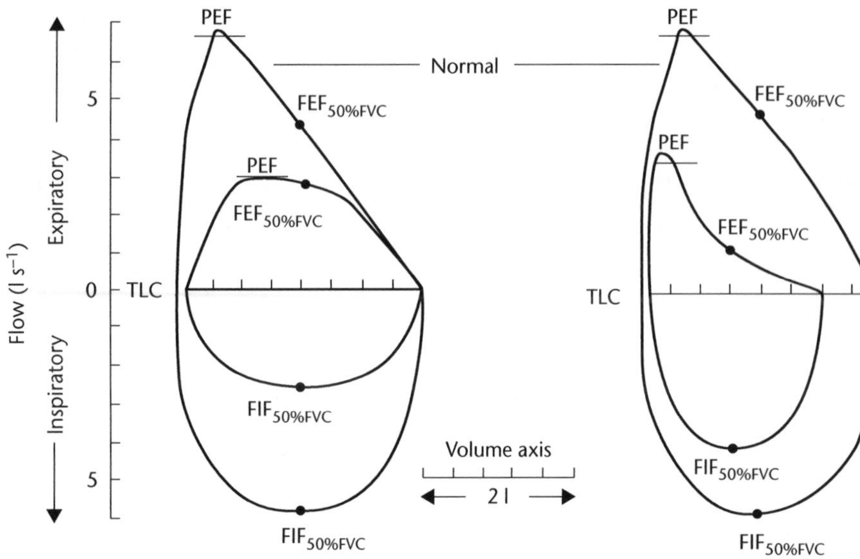

Fig. 12.3 Maximal flow–volume curves for a healthy subject (outer curves), a patient with moderate obstruction to the intrapulmonary airways (inner right-hand curve) and with obstruction to the extrathoracic airways (inner left-hand curve). PEF is peak expiratory flow. FEF_{50} and FIF_{50} are the forced expiratory and inspiratory flow at the lung volume (RV + 50%VC). On expiration at lung volumes less than 80% TLC the flows are relatively independent of the expiratory effort that is exerted (see Fig. 13.1, page 144). (Note that the scales for the two axes of the curves should preferably be in the ratio 2:1).

airways (Fig. 12.4). In this and some other circumstances the instantaneous lung volume can be less than its static counterpart [44] (also preceding paragraph).

The full inspiration that normally precedes the delineation of a flow–volume curve causes reflex bronchodilation. This can influence the outcome of an assessment of the response to a bronchodilator drug (Section 15.7.2). The error can be eliminated by measuring instead a partial expiratory flow–volume curve [45].

In patients with respiratory disorders, the several factors that influence the flow–volume curve give rise to curves of distinctive shape. Hence, inspection of the curves can contribute to clinical diagnosis (Section 38.3). The shape can indicate whether or not there is airflow limitation. Further information can be obtained by applying suction at the mouth during tidal expiration (negative pressure –0.3 to –0.5 kPa (–3 to –5 cm H_2O)). This amount of suction will normally increase the flow [46]. Manual compression of the abdomen can also be used [47]. The absence of a response is evidence for expiratory flow limitation (Section 13.6). However, interpretation of the findings may not be straightforward [46]. In terms of flow–volume spirometry, comparison of the curve obtained from a patient during maximal voluntary expiration with that during maximal exercise can illuminate the factors limiting exercise (Section 28.8.1).

Flow indices from the curves include peak expiratory flow and forced expiratory flow at the point when specified proportions of forced vital capacity have been expired, usually 25%, 50% or 75% [48]. These indices are designated, respectively, $FEF_{25\%FVC}$, $FEF_{50\%FVC}$ and $FEF_{75\%FVC}$ (see Fig. 12.4). They were formerly expressed as maximal expiratory flows (MEF) at a volume defined by the proportion of forced vital capacity *remaining to be expired.* Hence, in the absence of dynamic compression, $FEF_{75\%FVC}$ was equal to $MEF_{25\%FVC}$ etc [3]. However, the MEF terminology had to be abandoned on account of ambiguity in drafting, since where (as was intended) expiratory effort was

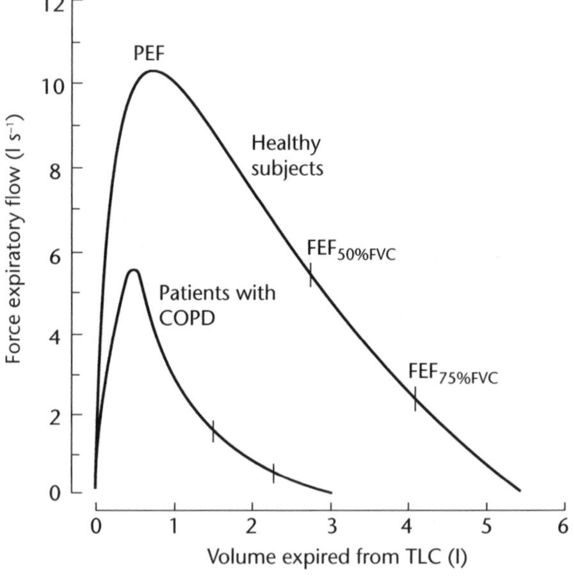

Fig. 12.4 Idealized flow–volume curve showing the principal indices. In practice the indices are the highest recorded from three technically satisfactory blows and need not all come from the same curve.

maximal, the resulting flow might be submaximal on account of dynamic compression [5].

The FEF indices are obtained from measurements of flow and of volume. As a result they are less reproducible than indices that entail the measurement of only one of these variables. In addition the reference values have a relatively wide dispersion (Tables 26.7 and 26.16, pages 339 and 347) and this can affect their usefulness. Changes in the indices are particularly difficult to interpret in circumstances when both volume and flow are affected, for example after inhalation of a broncho-active drug (Section 15.7.2).

Comment. The shape of the flow–volume curve has proved to be of value for diagnosis (Section 39.2.1) and for assessing the quality of measurements made by spirometry (Section 12.6.2). It can also be used to indicate the presence of expiratory flow limitation during exercise (Section 28.8.1). The $FEF_{75\%FVC}$ (formerly $MEF_{25\%FVC}$) has been found to be reduced amongst smokers and some shipyard welders and deep sea divers (Section 37.3 onwards). It can also be reduced following strenuous exercise. The relevance of these observations is unclear but point to possible future investigations. The index $FEF_{40\%TLC,\ pleth}$ provides an index of flow that is independent of dynamic compression. By contrast the flow indices $FEF_{25\%FVC}$ and $FEF_{50\%FVC}$ appear not to contain additional information compared with the related indices PEF and FMF; these latter indices should be used instead.

12.5.2 Inspiratory flow–volume curve

The inspiratory flow–volume curve reflects the force that is applied to the lung by maximal inspiratory effort. This expands the intrathoracic airways, so the maximal inspiratory flow is relatively insensitive to bronchoconstriction. However, it is sensitive to the calibre of extrathoracic airways including the nasopharynx. As a result the inspiratory flow is less during nose breathing compared with breathing through the mouth [49].

The inspiratory flow–volume curve is nearly symmetrical (Fig. 12.3) so its characteristics are adequately described by the mid-point, which is the forced inspiratory flow ($FIF_{50\%IVC}$). This index has replaced FIV_1 for assessing possible obstruction to extrapulmonary airways and weakness of the respiratory muscles (Sections 41.2 and 9.1). It may have a place in assessing the ventilatory response to exercise (Sections 28.8.1 and 29.8.2).

12.6 Measurement of single breath indices of ventilatory capacity

12.6.1 General considerations

The conditions of measurement, including those for serial observations and the equipment should meet the general requirements and technical specifications given in Chapter 7. The operator should have been trained [50] (Section 2.5). Equipment should be calibrated at the start of each measurement session (Section 7.15), and cleaned in the recommended manner (Section 7.13). Detailed recommendations have been made on these and other aspects of the measurements [3–5, 51], including the procedures to be adopted; standardisation is particularly important for patients with labile or narrowed airways [52, 53]. The recommendations are summarised in the following account.

12.6.2 Measurement of FEV_1 and other indices from volume–time curves

Equipment. The equipment may measure volume, e.g. a bellows or a rolling seal spirometer, or measure flow, e.g. a pneumotachograph or a rotating vane anemometer (turbine). Flow signals can be integrated to yield volume and most volume signals can be differentiated to yield flow. The apparatus should be used in accordance with the manufacturer's instructions.

Procedure. Subjects should be instructed to loosen any clothing that might restrict the movement of the chest or upper abdomen; dentures should be retained unless they are loose. A seated upright posture should normally be adopted, but standing is acceptable. A nose clip is needed for measurements on children, subjects who produce variable results and those, including some Australian aboriginals, who play musical instruments through the nose. For other subjects a nose clip is recommended, but not essential.

The subject takes the fullest possible inspiration through the mouth, then immediately puts the mouth round the mouthpiece and exhales forcibly. The operator should ensure that the initial inspiration is unhurried and continued up to total lung capacity. Maximal encouragement should be given. At this point the speed of the manoeuvre is increased. The subject quickly inserts the mouthpiece into his or her mouth and exhales with maximal effort. Any pause or loss of air around the mouthpiece is unacceptable. Again maximal encouragement is given (Fig. 12.5) and the expiration is continued to completion. Obstruction to the airway by the lips or teeth is a reason for repeating the test. Spirograms showing the derivation of some indices are given in Fig. 12.6.

Submaximal effort can lead to spuriously high values being recorded. This is illustrated in Fig. 12.1, where, with submaximal effort the FEV_1, indicated by the interrupted vertical line (left), is spuriously high (3.28 l compared with 2.81 l) due to there being less dynamic compression. As evidence for submaximal effort the apex of the flow–volume curve (right) is flattened and displaced to the right and the peak expiratory flow is submaximal (5.4 l s^{-1} compared with 6.2 l s^{-1}). Larger differences are observed in many patients with airflow limitation. Some mechanisms are discussed in Chapter 13. Some common faults are given in Table 12.4. They include failure to take a full inspiration, hesitation early in expiration and pursing the lips as if blowing into a trumpet. These faults should be corrected by dialogue with the subject. In addition, in some patients the completion of the expiration may provoke coughing which in turn can lead to reflex bronchoconstriction. This difficulty can be avoided if the operator instructs the subject to stop breathing out after the first second has been recorded. When this is done the forced vital capacity must be measured separately. Subjects performing the test for the first time should make two or more practice blows to develop a correct technique. Thereafter, three technically satisfactory blows are recorded.

In infants who of necessity cannot perform the respiratory manoeuvre this can be replaced by a procedure that includes rapid compression of the chest (Section 24.4.3). The procedure appears not to be applicable to older subjects.

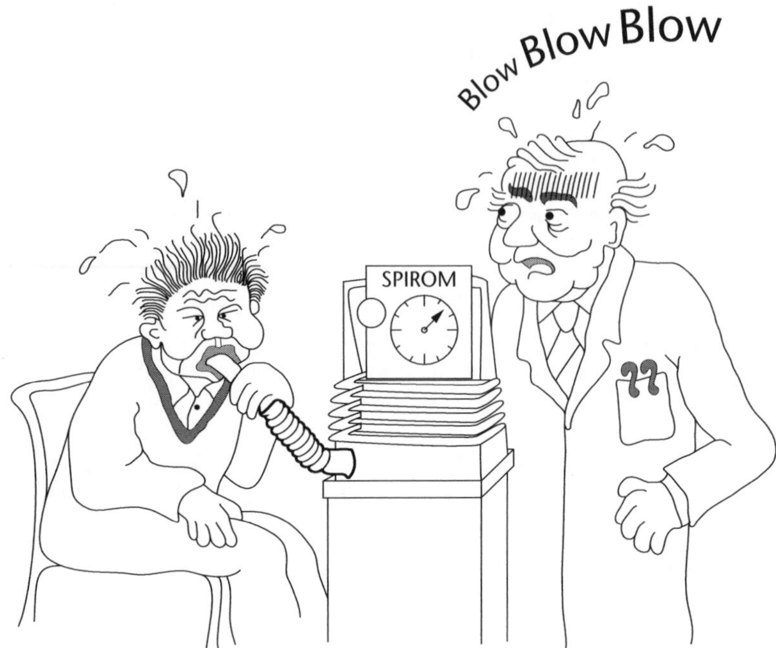

Fig. 12.5 Measurement of FEV_1 showing the effort required of both the subject and the operator.

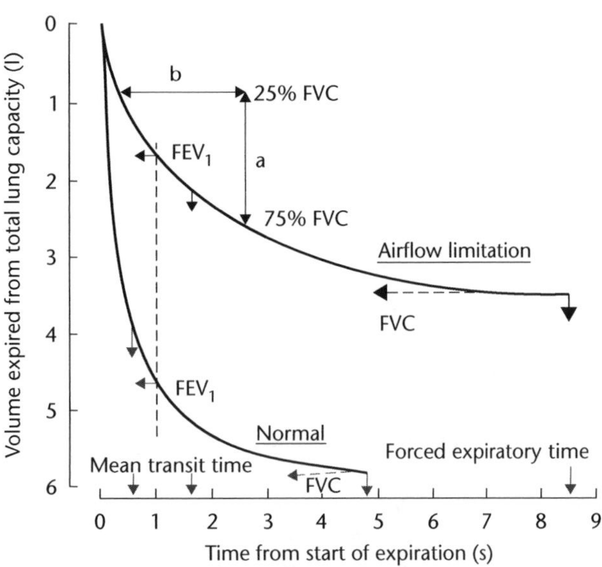

Fig. 12.6 Forced expiratory spirograms showing FEV_1, FVC, mean transit time and forced expiratory time in a healthy subject and a patient with chronic airflow limitation. Forced expiratory flow rate for expiration of the middle half of the forced vital capacity ($FEF_{25-75\%}$) is given by a/b.

Start and end of breath. When using a spirometer the start of expiration is usually defined by backward extrapolation of the steepest part of the volume–time curve to zero volume (Fig. 12.7). With computerised equipment the steepest slope is taken as that over a period of 80ms. The extrapolated volume should not exceed 5% of FVC or 150 ml whichever is the greater [5].

In many early studies the starting point was after 200 ml had been expired. In adults, values for FEV_1 obtained using this criterion are on average 179 ml less than by the backward extrapolation method [54]. For other methods a difference of 2.5% is fairly typical. The breath is usually considered to have ended when the subject cannot continue the exhalation or the volume change in 1.0 s does not exceed 25 ml and the duration of expiration exceeds 6 s (or 3 s in the case of children aged 10 years or less).

Which blow is best? When three technically satisfactory blows have been obtained the FEV_1 and FVC are usually taken as the highest recorded values; they need not have come from the same forced expiration. However, as a check on the stability of the results the highest FVC should not normally exceed the next highest value by more than 0.15 l (0.1 l if FVC < 1 l). In addition, in order to avoid error due to submaximal effort (Fig. 12.1) the flow–volume curve should preferably be recorded concurrently and be of acceptable quality (Section 12.6.3). The record should indicate the order in which the curves were obtained.

Reporting the results. Volumes and flows are reported at body temperature and pressure, saturated with water vapour (BTPS). For this purpose the apparatus temperature should be recorded to 1°C and an appropriate correction made (Section 6.6).

Reference values should take into account a subject's age, stature, gender and ethnic group (Section 26.2). A standard sheet should be used (e.g. Fig. 2.2, page 21, also [5]).

Table 12.4 Common faults in performance of a forced expiratory manoeuvre.

Previous inspiration not complete
Inspiration is from the instrument, not room air
Time between completion of inspiration and start of expiration >2 s
Expiration is hesitant or starts before the subject is connected to mouthpiece
Air escapes round the mouthpiece
Egress of air is hindered by pursed lips, tongue or partially closed teeth
Expiration is interrupted by coughing or premature inspiration
Expiration not maximally forced and sustained to residual volume (latter is not applicable to PEF)
Fault specific to PEF: airflow is generated by cheeks, not expiratory muscles

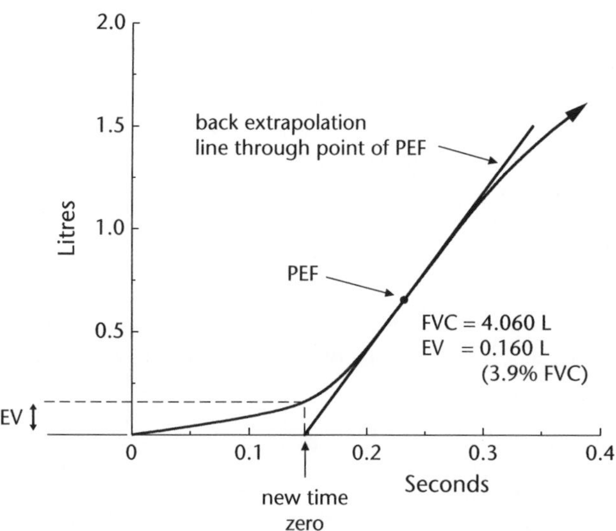

Fig. 12.7 Forced expiratory spirogram showing the backward extrapolation method for locating the start of forced expiration (i.e. t = 0). The extrapolated volume (EV) should not exceed 0.15 l or 5% of FVC whichever is greater.

12.6.3 Practical aspects of flow–volume spirometry

Equipment. The equipment should be suitable for measuring high flows and meet the other technical specifications for dynamic spirometry (Table 7.2, page 60). The curves can be registered and analysed on-line using an oscilloscope or other suitable recorder (Section 7.5) and a microprocessor. Alternatively, the information is recorded on magnetic tape then transcribed at reduced speed onto a relatively slow recorder after the test expiration has been completed.

Expiratory limb. The information used to construct an expiratory flow–volume curve from total lung capacity is obtained during measurement of FEV_1 and FVC by spirometry or by using a pneumotachograph; there are no additional requirements. At least three curves should be recorded.

Sub-maximal effort can distort the result by reducing the peak expiratory flow and hence the degree of dynamic compression. This leads to relatively high values for $FEF_{75\%FVC}$ and $FFF_{50\%FVC}$. To detect the error the appropriateness of the peak flow should be assessed by inspection of the flow–volume curve (Fig. 12.1). The start and end criteria should be met and the curve should not exhibit discontinuities. The three measurements of peak expiratory flow should not differ by more than 10%, and the curves should be of similar shape.

Accurate delineation of the expiratory limb of the curve without error from dynamic compression requires the use of a whole body plethysmograph (Section 12.5).

Partial expiratory limb. Partial expiratory flow–volume curves start from the end of a normal tidal inspiration. The procedure is best undertaken in a plethysmograph, but can be done by spirometry. In the latter event, the curves are assumed to terminate at residual volume; the percentages of vital capacity are then obtained by measuring the tracings from that point.

Inspiratory limb. Maximal inspiration from a spirometer or through a pneumotachograph can be disagreeable, so the reason for the test should be given in full and the procedure described. Inspiration is preceded by a full expiration and is continued with maximal effort through to total lung capacity. A nose clip should be used. The resulting curve should span the vital capacity and be smooth with a maximal flow at mid capacity (Fig. 12.3). However, the suction may lead to transient narrowing of extrathoracic airways early in inspiration that reduces the flow. The flow deficit can be eliminated by practice.

Flow–volume loops. Combining the maximal inspiratory and expiratory manoeuvres to produce a flow–volume loop can require considerable practice on the part of the subject. A satisfactory result is one which spans the vital capacity, the loop is closed without a volume deficit and the inspiratory and expiratory limbs are reproducible and of appropriate shape.

Derivation of flow–volume indices. The indices are in each case the highest observed value and need not all come from the same curve. The choice is made either from the numerical results [3] or the three curves are superimposed at total lung capacity (or for the partial curves at residual volume) and the outline is used for the derivation [55]. Flows are reported at the respective percentages of the largest FVC. Alternatively, the indices can all be derived from the curve having the highest value for FEV_1 plus FVC. This approach, which was formerly recommended by the American Thoracic Society, can lead to error if the PEF is submaximal indicating insufficient effort; the FEV_1 and flow indices can be spuriously high in consequence (Fig. 12.1).

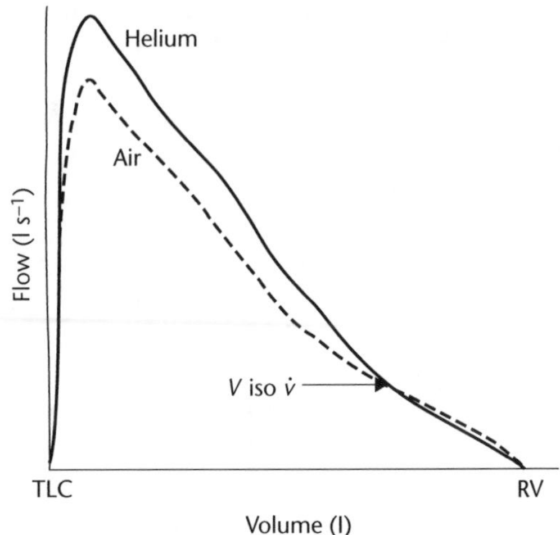

Fig. 12.8 Flow–volume curves in a healthy subject showing the effects of changes in gas density. The density affects the degree of turbulence and hence the flow rates at large lung volumes. When breathing air and a helium–oxygen mixture (F_I, He $= 0.8$), the volume of isoflow (V-iso $\dot{v}$) is the point where the two curves meet.

12.7 Density dependence

The density of the respired gas can be changed by altering the ambient pressure as in a pressure chamber, or by flushing the lungs with a gas mixture comprising helium or sulphur hexafluoride in 20% oxygen; the use of these gas mixtures also results in small changes in viscosity (Table 14.2, page 154) [56]. Changing the density alters the extent to which the flow in large airways is turbulent; it does not affect laminar flow (Section 14.3.4). The consequences for ventilatory capacity in healthy persons are illustrated in Fig. 14.2 (page 153) and for flow–volume curves in Fig. 14.3 (page 154). Superimposition of forced expiratory flow–volume curves obtained using two gases of different density provides a means of identifying the lung volume associated with the change from turbulent to laminar flow in these circumstances. This density dependence was envisaged as a test of small airway dysfunction, but the expectation has not been fulfilled [57, 58].

12.7.1 Volume of iso-flow

The difference from breathing air is mainly confined to flows at large lung volumes. Flows at small lung volume are entirely laminar and are not altered by changes in gas density. There is no change in vital capacity [59]. The proportion of vital capacity over which the flow is independent of gas density between breathing air and a helium mixture is called the *volume of iso-flow* (V-iso $\dot{v}$, Fig. 12.8); it indicates the lung volume during expiration at which the forced expiratory flow is no longer constrained by turbulence. Due to differences in viscosity a slightly different volume is obtained when the foreign gas is sulphur

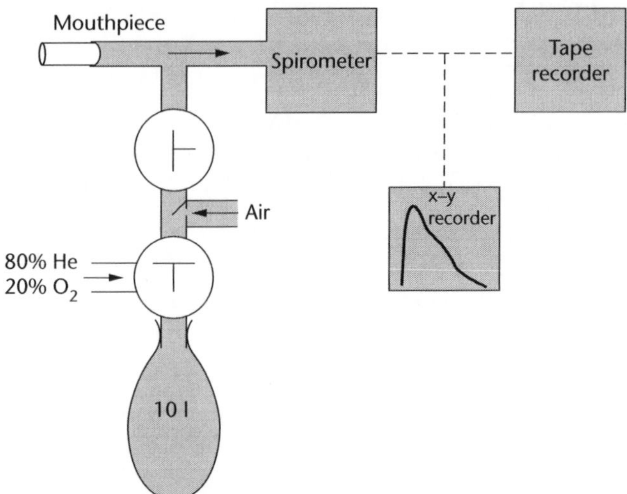

Fig. 12.9 Apparatus for recording the flow–volume curve breathing air and a helium–oxygen mixture. Prior to the test breath the subject inhales from the bag three full breaths of the appropriate gas, then exhales forcibly into the spirometer. If a pneumotachograph is to be used, the spirometer is replaced by a bag in box system. The pneumotachograph is then connected to the box. The curves are best recorded on magnetic media for subsequent reconstruction; they should also be displayed on an oscilloscope or an X–Y recorder having a time for full-scale response on the flow axis of not more than 0.3 s.

hexafluoride. The index is correlated with $\text{FEF}_{75\%\text{FVC}}$. It has rather poor reproducibility [60] and is used mainly in research.

12.7.2 Measurement of *V*-iso *v̇*

The helium is administered as three consecutive vital capacity breaths of 80% helium in oxygen, after which the forced expiration is performed immediately. Volume is recorded using a spirometer with facility for differentiation (Fig. 12.9) or a bag-in-box connected to a pneumotachograph and integrator. The result is reported as percentage changes in PEF and $\text{FEF}_{50\%\text{FVC}}$ and as the lung volume above RV at which the curves for air and helium first coincide. This volume of isoflow (V-iso$\dot{v}$) is reported as the per cent of forced vital capacity. Alternatively, where the lung volume is determined by plethysmography, the V-iso $\dot{v}$ is reported as per cent total lung capacity.

12.8 References

1. Eisen EA, Robins JM, Greaves IA, Wegman DH. Selection effects of repeatability criteria applied to lung spirometry *Am J Epidemiol* 1984; **120**: 734–742.
2. Ng'ang'a LW, Ernst P, Jaakkola MS et al. Spirometric lung function: distribution and determinants of test failure in a young adult population. *Am Rev Respir Dis* 1992; **145**: 48–54.
3. Quanjer PhH, Tammeling GJ, Cotes JE et al. Standardized lung function testing: lung volumes and forced ventilatory flows. 1993 update. *Eur Respir J* 1993; **6**(Suppl): 16: 4–40.

4. American Thoracic Society. Standardization of spirometry, 1994 update. *Am J Respir Crit Care Med* 1995; **152**:1107–1136.
5. Miller MR, Hankinson J, Brusasco V et al. Standardization of spirometry. Official statement of the American Thoracic Society and the European Respiratory Society Task Force. *Eur Respir J* 2005; **26**: 319–338.
6. Freedman S. Sustained maximum voluntary ventilation. *Respir Physiol* 1970; **8**: 230–244.
7. McKerrow CB. *The measurement of ventilatory capacity.* MD Thesis, University of Cambridge, 1955.
8. Kennedy MCS. A practical measure of the maximum ventilatory capacity in health and disease. *Thorax* 1953; **8**: 73–83.
9. McKerrow CB, McDermott M, Gilson JC. A spirometer for measuring the forced expiratory volume with a simple calibrating device. *Lancet* 1960; **1**: 149–151.
10. Gandevia B, Hughes-Jones P. Terminology for measurements of ventilatory capacity. *Thorax* 1957; **12**: 290–293.
11. Spiro SG, Hahn HL, Edwards RHT, Pride NB. An analysis of the physiological strain of submaximal exercise in patients with chronic obstructive bronchitis. *Thorax* 1975; **30**: 415–425.
12. Cotes JE, Posner V, Reed JW. Estimation of maximal exercise ventilation and oxygen uptake in patients with chronic lung disease. *Bull Eur Physiopathol Respir* 1982; **18**: 221–228.
13. Jones NL, Rebuck AS. Tidal volume during exercise in patients with diffuse fibrosing alveolitis. *Bull Eur Physiopathol Resp* 1979; **15**: 321–327.
14. Bernstein L, D'Silva JL, Mendel D. Effect of rate of breathing on maximum breathing capacity determined with a new spirometer. *Thorax* 1952; **7**: 255–262.
15. Quanjer PH, Lebowitz MD, Gregg I et al. Peak expiratory flow: conclusions and recommendations of a Working Party of the European Respiratory Society. *Eur Respir J* 1997; **10** (Suppl 24): 2s–8s.
16. Siafakas NM, Vermeire P, Pride NB et al. Optimal assessment and management of chronic obstructive pulmonary disease (COPD). *Eur Respir J* 1995; **8**: 1398–1420.
17. Wensley D, Pickering D, Silverman M. Can peak expiratory flow be measured accurately during a forced vital capacity manoeuvre? *Eur Respir J* 2000; **16**: 673–676.
18. Pedersen OF, Rasmussen TR, Omland O et al. Peak expiratory flow and the resistance of the mini-Wright peak flow meter. *Eur Resp J* 1997; **9**: 828–833.
19. Miller MR, Atkins PR, Pedersen OF. Inadequate peak flow meter characteristics detected by a computerised explosive decompression device. *Thorax* 2003; **58**: 411–416.
20. Pedersen OF, Rasmussen TR, Kjaergaard SK et al. Frequency response of variable orifice type peak flow meters: requirements and testing. *Eur Respir J* 1995; **8**: 849–855.
21. Miller MR, Dickinson SA, Hitchings DJ. The accuracy of portable peak flow meters. *Thorax* 1992; **47**: 904–909.
22. Pedersen OF, Miller MR, Sigsgaard T et al. Portable peak flow meters: physical characteristics, influence of temperature, altitude and humidity. *Eur Respir J* 1994; **7**: 991–997.
23. Hankinson JL, Filios MS, Kinsley KB, Petsonk EL. Comparing Mini-Wright and spirometer measurements of peak expiratory flow. *Chest* 1995; **108**: 407–410.
24. Folgering H, Brink W, Heeswijk O, Herwaarden C. Eleven peak flow meters: a clinical evaluation. *Eur Respir J* 1998; **11**: 188–193.
25. Ward DJ, Miller MR, Walters S et al. Impact of correcting peak flow for nonlinear errors on air pollutant effect estimates from a panel study. *Eur Respir J* 2000; **15**: 137–140.
26. Miles JF, Tunnicliffe W, Cayton RM et al Potential effects of correction of inaccuracies of the mini-Wright peak expiratory flow meter on the use of an asthma self-management plan. *Thorax* 1996; **51**: 403–406.
27. Hankinson JL, Reynolds JS, Das MK, Viola JO. Method to produce American Thoracic Society flow–time waveforms using a mechanical pump. *Eur Respir J* 1997; **10**: 690–694.
28. Kano S, Burton DL, Lanteri CJ, Sly PD. Determination of peak expiratory flow. *Eur Respir J* 1993; **6**: 1347–1352.
29. Hegewald MJ, Crapo RO, Jensen RL. Intraindividual peak flow variability. *Chest* 1995; **107**: 156–161.
30. Tiffeneau R, Pinelli A. Air circulant et air captif dans l'exploration de la fonction ventilatrice pulmonaire. *Paris Med* 1947; **37**: 624–628.
31. Gaensler EA. Analysis of the ventilatory defect by timed vital capacity measurements. *Am Rev Tuberc* 1951; **64**: 256–278.
32. Franklin W, Michelson AL, Lowell FC, Schiller IW. Clinical value of a tracing of forced expiration. I pulmonary disease. *New Eng J Med* 1955; **253**: 798–808.
33. Afschrift M, Clement J, van de Woestijgne KP. Maximal expiratory flows and effort independency in patients with airway obstruction. *J Appl Physiol* 1974; **37**: 599–569.
34. Krowka MJ, Enright PL, Rodarte JR, Hyatt RE. Effect of effort on measurement of forced expiratory volume in one second. *Am Rev Respir Dis* 1987; **136**: 829–833.
35. Tiffeneau R, Pinelli A. Régulation bronchique de la ventilation pulmonaire. *J Fr Med Chir Thorac* 1948; **2**: 221–244.
36. Leuallen EC, Fowler WS. Maximal mid-expiratory flow. *Am Rev Tuberc Pulm Dis* 1953; **72**: 783–800.
37. Chinn DJ, Cotes JE. Transit time analysis of spirograms: which blow is best? *Bull Europ Physiopathol Respir* 1986; **22**: 461–466.
38. Permutt S, Menkes HA. Spirometry. Analysis of forced expiration within the time domain. In: Macklem PT, Permutt S, eds. *The lung in the transition between health and disease.* New York: Marcel Dekker, 1979: 113–152.
39. Miller MR, Pincock AC. Repeatability of the moments of the truncated forced expiratory spirogram. *Thorax* 1982; **37**: 205–211.
40. Chinn DJ, Cotes JE. Transit time indices derived from forced expiratory spirograms: repeatability and criteria for curve selection and truncation. *Eur Respir J* 1994; **7**: 402–408.
41. Neuburger N, Levison H, Kruger K. Transit time analysis of the forced expiratory vital capacity in cystic fibrosis. *Am Rev Respir Dis* 1976; **114**: 753–759.
42. Fry DL. Theoretical considerations of the bronchial pressure–flow–volume relationships with particular reference to the maximum expiratory flow–volume curve. *Phys Med Biol* 1958; **3**: 174–194.
43. Coates AL, Desmond KJ, Demizio D et al. Sources of error in flow–volume curves: effect of expired volume measured at the mouth vs that measured in a body plethysmograph. *Chest* 1988; **94**: 976–982.
44. Clément J, van de Woestijne KP. Variability of maximum expiratory flow–volume curves and effort independency. *J Appl Physiol* 1971; **31**: 55–62.
45. Berry RB, Fairshter RD. Partial and maximal expiratory flow–volume curves in normal and asthmatic subjects before and after inhalation of metaproterenol. *Chest* 1985; **88**: 697–702.
46. Koulouris NG, Valta P, Lavoie A et al. A simple method to detect expiratory flow limitation during spontaneous breathing. *Eur Respir*

J 1995; **8**: 306–313. see also correspondence, *Eur Respir J* 1995; **8** 1624–1626.

47. Abdel KS, Serste T, Leduc D et al. Expiratory flow limitation during exercise in COPD: detection by manual compression of the abdominal wall. *Eur Respir J* 2002; **19**: 919–927.
48. Schrader PC, Quanjer PhH, Van Zomeren BC, et al. Selection of variables from maximum expiratory flow–volume curves. *Bull Europ Physiopathol Respir* 1983; **19**: 43–49.
49. Pertzse V, Watson A, Pride NB. Maximum airflow through the nose in humans. *J Appl Physiol* 1991; **70**: 1369–1376.
50. Gardner RM, Clausen JL, Epler GR et al. (on behalf of the ATS). Pulmonary function laboratory personnel qualifications. *Am Rev Resp Dis* 1986; **134**: 623–624.
51. Guidelines for the measurement of respiratory function; recommendations of the British Thoracic Society and the Association of Respiratory Technicians and Physiologists. *Respir Med* 1994; **88**: 165–194.
52. Brusasco V, Pellegrino R, Rodarte JR. Vital capacities in acute and chronic airway obstruction: dependence on flow and volume histories. *Eur Respir J* 1997; **10**: 1316–1320.
53. Koulouris NG, Rapakoulias P, Rassidakis A et al. Dependence of forced vital capacity manoeuvre on time course of preceding inspiration in patients with restrictive lung disease. *Eur Respir J* 1997; **10**: 2366–2370.
54. Smith AA, Gaensler EA. Timing of forced expiratory volume in one second. *Am Rev Respir Dis* 1975; **112**: 882–885.
55. Peslin R, Bohadana A, Hannhart B, Jardin P. Comparison of various methods for reading maximal expiratory flow–volume curves. *Am Rev Respir Dis* 1979; **119**: 271–277.
56. Staats BA, Wilson TA, Lai-Fook SJ et al. Viscosity and density dependence during maximal flow in man. *J Appl Physiol* 1980; **48**: 313–319.
57. Teculescu DB, Préfaut C. Why did density dependence of maximal expiratory flows not become a useful epidemiological tool? *Bull Europ Physiopathol Respir* 1987; **23**: 639–648.
58. Guillemi S, Wright JL, Hogg JC et al. Density dependence of pulmonary resistance: correlation with small airway pathology. *Eur Respir J* 1995; **8**: 789–794.
59. Dosman J, Bode F, Urbanetti J et al. The use of a helium–oxygen mixture during maximum expiratory flow to demonstrate obstruction in small airways in smokers. *J Clin Invest* 1979; **55**: 1090–l099.
60. McDonald JB, Cole TJ. The flow–volume loop: reproducibility of air and helium-based tests in normal subjects *Thorax* 1980; **35**: 64–69.

Further reading

See Historical references, Section 1.8.

CHAPTER 13

Determinants of Maximal Flows (Flow Limitation)

Maximal expiratory flows are determined by a number of factors. This chapter explains what they are and how they interact.

13.1 Overview

Maximal inspiratory and expiratory flows underlie ventilatory capacity and are of immense practical importance. They reflect all the features of the respiratory apparatus that have been described. In most circumstances inspiratory flows are adequate for whatever levels of ventilation the expiratory flows can sustain, and so attention focuses on expiration. The driving force for expiration comes from the respiratory muscles, both directly and via lung elasticity, which represents energy stored during the preceding inspiration.

During expiration from total lung capacity, the airflow up to peak flow is generated mainly by the muscles of expiration. At the peak, which occurs at a relatively large lung volume, the available muscle force, lung elastic recoil and airway calibre are all maximal. Beyond the peak the force comes mostly from lung elastic recoil and not directly from the expiratory muscles. This is due to the presence of flow-limiting mechanisms. High flows are now known to be limited to the speed at which a pulse wave of gas can be transmitted along the airway (*wave speed mechanism*). The point of limitation can then be in the trachea [1]. As expiration continues the limiting point moves peripherally up the airways.

The wave speed concept is a mathematical one that has helped our understanding of events pertaining to peak expiratory flow. Two earlier models are helpful for clarifying events later in the maximum forced expiratory manoeuvre. The equal pressure point theory of Mead et al. elegantly describes the interrelated contributions of lung elasticity and lung volume to maximal expiratory flow. Pride et al. represent the mechanism of expiratory flow limitation by a Starling resistor; this resembles a waterfall in that the flow is independent of the height of the fall. The theory can account for airway closure towards the end of expiration. All the theories are based on expiratory narrowing of airways that can be observed at bronchoscopy. In adults, but not in children, the narrowing can progress to closure of airways, which then determines residual volume (Section 10.1.3).

13.2 Relationship of expiratory flows to muscular effort

Evidence for most expiratory flows being independent of effort. The relationship of maximal flow to lung volume, and hence static recoil pressure, can be represented by a maximal flow–volume curve (e.g. Fig. 12.3, page 136). The curve has characteristic features that reflect the condition of the lungs. Within this constraint, the flow during *inspiration* is maximal at mid-volume. It varies directly with the applied pleural pressure (as measured in the oesophagus); hence, inspiratory flow is dependent on effort. It is not greatly influenced by airway resistance on account of the inspiratory pressure exerting traction on the airways, which keeps them open [2].

During maximal expiration from a position of full inspiration the flow rises to a peak early in the manoeuvre, and then exhibits a gradual decline as the volume of the lungs diminishes. This relationship is quite different from that on inspiration. The difference extends to the relationship of flow to applied pressure. Here, the relationship at constant lung volume, for example

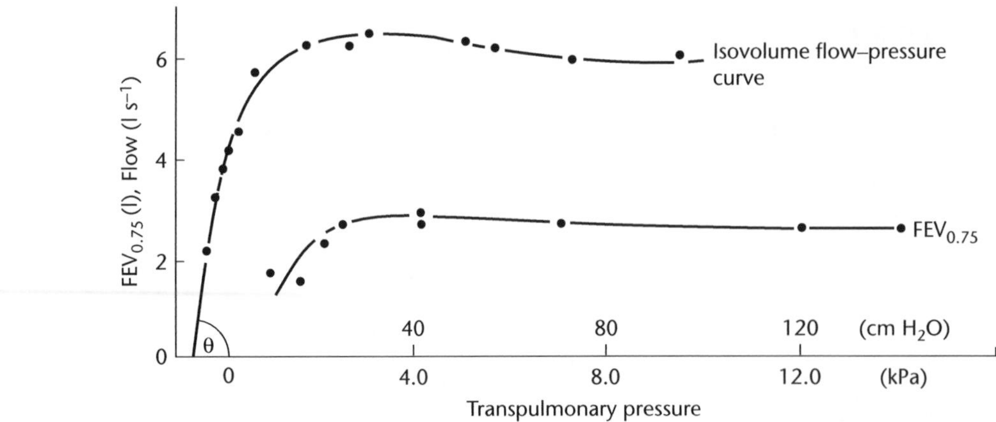

Fig. 13.1 The effect of variation in the force applied to the lungs on expiratory flow of normal subjects. The lower line shows the relationship of the $FEV_{0.75}$ to the maximal oesophageal pressure recorded during the expiration. The upper line is an isovolume flow–pressure curve: it shows the relationship of flow to pressure at the arbitrarily chosen volume of 50% of vital capacity above residual volume. The reciprocals of the initial slopes of these lines (θ) describe total lung resistance (*R*aw + *R*ti). The data were obtained from a series of vital capacity manoeuvres performed with varying effort; flow was recorded with a pneumotachograph, pressure with an intraoesophageal balloon and lung volume with a body plethysmograph. The latter cannot be replaced by a spirometer, since the relevant volume is that of the lungs when they are compressed during expiration and not total lung capacity minus the exhaled gas volume measured at atmospheric pressure. For interpretation see text. Sources: upper curve, [4]; lower curve, McKerrow CB, McDermott M, unpublished work, 1966.

50% of vital capacity, is particularly informative. The flow during the first three quarters of a second of expiration from total lung capacity ($FEV_{0.75}$) tells the same story (Fig. 13.1, lower and upper curves respectively). Under either set of circumstances, at the start of the expiration a rise in applied pressure initiates flow of air. However, once a modest pressure has been generated, a further increase *does not augment* the flow [3, 4]. Instead, there is a plateau level of flow that in healthy subjects is linearly related to lung volume. Hence, flow beyond the peak is driven not by respiratory muscles but by the elastic recoil of the lungs.

The finding provides an explanation for the remarkable stability and hence practical usefulness of the forced expiratory volume (FEV_1) as an index of ventilatory capacity (Section 12.4.1). It also opens the way to identifying that part of maximal expiratory flow that is effort dependent.

Flow that is dependent on effort. The effort-dependent part of a forced expiration extends from its commencement up to peak expiratory flow (Section 12.3). It can be displayed on a flow–volume curve, but is of too short duration to be shown on an isovolume flow–pressure curve. *Peak expiratory flow* is achieved with only a small displacement of air. Some of this represents air that is expelled from the airways by compression of their walls. The displacement is influenced by the compliance of the airways and other variables, as indicated in the following equation due to Clément et al. [5]. This describes the rate of change of the volume of the conducting airways with respect to time as a function (f) of other variables:

$$\mathrm{d}V\mathrm{aw}/\mathrm{d}t = f(C\mathrm{aw}, \dot{v}, C\mathrm{l}, \mathrm{d}P\mathrm{pl}/\mathrm{d}t) \qquad (13.1)$$

where the left-hand term is the rate of change of airway volume. *C*aw and *C*l are the compliance of the airways and of the lungs, which are normally quite similar, $\dot{v}$ is instantaneous flow and d*P*pl/d*t* is the rate of change with respect to time of the pleural pressure. On account of this multifactorial dependence, changes to peak flow caused by disease may be only weakly correlated with changes in other indices of forced expiratory flow (see, e.g., Fig. 38.1, page 533).

13.3 The equal pressure point theory of Mead et al. [6]

During the inspiration that precedes a forced expiration the pleural pressure is negative with respect to atmospheric pressure. This increases the lung volume and hence the elastic recoil pressure (*P*el). When the forced expiration starts, *P*pl becomes considerably positive and raises the alveolar pressure (*P*alv), and that pressure initiates the flow of air, i.e. *P*alv = *P*el + *P*pl. The flow creates a pressure drop down the airways because of frictional loss and linear acceleration of the gas molecules (convective acceleration; Section 14.3.4). At the mouth the pressure is zero because the entire *P*alv has been dissipated. Mead et al. separated the components *P*el and *P*pl by dividing the airway into two parts: an upstream segment where the pressure drop was equal to *P*el and a downstream segment where it was *P*pl. The resistance of the upstream segment was called *R*us and of the downstream segment *R*ds (see Fig. 13.2).

At the junction of the upstream and downstream segments the intraluminal pressure is *P*alv − *P*el = *P*pl, which is the same as the pressure surrounding the airway. The point separating these two segments was therefore called the equal pressure point (EPP).

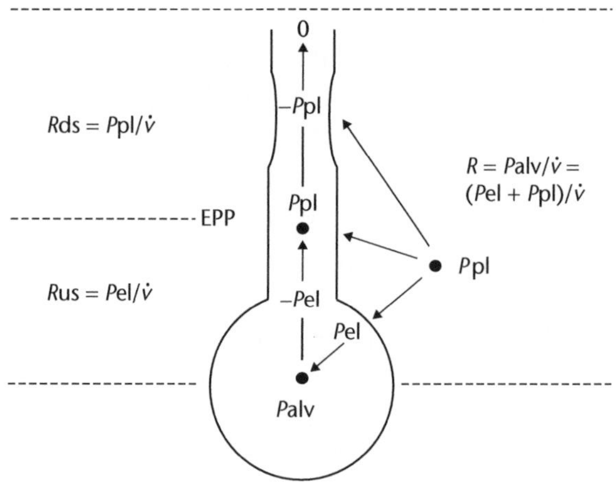

Fig. 13.2 Diagrammatic presentation of the equal pressure point theory by Mead et al. The lung is assumed to consist of a single alveolus emptying through an elastic airway. During the forced expiration the pressure in the alveolus (*Palv*) is positive and consists of two components, the elastic recoil pressure of the lungs (*Pel*) and the surrounding pleural pressure (*Ppl*), generated by the expiratory muscles ($Palv = Pel + Ppl$). The pressure drop along the airway from the alveolus to the mouth equals *Palv*; for flow to occur it must overcome the airway resistance (*Raw*). The airway is partitioned into two parts: an upstream part with the resistance *Rus*, across which the pressure drop is *Pel*, and a downstream part with the resistance *Rds*, across which the pressure drop is *Ppl*. At the transition between the two segments the intraluminal pressure is $Ppl = Palv - Pel$, and therefore equals the surrounding pressure *Ppl*. This point in the airway is called the equal pressure point (EPP). With flow analogous to current (*I*) and pressure analogous to electromotor force (*U*), the application of Ohm's law ($I = U/R$) on serial arrangement of two resistances provides the analogous equation:

$$\dot{v} = \frac{Palv}{Raw} = \frac{Pel}{Rus} = \frac{Ppl}{Rds}.$$

When *Ppl* exceeds a certain pressure (*Ppl#*) dynamic compression occurs and flow at a given lung volume levels off (Fig. 13.1). This empirical finding implies a proportional increase in *Ppl* and *Rds*, and hence their ratio stabilises; so flow is maximal and does not increase further with additional effort. The central part of the equation ($\dot{v}_{max} = Pel/Rus$) implies that $\dot{v}_{max}$ is independent of effort (*Ppl*), but decreases when *Pel* decreases and/or *Rus* increases. This is the case during expiration in both healthy subjects and patients with airways obstruction. In addition, in the patients, *Pel* may be small and/or *Rus* large at the start of expiration; hence, the flow axis of the expiratory flow–volume curve may be severely depressed. Source: Pedersen OF, unpublished work, 2001.

The flow through each segment is determined by the pressure drop (i.e. the driving pressure) and the resistance of the segment. Since the same flow obtains for the segments and for the whole lung it can be represented by a mechanical equivalent of Ohm's law (current = voltage/resistance) as follows:

$$\dot{v} = Palv/Raw = Pel/Rus = Ppl/Rds \qquad (13.2)$$

Downstream of the EPP the pressure within the airway will be less than that on the outside; this leads to the airway being compressed (dynamic compression). The larger the driving pressure (*Ppl*) the greater the compression, and vice versa. The segment then resembles a Starling resistor in which the flow is constant and independent of Ppl. Hence, in terms of the upstream segment:

$$\dot{v} = Pel/Rus \qquad (13.3)$$

The equal pressure point concept is based on the empirical finding that flow at a given volume ceases to increase when the pressure exceeds a limiting value. It does not provide an explanation. Instead, it illustrates that when effort is large enough, flow is determined by factors intrinsic to the lung, i.e. independent of effort. $\dot{v}_{max}$ is then determined by Pel and Rus. During the course of the expiration Pel decreases and Rus may increase; these changes cause $\dot{v}_{max}$ to decrease independent of effort. Similarly changes in Pel and Rus reduce the $\dot{v}_{max}$ in some diseases of the lung (Chapter 39). For example, airway obstruction, represented here by an increase in Rus, is a common cause for a reduced $\dot{v}_{max}$. A decrease in Pel, such as that occurs with emphysema or ageing of the lung, is equally important. The transmural pressure acts on the wall of the airway and so its distensibility (compliance) also influences the position of the equal pressure point [7]. With compliant airways the EPP is more peripheral than when the airway walls are rigid.

13.4 The waterfall concept of Pride et al. [8]

According to this hypothesis the intercept on the pressure axis of the graph relating maximal flow to elastic recoil defines a critical transmural pressure (Ptm'). The Ptm' reflects the ability of the airway to resist compression. The hypothesis assumes that Ptm' is independent of lung volume but this is unlikely to be true. A numerical example is given in Fig. 13.3.

In this theory, as in the EPP concept, the relationship between maximal flow and static elastic recoil pressure (the maximal flow–static recoil curve, i.e. MFSR curve) can be used to separate the respective contributions of Pel and Rus upon $\dot{v}_{max}$. A change in slope indicates a change in Rus, whereas displacement of $\dot{v}_{max}$ along the MFSR curve implies a change in Pel. This use of the MFSR curve identifies a site of flow limitation at which the transmural pressure need not be zero. In this event its location will differ from that of the equal pressure point.

13.5 Wave mechanics mechanism of Dawson and Elliott [9, 10]

Wave velocity is the maximal speed at which a pulse wave of gas molecules can be transmitted along an airway. According to

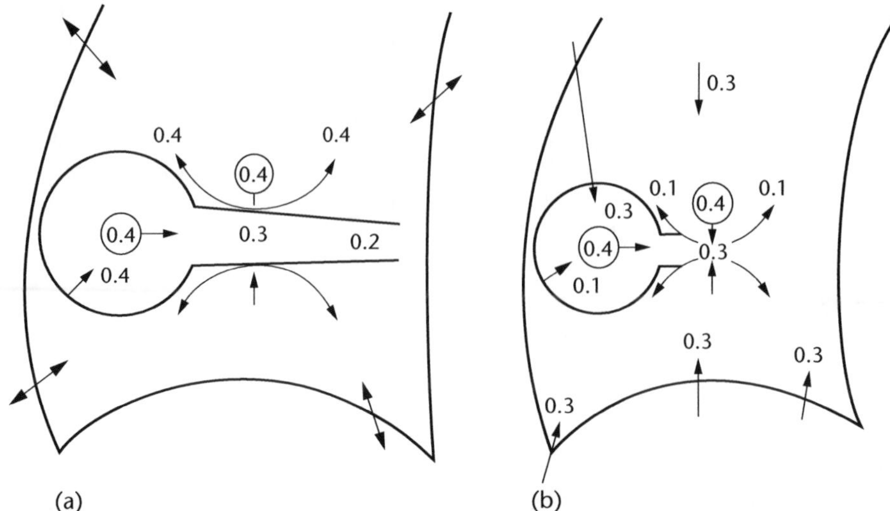

Fig. 13.3 Diagram illustrating waterfall concept of airway closure. (a) Passive expiration (pleural pressure assumed to be zero). Expiration is effected by the elastic recoil pressure of the lung (0.4 kPa). The thin-walled portion of the airway is held open by both the recoil pressure acting on its wall and the intraluminal pressure, i.e. that transmitted from the alveolus. Both forces act against the alveolar pressure (0.4 kPa) and the elastic forces of the airway (not shown in the diagram). (b) Active expiration. The *rise* in intrapleural pressure caused by contraction of the accessory muscles (+0.3 kPa) initially assists expiration. It also tends to collapse the airway especially as the opposing force, due to the traction of the lung tissue and the intraluminal pressure, decreases progressively as the lung gets smaller. The site of closure is located where the pressure within the airway (0.3 kPa) plus that required to deform the wall of the airway (here 0.1 kPa) is equal to the outside pressure (here 0.4 kPa). Source: Adapted from [8] with permission.

wave mechanics, flow limitation is due to interaction between the velocity, the compliance of the airway wall and the convective acceleration of the contained gas (Section 14.3.4). The latter process has the effect that as air is expired the velocity of the gas molecules, and hence the linear flow, increases progressively as gas passes from a large number of small airways to a small number of large airways. The driving pressure is the intraluminal pressure. In the airways this pressure is less than alveolar pressure because energy is used to overcome flow resistance and to accelerate the gas. The intraluminal pressure along the length of the airway then declines as does the transmural pressure, which is the force tending to keep the airways open.

A general equation has been derived for the transmural pressure at a certain point in the airway:

$$Ptm = Pel - Pfr - 0.5\rho(\dot{v}/A)^2 \quad (13.4)$$

where r and A are respectively the airway radius and cross-sectional area, *Pfr* is the frictional pressure loss and the other terms are as defined previously. The equation indicates that at any site or generation of airway, two variables reduce the transmural pressure below that of the elastic recoil pressure of the lungs. These are first the frictional pressure loss from the alveoli to that site, and second, the pressure needed to accelerate the gas molecules during expiration into larger airways that have a progressively smaller overall cross-sectional area. If the flow is maximal, the slope of the curve describing $\dot{v}$ as a function of Ptm (i.e. $d\dot{v}/dPtm$) must be zero. Differentiation gives:

$$\frac{dPtm}{dPtm} = \frac{dPel}{dPtm} - \frac{dPfr}{dPtm} - 0.5\rho \times \left(\frac{1}{A^2} \times 2\dot{V} \times \frac{d\dot{V}}{dPtm} - \frac{2}{A^3} \times \left(\dot{V}\right)^2 \times \frac{dA}{dPtm}\right) \quad (13.5)$$

where the first three terms are respectively one, zero and zero.

For $d\dot{V}/dPtm = 0$, $\dot{v} = \dot{v}_{max}$:

$$1 = \frac{\rho(\dot{v}max)^2}{A^3} \times \frac{dA}{dPtm}$$

or

$$\dot{v}max = A\left(\frac{A}{\rho} \times \frac{1}{\frac{dA}{dPtm}}\right)^{1/2} \quad (13.6)$$

This equation calculates the maximal flow that can traverse an airway segment having a given value for $Pel - Pfr$. It states that $\dot{v}_{max}$ decreases when airway area (A) decreases and when airway compliance ($dA/dPtm$) or gas density (ρ) increases.

The wave speed for gas molecules is given by $\dot{v}_{max}/A$. Both $\dot{v}_{max}$ and A have now been measured in human lungs, and so it has been possible to compare observed $\dot{v}_{max}$ with that predicted by eqn. 13.6. The ratio of the two velocities (i.e. $\dot{v}_{max}$ obs/$\dot{v}_{max}$ ws) is the wave speed index. This quantity has been found to

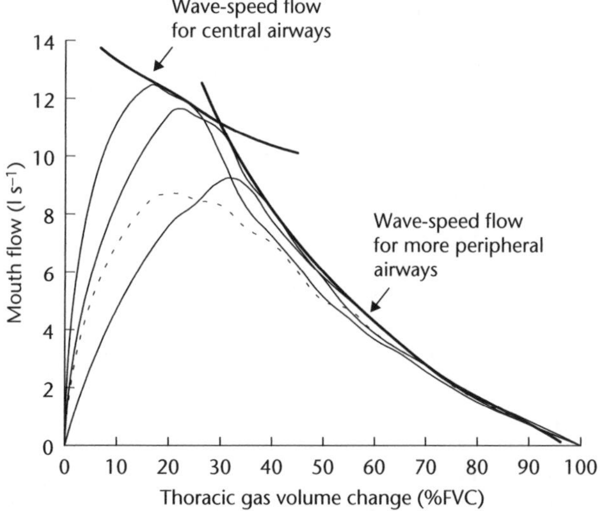

Fig. 13.4 Maximal expiratory flow–volume curves obtained with different degrees of effort. Volume changes were measured by whole body plethysmography in order to reduce gas compression artefacts compared with those measured at the mouth (Section 12.5.1). The initial flows were related to effort. The maximal flows at different volumes were achieved where and when the wave speed was reached (see text). Hence, peak flow was effort dependent and, with the exception of the dashed curve, wave speed limited. Source: Adapted from [13].

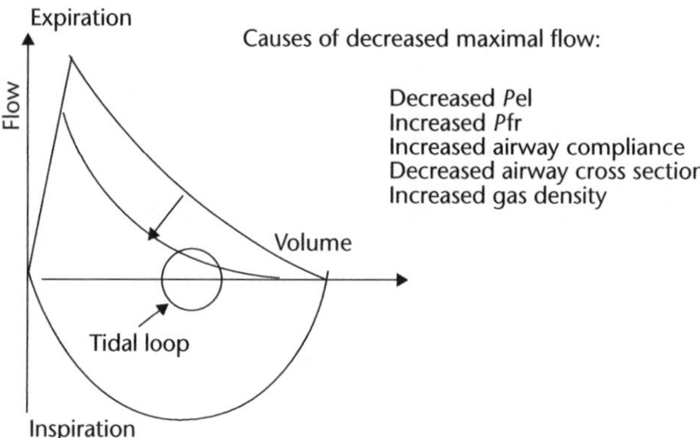

Fig. 13.5 Main factors determining maximal expiratory flow. The factors are listed in the figure. They are represented as having reduced the maximal expiratory flow to below the level required for normal tidal breathing. Source: Pedersen OF, unpublished work, 2001.

approach unity for the first three airway generations of intact excised human lungs [11]. In intact subjects this was also the case for 13 out of 15 healthy people and 4 of 10 asthmatics [12]. Thus, the maximal flow at high lung volumes is determined by the wave speed mechanism operating in large central airways (Fig. 13.4). Flow at lower volumes is determined by limitation in the peripheral airways where it is determined by both the wave speed and other mechanisms (e.g. Fig. 13.2). The site of airflow limitation acts as a choke point that determines the flow throughout the lungs. Downstream from the choke point the airway is compressed but high linear velocities can occur even exceeding wave speed (supra-critical velocity). The contributory factors have been analysed using models [14–19].

13.6 Practical implications of mechanisms for flow limitation

The existence of flow limiting mechanisms (at all but maximal lung volumes) has the effect that beyond a threshold level of effort the maximal expiratory flow reflects mainly the intrinsic mechanical properties of the lungs (Section 11.5.1), not the expiratory effort. Instead, from eqns. 13.4 and 13.6 the main factors determining the maximal flow are elastic recoil pressure (Pel), frictional pressure loss upstream from the flow-determining site (Pfr), gas density, cross-sectional area of the airway (A) and the slope of the relationship between the cross-sectional area and the distending transmural pressure (Ptm). The slope is the airway compliance ($C\text{aw} = \mathrm{d}A/\mathrm{d}P\text{tm}$).

Causes for a reduced $\dot{v}_{\max}$. As shown in Fig. 13.5, the maximal flow achievable breathing air decreases when lung elastic recoil (Pel) decreases, when resistance upstream to the choke point (Pfr) increases, when the airways get narrower (A decreases) and when the airways get more flaccid (Caw increases). Because of the density dependence, changes in gas density also affect the flow (Footnote 13.1).

Importance of lung volume. The limiting flow is critically dependent on lung volume because Pel decreases with volume. Hence, when flows obtained on two occasions in the same individual are to be compared, the measurements should relate to the same absolute lung volume (e.g. Section 15.7.2).

Relevance for flow–volume curves. As shown in Fig. 13.4, different parts of the expiratory flow–volume curve reflect properties of different airways. This is due to peripheral migration of the choke points with decreasing lung volume.

Relevance for coughing. The sequence of events in a cough is closure of the glottis, contraction of the abdominal muscles that raises the intrathoracic pressure, and opening of the glottis, leading to a sudden release of air. The upstream migration of the choke points and EPPs throughout expiration can contribute to the effectiveness of coughing by clearing progressively smaller airways as the cough continues. Thus, between two successive coughs the lung volume diminishes and the sites of flow limitation move upstream; in doing so they loosen secretions from

Footnote 13.1. Flow is reduced by breathing gas of increased density (as in diving) and increased when gas of low density is breathed (e.g. a mixture of helium in oxygen). However, the response to gas of low density may be counteracted by a simultaneous increase in Pfr if the viscosity of the gas is increased (Sections 12.7, 34.2 and 35.3.1).

more upstream airways, which the high flow velocity then expels. Since the downstream secretions are likely to have been removed by the earlier part of the cough there is now a clear path for the expulsion of secretions from the smaller airways. Premature collapse of airways, such as occurs in emphysema and probably in bronchiectasis, interferes with this mechanism and limits the cleansing action to the larger airways. It also leads to the development of high intrapleural pressures that contribute to cough syncope.

Flow limitation during tidal breathing. In cases of severe expiratory flow limitation, the expiratory flow may become so small that normal resting breathing is impeded. This is shown in Fig. 13.5.

The subject can compensate for insufficient tidal flow by shortening the inspiratory time, or breathing at a higher lung volume to increase Pel. As a result, functional residual capacity is increased in subjects with severe airways obstruction. The condition is known as *dynamic hyperinflation.* Its extent during exercise can be monitored by opticoelectronic plethysmography [20].

Expiratory flow limitation during tidal breathing can be detected by applying a sudden negative pressure to the mouth or positive pressure to the lower chest or abdomen. (See Footnote 13.2 for terminology.) If flow limitation is present, these procedures will fail to increase the flow (Section 12.5.1). Similar but less direct information can be obtained by impulse oscillometry (Section 14.4.4). During the inspiratory phase of the respiratory cycle the alveoli are in free communication with the mouth, whereas during expiration, in the presence of *expiratory airflow limitation* (EFL) the communication is effectively obstructed either functionally by a choke point or structurally by airway closure. In either event the reactance during expiration becomes much more negative and differs from that during inspiration [21].

Evidence for EFL can also be obtained during measurement of airway resistance in the body plethysmograph. In the presence of EFL the expiratory part of the loop cannot be closed. Instead, the alveolar pressure will continue to increase after maximal flow has been attained. Pressure and flow are then out of phase throughout expiration (cf. Section 16.1.9).

The presence of EFL and dynamic hyperinflation increase the work of the respiratory muscles, especially during expiration when the airway intraluminal pressure at end expiration can be positive (Footnote 13.2). The changes interfere with blood flow to the lungs and can contribute to breathlessness both at rest and during exercise (Sections 28.8.1, 38.2 and 38.3, *also* [21]).

Footnote 13.2. The application of suction at end expiration is designated NEEP (negative end-expiratory pressure) and the condition of positive end-expiratory intraluminal pressure associated with EFL as PEEPi (intrinsic positive end-expiratory pressure). The latter terminology differentiates the condition from therapeutic PEEP in which the raised intraluminal pressure is achieved by external means [21].

13.7 References

1. Melissinos CG, Mead J. Maximum expiratory flow changes induced by longitudinal tension on trachea in normal subjects. *J Appl Physiol* 1977; **43**: 537–544.
2. Aldrich TK, Shapiro SM, Sherman MS, Prezant DJ. Alveolar pressure and airway resistance during maximal and submaximal respiratory efforts. *Am Rev Respir Dis* 1989; **140**: 899–906.
3. Fry DL, Ebert RV, Stead WW, Brown CC. The mechanics of pulmonary ventilation in normal subjects and in patients with pulmonary emphysema. *Am J Med* 1954; **16**: 80–97.
4. Ingram RH Jr, Schilder DP. Effect of gas compression on pulmonary pressure, flow and volume relationship. *J Appl Physiol* 1966; **21**: 1821–1826.
5. Clément J, van de Woestijne KP, Pardaens J. A general theory of respiratory mechanics applied to forced expiration. *Respir Physiol* 1973; **19**: 60–79.
6. Mead J, Turner JM, Macklem PT, Little JB. Significance of the relationship between lung recoil and maximum expiratory flow. *J Appl Physiol* 1967; **22**: 95–108.
7. Smaldone GC, Bergofsky EH. Delineation of flow-limiting segment and predicted airway resistance by movable catheter. *J Appl Physiol* 1976; **40**: 943–952.
8. Pride NB, Permutt S, Riley RL, Bromberger-Barnea B. Determinants of maximal expiratory flow from the lungs. *J Appl Physiol* 1967; **23**: 646–662.
9. Dawson SV, Elliott EA. Wave-speed limitation on expiratory flow – a unifying concept. *J Appl Physiol* 1977; **48**: 493–515.
10. Dawson SV, Elliott EA. Use of the choke point in the prediction of flow limitation in elastic tubes. *Fed Proc* 1980; **39**: 2765–2770.
11. Hyatt RE, Wilson TA, Bar-Yishay E. Prediction of maximal expiratory flow in excised human lungs. *J Appl Physiol* 1980; **48**: 991–998.
12. Pedersen OF, Brackel HJ, Bogaard JM, Kerrebijn KF. Wave-speed determined flow limitation at peak flow in normal and asthmatic subjects. *J Appl Physiol* 1997; **83**: 1721–1732.
13. Pedersen OF. The Peak Flow Working Group: physiological determinants of peak expiratory flow. *Eur. Respir J* 1997; **10** (Suppl 24): 11s–16s.
14. Lambert RK, Wilson TA, Hyatt RE, Rodarte JR. A computational model for expiratory flow. *J Appl Physiol* 1982; **52**: 44–56.
15. Elad D, Kamm RD, Shapiro AH. Steady compressible flow in collapsible tubes: application to forced expiration. *J Fluid Mech* 1989; **203**: 401–418.
16. Pedley TJ, Schroter RC, Sudlow MF. Flow and pressure drop in systems of repeatedly branching tubes. *J Fluid Mech* 1971; **46**: 365–383.
17. Jan DL, Shapiro AH, Kamm RD. Some features of oscillatory flow in a model bifurcation. *J Appl Physiol* 1989; **67**: 147–159.
18. Schroter RC, Sudlow MF. Flow patterns in models of the human bronchial airways. *Respir Physiol* 1969; **7**: 341–355.
19. Tsuda A, Kamm R, Fredberg JJ. Periodic flow at airway bifurcations, II: Flow partitioning. *J Appl Physiol* 1990; **69**: 553–561.
20. Aliverti A, Stevenson N, Dellaca RL et al. Regional chest wall volumes during exercise in chronic obstructive pulmonary disease. *Thorax* 2004; **59**: 210–216.
21. Calverley PMA, Koulouris NG. Flow limitation and dynamic hyperinflation: key concepts in modern respiratory physiology. *Eur Respir J* 2005; **25**: 186–199.

Further reading

Hyatt RE. Forced expiration. In: Macklem PT, Mead J, eds. *Handbook of physiology, Vol. 3: Mechanics of breathing* (Section 3).Bethesda, MD: American Physiological Society, 1986: 295–314.

Ingram RH, Pedley TJ. Pressure–flow relationships in the lungs. In: Macklem PT, Mead J, eds. *Handbook of physiology, Vol. 3: Mechanics of breathing* (Section 3).Bethesda, MD: American Physiological Society, 1986: 277–293.

Wilson TA. The wave speed limit on expiratory flow. In: Chang HK, Paiva M, eds. *Respiratory physiology: an analytical approach.* New York: Marcel Dekker, 1989: 139–166.

CHAPTER 14

Theory and Measurement of Respiratory Resistance (Including Whole Body Plethysmography)

During breathing work is done in overcoming the resistance to movement of the lungs and chest cage. The present chapter explores this important subject. The mechanisms that control airway calibre and the assessment of changes in calibre are described in Chapter 15.

14.1 Introduction

In the absence of movement, the extent of lung inflation reflects a balance between the elastic recoils of the lungs and chest wall, gravitational force and tension in the respiratory muscles. Movement occurs when the equilibrium is disturbed. The rate of movement is influenced by the strength of the applied force and by the elasticity, resistance to movement and the inertia of the thoracic cage, lung tissue and gas contained in the lung. As a first approximation the elastance (i.e. the reciprocal of compliance, C) is related to volume (V), the resistance (R) to velocity of airflow and the inertia (I) to acceleration. The pressure difference across the lung (P) can be described in terms of these variables:

$$P = (1/C)V + R\,\mathrm{d}V/\mathrm{d}t + I\,\mathrm{d}^2V/\mathrm{d}t^2 \qquad (14.1)$$

This equation is an expression of Newton's third law of motion, stating that a force applied to a body is met by an opposing force of equal magnitude. The latter has components related to elasticity, resistance and inertia.

14.2 Inertia

According to the laws of physics, force (F) equals mass (M) times acceleration ($G = \mathrm{d}u/\mathrm{d}t$, where u is the velocity of the gas molecules). Pressure is F/A, where A is the area the force is acting on. The mass of a column of gas is $L \times A \times \rho$ where L is the length of the column, A its cross-sectional area and ρ the gas density. From this it follows that:

$$P = F/A = (L \times A \times \rho/A) \times G = L \times \rho \times \mathrm{d}u/\mathrm{d}t \qquad (14.2)$$

However, $u = \dot{V}/A$, and $\mathrm{d}u/\mathrm{d}t = (1/A) \times \mathrm{d}\dot{V}/\mathrm{d}t$, where $\dot{V}$ is the volumetric gas flow. $\mathrm{d}\dot{V}/\mathrm{d}t$ is the volume acceleration, which is the same as $\mathrm{d}^2V/\mathrm{d}t^2$, where V is volume. From this it follows that

$$P = (L \times \rho/A) \times \mathrm{d}^2V/\mathrm{d}t^2 \qquad (14.3)$$

The inertance I therefore equals $L \times \rho/A$. The pressure drop due to inertance is greatest when the flow increases rapidly, as occurs if the frequency of breathing rises. The work performed to achieve the acceleration is stored in the lung as kinetic energy.

Inertial forces are of negligible magnitude except when a high frequency oscillation is applied for purposes of assisting ventilation or for investigating the mechanical characteristics of the lung (Section 14.4.4).

14.3 Resistance

The force required to overcome the resistance to movement of the lungs and thorax is relatively large. Hence, when ventilation is increased the associated energy expenditure can represent a significant fraction of maximal uptake of oxygen. For this reason the frictional resistance of the lungs and chest wall can limit exercise. It can also influence the maximal rate at which air can move into and out of the lungs.

14.3.1 Total thoracic resistance

Total thoracic resistance is the sum of components attributable to the rib cage, the diaphragm, the abdominal wall and contents, the lung tissue and the gas in the lung airways. As with electrical resistances in series, these are additive in their effect. Hence,

$$P\text{total} = P\text{th} + P\text{ti} + P\text{aw} \quad (14.4)$$

where P is the force required to overcome the frictional resistance and th, ti and aw refer, respectively, to the thoracic rib cage and diaphragm, the lung tissue and the lung airways. For the thoracic cage the force is a simple function of the velocity of linear movement. The velocity cannot be measured directly, but can be described approximately in terms of the rate of airflow. Then, as a first approximation

$$P\text{th} = R\text{th} \times \dot{v}^{n1} \quad (14.5)$$

where Rth is the resistance of the thoracic cage, in kPa (or cm H_2O) l^{-1}s and $\dot{v}$ is the airflow (l s^{-1}). In most instances the value of the exponent $n1$ lies between 1.0 and 1.1. Hence, the relationship is effectively linear.

14.3.2 Total pulmonary resistance

Total pulmonary resistance is the sum of lung tissue resistance (Rti) and airway resistance (Raw):

$$R\text{l} = R\text{ti} + R\text{aw} \quad (14.6)$$

where Rl is the pulmonary flow resistance in kPa (or cm H_2O) l^{-1} s; it is therefore the pressure difference that must be applied between the pleural surface of the lungs and the lips in order to secure a velocity of flow of 1 l s^{-1}. This quantity can be derived from the slope of the initial part of the iso-volume flow–pressure curve, as illustrated in Fig. 13.1 (page 144).

14.3.3 Lung tissue resistance

Lung tissue resistance (Rti) normally represents approximately 10% of total pulmonary resistance (Table 14.1). Its relative contribution to pulmonary resistance is greater at large than at small lung volumes due to converse changes in airway resistance. The tissue resistance itself is increased in pulmonary fibrosis and other conditions where the quantity of interstitial lung tissue is increased. However, the increase can be simulated if different parts of the lung vary widely in their distensibility [2]. Tissue resistance cannot be measured; instead it is estimated rather inaccurately by subtracting airway resistance from total pulmonary resistance.

Table 14.1 Average values for the total thoracic resistance and its components at a flow of 0.5 l s^{-1} in healthy young men. The values in women are higher.

Site	Component	Resistance: SI units (kPa l^{-1}s)	Resistance: Traditional units (cm H_2O l^{-1}s)	Method of measurement
Mouth				Plethysmograph: Mouth to 2–3 mm airways; Interrupted: Mouth to Alveoli/Pleural space; Oesophageal balloon: Mouth to Pleural space; Forced Osscilation: Mouth to Chest surface
Larynx	Glottis	0.05*	0.5*	
2–3 mm airways	Raw (large)	0.05	0.5	
Alveoli	Raw (small)	0.02	0.2	
Pleural space	Rti	0.02	0.2	
Chest surface	Rth	0.12	1.2	
Sum	Rtotal	0.26	2.6	

* During gentle panting with the mouth wide open; higher values are obtained during normal breathing. Source [1].

14.3.4 Airway resistance

Airway resistance (*R*aw) is the sum of the resistances attributable to all airways individually. For each airway an important determinant of resistance is the airway diameter, which varies with lung volume (Section 11.4). Hence, airway resistance varies with lung volume. A theoretical basis is provided by Poiseuille's equation. This states that, for a simple tube, the resistance is related inversely to the fourth power of the radius [3]. Because in all airways the radius varies with lung size, the airway resistance varies throughout the respiratory cycle. The resistance is lower at large lung volumes when the airways are expanded; it rises during expiration as the airways diminish in size and becomes infinite at residual volume when some airways close (see Section 11.4). The relationship of the airway resistance to the lung volume is hyperbolic and illustrated for a healthy subject in Fig. 14.1. The reciprocal of airway resistance is conductance (*G*aw) and increases almost linearly with volume. Specific conductance (s*G*aw) is *G*aw/TGV, where TGV is thoracic gas volume. It varies less with lung volume than *G*aw.

The airway resistance is usually measured during inspiration, over a range of flows from 0 to 0.5 l s^{-1} and at a lung volume that is just above functional residual capacity (Section 14.4). The average value in adults is then approximately 0.13 kPa l^{-1} s (1.3 cm H_2O l^{-1}s, cf. Table 14.1).

The relative contributions to airway resistance made by airways of different size have been studied experimentally. This has been done using fine catheters inserted into the several classes of airway to obtain intraluminal pressures at different levels in the respiratory tract. The measurements demonstrated that during normal quiet respiration much of the resistance was provided by the nose, glottis and larynx (Table 14.1). Panting reduces these components of the resistance. Hence, during the measurement of lung resistance, panting can be used to focus attention on the airways (Section 14.6.3). Within the lungs, Macklem and others found that the resistance is mainly in the larger airways (diameter 3 mm to 8 mm) rather than the smaller ones [4, 5]. The finding has implications for assessment of the response to bronchodilator drugs (Chapter 15).

The resistance of the chest wall is of similar magnitude to that of the airways (*R*th, Table 14.1). However, the forces required to overcome these two resistances differ in their relationships to flow. In the chest wall the relationship is nearly linear (Section 14.3.1), but in the airways it is complex because the flow of air is laminar in some regions and turbulent in others.

Laminar and turbulent flow. In the periphery of the lungs the airways are of small diameter but, because there are many of them, their total cross sectional area is large. As a result, gas molecules travel relatively slowly. They move in lines parallel to the long axes of the airways, with molecules at the centre moving faster than at the periphery. This pattern of flow is described as streamlined or *laminar*. The force that is required to overcome

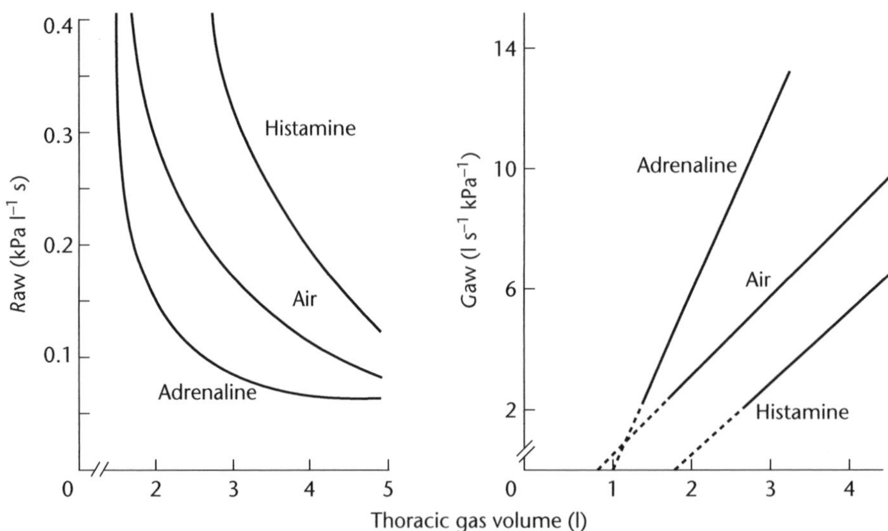

Fig. 14.1 Left: Relationship between airway resistance (*R*aw) and thoracic gas volume for a normal subject showing the effects of successive inhalations of aerosols of histamine and adrenaline; these, respectively, increase and decrease the resistance.
Right: Resistance varies inversely with the volume of gas in the thorax at the time of measurement. On this account, the relationship between airway conductance (*G*aw) and thoracic gas volume is effectively linear. However, due to airway closure there is a finite intercept on the x axis (Section 11.5.1), so the practice of expressing conductance per litre of lung volume (i.e. specific conductance) leads to error; the conductance at a specified volume can be used instead. Valid alternative methods of presenting such a result are given elsewhere. The data were obtained by McDermott and her colleagues (unpublished).

the frictional resistance is proportional to the flow (i.e. $P\text{aw} = R\text{aw} \times \dot{v}$) and the wave profile is parabolic (cf. Fig. 16.1, page 182).

The central airways are of larger diameter than the peripheral ones, but there are fewer of them so the total cross-sectional area is smaller. Thus, for a given volume flow of air the average forward velocity is higher, but the flow is often chaotic with gas molecules travelling transversely across the line of flow as well as longitudinally. This pattern is described as *turbulent*. With turbulent flow the wave profile is square and the frictional resistance is greater than with laminar flow, being proportional to the square of the mean forward velocity (i.e. $P\text{aw} = R\text{aw} \times \dot{v}^2$).

Contribution of pattern of flow to airway resistance. The airway resistance is the sum of its laminar and turbulent components. The first person to appreciate this was Rohrer, who used an additive model [6]:

$$P\text{aw} = k_1\,\dot{v} + k_2\,\dot{v}^2 \tag{14.7}$$

Subsequently, to allow for some flow being partly turbulent Ainsworth and Eveleigh proposed an exponential model [7, 8]:

$$P\text{aw} = R\text{aw} \times \dot{v}^n \tag{14.8}$$

Here, the exponent n varied between 1.0 and 1.9 depending on the degree of turbulence. To achieve greater precision entails allowing for the several factors that affect the transition from laminar to turbulent flow. This was done by Reynolds [9]:

$$\text{Reynolds number} = (\dot{v}\,D\,\rho)/(\eta\,A) \tag{14.9}$$

where, in appropriate units, $\dot{v}$ is the bulk flow of gas at a cross-sectional area A, D is the corresponding airway diameter and ρ and η are the gas density and viscosity. Reynolds numbers of less than 100 and more than 10,000 are associated, respectively, with completely laminar and fully turbulent flow, with other values intermediate. In the trachea during quiet breathing the Reynolds number is about 1500 so the flow is partly turbulent. With increasing minute ventilation it becomes progressively more turbulent and is completely turbulent during maximal ventilation. The airway resistance increases in consequence. In the bronchi the gas stream becomes turbulent at flows of approximately $5\,\text{l}\,\text{s}^{-1}$ but in the bronchioles at all levels of ventilation it is nearly laminar except at bifurcations where there are local eddies; these dissipate energy [10, 11]. In addition, because the total cross-sectional area of the larger airways is less than that of the smaller ones the speed of movement of individual gas molecules increases progressively as gas moves downstream towards the mouth. The process is described as *convective acceleration*. It has the effect that the total kinetic energy of the gas increases down the airway. However, the work of moving the gas, which is the product of the energy and the lateral pressure at the airway wall is only changed by the amount of frictional loss, so is nearly constant. Hence, as the velocity increases the lateral pressure decreases. The conditions are described by *Bernoulli's theorem*; this states that, neglecting frictional losses, the sum of the lateral pressure at the airway wall and the gas kinetic energy is independent of the cross-sectional area [12]. In the lung, if the flow–velocity profile is flat and allowing for frictional losses the conditions at the two sites can be represented by the following relationship due to Pedley [11]. The relationship is in traditional units.

$$P_1 + (1/2\,\rho)(\dot{v}/A_1)^2 = P_2 + (1/2\,\rho)(\dot{v}/A_2)^2 + P\text{fric} \tag{14.10}$$

where P_1 and P_2 are lateral pressures at two sites with the cross-sectional areas A_1 and A_2, and Pfric is the frictional pressure loss between these two sites.

Contributions of gas density and viscosity. The density and the viscosity of the respired gas (ρ and η in eqn. 14.9) affect, respectively, the numerator and denominator of the Reynolds number. The density varies directly with barometric pressure; hence turbulence in airways is reduced by ascent to altitude and increased by pressurisation or deep sea diving (Sections 34.2 and 35.3.1). Maximal flows at large lung volumes and maximal breathing capacity change correspondingly (Figs 14.2 and 14.3). The density is reduced and viscosity increased by breathing a gas mixture that contains helium. Gas mixtures that contain sulphur hexafluoride have an increased density but reduced viscosity (Table 14.2). These features can be used to partition the airflow into laminar and turbulent components (Section 12.7).

14.3.5 Some applied and clinical aspects

Factors that influence airway resistance. For the reasons stated above an increase in the airway resistance is usually due to narrowing of larger airways. The narrowing can be either

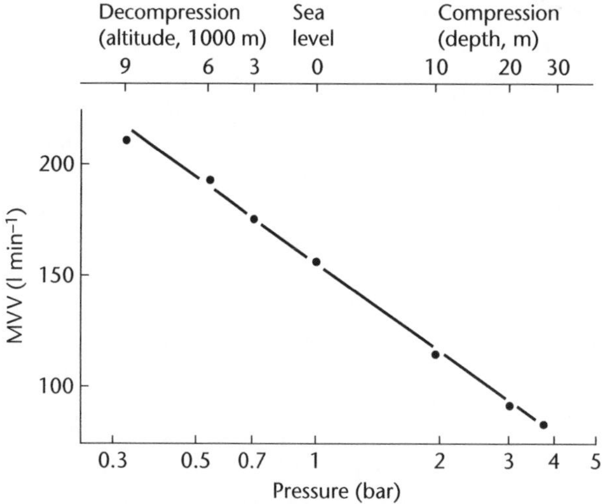

Fig. 14.2 The effect upon the maximal voluntary ventilation (MVV) of normal subjects of changes in the density and the kinematic viscosity of the respired gas caused by alterations in the ambient pressure in an altitude chamber. Source: [13].

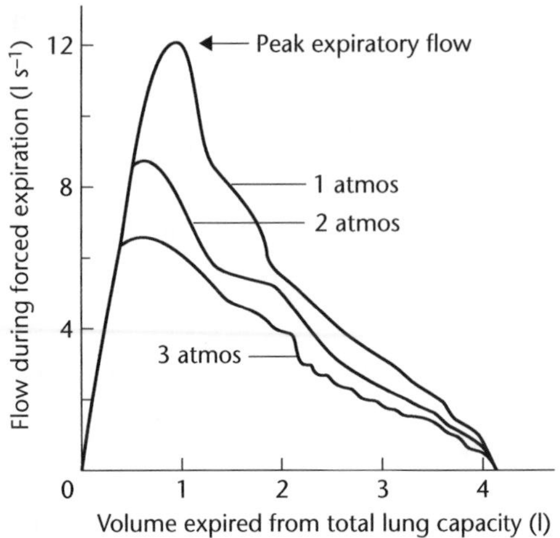

Fig. 14.3 Flow–volume curves for a healthy subject obtained under hyperbaric conditions in a compression chamber.

Table 14.2 Density and viscosity at 20°C of gas mixtures containing 80% nitrogen, helium or sulphur hexafluoride with 20% oxygen.

	Density (ρ, kg m^{-3})	Viscosity (η, kg m^{-1} s^{-1} × 10^{-9})	Kinematic viscosity (υ, m^2 s^{-1} × 10^{-9}) where $\upsilon = \eta/\rho$
N_2/O_2	1.286	1.792	1.393
He/O_2	0.429	1.952	4.550
SF_6/O_2	5.567	1.602	0.288

Note: in the lung the values are somewhat different due to the effects of temperature, CO_2 and water vapour.

extra- or intrathoracic and, if the latter, extrapulmonary or intrapulmonary. In all these situations obstruction may be due to the accumulation of material within the lumen (endomural obstruction), encroachment on the lumen by thickening of the epithelial or sub-epithelial tissue or to external compression by glands or by one or more space-occupying lesions. The intrathoracic airways are subject to a number of other factors including variation in bronchomotor tone from many causes, including the recent volume history of the lung (Section 15.2). In addition, the airways that are extrapulmonary are subject to compression if the intrathoracic pressure rises above atmospheric pressure. The airways that are intrapulmonary are narrowed if, for any reason, the traction that is exerted on their walls by the recoil of the lung tissue is reduced. This is the case in emphysema. The traction is increased in interstitial fibrosis; it is also increased if the resting respiratory level is raised through the subject breathing at nearer to total lung capacity. The larger lung volume can then compensate for loss of elastic recoil in emphysema or for an increase in bronchomotor tone, as occurs during an attack of asthma or following inhaling histamine. It can then partly reverse the reduction in airway calibre that occurs.

In all these circumstances the extent to which airways are deformed by external forces is determined by their rigidity and hence by the thickness of the sub-epithelial layer and the prevailing bronchomotor tone. Thus, the overall airway resistance is the resultant of a large number of processes, which between them operate at several sites in relation to individual airways (Table 14.3)

Obstruction in the periphery of the bronchial tree occurs with bronchiolitis or loss of lung elasticity. Conventional theory suggests that the obstruction needs to be intense if it is to exert a material effect upon the overall resistance (see Table 14.1). However, this may not be the whole story.

Small airways. Narrowing of small airways is not immediately obvious as the evidence is indirect and this is also the case for the methods used for its detection (Footnote 14.1). The methods do not distinguish between the principal causes of narrowing, namely inflammation, raised bronchomotor tone and loss of lung elasticity.

Loss of lung elasticity has two effects: it decreases the driving force for forced expiratory flow and, due to interdependence between lung parenchyma and intrapulmonary airways, it decreases airway cross-sectional area. The topic is potentially important on two grounds. First, as a result of interdependence, narrowing of small airways appears to impinge on the function of larger ones. Evidence for this has been found in the relationship between airway resistance and *P*st using measurements made at several lung volumes [18]. Second, the existence of narrowing of small airways could be a pointer to subsequent narrowing of larger ones [17]. So far, the evidence is not convincing [19].

Some direct consequences of an altered airway resistance. An increase in airway resistance reduces ventilatory capacity and hence the maximal ventilation during exercise. The changes depress the capacity for exercise and accentuate the associated breathlessness on exertion. A contributory factor is the premature closure of airways during expiration leading to an increase in residual volume without a commensurate increase in total lung capacity. As a result the vital capacity and exercise tidal volume are reduced and the shallow breathing interferes with the distribution of inspired gas (see below). The associated expiratory airflow limitation is considered in Section 13.6.

In the converse situation, subjects who have a low airway resistance tend to have a small residual volume. When the cause is interstitial fibrosis, the associated increase in recoil pressure reduces the size of the lungs but tends to preserve the airway calibre. This leads to the ventilatory capacity being larger than might be expected from the small size of the vital capacity (Section 40.4). The physiological picture can be complicated by defective gas

Footnote 14.1. The indices that have been used to identify narrowing of small airways have included $FEF_{75\%FVC}$, V-iso $\dot{v}$, dynamic compliance, derivatives of transit time analysis, single breath indices of lung gas distribution and lung reactance obtained by forced oscillometry [17], also see Sections 16.1.1 and 13.6.

Table 14.3 Types of generalised abnormality of airway calibre.

Endomural obstruction	Viscid mucus: polyp or foreign body in large airway
Mural encroachment on lumen	Sub-epithelial inflammation or oedema: mucus gland hyperplasia: stricture in large airway
Bronchomotor tone increased	Asthma, wheezy bronchitis, exposure to cotton dust, histamine and other causes of broncho-constriction.
	Stimulation of nasal epithelium [14]. Full inspiration in some circumstances [15, 16][†]
Extramural traction on intrapulmonary airways	*Reduced* at small lung volumes*, in the elderly and with emphysema (high lung compliance)
	Increased at large lung volumes* and with interstitial fibrosis (low lung compliance)
Mural deformability	*Reduced* with asthma and bronchitis
	Increased after bronchodilator drugs and with cylindrical bronchiectasis
Extramural compression of the lumen	*Static* by neoplasm or enlarged thyroid or lymph gland
	Transient with interstitial oedema
	Dynamic with coughing or during forced expiration

† see e.g. Section 12.5.1.
* Irrespective of cause and of lung compliance.

exchange across the alveolar capillary membrane. An additional factor is the excessive quantity of lung tissue; this contributes to the reduced size and increased stiffness of the lung and increases the work of breathing.

Some indirect consequences of an altered airway resistance. Through the mechanisms which have been described, a change in bronchomotor tone causes concurrent changes in airway resistance, lung volume and static recoil pressure. Interactions between these responses need to be taken into account when assessing bronchodilatation, bronchoconstriction and the effect of a chest illness. To this end, the measurements should be made at the same airflow and the same value of Pst, hence at the same absolute lung volume (Section 15.7.2).

When airway narrowing occurs it does not affect all airways equally. Instead, those regions where the airways are most affected incur the greatest reduction in ventilation. In this way, a high airway resistance, especially in the periphery, causes very uneven distribution of inspired air. The maldistribution reduces the effectiveness of gas exchange (Section 18.1).

14.3.6 Resistance of the upper airways

Prior to entering the thorax the air traverses the upper airways. These structures comprise either the nose or the mouth with its adjacent pharynx, together with the larynx and extrathoracic trachea. The calibres of the several structures are coordinated via the autonomic nervous system (Sections 3.3.10 and 3.3.11). The resistance of the oral pathway is included in the measurement of airway resistance. The additional resistance of the nasal pathway is high, roughly equal to that of the whole of the rest of the respiratory tract [20, 21]. The high resistance is a consequence of the nose functioning as a filter and air conditioner (Section 37.2). This role is abandoned during speech or moderately severe exercise in favour of breathing through the mouth. The nasal resistance is also bypassed during lung function testing.

The structures of the nose have a variable geometry (Fig. 37.1, page 506). This leads to a mixed flow pattern, with laminar and turbulent components in parallel. As a result, the flow resistance is only described approximately by Rohrer's simple model (eqn. 14.7) and the Reynolds number (eqn. 14.9) is not easily calculated. Hence, any measurement of nasal resistance is inevitably approximate [22, 23]. A high resistance is a predisposing factor for snoring and sleep apnoea (Sections 32.4 and 32.5).

14.4 Measurement of lung resistance

14.4.1 Introduction

The total lung resistance (Rl), which is the driving pressure divided by the flow, is equivalent to the pressure difference between the pleural surface of the lungs and the mouth when the flow at the lips is $1\ \text{l s}^{-1}$. It is the sum of the airway resistance (Raw) and the tissue resistance (Rti) for which the corresponding driving pressures are the pressure gradients between the alveoli and the mouth and between the pleura and the alveoli. Thus:

$$R\text{l} = R\text{aw} + R\text{ti} \tag{14.6}$$

The indices are calculated from measurements of velocity of airflow at the lips ($\dot{v}$) and pleural or alveolar pressure relative to pressure at the mouth (Ppl and PA, respectively). For laminar flow, such as occurs when velocity is less than $0.5\ \text{l s}^{-1}$, the relationship can be written in the form:

$$P\text{pl}/\dot{v} = P\text{A}/\dot{v} + (P\text{pl} - P\text{A})/\dot{v} \tag{14.11}$$

Flow is measured with a pneumotachograph (Section 7.3.2). Pressure at the pleural surface of the lungs is measured in the oesophagus; alveolar pressure is measured either at the mouth after interruption of the air stream or by application of Boyle's law using a body plethysmograph. These techniques form the basis for three distinct methods of estimating the lung resistance. The relationships between them are indicated in Table 14.1. In addition, the total thoracic resistance, which includes the resistance of the chest wall (eqn. 14.4), may be obtained by the method of forced oscillation, in which the pressure at the mouth is measured during the imposition of a pressure pattern, which is usually produced by a loudspeaker.

Lung resistance is usually reported in the units of resistance (i.e. kPa or cm $H_2O\,l^{-1}s$). However, the reciprocal of the resistance, which is the conductance (G), is often preferable because it is almost linearly related to the thoracic gas volume and to transpulmonary pressure (Fig. 14.1). In this instance the error due to neglecting the intercept is relatively small. The conductance is often expressed per litre of the thoracic gas volume when it is called specific conductance (sG). The term specific resistance sR is also used.

14.4.2 Choice of methods

Whole body plethysmography is the best way of measuring airway resistance because it is accurate, acceptable to most subjects and, in addition, yields thoracic gas volume; the latter is necessary for interpreting resistance measurements. Knowledge of thoracic gas volume also has other uses (e.g. Sections 15.6.1).

The forced oscillation (impedance) method measures total thoracic resistance. The technique does not require the active cooperation of the subject so is suitable for young children and during anaesthesia. It can be used to monitor rapid changes in airway calibre, for example those due to bronchodilation or bronchial provocation. However, the method is technically demanding, and it is subject to error caused by the mouth and pharynx absorbing some of the imposed oscillation. There is no concurrent estimate of thoracic gas volume.

The classical pressure–flow method measures pulmonary resistance. It requires oesophageal intubation, but can be applied in the absence of a plethysmograph. The method does not measure thoracic gas volume.

The interrupter method is a less sensitive guide to airways obstruction than the other methods, but has the advantage, for surveys, that it is readily portable [24].

14.4.3 Plethysmograph method

The method is described in Section 14.6 below.

14.4.4 Forced oscillation method

Outline. When the thorax is subjected to forced oscillation from a pump connected to the mouth a back pressure is developed. This is a function of both the amplitude of the oscillation and the total impedance of the respiratory system; the latter has three components: resistance, compliance and inertance. The component due to compliance (the elastic component) is a function of the change in volume of the thorax and is inversely related to the frequency of the oscillation that is imposed. The component due to inertance is a function of the acceleration of the thorax and is directly proportional to the frequency. Thus, when the frequency of the imposed oscillation is changed these two components of the total impedance are affected in opposite ways; there is then a frequency at which they are of equal magnitude and effectively neutralize each other. At this resonant frequency, which is normally about 9 Hz, the impedance of the lungs and thorax is almost entirely due to the resistive component. At other than the resonant frequency the sum of the elastic and inertial components is given by the reactance. The measurement that is usually made is of input impedance at the mouth in which both the forced oscillation and the volume change relate to the mouth. In transfer impedance the two relate to different sites with usually the pressure directed at the chest and the volume change measured from the mouth. The reverse is the case for the transfer impedance at the mouth (Fig. 14.4). The latter is the sum of the airway, lung tissue and chest wall resistances. Use may be made of the resonant frequency for measurement of the total thoracic resistance. The method was introduced by DuBois et al [26] and subsequently refined [25, 27–30].

Practical details. The measurement of input impedance at the mouth is made with the subject seated and the head in a vertical position; flexion of the neck should be avoided. The subject

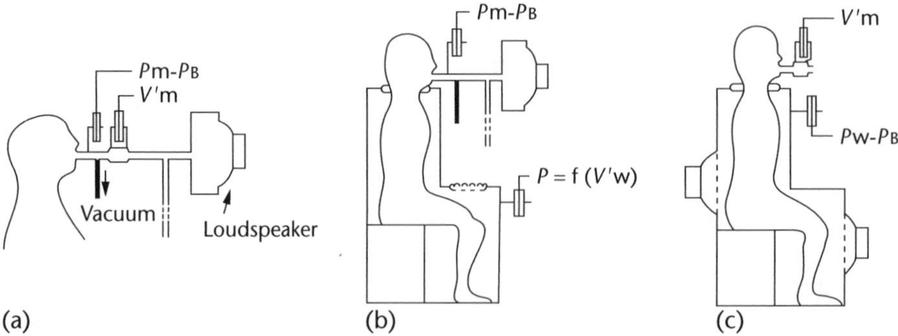

Fig. 14.4 Alternative approaches to measuring respiratory mechanical impedance. (a): pressure input at the mouth and flow measured at the mouth (input impedance at the mouth). (b): pressure input at the mouth and flow measured at the chest (transfer impedance at the mouth). (c): pressure input at the chest and flow measured at the mouth (transfer impedance at the chest); Pm, Pw, PB: mouth, body surface and barometric pressures, respectively; V'm, V'w: flows at the mouth and at the chest, respectively. Source: [25].

breathes through a pneumotachograph that is connected to a sine wave pump or loudspeaker. In order to straddle the resonant frequency the frequency of oscillation should cover the range 4–32 Hz. Very high frequencies (>100 Hz) can also be used. The amplitude of oscillation is usually 40 ml for adults and less for children. The pneumotachograph is continuously flushed with air (flow $\approx$ 12 l min^{-1}) to minimise accumulation of expired gas. The applied pressure is measured at the lips using a suitable transducer (Section 7.4). The pressure and the flow are displayed on the x and y axes of a computer screen or oscilloscope where convenient scales per cm of screen are, respectively, 0.16 kPa (1.6 cm H_2O) and 0.4 l s^{-1}. During the application of the forced oscillations the signal on the screen takes the form of an oblique loop; in normal subjects this reduces to a straight line at the resonant frequency. However, in patients with airways obstruction, because the compliance is frequency dependent, the resonant frequency can be very high and exceed the maximal frequency of the equipment. In these circumstances the looping can be reduced by subtracting from the pressure axis a signal that is proportional to either the integral or to the differential of the flow. These signals, which are proportional to the changes in volume and in acceleration of the imposed forced oscillation, relate, respectively, to the compliance and inertance components of the overall impedance. If the subject were not breathing spontaneously, the thoracic resistance would be the slope of the linear relationship that is obtained. In practice, the subject is breathing and this leads to variability in resistance between breaths. Averaging the separate pressures and flows over a series of breaths can reduce the variability. Averaging the individual resistances is less satisfactory.

Comment. The quality of the measurements depends on the transducers for pressure and flow having negligible impedance but similar phase and amplitude characteristics. In addition, an appropriate allowance should be made for the proportion of oscillatory flow that is taken up in the cheeks and upper airways. This proportion is increased in the presence of obstruction to intrathoracic airways and so the resistance is underestimated as a consequence. The error can be reduced by cupping the cheeks in the hands or by applying a compensatory oscillation externally. Alternatively, applying the oscillation to the trunk via a partial body plethysmograph that does not include the head can eliminate the error. The resulting transfer impedance at the chest has the further advantage that only the flow is measured at the mouth; the flow meter can then be opened to the atmosphere and have a less demanding specification than when the applied pressure and the flow are both measured at the mouth. The methodology for transfer impedance offers scope for further development.

The method has the advantages of only requiring minimal co-operation from the subject and, when performed at a single frequency, of having a short response time. It can therefore be used to monitor changes within breaths (e.g. Section 13.6) and during sleep, anaesthesia and mechanical ventilation of the lungs. There is an application for monitoring responses to bronchoactive drugs, particularly in children [30]. The method is of limited usefulness in population studies. This is due in parts to variation between subjects being related to the properties of the chest wall as well as to those of the lungs.

14.4.5 Pressure–flow method

Outline. The pressure–flow method for measuring the total lung resistance requires the intubation of the oesophagus and, if compliance is measured concurrently, it takes about 40 min of the subject's time. For these reasons it has been superceded by other methods except when measurement of the tissue resistance, or the resistance upstream of the equal pressure points (Section 13.3) is required.

To make the measurement, oesophageal intubation is performed in the manner described in Section 11.8.1 and the pressure and flow equipment are calibrated. The velocity of airflow and the oesophageal pressure in excess of mouth pressure are displayed as a pressure–flow diagram (Fig. 14.5).

The slope of the long axis of the diagram is the relationship of airflow velocity to total applied pressure; this is a first approximation to the desired relationship, which is between airflow velocity and *resistive* pressure. The latter is obtained by subtracting from the total pressure the component due to elastic recoil of the lung; this pressure is the product of the change in volume and the lung elastance.

Correction for compliance component of pressure. The correction is made using the relationship of lung volume to pressure

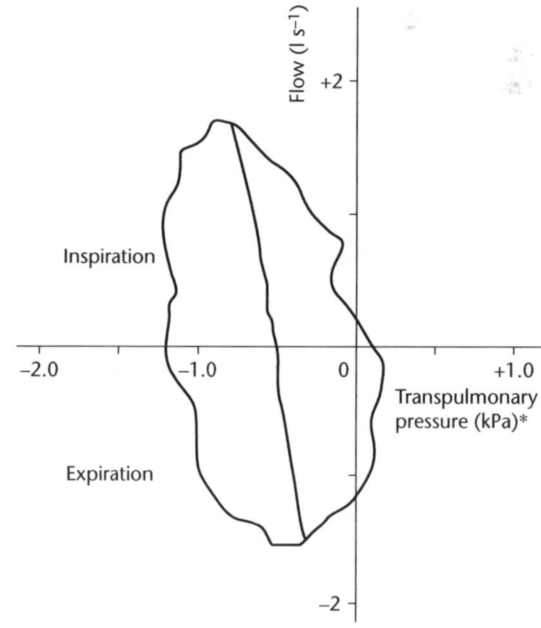

Fig. 14.5 Pressure–flow diagram obtained by the method of Mead and Whittenberger; this is described in the text. Source: [31].
*To obtain pressure in cm H_2O multiply these numbers by 10.

obtained concurrently with the flow–pressure curve (see Fig. 9.3, page 103). In this figure the resistive pressures at the points on the curves labelled Insp and Expn are represented by the horizontal distances from B. The corresponding total lung resistances are obtained by dividing the resistive pressures by the corresponding rates of airflow. The division can be performed electronically as, above functional residual capacity, the force that is required to overcome the elastic recoil of the lungs is nearly proportional to its volume. The volume is obtained by electrical integration of the output of the pneumotachograph. A component that is proportional to this volume is now subtracted from the pressure axis of the pressure–flow diagram.

This manoeuvre converts total pressure into resistive pressure; the slope of the long axis of the new diagram so obtained is the total lung conductance. The correction to the pressure axis is adjusted to minimise the area enclosed by the pressure–flow loop; in this circumstance the magnitude of the correction (i.e. the potentiometer setting) is a measure of the dynamic lung compliance (Section 11.8.4). The loop will reduce to a straight line as in Fig. 14.5 when both the airflow is entirely laminar (range of flows 0.5 l s^{-1} to 1.0 ls^{-1}) and the tidal excursion is small. The resistance is then unaffected by variations in lung volume during the procedure. However, it is affected by the average volume, which should also be reported (see Fig. 14.1).

Tissue resistance. Lung tissue resistance (Rti) is obtained as the difference between total lung resistance (Rl), which is measured by the pressure–flow method and the airway resistance (Raw), which is measured by the plethysmograph method:

$$R\text{ti} = R\text{l} - R\text{aw} \qquad (14.12)$$

On account of breath-to-breath variations it is essential that both resistances are measured during the same respiratory manoeuvre. Tissue resistance is normally small relative to airways resistance so the procedure is not particularly exact except when the tissue resistance is increased.

Upstream resistance. The concept of upstream resistance arises from equal pressure point theory, which is now superceded by a theory based on wave mechanics (Section 13.5). It is of theoretical interest but appears not to be of practical use. Upstream resistance is the resistance of peripheral airways under conditions of maximal flow, at which time the driving force is the static elastic recoil of the lung. At any lung volume it is given by the relationship:

$$R\text{us} = P\text{st}/\dot{v}\,\text{max} \qquad (14.13)$$

where Rus is the resistance of airways upstream of the equal pressure point. Pst is the static or elastic recoil pressure of the lungs at the lung volume specified, and $\dot{v}$max is the maximal airflow at that volume. The lung volume is measured by plethysmography. The appropriate values for pressure and flow are obtained from separate determinations of the relationship between recoil pressure and lung volume (Fig. 11.3, page 120), and that between maximal flow and volume (Fig. 12.4, page 136); the relationship between $\dot{v}$ max and Pst (Fig. 13.1, page 144) is linear over a wide range of lung volumes [32]. The slope (θ) is the upstream conductance and the intercept on the pressure axis is a measure of bronchial collapsibility.

14.4.6 Interrupter method

Outline. For this method of measuring airway resistance the alveolar pressure is measured at the mouth during interruption of the flow of gas by a shutter [7, 8]. When the shutter is closed the pressure equalises throughout the respiratory tract, so the pressure in the mouth rises to the level of that in the alveoli immediately prior to interruption. When the rate of airflow before the interruption is also known the airway resistance can be calculated. The measurement is usually made during a series of interruptions whilst the subject breathes through a resistance; this is adjusted to have a relationship of pressure to flow similar to that of the lung airways.

Practical details. The flow of gas down the airways is assumed to be partly turbulent to the extent that the pressure is proportional to the flow raised to the power of 1.6. Then, by analogy with eqn. 14.5:

$$P\text{aw} = R\text{aw} \times \dot{v}^{1.6} \qquad (14.14)$$

where Paw is the pressure difference between the alveoli and the mouth, $\dot{v}$ is the flow of gas and Raw is the airway resistance. The interruptions are effected by a rotating shutter that occludes then opens the airway for alternate periods of 0.05 s. This time is too brief to give rise to sensation so the subject is able to breathe through the apparatus at an apparently steady flow. The pressure in the mouthpiece when the shutter is open (P_1) reflects the airflow resistance of the apparatus. The pressure when it is closed (P_2) is that required to overcome the resistances of both the lung airways and the apparatus. The airway resistance (Raw) is then given by the following relationship:

$$R\text{aw} = \frac{(P_2 - P_1)}{P_1} \times R\text{c} \quad \text{kPa(or cm } H_2O)\text{l}^{-1}\text{s} \qquad (14.15)$$

where Rc is the resistance coefficient of the apparatus. The airway resistance is usually recorded at gas flows of 0.5 and 1.0 l s^{-1}.

Comment. The interrupter method yields a result that more nearly resembles the total lung resistance than its airway component. This is because, during the period of equalization of pressure after interruption, the pressure in the alveoli changes. An extrapolated initial value should be used [33]. In addition, when the airway resistance is high, the pressure that is measured at the mouth is not representative of that in the alveoli. This is due to distension of the cheeks and to movement of gas within the lungs

(Pendelluft effect, Section 16.1.9). The cheeks can be supported but the difficulty remains and affects the reliability of the result in this circumstance. Amongst the useful features of the method are that it is quick and simple for the subject, does not involve large or complex apparatus or tedious calculations and is appropriate for making serial measurements. It may have applications in studies of children too young to perform spirometry [34–36].

14.5 Nasal resistance (rhinomanometry)

The resistance is usually measured by anterior rhinomanometry. To this end a pressure transducer is inserted into one nostril through a nose plug or tape that is adjusted to occlude the airway. Pressure distal to the occlusion (postnasal pressure) is measured with respect to that in the mask used to measure airflow. The mask should fit closely round the nose or nose plus mouth. Flow is measured with a pneumotachograph connected to the mask. Because the relationship of resistance to flow is nonlinear (eqn. 14.8), resistance for each nostril separately can be expressed at constant transnasal pressure, usually 0.15 kPa (1.5 cm H_2O) or constant flow, usually 0.3 – 0.5 l s^{-1}. The reciprocal of the total nasal resistance is the sum of the reciprocal of the resistance for the two nares separately [22, 23]. The two measurements should have been made at the same transnasal pressure.

In posterior rhinomanometry the transnasal pressure is that between the mask and the postnasal space, obtained using a catheter. The method has the advantage that the pressure is common to both nostrils. Mouth pressure can be used as a surrogate, but this requires that the soft palate should be relaxed, which is not always the case.

By the forced oscillation technique the nasal resistance is the difference between total respiratory resistance measured through the nose and through the mouth. The method avoids the need to measure transnasal pressure, but the interpretation remains problematic because the relationship of nasal resistance to flow is not linear [37]. For most applications posterior rhinomanometry is the method of choice.

Nasal resistance is influenced by changes in the degree of vascular engorgement of the mucosa following, for example, alterations in inspired air temperature, changes in F_{I,CO_2} and inhalation of irritants. The resistance appears to be increased by hypoxia (Section 34.2).

14.6 Whole body plethysmography

14.6.1 Introduction

A typical whole body plethysmograph is an airtight box made of transparent plastic in which the subject sits. It can provide instantaneous values for the volume of gas in the thorax and intra-alveolar pressure. DuBois and colleagues introduced the procedure as a method for measuring airway resistance [38]. They used a box of constant volume. Subsequently, a constant pressure box was used by Mead for measurement of instantaneous lung volumes and hence of flow–volume curves based on thoracic gas volume [39]. As a result the curves reflect the true relationship of flow to lung volume. The relationship is not distorted by compression of intrathoracic gas, as affects the spirometric method (Section 12.5.1).

The plethysmograph lung volume differs from that measured by gas dilution because it includes any non-ventilated spaces, for example large emphysematous bullae [40]. It also includes intestinal gas [41]. The method is accurate but technically demanding and requires the use of sophisticated equipment [42]. It is an essential tool for the study of lung mechanics.

The *constant volume plethysmograph* is also called a pressure plethysmograph because the principal measurement is of pressure. It is used for measurement of airways resistance and thoracic gas volume. It can also be used to record gas uptake over fractions of the cardiac cycle (Section 17.3.3) and hence cardiac output. The system should have a high frequency response.

The *constant pressure plethysmograph* is also called a volume displacement plethysmograph; here the volume change is monitored using a spirometer or obtained by integration of the signal from a pneumotachograph of large cross-sectional area in the wall of the box. The spirometer should preferably have a high frequency response and the connection with the box should be of large diameter to avoid a resistance artefact. Electronic compensation for phase lag in the system is provided by a signal proportional to box pressure. The volume plethysmograph is used for delineation of flow–volume curves and also for measuring thoracic gas volume.

The principal source of error in the method is from changes in the humidity or temperature of air in the box during the procedure. Ways of reducing the error are described below. Error also arises as a consequence of gas exchange because, under normal circumstances, the amount of carbon dioxide that is produced is less than the amount of oxygen absorbed; this effect is usually small. In addition, the presence of material airflow obstruction, for example due to asthma, can slow down the transmission of alveolar pressure to the mouth. In this event the mouth pressure is not representative of alveolar pressure during the period when the airway is occluded. This can lead to overestimation of thoracic gas volume and underestimation of airway resistance [43, 44]. In this circumstance a more valid estimate of lung volume can be obtained by the radiographic method (Section 10.3.4).

14.6.2 Plethysmographic method for lung volume

Boyle's law states that if a given mass of gas is compressed at constant temperature, the product of pressure (P) and volume (V) is constant. This relationship is applied to the lung whilst the subject is sitting in the plethysmograph. The equipment is illustrated in Fig. 14.6. An important feature is the shutter; this is actuated by remote control to interrupt the flow of air through the mouth. To make the measurement the subject attempts to breathe in and out against the shutter with the glottis open; this is

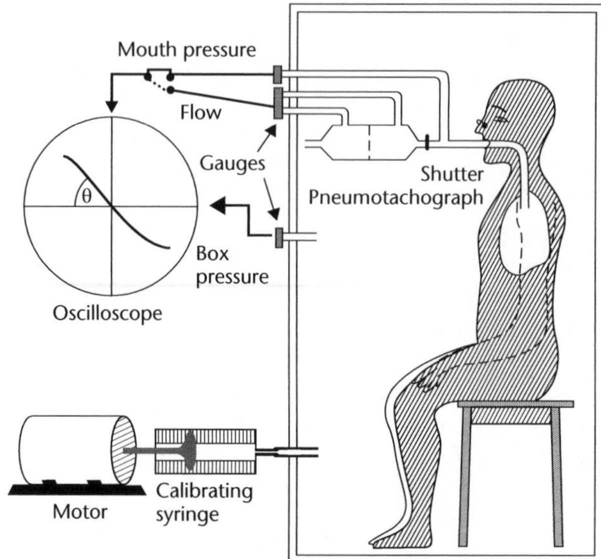

Fig. 14.6 Body plethysmograph (constant volume) and ancillary equipment for measuring the thoracic gas volume and airway resistance. The volume of the plethysmograph is about 700 l and full-scale deflection on the oscilloscope is obtained with a change in volume of 70 ml, equivalent to a change in pressure of 10 Pa (0.1 cm H_2O). Here tan θ is the pressure in the mouth during panting against the closed shutter expressed as a fraction of the pressure in the box. For calculation of thoracic gas volume tan θ is compared with the ratio of the signal due to movement of the calibrating syringe to the pressure in the box. For measurement of airway resistance tan θ is compared with the ratio of the signal from the pneumotachograph during gentle panting with the mouth open to the pressure in the box.

achieved by panting [45]. The panting movements vary the pressure and volume of gas present in the lungs. In this circumstance the following relationship applies:

$$PV = (P + \Delta P)(V - \Delta V) \qquad (14.16)$$

where P is alveolar pressure and ΔP is the change in pressure during panting against the shutter; V is the thoracic gas volume and ΔV is the change in volume due to compression of the chest by the respiratory movements. Cross-multiplying the terms within the brackets yields a product term $\Delta P \times \Delta V$. This is small relative to the other terms, so neglect of it only introduces an error equal to $\Delta P \times \Delta V$. The relationship then simplifies to:

$$V = P \times \Delta V/\Delta P \qquad (14.17)$$

Because water vapour condenses when compressed, its pressure remains constant and does not influence the result. Hence, the alveolar pressure (P) is effectively the barometric pressure less the pressure of water vapour in the lung (i.e. $P_B - P_{H_2O}$ at 37°C). The change in alveolar pressure during panting against the closed shutter (i.e. ΔP cm H_2O) is measured with a pressure transducer; this is arranged to record the pressure in the mouth. During closure the mouth pressure is equal to alveolar pressure. The change in lung volume (ΔV) is measured indirectly from the change in pressure of the air in the plethysmograph. The conversion of pressure change to volume change is calibrated by injecting a small measured volume of air (about 50 ml) into the plethysmograph and recording the ensuing rise in pressure within the box.

In practice, when the subject enters the plethysmograph the temperature of the air rises; this increases the pressure in the box. The pressure is released through a port to atmosphere. To make the measurement the subject breathes quietly through the pneumotachograph until, at the end of a normal expiration, the operator actuates the shutter to block off the mouthpiece. The same operation closes the port that permits the pressure to equalise between the box and air in the laboratory. The subject pants against the shutter with the cheeks supported by the hands to minimize any change in volume of the buccal cavity [46]. The mouth pressure and the box pressure are displayed on the two axes of the computer screen in the manner illustrated in Fig. 14.6 and the angle θ is recorded. Then, provided the transducers for mouth pressure and box pressure have similar calibrations,

$$\tan\theta = \Delta P/\Delta P\text{box} \qquad (14.18)$$

where ΔPbox is the change in pressure in the plethysmograph. If the calibrations differ a calibration factor will be required.

The box is now calibrated by determining the relationship of change in volume to change in pressure. This is done by noting the change in pressure that occurs when a measured volume of air is displaced into and out of the box. The air comes from a motor-driven calibrated syringe of capacity 50 ml (0.05 l) as in Fig. 14.6. The calibration is usually performed when the plethysmograph is empty. However, this practice introduces a small error due to the assumption that the changes in the box are isothermal (i.e. obey Boyle's law) when they are in fact adiabatic. The error is avoided if the subject remains in the box during the calibration. In either event the box pressure with respect to atmospheric pressure and the syringe volume are displayed, respectively, on the horizontal and the vertical axes of the screen, and the coefficient of proportionality, which is the tangent of the angle to the horizontal, is obtained. This coefficient is the change in volume of the air in the box per unit deflection on the pressure recorder (i.e. $\Delta V/\Delta P$box). In the absence of a subject it applies to the empty plethysmograph. An adjustment is then needed on account of the subject occupying some of the space. The coefficient is adjusted to the smaller volume of air during the measurement by means of the following relationship:

$$S_2 = S_1(V\text{box} - W/1.07)/V\text{box} \qquad (14.19)$$

where S_1 and S_2 are the initial and corrected coefficients of proportionality, Vbox is the volume of the plethysmograph in litres, W is the body weight of the subject in kilograms and the factor 1.07 is the average density of the human body. From these data the thoracic gas volume (V) is calculated as follows:

$$V = (P_B - P_{H_2O} \text{ at } 37°C)S_2/\tan\theta \times \text{BTPS correction} \quad (14.20)$$

The measurement of the thoracic gas volume requires only about 10 min of the subject's time and is readily performed when the airway resistance is recorded (see below). The residual volume and the total lung capacity can then be obtained by spirometry performed immediately after the period of panting. To this end the expiratory reserve volume and inspiratory capacity are measured and, respectively, subtracted from and added to the thoracic gas volume. For subjects with normal lungs the residual volume is equal to that recorded by the closed-circuit helium dilution method, except when much gas is present in the stomach or intestines. In the presence of airway obstruction a larger volume may be obtained by plethysmography [40]. The difference can reflect gas in non-ventilated parts of the lung. The method overestimates the lung volume when there is severe obstruction to airflow (cf. Section 16.1.9).

14.6.3 Plethysmographic method for airway resistance

Outline. The measurement is usually made using a constant volume plethysmograph (described above). The method using a constant pressure plethysmograph is similar. In the constant volume box, when the subject is present, the pressure fluctuates throughout the respiratory cycle. This is because the driving pressure needed to move the alveolar air along the airways affects the alveolar volume. On inspiration the volume increases and on expiration it decreases. These changes, respectively, compress and expand the air in the plethysmograph. The greater the airway resistance the greater are the pressure swings in both the lungs and the plethysmograph. With suitable calibration the alveolar pressures can be obtained from the box pressures. The calibration factor is the relationship between the two pressures. The factor is determined in the absence of airflow as this avoids the error that affects the measurement of alveolar pressure during interruption. It provides a true measure of the airway resistance, especially when obtained during panting. This pattern of breathing is adopted to minimise heating and cooling of the respired gas during breathing through the pneumotachograph. Alternatively, the need for panting can be reduced by the subject being provided with air at 37°C, saturated with water vapour. The measurement can then be made during quiet breathing. This procedure is more acceptable for the subject, but is associated with material loss of sensitivity in detecting changes in airway resistance because the resistance of the larynx is relatively larger and more variable during quiet breathing than during panting. The airway resistance should be related to the lung volume or the transpulmonary pressure at the time of measurement (see Fig. 14.1). The volume is measured concurrently in the plethysmograph; the method is described above.

Practical details. The pressure transducers should be capable of accurate measurement of pressure fluctuations of the order of 1 Pa (0.01 cm H_2O). The transducers should be in phase and their frequency responses should be at least 10 Hz (Section 7.3). Calibrations should be performed in relation to each batch of measurements and the appropriate calibration factor should be used in the calculation. The relationship of alveolar pressure to box pressure is obtained whilst the subject performs gentle panting movements against the closed shutter. In these circumstances, because of the absence of flow, the pressure is uniform throughout the respiratory tract, so can be measured in the mouthpiece. This pressure, and the pressure that is measured simultaneously in the box are displayed on the axes of an oscilloscope, computer screen or twin co-ordinate chart recorder. The slope of the resulting diagram ($\tan\theta$ in Fig. 14.6) is the ratio of the change in alveolar pressure to the change in box pressure ($\Delta P_A/\Delta P\text{box}$). The measurement of box pressure is repeated with the shutter open whilst the subject pants gently and shallowly through the pneumotachograph at flows of between 0 and 0.5 l s^{-1}. The pressure and the output from the pneumotachograph are displayed as before and the slope of the relationship is again determined ($\dot{v}/\Delta P\text{box}$). The airway resistance (Raw) is obtained from the ratio of the two slopes in the following manner:

$$Raw = \frac{\Delta P_A}{\Delta P\text{box}} \times \frac{\Delta P\text{box}}{\dot{v}} \text{ kPa (or cm } H_2O)l^{-1}s \quad (14.21)$$

The airway resistance is usually measured at a flow of 0.5 l s^{-1} but a flow of 1 l s^{-1} is sometimes adopted. During inspiration the resistances at the two flows are, in practice, similar. During expiration the resistance is higher at the higher flow because the airflow is partly turbulent and the lung volume is changing. An allowance can be made for the latter factor when the relationship of

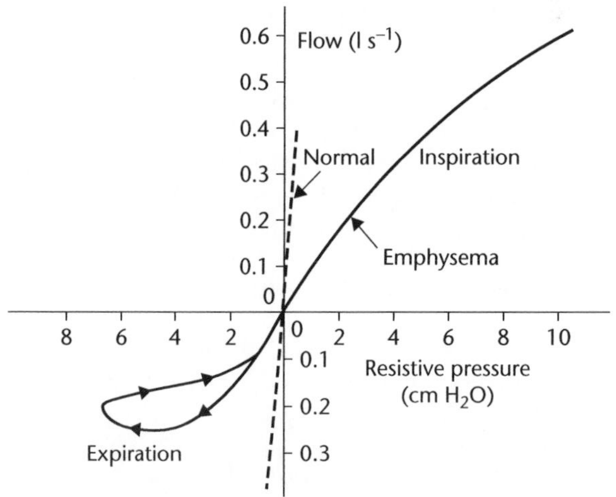

Fig. 14.7 Relationship of flow to resistive pressure during a representative maximal respiratory cycle in a healthy subject and a patient with emphysema. The record for the patient, but not the control subject, shows looping of the expiratory limb of the flow–pressure curve. Source: [47].

airway resistance to lung volume is known. However, the airway resistance during expiration is also affected by any undue rise in intrapleural pressure (Section 12.5.1). The compression is minimized by the subject performing the panting manoeuvre as gently and shallowly as possible; the frequency of panting should be less than 1 Hz and the expiratory flow should not exceed 0.5 l s^{-1}. A satisfactory result is then obtained in the majority of subjects, even though they may have no previous experience of the method. In a small number of subjects the result during expiration can be difficult to interpret because the relationship of flow to pressure ($\dot{v}/\Delta P$box) exhibits expiratory looping and is not linear (Fig. 14.7). This phenomenon is usually associated with obstruction to airflow.

14.7 References

1. Pride NB. The assessment of airflow obstruction. Role of measurements of airways resistance and tests of forced expiration. *Brit J Dis Chest* 1971; **65**: 135–169.
2. Gibson GJ, Pride NB. Pulmonary mechanics in fibrosing alveolitis: the effects of lung shrinkage. *Am Rev Respir Dis* 1977; **116**: 637–647.
3. Poiseuille JLM. Recherches expérimentales sur le mouvement des liquides dans les tubes de très petits diametres. *C R Acad Sci* 1840; **11**: 961–967, 1041–1048.
4. Macklem PT, Wilson NJ. Measurement of intra-bronchial pressure in man. *J Appl Physiol* 1965; **20**: 653–663.
5. Hughes JMB, Hoppin FG Jr, Mead J. Effect of lung inflation on bronchial length and diameter in excised lungs. *J Appl Physiol* 1972; **32**: 25–35.
6. Rohrer F. Der Stromungswiderstand in den menschlichen Atemwegen und der Einfluss der unregelmassigen Verzweigung des Bronchialsystems auf den Atmungsverlauf verschiedenen Lungenbezirken. *Pfluegers Arch Gesamte Physiol Menschen Tiere* 1915; **162**: 225–229.
7. Ainsworth MA, Eveleigh J. A method of estimating lung-airway resistance in humans. Porton technical papers 320 and 321. Wiltshire, UK: Chemical Defence Experimental Establishment, Porton, 1953.
8. Clements JA, Sharp JT, Johnson RP, Elam JO. Estimation of pulmonary resistance by repetitive interruption of airflow. *J Clin Invest* 1959; **38**: 1262–1270.
9. Reynolds O. An experimental investigation of the circumstances which determine whether the motion of water shall be direct or sinuous, and of the law of resistance in parallel channels. *Philos Trans R Soc Lond* 1883; **174**: 935–982.
10. Schroter RC, Sudlow MF. Flow patterns in models of the human bronchial airways. *Respir Physiol* 1969; **7**: 341–355.
11. Pedley TJ, Kamm RD. Dynamics of gas-flow and pressure–flow relationships. In Crystal RG et al, eds. *The lung: scientific foundations*, 2nd ed. Philadelphia: Lippincott-Raven, 1997: 1365–1382.
12. Bernoulli D. *Hydrodynamica*. Basel, Switzerland, 1738.
13. Miles S. The effect of changes in barometric pressure on maximum breathing capacity. *J Physiol* 1957; **137**: 85P–86P.
14. Kaufman J, Wright GW. The effect of nasal and nasopharyngeal irritation on airway resistance in man. *Am Rev Respir Dis* 1969; **100**: 626–630.
15. Lim TK, Pride NB, Ingram RH Jr. Effects of volume history during spontaneous and acutely induced airflow obstruction in asthma. *Am Rev Respir Dis* 1987; **135**: 591–596.
16. Nadel JA, Tierney DF. Effect of previous deep inspiration on airway resistance in man. *J Appl Physiol* 1961; **16**: 717–719.
17. Becklake MR, Permutt S. Evaluation of tests of lung function for screening for early detection of chronic obstructive lung disease. In: Macklem PT, Permutt S, ed. *The lung in the transition between health and disease*. New York: Marcel Dekker, 1979: 345–387.
18. Stanescu DC, Rodenstein DO, Hoeven C, Robert A. "Sensitive tests" are poor predictors of the decline in forced expiratory volume in one second in middle-aged smokers. *Am Rev Respir Dis* 1987; **135**: 585–590.
19. van de Woestijne KP, Jacquemin C, Atlan G, eds. Models in ventilatory mechanics. *Bull Physiopathol Respir* 1972; **8**: 179–430.
20. Hyatt RE, Wilcox RE. Extrathoracic airway resistance in man. *J Appl Physiol* 1961; **16**: 326–330.
21. Cockcroft DW, MacCormick DW, Tarlo SM, Hargreave FE. Nasal airway inspiratory resistance. *Am Rev Respir Dis* 1979; **119**: 921–926.
22. Eiser NM. The hitch-hiker's guide to nasal airway patency. *Respir Med* 1990; **84**: 179–183.
23. Liistro G, Rodenstein D, Stanescu D. Mechanics of the upper airways. In: Milic-Emili J., ed. *Respiratory mechanics. Eur Respir Mon* 1999; **12**: 92–111.
24. Frank NR, Mead J, Whittenberger JL. Comparative sensitivity of four methods for measuring changes in respiratory flow resistance in man. *J Appl Physiol* 1971; **31**: 934–938.
25. Peslin R. Methods for measuring total respiratory impedance by forced oscillations. *Bull Eur Physiopathol Respir* 1986; **22**: 621–631.
26. Dubois AB, Brody AW, Lewis DH, Burgess BF. Oscillation-mechanics of lungs and chest in man. *J Appl Physiol* 1956; **8**: 587–594.
27. Pride NB. Forced oscillation techniques for measuring mechanical properties of the respiratory system. *Thorax* 1992; **47**: 317–320.
28. Navajas D, Farre R. Oscillation mechanics. In: Milic-Emili J, ed. *Respiratory mechanics. Eur Respir Mon* 1999; **12**: 112–140.
29. Tomalek W, Peslin R, Duvivier C. Variations in airways impedance during respiratory cycle derived from combined measurements of input and transfer impedances. *Eur Respir J* 1998; **12**: 1436–1441.
30. Oostveen E, MacLeod D, Lorino H et al. The forced oscillation technique in clinical practice: methodology, recommendations and future developments. *Eur Respir J* 2003; **22**: 1026–1041.
31. Mead J, Whittenberger JL. Physical properties of human lungs measured during spontaneous respiration. *J Appl Physiol* 1953; **5**: 779–796.
32. Hyatt RE, Schilder DP, Fry DL. Relationship between maximum expiratory flow and degree of lung inflation. *J Appl Physiol* 1958; **13**: 331–336.
33. Sly PD, Lombardi E. Measurement of lung function in preschool children using the interrupter technique. *Thorax* 2003; **58**: 742–744.
34. Bridge PD, Lee H, Silverman M. A portable device based on the interrupter technique to measure bronchodilator response in schoolchildren. *Eur Respir J* 1996; **9**: 1368–1373.
35. Phagoo SB, Wilson NM, Silverman M. Evaluation of a new interruptor device for measuring bronchial responsiveness and the response to bronchodilator in 3 year old children. *Eur Respir J* 1996; **9**: 1374–1380.

36. Merkus PJFM, Mijnsbergen JY, Hop WCJ, de Jongste JC. Interruptor resistance in preschool children. Measurement characteristics and reference values. *Am J Respir Crit Care Med* 2001; **163**: 1350–1355.
37. Lorino AM, Lofaso F, Abi-Nader F et al. Nasal airflow resistance measurement: forced oscillation technique versus posterior rhinomanometry. *Eur Respir J* 1998; **11**: 720–725.
38. DuBois AB, Botelho SY, Comroe JH Jr. A new method for measuring airway resistance in man using a body plethysmograph: values in normal subjects and in patients with respiratory disease. *J Clin Invest* 1956; **35**: 327–335.
39. Mead J. Volume displacement body plethysmograph for respiratory measurements in human subjects. *J Appl Physiol* 1960; **15**: 736–740.
40. Bedell GN, Marshall R, DuBois AB, Comroe JH Jr. Plethysmographic determination of the volume of gas trapped in the lungs. *J Clin Invest* 1956; **35**: 664–670.
41. Brown R, Hoppin FG Jr, Ingram JH Jr et al. Influence of abdominal gas on the Boyle's law determination of thoracic gas volume. *J Appl Physiol* 1978; **44**: 469–473.
42. DuBois AB, van de Woestijne KP, eds. *Body plethysmography. Prog Resp Res*, vol 4. Basel: Karger, 1969.
43. Stanescu DC, Rodenstein D, Cauberghs M, van de Woestijne KP. Failure of body plethysmography in bronchial asthma. *J Appl Physiol* 1982; **52**: 939–948.
44. Brown R, Slutsky AS. Frequency dependence of plethysmographic measurement of thoracic gas volume. *J Appl Physiol* 1984; **57**: 1865–1871.
45. Stanescu DC, Pattijn J, Clément J, van de Woestijne KP. Glottis opening and airway resistance. *J Appl Physiol* 1972; **32**: 460–466.
46. Begin P, Peslin R. Influence of panting frequency on thoracic gas volume measurements in chronic obstructive pulmonary disease. *Am Rev Respir Dis* 1984; **130**: 121–123.
47. Mead J, Lindgren I, Gaensler EA. The mechanical properties of the lungs in emphysema. *J Clin Invest* 1955; **34**: 1005–1016.

CHAPTER 15

Control of Airway Calibre and Assessment of Changes

Assessment of the responses of airway calibre to treatment or provocation is an important function of any pulmonary laboratory. This chapter reviews the procedures against a background of the control mechanisms.

15.1 Introduction

Static dimensions. The diameter (calibre) of the airways is normally appropriate for the size of the lungs. It is related to body size and is less in children than in adults. Relative to lung size the calibre can be greater in females than in males (Section 25.7). It varies with the depth of inspiration as this affects the radial traction on airways from the surrounding lung tissue. For the same reason, under quiet resting conditions the calibre is influenced by posture (Section 16.1.8).

Tone of airway smooth muscle. Airway smooth muscle is contractile and this property if unrestrained can lead to closure of small airways. Restraint is normally exerted by the rhythmic stretching that occurs during the inspiratory phase of the breathing cycle and reinforced by periodic deep inspirations. The inspirations appear to act by increasing airway circumference, stretching the smooth muscle cells and loosening the intracellular bridges that attach myosin to actin [1]. Under normal circumstances this mechanism ensures that smooth muscle tone is minimal and is reduced further during a deep inspiration. This is not the case in asthma when a deep inspiration can result in bronchoconstriction (Section 12.5.1). In most normal persons the absence of meaningful muscle tone has the important consequence that airway calibre is determined by static forces and is not increased by administration of bronchodilator drugs. However, the amplitude of tidal breathing is reduced during sleep or anaesthesia and the change contributes to diurnal variation in airway calibre (Section 32.4.3). Snoring or sleep apnoea can also result in hypoxaemia that itself increases bronchomotor tone.

A reflex increase in bronchial tone occurs in response to stimulation of receptors in the airways by inhaled foreign bodies, mucus and other materials. The resulting bronchoconstriction enhances the effectiveness of the cough reflex (Section 37.2.1).

Disease processes that affect the airways can reduce the extent to which inspiration stretches the airway smooth muscle. When this happens the airways are more susceptible to constriction in response to provocation. The airway calibre is then reduced (see Section 15.4), but can usually be at least partly restored by administration of bronchodilator drugs.

Other determinants of airway calibre are mediated by the autonomic nervous system, the endocrine system, reflexes arising within the respiratory tract and processes that regulate body temperature. Many of these control systems are subject to diurnal variation that contributes to the airway calibre being less at night than during the day. The bronchoconstriction can be augmented by hypoxaemia (see below, Reflex hypoxic bronchoconstriction).

In most generalised diseases of the lung the amelioration of airflow limitation is a principal objective of respiratory therapy.

15.2 Physiological control of airway calibre

15.2.1 Parasympathetic nervous system

Bronchoconstriction occurs mainly through activation of the parasympathetic nervous system by receptors in airways. These supply information to the nucleus ambiguus in the brain stem. From there cholinergic motor nerves, that form part of the vagus nerves, activate ganglia in the airway walls (Section 3.3.10). The postganglionic fibres act by release of acetylcholine and this stimulates muscarinic receptors (M receptors) on airway smooth muscle cells and related structures. Activation of the receptors causes the muscle cells to contract.

The parasympathetic innervation is mainly to the large airways where, in the absence of reflex activation it maintains some residual bronchomotor tone. The smaller airways are sparsely innervated so any narrowing of these airways is mainly from inflammation or loss of lung elastic recoil (see emphysema, Section 40.4). Narrowing may be partly controlled by the autonomic nervous system through acetylcholine activating goblet cells to secrete mucus. The action of acetylcholine is potentiated by anticholinesterases and inhibited by atropine and other substances, including ipratopium bromide, that compete with acetylcholine to occupy M receptor sites on the smooth muscle cells. In addition to acetylcholine, the airway muscle tone can be increased in other ways, including by substance P, a neurotransmitter for non-cholinergic excitatory nerves and by calcitonin gene-related peptide [2, 3]. The pharmacological control of bronchomotor tone has features in common with that of pulmonary vasomotor tone (Section 17.2).

Intrapulmonary reflexes. Bronchomotor tone is modulated by reflexes arising from receptors located throughout the respiratory tract and mediated via the vagus nerves. The tone is decreased by activation of stretch receptors as occurs during inspiration. It is increased by stimulation of receptors in the nasal mucosa that respond to cold, and by receptors in the larynx that respond both to many chemical substances and to mechanical stimulation. Bronchomotor tone is also increased by stimulation of nerve endings that lie beneath the epithelium of the airways. The receptors in the larger airways contribute to the cough reflex and can usually adapt quickly. The receptors in the smaller airways often adapt slowly. They can be stimulated by inhalation of a bronchoconstrictor aerosol (e.g. histamine) and by airborne irritants such as particles of respirable dust, tobacco smoke and sulphur dioxide (Sections 37.2.1, 37.3 and 37.4).

Reflex hypoxic bronchoconstriction. Hypoxia stimulates the carotid body (Section 23.5) to cause reflex bronchoconstriction that is mediated via the vagus nerves. This reflex is inhibited by isoprenaline. It can occur in patients with chronic lung disease and differs from other types of bronchoconstriction in responding to oxygen enrichment of the inspired gas [4]. The reflex can summate with other stimuli to bronchoconstriction, for example methacholine [5]. Hypoxia also causes pulmonary vasoconstriction (Section 17.2.2).

Other systemic reflexes. The aortic baroreceptors can initiate bronchoconstriction in response to a fall in the systemic blood pressure. Strenuous exercise can exert a bronchodilator effect that is partly due to diminution of vagal tone. The converse phenomenon of post-exercise bronchoconstriction can occur in asthma (Section 15.8.3).

15.2.2 Bronchodilator nerves

The only bronchodilator innervation to the airways is provided by non-adrenergic, non-cholinergic nerves. These nerves extend from the larynx to the terminal bronchioles and stimulation causes long lasting dilatation, especially of the larger airways. Stimulation can also activate mucous glands. The neurotransmitter substance appears to be vasoactive intestinal peptide (VIP) or the related substance, peptide histidine isoleucine. The role of this system in controlling normal airway tone is unclear [2, 3].

15.2.3 Sympathetic nerves

The sympathetic nervous system appears not to innervate the airway smooth muscles directly. Instead there are nerves to the mucous glands, the blood vessels and ganglia in the airway walls. The innervation to the ganglia provides a pathway whereby an increase in sympathetic activity can inhibit parasympathetic bronchoconstriction caused by the action of the vagi. It also causes bronchodilatation by releasing adrenaline to act on β_2 receptors in the airway walls. This action, unlike that of the vagus nerves, affects all classes of airway. A reduction in bronchial tone following administration of catecholamine drugs can be inhibited by β_2 blocking drugs such as propranolol and atenolol.

15.2.4 Effect of carbon dioxide

Deficiency of carbon dioxide in the intraluminal gas causes bronchoconstriction both reflexly and by a direct effect on bronchial smooth muscle. When the hypocapnia is generalised, as with hyperventilation, the narrowing affects all classes of airway. However, if the hypocapnia is localised, e.g. after a small pulmonary embolus, the bronchoconstriction is usually localised as well (see also pulmonary embolism, Section 17.2.3). The bronchoconstriction is reversed by the inhalation of CO_2 in a fractional concentration of 0.06. This concentration also partly reverses the bronchoconstrictor action of some drugs, for example histamine and acetylcholine. Bronchoconstriction caused by hypocapnia is attenuated by atropine; this is evidence that the constrictor action is mediated in part via the vagus nerves [6]. The action is supplemented by a direct effect of CO_2 on bronchial smooth muscle. The mechanisms are under investigation [7]. These responses provide a mechanism whereby the ventilation to a part of the lung is adjusted in response to local variation in blood flow.

A material increase in the intraluminal concentration of carbon dioxide can cause paradoxical bronchoconstriction. This response is unaffected by atropine or isoprenaline and so appears to be a local reaction to a noxious stimulus, with the mechanism being unclear. It may arise in the bronchial muscle itself or be an axon reflex emanating from the larynx.

15.3 Atopy

Features. Some healthy persons respond to environmental allergens by producing increased quantities of immunoglobulin IgE. Such persons are said to be atopic. The condition has constitutional and environmental components [8] and puts an atopic individual at increased risk of IgE mediated diseases including infantile eczema, hay fever and some forms of asthma. The respiratory manifestations include an increased susceptibility to airflow limitation that gives rise to wheeze and breathlessness on exertion. These features may occur when exercising in cold air (Section 15.8.3), in response to provocation by inhalation of an aerosol containing histamine or methacholine (Section 15.8.2), or following exposure to occupational or environmental aerosols capable of causing asthma (Section 15.8.5, also 37.6.1 and 37.7.6). The same persons may also develop erythema and a weal on the skin following intradermal inoculation of a suspension of common allergens, such as house dust mite. The plasma concentration of immunoglobulin IgE is increased [9]. In many developed countries the prevalence of atopy has increased in recent years [10] but the incidence may now be levelling off. The reasons are unclear.

Assessment. Atopic status is usually assessed by skin testing using the anterior surface of the forearm. Drops containing antigen in suspension or solution are applied and each is then pricked into the skin with a clean needle. The needle is inserted obliquely to a depth just sufficient to lift the skin. A positive immediate reaction is the development of an itchy urticarial weal with diameter at 15 min usually in the range of 2–15 mm. Subsequently, after 10–40 min the weal temporarily becomes surrounded by erythema. A delayed reaction to a specific test antigen is likely to occur after 8–24 h, so if this is a possibility the site of innoculation should be reassessed at these times. Test antigens that might be used are: house dust mite, pollen of local grass and danders from dogs and cats to confirm atopic status, the suspected antigen (if there is one) and a saline control. In many circumstances a histamine (positive) control is used as well. To avoid an anaphylactic reaction developing in a highly sensitised subject, any non-standard antigen should be used initially in very low concentration along the lines described subsequently for inhalation challenge (Section 15.8.5).

15.4 Pathological causes of generalised airflow limitation

Increased tone in bronchial smooth muscle (bronchoconstriction). This abnormality causes narrowing that can affect any or all classes of airway. When present the change reduces the ventilatory capacity and gives rise to wheeze and breathlessness on exertion. Other features of airflow limitation are summarised in Section 14.3.5. The changes are reversible in response to treatment with broncho-active drugs.

Bronchoconstriction is an important feature of asthma (Section 40.2). It also occurs as a consequence of exposure to atmospheric or domestic air pollution (including tobacco smoke) or pollution of occupational origin. The effects of the different pollutants are cumulative and can cause severe limitation to airflow. However, much of the limitation can be due to associated structural changes arising from chronic inflammation in the airway walls. The latter condition is described as chronic obstructive pulmonary disease (COPD, see below and also Sections 37.3 and 40.3).

The increased bronchomotor tone is often due to stimulation of receptors that activate parasympathetic cholinergic nerves. This pathway responds to pharmacological interventions (Section 15.7.1). An additional stimulus to bronchoconstriction comes from substances that reach the environment of the muscle cells as part of a pathological response; the substances include some that emanate from the muscle cells themselves [11]. A role has also been suggested for inflammation in or around small airways interfering with the mechanism whereby respiratory movements lower the bronchomotor tone (see above Increased tone in bronchial smooth muscle). At the time of writing, the evidence is indirect [1, 12] and not fully worked out.

Structural changes in and around airways. Structural changes, described as *airway remodelling*, occur in response to inflammatory agents that are formed in the lung. The stimulus arises either from an allergic reaction, as in most cases of asthma, or is a result from release of mediators by neutrophils and other phagocytic cells as may occur in COPD (Section 40.3). Where the target is bronchial smooth muscle, this can generate further mediator substances. The inflammatory changes affect the small airways; they include vascular engorgement, interstitial oedema, infiltration of airway walls by inflammatory cells and extrusion of secretions and cell debris into the airways. These changes can occur in both asthma and COPD but the mechanisms, natural history and responses to treatment are different [13], see also Chapter 40. However, with passage of time the features of the airways in the two conditions may converge [14]. Differences in the lung parenchyma remain.

Asthma. The predominant inflammatory cells are eosinophils, lymphocytes and mast cells, the limitation to airflow is episodic and, except in the late stages can be expected to respond to therapy (Section 40.2).

COPD. The predominant inflammatory cells are neutrophils and macrophages. The airways obstruction is typically progressive and only partially responsive to bronchodilator therapy. As a result, acute episodes are usually superimposed on a progressive slow deterioration in function that often responds poorly to present standard treatment (Section 40.3). The condition can be preceded or accompanied by chronic bronchitis, but this is not invariable. In the longer term structural changes can occur in the lungs. Either fibrous tissue can be laid down that permanently constricts the affected airways or the lung parenchyma can be digested by proteolytic enzymes leading to weakening of its structural framework. This condition is emphysema (Section 40.4).

Combined abnormality. Some patients with airway narrowing that is mainly irreversible can have a significant reversible element to their airflow limitation, while in some asthmatics the flow limitation can become largely irreversible [14]. Patients who present at this stage in their illness can be described as having chronic non-specific lung disease (CNLD) or chronic airways obstruction (CAO).

15.5 Bronchodilatation as a diagnostic tool

From a clinical perspective a respiratory patient with variable airflow limitation that is reversed fully by bronchodilator and related therapy has asthma. One in whom the limitation is not fully reversible has COPD [15]. This classification includes amongst patients with COPD some in whom the reversible element is small and others in whom it is relatively large, verging on asthma. That the latter patients might actually have asthma has led some authorities to redraw the boundary between the two conditions. A reversibility that exceeds an arbitrary percentage of the reference or baseline value then becomes asthma whilst a lesser change is COPD. Changes in forced expiratory volume of 9%, 10% and 12% have been used for this purpose. The dichotomy assumes that the test expirations have been maximally forced since with submaximal effort the volume of gas expired in one second (relaxed expiratory volume) can be increased [Section 12.4.1]. In addition, patients vary in their susceptibility to individual bronchodilator drugs and to combinations of drugs, when the order of administration can influence the outcome. Thus, bronchodilator status should preferably be based on the optimal response not that to a single drug. However, for patients classified as apparently having COPD, the optimal bronchodilator response can cross and re-cross the diagnostic boundary during the course of the illness. The response appears to be normally distributed and does not reflect the lung pathology. Thus, an arbitrary responder status does not provide a sound basis for diagnosis where this is in doubt, nor for decisions on treatment [16, 17].

15.6 Physiological features of airflow limitation

Generalised narrowing of large airways (diameter >3 mm) is mainly due to an increase in bronchomotor tone, whilst narrowing of small airways is mainly a consequence of inflammation with or without a reduction in elastic recoil. The changes can sometimes be visualised by tomography (HRCT). They can be inferred from the results of physiological tests (Table 15.1).

Some consequences of bronchial provocation leading to narrowing of mainly the larger airways is shown in Fig. 15.1. The converse situation of bronchodilatation improving indices of forced expiratory flow is shown in Fig. 15.2 and Table 15.2.

Table 15.1 Some indices that reflect narrowing of lung airways.

Aspect	Mainly large airways	Mainly small airways
Ventilatory capacity	FEV_1, FVC, MVV, PEF & Tiffeneau Index reduced. (FEV% can be unchanged) Wheeze*	$FEF_{75\%\ of\ initial\ FVC}$ (flow at iso-volume) reduced Dispersion of transit times increased
Lung mechanics	Specific conductance (sGaw) reduced Dynamic compliance (Cdyn) reduced Other, including impedance*	
Lung volumes	Residual volume increased. VA′/VA reduced. Closing volume increased	
Gas distribution	Desaturation*	Lung mixing, including single breath N_2 index, aerosol bolus dispersion & N_2 slope increased
Gas exchange	Transfer factor unchanged (but reduced if calculated using VA′, Section 20.9.1)	R index of $\dot{V}_A/\dot{Q}$ inequality impaired Exercise ventilation increased (Section 28.4.7)

* particularly in children e.g. [18, 19]

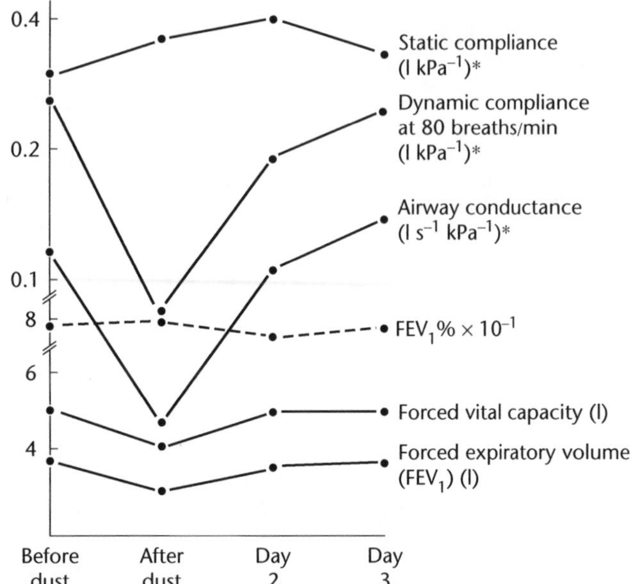

Fig. 15.1 Effect of mild bronchial obstruction caused by inhalation of cotton dust upon the lung function of a healthy subject. The semi-log scale indicates the relative magnitudes of the changes. In this instance, airway conductance and dynamic compliance were highly informative whereas FEV% and static compliance were not.
*To convert to traditional units (l and cm H_2O) multiply by 10.
Source: McDermott M, personal communication.

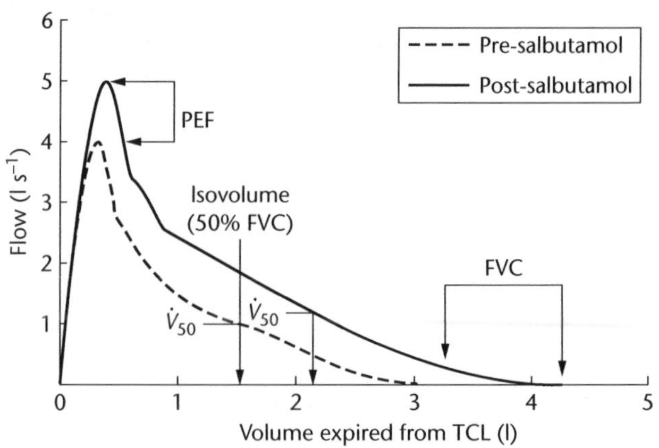

Fig. 15.2 Flow–volume curves before and after inhalation of a bronchodilator aerosol in a patient with airflow limitation that was partly reversible. The numerical results are given and interpreted in Table 15.2.

15.6.1 Calibre of larger airways

The above examples demonstrate that any of a number of lung function indices can be used to monitor variations in calibre of larger airways, including whole body plethysmography, dynamic spirometry and forced oscillometry.

Airway conductance. When the medical condition involves narrowing of large airways the best indicator of bronchodilatation is an increase in airway conductance (*G*aw) (Fig. 15.1). The measurement is made during tidal breathing so is not modified by reflex bronchodilatation from a prior full inspiration, as is an integral feature of most other tests. The conductance should be expressed at constant lung volume and not as specific conductance (s*G*aw = *G*aw/thoracic gas volume), since s*G*aw is not completely independent of lung volume (Section 14.3.4). Dynamic compliance can also be used (Fig. 15.1). The measurement of conductance (Section 14.3.4) is available at specialist centres where it is sometimes used for monitoring bronchial hyper-reactivity.

Single breath indices, FEV_1. This index is affected by narrowing of both large and small airways and is the index of choice in most circumstances. It is not suitable for young children or others who cannot cooperate in the measurement; for such subjects the impedance or other methods should be used instead (Table 15.1). FEV_1 has the disadvantage for some applications that the procedure may itself influence airway calibre, particularly in asthma, where both the initial inspiration to TLC and expiration to RV can increase bronchomotor tone [20]. Where these effects may be important, the conductance or indices from

Index	Before	After	% change*	Reference value
FEV_1 (l)	1.64	2.20	29	3.10
FVC (l)	3.24	4.34	29	4.43
$FEV_{1\%}$	50.6	50.7	0	66.1
IVC (l)	3.70	4.32	15	4.43
Tiffeneau index	44.3	50.9	16	66.1
PEF (l s^{-1})	4.1	5.1	22	8.9
$FEF_{50\% FVC}$ (l s^{-1})	1.0	1.2 †	18	3.0
TLC (l)	7.98	7.99	0	7.44
RV (l)	4.28	3.67	−15	2.68
Tl (mmol min^{-1} kPa^{-1})	9.81	9.84	0	9.5

* expressed as $100 \times \Delta x/\bar{x}$
† flow at isovolume = 1.9 l s^{-1}; change in flow at isovolume = 62%.

Table 15.2 Improvement in single breath indices of lung function following bronchodilatation in the patient with airflow limitation whose maximal expiratory flow volume curves are given in Fig. 15.2 (male, age 69 yr, height 1.84m, body mass 60 kg). The response was detected by FEV_1, PEF and flow at isovolume, but not by $FEF_{50\% FVC}$. Tiffeneau index (FEV_1/IVC) was informative whereas FEV% (FEV_1/FVC) was not.

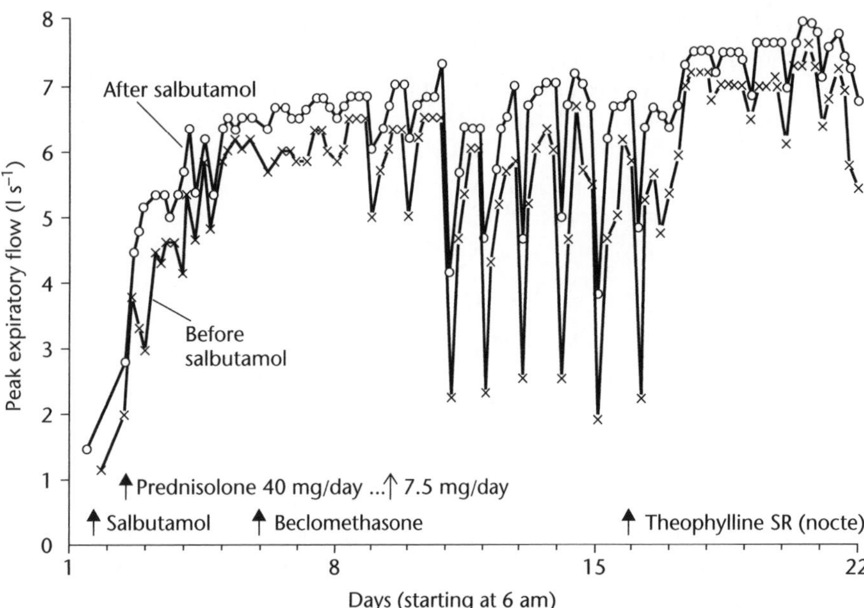

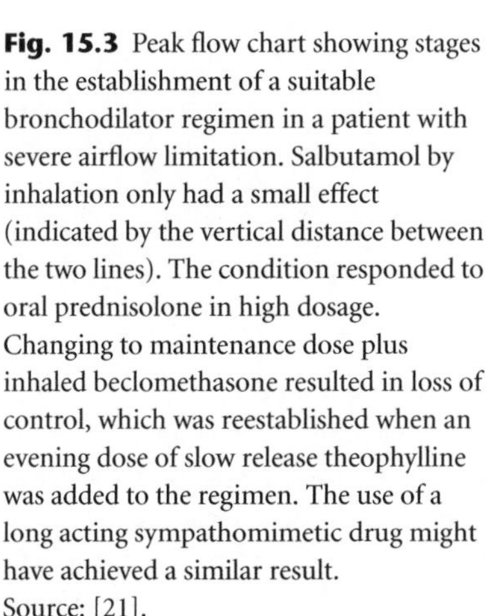

Fig. 15.3 Peak flow chart showing stages in the establishment of a suitable bronchodilator regimen in a patient with severe airflow limitation. Salbutamol by inhalation only had a small effect (indicated by the vertical distance between the two lines). The condition responded to oral prednisolone in high dosage. Changing to maintenance dose plus inhaled beclomethasone resulted in loss of control, which was reestablished when an evening dose of slow release theophylline was added to the regimen. The use of a long acting sympathomimetic drug might have achieved a similar result. Source: [21].

a partial expiratory flow–volume curve should be used instead (Section 12.5.1).

Peak expiratory flow. PEF is appropriate for serial measurements (Figs 15.3 and 15.7) and for home monitoring. However, peak flow can mislead if the calibration is alinear or the technique is incorrect (Section 12.3.2). The result can also mislead if the expiratory muscles are weak or if the compliance (flaccidity) of the walls of large airways is increased by the drug that is being assessed. The index does not detect narrowing of small airways.

Indices that relate to vital capacity. Some indices in this category, including FEV_1/FVC (FEV%) and forced mid-expiratory flow (FMF, also designated $FEF_{25-75\%FVC}$, Section 12.4.1), are invaluable for detecting the presence of airway obstruction but misleading for detecting changes. This is because an increase in airway calibre not only increases ventilatory capacity, but also reduces airway closure during expiration, so vital capacity is often increased as well (Fig. 15.2). As well as the above indices, similar considerations apply to forced expiratory flows when 50% or 25% of vital capacity remain to be expired. FEV% can paradoxically fall if the bronchodilator effect increases FVC more than the FEV_1 (Fig. 15.1). Indices based on flow (other than peak flow) should only be used when they can be measured at the same thoracic gas volume before and after administration of the bronchodilator drug [22]. The volume should then be measured by whole body plethysmography. This procedure is mainly of research interest.

15.6.2 Calibre of small airways

In some patients the main site of airflow limitation is the small airways. In this circumstance a change can usually be monitored using FEV_1, but not PEF or an index of airways resistance. However, some patients report an improved quality of life, reduced breathlessness on exertion or an increase in exercise capacity despite there being little change in FEV_1 [23–25]. In this circumstance the improvement appears to reside in small airways.

15.7 Bronchodilator therapy

15.7.1 Pharmacological and clinical aspects

Bronchodilator therapy is usually the most important component of treatment for airflow limitation. The treatment is likely to also include measures directed against both the cause of the limitation and the underlying medical condition, especially any accompanying inflammation in small airways. The latter can respond to anti-inflammatory drugs, usually a corticosteroid drug, so the two forms of therapy should be considered together.

The bronchodilators in current clinical use are short and long acting β-adrenoceptor agonists, anticholinergics and methylxanthines [26]. In acute childhood asthma intravenous magnesium sulphate can provide additional benefit. Agents that may sometimes prevent, but do not alleviate airflow limitation, such as sodium cromoglycate and leukotriene antagonists can be used as supplements.

β-adrenoceptor agonists. These drugs are derivatives of noradrenaline that binds to β_2 receptors on smooth muscle cells and some other structures. The principal action is to inhibit or reverse bronchoconstriction from any cause, of which the most common (in the absence of local inflammation) is increased parasympathetic activity mediated by acetylcholine. The mechanism entails increased intracellular production of cyclic AMP

and other changes that affect calcium-activated potassium channels on the cell membranes (maxi-K channels).

The β_2-agonists are administered preferably by inhalation, from a nebuliser, but can be taken orally. They have a good safety record unlike less selective drugs that can cause tachycardia and/or aggravate hypoxaemia [27]. A possible difficulty is that the bronchodilator response can become attenuated through the development of tolerance, but the change is seldom of sufficient magnitude to affect clinical management.

Anticholinergic drugs. These drugs compete with acetylcholine to occupy muscarinic receptors on smooth muscle cells. The process is dose dependent until all receptor sites are occupied. However, the receptors are of more than one type so there is a prospect of more selective blocking agents being developed. The mode of action is indicated under Parasympathetic nervous system above (Section 15.2.1). The drugs are administered by inhalation or nebulisation and side effects appear not to be a problem. Their action complements that of the β_2-adrenergic drugs and their effectiveness as bronchodilators is similar [28]. However, β_2-agonists are rather more effective in asthma, possibly because some bronchoconstriction is caused by leukotrienes or other inflammatory mediator, so is not of parasympathetic origin. Conversely, the anticholinergics may be better for COPD since both more of the bronchoconstriction is of reflex origin than in asthma and the action of the drug in suppressing the activity of goblet cells may be beneficial.

Methylxanthines. Over many years theophylline by mouth or intravenously has been found to be effective for relief of airflow limitation in some patients (e.g. Fig. 15.3). However, the mechanism is uncertain. The drug acts when given orally or intravenously, not by inhalation and its effectiveness is related to the plasma concentration. The action is on mast cells, suppressor T-lymphocytes (CD8+) and as an adenosine antagonist. Theophylline may also increase the contractility of fatigued diaphragm, but the evidence is inconclusive. It appears to act as an anti-inflammatory agent to increase the patency of small airways. Possibly on this account theophylline is widely used to increase the exercise capacity of some patients with COPD; the improvement occurs despite little change in ventilatory capacity [24].

Overview of treatment of airflow limitation. In most instances the immediate cause for acute limitation of airflow is an increase in the tone of bronchial smooth muscle. This is effected by the local parasympathetic nerves in response to stimulation by acetyl choline. It is reversed by inhalation of an aerosol containing an antidote; the most effective choice is usually a substance that activates sympathetic receptors in the airways (β_2 agonist), but an atropine analogue that blocks the muscarinic receptors for acetyl choline (e.g. ipratropium bromide) can also be used. The two classes of drug have different response times and can be used in combination. When the flow limitation is due to asthma the underlying inflammation in small airways is controlled with an anti-inflammatory corticosteroid drug. For recurring flow limitation the short acting bronchodilators can be replaced by longer acting analogues (e.g the β_2 agonists salmeterol or formoterol and the atropine analogue tiotropium). When the underlying cause is asthma a long-acting β_2 agonist can be combined with a corticosteroid drug in one preparation [29]. An anti-leukotriene drug may be of some help. In COPD a long acting atropine analogue can be the medication of first choice [30]. Inhaled corticosteroids, which reduce the frequency of exacerbations, can be tried under close observation, as can other classes of drugs including theophylline (Fig. 15.3, also [31]).

Disease severity as basis for treatment. The majority of patients with potentially reversible airflow limitation respond to one or more of the remedies that are listed in the previous paragraph. The treatments can be prescribed progressively, or the starting point can be selected in the light of clinical experience or from guidelines based on the initial limitation to airflow. The latter is usually graded in terms of forced expiratory volume (FEV_1), FEV/FVC or peak expiratory flow (PEF) [32]. However, use of PEF has disadvantages (Section 12.3.1), so in most circumstances, including in general practice, FEV_1 and FEV% should be used [14, 33]. The level can be the basis for treatment. This has the advantage of being unambiguous, but the guideline may lead to the initial treatment being sub-optimal if the patient's circumstances do not match those on which the algorithm was based. Where the algorithm has claims for universality further difficulties can arise [34, 35].

Administering a drug by inhalation. The objective is to deliver an effective dose to the bronchial epithelium with minimal deposition in the mouth, pharynx or lung parenchyma. This is best done using a monodispersed aerosol (Section 37.2.4), but appropriate dispensers are not widely available. Most patients use metered dose inhalers (MDI) which discharge into the mouth or into a spacer from which the aerosol is inhaled. The spacer, which can come in any of several sizes is a hollow vessel that is in series between the inhaler and the mouth. Its use reduces the need for accurate timing of the discharge from the inhaler and eliminates by sedimentation any large droplets of aerosol that might otherwise give rise to symptoms. Other aerosol dispensers are also used or the material can be delivered as a powder. In all instances the usage should be in accordance with the manufacturer's instructions (e.g. Table 15.3). Alternatively, the material can be inhaled during regular breathing from a nebuliser that is driven by a supply of compressed gas. This should preferably be air. When oxygen is used a watch should be kept for hypoventilation (Section 35.7.2). Nebulisers are popular with patients but expensive and give large doses. An MDI with spacer can deliver an equivalent dose of bronchodilator. Except for acute treatment, a nebuliser should only be used after an assessment based on objective criteria has been carried out.

Many patients coming for assessment will already have inhalers and approximately 30% are likely to use them incorrectly. Hence,

Table 15.3 Some practical aspects of aerosol administration.

To start. Shake dispenser Exhale to residual volume	
For MDI. Insert nozzle into open mouth. Actuate mechanism and concurrently make full inhalation at moderate rate Close mouth. Hold breath for at least 5 s Repeat once after 1 min	*For spacer.* Grip outlet with lips. Actuate mechanism, then make full inhalation at moderate rate

the assessment provides an opportunity to check the patient's technique and to provide retraining. A placebo inhalant can be used during training.

15.7.2 Measurement aspects

What constitutes a bronchodilator response? A decrease in airway calibre can be noticed as tightness of the chest, wheeze or increased breathlessness on exertion. The awareness is greatest if the change occurs rapidly and if the subject's sensory perception is above average. Under controlled conditions an improvement in FEV_1 of as little as 4% can be detected [36], so this increase or the equivalent reduction in symptoms or increase in exercise capacity [37] sets a lower limit to what might be considered a worthwhile improvement. Another limit is that the change should exceed the normal measurement error, which in the case of FEV_1 is of the order of 0.16 or 0.18 l [38, 39]. This is a trivial change for someone with a normal FEV_1 but in percentage terms can be a very large change for someone with a very low FEV_1. However, changes in symptoms are not experienced in absolute units but as proportional deviations from an existing level (Weber–Fechner law [40]), so the target change above a predetermined minimum is best expressed as a percentage. This might be an increase in FEV_1 of 12% of predicted value, as can be used for diagnosis of asthma, or 15%. Where there is little change in FEV_1 the criterion can be a comparable improvement in exercise capacity or other feature identifiable using a quality of life questionnaire (Section 8.2.6). A patient is unlikely to persist with a symptomatic treatment that he or she feels to be ineffective.

An intention to report an improvement as a percentage change raises the question as to how it should be expressed. For two determinations of FEV_1 before and after bronchodilator (x_1 and x_2, respectively), the usual format would be:

$$100(x_2 - x_1)/x_1 \qquad (15.1)$$

but this model in which the reference is to the initial level, has a poor reproducibility [41, 42]. The scatter is due to regression to the mean and can be avoided by relating the change due to the treatment not to the initial but to the mean level (see Section 5.4.2), hence:

$$100(x_2 - x_1)/0.5(x_2 + x_1) \qquad (15.2)$$

Unfortunately, this model is seldom used. Alternative denominators that have been suggested are the reference value for FEV_1 and either the maximal possible improvement in FEV_1 ($x_{pred} - x_1$) or the maximal attainable improvement ($x_{2,\max obs} - x_1$) [40, 41]. Results expressed in this form are an improvement on eqn 15.1, but do not meet the requirement of proportionality encapsulated in the Weber–Fechner law.

In addition, all these models describe the response in terms of a peak effect (possibly qualified by time from administration) but neglect the duration. The latter can be incorporated in the result by making serial measurements, then constructing a response–time curve and measuring the area under the curve. Alternatively, the curve should be represented mathematically and the overall result described by the parameters (coefficients) of the resulting equation [43]. This appears not to have been achieved in practice.

Assessment of individual patients

A routine assessment in a patient is usually performed by making measurements of FEV_1 before and after inhalation of an appropriate aerosol; this is usually a short acting β_2 adrenergic or anticholinergic drug (Section 15.7.1). The subject should not have used his or her inhaler and preferably not smoked a cigarette during the 4 h before the test. Where the assessment is for any evidence of reversibility of airflow limitation, the period of abstinence should reflect the time to nearly full response of all the drugs that the patient is receiving (e.g. 15–30 min or 9 h). Excitement or strenuous exercise are best avoided. The result is greatly influenced by the quality of the measurements, so these should be made in an unhurried manner by a recommended method.

Establishing a baseline. A positive result to a single test of bronchodilatation is usually an indication to start treatment, but this need not be so [44] and a negative response does not exclude this possibility. Greater certainty is achieved by first making base-line measurements over a few days then assessing the response to the drug at more than one time of day. When this is done the time between treatments should be at least 4 h.

Serial measurements. Serial measurements (e.g. Fig. 15.3) are essential when the bronchial tone is labile or the response is not immediate or uncertain, when the drug can cause euphoria and when the administration is prophylactic. For example, to assess the benefit from steroid drugs the assessment might be performed twice daily for three periods of 7 to 14 days with the drug administered during the second period only. In the case of prednisolone the dose might be 0.6 mg/kg daily for at least 14 days [45]. An assessment of at least over two weeks is required to test the effect of inhaled corticosteroids and can also then test whether the drug has helped to prevent bronchoconstriction in response to provocation with a specific antigen (Section 15.8.5).

Assessment involving groups of subjects

For a clinical trial that compares two drugs on a group of subjects the study design should be overseen by a statistician [46, 47]. The protocol should specify the class of patient, the state of health and the smoking status at the time of study. The airway calibre and amount of resting bronchomotor tone should be similar at the start of each period of treatment. The response should include the magnitude and the duration of bronchodilatation. This can be done by adjusting the doses so that both drugs produce the same initial response, then recording the subsequent amplitude and duration by serial measurements [48]. The measurements should be continued until the response has returned to its control level. Interpretation of the result should take account of circadian variation (Section 25.6). Where the trial is of a clinical nature, criteria involving symptoms and exercise tolerance should be included in addition to spirometry [49].

15.8 Bronchial hyper-responsiveness

15.8.1 Underlying considerations

Definitions. Airway *hyper-responsiveness* indicates that there is an increased tendency of the bronchi to constrict in response to stimulation. The term is a general one and has two notable components. The *sensitivity* of the airways indicates the threshold concentration of histamine or other substance that is required to initiate bronchoconstriction. In hyper-responsive subjects the threshold is diminished. The *reactivity* of the airways describes the change in airway calibre effected by a given increase in strength of the provoking stimulus (dose–response relationship). These features are apparent to variable extents in charts illustrating the response to inhalation challenge (Fig. 15.4 and Fig. 15.5). The *maximal response* is the plateau value seen in the dose–response relationship of most persons with healthy lungs. A plateau is uncommon in atopic individuals and seldom occurs in persons with asthma (see Fig. 15.5, also Tone of airway smooth muscle, Section 15.1). Where a plateau is achieved it is greater for histamine than for methacholine and if obtained with histamine is not affected by the additional presence of methacholine [51].

Biological variability. People differ in the responsiveness of their bronchial smooth muscle to agents that cause bronchoconstriction. The most important factor is atopic status; this dimension of a person's constitution and the method by which it is usually assessed are given in Section 15.3. Some 20% of most western

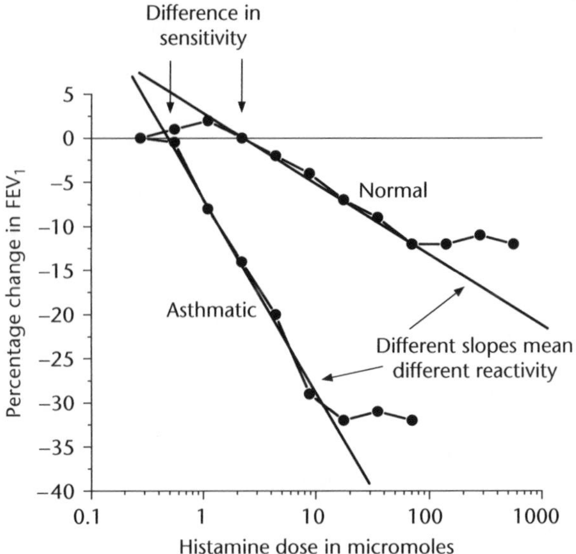

Fig. 15.4 Change in FEV_1 with increasing dose of histamine in two individuals. In the normal subject the FEV_1 did not start to fall until a dose of 4 μmol whereas in the patient with mild asthma the fall began at 1 μmol (a difference of sensitivity). The rate of drop in FEV_1 per unit dose was steeper in the asthmatic and so the asthmatic was more reactive.

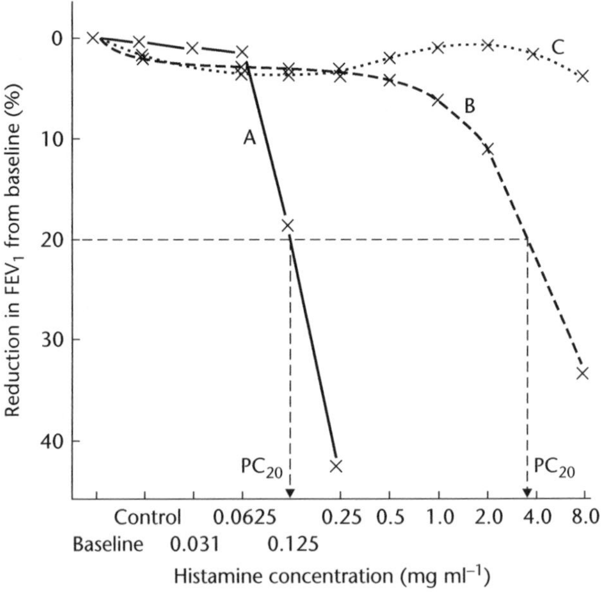

Fig. 15.5 Testing for bronchial hyper-reactivity in subjects suspected of having asthma. The FEV_1 was normal between attacks. The subjects inhaled saline and then graded doses of histamine solution from a Wright nebuliser for 2 min with 3 min intervals in between. Measurements of forced expiratory volume were made every 0.5 min. Subject A showed marked hyper-reactivity; subject B was moderately reactive; subject C did not react to histamine in the dosage used. The small reduction in FEV_1 occurring after the control inhalation of saline was probably physiological. Had the reduction been bigger the test would have had to be postponed as the challenge result could not have been interpreted satisfactorily. Source: [50].

Table 15.4 Aspects of respiratory sensitisation.

Aspect	Procedure for assessment (including outcome)	Comment
Atopy	Skin prick test weal diam >2mm Serum IgE >350 μg/ml	Responders at increased risk of sensitisation to some occupational allergens
Bronchial hyper-responsiveness	Non-specific bronchial challenge (histamine, methacholine, exercise, cold air)	Often accompanies occupational asthma
Temporal variation in PEF	Morning dip pattern (Fig. 15.6). Decline over working day or working week (Figs 15.7 and 8)	Measurements should extend over weekends and holidays
Asthma or alveolitis	Inhalation challenge test (Fig. 15.8) Radio allergosorbent (RAS) test	Can be confirmatory Carries small risk of sensitisation Identifies specific IgE in serum

populations are atopic [10]. Such persons have an increased sensitivity to some stimuli, e.g. to cold air (Sections 36.2 and 36.3). They readily become sensitised to antigenic dusts that cause extrinsic asthma, including occupational asthma (Section 37.7.6). Other than atopy, the susceptibility to bronchoconstriction is influenced by previous exposures to irritant or antigenic particles, inflammatory changes in the airways (such as occur with extrinsic allergic alveolitis), pulmonary congestion and possibly other factors. An increased response can be specific to one substance (e.g. an agent that causes occupational asthma), it can reflect interaction between stimuli (e.g. an allergen and oxides of nitrogen, Section 37.4.4) or be non-specific such that any constrictor stimulus can elicit an exaggerated response. Non-specific bronchial hyper-responsiveness also occurs in approximately 5% of persons who in other respects appear to have completely healthy lungs. Hyper-responders can be said to have 'twitchy' airways. Some aspects of respiratory sensitisation are indicated in Table 15.4.

The presence of sensitisation to a single substance is assessed by specific *bronchial challenge.* This entails the subject inhaling the relevant aerosol under controlled conditions. In other circumstances the assessment is of bronchial hyper-responsiveness to inhaled methacholine, histamine or other provoking agent. The extent of spontaneous variability in peak expiratory flow is not an adequate substitute [52].

15.8.2 Non-specific bronchial challenge

Indications. Non-specific bronchial challenge can be used as a screening test in epidemiology or occupational medicine. It can be a diagnostic tool for assessment of a patient whose medical features are consistent with asthma but in whom the response to bronchodilator therapy appears not to be compatible with that diagnosis. In this circumstance a negative response argues against asthma. A positive response can be confirmatory, but only when it is pronounced. The test is also used to confirm the effectiveness of prophylactic treatment with inhaled corticosteroids or other drug.

Contra-indications, precaution and side effects. A non-specific challenge test is normally considered safe when carried out according to a recommended protocol, provided the subject is not pregnant and does not have moderately severe asthma or another condition that might affect the outcome. (Table 15.5).

The procedure is considered to be safe when carried out according to the recommendations; these include the deployment

Table 15.5 Medical contra-indications to non-specific bronchial challenge testing.

Condition	Contra-indication Absolute	Relative
Asthma	FEV_1 < 50% predicted or < 1 l or 1.2 l*	FEV_1 <60% predicted or <1.5 l in men, 1.2 l in women
Other	Myocardial infarction or stroke in last 3 months Aortic aneurysm BP > 200/100 mm Hg Pregnancy	Nursing mother On cholinesterase inhibitor, e.g. for myasthenia gravis Epilepsy requiring treatment Upper respiratory tract infection in last 2 weeks

* Respectively from ATS and ERS guidelines. Sources: [53, 54, 55].

of trained personnel, and having medication for bronchospasm and equipment for resuscitation immediately available. After the test up to 25% of subjects may experience some chest tightness, cough or other symptom. The symptoms are usually mild and of short duration. They are probably less frequent after methacholine than after histamine. However, histamine is possibly safer as the induced bronchoconstriction appears to be more easily reversed by salbutamol. Staff may also be affected [56] and in order to protect them and prevent premature bronchoconstriction in patients the room should have good ventilation and contamination of the air should be minimised by use of a low resistance filter on the exhalation port from the equipment [53]. Reactive persons should not administer the test.

The results are influenced by the prevailing level of bronchomotor tone, the drug and the method of delivery that are used, the method of detecting bronchoconstriction and the index that is employed. These features should be standardised and taken into account when interpreting the findings [57]. Most laboratories follow the recommendation of ATS in administering methacholine and monitoring the response by spirometry [53].

Practical details. Monitoring the response is usually in terms of FEV_1. However, the index has the disadvantage that the full inspiration can elicit bronchodilatation (see below Problems with the measurement). Thus, for maximal accuracy airway conductance ($sGaw$) or total thoracic resistance ($Rtot$) [19] should be used instead. The last of these procedures is suitable for young children.

The reasons for performing the test, the condition of the subject, the safety precautions and related matters should conform to the conventions listed above. The subject should not currently be in receipt of bronchodilator therapy or be recovering from or have a viral infection. The initial FEV_1 should normally be greater than 70% of the reference value [54]. Smoking and drinks containing caffeine are best avoided during the 4 h prior to the test. Test solutions in appropriate concentrations made up in 0.9% saline (Table 15.6) should be at hand. They should be administered by inhalation, either for 2 min from a Wright nebuliser (5 ml of solution nebulised at a flow 8 l min^{-1}), five vital capacity breaths from a demand nebuliser (e.g. De Vilbiss) or five tidal breaths from a dosimeter. The drug delivery system should preferably have been calibrated in order that the results can be comparable between laboratories [57]. Further details and examples of the outcomes are shown in Figs 15.4 and 15.5.

To undertake the test a base line measurement is made in duplicate using the chosen index (usually FEV_1). The *lowest* of the chosen concentrations of methacholine (or histamine) is then administered as the *first* provoking dose. After 30 s and again after 90 s from the completion of the inhalation the physiological measurement is repeated; usually a single determination is sufficient but depending on its quality up to two repeats are permissible; in the case of FEV_1 the higher should be reported [53]. The next lowest concentration of aerosol is then administered

Table 15.6 Methacholine dosing schedule for 2-min tidal breathing method. Using the full procedure the first challenge is at level J (see also Short procedures below).

Designation	Dose (mg ml^{-1})*	Dilution
A	16	100 mg MetaCholine Chloride +6.25 ml 0.9% saline
B	8	50% of above
C	4	50% of above
D	2	50% of above
E	1.0	50% of above
F	0.5	50% of above
G	0.25	50% of above
H	0.125	50% of above
I	0.0625	50% of above
J	0.031	50% of above

* Interpretation of PC_{20}(expressed as dose of methacholine, mg ml^{-1}):
>16 normal bronchial reactivity;
4–16 borderline hyper-reactivity;
1–4 mild hyperactivity (positive test);
<1 moderate to severe hyperactivity.
Source: [53].

and this sequence is repeated until an endpoint is reached. The intervals between inhalations should not exceed 5 min. At the end of the test any airflow limitation is reversed with salbutamol or other β_2 stimulant drug.

The endpoint is when a 20% reduction in baseline FEV_1 or 35% reduction in sGaw has been achieved, or the maximal agreed concentration of aerosol has been administered. The endpoints are obtained by interpolation of a semi-log plot of FEV_1 or $sGaw$ on aerosol concentration or dose (Fig. 15.5). The result is in terms of either the last provoking concentration to be administered (PC_{20}, FEV_1 or PC_{35},$sGaw$), or the cumulative dose up to this point (PD_{20},FEV_1 or PD_{35},$sGaw$). If one subject is to be tested the procedure takes up to 1 h.

Short procedures and adaptations for respiratory surveys. The procedure can be shortened by using a lower end point (e.g. a 10% reduction in FEV_1), by leaving out alternate test concentrations or by omitting the lower test doses. The first two measures considerably reduce the sensitivity of the test, whilst the third can be hazardous in reactive subjects. In respiratory surveys, where a subject's answers to questions indicate they are unlikely to react, a higher starting dose can be administered. The procedure can also be shortened by monitoring the specific conductance instead of the forced expiratory volume.

Where a subject's FEV_1 fails to drop by 20% the test does not provide a quantitative score suitable for statistical analysis. This difficulty can be overcome by deriving an index of response using the slope of the relationship of the percentage reduction of FEV_1 on the final cumulative dose of the drug. This is called the log dose slope [59] and is calculated from

$$\text{LDSFEV}_1 = \log_{10}((\%\text{ change in FEV}_1)/(\text{total cumulative dose}) + 1) \tag{15.3}$$

Its use is recommended for population studies where estimates of bronchial hyper-responsiveness are required [60].

Interpretation. When the response is to methacholine, a PC_{20} FEV_1 of 16 mg ml^{-1} is normal and excludes a diagnosis of asthma, whilst a PC_{20} of 1 mg ml^{-1} or less on first assessment can be taken as evidence for the condition. However, with methacholine the effect can be cumulative, so a second test within 24 h of the first can yield a false positive result. Interpretations of intermediate results are given in Table 15.6. A false positive result can also be obtained when airway calibre is assessed by a method that does not entail full inspiration (see below). The sensitivity and specificity of the method have been reported [53, 54, 61].

Problem with the measurement. A bronchoconstrictor response to methacholine is not specific to persons who are atopic or have asthma. It can also occur but to a lesser extent in healthy subjects. This response is reduced if the challenge is repeated within 6 h [62]. It is apparent when monitoring is by measurement of airways conductance (PC_{35},s*G*aw) or when the forced oscillation method is used. An unambiguous result is also likely when the response is monitored using measurement of trans-cutaneous oxygen tension [53]. However, using FEV_1, the inspiration to total lung capacity initiates a bronchodilator reflex (Section 12.5.1). This can sometimes reverse the small degree of bronchoconstriction found in subjects who are not hyper-responsive. In this event the FEV_1 is unchanged and the response is negative [63]. In hyper-responsive subjects the constrictor stimulus is the stronger of the two and so FEV_1 falls, yielding a positive result [64]. Thus, the outcome of the test reflects a balance of forces and may not always be as conclusive as was thought to be at one time.

15.8.3 Exercise-induced airflow limitation

Background. Exercise can induce bronchoconstriction in persons with reactive airways and raised bronchomotor tone [54]. In such persons the cooling and drying of the airway epithelium that results from exercise can stimulate the release from mast cells of endogenous histamine, cysteinyl leukotrienes and other inflammatory mediators. A similar response can occur as a result of breathing cold air and the two effects summate. Hence, in the UK a typical initial manifestation of the condition is when the subject hurries out of the house on the first frosty morning of winter. However, in a hot dry environment, exercise leading to dehydration of the airways can cause bronchoconstriction in the absence of cooling. Thus, the two effects can occur independently.

Exercise-induced bronchoconstriction (EIB) is also called exercise-induced asthma (EIA). It is provoked by and develops shortly after a few minutes of near-maximal exercise of rapid onset. A period of warm up can provide protection and the obstruction can wear off if the exercise is prolonged [53]. A positive response is followed by a refractory period lasting up to 4 h [65]. These features need to be taken into account if a valid result is to be obtained.

Indications/contraindications. The usual application is to validate a diagnosis of EIB in a person with symptoms suggestive of the condition but who has a normal FEV_1. The test is also used to confirm the effectiveness of corticosteroid therapy. In children the test can be used to confirm a diagnosis of asthma [66] and as a method in epidemiological studies (Section 8.2.5). The contraindications include both those given in Table 15.5 and others that are specific to exercise, for example unstable cardiac arrhythmia, some arrhythmias and material hypertension (Table 29.3, page 421).

Procedure. Susceptibility to EIB is assessed by measurement of FEV_1 6 min before and 6 min after a period of moderately heavy exercise of duration 6–8 min. The FEV_1 should fall by at least 10% and be restored by a subsequent inhalation of salbutamol. Running, cycling or stepping exercise can be used, but not swimming as that exercise provides a less powerful constrictor stimulus [67]. On this account swimming is often a suitable recreation for persons with asthma.

Practical details. The medical condition of the subject and the facilities in the exercise laboratory should conform to the normal practices for exercise testing (Chapter 29). However, in the case of children who are reasonably active there is only need for a space where they can run or jump; a laboratory is not necessary [68]. The ambient temperature and relative humidity of the air should be on the low side of normal. If practicable the respired gas should have been dried or delivered from a source of compressed air. The subject should breathe through the mouth and wear a nose clip. No prior bronchodilator therapy and preferably no drink containing caffeine should have been taken on the day of the test. The FEV_1 should be measured prior to exercise. This should be of sufficient intensity to raise the exercise ventilation and cardiac frequency, respectively, to approximately 60% and 80% of the predicted maximum (e.g. Section 28.8.3). The appropriate level of exercise should be achieved within a time of 4 min; it should be maintained for 4 min (or 6 min if the onset is abrupt as when performing shuttle running). The total duration of exercise should be 6–8 min. The spirometry is repeated 6 min after the end of exercise.

Comment. The reproducibility of the reduction in FEV_1 for tests repeated within 4 weeks is of the order of 20%. The procedure is well tolerated by children and physically active adults.

15.8.4 Cold air provocation test

This test is usually performed at rest and does not entail pharmacologically active substances. In addition, when the response is monitored by the forced oscillation (impedance) method there is no need for the subject to perform respiratory gymnastics. Hence, the procedure is particularly suitable for elderly subjects and young children [69, 70]. The provoking agent is air which is cooled to –10°C by passage through a coil surrounded by a refrigerated sheath or a bucket of ice and salt. The subject breathes the air through the mouth for up to 10 min taking deep rapid breaths and hypocapnia is avoided by using a mouthpiece with a large deadspace or by providing 2% carbon dioxide as the respired gas. Other aspects of the procedure are as for exercise induced airflow limitation including the contraindications, the end-point and the refractory period [53, 54].

Fog produced by nebulising water [71, 72], or nebulised hypertonic agents such as mannitol [73] can also be used to test for bronchial hyper-responsiveness.

15.8.5 Specific bronchial challenge testing

Introduction

Bronchial challenge testing is used to establish whether or not a person's asthma or other symptoms are caused by sensitisation to a particular substance to which he or she has been exposed [74]. The exposure usually arises at work and the information can help to secure long-term respiratory health and/or financial compensation. The procedure is not without risk so, except when the context is a medical one, the case for obtaining the information should be reviewed impartially before the test is performed. The review is likely to include the results of other tests, e.g. some of those listed in Table 15.4.

Temporal variation

This can take the form of variation either between morning and evening (*circadian variation*) or over a working shift or working week. The presence of circadian variation is evidence for non-specific bronchial hyper-responsiveness, such as can occur with asthma, but not usually with COPD (e.g. Fig. 15.6). The information is obtained by having the patient record his or her peak expiratory flow (PEF) every 4 h except during sleep.

Variation in PEF over a shift or working week. This can be used to investigate a possible occupational cause for wheeze or other symptom. The procedure is of greatest use if the occupational exposure is of low intensity, for example as a result of inadequate occupational hygiene measures or if the asthmatic response is of the delayed onset type (e.g. Fig. 37.11, page 520). Occupational asthma of immediate onset is usually diagnosed by the patient.

Positive findings are likely to include (a) decline in PEF over a shift, (b) progressive deterioration over consecutive days at work, hence usually over the working week, (c) recovery during any period away from work, for example at week ends or after a holiday. The information is best obtained by the subject measuring the PEF every 2 h whilst at work, starting before entering the work place. However, measurements 4 times daily are nearly as good. Morning and evening measurements provide insufficient information [76]. The duration of measurements should be a minimum of 5 consecutive days, but usually the effects of breaks and a holiday should be included as well. The data points are displayed as graphs (Fig. 15.7); these are best interpreted by an experienced or trained observer or using a computer programme

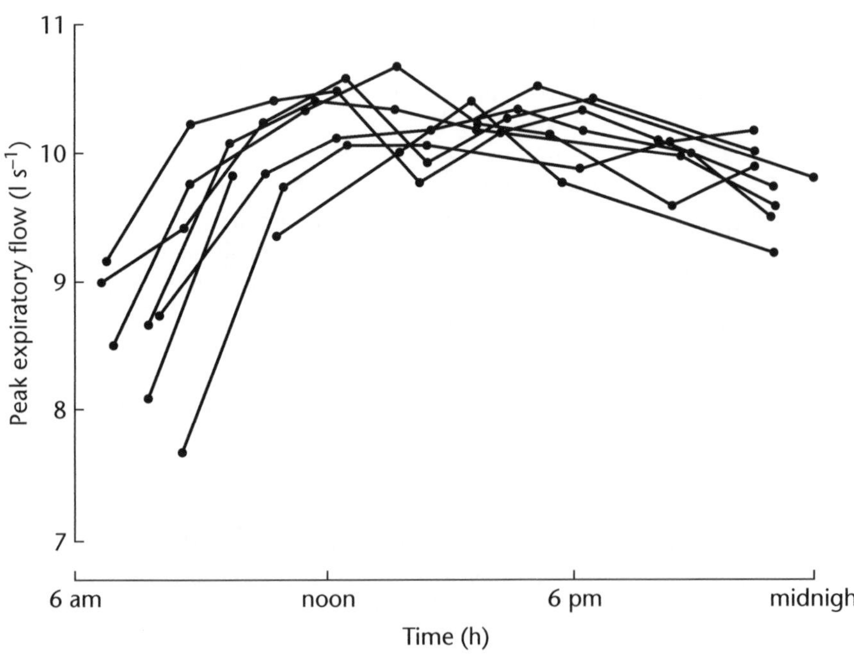

Fig. 15.6 Circadian measurements of peak expiratory flow rate in a pigeon fancier (precipitin positive) with exercise induced airflow limitation. There was a morning dip pattern which was reproducible from day to day. The morning dip was *not* reduced following 2 weeks away from pigeons; hence the airflow limitation was unlikely to have been related to that exposure. Source: [75].

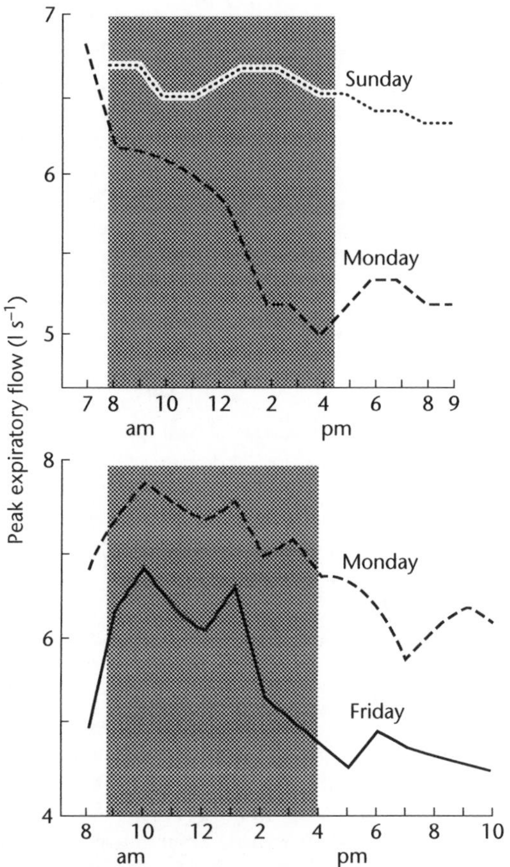

Fig. 15.7 Circadian values for peak expiratory flow in two electrical workers who became sensitised to colophony. The upper record shows progressive airways obstruction developing throughout the first working day after a rest day. The lower record shows further deterioration over subsequent days. Source: [77]

[78]. Investigators need to be alert to the possibility of subjects falsely recording their data [79] and so data logging meters are preferred for this form of testing.

Challenge with specific substances

Risks and benefits. During normal work any exposure to a specific antigen is usually mild, sensitisation builds up gradually and there is advance warning of possible future difficulties. The threat to health can be increased by failure of hygiene measures or if the exposure is unexpectedly increased by an incautious challenge, a spillage or other accident at work, or if an unfamiliar task is performed without due preparation. Any of these circumstances can threaten life.

Challenge away from the work place carries a particular risk when there is only minimal information on the susceptibility to the antigen of the person under test. Thus, challenge should be undertaken only if there is good reason for doing so. This might be (a) diagnosis or attribution in a person who is no longer exposed, (b) identification of a sensitising antigen from a mixture or (c) investigation of what appears to be a previously unidentified agent.

A positive challenge test is sometimes followed by nocturnal airway obstruction. This can be expected to respond to therapy and, in the absence of further occupational exposure, rarely lasts more than 2–3 days [74]. During this time there may be increased diurnal variation in airway calibre with a morning dip pattern. Its occurrence is further evidence for sensitisation to the substance being tested.

A person administering a challenge test is unlikely to be at risk since sensitisation appears not to develop as a result of a single exposure. However, technicians who administer the test frequently should be protected [56].

Preparations. The test is undertaken when the patient is in a stable state with no material airflow obstruction (e.g. $FEV_1 > 80\%$ predicted when off treatment) and not within a week of previous exposure to the suspected antigen or to histamine. The subject should not be taking bronchoactive drugs at the time. Challenge can be carried out either using graded doses from a dosimeter or in a manner that mimics exposure at work such as painting, welding, soldering, sifting or mixing. The manoeuvre should be performed within the hospital complex in a booth or small chamber ventilated to outside air. Full safety precautions should be available, including nebulised and intravenous bronchodilator drugs, intravenous hydrocortisone, oxygen and facilities for respiratory and cardiac resuscitation. The inhaled concentration of test substance should not exceed the hygiene standard and should be less than that experienced at work.

If the suspected allergen is soluble in water, the challenge can be undertaken using a nebulised aerosol. This should be prepared as a 10% weight-for-volume suspension in phosphate buffered saline. The suspension is agitated for 24 h at 4°C, filtered, dialysed against phosphate buffered saline, freeze-dried, resuspended at an appropriate concentration (which might be in the range 0.01–10 mg ml^{-1}) and sterilized using a multipore filter. The concentration for inhalation should initially be less than that which causes a positive intradermal reaction (Section 15.3).

Which measurements? When an immediate response to challenge is expected, this will involve the larger airways, so either the airway conductance or FEV_1 or peak expiratory flow should be monitored (e.g. Section 12.3.1). A delayed response can affect all classes of airway, or be confined to small ones. On this account the assessment should be based on a full forced expiration from which FEV_1 and flows at small lung volumes can be derived. Use of a constant pressure plethysmograph is recommended as an allowance can then be made for dynamic compression (Section 12.5.1). A late response is often accompanied by fever, leucocytosis, a fall in transfer factor and radiographic infiltrates. Thus, there is a case for monitoring some of these aspects as well.

The measurements of lung function are usually made throughout the day, initially at 5 min intervals and subsequently every hour. On day 1 the subject is instructed in the procedure and control measurements are made. On day 2, and if necessary on subsequent days, graded exposures are given and later these are repeated using a refined extract or after administration of

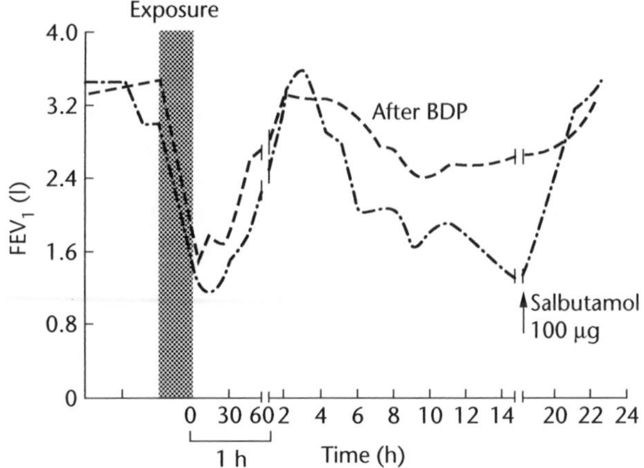

Fig. 15.8 Dual response of forced expiratory volume (FEV_1) to challenge with rye flour in a baker. The delayed but not the immediate asthmatic reaction was largely prevented by pre-treatment with beclomethasone diproprionate (BDP) but not by placebo treatment (not shown). Source: [80]

inhaled corticosteroid or other protective agent. Thus, in a study of the effects of colophony (pine resin) [77] Burge, Pepys and colleagues initially had their subjects inhale one natural breath of soldering fume, followed by three and six breaths at 15 min intervals if no reaction had occurred by then. On four subsequent days if no reaction had occurred the subjects breathed fumes on three occasions for 1 and 2 min, 5 min, 20 min and 60 min, with the subject reapplying the heated iron to the solder every 30 s throughout the exposure. In the case of an uncomplicated immediate response the measurements can be discontinued or made infrequently once the flow rate has returned to the initial value. If a delayed response is suspected the measurements should be continued into the following day. The results of the challenge tests are analysed graphically (Fig. 15.8) or used to construct a dose–response relationship; an immediate response is related to the logarithm of the dose but a late response may not be quantifiable and in this circumstance can be reported as present or absent. It can also be expressed in terms of a summary measurement, for example the mean peak expiratory flow for the 12 h following challenge or the average under the flow–time curve.

15.9 References

1. Seow CY, Fredberg JJ. Signal transduction in smooth muscle. Historical perspective on airway smooth muscle: the saga of a frustrated cell. *J Appl Physiol* 2001; **91**: 938–952.
2. Pendry YD. Neuronal control of airways smooth muscle. *Pharmacol Ther* 1993; **57**: 171–202.
3. Barnes PJ. Neural control of human airways in health and disease *Am Rev Respir Dis* 1986; **134**: 1289–1314
4. Libby DM, Briscoe WA, King TKC. Relief of hypoxia-related bronchoconstriction by breathing 30 per cent oxygen. *Am Rev Respir Dis* 1981; **123**: 171–175.
5. Dagg KD, Thomson LJ, Clayton RA et al. Effect of acute alterations in inspired oxygen tension on methacholine induced bronchoconstriction in patients with asthma. *Thorax* 1997; **52**: 453–457.
6. Sterling GM. Pharmacology of bronchoconstriction. *Bull Physiopathol Respir* (Nancy) 1972; **8**: 491–501.
7. Lai YL, Lee CF. Mediators and oxygen radicals in hyperpnea-induced airway constriction of guinea pigs. *Lung* 2000; **178**: 213–223.
8. Koppelman GH, Postma DS. The genetics of CD14 in allergic disease. *Curr Opin Allergy Clin Immunol* 2003; **3**: 347–352.
9. Jackola DR, Blumenthal MN, Rosenberg A. Evidence for two independent distributions of serum immunoglobulin E in atopic families: cognate and non-cognate IgE. *Hum Immunol* 2004; **65**: 20–30.
10. Williams HC. Is the prevalence of atopy increasing? *Clin Exp Dermatol* 1992; **17**: 385–391.
11. Amrani Y, Panettieri RA. Airway smooth muscle: contraction and beyond. *Int J Biochem Cell Biol* 2003; **35**: 272–276.
12. Fredberg JJ. Airway obstruction in asthma: does the response to a deep inspiration matter? *Respir Res* 2001; **2**: 273–275.
13. Sutherland ER, Martin RJ. Airway inflammation in chronic obstructive pulmonary disease: comparison with asthma. *J Allergy Clin Immunol* 2003; **112**: 819–827.
14. Silva GE, Sherrill DL, Guerra S, Barbee RA. Asthma as a risk factor for COPD in a longitudinal study. *Chest* 2004; **126**: 59–65.
15. Pauwels RA, Buist AS, Calverley PMA et al. Global strategy for the diagnosis, management, and prevention of chronic obstructive pulmonary disease: NHLBI/WHO global initiative for chronic obstructive lung disease (GOLD) workshop summary. *Am J Respir Crit Care Med* 2001; **163**: 1256–1276.
16. Brand PL, Quanjer PH, Postma DS et al. Interpretation of bronchodilator response in patients with obstructive airways disease. *Thorax* 1992; **47**: 429–436.
17. Calverley PM, Burge PS, Spencer S et al. Bronchodilator reversibility testing in chronic obstructive pulmonary disease. *Thorax* 2003; **58**: 659–664.
18. Godfrey S, Uwyyed K, Springer C, Avital A. Is clinical wheezing reliable as the endpoint for bronchial challenges in preschool children? *Pediatr Pulmonol* 2004; **37**: 193–200.
19. Delacourt C, Lorino H, Fuhrman C et al. Comparison of the forced oscillation technique and the interrupter technique for assessing airway obstruction and its reversibility in children. *Am J Respir Crit Care Med* 2001; **164**: 965–972.
20. Gayrard P, Orehek J, Grimaud C, Charpin J. Bronchoconstrictor effects of a deep inspiration in patients with asthma. *Am Rev Respir Dis* 1975; **111**: 433–439.
21. Pearce SJ cited in Cotes JE, Steel J. *Work-related lung disorders.* Oxford: Blackwell Scientific Publications, 1987: 408.
22. Afschrift M, Clement J, Peeters R, van de Woestijne KP. Maximal expiratory and inspiratory flows in patients with chronic obstructive pulmonary disease. Influence of bronchodilation. *Am Rev Respir Dis* 1969; **100**: 147–152.
23. Swinburn CR, Wakefield JM, Jones PW. Clinical improvement after treatment with prednisolone in chronic airways obstruction in absence of change in lung function. *Lancet* 1986; **1**(8475): 276.
24. Murciano D, Avclair M-H, Pariente R, Aubier M. A randomized controlled trial of theophylline in patients with severe chronic obstructive pulmonary disease. *N Engl J Med* 1989; **320**: 1521–1525.
25. Paggiaro PL, Dahle R, Bakran I et al. Multicentre randomised placebo controlled trial of inhaled fluticasone propionate in patients

with chronic obstructive pulmonary disease. International COPD Study Group. *Lancet* 1998; **351**: 773–780.

26. Barnes PJ. Bronchodilators: basic pharmacology. In: Calverley P, Pride N, eds. *Chronic obstructive pulmonary disease.* London: Chapman and Hall, 1995: 391–417.
27. Abramson MJ, Walters J, Walters EH. Adverse effects of beta-agonists: are they clinically relevant? *Am J Respir Med* 2003; **2**: 287–297.
28. MacNee W, Douglas NJ, Sudlow MF. Effects of inhalation of beta-sympathomimetic and atropine-like drugs on airway calibre in normal subjects. *Clin Sci* 1982; **63**: 137–143.
29. Barnes PJ. Scientific rationale for inhaled combination therapy with long-acting B2-agonists and corticosteroids. *Eur Respir J* 2002; **19**: 182–191.
30. Tashkin DP, Cooper CB. The role of long-acting bronchodilators in the management of stable COPD. *Chest* 2004; **125**: 249–259.
31. Barnes PJ. Theophylline: new perspectives for an old drug. *Am J Respir Crit Care Med* 2003; **167**: 813–818.
32. Randolph C. A review of asthma care guidelines in the United States. *Minerva Pediatr* 2003; **55**: 297–301.
33. Scottish Intercollegiate Network and British Thoracic Society. British guidelines on the management of asthma. 2003
34. Tsoumakidou M, Tzanakis N, Voulgarakaki O et al. Is there any correlation between the ATS, BTS, ERS and GOLD COPD's severity scales and the frequency of hospital admissions? *Respir Med* 2004; **98**: 178–183.
35. Celli BR, Halbert RJ, Isonaka S, Schau B. Population impact of different definitions of airway obstruction. *Eur Respir J* 2003; **22**: 268-273.
36. Redelmeier DA, Goldstein RS, Min ST, Hyland RH. Spirometry and dyspnea in patients with COPD. When small differences mean little. *Chest* 1996; **109**: 1163–1168.
37. Redelmeier DA, Bayoumi AM, Goldstein RS, Guyatt GH. Interpreting small differences in functional status: the six minute walk test in chronic lung disease patients. *Am J Respir Crit Care Med* 1997; **155**:1278–1282.
38. Tweeddale PM, Alexander F, McHardy GJR. Short term variability in FEV_1 and bronchodilator responsiveness in patients with obstructive ventilatory defects. *Thorax* 1987; **42**: 487–490.
39. Sourk RL, Nugent KM. Bronchodilator testing: confidence intervals derived from placebo inhalations. *Am Rev Respir Dis* 1983; **128**: 153–157.
40. Dehaene S. The neural basis of the Weber–Fechner law: a logarithmic mental number line. *Trends Cogn Sci* 2003; **7**: 147–147.
41. Dompeling E, van Schayck CP, Molema J et al. A comparison of six different ways of expressing the bronchodilator response in asthma and COPD; reproducibility and dependence of prebronchodilator FEV_1. *Eur Respir J* 1992; **5**: 975–981.
42. Waalkens HJ, Merkus PJFM, van Essen-Zandvliet EEM, et al. Dutch CNSLD Study Group. Assessment of bronchodilator response in children with asthma. *Eur Respir J* 1993; **6**: 645–651.
43. Oldham PD, Hughes DT. Analysis of the results of bronchodilator trials. *Bull Physiopathol Respir* 1972; **8**:693–699.
44. Guyatt GH, Townsend M, Nogradi S et al Acute response to bronchodilator: an imperfect guide to bronchodilator therapy in chronic airflow limitation. *Arch Intern Med* 1988; **148**: 1949–1952.
45. Webb JR. Dose response of patients to oral corticosteroid treatment during exacerbations of asthma. *Br Med J* 1986; **292**: 1047–1047.
46. Chinn S. Comparing and combining studies of bronchial responsiveness. *Thorax* 2002; **57**: 393–395.
47. Matthews JNS, Altman DG, Campbell MJ, Royston P. Analysis of serial measurements in medical research. *Br Med J* 1990; **300**: 230–235.
48. Freedman BJ. Principles of comparative drug trials with special reference to bronchodilators. In: Burley DM, Clarke SW, Cuthbert MF et al, eds. *Evaluation of bronchodilator drugs. Proceedings of an Asthma Research Council Symposium*, London, 1973. Trust for Education and Research in Therapeutics 1974.
49. van Schayck CP. Is lung function really a good parameter in evaluating the long-term effects of inhaled corticosteroids in COPD? *Eur Respir J* 2000; **15**: 238–239.
50. Keaney NP, King B. In Cotes JE, Steel J, eds. *Work-related lung disorders.* Oxford: Blackwell Scientific Publications, 1987: 357.
51. Sterk PJ, Timmers MC, Bel EH, Dijkman JH. The combined effects of histamine and methacholine on the maximal degree of airway narrowing in normal persons *in vivo. Eur Respir J* 1988; **1**: 34–40.
52. Douma WR, Kerstjens HAM, Roos CM et al. Changes in peak expiratory flow indices as a proxy for changes in bronchial hyerresponsiveness. *Eur Respir J* 2000; **16**: 220–225.
53. ATS. Guidelines for metacholine and exercise challenge testing – 1999. *Am J Respir Crit Care Med* 2000; **161**: 309–329.
54. Sterk PJ, Fabbri LM, Quanjer PhH et al. Airway responsiveness: standardized challenge testing with pharmacological, physical and sensitizing stimuli in adults. *Eur Respir J* 1993; **6**(Suppl 16): 53–83.
55. Joos GF, O'Connor B, Anderson SD et al. Indirect airway challenges. *Eur Respir J* 2003; **21**: 1050–1068.
56. Lundgren R, Soderberg M, Rosenhall L, Norrman E. Development of increased airway responsiveness in two nurses performing methacholine and histamine challenge tests. *Allergy* 1992; **47**: 188–189.
57. Ownby DR, Peterson EL, Johnson CC. Factors related to methylcholine airway responsiveness in children *Am J Respir Crit Care Med* 2000; **161**: 1578–1583.
58. Hartley-Sharpe CJ, Booth H, Johns DP, Walters EH. Differences in aerosol output and airways responsiveness between the DeVilbiss 40 and 45 hand held nebulisers. *Thorax* 1995; **50**: 635–638.
59. O'Connor G, Sparrow D, Taylor D et al. Analysis of dose response curves to metacholine. *Am Rev Respir Dis* 1987; **136**: 1412–1417.
60. Chinn S. Methodology of bronchial responsiveness. *Thorax* 1998; **53**: 984–988.
61. Godfrey S. Bronchial hyper-responsiveness in children. *Pediatr Respir Rev* 2000; **1**: 148–155.
62. Stevens WH, Manning PJ, Watson RM, O'Bryne PM. Tachyphylaxis to inhaled methacholine in normal but not asthmatic subjects. *J Appl Physiol* 1990; **69**: 875–879.
63. Brown RH, Croisille P, Mudge B et al. Airway narrowing in healthy humans inhaling methacholine without deep inspirations demonstrated by HRCT. *Am J Respir Crit Care Med* 2000; **161**: 1256–1263.
64. Beckett WS, Marenberg ME, Pace PE. Repeated methacholine challenge produces tolerance in normal but not in asthmatic subjects. *Chest* 1992; **102**: 775–779.
65. Reiff DB, Choudry NB, Pride NB, Ind PW. The effect of prolonged submaximal warm-up on exercise-induced asthma. *Am Rev Respir Dis* 1989; **139**: 479–484.
66. Godfrey S, Springer C, Novski N et al. Exercise but not methacholine challenge differentiates asthma from chronic lung disease in children. *Thorax* 1991; **46**: 488–492.

67. Fitch KD, Morton AR. Specificity of exercise in exercise-induced asthma. *Br Med J* 1971; **4**: 577–581.
68. Jones RS, Buston MH, Wharton MJ. The effect of exercise on ventilatory function in the child with asthma. *Br J Dis Chest* 1962; **56**: 78–86.
69. Schmekel B, Smith H-J. The diagnostic capacity of forced oscillation and forced expiration techniques in identifying asthma by isocapnic hyperpnoea of cold air. *Eur Respir J* 1997; **10**: 2243–2249.
70. Nielsen KC, Bisgaard H. Lung function response to cold air challenge in asthmatic and healthy children of 2–5 years of age. *Am J Respir Crit Care Med* 2000; **161**: 1805–1809.
71. Allegra L, Bianco S. Non-specific bronco-reactivity obtained with an ultrasonic aerosol of distilled water. *Eur J Respir Dis* 1980; **106**(Suppl): 41–49.
72. Lavorini F, Fontana GA, Pantaleo T et al. Fog-induced respiratory responses are attenuated by nedocromil sodium in humans. *Am J Crit Care Med* 2001; **163**: 1117–1120.
73. Andersen SD, Brannan J, Spring J et al. A new method for bronchial-provocation testing in asthmatic subjects using a dry powder of mannitol. *Am J Respir Crit Care Med* 1997; **156**: 758–765.
74. Vandenplas O, Malo JL. Inhalation challenges with agents causing occupational asthma. *Eur Respir J* 1997; **10**: 2612–2629.
75. Cotes JE, Steel J. *Work-related lung disorders.* Oxford: Blackwell Scientific Publications, 1987: 349.
76. Malo JL, Cote J, Cartier A et al. How many times per day should peak expiratory flow rates be assessed when investigating occupational asthma? *Thorax* 1993; **48**: 1211–1217.
77. Burge PS, Harries MG, O'Brien I et al. Bronchial provocation studies in workers exposed to the fumes of electronic soldering fluxes. *Clin Allergy* 1980; **10**:137–149.
78. Baldwin DR, Gannon P, Bright P et al. Interpretation of occupational peak flow records: level of agreement between expert clinicians and Oasys-2. *Thorax* 2002; 57: 860-864; *also Thorax* 2003; **58**: 461.
79. Verschelden P, CartierA, L'Archeveque J et al. Compliance with and accuracy of daily self-assessment of peak expiratory flow (PEF) in asthmatic subjects over a three month period. *Eur Respir J* 1996; **9**: 880–885.
80. Hendrick DJ, Davies RJ, Pepys J. Bakers' asthma. *Clin Allergy* 1976; **6**: 241–250.

CHAPTER 16

Distribution of Ventilation

Intrapulmonary distribution of gas can become deranged at an early stage of many lung diseases. This chapter describes the underlying physiology and how gas distribution can be assessed.

16.1 Determinants of distribution of gas

16.1.1 Overview

The principal determinants of the distribution of inspired gas are anatomical features that influence the bulk flow of gas, gravitational force and diffusion in the gas phase. Other factors include the extent of contraction of individual respiratory muscles and the tone of smooth muscle present in the walls of airways and pulmonary blood vessels. The tone is subject to regulatory mechanisms; these ensure that, so far as is practicable, the ventilation is appropriate for the perfusion (Section 18.1.2). However, some inspired gas only penetrates the lungs to the level of the bronchioles and so does not make a material contribution to gas exchange. In addition, even in normal lungs some gas is wasted in ventilating those alveoli that on account of inadequate perfusion contribute little to gas exchange. These features can be represented as constituting anatomical and physiological deadspaces, respectively (Sections 16.1.3 and 18.1.3).

16.1.2 Dilution factor

The alveoli are ventilated during each respiratory cycle by that part of the tidal volume that traverses the anatomical deadspace. In adults at rest the volume of this alveolar component of the tidal volume is about 0.4 l; the range is from 0.3 l during sleep to 6.0 l during respiratory manoeuvres. The gas is added to that present in the lungs (which is functional residual capacity); in an adult at rest this is approximately 2.5 l. Thus, under quiet resting conditions the dilution factor (expansion ratio) is normally about 1.2 [i.e.$(2.5 + 0.4) \div 2.5$].

16.1.3 Anatomical deadspace

On entering the lungs the inspired gas traverses the larger airways; these constitute an anatomical deadspace (Vd_{anat}). The movement of gas through this dead space is axial by bulk flow (convection), supplemented by lateral movement of molecules (Section 16.1.5). The anatomical deadspace is a zone of wasted ventilation that can be defined anatomically. It is an important component of physiological deadspace (Section 18.1.3).

Anatomical deadspace varies with the size of the lungs and hence the body size. It is also influenced by factors that determine the calibre of large airways (Table 14.3, page 155). The measurement of Vd_{anat} is by a single breath method (Section 16.2.3).

The mean Vd_{anat} in healthy young males is approximately 150 ml. In females it is rather less. A convenient reference value that allows for the variation with age and body size is the sum of age in years and body mass in pounds (kg × 2.2). This value is not reliable when the body composition is unusual (Section 4.7). The anatomical deadspace is seldom reported as such, but is used in the derivation of alveolar volume as part of the measurement of transfer factor by the single breath method (Section 20.4). It is also used for estimating the distensibility of the conducting airways (Section 11.9).

16.1.4 Bulk flow of gas along airways

Inspired gas enters the lungs by a process of bulk flow called convective ventilation. This has been studied using small particles (diameter 0.5–1.0 μm). They are of sufficiently small size such that few impact on the walls of airways, but not so small as to be subject to Brownian movement, and hence they do not enter the alveoli by diffusion (see below, also Section 19.2). The flow in the airways is mainly laminar (Section 14.3.4). The flow velocity is greatest at the centre of the airway and decreases progressively towards the periphery, so the flow profile is parabolic. On inspiration the axial stream of gas penetrates the gas resident in the airway which is to some extent displaced radially (Fig. 16.1, also below). The boundary layer between the resident gas and the newly inhaled gas is effectively washed away when the tidal volume exceeds 600 ml. With smaller tidal volumes the process of flushing becomes progressively less complete. However, the axial stream is preserved and still penetrates the lungs to the level of the alveolar ducts. On this account even very small tidal volumes, of the order of 60 ml in adults, can contribute to gas exchange.

16.1.5 Taylor laminar dispersion in airways

Under conditions of laminar flow the gas that is dispersed radially becomes a zone of nearly still air. This is partly due to it receiving molecules by diffusion; their migration is both radial and axial, against the direction of convective flow. The process was first investigated by Taylor, hence the designation *Taylor laminar dispersion* [2, 3].

Radial dispersion occurs particularly in medium sized airways corresponding to Weibel's generations 8 to 12, where the right and left main bronchi constitute generation 1 (Section 3.3.2).

Axial dispersion is mainly a feature of small airways and their attendant air spaces. The interrelations between radial and axial dispersion have been investigated using gas mixtures containing helium and sulphur hexafluoride. During inspiration the helium diffuses radially to a greater extent than the sulphur hexafluoride so the concentration of the latter gas in the small airways is relatively increased. Differences in axial diffusion also occur. Thus, for a given penetration by bulk flow the subsequent alveolar penetration by diffusion is much less for aerosol particles and greater for helium than for air. The difference in alveolar penetration between air and helium is increased when the diffusion pathway is lengthened by emphysema [4] and a similar change might be expected in diffuse interstitial fibrosis; the consequences for gas exchange are considered in Chapter 39. Alveolar penetration is also reduced when the environmental pressure, and hence the gas density are increased by a deep under water dive (Section 35.3).

16.1.6 Diffusion within acini

Gas molecules migrate by diffusion from parts of the lung reached by bulk flow out to the periphery of the lungs. This

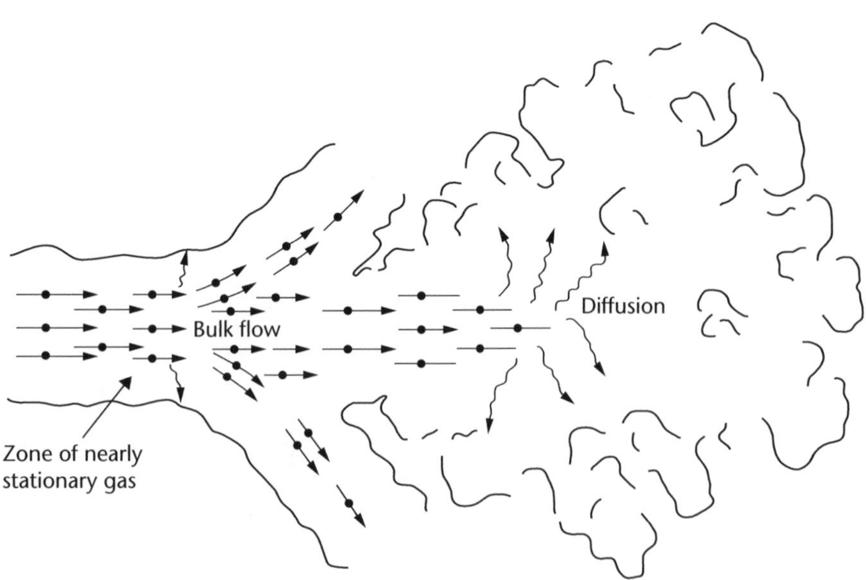

Fig. 16.1 Flow of gas molecules into an acinus during tidal breathing. Penetration into the alveolar ducts is by bulk flow. The alveoli and the zone of nearly stationary gas at the periphery of airways are ventilated by diffusion (cf. Fig. 3.5, page 26). Source [1].

process is almost instantaneous over distances of the order of one alveolar diameter, so is effective within an individual acinus. Diffusion over longer distances is enhanced by breath holding or adopting a slow respiratory frequency. These manoeuvres provide time for diffusion of gas to take place between adjacent lung units along both normal and collateral channels (Section 3.3.5); the latter is important during breath holding at small lung volumes when many small airways are occluded.

The role of diffusion within the acinus has been illuminated by use of gases of different diffusivity [5, 6]. Techniques have been devised to assess ventilation inhomogeneity in conductive and acinar zones of the lungs; these have clinical applications, e.g. to describe acinar involvement in asthma [7] and detect early obliterative bronchiolitis after double lung transplantation [8].

16.1.7 Pleural fluid pressure

The lungs are free to move within the thoracic cavity except at the hilum where they are attached to the mediastinum. Elsewhere the structures are separated by a layer of fluid between the visceral and parietal pleura. The pleural space does not contain gas. This is because the sum of the tissue gas tensions is considerably less than atmospheric pressure, so any gas in the pleural space is reabsorbed (Section 34.7).

The pleural fluid, like the interstitial fluid, is formed by ultrafiltration from serum. The fluid contains relatively little protein (concentration in the range 1%–2%) so the osmotic pressure is less than that of plasma. This causes fluid to be reabsorbed and as a result the pleural space is relatively dry (fluid volume approximately 10 ml). The small volume reflects a balance of forces that include the capillary osmotic and hydrostatic pressures, the recoil pressures of the lung and chest wall (sub-atmospheric pressure throughout most of the respiratory cycle, Section 11.2), gravitational force acting in the vertical plane of the lung and traction or support from the lung hilum.

In any posture the pleural fluid pressure with respect to atmospheric pressure is more negative at the top than at the bottom of the lung. Under static conditions the gradient reflects the pyramidal shape of the lung and the density of pleural fluid; this is effectively unity and greater than that of the lungs, where the density is approximately 0.22 kg dm^{-3} due to the presence of air (see below). Under dynamic conditions pleural fluid is in motion, and this leads to the vertical pressure gradient being the same in pleural liquid and at the pleural surface of the lungs [9, 10].

16.1.8 Gravitational force

Effect of pleural surface pressure on lung expansion. In an upright posture the surface gradient down the lungs (distance approximately 0.3 m) is about 0.75 kPa (7.5 cm H_2O). This has the effect that the expansion of the lungs is not uniform, but exhibits a vertical gradient. The gradient has been investigated using inert gases labelled with radioactive tracers [11–14]. The simplest technique entails recording the distribution of inhaled xenon gas with scintillation counters placed outside the chest (Section 7.12). In this and other ways it has been shown that during slow inspiration from residual volume, the first gas to be inhaled goes to the upper part of the lungs; in the middle range of inspiration the air is distributed between the regions. As inspiration continues, a larger proportion goes to the lower region until, at near to total lung capacity, the apex is almost fully inflated and the last air to be inhaled goes mainly to the lung bases. The bases are also the recipients of most of the tidal volume during normal breathing. The regional distribution of the respired gas is greatly influenced by the slope of the volume–pressure curve and by the point on the curve where inspiration begins. The probable mechanism is illustrated in Fig. 16.2.

For a given vertical pressure gradient, a lung of high compliance will exhibit larger regional differences in ventilation than a lung of low compliance. The perfusion of the lungs is distributed similarly (Section 17.1.3).

During expiration, the existence of a pressure gradient leads to the different lung regions emptying in the reverse order from inspiration. The bases tend to empty before the apices, hence *first in is last out.* The regional differences are less clear than during inspiration, especially at large lung volumes. The more uniform emptying is contributed to by the absence of hysteresis during expiration and by a paradoxical increase in tone of the muscle of the diaphragm that tends to reduce the gradient of pleural pressure. However, the regional differences become more pronounced at near to residual volume due to the closure of airways that serve the lung bases. The lung volume at which closure becomes detectable by current methods is called the *closing capacity* [15, 16]. It is the resultant of all the factors that determine the calibre of the intrapulmonary airways (Table 14.3, page 155). The measurement is given below (Section 16.2.5).

The vertical gradient in lung expansion affects the diameters of alveoli. These are normally more expanded in the upper than in the lower regions, especially at small lung volumes. The difference disappears at total lung capacity when all alveoli are fully expanded. Below total lung capacity the alveolar size is related to the pressure tending to expand the lungs. This may be represented in the form:

$$P = W \div A \tag{16.1}$$

where P is the gravitational pressure at any horizontal plane across the lung, A is the cross sectional area of the plane and W is the weight of the lung below it [17]. This relationship points to the mechanical stresses on the lungs being less at the lung bases than in the superior lobes and at the apices of the inferior lobes; it is probably no coincidence that these places are also the commonest sites of emphysema [18].

16.1.9 Uneven distribution of compliance and resistance

Lung units of high compliance (i.e. a steep volume–pressure curve) tend to have a high expansion ratio, and vice versa; such

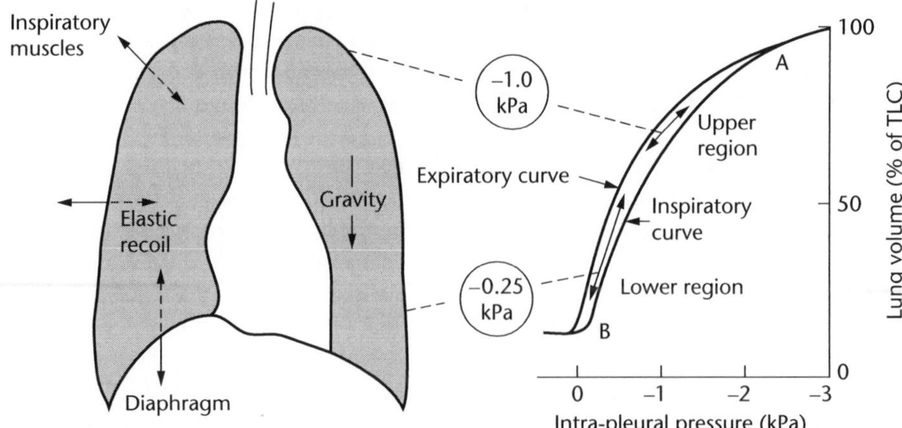

Fig. 16.2 The effect of pleural surface pressure on regional distribution of ventilation. The lungs (left) has superimposed on them the forces that are applied during inspiration; these are opposed by the elastic recoil of lung tissue that varies with volume. The relationship of volume to pressure is shown on the right-hand side of the diagram (cf. Fig. 11.4, page 120); it is assumed to be the same for upper and lower regions. At functional residual capacity the alveoli of the upper region, due to their position on the volume–pressure curve, are more expanded than those of the lower region. As a result their potential for further expansion is limited. A more negative pleural pressure then leads to a smaller volume change than in the lower region, which is on the steeper part of the curve. On inspiration at near to total lung capacity (TLC) the upper region is on the nearly horizontal part of the curve (A in the diagram), so does not expand at all. By contrast, on inspiration from residual volume, the upper region (intrapleural pressure −0.4 kPa) has a large expansion ratio, but the lower region (intrapleural pressure + 0.35 kPa) is on the flat tail of the curve where there is no expansion (B in the diagram). Source: [12].

variation contributes to *spatial* inequality of ventilation. Differences in lung resistance give rise to *temporal* inequality when lung units fill and empty sequentially. Alveoli served by airways that are wide and short tend to fill quickly and hence early in inspiration whereas those that are served by relatively long and narrow airways take longer to fill and so, on average, fill later in inspiration. Similar differences obtain on expiration when the alveoli served by the wider airways empty sooner than those served by the narrower ones, hence, within a lung unit, *first in is first out.* This is in contrast to the effect of gravity, *first in is last out* (above).

A lung composed of units of equal compliance but unequal airway resistance may be expected to exhibit temporal inequality of ventilation. Whether or not there is also spatial inequality will depend on the duration of inspiration. If it is prolonged then, for a given change in pleural surface pressure, all alveoli will achieve the same expansion ratio but if it is brief the lung units having a high resistance will expand less than the lower resistance units. The behaviour of the lungs in these terms has been investigated theoretically and from experiments on models. In that of Otis and colleagues [19] the lungs are considered as a series of parallel units each consisting of a tube of resistance R leading into a container having a compliance C. When such a system is ventilated using a pump that delivers a sine wave, the extent to which the pressure applied to the lungs is out of phase with flow can be expressed in degrees as the phase angle θ (Fig. 16.3). By analogy with electrical alternating current theory:

$$\tan\theta = \frac{1}{2\pi fCR} \tag{16.2}$$

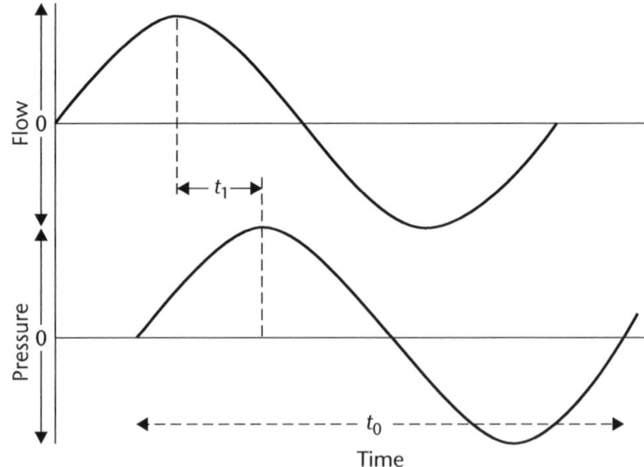

Fig. 16.3 Diagram illustrating the derivation of the phase angle from the pneumotachograph record of airflow and the pressure applied across the lungs between the pleural surface and the mouth. The phase angle is the segment of the respiratory cycle between peak flow and peak pressure (t_1) expressed as a fraction of the complete cycle (t_o), when the latter is 360°. Then $\theta = t_1/t_o \times 360°$. Source: [19].

where f is respiratory frequency. The product of the compliance and the resistance (C × R) is the 'time constant of the lungs'. This is the time after the sudden application of a pressure gradient across the lung for the flow to arrive at within $1/e$ or 36.8% of its equilibrium value. For the model, the time constant is larger when either the resistance or the compliance is increased. In practice an increase in resistance is the more relevant as it is associated with a reduced rate of airflow. According to the model the phase angle is small when pressure and flow are nearly in phase. When two compartments have different phase angles due to differences in resistance, gas can be flowing out of one at a time when it is flowing into the other and vice versa. This 'Pendelluft' phenomenon has been demonstrated in the lungs (Fig. 18.6, page 220). It reduces the effective tidal volume and the accuracy of measurements of resistance and compliance for the lungs, especially when these are made at high frequencies of breathing. For the model in such circumstances, the dynamic compliance is less than, and the airway resistance is greater than that given by summation of the resistance and compliance of the component units. Similarly in man, when the airway resistance is increased, the dynamic compliance is lower than the static compliance (Section 11.6). In this circumstance the distribution of ventilation is uneven. The time constant is short when the resistance and compliance are reduced. This combination can occur in diffuse interstitial fibrosis. It is associated with a reduced ability to expand the lungs but the proportion of vital capacity that can be expired in 1 s (i.e. $FEV_1\%$) is usually increased and the peak expiratory flow may be within normal limits (Section 40.4). A reduction in compliance has relatively little effect upon those indices of inequality of distribution of gas that assess temporal rather than spatial inequality. On this account the spatial component of the inequality is sometimes overlooked.

16.1.10 Uneven contraction of respiratory muscles

In any posture except the lateral one the vertical gradient of pleural surface pressure and the wide range of regional time constants explain most of the observed variations in regional lung gas distribution. However, discrepancies have been identified in a number of circumstances (Table 16.1), and their diversity illustrates the ingenuity and persistence of respiratory physiologists. The observations were often made initially using single breath techniques in which either the nitrogen present in the lungs was diluted by a single breath of oxygen or the test breath was tagged using a bolus of radioactive gas such as xenon (^{133}Xe) (Section 7.12).

Table 16.1 Experimental situations used to study lung gas distribution [20–25].

Experimental situations
Different postures (supine, prone or lateral)
Inspiratory effort varied in intensity
Subject uses different muscles (intercostals, accessory muscles or diaphragm)
Gas density or viscosity modified by breathing helium or sulphur hexafluoride
Mechanical ventilation with muscular action suppressed
Lung expansion reduced by strapping the lower rib cage
Immersion in water
Transpulmonary pressure increased by breathing through a resistance
Gravitational force modified in a human centrifuge, spacecraft or aircraft accelerating or moving in a parabolic trajectory.

The unifying theme through many of the studies is that the vertical gradient of pleural surface pressure can be modified locally by selective contraction of individual groups of respiratory muscles. In any posture forced inspiration from residual volume but not from functional residual capacity usually augments the flow of gas to the apex of the lungs (cf. Fig. 16.2); this is a consequence of increased contraction of the intercostal and accessory muscles and is associated with local distortion of the rib cage [26]. Accentuated contraction of the diaphragm increases the flow to the lung bases in all postures but particularly when lying on the side (lateral decumbent position) when the piston-like action of the diaphragm is enhanced by the structure forming much of the lateral boundary of the lungs (cf. Fig. 9.1, page 101). [27].

16.1.11 Effects of cardiac systole

Contraction of the heart redistributes blood both within the thorax and between the thorax and the systemic circulation; it also generates a pulse wave that is transmitted to lung tissue via the pulmonary circulation. These perturbations contribute to the mixing of gas within the lungs; the effect varies directly with the mass of the molecules and on this account differs from mixing by diffusive conductance in being greater for sulphur hexafluoride than for helium. The mixing effect might be expected to be greater for carbon dioxide than for oxygen but in practice the opposite is the case [28]. Cardiac systole also draws gas along the airways [29]. At rest the volume displaced is about 60 ml per heartbeat. The changes lead to oscillations in the alveolar concentrations of oxygen and carbon dioxide in the expired gas (cardiogenic oscillations): the changes are illustrated in Fig. 16.7 (page 188). The amplitude of the oscillations reflects the unevenness of distribution of ventilation–perfusion ratios within the lungs [30] (see also Fig. 18.7, page 220).

16.1.12 Perspective

During normal tidal breathing intrapulmonary mixing of gas is optimal at lung volumes just above those associated with airway closure. The mixing is mainly due to convection and the most important determinant is tidal volume. During controlled breathing with a tidal volume of 1 l the mixing within the acinus is normally complete within five breaths. During the first breath diffusion also contributes to gas mixing. The changes during subsequent breaths reflect sequential emptying of larger regional units containing gas at different concentrations [31]. The role of diffusion is largely confined to events within the acinus. This has been demonstrated using gases of different diffusivity to separate the diffusive component of lung mixing from that due to convection [31]. The method has for the first time provided quantitative information on the condition of the alveolar ducts in pulmonary

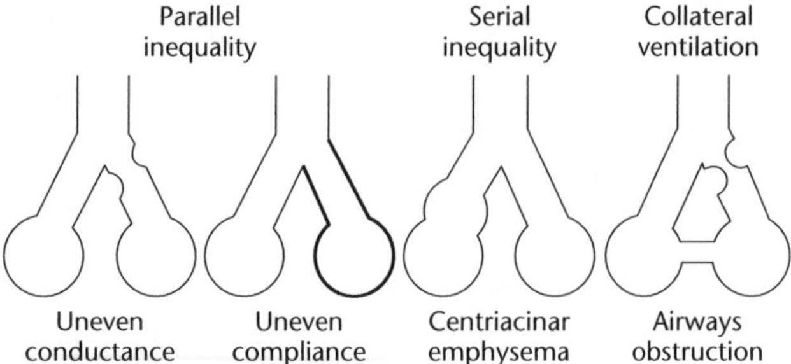

Fig. 16.4 Examples of uneven lung function. The effects of parallel and serial inequality can be described in terms of parallel and serial deadspaces; the latter can also be represented as stratified inhomogeneity.

diseases [7, 8]. Models illustrating some types of functional abnormality to which the new technique can be applied are shown in Fig. 16.4.

Lung mixing by diffusion is of increased importance when the local delivery of gas by bulk flow is for any reason impaired [32, also Section 19.2.4]. Distribution is also affected by any local scarring in the lungs or pleura. Such changes can distort the movement of the lungs but their overall effect on gas exchange is usually small.

16.2 Assessment of distribution of ventilation

16.2.1 Overview

The extent of uneven distribution of ventilation is usually assessed using a single breath procedure in which the subject inhales a test breath of 100% oxygen that dilutes the nitrogen already present in the lungs. The extent of uneven distribution is inferred from changes in concentration of nitrogen in gas sampled at the mouth during the subsequent exhalation. Somewhat different information is obtained if, instead of using nitrogen, (i.e. the resident gas), the procedure employs an inert gas that is foreign to the lungs, for example a test breath or bolus of helium, argon, neon or radioisotope such as xenon, nitrogen or krypton (Sections 7.12 and 18.6). A radioactive isotope can also be used to assess the regional distribution of gas. Localisation on an anatomical basis can be achieved by sampling gas from a bronchoscope with its tip placed in a lobar bronchus (Section 18.5). Changes in distribution of ventilation with respect to time can be assessed by analysis of a series of breaths (multibreath tests). Distribution by bulk flow can be investigated using aerosol particles (Section 16.2.8) and distribution by diffusion using gases of different diffusivity (density dependency analysis). Indices of uneven distribution of ventilation with respect to perfusion ($\dot{V}A/\dot{Q}$) are considered in Chapter 18, and the consequences of gas exchange for oxygen and carbon dioxide in Chapters 21 and 22.

16.2.2 Single breath nitrogen tests of uneven ventilation

For epidemiological and occupational surveys a single breath nitrogen test is often used because it is a simple and sensitive indicator of slight abnormalities of ventilation not reflected in the forced expiratory volume.

The procedure yields the anatomical deadspace (Fowler deadspace), the Fowler index of uneven ventilation, the slope of the alveolar plateau (phase 3), the closing volume and an estimate of residual volume from which the closing capacity can be calculated. The methods were introduced by Ward Fowler following the development by Lilly of a rapid ultraviolet emission analyser for nitrogen [33]. Alternative indicator gases are given above.

Apparatus. Volume is measured in a spirometer or, if the gases of interest are oxygen and nitrogen, from integration of the output of a pneumotachograph that is calibrated appropriately for 100% oxygen. Nitrogen concentration is measured with a nitrogen meter or respiratory mass spectrometer. With the latter a small error in the nitrogen signal occurs from the presence of carbon monoxide, as that gas has the same mass as nitrogen (28). The CO can be present in exhaled breath. It is also formed from carbon dioxide in the instrument's measuring chamber. Gas volume and concentration are displayed on an XY recorder. Oxygen is delivered from a demand valve, bag or spirometer. A convenient tap assembly is illustrated in Fig. 16.5. It should include a means of registering the flow during expiration. The apparatus is arranged so that the subject is studied seated in an upright posture. A nose clip is worn.

16.2.3 Measurement of anatomical deadspace

The subject breathes normally through the mouthpiece to air, then at the end of an expiration is switched to the oxygen reservoir (this is labelled 'diluent gas' in Fig. 16.5). A single tidal breath of oxygen is inhaled and the subject then exhales normally. The time between the end of inspiration and the start of expiration should be standardised at 0.4–0.6 s [34]. During expiration the nitrogen concentration is recorded. A schematic result is illustrated in Fig. 16.6. The curve has three parts (phases) of which the first represents oxygen in the anatomical deadspace down to the level of the terminal bronchioles. This gas is expired unaltered and does not contain nitrogen. The second phase represents the transition from sampling deadspace gas to sampling gas from alveoli. This phase is used to measure the deadspace (Fig. 16.6). The start of the third phase defines the beginning of the alveolar plateau. The properties of the plateau are considered subsequently.

The shape of phase 2 is influenced by the degree of turbulence (Section 14.3.4) and by the extent of diffusive mixing in the airways. The latter is increased by any delay between completing the inhalation of oxygen and starting to breathe out.

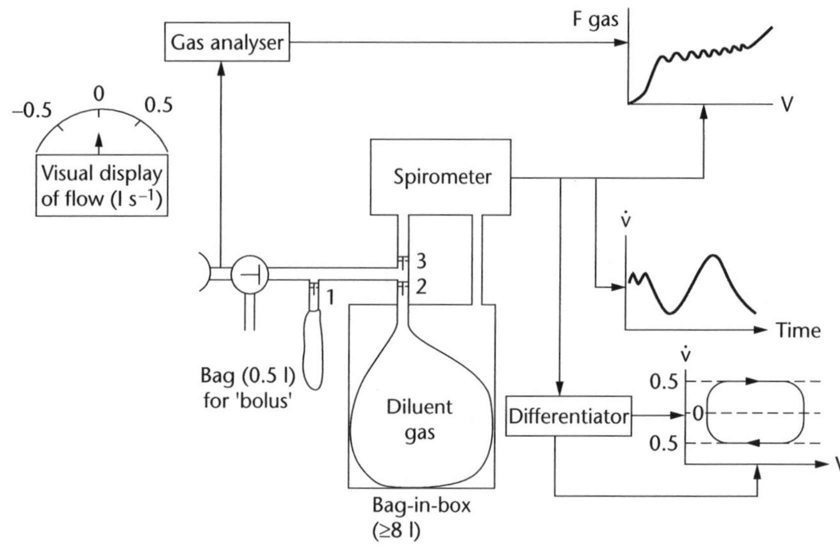

Fig. 16.5 Apparatus for single breath tests of uneven lung function. The valves 1 and 2 are adjusted so that the bag containing the bolus of test gas empties before the subject inhales from the bag-in-box (Donald, Christie box). The respiratory flows during inspiration and expiration should be in the range 0.3–0.5 l s^{-1} for 95% of the expiration. The display should be visible to the subject. The instruments should have response times of less than 0.1 s and the records of volume and of concentration should be synchronous; when two gases are to be analysed this is best done using a mass spectrometer and not separate analysers. F_{gas} is fractional concentration of test gas.

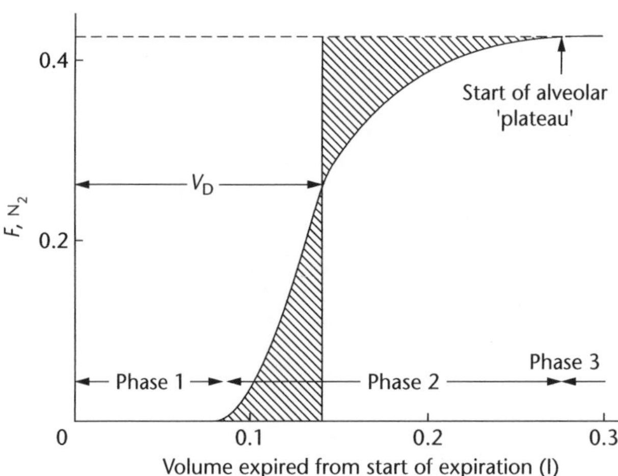

Fig. 16.6 Method for obtaining the anatomical deadspace following the inhalation of a single tidal breath of oxygen. The fractional concentration of nitrogen at the lips and the volume expired are recorded. The time between the end of inspiration and the start of expiration should be standardised at 0.4–0.6 s. The anatomical deadspace is obtained by dividing the rising part of the curve so that the two shaded areas are equal.

Hence, the post-inspiratory pause should be standardised at 0.4–0.6 s. The anatomical deadspace varies with body size and lung volume so the tidal volume and functional residual capacity or thoracic gas volume should be recorded. The deadspace is, for practical purposes, equal for all gases except those that are very soluble in an aqueous medium, hence helium in oxygen ($F_{He} = 0.8$) or carbon dioxide in air can also be used as the indicator gas.

Measurement of anatomical deadspace as part of the procedure for estimating the distensibility of the conducting airways is described in Section 11.9.

16.2.4 Procedures for nitrogen indices of gas mixing within the lungs

For the standard procedure, the subject breathes quietly through the mouthpiece to air, takes two deep breathes, then makes a full, relaxed expiration to residual volume. He or she signals that expiration is complete, the operator turns the tap connecting the mouthpiece to the oxygen reservoir and the subject makes a slow full inspiration to total lung capacity. This is followed immediately and without breath holding by a slow full expiration to residual volume. During these manoeuvres the flow should not deviate outside the range 0.3–0.5 l s^{-1}. Alternatively if flow is monitored using a 4-mm diameter constriction in the mouthpiece the pressure proximal to the constriction should not exceed 0.7 kPa (7 cm H_2O).

The *Fowler nitrogen index* is the difference between the concentration of nitrogen in gas sampled at 750 ml and at 1250 ml after the start of expiration. The index has the disadvantage that the starting point is often in phase 2, so the reproducibility is poor.

Single breath nitrogen index (slope of phase 3). This index is the slope of the alveolar plateau as depicted by the linear part of phase 3 (Fig. 16.7).

The slope is usually taken from when 30% of vital capacity has been expired to the start of phase 4. The latter is defined below under 'closing volume and capacity'. The position of the best fitting line is usually determined by eye. Alternatively, a computer programme can be used. However, errors in commercial programmes have been reported so these should be checked carefully. The units are $N_2\%\ l^{-1}$. The measurement should be repeated with a view to obtaining three technically satisfactory results (Table 16.2). The mean result should be accepted. However, if the subject has difficulty with the procedure the mean of two or even a single result should be used, as repeated attempts (e.g. more than six) can be counterproductive. The interval between tests

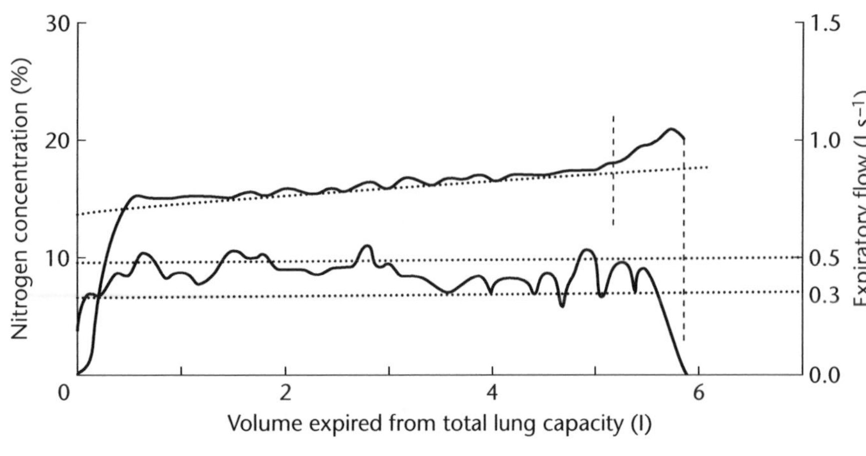

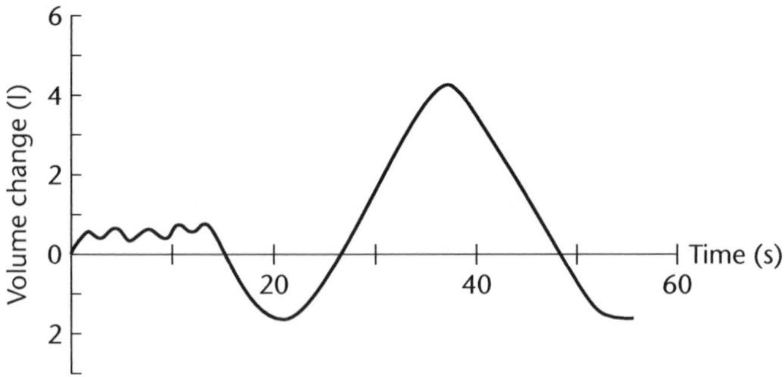

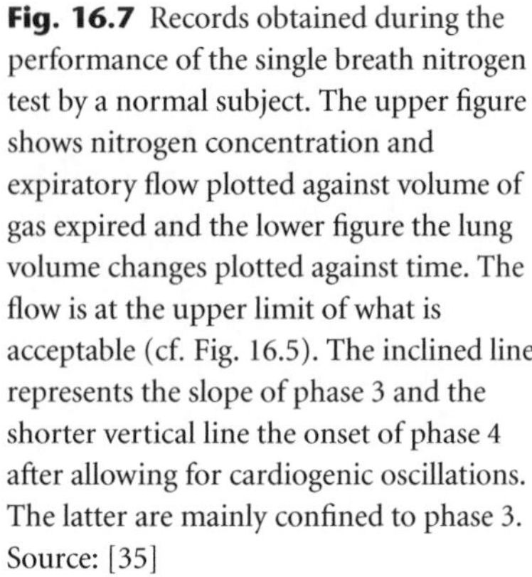

Fig. 16.7 Records obtained during the performance of the single breath nitrogen test by a normal subject. The upper figure shows nitrogen concentration and expiratory flow plotted against volume of gas expired and the lower figure the lung volume changes plotted against time. The flow is at the upper limit of what is acceptable (cf. Fig. 16.5). The inclined line represents the slope of phase 3 and the shorter vertical line the onset of phase 4 after allowing for cardiogenic oscillations. The latter are mainly confined to phase 3. Source: [35]

Table 16.2 Criteria for acceptability of single breath nitrogen test [36].

Test criteria
Inspired and expired volumes should agree to within 5%
Expired volume should be within 10% of vital capacity
The curve should not be interrupted by step changes in N_2
Inspiratory and expiratory flows should be within the prescribed limits.

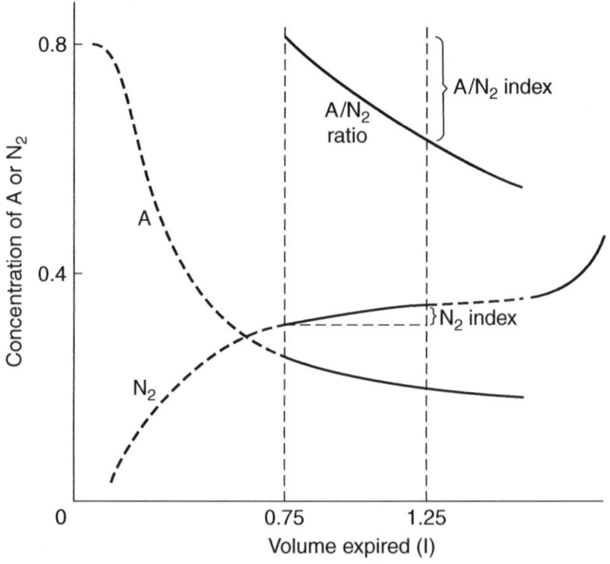

Fig. 16.8 Argon/nitrogen index of uneven ventilation. For this test the inspirate is 80% argon, 20% oxygen. The gases are analysed using a mass spectrometer. Source: [37].

should be sufficient to wash out the additional oxygen from the lungs, this is 3–5 min in healthy subjects but up to 10 min in some patients.

Strict criteria for performance of the test are necessary because the nitrogen slope is greatly influenced by the pre-inspiration lung volume, the volume of oxygen inhaled, uneven lung expansion (such as can accompany rapid inspiration or contraction of accessory muscles) and the rate of expiration. In one study, the results for 22% of untrained shipyard workers were rejected because they could not inhale from residual volume at the optimal slow rate [35]. An additional source of error is gas exchange continuing during the test expiration; this leads to a progressive rise in concentration of nitrogen throughout expiration (Section 21.5.2) equivalent to approximately 10% of the normal nitrogen difference. The error can be avoided by adding helium or argon to the inhaled oxygen and expressing the result in terms of the ratio of the concentration of nitrogen to that of the foreign gas (Fig. 16.8). Gas exchange affects both gases to the same extent so the ratio is independent of this effect.

Comment. The numerical values for nitrogen slope ($N_2\%\ l^{-1}$) and the Fowler index ($N_2\%$) are similar despite the units being different. Reference values are available (Fig. 26.10, page 351).

The nitrogen slope is increased by narrowing of small airways and by structural changes within the acinus altering the path length for diffusion, for example in emphysema.

Modified single breath methods. These methods focus on the contributions to lung mixing of convection within lung regions and of diffusion. The first step is to start the test inspiration at a volume above closing volume so that all the airways are open [38]. The simplest modified procedure entails a test inspiration of 1l of oxygen starting from functional residual capacity (FRC). The inspiration is preceded by two deep breaths to establish that all airways are open, then three normal tidal breaths to define the FRC. The inspiration and subsequent complete expiration are made slowly with minimal delay between them. The nitrogen slope is higher than by the standard method; it is calculated in the manner described. The procedure is sensitive and has few lapses, but does not yield a closing volume. This can be obtained if the test inspiration is not limited to 1 l but is continued to total lung capacity. The result is then somewhat influenced by regional differences and the closing volume is higher than that obtained by the standard method.

Density dependency analysis. Additional information on gaseous diffusion can be obtained by extending the modified procedure to several controlled breaths and using gases of different diffusivity, for example helium and sulphur hexafluoride (Table 14.2, page 154). From these data the component of the slope of phase 3 that is due to gaseous diffusion can be separated from that due to convection. The former reflects the condition of alveolar ducts and other structures within the acinus [5, 6, 31]. The method can illuminate lung function at the level of the acinus [7, 8] and further work is indicated.

16.2.5 Closing volume and capacity

Closing volume is the volume of gas exhaled from the onset of phase 4 to residual volume [15, 16]. It is usually reported as a percentage of vital capacity and designated CV%. Alternatively, it can be reported as *closing capacity* which is the lung volume at which closure can be detected, expressed as a percentage of total lung capacity:

$$CC(\%) = 100(CV + RV)/(VC + RV) \qquad (16.3)$$

where CC is closing capacity, CV is closing volume, RV is residual volume and VC is vital capacity, all expressed in litres. Thus, the denominator is total lung capacity.

In healthy subjects the presence of phase 4 and hence of a closing volume, is evidence for regional differences in lung filling and emptying. This is because during inspiration from residual volume the upper zones have a lower expansion ratio than the lower zones (Fig. 16.2). Hence, at the end of the test inspiration, the oxygen concentration in the upper zone is lower and nitrogen concentration higher than in the bases. Both zones contribute gas to the subsequent expiration; however, towards the end of expiration some basal airways close. Thereafter the gas that is expired comes mainly from the upper zones that are relatively rich in nitrogen; hence, the recorded concentration rises.

The closing volume is relatively large in early childhood, falls to an average of less than 10% in early adulthood, and then rises nearly linearly to an average of 30% in older subjects (Figs 26.4 and 26.10, pages 343 and 351). CV% is increased in most smokers and persons with airflow limitation.

Measurement of CV

Single breath nitrogen method. The closing volume is usually obtained during the course of estimating the slope of phase 3 of the single breath nitrogen curve by the vital capacity method. The phase 3 occupies most of expiration. It is followed by a rise (phase 4, see Fig. 16.7). In some subjects the rise is followed by a sharp fall in concentration, designated as phase 5.

The onset of phase 4 is the point at which the nitrogen concentration rises above the inclining phase 3; in its identification allowance needs to be made for the cardiogenic oscillations. Closing volume extends from this point to residual volume which, therefore, should be delineated correctly. This is particularly important in adolescents and young adults in whom closing volume may occur near the end of the vital capacity manoeuvre. For such subjects acceptance of the criterion that the expired volume should be at least 90% of vital capacity can lead to the closing volume being missed. A 99% criterion increases the yield. In addition, identification of the onset of phase 4 can be assisted by administration of a bolus of air at the start of the test inspiration of oxygen [39]. Manual compression of the thorax at the end of expiration can also be considered but this manoeuvre needs to be validated.

Bolus method. The method differs from that described above in that a foreign indicator gas is used instead of nitrogen. Radioactive xenon (^{133}Xe) was first used for this purpose [40] but helium, argon or neon are preferable as they do not emit ionising radiation. The procedure is exactly as described except that the test inspiration from residual volume is a bolus of approximately 0.3 l of the chosen gas followed by air. An appropriate analyser is used, for example a respiratory mass spectrometer or a critical orifice helium analyser [41].

Limitations of bolus method. By the bolus method the phase 3 usually exhibits marked cardiogenic oscillations but these disappear at the onset of phase 4 due to the closure of airways. The closing volume is apparent in all subjects including those in whom it is not detectable by the nitrogen method. However, compared with the nitrogen method the closing volume is invariably higher [16]. It can also respond differently to acute airflow obstruction. This is due to the mechanism for producing a closing volume being different in the two situations. By the nitrogen method any inequality is detected in terms of expansion ratios (Section 16.1.2). By the bolus method the separation is anatomical with the test gas being inhaled mainly into the upper zones which normally fill earlier and empty later than the lower zones

[16] (also Section 16.1.8). Phase 3 obtained by the bolus method should not be used because it is greatly influenced by technical and other factors associated with the measurement.

Other methods for closing volume. A closing volume is demonstrable in the relationship of transpulmonary pressure to lung volume [42] and of airflow resistance to thoracic gas volume (Fig. 14.1, page 152). The volumes are larger than those seen by gas dilution methods.

Derivation of closing capacity. Using equation 16.3 the closing capacity is calculated from closing volume, vital capacity and residual volume. The first two are obtained during measurement of closing volume. The residual volume is often calculated using additional information obtained during the same test. This is acceptable for subjects with normal or only slightly impaired gas mixing. The following relationship is used:

$$V_A = \frac{V_I,\ F_{A,N_2} - (V_{E,N_2})(Vd/(V_E - Vd))}{F_{A,N_2} - (V_{E,N_2})/(V_E - Vd)} \text{ litres} \qquad (16.4)$$

where V_A, V_I, V_E and Vd are, respectively, the alveolar volume, the inspired and expired volume and the volume of the anatomical deadspace in litres BTPS. F_{A,N_2} is the fractional alveolar concentration of nitrogen before the test breath and V_{E,N_2} is the volume of nitrogen expired; this is equal to the area under the single-breath curve determined either by planimetry or by electrical integration. The method can underestimate the alveolar volume when there is airways obstruction (cf. Section 10.3.2). For such subjects residual volume should be measured by an independent procedure (see Chapter 10).

16.2.6 Nitrogen slope and closing volume in epidemiology

The nitrogen slope arises mainly from local variations in ventilation and gaseous diffusion within and between acini whereas the closing volume arises from regional differences in expansion ratios. As a result the two indices are complementary. In different circumstances both have been found useful in epidemiological surveys [e.g. 43–45], but there are snags. A proportion of subjects cannot perform the slow vital capacity that the unmodified nitrogen method requires [46] and some young adults do not have a closing volume (Section 10.2). Furthermore, the several methods for measuring closing volume give different results. Closing volume is also strongly associated with smoking and this can be assessed more directly in other ways. Thus, closing volume appears to be of limited usefulness except in those who have never smoked, or where an environmental factor such as welding fumes interacts with smoking. The nitrogen slope can detect narrowing of small airways and, possibly, the early effects of emphysema but these abnormalities are usually considered to be indicated with greater certainty by the flow–volume curve or frequency dependence of dynamic compliance [47–50] and by a reduced transfer factor. In addition, the nitrogen indices are not consistently good predictors of a subsequent accelerated decline in forced expiratory volume [51, 52]. Thus, despite early promise [53], the single breath nitrogen test using a vital capacity breath of oxygen appears to be of limited usefulness for respiratory surveys. A method that incorporates a density dependency analysis is likely to be more informative.

16.2.7 Multi-breath indices of gas mixing

Lung volume index of uneven ventilation. This index is the ratio of the alveolar volume (i.e. total lung capacity minus anatomical deadspace) estimated by a single breath technique to that by a multi-breath or plethysmographic method. It is designated $V_{A,eff}/V_A$ and is available whenever a reasonably full lung function assessment is carried out. In young healthy subjects the two volumes are nearly identical ($V_{A,eff}/V_A$ in the range 0.9–1.0). The $V_{A,eff}$ is less when the volume accessible to a single inspiration is reduced. On this account the index decreases with age (Table 26.23, page 358) and when distribution of inspired gas is uneven (e.g. Table 40.4, Case F vs Case E, page 556). A value above 1.0 indicates technical error in one of the component measurements.

The $V_{A,eff}/V_A$ is correlated with forced expiratory volume as a percentage of vital capacity (FEV_1%) and residual volume as a percentage of total lung capacity (RV %). The three indices can be combined in an empirical index of airflow obstruction:

$$COI = 75 + 0.5\,RV\% - 40\,V_{A,eff}/V_A - 0.3\,FEV_1\%. \qquad (16.5)$$

where COI is *combined obstruction index* [54]. Reference values are available (Table 26.16, page 347).

Closed circuit mixing index. The index is obtained during measurement of functional residual capacity by the closed circuit helium dilution method. It is the number of breaths completed by the subject up to the point when the concentration of helium in the circuit has fallen to within 10% of the equilibrium value. The index is not recommended.

Open circuit indices of gas mixing. The open circuit method for measuring functional residual capacity (Section 10.3.3) yields several mixing indices. These relate to quiet resting conditions. The *7-min nitrogen concentration* is the alveolar concentration obtained after most of the nitrogen has been flushed from the lungs by breathing oxygen for 7 min. The concentration is normally less than 1.5% at age 20, increasing to less than 2.5% at age 60. Higher values are obtained when gas mixing is impaired. The index is influenced by the ventilation minute volume and pattern of breathing.

The *lung clearance index* (*LCI*) is the volume of oxygen that must be breathed in order to lower the concentration of nitrogen in end tidal gas to 2% [55, 56]. The volume is expressed as a multiple of functional residual capacity. In healthy young adults

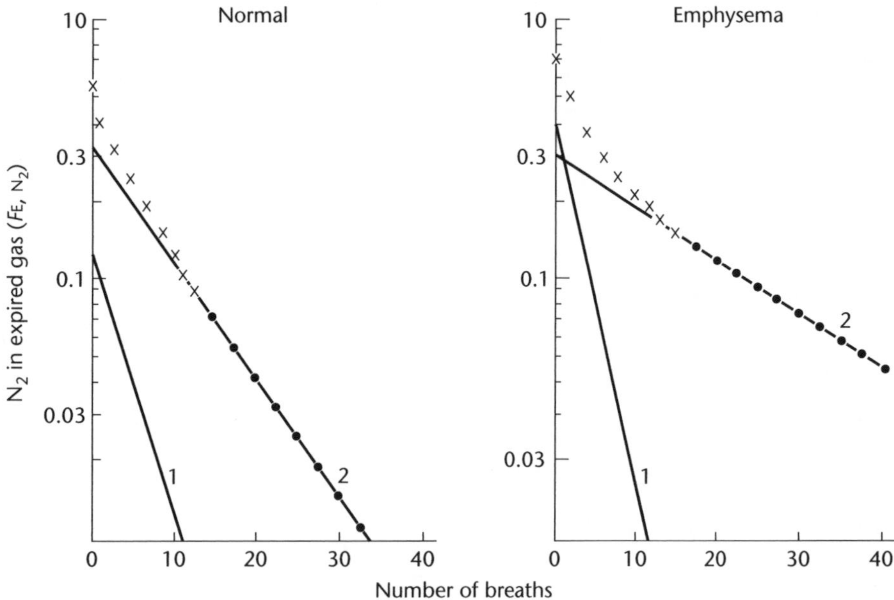

Fig. 16.9 Nitrogen washout curves obtained during breathing oxygen by a healthy subject and a patient with emphysema. The curves are subdivided into two components which represent alveoli that are well and poorly ventilated; these, respectively, have a high and low expansion ratio. To perform the analysis the slow mixing compartment of the lung is defined by the best fit for the tail of the curve where it is marked with dots. This is designated line 2. The fast mixing compartment is then defined by line 1 that is obtained by replotting the difference between the upper end of line 2 and the proximal part of the curve where it is marked with crosses. The rate of gas replacement in each compartment is described by the slope of the appropriate line; the rate for the poorly ventilated alveoli is slower in the patient with emphysema than in the healthy subject.

the LCI is in the range 5.0–9.0. Higher values are obtained in older subjects and when the effectiveness of gas mixing is impaired. [57].

Moment analysis applied to the nitrogen washout curve yields two indices that are uninfluenced by differences in breathing pattern and lung size between subjects [58]. The ratio of the first-to-zero moments (μ_1/μ_0) and the second-to-zero moments (μ_2/μ_0) are weighted, dimensionless integral measures that have a small variability between subjects, require fewer breaths for their computation and are more sensitive to mild degrees of ventilation inhomogeneity than the 7-min nitrogen concentration or LCI [59]. The μ_1/μ_0 is significantly higher in healthy, preschool children (mean $= 2.14$) than in older children (mean $=$ 1.97) or young adults (mean $= 2.04$) suggesting that washout is less homogenous in the very young, prior to cessation of alveolar multiplication [60].

Mixing compartments. The compartments are obtained by exponential analysis of the relationship of nitrogen concentration to breath number during the washout period. The fall in concentration of nitrogen per breath is proportional to the concentration present and is linear when the log of the concentration is related to the number of breaths, provided the breaths are of equal volume. In healthy young adults the semilog plot is slightly curvilinear (Fig. 16.9); this is evidence for the presence of a range of expansion ratios. The range is widened by ageing or airway narrowing. For purposes of analysis the washout curve can be partitioned into two or more exponentials. These represent hypothetical chambers of different size and different expansion ratios which, if they were connected in parallel, would yield a washout curve similar to that which is observed for the intact subject. The analysis does not provide a unique description but it permits the construction of a model of lung mixing on which can be grafted similar descriptions of the perfusion and diffusion characteristics of the lungs [61].

In nitrogen decay curves, the quantity of nitrogen remaining in the lungs is related to the volume of oxygen that has been inhaled (Fig. 16.10). Linear deviation from the relationship for an ideal single chamber lung (as for bronchitis in the figure) is then evidence for impaired mixing between the inhaled gas and the alveolar gas within lung units (stratified inhomogeneity, cf. Fig. 16.4). Curvilinearity in the relationship is due to differences in time constants between the units [57].

Multiple breath washout techniques can sometimes detect early airway narrowing at a time when the results of spirometry are still within normal limits [62, 63].

16.2.8 Airspace diameter from aerosol recovery

An aerosol of small inert particles suspended in air can be used to indicate the average diameters of the air spaces into which they are inhaled. The method makes use of the normal protective process whereby inhaled particles of diameter 0.5 to 2 μ deposit on the respiratory epithelium by sedimentation and are subsequently

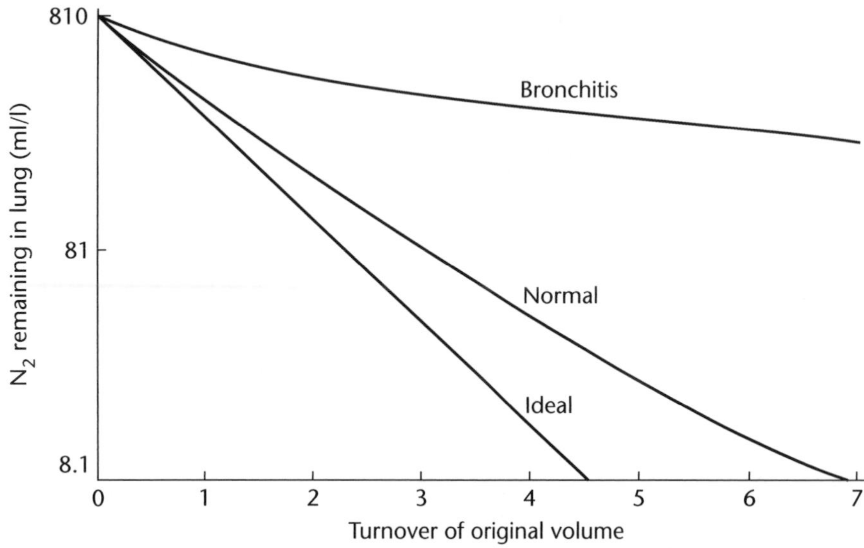

Fig. 16.10 Lung decay curves showing the washout of nitrogen by breathing oxygen. The ordinate is the volume of nitrogen remaining in the lung expressed per litre of lung volume. The abscissa is the volume of oxygen inhaled, expressed per litre of lung volume. For interpretation see text. Source: [57]

cleared (Section 37.2.2). The rate of deposition depends on the mean settling velocity of the particles, their residence time in the lung and the diameter of the air spaces. The settling velocity is determined by the physical characteristics of the particles with respect to those of alveolar gas (eqn 37.2, page 507). The residence time reflects the time of breath holding and the penetration into the lung as determined by the depth of inspiration. All these variables are under the control of the operator.

Method. For studies of alveolar deposition, particles of diameter 0.5μm–1.0 μm can be used. Their nuclei are of sodium chloride and they are coated with di 2-ethylhexyl sebacate prepared in a modified La Mer-Sinclair generator. The particles are produced by volatilising the salt in an atmosphere of nitrogen and heating it with the sebacate vapour at 400°C. Alternatively, triphenyl phosphate particles can be used. The concentration of particles in inhaled and exhaled air is determined using a Tyndallometer in which a light beam from a quartz halogen lamp illuminates the aerosol as it enters and leaves the mouth. The scatter of light at right angles to the beam is monitored using a photomultiplier.

The particles are inhaled from the bag-in-box during a single test inhalation made under controlled conditions of flow and volume; the subsequent expiration can be either immediate (Fig. 16.11) or after breath holding for up to 30 s. The deposition of particles in the alveoli increases exponentially with time of breath holding, so the proportion of particles that are recoverable in the expired gas declines. The half-time for recovery ($t_{1/2}$) can be calculated by making the measurement after different times, with an allowance made for loss of particles by deposition during expiration. Under standard conditions the $t_{1/2}$ varies with total lung capacity, age and gender and is increased in smokers, subjects with chronic bronchitis and men exposed to coal mine dust [66–68].

The $t_{1/2}$ varies inversely with distance over which sedimentation is taking place, so can be used to estimate the effective

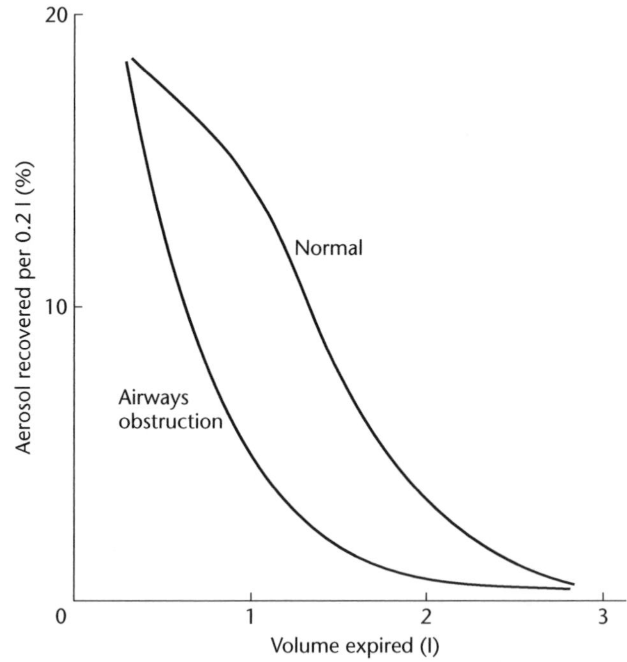

Fig. 16.11 Aerosol recovery curves for a healthy subject and a patient with airways obstruction showing the decline in concentration of aerosol particles (diameter 0.5μm) during exhalation following a single test inhalation. The separation between the curves reflects the degree of airways obstruction. The procedure was that of Muir [64]. Source: [65]

airspace diameter (EAD) [69]. The estimates of size and the magnitude of the changes with age are concordant with those from morphological data [70].

Aerosol dispersion and mean airspace diameter are increased in the presence of conditions commonly associated with emphysema. The change in EAD is then similar to that estimated by high-resolution computer assisted tomography (HRCT) [71]. It is inversely related to the change in transfer factor (Tl,co), but not to that in other indices of lung function [72]. The technique may be applied when screening patients with chronic bronchitis to identify those in whom there is additional airspace enlargement [73]. In patients with pulmonary fibrosis mean airspace size is increased but aerosol dispersion is not different from that in healthy subjects [74].

The method provides information on abnormalities at the level of the acinus that can be detected at a stage in the illness when the results of most screening tests are within normal limits.

16.2.9 Methods using radioisotopes

See Sections 7.12 and 18.6.

16.3 Critical comment

For respiratory epidemiological surveys the traditional single breath nitrogen indices of lung mixing appear to have outlived their usefulness [75]. If they are to have a place, for example in occupational surveys, a modified procedure may be appropriate, e.g. [46]. Information to supplement that from spirometry is more likely to come from the use of gases of different density (*density dependency analysis*, page 189) and of monodispersed aerosol particles that can indicate the effective airspace diameter (*EAD*). These tests might now be tried out epidemiologically. In the lung function laboratory more consideration might be given to the use of multiple-breath inert gas washouts [62, 63].

16.4 References

1. Muir DCF. Bulk flow and diffusion in the airways of the lung. *Brit J Dis Chest* 1966; **60**: 169–176.
2. Taylor GI. Dispersion of soluble matter in solvent flowing slowly through a tube. *Proc R Soc Lond Ser A* 1953; **219**: 186–193.
3. Piiper J, Scheid P. Diffusion and convection in intrapulmonary gas mixing. In: Farhi LE, Tenney SM, ed. *Handbook of physiology, Vol 4: gas exchange* (Section 3). Bethesda, MD: American Physiological Society, 1987: 51–70.
4. Georg J, Lassen NA, Mellemgaard K, Vinther A. Diffusion in the gas phase of the lungs in normal and emphysematous subjects. *Clin Sci* 1965; **29**: 525–532.
5. Dutrieue B, Lauzon A-M, Verbanck S et al. Helium and sulfur hexafluoride bolus washin in short-term microgravity. *J Appl Physiol* 1999; **86**: 1594–1602.
6. Dutrieue B, Vanholsbeeck F, Verbanck S, Paiva M. A human acinar structure for simulation of realistic alveolar plateau slopes. *J Appl Physiol* 2000; **89**: 1859–1867.
7. Verbanck S, Schuermans D, Noppen M et al. Evidence of acinar airway involvement in asthma. *Am J Respir Crit Care Med* 1999; **159**: 1545–1550.
8. Estenne M, Van Muylem A, Knoop C, Antoine M. Detection of obliterative bronchiolitis after lung transplantation by indexes of ventilation distribution. *Am J Respir Crit Care Med* 2000; **162**: 1047–1051.
9. Agostoni E, D'Angelo E. Pleural liquid pressure. *J Appl Physiol* 1991; **71**: 393–403.
10. Lai-Fook SJ, Rodarte JR. Pleural pressure distribution and its relationship to lung volume and interstitial pressure. *J Appl Physiol* 1991; **70**: 967–978.
11. Milic-Emili J, Henderson JAM, Dolovich MB et al. Regional distribution of inspired gas in the lung. *J Appl Physiol* 1966; **21**: 749–759.
12. Milic-Emili J. Static distribution of lung volumes. In: Macklem PT, Mead J, ed. *Handbook of Physiology, Vol. 3: Mechanics of breathing* (Section 3). Bethesda, MD: American Physiological Society, 1986: 561–574.
13. Senda M, Murata K, Itoh H et al. Quantitative evaluation of regional pulmonary ventilation using PET and nitrogen-13 gas. *J Nucl Med* 1986; **27**: 268–273.
14. Zwijnenburg A, Klumper A, Roos CM et al. Lung volume calculations from 81Krm SPECT for the quantitation of regional ventilation. *Clin Physiol Meas* 1988; **9**: 147–154.
15. Anthonisen NR, Danson J, Robertson PC, Ross WRD. Airway closure as a function of age. *Respir Physiol* 1970; **8**: 58–65.
16. Knudson RJ, Lebowitz MD, Burton AP, Knudson DE. The closing volume test: evaluation of nitrogen and bolus methods in a random population. *Am Rev Respir Dis* 1977; **115**: 423–434.
17. Glazier JB, Hughes JMB, Maloney JE, West JB. Vertical gradient of alveolar size in lungs of dogs frozen intact. *J Appl Physiol* 1967; **23**: 694–705.
18. West JB. Distribution of mechanical stress in the lung, a possible factor in localisation of pulmonary disease. *Lancet* 1971; **1**: 839–841.
19. Otis AB, McKerrow CB, Barlett RA et al. Mechanical factors in distribution of pulmonary ventilation. *J Appl Physiol* 1956; **8**: 427–443.
20. Greene R, Hughes JMB, Sudlow MF, Milic-Emili J. Regional lung volumes during water immersion to the xiphoid in seated man. *J Appl Physiol* 1974; **36**: 734–736.
21. Sybrecht G, Landau L, Murphy BG et al. Influence of posture on flow dependence of distribution of inhaled ^{133}Xe boli. *J Appl Physiol* 1976; **41**: 489–496.
22. Jones RL, Overton TR, Sproule BJ. Frequency dependence of ventilation distribution in normal and obstructed lungs. *J Appl Physiol* 1977; **42**: 548–553.
23. Chevrolet JC, Emrich J, Martin RR, Engel LA. Voluntary changes in ventilation distribution in the lateral posture. *Respir Physiol* 1979; **38**: 313–323.
24. Amis TC, Jones HA, Hughes JMB. Effect of posture on interregional distribution of pulmonary ventilation in man. *Respir Physiol* 1984; **56**: 145–167.
25. Paiva M. Uneven ventilation. In: Crystal RG, West JB, Weibel ER, Barnes PJ, eds. *The lung: scientific foundations.* 2nd ed. Philadelphia, Lippincott-Raven 1997; 1403–1413.
26. Crawford, AB, Dodd D, Engel LA. Changes in rib cage shape during quiet breathing, hyperventilation and single inspirations. *Respir Physiol* 1983; **54**: 197–209.
27. Roussos CS, Martin RR, Engel LA. Diaphragmatic contraction and the gradient of alveolar expansion in the lateral posture. *J Appl Physiol* 1977; **43**: 32–38.
28. Kelly SM, Brancatisano AP, Engel LA. Effect of cardiogenic gas mixing on arterial O_2 and CO_2 tensions during breath holding. *J Appl Physiol* 1987; **62**: 1453–1459.
29. Cybulsky IJ, Abel JG, Menon AS et al. Contribution of cardiogenic oscillations to gas exchange in constant-flow ventilation. *J Appl Physiol* 1987; **63**: 564–570.
30. Fowler KT, Read J. Cardiogenic oscillations in expired gas tensions, and regional pulmonary blood flow. *J Appl Physiol* 1961; **16**: 863–868.

31. Crawford AB, Makowska M, Kelly S, Engel LA. Effect of breath holding on ventilation maldistribution during tidal breathing in normal subjects. *J Appl Physiol* 1986; **61**: 2108–2115.
32. Menkes HA, Macklem PT. Collateral flow. *Handbook of physiology, the respiratory system 3.* Bethesda MD: American Physiological Society, 1984: 337–353.
33. Fowler WS. Lung function studies. II. The respiratory dead space. *Amer J Physiol* 1948; **154**: 405–416.
34. Norris RM. Effect of breath-holding on anatomical deadspace. *Clin Sci* 1967; **33**: 549–557.
35. El-Gamal FM. PhD Thesis, University of Newcastle upon Tyne, 1986
36. National Heart and Lung Institute. Suggested standardized procedures for closing volume determinations. (Nitrogen Method). Bethesda MD: National Heart and Lung Institute, 1973.
37. Sikand R, Cerretelli P, Farhi LE. Effects of Va and Va/Q distribution and of time on the alveolar plateau. *J Appl Physiol* 1966; **21**: 1331–1337.
38. Crawford AB, Cotton DJ, Paiva M, Engel LA. Effect of airway closure on ventilation distribution. *J Appl Physiol* 1989; **66**: 2511–2515.
39. Hamosh P, Taveira da Silva AM. Air bolus method compared to single breath method for determination of closing volume. *Am Rev Respir Dis* 1974; **110**: 518–520.
40. Dollfuss RE, Milic-Emili J, Bates DV. Regional distribution of ventilation of the lung studied with boluses of ^{133}Xenon. *Resp Physiol* 1967; **2**: 234–246.
41. Green, M, Travis DM, Mead J. A simple measurement of phase IV (closing volume) using a critical orifice helium analyser. *J Appl Physiol* 1972; **33**: 827–830.
42. Demedts M, Clément J, Stanescu DC, van de Woestijne KP. Inflection point on transpulmonary pressure–volume curves and closing volume. *J Appl Physiol* 1975; **38**: 228–235.
43. Olsen HC, Gilson JC. Respiratory symptoms, bronchitis and ventilatory capacity in man. *Br Med J* 1960; **1**: 450–456.
44. Lapp NL, Block J, Boehlecke B et al. Closing volume in coal miners. *Am Rev Respir Dis* 1976; **113**: 155–161.
45. Chinn DJ, Cotes JE, El Gamal FM, Wollaston JF. Respiratory health of young shipyard welders and other tradesmen studied cross sectionally and longitudinally. *Occup Environ Med* 1995; **55**: 33–42.
46. Teculescu DB, Damel MC, Costantino E et al. Computerised single-breath nitrogen washout: predicted values in a rural French community. *Lung* 1996; **174**: 43–55.
47. Martin RR, Lindsay D, Despas P et al. The early detection of airway obstruction. *Am Rev Respir Dis* 1975; **111**: 119–125
48. Abboud RT, Morton JW. Comparison of maximal mid-expiratory flow, flow volume curves, and nitrogen closing volumes in patients with mild airway obstruction. *Am Rev Respir Dis* 1975; **111**: 405–417.
49. Oxhøj H, Bake B, Wilhelmsen L. Ability of spirometry, flow–volume curves and the nitrogen closing volume test to detect smokers. *Scand J Respir Dis* 1977; **58**: 80–96.
50. Viegi G, Paoletti P, Di Pede F et al. Single breath nitrogen test in an epidemiologic study in North Italy. Reliability, reference values and relationships with symptoms. *Chest* 1988; **93**: 1213–1220.
51. Stanescu DC, Rodenstein DO, Hoeven C, Robert A. "Sensitive tests" are poor predictors of the decline in forced expiratory volume in one second in middle-aged smokers. *Am Rev Respir Dis* 1987; **135**: 585–590.
52. Buist AS, Vollmer WM, Johnson LR, McCamant LE. Does the single-breath N_2 test identify the smoker who will develop chronic airflow limitation? *Am Rev Respir Dis* 1988; **137**: 293–301.
53. Buist AS. Early detection of airways obstruction by the closing volume technique. *Chest* 1973; **64**: 495–499.
54. Cotes JE. Lung volume indices of airway obstruction: a suggestion for a new combined index. *Proc R Soc Med* 1971; **64**: 1232–1235.
55. Becklake MR. A new index of the intrapulmonary mixture of inspired air. *Thorax* 1952; **7**: 111–116.
56. Bouhuys A. Pulmonary nitrogen clearance in relation to age in healthy males. *J Appl Physiol* 1963; **18**: 297–300.
57. Prowse K, Cumming G. Effects of lung volume and disease on the lung nitrogen decay curve. *J Appl Physiol* 1973; **34**: 23–33.
58. Saidel GM, Salmon RB, Chester EH. Moment analysis of multibreath lung washout *J Appl Physiol* 1975; **38**: 328–334
59. Fleming GM, Chester EH, Saniie J, Saidel GM. Ventilation homogeneity using multibreath nitrogen washout: comparison of moment ratios and other indices. *Amer Rev Resp Dis* 1980; **121**: 789–794.
60. Wall MA, Misley MC, Brown A. Changes in ventilation homogeneity from preschool through young adulthood as determined by moment analysis of nitrogen washout *Paediatric Res* 1988; **23**: 68–71.
61. Gilson JC, Hugh-Jones P, Oldham PD, Meade F. Lung function in coal workers' pneumoconiosis. Gas-distribution and transfer. *Spec Rep Med Res Coun (Lond)* 1955; **290**: 114–124 and 150–201.
62. Verbanck S, Schuermans D, Paiva M, Vincken W. Nonreversible conductive airway ventilation heterogeneity in mild asthma. *J Appl Physiol* 2003; **94**: 1380–1386.
63. Gustafson PM, Aurora P, Lindblad A. Evaluation of ventilation maldistribution as an early indicator of lung disease in children with cystic fibrosis. *Eur Respir J* 2003; **22**: 972–979.
64. Muir DCF, The production of mono-dispersed aerosols by a La Mer-Sinclair generator. *Ann Occup Hyg* 1965; **8**: 233–238.
65. Cotes JE, Houston K, Saunders MJ. Interpretation of aerosol recovery curves following inhalation of monodispersed particles. *J Physiol (Lond)* 1971; **213**: 22p.
66. McCawley M, Lippmann M. Development of an aerosol dispersion test to detect early changes in lung function. *Am Ind Hyg Assoc J* 1988; **49**: 357–366.
67. Lapp NL, Hankinson JL, Amandus H, Palmes ED. Variability in the size of airspaces in normal human lungs as estimated by aerosols. *Thorax* 1975; **30**: 293–299.
68. Hankinson JL, Palmes ED, Lapp NL. Pulmonary air space size in coal miners. *Am Rev Respir Dis* 1979; **119**: 391–397.
69. Blanchard JD, Heyder J, O'Donnell CR, Brain JD. Aerosol-derived lung morphometry: comparisons with a lung model and lung function indexes. *J Appl Physiol* 1991; **71**: 1216–1224.
70. Brand P, Rieger C, Beinert T, Heyder J. Aerosol derived airway morphometry in healthy subjects. *Eur Respir J* 1995; **8**: 1639–1646.
71. Kohlhaufl M, Brand P, Rock, C et al. Non-invasive diagnosis of emphysema. Aerosol morphometry and aerosol bolus dispersion in comparison to HRCT. *Am J Respir Crit Care Med* 1999; **160:** 913–918.
72. Bennett WD, Smaldone GC. Use of aerosols to estimate mean air-space size in chronic obstructive pulmonary disease. *J Appl Physiol* 1988; **64**: 1554–1560.
73. Kohlhaufl M, Brand P, Selzer T et al. Diagnosis of emphysema in patients with chronic bronchitis: a new approach. *Eur Respir J* 1998; **12:** 793–798.
74. Brand P, Kohlhaufl M, Meyer T et al. Aerosol-derived airway morphometry and aerosol bolus dispersion in patients with lung fibrosis and lung emphysema. *Chest* 1999; **116**: 543–548.
75. Pedersen OF, Miller MR. Lung function. In: Anesi-Maesano, Gulsvik A, Viegi G, eds. *Respiratory epidemiology in Europe Eur Respir Mon* 2000, **5**: 167–198.

Further reading

Becklake MR, Permutt S. Evaluation of tests of lung function for screening for early detection of chronic obstructive lung disease. In: Macklem PT, Permutt S, ed. *The lung in the transition between health and disease.* New York: Marcel Dekker, 1979: 345–387.

Verbanck S, Schuermans D, Vincken W, Paiva M. Saline aerosol bolus dispersion. I. The effect of acinar airway alteration. *J Appl Physiol* 2001; **90**: 1754–1762.

Verbanck S, Schuermans D, Paiva M, Vincken W. Saline aerosol bolus dispersion. II. The effect of conductive airway alteration. *J Appl Physiol* 2001; **90**: 1763–1769.

Vollmer WM, McCamant LE, Johnson LR, Buist SA. Long-term reproducibility of tests of small airways function. *Chest* 1990; **98**: 303–307.

CHAPTER 17

Distribution and Measurement of Pulmonary Blood Flow

This chapter describes the distribution within the lungs and measurement of pulmonary blood flow; the flow is normally the same as cardiac output. The adjustment of blood flow with respect to ventilation is discussed in Chapter 18.

17.1 Distribution of pulmonary blood flow: mechanical and structural factors

17.1.1 Overview

In healthy persons the distribution of blood flow within the lungs is determined mainly by two mechanisms. The first is the vertical gradient of pressure due to the operation of gravitational force. The gradient influences the relative perfusion of superior and inferior zones of the lung; a related mechanism influences the distribution of ventilation (Section 16.1.8). These regional differences extend to affect gas exchange (e.g. Section 21.5.2). The second is the local anatomy. This leads to the flow within individual lobes being distributed unevenly. The unevenness is likely to be of little consequence if, as appears to be the case, the ventilation is distributed similarly. Subsidiary mechanisms include the extent of lung expansion and critical closure of arterioles.

17.1.2 Pulmonary capillaries

Pulmonary capillary blood volume. The volume is defined as that which participates in gas exchange. For an adult in a seated posture it is normally in the range 50–100 ml. The distribution is not uniform, but exhibits a vertical gradient; this is reduced on lying down when the distribution is more uniform in a prone than in a supine posture [1].

The volume increases during exercise to accommodate the increased metabolic demand. In addition the pulmonary capillary bed is a store for blood that is not required elsewhere in the body. The store is drawn on by the gastrointestinal tract in relation to meals and by the skin when there is a need to disperse heat. These and other determinants of pulmonary capillary blood volume and the method of measurement are given in Section 20.9 (e.g. Tables 20.11 and 20.12).

Pulmonary capillary blood flow. Blood flows through the lungs in pulses generated by contractions of the right ventricle. The pulses raise the pulmonary arterial pressure, distend the blood vessels of the lung and displace blood from pulmonary arterioles into alveolar capillaries where the flow is also pulsatile. Direct evidence that this affects the lung function has been obtained from two sources. For the lungs as a whole, measurements by body plethysmography have shown that instantaneous gas exchange oscillates at the frequency of the heartbeats (Section 17.3.3). At the local level, inspection of alveolar capillaries by light microscopy has shown that most capillaries contain blood that is in motion, in some the blood is stationary, whilst others contain only plasma. The proportion in the first category varies with cardiac output. The spare capacity ensures that the bed can accommodate the stroke volume during exercise and act as a blood depot in the manner described above.

17.1.3 Vertical gradient in blood flow

Studies using radioactive gases point to the perfusion varying down the vertical axis of the lung [2, 3]. Four zones have been identified (Fig. 17.1). Their location is determined mainly by the perfusion gradient. This is the resultant of the pulmonary arterial and venous pressures, both of which are subject to the influence of gravity, and the pressure in the alveoli (alveolar pressure) that in the absence of airflow obstruction is nearly uniform throughout the lungs.

Zone 1. For blood to flow, the intravascular pressure or the traction exerted on the vessel walls must exceed intraalveolar pressure. If not, the alveolar capillaries will be compressed and emptied of blood. Compression occurs at the apex of the lung (zone 1) when the subject is at rest in an upright posture. It affects the capillaries in the alveolar septa and is due to the local pulmonary arterial pressure falling below the alveolar pressure. The capillaries reopen if the pulmonary arterial pressure is increased, as occurs with exercise (Fig. 28.4, page 400), hypoxia or the subject adopting a supine posture. The closure does not affect the alveolar corner vessels as they are distended by inflation of the lung (cf. Fig. 11.2, page 119). These vessels provide a pathway for perfusion of superior parts of the lung [5].

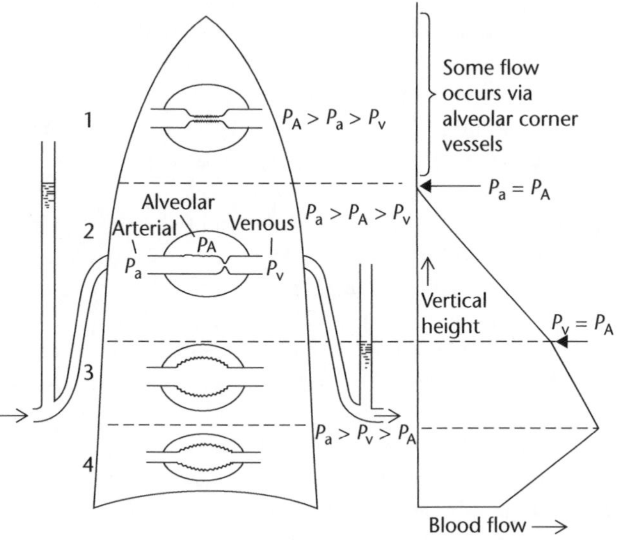

Fig. 17.1 Diagram showing the distribution of blood flow in the lung. In zone l the alveolar pressure (*P*a) exceeds the pulmonary arterial pressure (*P*a), so the alveolar septal vessels, but not the alveolar corner vessels, are collapsed. In zone 2 the arterial pressure exceeds the alveolar pressure, which in turn exceeds the venous pressure (*P*v); hence, the distal parts of the alveolar vessels are compressed and flow is reduced. The intravascular pressure then builds up and flow is resumed intermittently. This is the principle of the Starling resistor. On account of gravity affecting the venous pressure, the compression is greater and hence the flow is less at the top than at the bottom of this zone. Throughout zone 3 the driving pressure is the difference between the arterial and venous pressures. The intravascular pressure increases down the zone and the flow increases accordingly. The intravascular pressure is highest in zone 4 where it contributes to a rise in the interstitial pressure; this is of little consequence except when the interstitial pressure is also increased from other causes (see discussion of zone 4 in text). Source: [4]

Zone 2. In the upper part of the perfused region (zone 2) the pulmonary arterial pressure exceeds the alveolar pressure during systole but not during diastole. Both these designated pressures exceed those in pulmonary veins. In this circumstance the flow is intermittent or pulsatile and is determined by the arterial to alveolar pressure difference, not the absolute level. The conditions resemble a waterfall or weir in which the flow of water is independent of the height of the fall [6, 7]. Similar conditions obtain in a Starling resistor (Fig. 17.1).

Zone 3. This is the principal perfused region of the lung. Here the pulmonary venous pressure exceeds the alveolar pressure, so the vessels are distended with blood throughout their length. The flow is determined by the arterial to venous pressure gradient [8].

Zone 4. In the most dependent part of the lungs the intravascular hydrostatic pressure is relatively high. This can lead to fluid passing into the interstitial tissue. In normal circumstances the quantity of fluid is small. It can increase dramatically if pulmonary venous pressure and/or the permeability of the pulmonary capillary membrane are increased or the plasma osmotic pressure is reduced, thus causing alveolar interstitial oedema (Section 41.12). In any of these circumstances the blood flow at the base of the lung (zone 4) is reduced. In addition, the lung becomes stiffer and this impairs the function further (e.g. Section 38.3.2).

17.1.4 Lung expansion

As well as being influenced by gravitational force, the distribution of blood flow is affected by the degree of lung expansion because this contributes to the traction across the various structures. Estimates of the magnitude of the response are subject to the limitations of isotope methodology (Sections 7.12 and 18.6). The response is best expressed as blood flow per alveolus; this varies with the depth of inspiration (Fig. 17.2). Flow to the bases of the lung is reduced following expiration to residual volume.

17.1.5 Flow across defined planes within the lungs

Understanding of the anatomical component of distribution of blood flow is of recent origin. This is due to the earlier radioisotope studies employing radiation detectors that averaged over

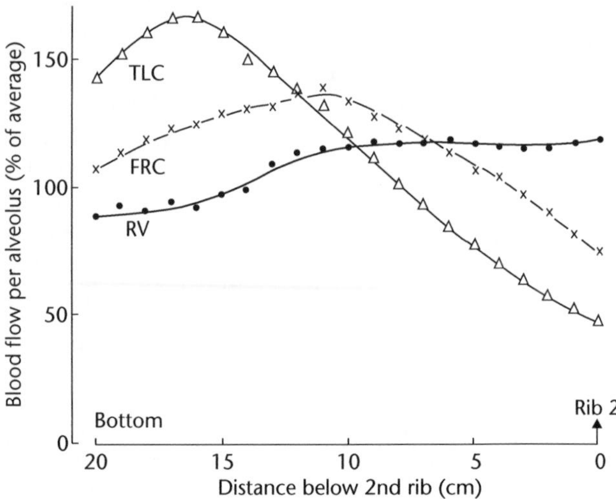

Fig. 17.2 Relationship of blood flow per alveolus to distance below the second rib in seated subjects holding the breath at different lung volumes. Blood flow is expressed relative to the average. TLC: total lung capacity, FRC: functional residual capacity, RV: residual volume. Source: [9], see also Section 18.6.

transverse planes in the lung. Using this approach, variability within planes is not detectable.

The local distribution of pulmonary blood flow in 2-cm cubes of lung tissue has been examined following injection of microspheres into the pulmonary circulation [10]. Different postures have been used and several species of mammal investigated. The results show that two thirds of the variability in regional perfusion is due to a factor common to all postures, probably the anatomical structure of the lungs. This finding has been confirmed in studies during weightlessness [11].

17.1.6 Critical closure of arterioles

In the systemic circulation an arteriole closes if the pressure within its lumen is reduced suddenly to below a critical level [12]. The initiating mechanism is that the smooth muscle in the wall of the artery does not immediately relax to a comparable extent. Instead the excess tension summates with the elastic recoil of the wall of the vessel to cause abrupt obliteration of the lumen. The pressure proximal to the closure then rises until it exceeds the critical closing pressure. When this happens the patency is restored.

Critical closure appears to be an intrinsic property of arterioles. In the lung it provides a mechanism for stabilising the level of pulmonary arterial pressure by permitting rapid adjustment to the number of arterioles that are perfused with blood.

17.1.7 Measurement of distribution of blood flow

Go to Section 18.6

17.2 Pulmonary vasomotor tone

17.2.1 Introduction

The pulmonary circulation differs from the systemic circulation in operating with relatively low systolic and diastolic pressures (normal levels approximately 25 and 10 mm Hg, respectively). The normal mean pressure is approximately 15 mm Hg (2 kPa) and the driving force to maintain the pulmonary circulation is only about 10 mm Hg (1.3 kPa) compared to about 80 mm Hg (10.6 kPa) in the systemic circulation. The low flow resistance is associated with the walls of small pulmonary arteries containing a relatively thin layer of smooth muscle and having little by way of muscle tone. The muscle tone is increased by a reduced oxygen tension; this can be either local when it reduces the local blood flow or generalised throughout the lungs when it raises pulmonary arterial pressure. Persistent hypertension leads to progressive hypertrophy of smooth muscle cells in the walls of small pulmonary arteries. This has clinical implications (Section 17.2.4).

The residual tone represents mainly a balance within the sympathetic nervous system between the activities of α_1 adrenoceptors that promote contraction of vascular smooth muscle and α_2 and β adrenoceptors that promote relaxation [13]. The pharmacological control mechanisms have features in common with those that regulate bronchomotor tone (Section 15.2).

The α_1 adrenoceptors respond to hypoxia, severe hypercapnia and some chemicals via stimulation of chemoreceptors in the carotid body. This reflex is weaker in man than in some other mammals. It is subsidiary to the direct response of vascular smooth muscle to hypoxia that is described below. The α_1 receptors may also be the final common path for reflexes arising from the vascular regulatory area in the medulla. Nonadrenergic noncholinergic nerves may also be involved, but their role appears not to have been established *in vivo*.

Stimulation of cholinergic nerves can cause vasodilatation. This mechanism appears to operate only when the vasomotor tone is increased. In this circumstance, acetylcholine stimulates the release of nitric oxide; the latter then promotes vasodilatation through a mechanism that is described below.

17.2.2 Hypoxic vasoconstriction

In 1946 von Euler and Liljestrand made the important observation that ventilation of the lungs with gas deficient in oxygen or containing carbon dioxide raised the pressure in the pulmonary artery [14]. They suggested that the rise was the sum of local pulmonary vasoconstrictor responses throughout the lungs. If so, the constriction provided a mechanism for reducing the perfusion to parts of the lung that were poorly ventilated and hence for minimising hypoxaemia due to local hypoventilation. Subsequent work has confirmed this hypothesis and shown that local hypoxia acts in this way in man. The control mechanism

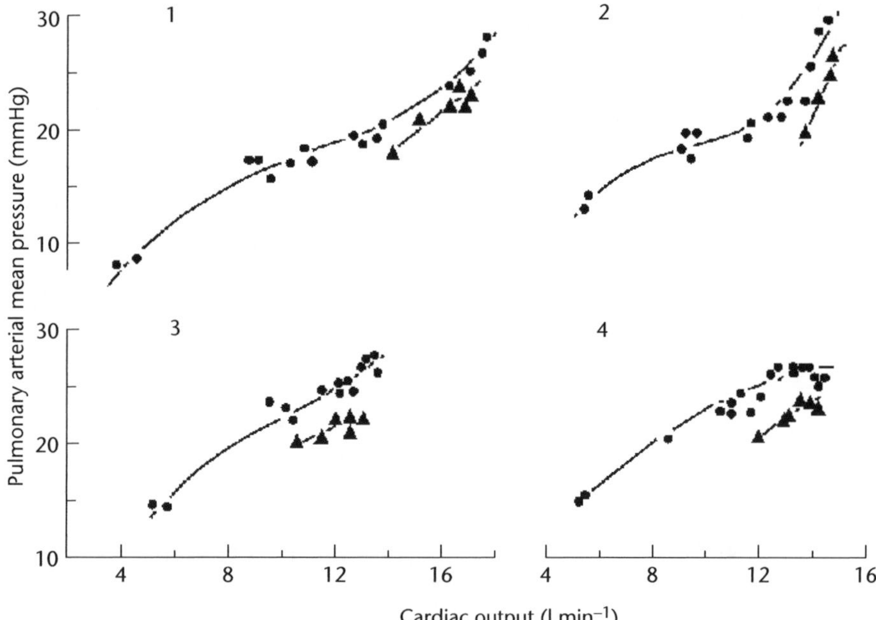

Fig. 17.3 Parallel shifts in the relationship of pulmonary arterial mean pressure to cardiac output in response to breathing oxygen instead of air during exercise (▲ and ●, respectively). The subjects were four asymptomatic working coal miners with normal lung function and pulmonary arterial mean pressures. Source: [18]

is independent of local hypercapnia and acidaemia. These circumstances can affect the vasomotor tone, but, whereas a fall in pH stimulates vasoconstriction, the response is less when the acidaemia is caused by carbon dioxide.

Contraction of pulmonary vascular smooth muscle is normally controlled by the local tension of oxygen within the muscle cells [15]. The tension is the resultant of diffusion of oxygen from adjacent sources; these are alveolar gas, mixed venous blood and bronchial arteries that supply blood vessels (vasa vasorum) in the walls of pulmonary arteries. Hypoxic vasoconstriction occurs at oxygen tensions in the range 13 kPa down to 2.7 kPa (100 to 20 mm Hg). More severe hypoxia causes vasodilatation.

Hypoxic vasoconstriction is due in part to oxidative stress associated with an increase in concentration of phosphatidylcholine hydroperoxide. This follows a rise in the local concentration of xanthine oxidase and can be reversed by the anti-oxidant substance N-acetylcysteine [16]. However, the normal corrective is to increase the local tension of oxygen in the muscle cell. This leads to immediate relaxation; its extent varies with the local oxygen tension up to the normal level of breathing air. In healthy people higher oxygen tensions do not have any additional effect [17]. However, in patients with lung disease the critical local oxygen tension may only be achieved by breathing air enriched with oxygen. In addition, if the vasoconstriction has been of long duration the full response will not occur until the associated muscle hypertrophy has been reversed (see below: Clinical aspects). Hypoxic vasoconstriction can also be reversed by some sympathomimetic drugs including aminophylline and isoprenaline.

Vasodilatation due to release of hypoxic vasoconstriction influences the relationship of pulmonary vascular pressure to pulmonary blood flow; this exhibits a nearly parallel shift (Fig. 17.3). Several explanations have been suggested [19]. One is that the shift is due to the opening of vessels via the Starling resistor mechanism illustrated in Fig. 17.1.

Susceptibility to hypoxic pulmonary vasoconstriction is an inherited characteristic that varies between people and between different species of mammal. Some creatures that live at high altitude, including the llama and bar-headed goose, are not affected. In man the susceptible individuals are at increased risk of pulmonary hypertension if they ascend to high altitude or develop a generalised lung disease [20]. Such persons may have low efficiency sodium pumps in the cells lining their alveoli [21].

17.2.3 Local pharmacological mechanisms

The smooth muscle cells in the walls of small pulmonary arteries are subject to a number of local influences of which the most important are the prevailing concentrations of guanosine and adenosine 3′–5′ cyclic monophosphate (respectively, cGMP and cAMP). Both these substances dilate vascular smooth muscle. They act by reducing the local concentration of calcium ions (Ca^{2+}) within the muscle cells and hence the extent of contraction of myosin. The cAMP mechanism is brought into play by stimulation of β-adrenergic or prostaglandin PGI2 receptors. The cGMP mechanism is activated by a pathway that includes nitric oxide; this substance is the principal and, in man, possibly the only constituent of endothelium-derived relaxing factor (EDRF). It is formed from l-arginine through a reaction that is mediated via an increase in oxygen tension. This pathway increases the formation and hence the local concentration of cGMP. The latter substance is normally inactivated through the action

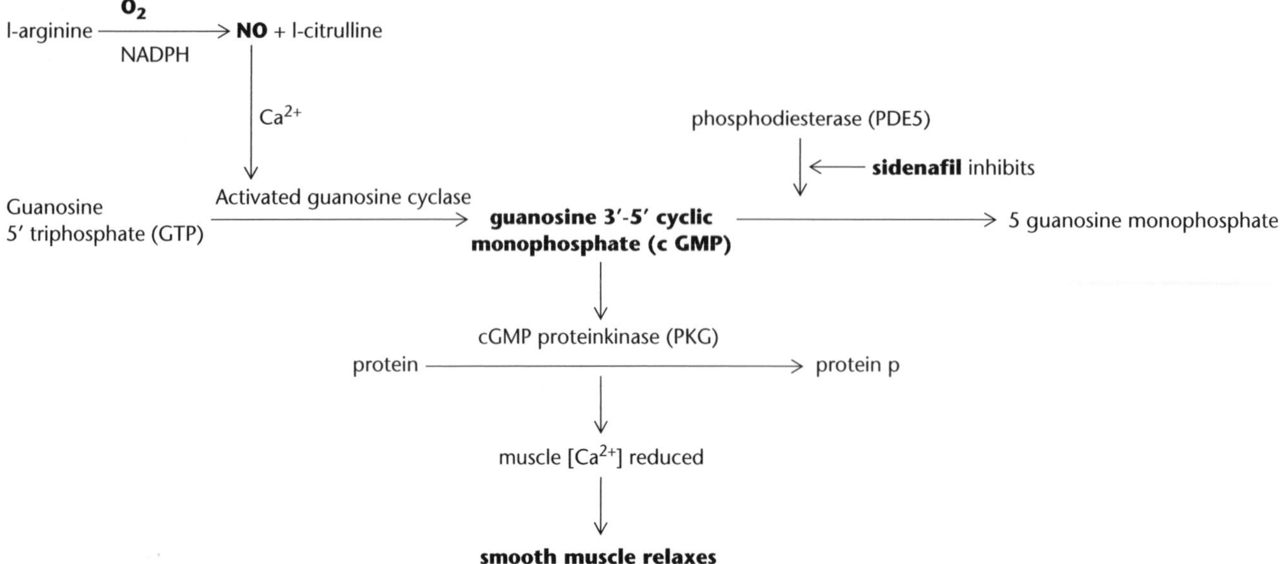

Fig. 17.4 Model illustrating the roles of nitric oxide, oxygen and sildenafil in reversing hypoxic pulmonary vasoconstriction. Source: [22]

of phosphodiesterase (PDE5). Inhibition of this reaction leads to vasodilatation (see Fig. 17.4). The related features are currently the subject of intensive research [e.g. 23–26].

Other substances can also change the pulmonary vasomotor tone. However, the extent and direction of any effect can vary between species and with circumstances; these include the prevailing oxygen tension and the presence of other active substances. Thus, the relevance of the observations is often uncertain and the full picture has still to emerge [27].

Amongst substances that are predominantly vasodilators, calcitonin-generated peptide and vasoactive intestinal peptide act directly on the smooth muscle cells. The actions of superoxide dismutase, bradykinin and substance P are mediated through the release of nitric oxide. One or more of these compounds may contribute to pulmonary vasodilatation in patients with portal hypertension. Platelet activating factor can cause dilatation, but more often it is a vasoconstrictor. Vasoconstriction can also occur in response to angiotensin II, histamine, prostaglandin F2α and opioid peptides; some of these substances can contribute to the responses to lung injury.

17.2.4 Clinical aspects

Pulmonary vasomotor tone is high during foetal life and falls at birth; the change is mediated by nitric oxide (Section 24.2). Subsequently, the tone is generally low, but local vasoconstriction in response to local hypoxia secondary to hypoventilation is of crucial importance for gas exchange (Section 18.1.1). The vasoconstriction improves the oxygenation of the blood by reducing the contribution from lung units with a low $\dot{V}_A/\dot{Q}$ ratio. It also raises the pressure in the pulmonary circulation. Persistence of this condition can lead to hypertrophy of smooth muscle cells in the walls of small pulmonary arteries, severe pulmonary hypertension and right heart failure. The condition responds gradually to long-term oxygen therapy (Section 35.7.1). In addition to oxygen the vasoconstriction can be reduced by other vasodilator drugs such as nitric oxide [28], but at the cost of aggravating the $\dot{V}_A/\dot{Q}$ imbalance. For this reason hypoxaemia can complicate the relief of bronchoconstriction by a non-selective or partially selective drug that also relaxes pulmonary blood vessels [29].

Generalised pulmonary vasoconstriction occurs in persons exposed to a reduced barometric pressure at altitude or in a decompression chamber. In these circumstances vasodilator drugs are irrelevant as the hypoxaemia affects all organs, not only the lungs. The appropriate response is to raise the barometric pressure or administer oxygen.

17.3 Measurement of cardiac output and pulmonary blood flow

17.3.1 Introduction

The outputs of the right and left ventricles only differ by the amount of any intravascular shunt and this is normally small. Hence, in most circumstances either quantity can provide an estimate of cardiac output and pulmonary blood flow. If there is a shunt, the choice of procedure and interpretation should be considered carefully.

Cardiac output is traditionally measured by application of the law of conservation of mass (Fick principle) to an indicator substance that traverses the pulmonary circulation. It can also be measured by physical methods of which the most satisfactory is that of aortic blood flow velocity by the Doppler ultrasound technique with separate estimation of aortic diameter. Electrical bio-impedance, ballistocardiography and other techniques can be used but their accuracy is lower.

17.3.2 Fick methods for gases and indicator substances

The Fick methods entail measuring over a timed interval the dilution of a known amount of indicator material and accounting for all of it. The relationship has the form

$$F \times C\alpha.\text{out} = j + F \times C\alpha.\text{in} \qquad (17.1)$$

where F is the flow, $C\alpha$ is the equilibrium concentration of indicator material entering or leaving the mixing chamber and j is the rate at which the indicator is added to or removed from the system. Hence for oxygen

$$\dot{Q}\text{t}\,(1\ \text{min}^{-1}) = \frac{\dot{n}\text{o}_2}{44.6}/(\text{Ca, o}_2 - C\bar{\text{v}},\text{o}_2) \qquad (17.2)$$

where $\dot{Q}$t is cardiac output and $\dot{n}$ o_2 is oxygen consumption (mmol min^{-1}). When oxygen consumption is in l min^{-1} the conversion factor (44.6) is omitted. The term within the bracket is the difference between the quantities of oxygen in arterial (a) and mixed venous blood ($\bar{v}$) in litres STPD per litre; it is the volume of oxygen added to 1 l of blood in the lungs. Other gases that can be used include carbon dioxide and the moderately soluble gases acetylene, nitrous oxide and freon-22. For acetylene a correction of approximately 10% is made for the quantity which dissolves in lung tissue. Highly soluble gases, for example diethyl ether, cannot be used because uptake occurs into the epithelium of the upper respiratory tract. Insoluble gases, such as helium or argon, are unsuitable because the quantity exchanged is too small to be measured accurately. The principle of mass balance also applies to substances administered by injection including indocyanine green dye and cold saline. For the latter substance the resulting temperature change provides a nearly unique signal in not being affected by recirculation of blood back to the lungs from the systemic circulation.

Direct Fick method for oxygen. This is the standard against which other methods are compared. The procedure entails cannulation of a peripheral artery (Section 7.9) and catheterisation of the right heart for placement of a catheter in a pulmonary artery. The catheter has a double lumen and is fitted with an inflatable balloon. It is inserted into a peripheral vein and allowed to float with the flow of blood returning to the heart. When the balloon reaches the right atrium it is inflated and this leads to the catheter being carried into a pulmonary artery [30]. Collections of systemic arterial blood, mixed venous blood from the pulmonary artery and mixed expired gas for measurement of oxygen consumption (Section 7.8.1) are made concurrently under steady state conditions usually over a 2-min period. The calculation is given in eqn. 17.2.

Rebreathing method using oxygen. By this method [31] the content of oxygen in arterial blood is estimated from that in end tidal gas sampled at the lips. The latter quantity (Pet,o_2) exceeds the tension in arterial blood (Pa,o_2) by an amount (a) that is approximately 1.6 kPa (12 torr). Hence,

$$P\text{a,o}_2 = P\text{et,o}_2 - \text{a} \qquad (17.3)$$

The oxygen tension of pulmonary pre-capillary blood is obtained by a rebreathing method. The corresponding oxygen contents are obtained via the oxygen dissociation curve; hence the method is invalid if there is a shunt of blood across the lungs. The calculation of cardiac output is made using eqn. 17.2.

The capacity of the rebreathing bag is usually 6 l and it initially contains a volume of gas equal to the functional residual capacity of the subject. The gas composition is carbon dioxide in a fractional concentration of 0.09 with the remainder gas nitrogen, but the composition is subject to adjustment. Rebreathing is for 10 s and the subject rebreathes deeply and rapidly. The oxygen concentration at the lips is monitored using a respiratory mass spectrometer. During rebreathing the oxygen tensions of gas from the lungs and from the bag converge towards a plateau value. This is usually reached within 4 s and persists thereafter (Fig. 17.5).

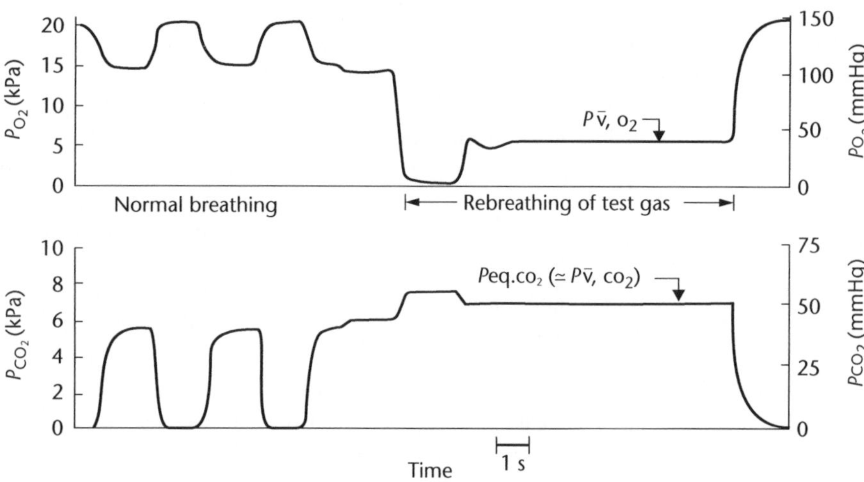

Fig. 17.5 Measurement of mixed venous gas tensions by rebreathing. The record was obtained using a respiratory mass spectrometer and shows sustained equilibria for both oxygen and carbon dioxide. The rebreathing bag initially contained carbon dioxide in the fractional concentration 0.08 with the remainder nitrogen. However, a plateau for oxygen is attained more readily if some oxygen is added to the gas mixture. For details see text. Source: [31]

At this point the oxygen tension is equal to that of mixed venous blood [32]. In some circumstances the venous tension can fall to a dangerously low level, for example during strenuous exercise and in subjects who are anaemic or have atherosclerosis. The method is used mainly for young adults. In other circumstances the carbon dioxide method is preferable.

Rebreathing method using carbon dioxide. This method resembles that for oxygen so is affected by poor lung mixing or the presence of a blood shunt across the lungs. Fluctuations in the quantity of carbon dioxide dissolved in lung tissue can also influence the result, but in practice this is unimportant. The carbon dioxide output is obtained by collection and analysis of expired gas (Section 7.8).

The CO_2 tension in systemic arterial blood is obtained in one of three ways:

1 Analysis of arterialised blood from an ear lobe (Section 7.11.1),

2 Calculation from that in mixed expired gas assuming a value for the physiological deadspace (Section 18.4.1). In the method of Jones and colleagues [33] the following relationship is used:

$$Pa,CO_2 = Pet,CO_2 - 0.133\,[(4 \times \dot{n}\,CO_2/44.6) - 0.13\,f\mathrm{R} + 0.75] \tag{17.4}$$

where Pa,CO_2 and Pet,CO_2 are, respectively, the tensions of carbon dioxide in arterial blood and end-tidal gas in kPa, $\dot{n}\,CO_2$ is the output of carbon dioxide in mmol min^{-1} and $f\mathrm{R}$ is the frequency of breathing per min. When the measurement is made in l min^{-1} and mm Hg the conversion factors 0.133 and 44.6 should be omitted.

3 Derivation from the mean alveolar or end tidal CO_2 tension. The latter is obtained by continuous analysis of expired gas at the lips using a rapid infrared gas analyser or respiratory mass spectrometer.

The tension of CO_2 in pulmonary pre-capillary blood (i.e. mixed venous blood, $P\bar{v}, CO_2$, Fig. 17.5) is obtained by rebreathing a gas mixture containing 30% O_2 and 9–13% CO_2. Some subjects experience discomfort during the rebreathing.

The blood–gas tension difference ($P\bar{v},CO_2 - Pa,CO_2$) is used to calculate the corresponding content difference ($C\bar{v},CO_2 - Ca,CO_2$) which in turn is inserted into the Fick equation for cardiac output:

$$\dot{Q}t\,(1\,min^{-1}) = \frac{\dot{n}\,CO_2}{44.6}/(C\bar{v},CO_2 - Ca,CO_2) \tag{17.5}$$

In this equation the terms, units and conversion factor are as for eqn. 17.2 but with carbon dioxide substituted for oxygen.

Practical detail of the rebreathing method for $P\bar{v},CO_2$. The capacity of the rebreathing bag should normally be 5 l, the volume of test gas 1.5 times the tidal volume of the subject and the rebreathing time at least 12 s. The composition of the test gas is that needed to achieve equilibrium and is determined by trial and error. For the initial trial the gas composition should be 0.3 ($F\mathrm{I},O_2$), 0.11 ($F\mathrm{I},CO_2$), 0.59 ($F\mathrm{I},N_2$) and during rebreathing the fluctuations in carbon dioxide tension between inspiration and expiration should narrow to less than 0.1 kPa (1 torr). If, instead of a plateau, the concentration rises or falls throughout the rebreathing then the procedure should be repeated using, respectively, a $F\mathrm{I},CO_2$ of 0.09 or 0.13. The interval between trials should be at least 3 min. Alternatively, the linear part of the record can be extrapolated to 20 s from the start of rebreathing and the corresponding CO_2 tension used instead [34, 35]. The equilibrium tension of carbon dioxide should, theoretically, be equal to that in pulmonary pre-capillary blood and this is usually the case at rest. However, on exercise the equilibrium gas tension exceeds the blood tension by a small amount. This difference is technical and can be allowed for using the following empirical equation [36]:

$$Pox, \bar{v}, CO_2 = Peq,CO_2 - 0.133(1.4 + 2.6\,\dot{n}\,CO_2/44.6)\,k\mathrm{Pa} \tag{17.6}$$

where $Pox,\bar{v},CO_2$ is the tension of carbon dioxide in oxygenated mixed venous blood, Peq,CO_2 is the equilibrium tension of carbon dioxide and $\dot{n}\,CO_2$ is output of carbon dioxide in mmol min^{-1}. The constant terms 0.133 and 44.6 are omitted when traditional units are used.

The conversion from blood gas tensions to the corresponding contents of carbon dioxide is best done using the following relationship:

$$CCO_2,\text{blood} = CCO_2,\text{plasma} \times \left(1 - \frac{0.0289[\mathrm{Hb}]}{(3.352 - 0.456 \times SO_2) \times (8.142 - \mathrm{pH})}\right) \tag{17.7}$$

where CCO_2, plasma $= 2.226 \times s \times$ plasma $PCO_2 \times (1 + 10^{pH - pK'})$, CCO_2 is CO_2 content, SO_2 is O_2 saturation, s is the plasma CO_2 solubility coefficient, and pK' is the apparent pK from the equations of Kelman [see 37]. Alternatively the nomogram of McHardy (Fig. 17.6) can be used instead.

Intra-breath method for carbon dioxide. By this method the tensions of carbon dioxide in systemic arterial and mixed venous blood are obtained from an analysis of gas sampled at the lips during a single slow expiration. The gas tension difference is converted to a content difference and is used in the Fick equation as described above. The method has the advantages that all the data required for the calculations are obtained during the test expiration and measurements can be repeated at intervals of approximately 40 s. Hence, it can be used to follow changes in cardiac output at the start or end of exercise. The method is unreliable in the presence of uneven lung function. The basic procedure [39] is described in Fig. 17.7. It can be improved without introducing a second stage into the procedure by the subject

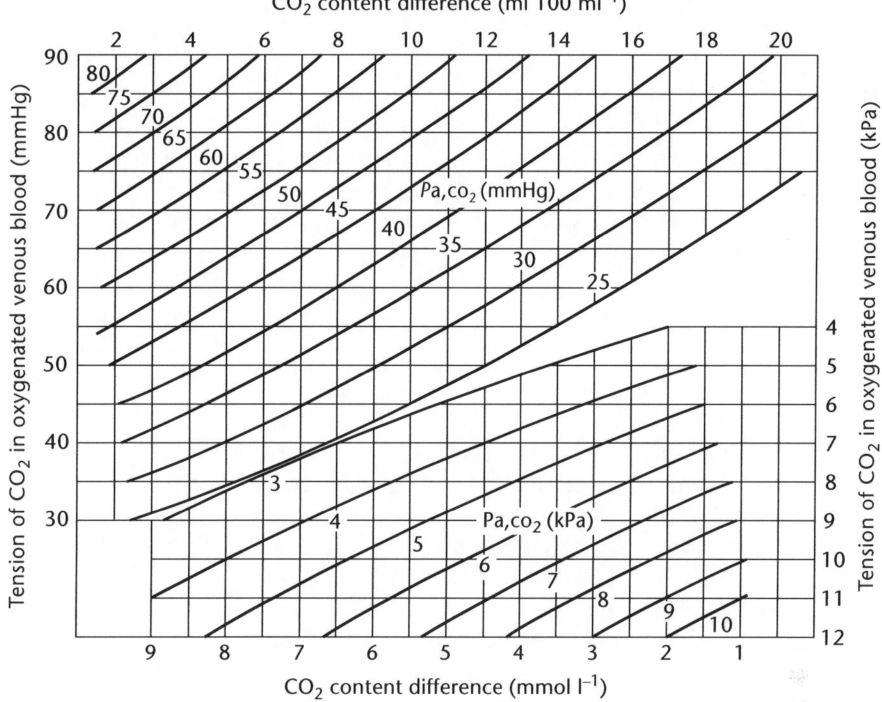

Fig. 17.6 Differences in content of carbon dioxide between venous and arterial blood ($C\bar{v},co_2 - Ca,co_2$) for a range of tensions of carbon dioxide in arterial and oxygenated venous blood. They are calculated for a saturation of oxygen in arterial blood (Sa,o_2) of 95% and a blood concentration of haemoglobin monomer of 9.2 mmol l^{-1} (15 g dl^{-1}). Where one or both of these quantities deviate materially from the assumed values, the true CO_2 content difference may be obtained by addition of a factor (f); in traditional units this is calculated as follows:

$f = 0.015\ (\mathrm{Hb} - 15)\ (P\bar{v},co_2 - Pa,co_2) - 0.064\ (95 - Sa,o_2)$ ml dl^{-1}

[e.g. Pa,co_2 and $P\bar{v},co_2$, respectively 40 and 55 torr, Hb 10 g dl^{-1}, Sa,o_2 100%. The factor is then –0.8 and the corrected difference 5.3 ml dl^{-1}]. Source: [38]

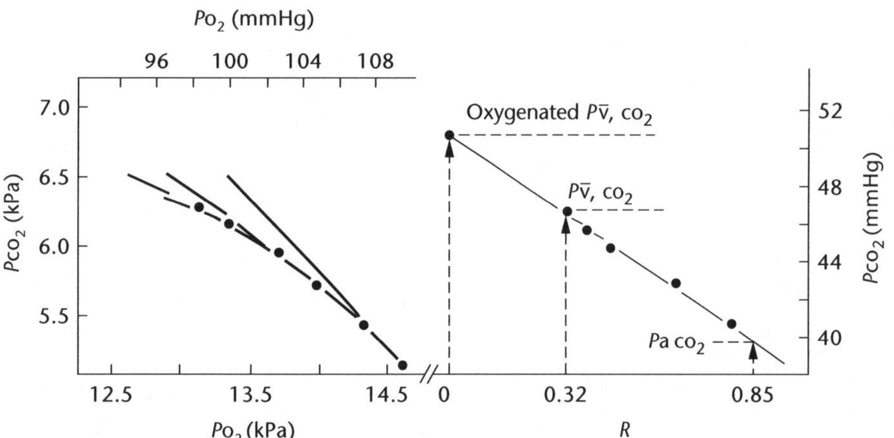

Fig. 17.7 Derivation of the tensions of carbon dioxide in arterial and mixed venous blood from analysis of expired gas for oxygen and carbon dioxide during a single expiration. The data are plotted in the form of an O_2–CO_2 diagram (Fig. 21.6, page 270) and the best curve is fitted. The slopes (S) at successive points on the curve are used to calculate values for respiratory exchange ratio (R) using the alveolar air equation (Eqn. 18.6, page 217) rearranged into the form

$$S = [R + (1 - R)F_{I,CO_2}]/[1 - (1 - R)F_{I,O_2}]$$

Pco_2 is plotted against R, where a linear relationship is obtained. The Pco_2 of arterial blood is that associated with the steady state R (usually 0.85). The Pco_2 of mixed venous blood is that associated with an R of 0.32. This is because at $R = 0.32$ the CO_2 output relative to the oxygen uptake (0.32:1.0) is due solely to oxygen displacing CO_2 from combination with haemoglobin (Haldane effect, Section 21.2.2); the Pco_2 remains constant and equal as between arterial and mixed venous blood. The Pco_2 of the oxygenated mixed venous blood is similarly defined by $R = 0$, when there are equal *contents* of carbon dioxide in arterial and mixed venous blood.
Source: [39]

performing controlled rebreathing during the expiration (Ohta Y unpublished, also [40]).

Methods using inert gas. Advances in mass spectrometry have facilitated the use of soluble gases that are inert and do not react with blood as alternatives to resident gases for measurement of cardiac output. The gases include acetylene, nitrous oxide and freon-22. For such gases the Fick equation has the form:

$$\dot{Q} = \dot{n},\mathrm{tg}/a(P_{\mathrm{A}} - P_{\bar{v}})\,\mathrm{l\ min^{-1}} \quad (17.8)$$

where $\dot{Q}$ is cardiac output ($\mathrm{l\ min^{-1}}$), $\dot{n}$, tg is the uptake of test gas ($\mathrm{mmol\ min^{-1}}$) and P_{A} and $P_{\bar{v}}$ are, respectively, the tensions (kPa) in alveolar gas and mixed venous blood. The factor (a) is the solubility of the gas in blood at 37°C (Table 19.1, page 225).

The tension in alveolar gas is usually obtained by analysis of a gas sample obtained after exhalation of 750 ml to flush the deadspace. The tension in mixed venous blood is initially zero. It rises after about 20 s on account of recirculation of blood containing gas absorbed during the previous passage through the lungs. Hence, the breath hold or rebreathing must be completed within this time [41–45]. When freon is used the concentration in the indicator should be 4% and its alveolar concentration analysed using a respiratory mass spectrometer. The pulmonary blood flow is given by

$$\dot{Q}_{\mathrm{C}} = \frac{V_{\mathrm{A}}.P_{\mathrm{B}}/(P_{\mathrm{B}} - P_{\mathrm{H_2O}})}{S\beta \times t[V_{\mathrm{A}}/(V_{\mathrm{A}} + \mathrm{Sti}\,V\mathrm{ti})] \times \log_e[V_{\mathrm{A}}/(V_{\mathrm{A}} + \mathrm{Sti}\,V\mathrm{ti}) \times (F_{\mathrm{A}},\mathrm{fr_O}/F_{\mathrm{A}},\mathrm{fr}_t)]} \quad (17.9)$$

where V_{A} is alveolar volume estimated from the dilution of the inert gas (eqn. 20.16, page 225), t is breath-holding time, P_{B} is barometric pressure, Vti is lung tissue volume (approximately 11.5% of V_{A}), S is Bunsen solubility coefficient for freon, respectively, in blood (β) and lung tissue (ti) and F_{A},fr is the alveolar concentration of freon-22. The concentration at time 0 is calculated from the inspired concentration and the initial and alveolar concentrations of the inert gas, that at time t is obtained from the alveolar gas sampled at the end of breath holding. The intermediate calculations are as for the measurement of transfer factor (Section 20.4), hence the two can be combined in a single manoeuvre [46].

In one study [43] the reproducibility, expressed as the standard error of the estimate, was reported as approximately 0.7 $\mathrm{l\ min^{-1}}$. The relationship to the direct Fick method was given by

$$\dot{Q}\ \text{freon-22} = 1.37 + 0.77\dot{Q}\ \text{Fick}\ \pm 0.49 \quad (17.10)$$

Plethysmograph method. The measurement is made at rest or during cycle ergometry in a whole body plethysmograph (Section 14.6). The subject inhales first a vital capacity breath of oxygen to raise the alveolar oxygen tension, then a vital capacity breath of 100% nitrous oxide. This is followed immediately by partial exhalation, then breath holding for 15 s at functional residual capacity. The subject then breathes out. During the exhalations the expired gas is analysed for nitrous oxide. To obtain cardiac output the mean of the two alveolar concentrations is inserted into a version of eqn. 17.1, together with the gas uptake measured by plethysmography. The procedure is then repeated with air as the test gas.

When a constant volume plethysmograph is used the uptake of nitrous oxide by blood causes a fall in pressure. This is converted to volume by use of the calibration factor for the box. Using a constant pressure box the change in volume is obtained using a pneumatic servo-system that adds gas at the rate needed to keep the pressure constant.

The signal that is obtained has a steady component that reflects changes in temperature. There is also a variable component with a pronounced cardiac rhythm. The procedure can be modified to show a respiratory rhythm as well. After allowing for the effects of temperature, the signal reflects uptake of nitrous oxide and also variations in respiratory exchange ratio due to different rates of uptake and evolution of oxygen and carbon dioxide in the lungs (R effect). The observations are evidence that the pulsations of alveolar capillary blood flow are imparted to gas exchange across the alveolar capillary membrane [47, 48]. Pulsatility has also been demonstrated for other gases [e.g. 49].

Indicator dilution methods. For this application of the Fick principle the cardiac output is determined from the dilution of a measured quantity of indicator substance that is injected rapidly into the superior vena cava or pulmonary artery. The method has the advantage for respiratory patients of being independent of uneven lung function. It can also be repeated after a brief period (40 s to 2 min depending on the indicator) so can be used for studying responses to exercise or other stimuli.

Immediately following the injection, the concentration of indicator in blood is recorded at a site distal to where mixing with resident blood has taken place. The sampling site is usually a systemic artery, but for material injected into the superior vena cava the pulmonary artery is sampled instead. The concentration of indicator is initially zero. Then as indicator reaches the sampling site its concentration rises. Subsequently, the concentration falls exponentially towards the initial value. The decline may be interrupted by a secondary rise due to some of the indicator material traversing the lungs a second time. The effect on the dilution curve of recirculation of indicator material is eliminated by replotting the exponential portion of the curve on semi-log paper when the decline is effectively linear and can be extrapolated to zero. The cardiac output is calculated from the quantity of indicator and the total area under the dilution curve expressed in log normal units (Fig. 17.8).

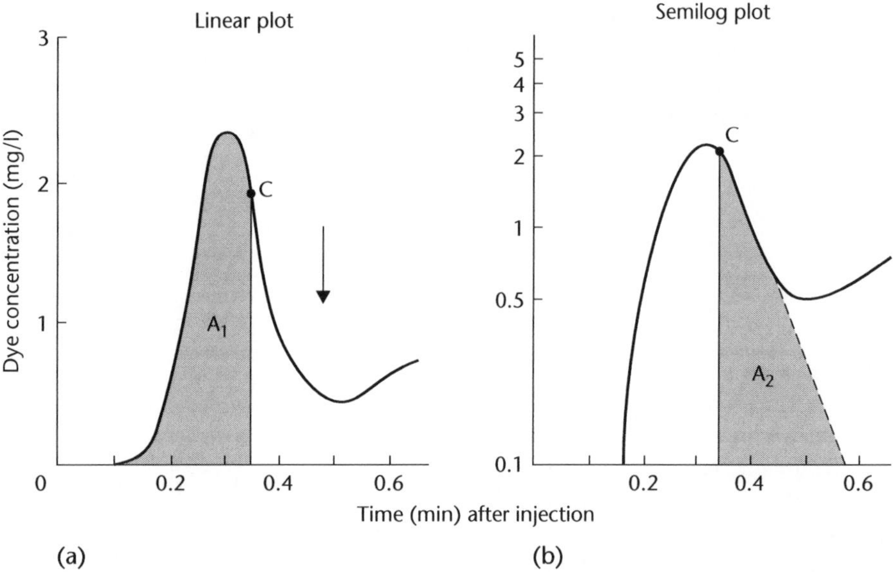

Fig. 17.8 Measurement of cardiac output by the indicator dilution method. In this instance the indicator was indocyanine green. The dye concentration in blood was obtained using a spectrophotometer and lamp mounted, respectively, above and below a cuvette through which blood from the brachial artery was drawn at a constant rate. The light absorption at a wavelength of 805 nm (8050 Å) was compared with that of samples of the subject's blood containing known concentrations of dye. These were prepared by a serial dilution method. Graph (a) shows the changes in concentration following rapid injection of 3 mg of dye into the superior vena cava. The arrow marks the recirculation of dye through the systemic circulation. In graph (b) the data have been replotted on a semi-log scale. The interrupted line is a linear extrapolation of the descending exponential portion of the curve before recirculation of dye has taken place. The area under this part of the curve (A_2) is given by

$$\text{Area}\,(A_2) = \frac{\text{Concentration of dye at C}}{\text{Slope of exponential}}$$

The area (A_1) is obtained by planimetry. The total area is the product of time (min) and mean concentration of dye (mg l^{-1}); when the dose of dye is also in mg the cardiac output ($\dot{Q}t$) is given by

$$\dot{Q}t = \frac{\text{Dose of dye}}{A_1 + A_2}\ \text{l min}^{-1}$$

Indicators in current use include the dye indocyanine green, human albumen labelled with iodine-133 or Tc-99 and cold saline solution. Indocyanine green can be monitored using an ear oximeter, but use of a cuvette as in Fig. 17.8 has the advantage for exercise studies that there is no movement artefact. Indocyanine green has the advantage over other dyes (e.g. Coumassie blue) that the quantity of dye is small so the skin is not discoloured. In addition, excretion into the bile is rapid so measurements can be repeated at 2-min intervals, and the method is independent of the arterial oxygen saturation. Labelled albumen is detected using a scintillation counter. This can be placed over the precordium. More reproducible results are obtained by analysing samples of blood obtained from an arterial cannula. The samples are collected serially every half second. With the cold saline method the changes in temperature are recorded with a thermistor that is inserted through a needle into the pulmonary artery or a large systemic artery. The reproducibility and accuracy of the methods have been scrutinised [e.g. 50, 51].

17.3.3 Physical methods

Doppler echocardiography. This procedure measures mean blood flow in the ascending aorta. It is less suitable for measuring absolute output and does not measure pulmonary blood flow if there are shunts. The method is based on the twin assumptions that the probe is in the line of flow and the flow is uniform across a cylinder of blood extending outwards from the aortic orifice. In practice there is good agreement with other methods [52]. A related procedure can be used to measure cardiac volume [53]. Echocardiography cannot be used when there is movement of the trunk, as, for example, during treadmill walking or stepping exercise.

To make the measurement the blood flow in the aorta is measured by ultrasound and aortic cross-sectional area by echocardiography. Then,

$$\dot{Q} = f \times \dot{v} \times A \qquad (17.11)$$

where $\dot{Q}$ is cardiac output, f is the fraction of the cardiac cycle occupied by systole, $\dot{v}$ is mean aortic flow velocity during systole and A is aortic cross-sectional area. The instantaneous velocity is measured by the change in frequency when pulses of ultrasound waves of frequency 2 mHz from an emitter in the suprasternal notch are directed into the line of flow. The direction should be that associated with a smooth velocity–time curve that rises to a peak early in systole, a high frequency whistling sound when listening to the audible signal and the highest obtainable mean velocity when the signal is integrated over the duration of systole. The duration can be obtained separately by phonocardiography. The cross-sectional area is usually that measured 2 cm above the aortic orifice. At this site the area in an adult is approximately 3 cm^2. The area should be estimated directly. Calculation of the area from the diameter is inaccurate since the cross section is not circular. Valid dimensions are those between the leading edges of the anterior and posterior echoes.

Electrical bio-impedance cardiography. The method estimates stroke volume for both ventricles from the rate of change of thoracic impedance over the cardiac cycle. The method is not invalidated by exercise, is convenient and of good reproducibility; it is suitable for monitoring changes in cardiac output but the absolute accuracy is poor.

To make the measurement, input electrodes are applied bilaterally to the side of the neck and to the lower thoracic cage and supplied by a constant current sinusoidal field generator. The impedance signal is recorded through pairs of electrodes placed, respectively, 5 cm below and above the input electrodes. The stroke volume is calculated using the relationship

$$\mathrm{SV} = \frac{\mathrm{d}z/\mathrm{d}t\ \max}{z}\, t \times \mathrm{PF} \tag{17.12}$$

where z is the thoracic base impedance in ohms (Ω), $\mathrm{d}z/\mathrm{d}t$ max the maximal rate of change of impedance during systole (Ω/s), t the ventricular ejection time (s) and PF an empirical personal factor which reflects the distance between the electrodes and other variables; it can be expressed in terms of age, sex, stature and body mass.

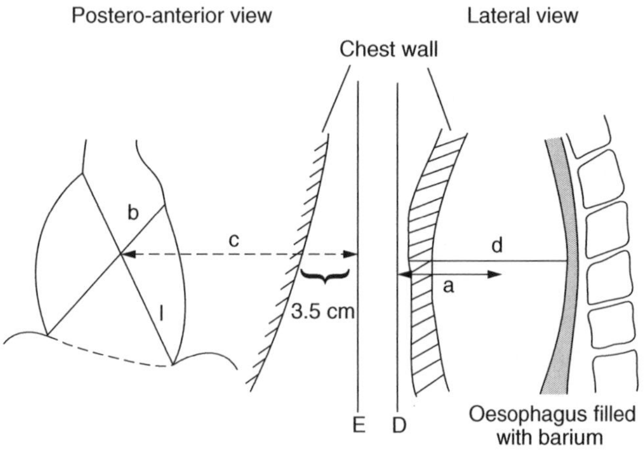

Fig. 17.9 Radiographic method for estimating heart volume. Only X-rays showing a clearly defined cardiac outline should be used. Dimensions are measured in centimetres. The length of the heart (l) is taken from the apex to the junction with the great vessels and the breadth (b) (which is nearly at right angles to the length) from the junction with the pulmonary conus to the junction with the diaphragm; the depth (d) is the maximal horizontal distance. The heart volume (HV) is given by

$$HV = l \times b \times \left(\frac{A-a}{A}\right)^2 \times d\left(\frac{A-c}{A}\right) \times \frac{\pi}{6}\ \mathrm{cm}^3$$

where A is the anode to film distance, a and c are, respectively, the distances from the centre of the heart to the film as seen end-on in the lateral and the posterio-anterior projections (D and E, respectively). The chest wall to film distances are taken, respectively, as 0.5 and 3.5 cm.

17.4 Radiographic heart volume

The volume of the heart can be estimated from its dimensions on postero-anterior and lateral chest radiographs. For optimal accuracy the exposures should be triggered by the electrocardiogram. They are made after a full inspiration with the heart in diastole and, for the lateral view, the posterior border is delineated with barium sulphate gruel. The method is shown in Fig. 17.9. The volume includes the epicardial fat.

17.5 References

1. Jones AT, Hansell DM, Evans TW. Pulmonary perfusion in supine and prone positions: an electron-beam computed tomography study. *J Appl Physiol* 2001; **90**: 1342–1348.
2. West JB, Dollery CT, Naimark A. Distribution of blood flow in isolated lung; relation to vascular and alveolar pressures. *J Appl Physiol* 1964; **19**: 713–724.
3. Anthonisen NR, Milic-Emili J. Distribution of pulmonary perfusion in erect man. *J Appl Physiol* 1966; **21**: 760–766.
4. West JB. *Ventilation/blood flow and gas exchange.* 3rd ed. Oxford: Blackwell Scientific Publications, 1977.
5. Lamm WJ, Kirk KR, Hanson WL et al. Flow through zone 1 lungs utilizes alveolar corner vessels. *J Appl Physiol* 1991; **70**: 1518–23.
6. Lopez-Muniz R, Stephens NL, Bromberger-Barnea B et al. Critical closure of pulmonary vessels analyzed in terms of Starling resistor model. *J Appl Physiol* 1968; **24**: 625–635.
7. Rickaby DA, Dawson CA, Linehan JH, Bronikowski TA. Alveolar vessel behavior in the zone 2 lung inferred from indicator-dilution data. *J Appl Physiol* 1987; **63**: 778–784.
8. Glazier JB, Hughes JMB, Maloney JE, West JB. Measurements of capillary dimensions and blood volume in rapidly frozen lungs. *J Appl Physiol* 1969; **26**: 65–76.
9. Hughes JBM, Glazier JB, Maloney JE, West JB. Effect of lung volume on the distribution of pulmonary blood flow in man. *Resp Physiol* 1968; **4**: 58–72.
10. Glenny RW, Bernard S, Robertson HT, Hlastala MP. Gravity is an important but secondary determinant of regional pulmonary blood flow in upright primates. *J Appl Physiol* 1999; **86**: 623–632.

11. Glenny RW, Lamm WE, Bernard SL et al. Selected contribution: Redistribution of pulmonary perfusion during weightlessness and increased gravity. *J Appl Physiol* 2000; **89**: 1239–48.
12. Burton AC, Stinson RH. The measurement of tension in vascular smooth muscle. *J Physiol (Lond)* 1960; **153**: 290–305.
13. Barnes PJ, Liu SF. Regulation of pulmonary vascular tone. *Pharmacol Rev* 1995; **47**: 87–131.
14. von Euler US, Liljestrand G. Observations on the pulmonary arterial blood pressure in the cat. *Acta Physiol Scand* 1946; **12**: 301–320.
15. Murray TR, Chen L, Marshall BE, Macarak EJ. Hypoxic contraction of cultured pulmonary vascular smooth muscle cells. *Am J Respir Cell Mol Biol* 1990; **3**: 457–465.
16. Hoshikawa Y, Ono S, Suzuki S et al. Generation of oxidative stress contributes to the development of pulmonary hypertension induced by hypoxia. *J Appl Physiol* 2001; **90**: 1299–306.
17. Hambraeus-Jonzon K, Bindslev L, Mellgard AJ, Hedenstierna G. Hypoxic pulmonary vasoconstriction in human lungs. A stimulus-response study. *Anesthesiology* 1997; **86**: 308–315.
18. Field GB, Cotes JE. Lability of pulmonary pressure–flow curves during exercise in clinically mild bronchitis; evidence for a pulmonary vascular sluice in man. *Clin Sci* 1970; **38**: 461–77.
19. Mitzner W,Huang I. Interpretation of pressure–flow curve in the pulmonary vascular bed. In: Wills JA, Dawson CA, Weir EK, Buckner CK, eds. *Pulmonary circulation in health and disease.* Orlando, Academic Press, 1987; 215–230.
20. Read J, Lee JH, Pain MCF. Two groups of subjects with obstructive lung disease, defined by pulmonary vascular reactivity. *Proc Aspen Emphysema Conference U.S.* Dept. Health Education and Welfare 1967; **10**: 229–239.
21. Sartori C, Duplain H, Lepori M et al. High-altitude impairs nasal transepithelial sodium transport in HAPE-prone subjects. *Eur Respir J* 2004; **23**: 916–920.
22. Corbin JD, Francis SH. mini review. Cyclic GMP Phosphodiesterase-5: Target of Sildenafil* *J Biol Chem* 1999; **274**:13729–13732.
23. Hoshikawa Y, Voelkel NF, Gesell TL et al. Prostacyclin receptor-dependent modulation of pulmonary vascular remodeling. *Am J Respir Crit Care Med* 2001; **164**: 314–318.
24. Dukarm RC, Russell JA, Morin FC et al. The cGMP-specific phosphodiesterase inhibitor E4021 dilates the pulmonary circulation. *Am J Respir Crit Care Med* 1999; **160**: 858–865.
25. Hambraeus-Jonzon K, Chen L, Freden F et al. Pulmonary vasoconstriction during regional nitric oxide inhalation: evidence of a blood-borne regulator of nitric oxide synthase activity. *Anesthesiology* 2001; **95**: 102–112.
26. Rybalkin SD, Rybalkina IG, Feil R et al. Regulation of cGMP-specific phosphodiesterase (PDE5) phosphorylation in smooth muscle cells. *J Biol Chem* 2002; **277**: 3310–3317.
27. Rodman DM, Voelkel NF. Regulation of vascular tone. In: Crystal RG et al, ed. *The lung: scientific foundations.* 2nd ed. Philadelphia: Lippincott-Raven, 1997: 1473–1492.
28. Krasuski RA, Warner JJ, Wang A et al. Inhaled nitric oxide selectively dilates pulmonary vasculature in adult patients with pulmonary hypertension, irrespective of etiology. *J Am Coll Cardiol* 2000; **36**: 2204–2211.
29. Halmagyi DF, Cotes JE. Reduction in systemic blood oxygen as a result of procedures affecting the pulmonary circulation in patients with chronic pulmonary disease. *Clin Sci* 1959; **18**: 475–489.
30. Ganz W, Donoso R, Marcus HR et al. A new technique for measurement of cardiac output by thermodilution in man. *Am J Cardiol* 1971; **27**: 392–396.
31. Cerretelli P, Cruz JL, Farhi LE, Rahn H. Determination of mixed venous O_2 and CO_2 tensions and cardiac output by a rebreathing method. *Respir Physiol* 1966; **1**: 258–264.
32. Kelman GR. $P\bar{v}{,}O_2$ by nitrogen rebreathing – a critical, theoretical analysis. *Respir Physiol* 1972; **16**: 327–336.
33. Jones NL, Campbell EJM, McHardy GJR et al. The estimation of carbon dioxide pressure of mixed venous blood during exercise. *Clin Sci* 1967; **32**: 311–327.
34. Denison D, Edwards RHT, Jones G, Pope H. Estimates of the CO_2 pressures in systemic arterial blood during rebreathing on exercise. *Respir Physiol* 1971; **11**: 186–196.
35. Godfrey S, Davies CTM. Estimates of arterial P_{CO_2} and their effect on the calculated values of cardiac output and deadspace on exercise. *Clin Sci* 1970; **39**: 529–537.
36. Jones NL, Robertson DG, Kane JW, Campbell EJM. Effect of P_{CO_2} level on alveolar-arterial P_{CO_2} difference during rebreathing. *J Appl Physiol* 1972; **32**: 782–787.
37. Douglas AR, Jones NL, Reed JW. Calculation of whole blood CO_2 content. *J Appl Physiol* 1988; **65**: 473–477.
38. McHardy GJ. The relationship between the differences in pressure and content of carbon dioxide in arterial and venous blood. *Clin Sci* 1967; **32**: 299–309.
39. Kim TS, Rahn H, Farhi LE. Estimation of true venous and arterial PCO_2 by gas analysis of a single breath. *J Appl Physiol* 1966; **21**:1338–1344.
40. Farhi LE, Nesarajah MS, Olszowka AJ et al. Cardiac output determination by simple one-step rebreathing technique. *Respir Physiol* 1976; **28**: 141–159.
41. Rosenthal M, Bush A. The simultaneous comparison of acetylene or carbon dioxide flux as a measure of effective pulmonary blood flow in children. *Eur Respir J* 1997; **10**: 2586–2590.
42. Bush A, Busst CM, Johnson S, Denison DM. Rebreathing method for the simultaneous measurement of oxygen consumption and effective pulmonary blood flow during exercise. *Thorax* 1988; **43**: 268–275.
43. Kendrick AH, Rozkovec A, Papouchado M et al Single-breath breath-holding estimate of pulmonary blood flow in man: comparison with direct Fick cardiac output. *Clin Sci* 1989; **76**: 673–676.
44. Hoeper MM, Maier R, Tonjers J et al Determination of cardiac output by the Fick method, thermodilution and acetylene rebreathing in pulmonary hypertension. *Am J Respir Crit Care Med* 1999; **160**: 535–541.
45. Clark JS, Lin YJ, Criddle MJ et al. Cardiac output and mixed venous O_2 content measurements by a tracer bolus method: animal validation study. *J Appl Physiol* 1998; **85**: 459–464.
46. Johnson RL Jr, Spicer WS, Bishop JM, Forster RE. Pulmonary capillary blood volume, flow and diffusing capacity during exercise. *J Appl Physiol* 1960; **15**: 893–902.
47. Lee G de J, Dubois AB. Pulmonary capillary blood flow in man. *J Clin Invest* 1955; **34**: 1380–1390.
48. Dubois AB, Marshall R. Measurements of pulmonary capillary blood flow and gas exchange throughout the respiratory cycle in man. *J Clin Invest* 1957; **36**: 1566–1571.
49. Menkes HA, Sera K, Rogers RM et al. Pulsatile uptake of CO in the human lung. *J Clin Invest* 1970; **49**: 335–345.

50. Wessel HU, Paul MH, James GW, Grahn AR. Limitations of thermal dilution curves for cardiac output determinations. *J Appl Physiol* 1971; **30**: 643–652.
51. Bate H, Rowlands S, Sirs JA. Influence of diffusion on dispersion of indicators in blood flow. *J Appl Physiol* 1973; **34**: 866–872.
52. Ihlen H, Endresen K, Golf S, Nitter-Hauge S. Cardiac stroke volume during exercise measured by Doppler echocardiography: comparison with the thermodilution technique and evaluation of reproducibility. *Br Heart J* 1987; **58**: 455–459.
53. Ota T, Kisslo J, von Ramm OT, Yoshikawa J. Real-time, volumetric echocardiography: usefulness of volumetric scanning for the assessment of cardiac volume and function. *J Cardiol* 2001; **37**(Suppl 1): 93–101.

Further reading

Merrill EW. Rheology of blood. *Physiol Rev* 1969; **49**: 863–888.

CHAPTER 18

Inter-Relations between Lung Ventilation and Perfusion ($\dot{V}A/\dot{Q}$)

Gas exchange occurs when fresh air and venous blood come together in the lungs. The matching between ventilation and perfusion ($\dot{V}A$ and $\dot{Q}$) is quite good in healthy persons, but less so in disease when any mismatch causes hypoxaemia and excessive ventilation. This chapter elaborates on $\dot{V}A/\dot{Q}$ relationships.

18.1 Introduction

18.1.1 Distribution of gas and blood

Proximity of gas and blood. The bronchial and vascular trees of the lungs share common terminations in individual acini. Here gas is separated from blood by the alveolar capillary membrane that is both thin and permeable to gases. For gas exchange to be efficient each acinus should receive fresh air and venous blood from the right atrium in appropriate proportions [1]. This depends on having control mechanisms. In normal circumstances the mechanisms operate effectively and as a result the tensions of oxygen and carbon dioxide in pulmonary venous blood are nearly equal to those in expired alveolar gas. Gas exchange becomes imperfect if the membrane is damaged causing a transfer defect (Chapter 19) or the flows of incoming gas and blood to different parts of the lungs are poorly matched, so there is ventilation–perfusion inequality (e.g. a part may have high ventilation but low perfusion or vice versa).

Distribution of blood flow. The flow is subject to gravitational force. As a result, blood is delivered preferentially to dependent parts of the vascular bed. The distribution is most uniform when the subject is in a prone position [2, 3]. The perfusion has been analysed in terms of four zones with different characteristics (Section 17.1.3). The zones reflect the respective relationships of alveolar pressure to the intravascular pressures at the two ends of the pulmonary capillaries. These in turn are influenced by the condition of the surrounding lung, cardiac output and other factors. Within the different zones the lung anatomy is not uniform, but exhibits variations that largely determine how the local blood flow is distributed.

Distribution of ventilation. The distribution is determined by the many physical features of the lungs. They include the rheological characteristics of airways of different calibre, the amounts and sites of application of inspiratory force, the extent of lung expansion and the effects of gravitational force on pleural fluid pressure and lung distensibility (see e.g. Chapters 11 and 14). The gradient of pleural pressure is least and the uniformity of ventilation greatest when the subject is in a prone position [3, 4]. The physical factors can interact. They influence the extent to which fresh air enters and is distributed uniformly within the lungs

(Chapter 16). The pattern can be modified by environmental factors and by lung disease; these can superimpose any of a range of abnormalities from transient changes in bronchomotor tone to gross structural deformity.

Physical matching of ventilation to perfusion. Two physical processes contribute to the matching of ventilation to perfusion. The first is adopting a prone position. This improves the homogeneity of the distributions of both ventilation and perfusion, and hence that of $\dot{V}_A/\dot{Q}$ ratios [4]. The second is the redistribution during inspiration of gas present in the anatomical deadspace at the end of the preceding expiration (Section 16.1.3). However, the beneficial effect of the redistribution is small. In most circumstances this is also the case for the passive effects of posture [5].

Physiological matching of ventilation to perfusion. Matching is effected mainly by adjustments to the calibre of airways and small pulmonary blood vessels. This entails regulating the tone of smooth muscle in the walls of the two sets of structures [6]. The overall control mechanisms have been described in previous chapters (Sections 15.2 and 17.2). There are also specific feedback mechanisms. The mechanism for blood vessels is vasoconstriction in response to local hypoxia (Section 17.2.2). This mechanism directs mixed venous blood in the pulmonary arteries away from parts of the lungs that are ventilated inadequately. If there are many such sites the compensation is achieved at the cost of a rise in pressure in the pulmonary artery that can precipitate right heart failure. The mechanism for the airways is based on the local tension of carbon dioxide and to a lesser extent on other substances. A low CO_2 tension promotes bronchoconstriction and a relatively high-tension bronchodilatation (Section 15.2.4). This mechanism diverts ventilation away from locations where there is relatively little perfusion and towards those where more ventilation is appropriate.

The physical processes that determine the separate distributions of ventilation and perfusion are of limited scope, so the regulatory mechanisms have much to do and in general they are effective [7, 8]. As a result the mean alveolar to arterial gas tension differences for oxygen and carbon dioxide are normally very small (Section 21.5.2, also Table 26.23, page 358). They become larger when the lungs deteriorate as a result of wear and tear consequent on increasing age, environmental insults or disease. In most respiratory patients the distribution is sub-optimal. This gives rise to hypoxaemia, some hypercapnia and ineffectual ventilation of the lungs; the ventilatory cost of activities is increased in consequence (Section 28.4.7).

18.1.2 Ventilation–perfusion ratios

In a normal subject at rest, the ventilation that penetrates to the level of the alveolar ducts (alveolar ventilation, $\dot{V}_A$) and the corresponding flow of blood ($\dot{Q}$) are, respectively, approximately 4.5 l min^{-1} and 5 l min^{-1}. Hence, in this instance the ratio of ventilation to perfusion ($\dot{V}_A/\dot{Q}$ ratio) for the two lungs is 0.9 (i.e. 4.5/5.0). Haldane was probably the first person to recognize that for effective gas exchange the matching of ventilation to perfusion should extend to individual alveoli [9]. For example, an alveolus where the levels of ventilation and perfusion are both below the average can make a small but appropriate contribution to gas exchange. By contrast, one that is well ventilated but poorly perfused cannot.

Early studies into the effects of imperfect matching of ventilation to perfusion ($\dot{V}_A/\dot{Q}$) were made for oxygen (e.g. [10]). They depended on finding acceptable definitions of alveolar oxygen and carbon dioxide tension [11] and on being able to make accurate measurements in blood [12], see also Section 7.10.2. Rahn and Fenn produced an all-embracing O_2–CO_2 diagram of beauty and deceptive simplicity [13] (Fig. 21.6, page 270). Riley developed a five-compartment model for describing uneven lung function that still has clinical relevance [14]. Farhi considered the interrelation between gas solubility and $\dot{V}_A/\dot{Q}$ in determining the uptake and elimination of inert gases in the lungs [15, 16]. This work led West and Wagner to develop a sophisticated model of gas exchange with 50 compartments; these spanned the whole range of possible $\dot{V}_A/\dot{Q}$ ratios from zero to infinity [17–19]. The sizes of the compartments were assessed using a multiple inert gas elimination technique (MIGET, see below). The method gave new life to a single breath index of $\dot{V}_A/\dot{Q}$ inequality based on instantaneous respiratory exchange ratio (Section 18.3). The index can be applied epidemiologically.

None of these models fully described the extent of uneven lung function in different circumstances, but all can make useful contributions.

18.1.3 Five-compartment model

This model treats the mixed expired gas as if it is made up of two parts, the *alveolar ventilation* and the *deadspace ventilation* [11]. The alveolar ventilation participates in gas exchange. The deadspace ventilation is wasted in ventilating both the anatomical deadspace and an alveolar deadspace comprising alveoli that are poorly perfused. The two make up the *physiological deadspace* [20]. Similarly, the mixed arterial blood is partitioned into a gas-exchanging compartment that is involved in gas exchange and a *blood shunt compartment* [14]. The latter is the sum of the blood flow that bypasses the lungs (anatomical shunt) and the blood perfusing alveoli that are poorly ventilated. Their combined effects on gas exchange is given by the proportion of mixed venous blood that, if added to oxygenated blood from the gas-exchanging compartment, would yield the observed arterial oxygen saturation.

The analysis has five points of reference; of these the first four are the gas tensions in inspired and mixed expired gas and arterial and mixed venous blood. These quantities together with respiratory exchange ratio are used to identify the composition of a single chamber gas-exchanging compartment (*ideal alveolar air*) that is compatible with the deadspace and shunt compartments described above. The five compartments are illustrated in

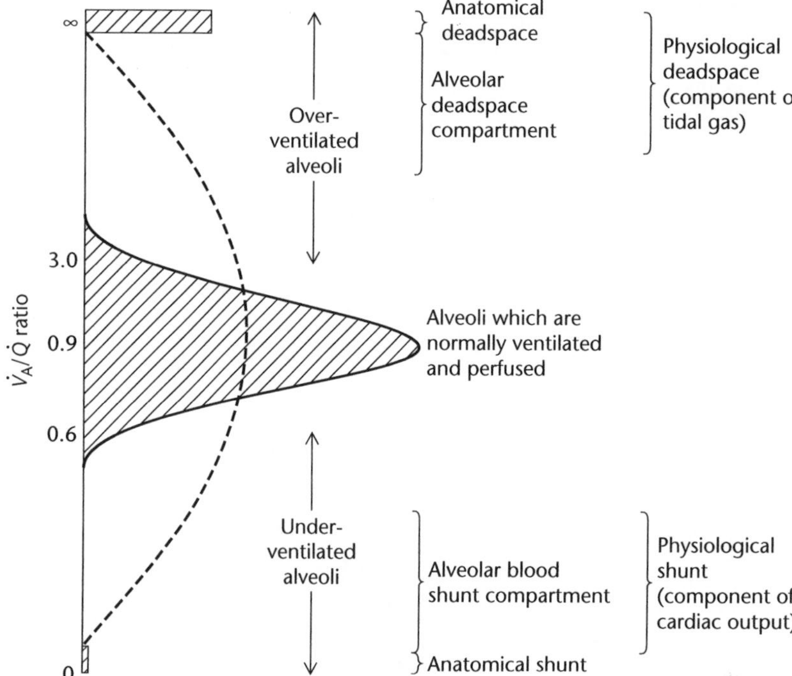

Fig. 18.1 Terminology for the five-compartment model of lung ventilation–perfusion ratios of Riley and others. This places all $\dot{V}_A/\dot{Q}$ ratios from zero to infinity into one of five compartments. The shaded areas are for a normal subject. The interrupted line indicates a wide range of $\dot{V}_A/\dot{Q}$ ratios. The diagram is schematic (see also Table 18.1, page 215).

Fig. 18.1. The measurement of the compartments is described in Section 18.4.

18.1.4 Overview of methods

The five-compartment model can be used to partition the difference in tension of oxygen between alveolar gas and arterial blood ($A - aD_{O_2}$) into two parts. Of these one component reflects the proportions in which gas and blood from different parts of the lungs mix to form, respectively, mixed expired gas and mixed arterial blood. In the presence of uneven lung function (wide range of $\dot{V}_A/\dot{Q}$ ratios) the gas tensions in the two media are inevitably different. The contribution of this process to the ($A - aD_{O_2}$) is called the *distribution effect.* The second component of the $A - aD_{O_2}$ is due to the blood dissociation curve for oxygen not being linear (Fig. 21.1, page 260). As a result when streams of blood from differently ventilated parts of the lungs are mixed the final oxygen tension is influenced by their respective positions on the oxygen dissociation curve. These features of the Riley model are elaborated subsequently. The distribution effect can be investigated independent of the dissociation curve effect by using foreign inert gases for which the relationship between the tension of the gas and content when in equilibrium with blood is linear. This principle is employed in the multiple inert gas elimination technique (MIGET) that is described next.

Impaired gas exchange due to ventilation–perfusion inequality can also be described in other ways. These include the $A - aD_{O_2}$ referred to above and changes in respiratory exchange ratio during a single expiration (*intra-breath R* below). Regional differences can be visualised using isotopes (Section 18.6) and differences between lobes can be studied using samples of gas obtained from individual lobes (Section 18.5).

18.2 Multiple inert gas elimination technique

18.2.1 Description

The multiple inert gas elimination technique for exploring uneven lung function (MIGET) was proposed by Farhi and developed by West and Wagner [15–19]. It is based on the assumptions that gaseous equilibrium is achieved between pulmonary capillary blood and alveolar gas during one passage through the lungs and ventilation and perfusion are continuous processes.

By this method six gases that have different solubilities in saline are infused into a peripheral vein. Gases of high solubility tend to be retained in the blood and are only removed in significant quantities when the ventilation is high relative to the perfusion; such gases have a high blood–gas partition coefficient (Section 19.3.1). Gases of low solubility are completely removed from blood and enter the alveolar gas at a relatively low level of ventilation; they have a low blood–gas partition coefficient. From the relative extents to which the six gases are retained in or lost from the blood, the proportions of ventilation and blood flow going to the lung units having any of 50 $\dot{V}_A/\dot{Q}$ ratios from zero to infinity can be identified.

In persons with healthy lungs most lung units have $\dot{V}_A/\dot{Q}$ ratios that are close to the mean value for sedentary subjects of approximately 0.9 litres per litre. Thus, the distribution of $\dot{V}_A/\dot{Q}$ is unimodal with a relatively small standard deviation.

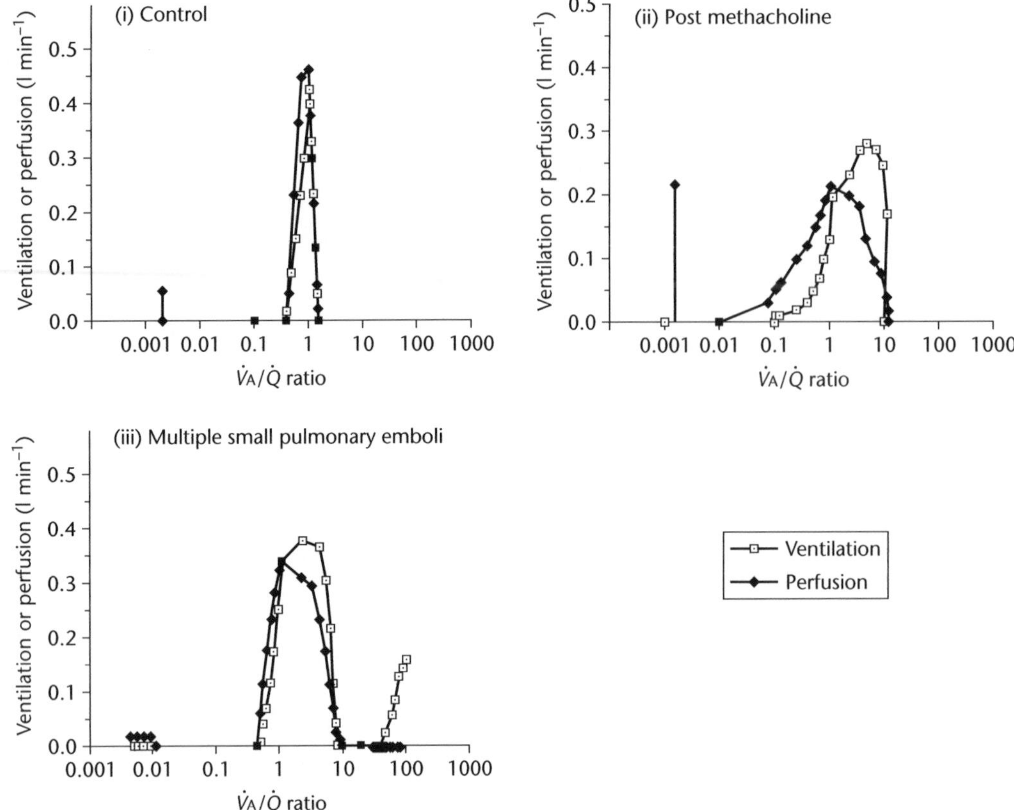

Fig. 18.2 Distributions of $\dot{V}_A/\dot{Q}$ ratios in two dogs.
Panel (i): Control observation. The distribution was normal. There was a small blood shunt compartment.
Panel (ii): Inhalation of metacholine. This reduced the ventilation to parts of the lung and caused a compensatory reduction in perfusion. The dispersion of $\dot{V}_A/\dot{Q}$ ratios was increased. The blood shunt compartment was increased on account of some lung units receiving little ventilation.
Panel (iii): Injection of glass microspheres into the pulmonary circulation. Part of the lung became under-perfused so had a high $\dot{V}_A/\dot{Q}$ ratio, whilst part was relatively normal. As a result the distribution of ventilation was bimodal. In the perfused lung (closed circles) part was not ventilated at all, indicating the opening up of anastomotic channels (low $\dot{V}_A/\dot{Q}$ ratio). Source: [Reed JW, Guy H unpublished].

In the presence of airflow limitation the dispersion is increased whilst if a part of the lungs is not ventilated or not perfused its $\dot{V}_A/\dot{Q}$ ratio approaches a limiting value that is, respectively, either zero or infinity (Fig. 18.2).

The multiple inert gas elimination technique (MIGET) has the advantages that the contributions to gas exchange of differently ventilated and perfused lung regions are assessed concurrently not consecutively and the procedure, unlike that using oxygen (Section 21.4), does not itself alter what is being measured. The method can also illuminate other features of gas exchange.

Changes in cardiac output influence the mixed venous oxygen tension and hence the extent to which blood from poorly ventilated alveoli and the anatomical shunt lower the arterial oxygen tension. Impaired diffusion results in the arterial oxygen tension being lower than would be expected on the basis of ventilation–perfusion inequality alone [21], see also Section 21.4.4. The method yields intuitively sensible distributions and shows change in the expected directions as a result of interventions (Fig. 18.2).

The model has the disadvantage of not including anatomical features of the lungs, including any lung pathology. It neglects possible mitigating factors including the distribution of deadspace gas (Section 18.1.1), collateral ventilation, cardiogenic mixing, and oscillations due to ventilation and perfusion not being continuous processes. It also overlooks blood that is oxygenated via the bronchial circulation when there is pulmonary vascular occlusion. Some of these limitations are only of theoretical interest whilst others have been largely resolved [22–27]. The method has illuminated many aspects of gas exchange including those associated with asthma, pulmonary embolism, cirrhosis of the liver and haemodialysis [28–30]; see also Chapter 42. MIGET is a useful if expensive tool for evaluating intervention studies. Its features have been summarised [31].

18.2.2 Making the measurement

Extended theory. For a lung compartment that is homogeneous with respect to its ventilation–perfusion ratio the quantity of gas being exchanged between the alveoli and the pulmonary capillary blood is the same as that exchanged between the alveoli and the atmosphere. This quantity, expressed as a fraction of that in the mixed venous blood, is a function of the ventilation–perfusion ratio and the blood–gas partition coefficient for the gas in question. It is given by the following equation of Kety [32]:

$$P\text{A}/P\bar{\text{v}} = P\text{c}'/P\bar{\text{v}} = \lambda/(\lambda + \dot{V}\text{A}/\dot{Q}) \qquad (18.1)$$

where the three partial pressure terms refer, respectively, to the alveolar gas, the mixed venous blood and the blood leaving the alveolar capillaries; λ is the blood–gas partition coefficient for the inert gas in question and $\dot{V}\text{A}/\dot{Q}$ is the ventilation–perfusion ratio for the particular compartment. Then, on rearrangement and after substituting arterial for end-capillary gas tension:

$$\dot{V}\text{A}/\dot{Q} = \lambda(P\bar{\text{v}}/P\text{a} - 1) \qquad (18.2)$$

where the ratio of the gas tensions in the arterial and mixed venous blood ($P\text{a}/P\bar{\text{v}}$) is the fraction of the gas retained by the blood during its passage through the lungs. In practice six gases having different blood–gas partition coefficients are used (Fig. 18.3).

Procedure. The six gases are dissolved in saline and infused into a vein in one arm or hand. The infusion rate in a resting subject is 3 ml of saline per minute, or more during exercise, and the measurements of gas concentration in expired gas and arterial and mixed venous blood are normally made after 30 min. Expired gas and arterial blood are sampled directly. Mixed venous blood is sampled from a catheter in the pulmonary artery and cardiac output is measured using indocyanine green as an indicator (Section 17.3.2). The collection of so much data permits some flexibility in the arrangements, for example gas concentrations in mixed venous blood can be calculated by application of the Fick principle instead of being sampled directly, and with suitable precautions systemic venous blood can substitute for systemic arterial blood. Gas analysis is performed using gas chromatography. This process should preferably be automated with the analyser connected in line to the computer.

Calculation. The results are analysed in terms of a 50-compartment model lung in which the ventilation–perfusion ratios range from zero (i.e. pure shunt) to nearly infinity. In this circumstance, the mixed arterial concentration of each of the gases is a blood flow weighted mean of the values for the several compartments. Similarly, the mean concentration in expired gas is the ventilation weighted mean for the same compartments. The analysis identifies a numerical distribution of ventilation–perfusion that is compatible with the arterial and alveolar concentrations of all gases concurrently.

The programme for the calculation includes an algorithm for enforced smoothing of the $\log_e$ $\dot{V}\text{A}/\dot{Q}$ distribution curve and calculation of its mean and standard deviation or dispersion (respectively, the first and second moments) [23]. The reproducibility of the dispersion expressed as the coefficient of variation has been found to be approximately 8.5% when based on a single estimate and 6.1% for duplicates. The log dispersions of $\dot{V}\text{A}/\dot{Q}$ with respect to both perfusion and ventilation (designated log SD $\dot{Q}$

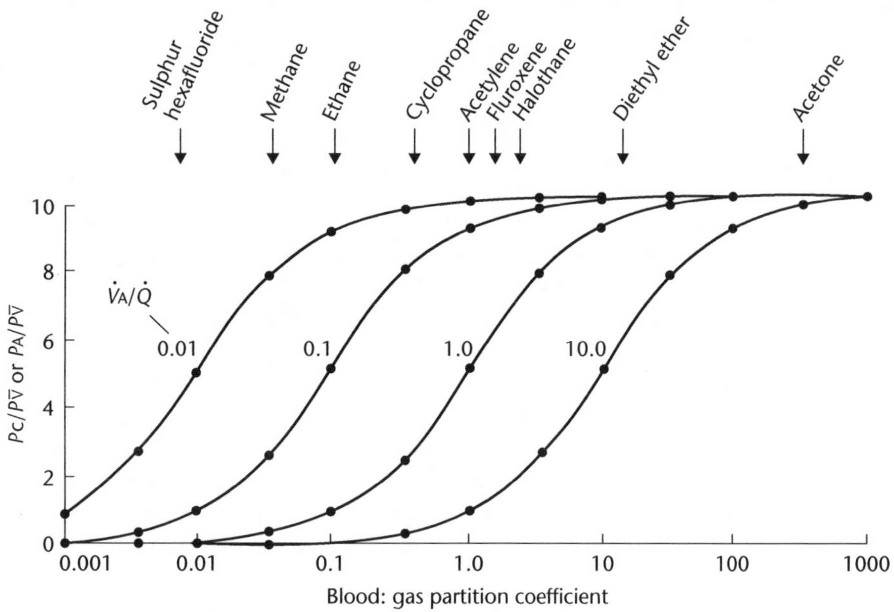

Fig. 18.3 Relationship between inert gas retention $P\text{c}/P\bar{v}$ (or excretion $P\text{A}/P\bar{v}$) and blood–gas partition coefficient, using a logarithmic scale for the abscissa. Four curves are drawn, each for homogeneous lung units with different $\dot{V}\text{A}/\dot{Q}$ ratios. Source: [18]

and log SD $\dot{V}$A) are reported together with the standard deviation of the difference between the measured gas retentions and excretions; this overall index of heterogeneity of lung function is given by

$$\text{Disp } R - E = 100\sqrt{\sum_{1}^{n}(R - E)^2/n} \qquad (18.3)$$

where R and E are, respectively, the retentions and the excretions corrected for the physiological deadspace. The correction is made using a calculated deadspace that is compatible with the observed gas retentions and partition coefficients, cardiac output and ventilation minute volume [33].

Comment. The method is limited by the accuracy of present chromatographic techniques for gas analysis. In addition, it does not provide a unique answer as the same arterial and alveolar concentrations could result from other distributions of ventilation and perfusion in the lung. However, these limitations are no greater than for other methods that attempt to describe in simple terms the complex gas-exchanging function of the lung. This method is the most successful so far.

18.3 Intra-breath R index of $\dot{V}$A/$\dot{Q}$ inequality

During a single expiration, after exhalation of deadspace gas, the tensions of oxygen, carbon dioxide and nitrogen measured at the mouth each attain a nearly constant level; this was formerly called the alveolar plateau for the gas in question. However, the term phase 3 is preferable as the "plateau" usually has a significant slope (e.g. Fig. 16.7, page 188). This is because, for each gas, the alveoli that empty later in expiration usually have a lower ventilation–perfusion ratio than those that empty earlier. Because high $\dot{V}$A/$\dot{Q}$ ratios are associated with high respiratory exchange ratios (RER) and vice versa, the slope of phase 3 for respiratory exchange ratio is affected by the uneven distribution of time constants within the lung. Other factors contribute as well because the slope is also influenced by uneven distribution of compliance (e.g. Fig. 18.4).

The intra-breath R is the proportional change in $\dot{V}$A/$\dot{Q}$ ratio per litre of expired gas over the middle half of a slow expiration from total lung capacity [34]. The change is calculated from that in the instantaneous respiratory exchange ratio (R). The test preceded the development of the multiple inert gas elimination technique (MIGET) by which it has been validated [35]. The test is not invasive and is easy and quick to perform. It requires a respiratory mass spectrometer and a computer programme that can adjust for changes in gas exchange taking place during the expiration [36, 37]. The former is now available in most lung function laboratories and the latter can be obtained from those who have worked with the method.

Derivation. The respiratory exchange ratio is calculated from the alveolar air equation (eqn. 18.17, below); this can be rearranged in the form:

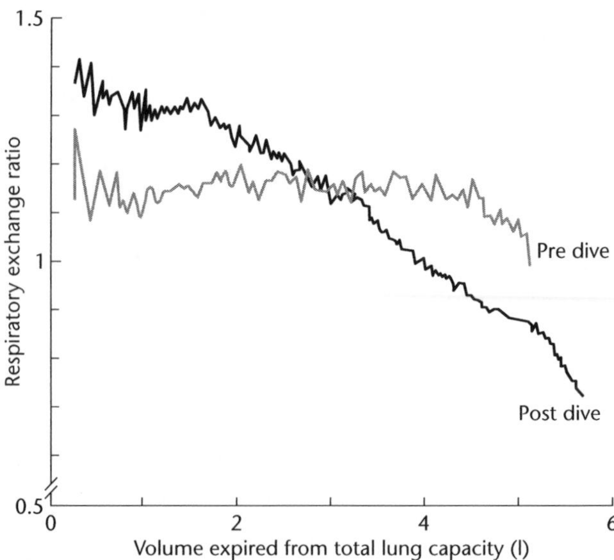

Fig. 18.4 Intra-breath R in a healthy man before and after onset of ventilation–perfusion inequality; this was caused by intravascular bubbles accumulating in the pulmonary circulation during decompression following a saturation dive. Source: [Thorsen I, Reed JW unpublished.]

$$R = P_{A,CO_2}(1 - F_{I,O_2})/(P_{I,O_2} - P_{A,O_2} - F_{I,O_2} \times P_{A,CO_2}) \qquad (18.4)$$

The corresponding ventilation–perfusion ratios are then calculated using the mass balance equation for oxygen passing from alveolar gas to pulmonary capillary blood.

$$\dot{V}_A/\dot{Q} = bR(C_{a,O_2} - C_{\bar{v},O_2})/P_{A,CO_2} \qquad (18.5)$$

where $\dot{V}$A/$\dot{Q}$ is the ventilation–perfusion ratio that corresponds to the measured respiratory exchange ratio (R). The term within the bracket is the difference in content of oxygen between arterial and mixed venous bloods; this is usually assumed to be 2 mmol l^{-1} (44 ml l^{-1}), equivalent to a difference in saturation of 22%. P_{A,CO_2} is the tension of carbon dioxide in alveolar gas; it is assumed to be equal to that in oxygenated venous blood. The constant term (b) is a factor that makes the different terms compatible; in SI units it is 2.58 and in traditional units 0.863.

The result can be displayed graphically as instantaneous respiratory exchange ratio against volume expired from total lung capacity (Fig. 18.4). The contribution of uneven gas exchange can be indicated by superimposing on the basic diagram a curve calculated using the subject's total lung capacity and a measured or assumed overall $\dot{V}$A/$\dot{Q}$ ratio.

Procedure. The subject breathes through a mouthpiece connected to a flow transducer, then slowly inhales air to total lung

Table 18.1 Five-compartment model: summary.

Compartment	Sub-divisions	Derivations
Physiological deadspace (V_{DS})	Anatomical deadspace ($V_{D,anat}$) Alveolar deadspace ($V_{D,alv}$)	Fowler method (Section 16.2.3) $V_{D,alv} = V_{DS} - V_{D,anat}$.
Ideal gas-exchanging compartment		Alveolar air equation (Section 18.4.3)
Physiological shunt ($\dot{Q}s$) also called venous admixture effect ($\dot{Q}va$), see Section 18.4.4	Alveolar shunt compartment ($\dot{Q}s,alv$) Anatomical shunt compartment ($\dot{Q}s,anat.$)	$\dot{Q}s,alv = \dot{Q}s - \dot{Q}s,anat.$ Oxygen method (Section 18.4.5) Inert gas methods

capacity and immediately exhales completely at a slow rate; this procedure resembles that for the single breath nitrogen test of uneven lung function (Section 16.2.4). The respired gas is sampled continuously from the mouthpiece and analysed for oxygen, carbon dioxide and nitrogen using a respiratory mass spectrometer. The output from the mass spectrometer should be processed by a computer. If it is intended to compare the two tests, the controlled inspiration should be preceded by the subject breathing out to residual volume, then inhaling a bolus of argon with the air (see single breath argon–nitrogen test, Fig. 16.8, page 188). To obtain instantaneous $\dot{V}_A/\dot{Q}$ ratios (eqn. 18.5) there is need to know the arterio-venous oxygen content difference. To this end the oxygen uptake is measured (Section 7.8.1) and the cardiac output is either estimated (eqn. 28.1, page 399), or measured by the carbon dioxide rebreathing method (Section 17.3.2).

18.4 Derivation of the classical five-compartment model

This model is described on page 210 above. Its derivation requires knowledge of the gaseous composition of inspired and mixed expired gas and of arterial and mixed venous blood. These quantities are used to calculate values for three principal compartments of which two are subdivided to yield five in all; the stages are summarised in Table 18.1.

18.4.1 Physiological deadspace

This compartment comprises parts of the lungs where there are either no perfused alveoli or where the alveoli are under-perfused with respect to their ventilation. The $\dot{V}_A/\dot{Q}$ ratios of these compartments are, respectively, infinity and above the average for the lung as a whole (see Fig. 18.1). The two compartments form an anatomical deadspace and a hypothetical alveolar deadspace chosen to be compatible with ideal alveolar air. The ideal alveolar air is described below and the measurement of anatomical deadspace is in Section 16.2.3.

In the derivation of physiological deadspace the carbon dioxide content of mixed expired gas is represented as comprising carbon dioxide from deadspace gas that has the composition of inspired gas (so is effectively zero) and ideal alveolar gas in which the tension of carbon dioxide is that of the mixed arterial blood (Pa,CO_2). Then, by the mass balance equation and including a term for carbon dioxide in the mouthpiece and valve box:

$$Vt \times F_{E,CO_2} = V_{A,t} \times F_{A,CO_2} + (Vd + \alpha Vid) \times F_{I,CO_2} \tag{18.6}$$

where Vt is tidal volume, Vd is the physiological deadspace and $V_{A,t}$ is the alveolar component of the tidal volume. Vid is the deadspace of the mouthpiece, value box and related apparatus and α is the fraction of Vid that enters the alveolar compartment. F_{CO_2} and P_{CO_2} (used subsequently) are, respectively, the fractional concentrations and tensions of carbon dioxide in inspired gas (I) and expired gas (E). (A) refers to ideal alveolar air, where the gas tension is that of mixed arterial blood (see Pa,CO_2 above).

But

$$V_{A,t} = Vt - (Vd + \alpha Vid) \tag{18.7}$$

and, when breathing air, F_{I,CO_2} is zero. On substitution and elimination the relationship then becomes:

$$Vt \times F_{E,CO_2} = (Vt - Vd - \alpha Vid) \times F_{A,CO_2} \tag{18.8}$$

or, multiplying both sides by the dry gas pressure in the lungs ($P_B - P_{H_2O}$)

$$Vt \times P_{E,CO_2} = (Vt - Vd - \alpha Vid) \times P_{A,CO_2} \tag{18.9}$$

then, on rearrangement:

$$Vd/Vt = (P_{A,CO_2} - P_{E,CO_2})/P_{A,CO_2} - \alpha Vid/Vt \tag{18.10}$$

The fraction α normally approaches unity but is reduced when, as in pulmonary embolism, there is a large alveolar deadspace (see Footnote 18.1).

Footnote 18.1. Value for α [38]:

$$\alpha = \left(\frac{P_{A,CO_2}}{Pa,CO_2}\right)^2 = \left(\frac{P_{E,CO_2}, Vt}{Pa,CO_2(Vt - Vd,anat - Vid)}\right)^2 \tag{18.11}$$

where $Vd,anat$ is anatomical deadspace and the other terms are defined in the text.

The basic methods are described in Chapter 7 and the measurement of anatomical deadspace is in Section 16.2.3. Formerly the composition of alveolar gas was obtained by the method of Haldane and Priestley or by on-line continuous sampling of expired gas at the lips. If this is done the relevant concentration is that one third of the way along the alveolar plateau (phase 3). The instrument deadspace is estimated from its dimensions, or volumetrically by water displacement, and the tidal volume by a standard method (Section 7.3.1).

18.4.2 Alveolar ventilation

By the traditional method alveolar ventilation is calculated from the ratio *Vd*/*Vt*, also called the deadspace effect. This is the amount by which the alveolar gas expired in each breath is diluted by gas in the physiological deadspace (*Vd*), neglecting the instrument deadspace. Then Eqn 18.10 becomes:

$$Vd/Vt = 100 \times (F_{A,CO_2} - F_{E,CO_2})/F_{A,CO_2} \qquad (18.12)$$

where *F* is fractional gas concentration.

For example, if alveolar $CO_2 = 6\%$ and mixed expired $CO_2 = 4.2\%$,

$$Vd/Vt = (6 - 4.2)/6 \times 100 = 30\%.$$

In this instance the remaining 70% is the alveolar component of the tidal breath (i.e. $Vt - Vd$). It is used to obtain the alveolar ventilation per minute ($\dot{V}_A$).

$$\dot{V}_A = f_R(Vt - Vd),$$

where fR is respiratory frequency. The units are l BTPS min^{-1}.

In healthy young men the average physiological deadspace when seated is about 180 ml, which is 25–30% of the tidal volume. The *Vd*/*Vt* rises to 40% in middle age. During exercise the average lung volume increases. This expands the anatomical deadspace but the alveolar component of the breath increases relatively more, so the ratio *Vd*/*Vt* falls (Fig. 18.5). The reduction is accentuated by the exercise also increasing the cardiac output. This leads to the perfusion of the lungs becoming more uniform; the change shrinks the alveolar deadspace.

The alveolar deadspace expands when one or more branches of the pulmonary artery are obstructed by a pulmonary embolus or by thrombosis. It is also increased by uneven lung function from any cause as this interferes with the distribution of ventilation (Section 18.1.1).

18.4.3 Ideal alveolar air

The concept of ideal alveolar air is central to the five-compartment model of gas exchange in the lungs [11, 13]. The model assumes a single chamber gas exchanger in which the respiratory exchange ratio is that of mixed expired gas and the tension of carbon dioxide is that for arterial blood. The oxygen tension of ideal alveolar air is one that is compatible with these two quantities. It is calculated using the alveolar air equation. This is based on the mass balance equation for the respired gases (eqn. 7.7, page 66). Allowance is made for movement of gas into or out of the lung on account of the volumetric transfers of oxygen and carbon dioxide seldom being equal (*R* effect).

From eqn. 7.7:

$$\dot{V}_I = \dot{V}_E \times F_{E,N_2}/F_{I,N_2} \qquad (18.13)$$

where *F* is fractional concentration of gas, in this case nitrogen, and $\dot{V}$ is ventilation minute volume, I and E refer to inspired and expired gas, respectively.

But, neglecting the rare gases and inspired CO_2 the term F_{E,N_2} can be replaced by $(1 - F_{E,O_2} - F_{E,CO_2})$, and F_{I,N_2} by $(1 - F_{I,O_2})$. The relationship then becomes:

$$\dot{V}_I = \dot{V}_E(1 - F_{E,O_2} - F_{E,CO_2})/(1 - F_{I,O_2}) \qquad (18.14)$$

Similarly, the respiratory exchange ratio (R), can be written in the form:

$$R = (\dot{V}_E \times F_{E,CO_2})/(\dot{V}_I \times F_{I,O_2} - \dot{V}_E \times F_{E,O_2}) \qquad (18.15)$$

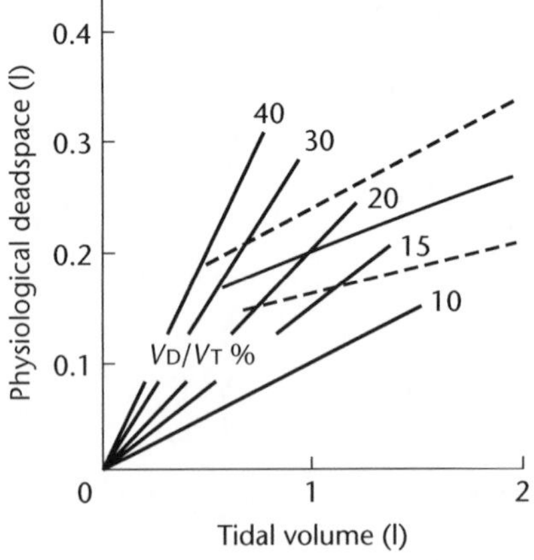

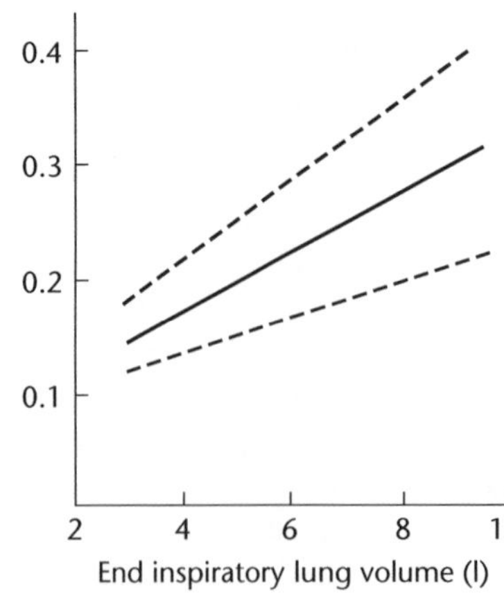

Fig. 18.5 Relationship of physiological deadspace to tidal volume and to end-inspiratory lung volume at rest and during exercise in healthy young adults. Higher values are observed in older subjects. The isopleths are for deadspace as a percentage of tidal volume (*Vd*/*Vt*%). Sources: [39–41]

By combining eqns. 18.14 and 18.15 the ventilation terms can be eliminated. In addition, the present model assumes that the respiratory exchange ratios for alveolar and expired gas are equal, so fractional concentrations in alveolar gas (FA) can be substituted for those in expired gas (FE). Then, on rearrangement:

$$F\text{A},O_2 = F\text{I},O_2 - \frac{F\text{A},CO_2}{R} + \frac{F\text{A},CO_2}{R} \times F\text{I},O_2(1 - R) \tag{18.16}$$

Or, in terms of partial pressures:

$$P\text{A},O_2 = F\text{I},O_2 \times (P\text{B} - P\text{H}_2\text{O}) - \frac{P\text{A},CO_2}{R} + \frac{P\text{A},CO_2}{R} \times F\text{I},O_2(1 - R) \tag{18.17}$$

The respiratory exchange ratio is obtained by analysis of expired gas (Section 7.8). The inspired fractional concentration of oxygen is 0.2093 when breathing air and is otherwise obtained by analysis. The alveolar tension of carbon dioxide is the tension present in arterial blood, hence is the same as that used for calculating physiological deadspace (see above).

The composition of ideal alveolar air is used in the calculation of the venous admixture effect (see below). It is also the starting point for graphical analysis of lung gas exchange by means of the O_2–CO_2 diagram (Fig. 21.6, page 270) [13].

18.4.4 Physiological shunt (venous admixture effect)

The physiological shunt is the mirror image of the physiological deadspace. By its use, the saturation of arterial blood with oxygen is represented as a mixture of blood exposed to ideal alveolar air (about 98% saturated) and mixed venous blood (approximately 75% saturated at rest). No allowance is made for any contribution from impaired diffusion. The component attributed to mixed venous blood includes some from alveoli that are poorly ventilated with respect to their perfusion (Fig. 18.1). Hence, the compartment is strictly not a blood shunt, but a *venous admixture effect*. On this account it is usually designated $\dot{Q}$va, or, with respect to cardiac output as $\dot{Q}$va/$\dot{Q}$t (see Footnote 18.2).

Derivation of venous admixture effect

The derivation is via the mass balance equation:

$$\dot{Q}\text{t} \times C\text{a},O_2 = \dot{Q}\text{s,air} \times C\bar{\text{v}},O_2 + (\dot{Q}\text{t} - \dot{Q}\text{s,air}) \times Cc',O_2 \tag{18.18}$$

where C is content of oxygen and c′, a and v̄ refer, respectively, to the end-capillary, arterial and mixed venous blood. The physiological shunt as a percentage of cardiac output is obtained by rearrangement:

$$\dot{Q}\text{s,air}/\dot{Q}\text{t}(\%) = [(Cc',O_2 - C\text{a},O_2)/(Cc',O_2 - C\bar{\text{v}},O_2)] \times 100 \tag{18.19}$$

It is expressed in terms of saturation of haemoglobin (S) by dividing numerator and denominator by the capacity of the blood for oxygen, then:

$$\dot{Q}\text{s,air}/\dot{Q}\text{t}(\%) = [(Sc',O_2 - S\text{a},O_2)/(Sc',O_2 - S\bar{\text{v}},O_2)] \times 100 \tag{18.20}$$

Comment. The concept of venous admixture arose at a time when measurement of blood oxygen saturation was widely available, but measurement of gas tensions was still a specialist procedure. The two are linked through the oxygen dissociation curve (Section 21.2.2). Due to the shape of the curve the index $\dot{Q}$va/$\dot{Q}$t is insensitive to small reductions in oxygen tension.

Subdivisions of $\dot{Q}$va/$\dot{Q}$t. The physiological shunt is made up of blood from two sources. The first is that which enters the left atrium without participating in gas exchange. The blood constitutes an *anatomical shunt* across the ventilated alveoli. It is designated $\dot{Q}$s and can be intrapulmonary or extrapulmonary. Some causes are given below. The defining feature of this compartment is that the saturation of the shunted blood does not increase when the subject breathes oxygen (see below). The second component of the physiological shunt is blood that traverses capillaries in the walls of alveoli that are poorly ventilated. It is usually referred to as the *alveolar blood shunt compartment.* Strictly the term venous admixture effect should be allocated to this compartment, but historically it is used for $\dot{Q}$va/$\dot{Q}$t as a whole.

Values for $\dot{Q}$va/$\dot{Q}$t in different circumstances. In a healthy young adult at rest representative values for Sc',O_2, $S\text{a},O_2$ and $S\bar{\text{v}},O_2$ might be, respectively, 98%, 97.5% and 75%. Inserting these values in eqn. 18.20 then gives:

$$\dot{Q}\text{va}/\dot{Q}\text{t} = 100(98 - 97.5)/(98 - 75) = 2.2\%$$

Hence, 2% of cardiac output could be said not to participate in gas exchange. At age 60 the average proportion is approximately 4% [42].

Amongst the intrapulmonary causes for an increased venous admixture effect, an enlarged anatomical shunt occurs in some cases of bronchiectasis, atelectasis and pulmonary oedema. An enlarged alveolar blood shunt occurs when some physical attribute of the lungs is not functioning normally. For this to affect $\dot{Q}$va/$\dot{Q}$t, the abnormality must be either distributed unevenly, or be so severe as to cause respiratory failure. Examples are generalised airflow limitation and localised obstruction of

Footnote 18.2. The symbol $\dot{Q}$s is sometimes used in this context, but the usage is not correct (see subdivisions of $\dot{Q}$va/$\dot{Q}$t below).

airways at the base of the lungs (dependent obstruction). The latter can occur at low lung volumes from any cause (including posture and obesity) or be secondary to interstitial oedema, for which the cause might be a rise in pulmonary venous pressure or fall in plasma osmotic pressure. Extrapulmonary causes for an increased venous admixture include cyanotic congenital heart disease and portal cirrhosis (Sections 41.18.2 and 41.20.2).

From its derivation (above) the contribution of venous admixture to hypoxaemia is greatest when $C\bar{v},O_2$ is reduced by exercise, cardiac output is low (e.g. because of bradycardia, vascular obstruction or shock) or oxygen transport is impaired by anaemia (see Footnote 18.3).

Measurement of $\dot{Q}va/\dot{Q}t$. The $\dot{Q}va/\dot{Q}t$ is calculated from values for blood oxygen saturation at the three sites given in eqn. 18.20. The saturation in arterial blood ($S\bar{v},O_2$) is measured directly. The saturation in the mixed venous blood ($S\bar{v},O_2$) is obtained in one of the following ways: (i) by analysis of mixed venous blood obtained at cardiac catheterization, (ii) from the dissociation curve following a rebreathing procedure for measurement of tension of oxygen in mixed venous blood (Section 17.3.2), (iii) by calculation via the Fick relationship (eqn. 17.1, page 201) from measurements of consumption of oxygen, content of oxygen in systemic arterial blood and cardiac output, (iv) from an assumed value for the difference in saturation between arterial and mixed venous bloods; the difference is assumed to be 22% at rest and rather more on exercise.

The saturation in pulmonary end-capillary blood (Sc',O_2) cannot be measured directly; however, the corresponding tension of oxygen when the subject is breathing air is almost the same as that in the alveolar gas (see opening paragraph above). The tension in alveolar gas is obtained by use of the alveolar air equation; it is assumed to exceed by 0.1 kPa (1 torr) the tension in blood as it leaves the pulmonary capillaries so the latter is obtained by difference. The corresponding oxygen saturation is obtained from the blood dissociation curve for oxygen (Fig. 21.1, page 260). The validity of the assumed gradient for oxygen between alveolar gas and pulmonary end-capillary blood (in this case 0.1 kPa) is subsequently tested in the way described in Section 21.4.4.

18.4.5 Measurement of the anatomical shunt

Introduction. The physiological shunt is partitioned into its anatomical and alveolar blood shunt compartments by observing the effect of the subject breathing 100% oxygen. This raises the tension in all ventilated alveoli to a level in excess of 13 kPa (100 torr); hence pulmonary exchange of oxygen takes place on the flat linear part of the dissociation curve and the alveolar blood shunt compartment is eliminated. Most of the difference in tension of oxygen between mixed alveolar gas and systemic arterial blood is then due to the anatomical shunt.

Essential preliminaries. Prior to measurement of arterial oxygen tension the subject should have breathed oxygen for sufficient time to eliminate nitrogen from the lungs. Deep breaths should be taken to avoid atelectasis [43] (see also Section 35.7.2). The measurement itself should be performed using a polarograph that has been calibrated over the whole range. The analysis is best performed *in situ* using an intra-arterial electrode. Alternatively, if drawn blood is used it should be taken using glass syringes, (not plastic) and analysed immediately [44, 45].

Calculation. This can be calculated using a version of equation 18.20 in which allowance is made for the quantity of oxygen dissolved in alveolar capillary plasma:

$$\frac{\dot{Q}s,O_2}{\dot{Q}t}(\%) = \frac{h(Sc',O_2 - Sa,O_2) + s(Pc',O_2 - Pa,O_2)}{h(Sc',O_2 - S\bar{v},O_2) + s(Pc',O_2 - P\bar{v},O_2)} \times 100 \qquad (18.22)$$

where $\dot{Q}s,O_2/\dot{Q}t$ is the anatomical shunt as percentage of cardiac output, h is a factor which converts from saturation to quantity of oxygen combined with haemoglobin, s is the solubility of oxygen in plasma and the other terms are as defined above. When breathing oxygen Sc',O_2 is approximately 100% and Pc',O_2 is effectively alveolar oxygen tension. Hence, in the absence of nitrogen:

$$Pc',O_2 \approx P\text{B} - P\text{H}_2\text{O} - Pa,CO_2 \qquad (18.23)$$

where $P\text{B}$, $P\text{H}_2\text{O}$ and Pa,CO_2 are respectively barometric pressure, the pressure of water vapour in the lung and the tension of carbon dioxide in arterial blood. This quantity, which is nearly equal to alveolar carbon dioxide tension, is obtained from analysis of systemic arterial blood. The arterial oxygen tension is measured concurrently.

If the anatomic shunt is relatively small then the tension of oxygen in the systemic arterial blood exceeds about 20 kPa (150 torr) and the term ($Sc',O_2 - Sa,O_2$) is effectively zero. The relationship

---

Footnote 18.3. From the Fick equation (page 201), cardiac output is given by

$$\dot{Q}t = \dot{n}\,O_2/(Ca,O_2 - C\bar{v},O_2)$$

where $\dot{Q}t$ is cardiac output, $\dot{n}\,O_2$ is oxygen uptake and the term within the bracket is the difference in oxygen content between arterial and mixed venous blood. $\dot{Q}t$ is the product of cardiac frequency (fc) and stroke volume (SV) whilst Ca,O_2 is a function of the oxygen dissociation curve (f), haemoglobin concentration [Hb] and arterial oxygen saturation (Sa,O_2). Then, on substitution and rearrangement:

$$C\bar{v},O_2 = f \times [Hb]\,Sa,O_2 - \dot{n}\,O_2/(fc \times SV) \qquad (18.21)$$

thus becomes:

$$\frac{\dot{Q}s,o_2}{\dot{Q}t}(\%) = \frac{s(P\text{B} - P\text{H}_2\text{O} - Pa,\text{CO}_2 - Pa,\text{O}_2)}{h(100 - S\bar{v},\text{O}_2) + s(P\text{B} - P\text{H}_2\text{O} - Pa,\text{CO}_2 - P\bar{v},\text{O}_2)} \times 100 \qquad (18.24)$$

In addition to the gasometric method, the physiological shunt can be obtained from the proportion of the dose of a tracer gas that traverses the lung after injection in solution into the superior vena cava. Krypton-85 or xenon-133 can be used for this purpose (Section 18.6).

18.4.6 Measurement of the pulmonary blood shunt

The pulmonary blood shunt comprises intracardiac and related shunts but not post-pulmonary shunts through bronchial veins, thebesian veins, anterior cardiac veins and portal-pulmonary venous anastomoses. The two types of shunt are included in the anatomical shunt as estimated by the oxygen method (Section 18.4.5).

Derivation. Pulmonary blood shunt is the difference between cardiac output measured by a non-volatile indicator (e.g. indocyanine green, page 204) and pulmonary blood flow. The latter is estimated from the proportion of an inert gas that remains in the blood during its passage through the lungs and is not lost into the alveoli. The volatile indicator is a gas dissolved in saline. Ideally it should disappear without trace on entering the alveoli. In this circumstance the proportion of the indicator present in arterial blood is determined solely by the size of the shunt. In practice, removal from the alveoli is incomplete; the remainder then exerts a back pressure which contributes to the gas present in the arterial blood drawn for analysis. The contribution of the back pressure can be determined by using two indicators having different partition coefficients, for example tritium (T_2) and krypton-85. However, the procedure is then too complicated for regular use except as part of the multiple inert gas technique for ventilation perfusion inequality. As an alternative, Murray and colleagues suggested using a single volatile indicator and making an empirical correction for backpressure [46]. These workers employed Xenon-133 which is widely used for study of regional lung function (Section 18.6). Where that information is not required the indicator of choice is krypton-85 which has a low blood–gas partition coefficient and the energy of the emission is also low. Acetylene, nitrous oxide and freon-22 are other possibilities.

Procedure. The solution of indocyanine green is equilibrated with xenon-133 in a 30-ml syringe for long enough to raise the activity to 0.5 mc/ml. The material is transferred to a smaller syringe through a millipore filter and 3 ml is injected rapidly into the superior vena cava from a catheter in a brachial vein. The dye dilution curve is obtained from the output of a densitometer attached to an arterial cannula and concurrently blood is collected in a 30 ml syringe over a period of 1 min. Two similar blood samples are collected sequentially, the first after 10 min for determining residual circulating radioactivity and the second after the subject has inhaled a 3 ml bolus of xenon-133 administered by injection into the mouthpiece whilst the subject is breathing air. The latter sample is used to estimate the relationship of the back pressure to the dose of xenon-133. The radioactivity of the delivery syringe before and after the injection, and of the three collecting syringes are determined using a scintillation counter. The blood is then used to make serial dilutions of a further sample of dye, the densitometer is calibrated and cardiac output calculated (Section 17.3). The pulmonary blood shunt is then given by

$$\dot{Q}s/\dot{Q}t = \frac{\text{SC measured} - \text{SC back pressure}}{\text{SC calculated}} \qquad (18.25)$$

where SC is scintillation count in the relevant blood sample or in the case of the denominator the count which would have obtained if none of the gas had passed into the alveoli; the latter is given by SC injected/ $\dot{Q}t$ (dye). The limitations to the procedure have been discussed [46].

18.5 Lobar $\dot{V}_A/\dot{Q}$ inequality

The separate function of the right and left lungs was formerly assessed by bronchospirometry using a Carlens catheter [47]. Fibre optic bronchoscopy and bronchial catheterisation are now used instead. The sampled gas is analysed using a respiratory mass spectrometer (Section 7.7) [48]. This can be in the lung function laboratory, with a connection provided by a long sampling line (up to 30 m). By using a number of indicator gases many aspects of lung function can be assessed, including the range of the ventilation–perfusion ratios. In Fig. 18.6 and in some other studies [e.g. 49] the indicator was carbon dioxide. Argon or helium is appropriate for alveolar ventilation, freon-22 or acetylene for blood flow and carbon monoxide ($C^{18}O$) for transfer factor (e.g. Fig. 18.7). In unilateral lung disease additional information can be obtained from measurements made with the subject lying in the left or right lateral positions. The arterial oxygen tension is often higher when the diseased lung is uppermost, whilst in this position the increase in resting respiratory level compared with the supine position is less than that when the diseased lung is dependent.

The proportion of lobar volume that is accessible to the respired gas can be estimated using a catheter located in the appropriate bronchus. A 20 ml bolus of argon is injected via the catheter during a slow inspiration from residual volume. The catheter is then connected to the respiratory mass spectrometer for analysis of the local argon concentration during the subsequent expiration. The accessible volume is calculated from the dilution of the argon. Alternatively, a balloon catheter

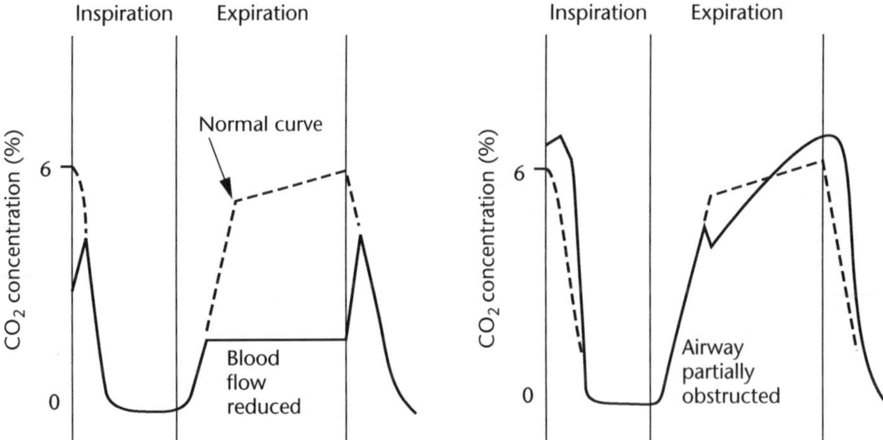

Fig. 18.6 Capnigram obtained by sampling from a lobar bronchus. The normal fluctuations during the respiratory cycle are shown by the interrupted line. When the lobar blood flow is reduced (left hand diagram) the alveolar concentration during expiration is diminished. At the start of inspiration the concentration rises briefly due to the entry into the lobe of deadspace gas which has come from normally perfused regions of the lung. When the airway is partly obstructed (right hand diagram) the concentration during expiration rises to an initial peak, declines and then rises again. The initial peak is due to the affected lobe continuing to inspire gas from adjacent lobes which are starting to expire (Pendelluft effect). The high alveolar plateau is due to the lobar ventilation being reduced and the continuation of the plateau into the subsequent inspiration is due to the affected lobe ventilating out of phase with the rest of the lung. Source: [47]

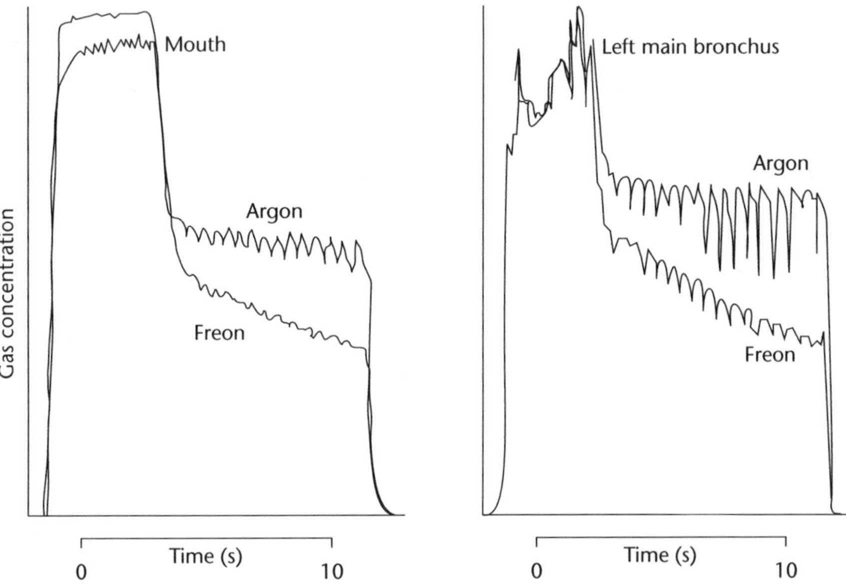

Fig. 18.7 Effect of lying on the left side on the distribution of ventilation and blood flow between the two lungs. The subject exhaled to residual volume, inhaled a single breath of gas comprising argon (A) and freon-22 ($CH_2F^{22}Cl$) in air, held the breath for 10 s, then exhaled. Gas was sampled at the mouth and in the left main bronchus and analysed in a mass spectrometer. Separation of the two samples was effected by using sampling lines of different lengths. Compared with mixed gas sampled at the mouth, that from the left lung contained more argon and less freon-22; this was evidence for the lower left lung being better ventilated and perfused than the right lung. Source: [48]

(e.g. Swann–Ganz 4F) can be placed in the lobar or segmental bronchus. The subject then inhales a vital capacity breath of a gas mixture containing argon in appropriate concentration, after which the balloon is inflated and the subject makes a full expiration. Subsequently, the balloon is deflated and expiratory effort continued. The additional volume expired and the local argon concentration during expiration are used to calculate the accessible gas volume. In the presence of airway obstruction this volume can be less than that obtained by an alternative method (Section 16.2.7).

In a similar manner the contribution of a part of the lung to ventilatory capacity or gas exchange for the lungs as a whole can be obtained by the subject performing the requisite measurements without and with occlusion of the appropriate bronchus.

18.6 Isotope-based indices of regional $\dot{V}_A/\dot{Q}$

Gamma (γ) radiation from some radioisotopes has the valuable attribute of penetrating body tissue, including that of the lungs and chest wall. On this account the isotopes are used to visualise lung ventilation and perfusion. In most instances the distribution is viewed in an antero-posterior projection (as are most chest X-rays), but lateral projections are also possible. The definition is critically dependent on the γ energy of the radiation. Where this is high, as with isotopes that emit positrons, coincidence counting can be used (Section 7.12) and the display then reflects the radioactivity throughout the plane of the lungs that is being investigated. Positron-emitters are mostly produced in a cyclotron and have a very short half-life (e.g. Table 7.10 page 74); this limits their availability to a few sites.

In order to match ventilation and perfusion the energy levels of the labels used for the two media should be similar. This can be achieved in the case of ^{133}Xe (Fig. 7.9, page 73) and the gas is convenient to use on account of having a half-life of 5.3 days. Unfortunately, the γ energy of the radiation is relatively low (80 KeV), so some is absorbed within the lungs and that which reaches an external counter is mainly from superficial levels of the projection. The depth can be increased by placing counters on both sides of the chest (Fig. 7.8, page 73). A higher energy emission is preferable, for example 140 KeV as obtains for Technetium (^{99m}TC) that is commonly used for perfusion scans (see below). The same substance, in the form of an ultrafine aerosol (Technigas) can then be used for the ventilation scan. In subjects with normal lungs the aerosol has virtually the same pulmonary distribution as a conventional gas; this may not always be the case in patients with lung disease. A technically better option for ventilation scans is to use locally produced ^{81m}K. This gas has a half-life of 13 s so most of it disappears from the body in less time than is taken for blood from the lungs to recirculate to the chest wall. As a result, the signal is specific to lung tissue, the dose of radiation is small and the measurement can be repeated within a minute. As normally obtained the method provides information on ventilation per unit of ventilated lung volume ($\dot{V}E/V$). This can be compared with the regional perfusion (see below).

Measurement of local ventilation ($\dot{V}E/V$). The isotope (^{81m}Kr) is generated on site by elutriation from an ion exchange resin column containing 81Rb. The flow of air through the column is approximately 1 l min^{-1}; the isotope is delivered through a disposable face mask to the patient who will normally be breathing quietly, sitting in front of a gamma camera (Fig. 7.9, page 73). In equilibrium, under quiet resting conditions the ^{81m}Kr count rate reflects the balance between the arrival and removal of radioactivity, i.e.

$$^{81m}\mathrm{Kr} = \dot{V}\mathrm{I} \times \mathrm{C\,I}/(\dot{V}\mathrm{E}/V + \lambda) \qquad (18.26)$$

when $\dot{V}$I and CI are, respectively, inspired ventilation (l min^{-1}) and inspired radioactive concentration, representing regional isotope arrival; $\dot{V}$E/V is expired ventilation per unit volume (l min^{-1}l^{-1}) which, with the radioactive decay constant λ represents the removal processes. The normal values at rest for $\dot{V}$E/V is 1–1.8 min^{-1} and for λ 3.2 min^{-1}. During hyperventilation the ^{81m}Kr signal tends to reflect the local lung volume.

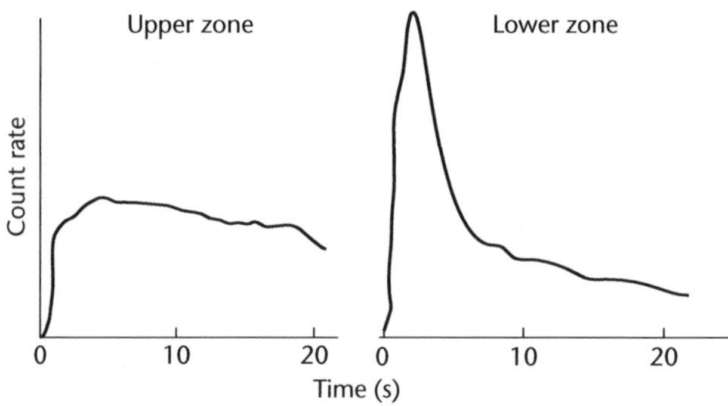

Fig. 18.8 Regional count rates for the upper and lower zones of a healthy lung during the inhalation of c^{15}o$_2$ followed by breath holding. The initial rise reflects the arrival of the isotope by ventilation bulk flow, the subsequent clearance reflects the blood flow per unit of tissue volume; this is greater for the lower than for the upper zone. An arrangement for counting is shown in Fig. 7.8, page 73. Source: [50]

Regional pulmonary blood flow. The optimal method for regional blood flow entails the use of C^{15}O$_2$ that is generated locally in a cyclotron. The oxygen molecules rapidly enter the lung water pool as $H_2^{15}O$ via the mediation of carbonic anhydrase. As a result the initial slope of the clearance curve is proportional to the blood flow per unit volume of parenchymal tissue including the interstitial tissue and the blood in alveolar capillaries (Fig. 18.8). A delayed C^{15}O$_2$ clearance may be an early sign of oedema or reflect a reduction in local blood flow. Most centres do not have access to a cyclotron so instead they use ^{99m}Tc labelled microspheres. These particles can provide similar information (HMPAO, Table 7.11, page 74).

The method entails the intravenous injection of microspheres of human serum albumen labelled with technetium-99m. The particles (diameter 20–50 μm) impact in the small pulmonary vessels in proportion to the local perfusion. The resulting radioactivity can be compared with that for local ventilation obtained using ^{81m}Kr. In both instances the volume of lung in the counting field influences the measurement. It is also influenced by the g energy of the emission as this determines the volume of lung that contributes to the signal reaching the detector. It is therefore important that the energies of the two emissions are similar (Table 7.10, page 74).

The particles obstruct some pulmonary blood vessels so the procedure is not without risk for patients with severe restriction of the pulmonary vascular bed. In addition some particles enter the systemic circulation, through right to left intrapulmonary or intracardiac shunts. However, these emboli appear not to cause side effects. The size of the shunt can be estimated by scanning the kidneys to obtain the lung–kidney activity ratio. This correlates with the shunt measured by the oxygen method (Section 18.4.5) but in absolute terms may exceed it because some channels allow the passage of 30 μm particles whilst at the same time being small enough to take part in gas exchange. Similar information can be obtained using ^{133}Xe; the methods are indicated in Fig. 7.8, page 73.

These techniques are widely used to assess regional $\dot{V}_A/\dot{Q}$ in a range of circumstances [2, 51–55] and are applied extensively for investigating suspected pulmonary embolism. However, they underestimate the full extent of uneven lung function since without additional information, e.g. [56], intraregional differences in $\dot{V}_A/\dot{Q}$ are not taken into account.

Regional $\dot{V}_A/\dot{Q}$ relationships. The development of positron emission Tomography (PET) using the nitrogen isotope N-13 has introduced a new dimension into the investigation of regional lung function. A bolus of the gas dissolved in saline is injected intravenously and that part which enters perfused alveoli then passes into the gas phase from where its washout is monitored. The method can provide rapid and repeated estimates of regional $\dot{V}_A/\dot{Q}$ [57, 58].

18.7 Conclusions

In respiratory patients uneven lung function is the commonest cause of hypoxaemia and a contributory factor in hypercapnia (Section 21.5.2). It is also the principal cause for increased ventilation during daily activities (Section 28.4.7) and on this account contributes to breathlessness on exertion. The hypoxaemia initiates changes in the pulmonary circulation, erythropoietic system, brain and other organs that can be responsible for extensive damage throughout the body. Hence, $\dot{V}_A/\dot{Q}$ inequality is important. In a clinical setting it is assessed in terms of the arterial blood gases and indices that are based on them, including the venous admixture effect and its subdivisions. The underlying mechanisms can be investigated using the distribution of ventilation–perfusion ratios obtained by the multiple inert gas elimination technique. The method is used mainly in research investigations.

For patients in whom there may be localised areas of hypoventilation or pulmonary thrombo-embolism, or where a lobectomy or pneumonectomy is contemplated, regional lung function should be investigated. This is usually done using a ventilation scan with ^{81m}Kr and a perfusion scan with ^{99m}Tc. Magnetic resonance imaging can also be used [59]. However, these methods are now being superceded by that using nitrogen-13.

For screening populations, including those that may be exposed to occupational hazards, the initial focus of interest is usually in the airways. For this application, an assessment can often usefully include indices of uneven distribution of ventilation (Section 16.2.1). If there is likely to be a vascular component, strong consideration should be given to the intra-breath R index of uneven lung function (Section 18.3).

18.8 References

1. Butler C, Kleinerman J. Capillary density: alveolar diameter, a morphometric approach to ventilation and perfusion. *Am Rev Respir Dis* 1970; **102**: 886–894.
2. Amis TC, Jones HA, Hughes JMB. Effect of posture on inter-regional distribution of pulmonary perfusion and VA/Q ratios in man. *Respir Physiol* 1984; **56**: 169–182.
3. Nyren S, Mure M, Jacobsson H et al. Pulmonary perfusion is more uniform in the prone than in the supine position: scintigraphy in healthy humans. *J Appl Physiol* 1999: **86**: 1135–1141.
4. Mure M, Domino KB, Lindahl SGE et al. Regional ventilation-perfusion distribution is more uniform in the prone position. *J Appl Physiol* 2000; **88**: 1076–1083.
5. Glenny RW, Lamm WJE, Albert RK, Robertson HT. Gravity is a minor determinant of pulmonary blood flow distribution. *J Appl Physiol* 1991; **71**: 620–629.
6. Hughes JMB. Lung gas tensions and active regulation of ventilation/perfusion ratios in health and disease. *Br J Dis Chest* 1975; **69**: 153–170.
7. Glenny RW, Bernard SL, Robertson HT. Pulmonary blood flow remains fractal down to the levels of gas exchange. *J Appl Physiol* 2000, **89**: 742–748.
8. Wagner WW Jr, Todoran TM, Tanabe N et al. Pulmonary capillary perfusion: intra-alveolar fractal patterns and inter-alveolar independence. *J Appl Physiol* 1999; **86**: 825–831.
9. Haldane JS. *Respiration.* New Haven, CT: Yale University Press, 1922.
10. King TKC, Briscoe WA. Blood gas exchange in emphysema: an example illustrating method of calculation. *J Appl Physiol* 1967; **23**: 672–682.
11. Riley RL, Cournand A. "Ideal" alveolar air and the analysis of ventilation–perfusion relationships in the lungs. *J Appl Physiol* 1948–49; **1**: 825–847.
12. Riley RL, Campbell EJM, Shephard RH. A bubble method for estimation of $P\text{CO}_2$ and $P\text{O}_2$ in whole blood. *J Appl Physiol* 1957; **11**: 245–249.
13. Rahn H, Fenn WO. *A graphical analysis of the respiratory gas exchange. The O_2–CO_2 diagram.* Washington DC: American Physiological Society, 1955.
14. Riley RL, Permutt S. Venous admixture component of the A-a $P\text{O}_2$ gradient. *J Appl Physiol* 1973; **35**: 430–431.
15. Farhi LE, Yokoyama T. Effects of ventilation–perfusion equality on elimination of inert gases. *Respir Physiol* 1967; **3**: 12–20.
16. Farhi LE, Olszowka AJ. Analysis of alveolar gas exchange in the presence of soluble inert gases. *Respir Physiol* 1968; **5**: 53–67.
17. West JB. Ventilation-perfusion inequality and overall gas exchange in computer models of the lung. *Respir Physiol* 1969; **7**: 88–110.
18. Wagner PD, Saltzman HA, West JB. Measurement of continuous distributions of ventilation–perfusion ratios: theory. *J Appl Physiol* 1974; **36**: 588–599.
19. Wagner PD. Calculation of the distribution of ventilation-perfusion ratios from inert gas elimination data. *Fed Proc* 1982; **41**: 136–139.
20. Riley RL, Permutt S, Said S et al. Effect of posture on pulmonary dead space in man. *J Appl Physiol* 1959; **14**: 339–344.
21. Rice AJ, Thornton AT, Gore GJ et al. Pulmonary gas exchange during exercise in highly trained cyclists with arterial hypoxaemia. *J Appl Physiol* 1999; **87**: 1802–1812.

22. Jaliwala SA, Mates RE, Klocke FJ. An efficient optimization technique for recovering ventilation-perfusion distributions from inert gas data. *J Clin Invest* 1975; **55**: 188–192.
23. Olszowka AJ. Can *V*A/Q distributions in the lung be recovered from inert gas retention data? *Respir Physiol* 1975; **25**: 191–198.
24. Evans JW, Wagner PD. Limits on *V*A/Q distribution from analysis of experimental inert gas elimination. *J Appl Physiol* 1977; **42**: 889–898.
25. Hlastala MP, Robertson HT. Inert gas elimination characteristics of the normal and abnormal lung. *J Appl Physiol* 1978; **44**: 258–266.
26. Kapitan KS, Wagner PD. Information content of multiple inert gas elimination measurements. *J Appl Physiol* 1987; **63**: 861–868.
27. Whiteley JP, Gavaghan DJ, Hahn CEW. A tidal breath model for the multiple inert gas elimination technique. *J Appl Physiol* 1999; **87**: 161–169.
28. Wagner PD, Laravuso RB, Uhl RR, West JB. Continuous distributions of ventilation-perfusion ratios in normal subjects breathing air and 100% O_2. *J Clin Invest* 1974; **54**: 54–68.
29. Rodriguez-Roisin R. *Series editor*. Contribution of multiple inert gas elimination technique to pulmonary medicine. *Thorax* 1994; **49**: 813–814, 924–932, 1027–1033, 1169–1174, 1251–1258.
30. West JB, Wagner PD. Pulmonary gas exchange. *Am J Respir Crit Care Med* 1998; **157**: S82–87.
31. Roca J. Wagner PD. Principles and information content of the multiple inert gas elimination technique. *Thorax* 1993; **49**: 815–824.
32. Kety SS. The theory and applications of the exchange of inert gas at the lungs and tissues. *Pharmacol Rev* 1951; **3**: 1–41.24.
33. Fortune JB, Wagner PD. Effects of common dead space on inert gas exchange in mathematical models of the lung. *J Appl Physiol* 1979; **47**: 896–906.
34. West JB, Fowler KT, Hugh-Jones P, O;Donnell TV. Measurement of the ventilation-perfusion ratio inequality in the lung by the analysis of a single expirate. *Clin Sci* 1957; **16**: 529–547.
35. Prisk GK, Guy HJB, West JB, Reed JW. Validation of measurements of ventilation-to-perfusion ratio inequality in the lung from expired gas. *J Appl Physiol* 2003; **94**: 1186–1192.
36. Meade F, Pearl N, Saunders MJ. Distribution of lung function (*V*A/Q) in normal subjects deduced from changes in alveolar gas tensions during expiration. *Scand J Respir Dis* 1967; **48**: 354–365.
37. Guy HJ, Gaines RA, Hill PM et al. Computerized, non-invasive tests of lung function. A flexible approach using mass spectrometry. *Am Rev Respir Dis* 1976; **113**: 737–744.
38. Singleton GJ, Olsen CR, Smith RL. Correction for mechanical deadspace in the calculation of physiological deadspace. *J Clin Invest* 1972; **51**: 2768–2772.
39. Asmussen E, Nielsen M. Physiological dead space and alveolar gas pressures at rest and during muscular exercise. *Acta Physiol Scand* 1956; **38**: 1–21.
40. Lifshay A, Fast CW, Glazier JB. Effects of changes in respiratory pattern on physiological deadspace. *J Appl Physiol* 1971; **31**: 478–483.
41. Bradley CA, Harris EA, Seelye ER, Whitlock RML. Gas exchange during exercise in healthy people. (i) The physiological deadspace volume. *Clin Sci* 1976; **51**: 323–333.
42. Harris EA, Seelye ER, Whitlock RML. Gas exchange during exercise in healthy people. II Venous admixture. *Clin Sci* 1976; **51**: 335–344.
43. Dantzker DR, Wagner PD, West JB. Instability of lung units with low VA/Q ratios during O_2 breathing. *J Appl Physiol* 1975; **38**: 886–895.
44. Pretto JJ, Rochford PD. Effects of sample storage time, temperature and syringe type on blood gas tensions in samples with high oxygen partial pressures. *Thorax* 1994: **49**: 610–612.
45. Smeenk FWJM, Janssen JDJ, Arends BJ et al. Effects of four different methods of sampling arterial blood and storage time on gas tensions and shunt calculation in the 100% oxygen test. *Eur Respir J* 1997; **10**: 910–913.
46. Murray JF, Davidson FF, Glazier JB. Modified technique for measuring pulmonary shunts using xenon and indocyanine green. *J Appl Physiol* 1972; **32**: 695–700.
47. Hugh-Jones P, West JB. Detection of bronchial and arterial obstruction by continuous gas analysis from individual lobes and segments of the lung. *Thorax* 1960; **15**: 15–64.
48. Williams SL, Pierce RJ, Davies NJH, Denison DM. Methods of studying lobar and segmental function of the lung in man. *Br J Dis Chest* 1979; **73**: 97–112.
49. Hoffbrand BI. The expiratory capnogram: a measure of ventilation-perfusion equalities. *Thorax* 1966; **21**: 518–523.
50. West JB, Dollery CT. Distribution of blood flow and ventilation in the lung, measured with radioactive carbon dioxide. *J Appl Physiol* 1960; **15**: 405–410
51. Kaneko K, Milic-Emili J, Dolovich MB et al. Regional distribution of ventilation and perfusion as a function of body position. *J Appl Physiol* 1966; **21**: 767–777.
52. Holland J, Milic-Emili J, Macklem PT, Bates DV. Regional distribution of pulmonary ventilation and perfusion in elderly subjects. *J Clin Invest* 1968; **47**: 81–92.
53. Ewan PW, Jones HA, Nosil J et al. Uneven perfusion and ventilation within lung regions studied with nitrogen-13. *Respir Physiol* 1978; **34**: 45–59.
54. Harf A, Pratt T, Hughes JMB. Regional distribution of *V*A/*Q* in man at rest and with exercise measured with krypton-81m. *J Appl Physiol* 1978; **44:** 115–123.
55. Orphanidou D, Hughes JMB, Meyers MJ et al. Tomography of regional ventilation and perfusion using krypton 81m in normal subjects and asthmatic patients. *Thorax* 1986; **41**: 542–551.
56. Kreck TC, Krueger MA, Altemeier WA et al. Determination of regional ventilation and perfusion in the lung using xenon and computed tomography. *J Appl Physiol* 2001; **91**: 1741–1749.
57. Galletti GG, Venegas JG. Tracer kinetic model of regional pulmonary function using positron emission tomography. *J Appl Physiol* 2002; **93**: 1104–1114.
58. Richter T, Bellani G, Harris RS, et al. Effect of prone position on regional shunt, aeration and perfusion in experimental acute lung injury. *Am J Respir Crit Care Med* 2005; **172**: 480–487.
59. Hatabu H, Chen Q, Levin DL *et al* Ventilation-perfusion MR imaging of the lung. *Magn Reson Imaging Clin N Am* 1999; **7**: 379–392.

Further reading

Jones NL, McHardy GJR, Naimark A, Campbell EJM. Physiological deadspace and alveolar–arterial gas pressure differences during exercise. *Clin Sci* 1966; **31**: 19–29.

CHAPTER 19

Transfer of Gases into Blood in Alveolar Capillaries

Gases enter the lungs by bulk flow and pass by diffusion into the lung parenchyma. Here oxygen and some other gases combine with haemoglobin. The present chapter describes these processes and explains why carbon monoxide and nitric oxide are used to measure the gas transfer properties of the lungs.

19.1 Introduction

The act of breathing introduces fresh air into the respiratory bronchioles, alveolar ducts and atria of the lungs. From these structures there is a net flow of oxygen by diffusion up to the alveolar capillary membrane. Carbon dioxide from the pulmonary capillaries moves in the reverse direction. Gas uptake proceeds by the gas dissolving in interstitial fluid and traversing the gas-to-tissue interface. Subsequently, there is a net migration of oxygen molecules across the cytoplasm of the alveolar type 1 cells, the plasma in alveolar capillaries and the membrane surrounding the red cells. The oxygen then combines reversibly with haemoglobin and the resulting compound is dispersed throughout the body by circulation of blood. The overall rate constant for the whole process is the transfer factor of the lungs for oxygen, also called diffusing capacity (Section 19.3.5).

The transfer factor (*T*l) can be modelled using a simple equation, applicable to all gases entering the lungs, including carbon monoxide that is commonly used for measurement (hence *T*l,CO) and nitric oxide that may be used increasingly in future. The subdivisions of *T*l,CO (and also of *T*l,NO) are the diffusing capacity of the alveolar capillary membrane (*D*m) and the ability of haemoglobin present in alveolar capillaries to take up the relevant gas. The latter is the transfer factor for the blood in alveolar capillaries and is the product of the rate of reaction (θ) and the quantity of haemoglobin. The quantity can be expressed in terms of the haematocrit and the volume of blood in the capillaries (*V*c). The procedures for measurement are described in the next chapter.

19.2 Diffusion in the gas phase

19.2.1 Directional velocity

Respirable gases are molecules having a diameter of approximately 3×10^{-10}m. The average distance between the molecules is about 10 diameters at atmospheric pressure, but the range is wide as the molecules move in random directions at high speed. Their movement is due to kinetic energy; this is the product of mass and velocity squared ($1/2\ MV^2$, where V is instantaneous velocity) and at a given temperature is the same for all

Table 19.1 Molecular weight (MW), capacitance coefficient (mmol l^{-1} kPa^{-1}) and solubility (vol STPD, vol^{-1} atm^{-1}) in water at 37°C (β and s, respectively), oil-to-water partition coefficient and the rate of diffusion (from eqn. 19.4) relative to that of oxygen for some respired gases. Sources: [1–6].

Substance	MW	β	s	Partition coefficient	Rate of diffusion
O_2	32	0.0105	0.0239	5.0	1.00
C_2H_2	26	0.3301	0.749	–	34.8
CH_4	16	0.0137	0.0312	–	1.84
Ar	40	0.0114	0.0259	5.3	0.97
CO_2	44	0.2514	0.567	1.6	20.3
CO	28	0.0081	0.0184	–	0.83
He	4	0.0037	0.0085	1.7	1.01
Kr	85*	0.0198	0.0449	9.6	1.15
N_2	28	0.0054	0.0123	5.2	0.55
NO	30	0.0180	0.041	-	1.76
N_2O	44	0.1710	0.388	3.2	13.9
Xe	133*	0.0375	0.085	20.0 †	1.75

* Radioactive isotope.

† Fat-to-blood partition coefficient 8.0–9.8:1.

Note: In the gas phase the value for β for an ideal gas at 37°C is 0.388 mmol l^{-1} kPa^{-1}. In blood, for gases which combine chemically, β is determined mainly by the slope of the dissociation curve.

gases. Hence, the rate of diffusion of a gas is inversely proportional to the square root of its mass or density (see Graham's Law, Section 6.7). The mass is described in terms of molecular weight relative to hydrogen (H_2) that has a molecular weight of 2 (Table 19.1). The rate of diffusion also varies inversely with barometric pressure. At constant temperature and pressure, gas molecules of similar mass have similar average velocities, for example under normal ambient conditions the velocities of oxygen and carbon dioxide are both approximately 4 m s^{-1}. The velocities of nitrogen and carbon monoxide are only slightly greater than that of oxygen; the velocity of helium is about 4 times greater and that of sulphur hexafluoride correspondingly less. The close proximity of the molecules leads to collisions. These occur with a frequency of approximately 5×10^9 s^{-1}; the frequency is independent of the mass so the distance a particle travels between collisions, which is the mean free path, is a function of velocity. Compared with oxygen, helium has a long mean free path so diffuses relatively rapidly whilst sulphur hexafluoride has a short path and diffuses slowly. The collisions lead to the movement of individual molecules being in random directions, so where there is a flow in one direction due to gas exchange, it is slow relative to the average velocity of the molecules (Fig. 19.1).

For oxygen the directional velocity is approximately 10 mm s^{-1}. This is rapid with respect to the distance between the respiratory bronchiole and the attendant alveoli, which is usually less than 1 mm. As a result, mixing of inhaled air with gas present in the alveoli takes place rapidly, with a mean mixing time in the range 2.4–3.1 s [7].

19.2.2 Diffusion coefficient

The concept of diffusion coefficient was developed by Fick who postulated that, under steady-state conditions, the diffusional flux was proportional to the concentration gradient:

$$Jz = -D\,dC/dz \qquad (19.1)$$

where J is mass flux, dC/dz is the concentration gradient in direction z and the constant term D is the diffusion coefficient. In practice, gas concentration (C) is often expressed in terms of partial pressure (P) or fractional concentration (F): then, for gas species y:

$$Py = Cy/\beta g \qquad (19.2)$$

$$Fy = Cy/(\beta g \times P\text{tot}) \qquad (19.3)$$

where Ptot is total pressure and βg is the capacitance coefficient which is the quantity of substance in undiluted gas in the units mmol/(volume × pressure). Values for βg are given in Table 19.1.

Equation 19.1 is now known as Fick's first law [8]. His second law is for non-steady-state conditions when the concentration varies with time. Under these circumstances the principle enshrined in the law is that of conservation of mass (Sections 17.3.1 and 17.3.2).

19.2.3 Behaviour of gas mixtures

Gases in a mixture influence each other's behaviour through attraction, repulsion and collision [9]. In a mixture of two gases,

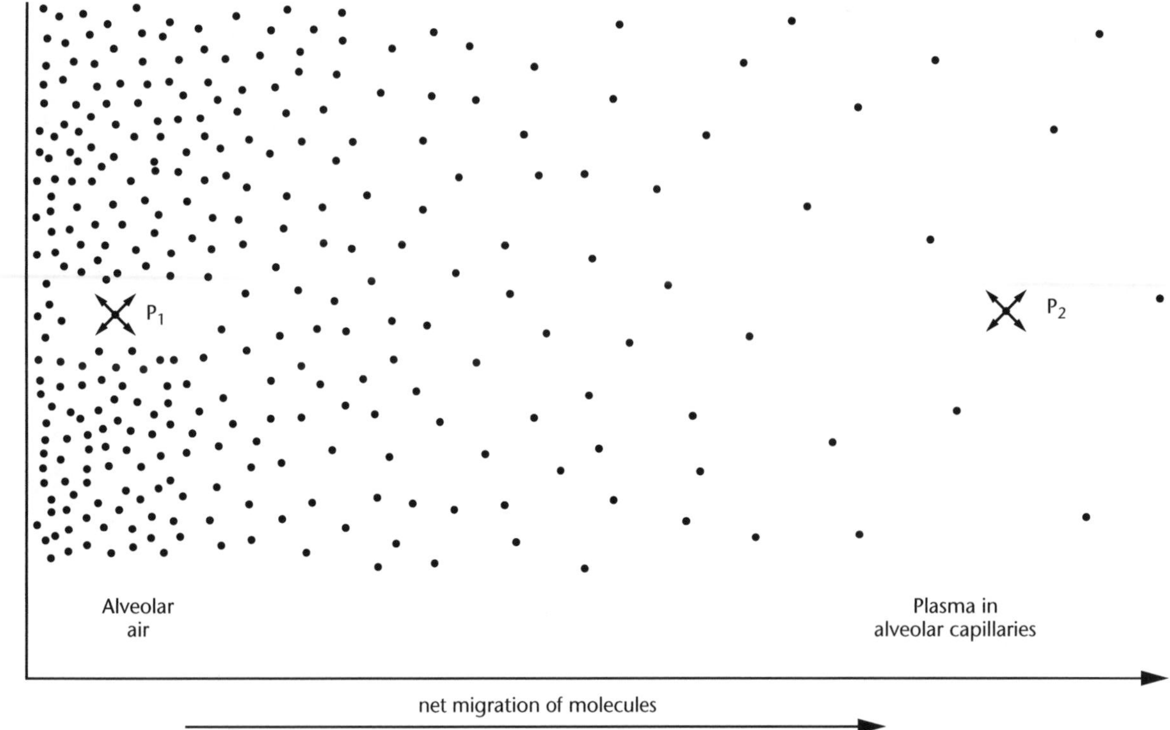

Fig. 19.1 Migration of gas molecules by diffusion from a respiratory bronchiole to the alveolar membrane. The illustration is for carbon monoxide as this gas is commonly used for measurement of the rate constant.

the gas that diffuses faster speeds up the slower one and is itself slowed in the process. As a result the binary diffusion coefficient is the same for both the constituents. Its magnitude depends on the respective molecular weights. Thus, for oxygen at 37°C the binary diffusion coefficients in mixtures with nitrogen, helium and sulphur hexa-fluoride are, respectively, 0.22, 0.79 and 0.10 cm^2 s^{-1} [1]. The presence of a third gas exerts separate influences on the diffusivity of the other two gases. In the example cited, the introduction of carbon dioxide reduces the diffusivity of oxygen, but the latter is then no longer the same as that of the carrier gas.

19.2.4 Applications

Normal gas exchange. Within alveoli the movement of gas molecules ensures that they mix almost instantaneously. There is no significant concentration gradient or boundary layer at the gas-to-tissue interface such as might hinder gas flow. Instead, the conditions are optimal for exchange of gas across the alveolar capillary membrane.

Diffusion also contributes to gas mixing within terminal lung units and dispersion of gas in lung airways (Section 16.1.5). These processes contribute approximately 10% of the overall resistance to diffusion within the lungs.

Investigative techniques. The relationship of the diffusivity to the mass of a gas can be used to investigate aspects of gas distribution (e.g. Section 16.2.1).

Diffusion respiration. In the absence of ventilation, gas exchange within alveoli leads to the alveolar tension of carbon dioxide rising to that in the capillary blood. Thereafter, in the absence of ventilation the movement of CO_2 ceases. By contrast, for oxygen the molecules that are taken up into the blood are replaced by others from the airways. As a result, during breathing air, the absence of ventilation leads to the selective accumulation of nitrogen. However, during breathing oxygen the replacement molecules are also oxygen, so gas uptake can continue until the oxygen in the anatomical deadspace is used up. This process is called *diffusion respiration*; it is of use in the management of patients receiving assisted ventilation since, after the lungs have been flushed with oxygen, the respirator can be disconnected safely for short periods without the patient becoming hypoxaemic.

19.3 Transfer of gas across the alveolar capillary membrane

The alveolar epithelium is made up of cells that fit closely together so gas exchange is by penetration, not by finding holes (Section 3.3.6). The epithelium is lined by a net made up of lipoprotein molecules and has water repellent properties. It is coated with dipalmitoyl lecithin and this substance lowers the surface tension of the boundary layer (Section 11.3). Gases pass across the membrane either by dissolving in the lipid layer or passing through gaps in the lipid to dissolve directly in the aqueous compartment of the epithelial cells [10]. The size of the gaps, hence the permeability, appears to be related to lung volume [11, 12]. The uptake is practically instantaneous. The quantity of gas that dissolves depends on its solubility. This varies for different gases from a very low value for helium and other insoluble gases to a relatively high value for diethyl ether, with most other gases being intermediate (e.g. Section 18.2.1). For a given partial pressure a soluble gas builds up a bigger surface concentration within the alveolar cell than one which is insoluble; other factors being equal its rate of diffusion in solution is greater in consequence. Once within the epithelial cells the molecules are in an aqueous medium and can diffuse freely into the lung interstitial fluid, the interior of the endothelial cells of the alveolar capillaries and the blood plasma. The volume of intra- and extracellular fluid in pulmonary tissue (lung water) is normally in the range 0.2 l–0.25 l [13].

Exchanges between lung water and blood plasma takes place where the alveolar capillary membrane is bounded on the one side by alveoli that are ventilated and on the other by capillaries and small arterioles that contain blood. Approximately half the alveolar membrane normally meets this requirement; the other half either adjoins the interstices between the alveolar capillaries or constitutes those alveoli that are devoid of either ventilation or perfusion. However, some oxygen enters the blood in the pulmonary arterioles [14]; similarly blood may exchange gas with respiratory bronchioles as well as with alveoli. Thus, the site of gas exchange is difficult to define anatomically. Instead it is convenient to define alveolar vessels as those that exchange gas with the air-containing spaces of the lung. For the vessels to make a useful contribution the blood should be flowing, but blood that is stationary also contributes up to the time when it becomes fully saturated with gas. This is the case during measurement of transfer factor by the single-breath method (Section 20.4).

The rapid flow of gas across the alveolar capillary membrane reflects the short distances that are involved (0.15 μm to 0.5 μm). The flow is assisted by factors that promote circulation of lung tissue fluid, for example thermal gradients due to variations in metabolic activity within the cells and movement imparted by respiration and the pulsatile flow of blood. The hypothesis that a chemical mediator contributes to the exchange of gas was suggested by Bohr (Section 19.5) and revived subsequently [15], but has little evidence to support it [16].

The rate constant for the transfer of gas across the alveolar capillary membrane depends on the physiological conditions at the time and on the physical and chemical properties of the gas. The former include the area and thickness of the membrane and the latter the molecular weight and solubility of the gas. Then for the whole lung:

$$D\text{gas}, x = k \frac{\mathrm{A}}{\mathrm{d}} \frac{sx}{\sqrt{\mathrm{MW}x}} \tag{19.4}$$

where Dgas,x is the overall rate of transfer of gas x in vols per unit of pressure gradient per unit time, k is the diffusion coefficient of the gas in the alveolar membrane (cm^2 per unit time, from eqn. 19.1 above). A and d are, respectively, the area and thickness of the membrane (cm), sx is the solubility of gas x in the lung tissue (vols/vol per unit gas partial pressure) and MWx is molecular weight (Graham's law, Section 6.7). Values of s for different gases are given in Table 19.1.

The quantity Dx in appropriate units is the diffusive conductance of the alveolar capillary membrane for substance x [17]. It is also called the diffusing capacity or transfer factor (Section 19.3.5).

The rapidity with which gas traverses the alveolar capillary membrane contributes to the time to achieve nearly complete equilibrium after a stepwise change in alveolar gas concentration. Thus, from eqn. 19.4, for an inert gas that moves by diffusion and does not react chemically in the blood, the time to 99% equilibrium varies with the square root of the molecular weight for the gas in question. Based on eqn. 19.7 which is given below, the half time for halothane (molecular weight 197.5) is of the order of 0.04 s and for hydrogen (molecular weight 2) approximately 0.004 s; these times are in the ratio $\sqrt{(197.5/2)}$:1 which is effectively 10:1. The times to equilibrium for most other inert gases lie within these limits. The times are very short compared with the transit time for blood through alveolar capillaries that is about 0.75 s at rest and 0.3 s during maximal exercise. The times to equilibrium for oxygen and carbon dioxide are somewhat longer on account of these gases also reacting chemically with blood. This aspect is considered below.

19.3.1 Role of gas solubility in blood

The instantaneous flow of gas across the alveolar membrane is described by the Fick equation (eqn. 19.1). For a gas x this can be written in the form:

$$\mathrm{d}Q/\mathrm{d}t = Dx[P_{\mathrm{A}},x_t - P_{\mathrm{c}}, x_t] \tag{19.5}$$

where dQ/dt is the quantity of gas transferred instantaneously at time t. Dx is the diffusive conductance and the term within the bracket is the instantaneous partial pressure gradient for gas x. The quantity of gas can also be expressed in terms of solubility and partial pressure. Hence,

$$\mathrm{d}Q/\mathrm{d}t = sx, \text{blood} \times \mathrm{d}Px/\mathrm{d}t \times 10^{-2}\, V\mathrm{c} \tag{19.6}$$

where sx,blood is the solubility of gas x in red cells and plasma (ml/ 100 ml per unit of gas partial pressure), dPx/dt is the rate of change of capillary partial pressure with time and Vc is capillary blood volume (ml). Equations 19.4 to 19.6 can be combined and integrated with respect to time, then

$$Pxt = P_{\mathrm{A}},\mathrm{x} + (P\bar{\mathrm{v}}, x - P_{\mathrm{A}}, x) \times \exp - \frac{(100kA \times sx\,\text{tissue})}{60\mathrm{d}V\mathrm{c} \times sx\,\text{blood}\sqrt{(\mathrm{MWx})}}t \tag{19.7}$$

where $P\bar{v},x$ is the partial pressure of gas x in mixed venous blood as it enters the alveolar capillaries at time zero and the other terms are as defined above. This derivation is due to Forster and the intermediate steps are given by Wagner [18, 19]. The equation describes the change with time in the partial pressure of a gas entering or leaving the alveolar capillaries as an exponential function of the driving pressure (i.e. the alveolar-mixed venous partial pressure difference). The exponent term includes the ratio of the solubilities of the gas in lung tissue and blood. It is independent of both the individual solubilities and the alveolar partial pressure provided that these are independent of each other. This is the case for most inert gases. The ratio of the solubilities (expressed in the same units) is close to unity except for gases that are very soluble in fat. For carbon dioxide, which combines chemically with constituents of blood, the ratio of the solubilities is also nearly independent of the partial pressure because the whole blood dissociation curve is effectively linear (Section 22.2.2). When solubility is expressed in the units ml per 100 ml per mm Hg, $s\text{CO}_2$ is approximately 0.07. Wagner has expressed βCO_2 as the ratio of the arterio-venous CO_2 content difference to the corresponding difference in partial pressure; these differences are, respectively, approximately 4 ml/100 ml and 5 mm Hg giving a value for βCO_2 of 0.8. Hence, the solubility ratio is of the order of 1/11. Based on this figure and after allowing for molecular weight the estimated time to 99% equilibrium of carbon dioxide across the alveolar capillary membrane comes out at 0.21 s. For oxygen $s\text{O}_2$ is approximately 0.003. The value of βO_2 at rest obtained using the same procedure as for βCO_2 comes out at 0.083; this results in a value for the ratio $s\text{O}_2/\beta\text{O}_2$ of 1/27 which is approximately 40% of that for carbon dioxide but only about 4% of those for inert gases that have a ratio of unity. Assuming this ratio and, if the dissociation curve were linear, the time to 99% equilibrium of oxygen across the alveolar capillary membrane in a resting subject comes out at 0.43 s. However, Forster and Wagner point out that the equilibrium time for oxygen is reduced by the curvilinearity of the dissociation curve and its dependence on other factors in blood. Carbon dioxide does not share these advantages; its dissociation curve is effectively linear and the chemical reaction with blood has several components some of which are relatively slow.

Thus, despite the high diffusivity of the carbon dioxide in solution the time to equilibrium across the alveolar capillary membrane exceeds that for oxygen. The process of transfer is described below.

19.3.2 Transfer involving chemical reaction with blood

Transfer of gases by diffusion alone severely limits the volume of tissue that can be supplied and the quantity of gas that can be transferred. The limitation was eased some 450 million years ago by the evolution of haemoglobin and the development of a system for its circulation round the body. In resting man the transfer of oxygen into the blood in the alveolar capillaries is confined to an aliquot of some 70 ml (Vc) that is replaced with each contraction of the heart; the average residence time is 0.75 s. On exercise the volume of blood is greater but its residence time is less (about 0.3 s at maximal exercise).

The transfer of oxygen from plasma to erythrocytes occurs by diffusion. This process is supplemented by convective mixing of the plasma as a consequence of respiratory movements and the pulsatile flow of blood.

Penetration of the red cell membrane is assisted by its large surface area and by migration of haemoglobin molecules between the surface and interior of the cells; the process has been described as facilitated diffusion [16]. In addition, the corpuscles change their shape as they traverse the capillaries. This stirs the contents of the cells and causes changes in pressure that lead to movement of water and hence of gases in solution between the cells and plasma. By these means the penetration of the red cell membranes by gas molecules takes place rapidly and the cell contents are mixed effectively.

Gases combine chemically with haemoglobin at finite rates. The reactions are reversible so may said to be opposed by back reactions that also have specific reaction rates [20, 21]. The rates of the forward reactions for oxygen, carbon monoxide and nitric oxide (designated θ_x, where x is the gas under consideration) have been determined *in vitro* for both haemoglobin in solution (Table 19.2) and for intact red blood corpuscles. However, the

Table 19.2 Some features of oxygen, carbon monoxide and nitric oxide that are relevant for gas exchange.

	Molecular weight	Solubility at 37°C (s)	Rate of diffusion (a)	$P\bar{v}$ (kPa) (b)	P_{50} (kPa) (c)	Combination velocity (d)
O_2	32	0.024	1.0	5.3	3.5	47
CO	28	0.018	0.83	(2-100) $\times 10^{-4}$	1.5×10^{-3}	0.9
NO	30	0.041	1.76	8×10^{-7}	3.9×10^{-7}	255

(a) rate relative to oxygen (from Table 19.1).
(b) mixed venous tension at rest: range for CO includes smokers.
(c) tension for 50% saturation reflects affinity for haemoglobin.
(d) with haemoglobin in solution (units $M^{-1}\ s^{-1} \times 10^{-5}$) [5].

Table 19.3 Summary of factors that limit alveolar capillary gas transfer.

	Anatomical dimensions (Dm)	Diffusion within blood	Rate of reaction with haemoglobin (θVc)	Rate of back reaction (ϕCVc)
Oxygen	√	(√)	(√)	√
Carbon monoxide	√	(√)	√	–
Nitric oxide	√	(√)	–	–

measurements are technically difficult to perform and the confidence limits are wide. Values for θ_{co} are given in eqn. 20.29 and Table 20.9 (pages 248 and 249).

In the SI system the rates are expressed as conductances, in the units mmol min^{-1} per litre of blood per kPa of plasma tension. The overall rate for both lungs is then the product of the reaction rate, the driving pressure (i.e. the partial pressure difference) and the volume of blood (Vc). Variation in the latter quantity or in the concentration of haemoglobin will affect the rates of combination of oxygen, carbon monoxide and possibly nitric oxide. The reported rates are for normal haemoglobin; those for atypical haemoglobins (Tables 21.3, page 262 and 27.2, page 367) are likely to be different. In addition, the reaction rates vary with the temperature and acidity of the blood. For carbon monoxide the rate is also a function of the tension of oxygen in the plasma which therefore affects the rate at which carbon monoxide displaces oxygen and combines with haemoglobin (Section 19.4.2). This interaction between oxygen and carbon monoxide in their reactions with haemoglobin is used to estimate the diffusing capacity of the alveolar capillary membrane and the volume of blood in alveolar capillaries (Section 20.8).

Blood that has been conditioned in the alveolar capillaries is replaced by mixed venous blood at a rate that is a function of the cardiac output. This quantity together with the metabolic demand, determine the oxygen content of the venous blood and hence the back tension exerted by gas entering the alveolar capillaries. Subsequently, the cardiac output influences the plasma back tension along the length of the capillaries by determining the rate at which the plasma is replaced. Thus, even in ideal lungs the rate of gas exchange is determined by a number of factors.

19.3.3 General gas equation

When a unit of blood plasma enters an alveolar capillary a very rapid exchange of gas occurs with that in the adjacent alveolus. In the case of an inhaled gas that is chemically inert the rate of gas transfer is determined by the diffusion gradient, the solubility and the flow of blood. Gaseous equilibrium is attained within about 20 ms and thereafter the plasma tension remains virtually constant. For a gas that combines with haemoglobin a similar initial rise in the plasma tension occurs. However, the gas tension does not immediately reach the level of the alveoli. Instead, a dynamic equilibrium is established in which the rate at which the gas traverses the alveolar membrane is balanced by the rate at which it combines with blood. In the case of oxygen this occurs within about 10 ms. The compound that is formed then tends to dissociate. For carbon monoxide and nitric oxide the back reaction is minimal (Table 19.3). For oxygen the back reaction is material and raises the plasma gas tension. The extent of the back reaction is proportional to the concentration of the compound with haemoglobin; this increases during the transit of the blood along the capillary. Consequently, the tension of oxygen in plasma rises progressively up to an equilibrium value that is usually attained within about 0.3 s (Fig. 21.2, page 263).

The principal factors that contribute to the transfer of gas are indicated in Fig. 19.2. Additional factors not included in the model include secretion of gas by tissue and reaction of gas with compounds other than oxyhaemoglobin [22]. In the case of nitric oxide, provided the alveolar gas is not contaminated by nasal or deadspace gas the model can still be applied.

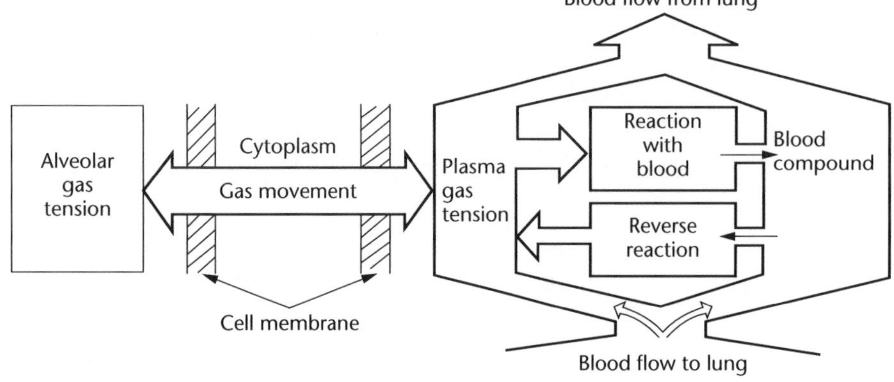

Fig. 19.2 Schematic representation of the processes that determine the transfer of gases from alveolar gas to alveolar capillary plasma. The processes are represented mathematically in eqn. 19.8. The special case of carbon monoxide during breath holding is shown in Fig. 19.3.

For a single chamber lung the overall rate of transfer at one point in time can be described by a unitary equation [23] given here in SI units, in which at any point in time

$$\mathrm{Dm}(P_{\mathrm{A}} - P_{\mathrm{c}}) = P_{\mathrm{c}}(\beta \dot{Q} + \theta V_{\mathrm{c}}) - (\phi C V_{\mathrm{c}} + P_{\bar{v}}\beta \dot{Q})\ \mathrm{mmol\ min^{-1}} \quad (19.8)$$

where Dm is diffusing capacity of the alveolar capillary membrane in mmol min^{-1} per kPa of diffusion gradient. (For traditional units see Footnote 19.1)

P_A, P_c and $P_{\bar{v}}$ are, respectively, the tensions in kPa of gas in the alveoli, the alveolar capillary plasma and the mixed venous blood entering the alveolar capillaries; $\dot{Q}$ is the cardiac output in $l\ min^{-1}$; β is the capacitance coefficient at 37°C in mmol per litre of blood per kPa of pressure; θ and ϕ are the rates of combination of the gas with blood and of breakdown of the compound which is formed, the units are for θ mmol $min^{-1} l^{-1}$ per kPa of plasma tension and for ϕ per unit of concentration of compound; C is concentration of the blood compound; Vc is the volume of blood in the alveolar capillaries in litres.

The term on the left side of the equation is the rate at which gas enters the alveolar capillary plasma from the alveoli. On the right side of the equation the first term is the rate at which gas is removed from the plasma by circulation of plasma and by reaction with haemoglobin. The second term is the rate at which gas is added to the alveolar capillary plasma. The sources of the gas are breakdown of the compound with haemoglobin and circulation of blood bringing in additional gas that is present in solution in the mixed venous plasma. The mean plasma tension cannot be measured directly; it can, however, be described in terms of the other variables.

19.3.4 Concept of resistance to transfer of gas

The transfer of gas from the alveoli to the haemoglobin in the alveolar capillaries entails overcoming a series of hurdles or resistances. First, that imposed by the alveolar capillary membrane, next, the resistances imposed by diffusion within the blood and by the relatively slow combination of the gas with haemoglobin and lastly, the resistance set up by the back pressure of gas dissolved in the plasma. The latter comes from gas that has passed through the membrane and from that evolved in the red cells by breakdown of the haemoglobin compound (*back reaction*). These resistances act one after another and therefore summate, in series. By analogy with electric current, resistance is given by pressure (voltage) divided by the flow (current) so resistance is equal to pressure per unit of flow. The diffusing capacity of the alveolar capillary membrane (Dm) is flow per unit of pressure, so that $1/Dm$ has the dimensions of resistance. Similarly, when blood is flowing, $\beta\dot{Q}$ is measured in terms of flow per unit of pressure, and so is θVc. The resistances set up by the latter two factors are $1/\beta\dot{Q}$ and $1/\theta Vc$, respectively. The resistance $1/Dm$ is that across the alveolar membrane. The other two resistances act between the membrane and the red cell, both maintaining a raised plasma tension of gas. Therefore, they act simultaneously and, as a first approximation, can be added together as $1/(\beta\dot{Q} + \theta Vc)$. The overall resistance to transfer of gas across the lungs from respiratory bronchioles to haemoglobin ($1/Tl$) is the sum of the three individual resistances:

$$\frac{1}{Tl} = \frac{1}{Dm} + \frac{1}{(\beta\dot{Q} + \theta Vc)} \quad (19.9)$$

where Tl is the conductance or transfer factor of the lung. The relationship is an exponential one and can also be given in this form. (see Footnote 19.2)

The overall rate of transfer of gas from alveoli to blood is the product of the transfer factor (also described as capacitance coefficient) and the alveolar tension in excess of the back tension. Hence, from eqn. 19.9:

$$\text{Rate of transfer of gas from alveoli to blood} = \frac{1}{\dfrac{1}{Dm} + \dfrac{1}{(\beta\dot{Q} + \theta Vc)}} \times \text{(Alveolar tension} - \text{back tension)} \quad (19.10)$$

The back tension is considered below. It contributes to the effective gas–pressure gradient (or *transfer gradient*) between the alveolar gas and the capillary blood. The gradient for oxygen is also called the diffusion gradient but this usage is not strictly correct since the gradient is the resultant of several processes and is not solely due to diffusion (see below). For carbon monoxide, transfer gradient is sometimes called effective alveolar tension or alveolar drive.

19.3.5 Terminology: transfer factor or diffusing capacity?

The term diffusing capacity (Do_2) was introduced at a time when combination of oxygen with haemoglobin was believed to be practically instantaneous. In this circumstance eqn. 19.9 indicates that the reaction rate θ would be very large, the term $1/(\beta\dot{Q} + \theta Vc)$ very small and the diffusing capacity of the lung equal to Dm (the diffusing capacity of the alveolar capillary

---

Footnote 19.1. In traditional units the rate of transfer of gas substance is in ml STPD min^{-1} mm Hg^{-1}, volume is in ml and the capacitance coefficient (β) is replaced by $s/760$ where s is the Bunsen solubility coefficient (Table 19.1).

Footnote 19.2. The corresponding exponential equation describing the total conductance across the alveolar capillary membrane is given by

$$G = \dot{Q}\beta(1 - e^{-(Tl/Q\beta)})$$

where G is conductance and the other terms are as defined in the text [24].

membrane). In practice, the term $1/(\beta\dot{Q} + \theta Vc)$ is of material magnitude for oxygen on account of the back tension that develops, and for carbon monoxide on account of the reaction with haemoglobin taking place relatively slowly (Table 19.2). For both gases the capacitance coefficient can be described correctly by transfer factor, a term used by chemical engineers to describe the migration of a chemical substance involving more than one process. The rate of migration need not be maximal. The substance and the starting and finishing points of the migration should be defined. For the lung the term Tl,co meets this requirement (see also Section 20.1.1). By contrast, the historical term 'diffusing capacity' which implies a maximal rate of migration by diffusion alone clearly does not. The historical concept more nearly applies to nitric oxide as the reaction with haemoglobin is rapid (Table 19.2) and consequently Tl,NO closely approximates to Dm,NO (Section 19.4.4).

19.4 Application of general gas equation (eqn.19.8) to individual gases

Introduction. The equation takes into account a number of properties of gases that can affect gas exchange, but gases differ in the extent to which the properties are relevant. The simplest circumstance is when the gas is inert. The circumstances for carbon monoxide and nitric oxide are more complex, but less so than for oxygen, where all the properties in the model make a contribution. Some differences between the principal gases that combine with haemoglobin are indicated in Tables 19.2 and 19.3. Some numerical values are given in Table 19.2.

19.4.1 Gases that do not combine with haemoglobin

In this circumstance θ is zero. Dm is large relative to $\beta\dot{Q}$, so $1/Dm$ is relatively very small and may as a first approximation be neglected. The transfer factor then simplifies to $Tl = \beta\dot{Q}$. The appropriate back tension for the calculation of the effective alveolar tension in these circumstances is the tension of gas in the mixed venous blood entering the alveolar capillaries. These quantities may be substituted in eqn. 19.10, which then becomes the Fick equation for determining cardiac output (Section 17.3.2).

19.4.2 Carbon monoxide

Carbon monoxide resembles oxygen in its solubility and molecular weight (Table 19.1) and its ability to enter into reversible combination with haemoglobin. However, compared with oxygen the reaction takes place at low partial pressures, hence haemoglobin can be said to have a high affinity for carbon monoxide. The relative affinities of the two gases are defined by the Haldane constant, which, in terms of gas tensions is approximately 230 (range 200–250). (see Footnote 19.3)

The high avidity of carbon monoxide for partially oxygenated haemoglobin is complemented by the reverse reaction being extremely slow. This feature has two important consequences that form the basis for measurement of transfer factor for carbon monoxide by the single breath and rebreathing methods. First, during a short period of breath holding the haemoglobin binds almost all the carbon monoxide that enters the alveolar capillaries and the plasma tension of co (Pc, co) does not rise much above that in mixed venous blood. Consequently, the allowance for the back tension of carbon monoxide in the blood is straight forward and, as normally carried out the procedure carries no risk of carbon monoxide poisoning (cf. Section 37.4.1). Second, except in rare circumstances (e.g. Footnote 19.4), the Pc, co is not dependent on CO being removed from alveolar capillaries by convection in circulating blood. Hence, the term $\beta\dot{Q}$ in eqn. 19.10 is normally small compared with the term θVc and may, as a first approximation, be neglected. Roughton and Forster have pointed out that in this circumstance the relationship for transfer factor for CO simplifies to

$$\frac{1}{Tl,\,\text{co}} = \frac{1}{Dm,\,\text{co}} + \frac{1}{\theta Vc} \tag{19.13}$$

In this form the resistance of the lung parenchyma to the transfer of carbon monoxide is the sum of the resistances of the membrane to diffusion ($1/Dm$) and of the blood to taking up carbon monoxide ($1/\theta Vc$) [20]. The relationship is illustrated in Fig. 19.3.

The relationship has two important applications:

1 Carbon monoxide competes with oxygen for places on the haemoglobin molecule. As a result the reaction rate θco varies

Footnote 19.3. The Haldane constant (M) is given by

$$\frac{[\text{co Hb}]}{[\text{o}_2\,\text{Hb}]} = M\frac{P\text{co}}{P\text{o}_2} \tag{19.11}$$

where the left-hand term is the ratio of the concentrations of carboxy- and oxyhaemoglobin, and that on the right is the product of the ratio of the gas tensions and the Haldane constant [25]. When the gases are described in terms of their concentrations, the value for M is increased by the factor 1.3, which is the ratio of the solubilities (s) of the two gases (Table 19.1) i.e.:

$$\frac{[\text{co}]}{[\text{o}_2]} = \frac{s\text{co}P\text{co}}{s\text{o}_2 P\text{o}_2} = \frac{1}{1.3}\frac{P\text{co}}{P\text{o}_2} \tag{19.12}$$

M is determined mainly by the ratio of the rates of association and dissociation of carbon monoxide with the intermediate compound of haemoglobin and oxygen Hb_4o_6 (Section 21.2.1).

Footnote 19.4. The residence time for blood traversing alveolar capillaries may be reduced in some patients with portal cirrhosis (Section 41.20). On this account the term $\beta\dot{Q}$ contributes to the transfer resistance and Tl is reduced [26].

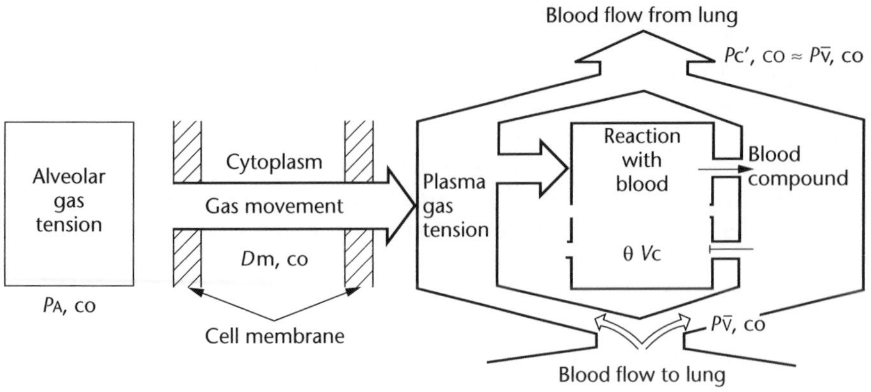

Fig. 19.3 Model of gas exchange in the lungs (Fig. 19.2) modified to illustrate the uptake of carbon monoxide. The virtual absence of a back reaction leads to the partial pressure of co in alveolar capillary plasma being nearly the same as that in mixed venous blood. This simplifies the measurement of Tl,co compared with measurement of Tl,O_2.

inversely with oxygen tension (Section 20.7.4). This inverse relationship is the basis of the Roughton, Forster method for measuring Dm and Vc (Section 20.8).

2 At any oxygen tension, the reaction rate for the lungs is dependent on the quantity of haemoglobin that participates in gas exchange. The quantity is contained in θVc. The contribution of [Hb] can be made explicit by redefining the other terms and in this form eqn. 19.13 can be used to interpret values of transfer factor in circumstances when the haemoglobin concentration is abnormal (Section 20.7.2).

19.4.3 Oxygen

The two-way nature of the reaction of oxygen with haemoglobin leads to the plasma oxygen tension rising down the length of the capillary and being greatly influenced by the rate of blood flow. Hence, all the terms in eqn. 19.8 contribute to the outcome. This has the effect that measurement of transfer factor for oxygen is relatively complicated, except when an isotope is used [27]. The difficulty has led to the alternative use of carbon monoxide and nitric oxide for measuring the gas exchanging properties of the lungs (Chapter 20). The methods used to measure Tl,O_2 are described in (Section 21.4).

19.4.4 Nitric oxide

Nitric oxide is a sparsely soluble gas that combines with haemoglobin to form nitrosyl-haemoglobin and with oxyhaemoglobin to form methaemoglobin; the rate constants for these two reactions are similar [28]. As a result, the rate of combination of nitric oxide with haemoglobin is independent of oxygen tension [29]. It is also relatively rapid, approximately 280 times that of carbon monoxide (Table 19.2), so the term $1/\theta Vc$ in eqn. 19.9 is very small. In addition, the rate of dissociation of nitrosyl-haemoglobin is extremely slow so there is no significant back tension in the capillary plasma on this account and hence the term $1/\beta \dot{Q}$ in eqn. 19.9 is negligible as well. In these circumstances the transfer factor for nitric oxide (Tl,NO) should be a measure of the diffusing capacity of the alveolar capillary membrane (Dm). This was first pointed out by Borland and Higenbottam [30, 31]. If no other factors are involved, Dl, NO should then be twice Dm, CO since, whilst the molecular weights of the two gases are similar, the solubilites are in the ratio 2:1 (Table 19.1). The values are for water at 37°C, but those in lung tissue are likely to be similar. However, the reaction rate *in vivo* may not be infinite and diffusion of the gas from the plasma to the interior of the red cells (which is the diffusive resistance of the blood) may also contribute to the rate of gas exchange [28]. If so, whilst the ratio Dm,NO/Dm,CO should approximate to 2.0 this will not be the case for Dl,NO/Dm,CO [32]. In a recent study the ratio was found to be 2.49 ± 0.28 [33] but an alternative value for the reaction rate θCO would have given a different result (Section 20.7.4).

Nitric oxide is not an easy gas to investigate on account of its many biological properties. However, the difficulties are being overcome and the measurements that have been made point to Dl, NO illuminating the gas exchanging properties of the lungs. In addition, the level of Dl, NO influences the extent to which nitric oxide produced in the lungs migrates inwards into the blood rather than outwards to the mouth [22, 34, 35]. This has practical relevance for interpreting the level of alveolar production of NO [36]. The level is increased with acute inflammation of the lung, for example in asthma, and accompanying acute lung injury (*q.v.*). Measurement of Dl,NO is discussed in Section 20.10.

19.5 Practical consequences

Present views on the processes whereby oxygen and related gases enter the blood emerged from experiments, initiated by JS Haldane and Christian Bohr into the possible secretory role of alveolar cells (Section 19.3). These investigations led progressively to the current position in which transfer factor (diffusing capacity) for carbon monoxide, measured by a single breath (breath holding) method is the recommended index of lung gas exchange. The considerable merits and the limitations to this approach and the alternatives that are available are considered in the next chapter (Chapter 20). Gas exchange for oxygen is discussed in Chapter 21.

19.6 References

1. Chang HK, Farhi LE. Ternary diffusion and effective diffusion coefficients in alveolar spaces. *Respir Physiol.* 1980; **40**: 269–279.
2. Hardewig A, Rochester DF, Briscoe WA. Measurement of solubility coefficients of krypton in water, plasma and human blood, using radioactive Kr85. *J Appl Physiol* 1960; **15**: 723–725.
3. Andersen AM, Ladefoged J. Partition coefficient of 133Xenon between various tissues and blood in vivo. *Scand J Clin Lab Invest* 1967; **19**: 72–78.
4. Wagner PD, Saltzman HA, West JB. Measurement of continuous distributions of ventilation-perfusion ratios: theory. *J Appl Physiol* 1974; **36**: 588–599.
5. Meyer M, Schuster K-D, Schulz H et al. Pulmonary diffusing capacities for nitric oxide and carbon monoxide determined by rebreathing in dogs. *J Appl Physiol* 1990; **68**: 2344–2357.
6. Wilhelm E, Battino R, Wilcock J. Low pressure solubilities of gases in liquid water. *Chem Rev* 1977; **77**: 219–262.
7. Chang HK, Paiva M, ed. *Respiratory physiology. Analytical approach.* Lung biology in health and disease 40. New York: Marcel Dekker, 1989.
8. Fick A. Ueber die messung des blutquantums in den herzvent rikeln. S B. Phys-med Ges Wurgburk July 9, 1870.
9. Chang HK. General concepts of molecular diffusion. In: Engel LA, Paiva M, eds. *Gas mixing and distribution in the lung.* New York: Marcel Dekker, 1985: 1–22.
10. Taylor AE, Gaar KA. Estimation of equivalent pore radii of pulmonary capillary and alveolar membranes. *Am J Physiol* 1970; **218**: 1133–1140.
11. Staub NC. Respiration. *Annual Rev Physiol* 1969; **31**: 173–202.
12. Davidson MR, Fitzgerald JM. Transport of O_2 along a model pathway through the respiratory region of the lung. *Bull Math Biol* 1974; **36**: 275–303.
13. Charan NB Regulation of lung water. *Cardiologia* 1998; **43**: 1305–1314.
14. Jameson AG. Gaseous diffusion from alveoli into pulmonary arteries. *J Appl Physiol* 1964; **19**: 448–456.
15. Sybert A, Ayash R, Chatham M, Gurtner GH. CO concentration-dependent changes in pulmonary diffusing capacity in humans. *J Appl Physiol* 1982; **53**: 505–509.
16. Kreuzer F, Hoofd L. Facilitated diffusion of oxygen and carbon dioxide. In: Fahri LE, Tenney SM, eds. *Handbook of physiology, Vol. 4: Gas exchange* (Section 3). Bethesda, MD: American Physiological Society, 1987: 89–111.
17. Bartels H, Dejours P, Kellogg RH, Mead J. Glossary on respiration and gas exchange. *J Appl Physiol* 1973; **34**: 549–558
18. Forster RE. Exchange of gases between alveolar air and pulmonary capillary blood: pulmonary diffusing capacity. *Physiol Rev* 1957; **37**: 391–452.
19. Wagner PD. Diffusion and chemical reaction in pulmonary gas exchange. *Physiol Rev* 1977; **57**: 257–312.
20. Roughton FJW, Forster RE. Relative importance of diffusion and chemical reaction rates in determining rate of exchange of gases in the human lung, with special reference to true diffusing capacity of pulmonary membrane and volume of blood in the lung capillaries. *J Appl Physiol* 1957; **11**: 290–302.
21. Sirs JA. The egress of oxygen from human HbO_2 in solution and in the erythrocyte. *J Physiol* 1967; **89**: 461–473.
22. Tsoukias NM, George SC. A two-compartment model of pulmonary nitric oxide exchange dynamics. *J Appl Physiol* 1998; **85**: 653–666.
23. Cotes JE, Meade F. Contributions to discussion. In: Dickens F, Neil E, eds.. *Oxygen in the animal organism. Symposium of International Unions of Biochemistry and Physiological Sciences*, London 1–5 Sept 1963. Oxford: Pergamon 1964, 47.
24. Scheid P, Piiper J. Blood gas equilibrium in lungs and pulmonary diffusing capacity. In: Chang HK, Paiva M, eds. *Respiratory physiology an analytical approach.* New York: Marcel Dekker, 1989: 453–497.
25. Douglas CG, Haldane JS, Haldane JBS. The laws of combination of haemoglobin with carbon monoxide and oxygen. *J Physiol (Lond)* 1912; **44**: 275–304.
26. Cotes JE, Field GB, Brown GJA, Read AE. Impairment of lung function after portacaval anastomosis. *Lancet* 1968; **1**: 952–955.
27. Hyde RN, Forster RE, Power GG et al. Measurement of O_2 diffusing capacity of the lung with a stable O_2 isotope. *J Clin Invest* 1966; **45**: 1178–1193.
28. Liu X, Samouilov A, Lancaster JR Jr, Zweier JL. Nitric oxide uptake by erythrocytes is primarily limited by extracellular diffusion not membrane resistance. *J Biol Chem* 2002; **277**: 194–199.
29. Borland CDR, Cox Y. Effect of varying alveolar oxygen partial pressure on diffusing capacity for nitric oxide and carbon monoxide, membrane diffusing capacity and lung capillary blood volume. *Clin Sci* 1991; **81**: 759–765.
30. Borland C, Chamberlain A, Higenbottam TW. The fate of inhaled nitric oxide *Clin Sci* 1983; **65**: 37P.
31. Borland CDR, Higenbottam TW. A simultaneous single breath measurement of pulmonary diffusing capacity with nitric oxide and carbon monoxide. *Eur Respir J* 1989; **2**: 56–63.
32. Borland C, Mist B, Zammit M, Vuylstreke A. Steady-state measurement of NO and CO lung diffusing capacity on moderate exercise in men. *J Appl Physiol* 2001, **90**: 538–544.
33. Tamhane RM, Johnson RL Jr, Hsia CCW. Pulmonary membrane diffusing capacity and capillary blood volume measured during exercise from nitric oxide uptake. *Chest* 2001; **120**: 1850–1856.
34. DuBois AB, Douglas JS, Stitt JT, Mohsenin RM. Production and absorption of nitric oxide gas in the nose. *J Appl Physiol* 1998; **84**: 1217–1224.
35. Pietropaoli AP, Perillo IB, Torres A et al. Simultaneous measurements of nitric oxide production by conducting and alveolar airways of humans. *J Appl Physiol* 1999; **87**: 1532–1542.
36. Perillo IB, Hyde RW, Olszowka AJ et al. Chemiluminescent measurements of nitric oxide pulmonary diffusing capacity and alveolar production in humans. *J Appl Physiol* 2001; **91**: 1931–1940.

Further reading

Chinnard FP, Enn T, Nolan MF. The permeability characteristics of the alveolar capillary barrier. *Trans Assoc Am Physicians* 1962; **75**: 253–261.

Effros RM, Mason GR. Measurements of pulmonary epithelial permeability in vivo. *Am Rev Respir Dis* 1983; **127**: S59–S65 (Review article).

Weibel ER. How does lung structure affect gas exchange? *Chest* 1983; **83**: 657–665.

Bachofen H, Weber J, Wangensteen D, Weibel ER. Morphometric estimates of diffusing capacity in lungs fixed under zone II and zone III conditions. *Respir Physiol* 1983; **52**: 41–52.

CHAPTER 20

Transfer Factor (Diffusing Capacity) for Carbon Monoxide and Nitric Oxide (*T*l,CO, *T*l,NO, *D*m and *V*c)

*Ability to transfer oxygen from alveolar gas to blood in alveolar capillaries is usually assessed by measurement of transfer factor (diffusing capacity) for carbon monoxide (*T*l,CO) and its subdivisions. The present chapter describes the methods.*

20.1 Introduction

20.1.1 Terminology

Transfer factor. The transfer of oxygen from alveolar gas to blood in alveolar capillaries involves a number of stages. The principal ones are diffusion within the alveolar ducts, atria and alveoli, solution of oxygen in the fluid compartment of the lungs, passage across the alveolar capillary membrane, diffusion within blood plasma and red cells and chemical combination with haemoglobin. The rate constant for this complex sequence of events varies with circumstances. It is described appropriately by *transfer factor*, a term used by chemical engineers [1, 2]. To be unambiguous, the gas being transferred, the sites between which the movement takes place and the method of measurement should be indicated Thus, *T*l,O_2.ss is the rate constant for the transfer of oxygen across the lung membrane measured by a steady state method. The term describes the average migration of gas molecules, but an individual molecule may move in any direction that is available. The measurement is usually made with the subject seated in a chair. If the posture or level of activity is different the circumstances should be indicated.

Diffusing capacity. Diffusing capacity is an earlier name for transfer factor, still used in some centres. It is inappropriate for two reasons. The index is usually obtained at rest when the index is submaximal so it is not a *capacity* measurement. In addition, several processes contribute to the rate constant, not only diffusion. These features are not in dispute so the term diffusing capacity is likely to be replaced progressively by transfer factor [3]. *Diffusive conductance* is also used [4] but this term is more appropriate for what is now designated *D*m (see below)

*Diffusion constant, K*co. The transfer factor per litre of alveolar volume was used by Marie Krogh [5] who called it diffusion constant (*K*co). The term has the same limitations as 'diffusing capacity' (see above also Section 20.4.2). The more precise alternative is Tl/V_A.

20.1.2 Why use carbon monoxide for the measurement?

The transfer factor can be measured for oxygen, carbon monoxide or nitric oxide. That for oxygen has over-riding biological importance, but oxyhaemoglobin dissociates readily so there is a material back tension of oxygen in the alveolar capillary plasma. The tension rises along the length of the capillaries (e.g. Fig. 21.2, page 263) and can only be measured indirectly (Section 21.4). The transfer factor for nitric oxide is of recent origin and holds promise for the future (Sections 19.4.4 and 20.10)

Currently, the methods of choice are those that use carbon monoxide (Tl,co). This is because the gas is not normally present in the body in meaningful quantities except as a result of inhalation and the compound with haemoglobin (COHb) does not readily dissociate. As a result the mean tension of CO in alveolar capillary blood ($P\bar{c}$,co), also called the back tension, can usually be taken as zero. Where this is the case, the transfer gradient for carbon monoxide (cf. Section 21.3.1) is the mean tension in alveolar gas (P_A,co). Where $P\bar{c}$,co is not zero, the back tension is that in the mixed venous blood (Section 20.2).

Carbon monoxide is harmless in low concentrations (Section 37.4.1), the gas can be analysed satisfactorily using a dedicated analyser (though not normally with a respiratory mass spectrometer) and the measurement of Tl,co by any of the widely used methods fulfils the criteria for a satisfactory test (Table 2.1, page 15). The measurement can be extended to include measurement of the component variables (*D*m and *V*c, see below) and reference values are widely available. The procedure is routine in most lung function laboratories.

20.1.3 *Dm* and *Vc*, components of transfer factor (diffusing capacity)

The transfer of carbon monoxide into the blood entails the gas molecules migrating by diffusion from alveolar gas to alveolar capillary plasma followed by their combining with haemoglobin (Section 19.4.2). There is no material back reaction (Fig. 19.3, cf. Fig. 19.2, pages 232 and 229) and this greatly simplifies the measurement. The rate constant for the diffusive component is designated *D*m, where *D* represents the process of diffusion across m, the alveolar capillary membrane. By tradition the index is designated *diffusing capacity of the alveolar capillary membrane*, implying that it is a maximal measurement. This is usually the case when the measurement is made at total lung capacity (Section 20.9.1). *D*m for carbon monoxide exceeds that for oxygen by a small amount that reflects the different molecular weights and solubilities of the two gases (Section 21.4.2).

The rate constant for the combination of carbon monoxide with haemoglobin is for the lungs as a whole; hence, it depends on the quantity and chemical characteristics of the haemoglobin present in alveolar capillaries. The quantity can be represented by the product of the haemoglobin concentration and the volume of blood that is participating in gas exchange. This concept defines the *volume of blood in alveolar capillaries* in terms of gas exchange and not anatomical structures. It is designated *V*c. The chemical rate constant then becomes θVc, where θ is the reaction rate of the gas with haemoglobin, expressed in appropriate units. For carbon monoxide the reaction rate is greatly influenced by the prevailing oxygen tension (Section 20.7.4). The physiological features and measurement of *D*m and *V*c are described later in the chapter.

20.2 Methods for measuring *Tl*,co

Introduction. The basic relationship describing gas uptake in the lung is:

$$\text{Uptake of gas G per unit time} = Tl,_G(P_{A,G} - P\bar{c},_G) \quad (20.1)$$

where Tl,G is the rate constant (transfer factor) for the lung for gas G and $P_{A,G}$ and $P\bar{c}$,G are the corresponding mean tensions of the gas in alveoli and alveolar capillaries, respectively. The difference between the two tensions is the transfer gradient.

The basic model and its limitation. The transfer factor for CO (Tl,co) is the quantity of the gas that is transferred from alveolar gas to blood in alveolar capillaries per minute per unit gas tension difference between these two sites. It is given by a version of eqn. 20.1

$$Tl,\text{co} = \frac{\text{uptake of CO per min}}{(P_{A,\text{co}} - P\bar{v},\text{co})} \quad (20.2)$$

where P_A,co and $P\bar{v}$,co are the mean tensions of carbon monoxide in the alveoli and in mixed venous blood. The last term ($P\bar{v}$,co) replaces the term $P\bar{c}$,co in eqn. 20.1, (for explanation, see Section 20.1.2). The model represents the lung as a simple gas exchanger where the gases are perfectly mixed so all parts contribute equally to the result. Yet the ventilation is uneven with respect to lung volume in that, even in a healthy subject, a single inspirate is not distributed uniformly between different regions of the lungs (Section 16.1). In patients with airways obstruction the distribution is uneven with respect to time, since the obstructed parts fill and empty relatively slowly. The function is also uneven with respect to gas exchange in that differences in expansion ratio can reflect variations in thickness of the alveolar

Table 20.1 Methods for measuring Tl,co.

Method	Lead author(s)	Some features
Steady state (on exercise)	Filley [6], Bates* [7], Leathart [8]	$V_A = FRC + 0.5\ Vt$. Error from uneven lung function especially at rest
Single breath	Forster [9]	$V_A = 0.95$ TLC. Method minimises regional inequality
Single expiration	Nadel [10]	Amplifies regional inequality
Open circuit wash in	Gilson & Meade [11]	Allows for uneven ventilation. Is technically demanding
Rebreathing	Lewis [12]	Allows for uneven ventilation. Breathing manoeuvre is not easy
Multiple inert gas†	West & Wagner [13]	Method is technically demanding

* Bates also used Fractional CO uptake ($1 - F_{E,CO}/F_{I,CO}$), called 'ductance de CO' by Lacoste.
† the method was used initially to obtain Tl,O_2.

capillary membrane. Additional factors affect the amount and flow of blood in different alveolar capillaries. Consequently, gas exchange is not uniform throughout the lung. Instead, there is inequality with respect to lung volume, ventilation–perfusion and diffusive characteristics. These features introduce different approximations into the measurement depending on which method is used; each represents a compromise with its own advantages and limitations (Table 20.1).

Components of the model (eqn. 20.2). Steady state methods. The uptake of carbon monoxide is measured during regular breathing of air to which carbon monoxide has been added. The relevant variables are the ventilation minute volume and the concentrations of carbon monoxide in inspired and mixed expired gas. The denominator of eqn. 20.2 usually comprises only the term $P_{A,CO}$, since, in most circumstances $P\bar{v},co$ is effectively zero. Exceptions include heavy smokers, persons who have recently smoked a cigarette and those on whom multiple determinations are being carried out. In any of these circumstances the back tension should be measured (Section 20.7.1). The alveolar carbon monoxide tension is calculated from the tension in the expired gas and the physiological deadspace for carbon monoxide. The latter is assumed to be the same as for carbon dioxide which, in turn, is calculated in one of several ways, each with its own features (Section 20.3). The resulting estimate of Tl,co is very susceptible to uneven lung ventilation especially when ventilation is low on account of the measurement being made at rest. The method is more reliable during exercise. It is used at rest if the subject cannot cooperate in the measurement, for example an infant or a patient who is unconscious.

Breath holding and related methods. The uptake of CO is measured during a controlled breathing manoeuvre, either breath holding for 10 s, rebreathing from a bag or making a single slow expiration. In each instance the lungs have access to a finite quantity of carbon monoxide in a defined space, so on the assumption that the gas is perfectly mixed the rate at which CO disappears from the space is proportional to the amount present (i.e. the disappearance from the space is exponential). Then, at one point in time the rate is given by Krogh's equation [5]:

$$dF,co/dt = -F,co \times (Tl,co/V) \qquad (20.3)$$

where F,co is mean alveolar concentration of CO at time t and V is the volume of the space (the lung or lung plus rebreathing bag). Krogh worked in absolute units (Section 20.9.1). The equation in present day units is given as eqn. 20.11 (below).

The uptake of CO over time is represented graphically in Fig. 20.1. When a linear scale is used the decline in alveolar concentration is curvilinear, but it is linear on a semi-log scale

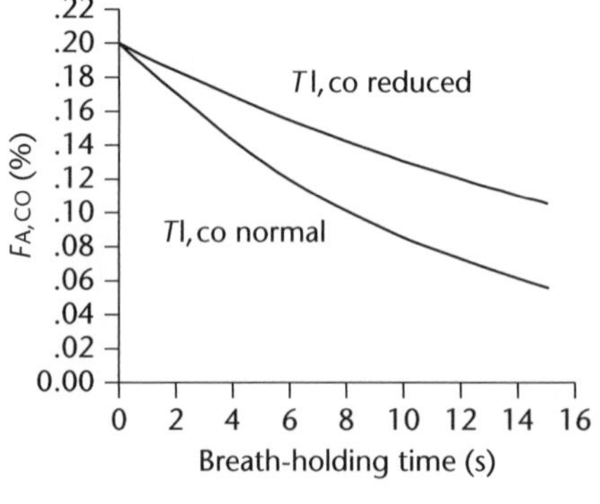

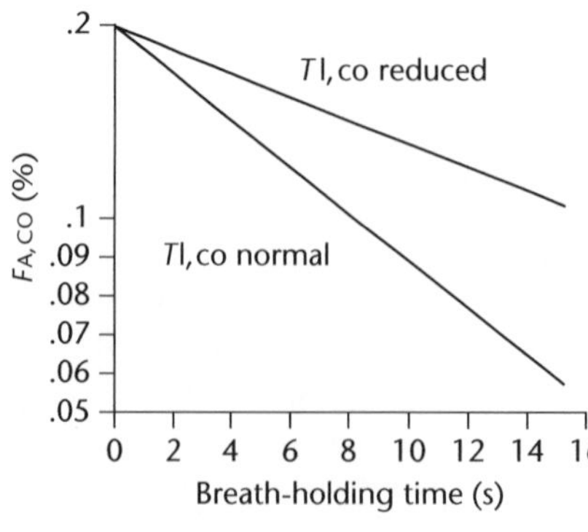

Fig. 20.1 Uptake of carbon monoxide from the lung during breath holding, showing typical relationships for a healthy young man and a patient with defective gas transfer (transfer factor, respectively, 12 and 6 in SI units, 36 and 18 in traditional units). The CO uptake is linear when expressed using a log scale (semi-log plot, right hand graph).

(Fig. 20.1). The logarithmic transformation makes possible the measurement of transfer factor by these methods.

Choice of methods. Of the methods listed in Table 20.1, the single-breath (breath holding) method has the merit of minimising regional inequality as it is measured at total lung capacity, and is simple to perform by all but the most disabled subjects (vital capacity >1.5 l). The method is suitable for respiratory surveys so reference values are available and it is used in a majority of lung function laboratories. The method is recommended internationally [14, 15, 16]. The rebreathing method is particularly suitable for patients with a small vital capacity or where there is a risk of cross-infection. It is suitable for patients with uneven lung function because rebreathing improves the lung mixing [17]. However, this advantage can be offset by such patients often not being able to perform the breathing manoeuvre adequately. The single expiration method has potential for exploring regional differences in gas exchange, but this aspect has still to be developed. It can be applied during maximal exercise.

20.3 Measurement of *Tl,co.ss* (steady state method)

The method is suitable for young children and subjects who are anaesthetised. It can be used during exercise.

20.3.1 Practical details

The measurement is made whilst the subject breathes a gas mixture containing a low concentration of carbon monoxide ($F_{I,CO} \approx 0.001$) made up in air. Breathing is continued for long enough to achieve a steady state in which the quantity of carbon monoxide entering the alveoli from the inspired gas is equal to that taken up from the alveolar gas by the blood. One or two minutes is usually sufficient time. The expired gas is then collected for 1 min. The expired carbon monoxide concentration is obtained by analysis and this quantity, together with the ventilation minute volume, are used to calculate the carbon monoxide uptake.

In most versions of the method, the alveolar carbon monoxide tension is calculated from the mixed expired concentration by making an allowance for the physiological deadspace. The deadspace is that for carbon dioxide but is effectively the same for carbon monoxide. Then:

$$Vd/Vt = (P_{A,CO_2} - P_{E,CO_2})/(P_{A,CO_2} - P_{I,CO_2}) \quad (20.4)$$

$$= (P_{E,CO} - P_{A,CO})/(P_{I,CO} - P_{A,CO}) \quad (20.5)$$

hence,

$$P_{A,CO} = P_{I,CO} - \frac{P_{A,CO_2} \times (P_{I,CO} - P_{E,CO})}{P_{E,CO_2}} \quad (20.6)$$

where *Vd* and *Vt* are physiological deadspace and tidal volume; P_I, P_A and P_E refer to the tensions of the designated gases (carbon dioxide and carbon monoxide) in inspired, alveolar and expired gas.

The tensions of carbon monoxide and carbon dioxide in the inspired and the expired gas are obtained by analysis; the tension of carbon dioxide in the alveolar gas is estimated in one of several ways. In the *Filley method* the tension of carbon dioxide is that in arterial blood [6]. This is effectively the same as in the mixed alveolar gas, except when the range of ventilation–perfusion ratios is increased (see below). In the *Bates method* the alveolar gas concentrations are obtained by sampling the expired gas at the lips into a rapid analyser for carbon dioxide or carbon monoxide [7]. The required gas concentration is that in the early part of the alveolar plateau (shown by arrow in Fig. 18.6, page 220). This procedure is unreliable at rest on account of the tidal volume being relatively low. It can yield a representative value for the alveolar concentration during exercise, provided the distribution of lung function is fairly uniform. In the *Leathart method* the effect of uneven lung function is allowed for by obtaining the alveolar carbon dioxide tension during rebreathing (Section 17.3.2) [8]. The corresponding tension for carbon monoxide is that calculated using eqn. 20.6.

20.3.2 Limitations of steady state methods

Uneven lung function is an important source of error in steady state methods. This is especially so at rest as the range of uncertainty in estimating the alveolar carbon monoxide tension is large relative to the transfer gradient. The error is less on exercise because the lung function is then more uniform [18]. This improves the accuracy of estimation of $P_{A,CO}$ and increases the transfer gradient. The result is still inaccurate if lung function is uneven. A low result by the method involving sampling the expired gas (Bates' method) is then evidence for either a transfer defect or uneven lung function. A low result by the method based on arterial blood (Filley method) is usually evidence for a transfer defect; however, the abnormality can be exaggerated if the lung function is uneven [19, 20, 21]. The result can also be influenced by hyperventilation and by changes in airway calibre from any cause [22–25]. A measurement of back tension must form part of the procedure as the concentration of carbon monoxide in the test gas is relatively low.

20.4 Measurement of *Tl,co.sb* (single breath, breath-holding method)

The single-breath method was proposed by Bohr [2] and developed by Marie Krogh who obtained alveolar samples at the beginning and end of a period of breath holding [5]. However, the samples came from parts of the lungs having different expansion ratios, so the method was unsound. The difficulty was overcome by Forster, Fowler and colleagues on advice from Kety that the initial gas concentration could be calculated from the dilution of an inert gas added to the test gas mixture [9, 26]. The method of Forster is widely used on account of its good reproducibility and convenience for the subject [27]. The method has been subject to standardisation by international organisations [14, 15, 16]; their recommendations are incorporated in the present account.

Outline. A single vital capacity breath of test gas containing carbon monoxide and an inert gas (usually helium or methane) is inhaled and held in the lung for a timed period (usually 8 s). During the subsequent exhalation a sample of alveolar gas is taken for analysis. The rate of uptake of CO (hence its disappearance from the lungs during breath holding) is proportional to the amount present, so is obtained from the exponential decline in (CO); the decline is linearised by using a semi-log plot (Fig. 20.1). The initial alveolar concentration of CO is obtained by measuring the dilution in the lungs of the inert gas present in the test gas and making the assumption that the CO is diluted to the same extent. The final alveolar concentration of CO is obtained from the alveolar sample. The method has the advantage of only requiring the analysis of the inspired gas and one alveolar sample; in addition, the procedure compensates for the distribution of CO in the lungs being uneven because the inert gas is distributed in a similar manner.

For routine measurements the optimal alveolar oxygen tension during breath holding is that normally present at sea level [16]. The test is sometimes extended by making an additional measurement at a higher tension. The two sets of results are then used to calculate the respective contributions to gas exchange of the diffusing capacity of the alveolar capillary membrane (Dm) and the volume of blood in alveolar capillaries (Vc). Dm and Vc can also be obtained from the concurrent measurement of Tl,co and Tl,NO (Section 20.10).

Which lung volume? As originally developed the Tl,co.sb was for the lungs as a whole, so the volume used to calculate uptake of carbon monoxide was the volume of the test breath plus residual volume measured separately [28]. This convention made a full allowance for uneven lung function as the whole of the lung volume (VA) was assumed to take part in gas exchange, not merely the part into which the test gas was distributed. The assumption appears to be valid for cases of chronic bronchitis or asthma, without emphysema as the alveoli are intact. Some of these patients may have alveolar capillaries that are poorly perfused as a result of hypoxic vasoconstriction, but this has little effect on the uptake of CO during breath holding, provided the capillaries contain their usual quantity of blood (Fig. 19.3, page 232).

The assumption of normal gas exchange with respect to lung volume is not valid when the lung contains emphysematous spaces that do not take part in gas exchange. Thus, the derivation using VA provides an upper limit for the transfer factor in the prevailing circumstances. A lower limit is provided by basing the calculation on the lung volume measured by the dilution in the lung of the helium (or other inert gas) contained in the test breath (effective VA, designated VA,eff [14]). This practice has the advantage for a busy laboratory that only one procedure is needed [29]. When the lung function is relatively uniform, the result represents the transfer characteristics of the whole lung, but is an underestimate in the presence of airway narrowing, as when the subject is not fully bronchodilated at the time of measurement [30]. In this circumstance part of the reduction in transfer factor reflects the use of too small a VA and does not necessarily indicate defective alveolar capillary function. Interpretation can be assisted by correction of any reversible bronchoconstriction prior to the measurement and by reporting the range of uncertainty as between using in the calculation the single-breath and multi-breath (or plethysmographic) estimate of lung volume during breath holding. The ratio of the volumes (VA,eff/VA) constitutes the lung volume index of uneven ventilation (Section 16.2.7). A low ratio relative to the reference value (e.g. 0.7) is usually evidence for uneven lung function contributing to the result. A value exceeding unity is always due to one or other measurement being defective (e.g. Fig. 20.4 below). Where the volume inspired is sub-maximal or the vital capacity is abnormal the use of a correction factor is sometimes informative [31]. In addition, in some circumstances there may be a case for estimating the alveolar volume from the dilution of nitrogen instead of helium (see Nitrogen recovery method for measuring VA, page 242).

Time of breath holding. The breath-holding time is a compromise between the convenience of the subject and the need for a measurable change in alveolar concentration of carbon monoxide [32]. Ten seconds is optimal. Ideally its limits should be clearly defined by the subject inhaling and exhaling the test gas with infinite speed. In practice this is an unrealistic expectation, so allowance must be made for gas exchange taking place during inspiration and expiration as well as during breath holding. Early protocols to this effect [28, 33] were to varying extents unsatisfactory, so should not be used [30]. The difficulty was first addressed in depth by Jones & Meade [34], whose method is recommended for routine use (see below Fig. 20.3). An alternative approach is to estimate separately the uptake of CO during the three distinct phases of the manoeuvre [35, 36]. Hence,

during inhalation:

$$d[V_A(t)F_{A,co}(t)]/dt = -Tl,co(t)(P_B - P_{H_2O}) \times F_{A,co}(t) + F_{I,co}\, dV_A(t)/dt \quad (20.7)$$

during breath holding:

$$V_A(BH) dF_{A,co}(t)/dt = -Tl,co(P_B - P_{H_2O}) \times F_{A,co}(t) \quad (20.8)$$

during exhalation:

$$V_A(t) dF_{A,co}(t)/dt = -Tl,co(P_B - P_{H_2O}) \times F_{A,co}(t) \quad (20.9)$$

where $V_A(t)$ is alveolar volume and $F_{A,co}(t)$ is fractional concentration of alveolar CO at time t, $F_{I,co}$ is fractional concentration of CO in inspirate, $(P_B - P_{H_2O})$ is the pressure of dry gas in the lungs and $V_A(BH)$ is the alveolar volume during breath holding. In SI units P_{H_2O} is 6.3 kPa and in traditional units 47 mm Hg. In the calculations a value is assumed for *T*l,co and used to compare the predicted $F_{A,CO}$ with that observed in the sample volume. An iterative process is used to determine a value for *T*l,co (the *T*l,co.3EQ) that results in the predicted and observed $F_{A,CO}$ falling within a tolerance of 0.01% of the measured alveolar CO.

The three-equation method makes individual allowances for inhaled flow, breath-holding time, exhaled flow and the volume and timing of the alveolar gas sample. However, the model is based on the inexact assumption that *T*l,co is independent of lung volume. The method requires rapid responding gas analysers. When compared with other empirical corrections for breath-holding time the method gives more reliable estimates of *T*l,co in conditions when exhaled flow is prolonged by airflow limitation [37]. It also results in a more accurate estimate of single-breath alveolar volume when ventilation is non-uniform [38].

Apparatus. The equipment used for measuring *T*l,co.sb has changed over time, from simple combinations of valves, taps and bags, through semi-automatic equipment [39] to sophisticated automated apparatus that combine the measurement of gas transfer with that of other aspects of lung function (see also Section 2.5). The changes have reduced the bulk and increased the versatility and ease of use of the equipment. However, the conventions and calculations are often predetermined, sometimes inappropriate and not always as transparent as is now considered necessary. Equipment should conform to accepted standards for accuracy of gas volume, flow, time and gas composition (Chapter 7). In addition, the operator and the subject should be provided with feedback on how well the requisite breathing manoeuvres have been carried out (Section 7.16).

The gases and how they are analysed. The test gas comprises carbon monoxide (fractional concentration usually 0.003), an inert gas and some oxygen, with the residual gas nitrogen. In the cases of the first two of these gases the method requires that the ratios of their concentrations in samples of inspired and alveolar gas are measured accurately. To achieve this the two samples should always be analysed concurrently. It is not sufficient to rely on the composition of the inspirate as recorded on the gas cylinder.

(i) Carbon monoxide. Carbon monoxide is analysed by infrared absorption, a chemical method or gas chromatography. The former method is well established and yields accurate results when care is taken to calibrate and maintain the detector. The detector has a useful life of, on average, 10 years. The gas mixtures used for the calibration should have been stored in a cylinder lined with tin as the gas reacts with iron. Alternatively, fresh mixtures can be prepared in the laboratory using a gas burette, a Wösthoff pump which has been calibrated (Section 7.15), or a closed-circuit apparatus. The linearity of the analyser is more important than the accuracy because the principal objective is to obtain the ratio of the expired to the inspired carbon monoxide concentration. The absolute concentration is only needed when it is proposed to allow for the back pressure of carbon monoxide in blood (Section 20.7.1). The procedure for checking the linearity is illustrated in Fig. 20.2. Infrared analysers are sensitive to carbon dioxide and to water vapour so these gases should be absorbed from the test gas prior to analysis (see above). Some analysers are also sensitive to oxygen due to its presence causing broadening of the spectral absorption bands for carbon monoxide. Spectral broadening can be allowed for by including an appropriate amount of oxygen in the calibration gas. The correction may also be required when measuring the alveolar concentration and hence the back tension of carbon monoxide in the lungs of smokers. In such circumstances the alveolar oxygen tension should be measured concurrently.

(ii) Inert gas. The inert gas is usually helium (fractional concentration in the range 0.02–0.14) or methane (FCH4 < 0.01), but neon or other non-reactive gas can also be used. Helium is commonly measured using a katharometer because the instrument is stable and provides a reliable means of calibrating other analysers. Alternative methods are also available (Table 7.6, page 65). The katharometer should be fitted with a control unit to maintain a constant current through the detector. The instrument is slightly sensitive to carbon dioxide and water vapour and also responds to the ratio of the concentrations of oxygen and nitrogen in the gas samples. To enhance the specificity of the analysis, first the carbon dioxide and then the water vapour should be absorbed, respectively, by soda lime $[Ca(OH)_2]$ and anhydrous calcium chloride or copper sulphate. The order is important as the reaction of CO_2 with $Ca(OH)_2$ liberates water vapour that is then removed by the drying agent. The treatment reduces the volume of the sample and this, in turn, increases the concentrations of helium and carbon monoxide. However, both gases are concentrated to the same extent so their ratio is not affected. The ratio is needed for the measurement of transfer factor. In addition, if helium is used for calculating the effective (single breath) alveolar volume, its absolute concentration is also required. To obtain the latter, the measured concentration of helium is reduced in proportion to the amount of carbon dioxide that was absorbed (usually 5%). An allowance should also be made for contamination of the alveolar sample by gas (usually air) in the deadspace of the sample bag.

For routine measurements of *T*l,co the katharometer is calibrated for helium in dry air. However, when the alveolar sample contains a high concentration of oxygen, as for determining the diffusing capacity of the alveolar capillary membrane, the reading from the katharometer should be adjusted to allow for the oxygen–nitrogen ratio of the mixture. The correction factor varies between instruments so it should be obtained by calibration or from the manufacturers.

Methane is analysed by an infrared method that is also used for carbon monoxide. Regular calibration is necessary

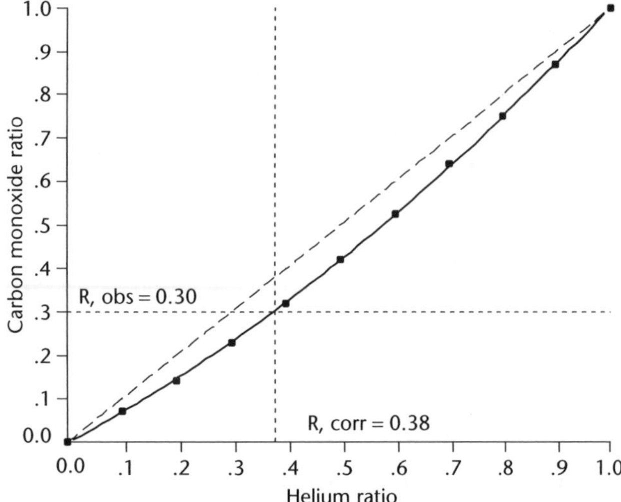

Fig. 20.2 Calibration of CO analyser. This diagram illustrates the procedure for calibrating a carbon monoxide analyser against a katharometer that has itself been calibrated for helium in air (see Section 7.15.2). An analogous procedure should be used for a meter calibrated for helium in oxygen. The CO analyser is zeroed on room air and a large bag filled with the gas mixture used for the measurement of transfer factor. The initial concentration is recorded and then the mixture is diluted with air from a syringe or cylinder of medical air. The mixture is reanalysed and the concentrations of helium and carbon monoxide are expressed as a ratio of their respective initial values. The dilution is repeated serially and the ratios tabulated and plotted against one another. A linear relationship is evidence that the calibration is satisfactory and may be used without correction. A curvilinear relationship is evidence of the need for correction. For the ratio of the expired alveolar to the inspired CO concentration (R,obs) the corresponding helium ratio (R,corr) should be used. In the example above:

Observed gas concentrations:
Inspired CO, $F_{I,CO} = 0.28\%$, alveolar CO, $F_{A,CO} = 0.084\%$
Observed CO ratio (R, obs) = 0.084/0.28 = 0.30
Corrected CO ratio (R, corr) = 0.38

Therefore, corrected $F_{A,CO} = 0.38 \times$ Inspired CO = 0.106%

For the calculation of the diffusing capacity of the alveolar capillary membrane where a correction for back tension is required the true ratio of the initial to the final alveolar concentration of CO is given by:

$$F_{A,CO_0}/F_{A,CO_t} = (F_{A,He}/F_{I,He} \times F_{I,CO}/F_{A,CO}) = (F_{A,He}/F_{I,He} - R_B) \div (R_{,corr} - R_B) \quad (20.10)$$

where R_B is the helium ratio to the measured back tension of CO expressed as a fraction of the inspired CO tension. Once a dilution curve has been constructed it can be used repeatedly provided the calibration is constant. This can be assessed by setting the meter on the inspirate mixture then performing one spot check at the dilution of maximal deviation from linearity.

(Section 7.15.2). The method is suitable for use with a mass flow detector. The measurement can then be combined with others, including ventilatory capacity and transfer factor by the single-expiration method.

(iii) Oxygen. The optimal fractional concentration of oxygen for routine measurement of $Tl_{,CO}$ at sea level is 0.17–0.18 [14, 16]. This maintains a nearly normal alveolar O_2 tension irrespective of the volume of test gas that the subject is able to inspire. The gas mixture can be prepared by adding air in the ratio 7:1 to a mixture of 2% carbon monoxide in helium. The latter is decanted from a master cylinder; the cylinder should be tin lined (see above). Many laboratories, particularly in North America use a test gas containing 21% oxygen ($F_{I,O_2} = 0.21$) [15]; this is appropriate for measurements made at an altitude of 1500 m. When used at sea level the reference values should have been measured at the same oxygen tension [16].

The concentration of oxygen in alveolar gas is not normally required for routine measurement of $Tl_{,CO}$. It is needed if alveolar volume is calculated from the dilution of nitrogen in alveolar gas. In this circumstance the nitrogen concentration is usually obtained by difference (as in Section 7.8.1). The F_{A,O_2} is also used in the determination of *Dm* and *Vc* by the Roughton–Forster method (Section 20.8) and for interpreting values for $Tl_{,CO}$ obtained during conditions of hypoxia at high altitude.

Procedures. The transfer factor is influenced by the quantity of blood in the lungs and the lung temperature. These effects are minimised by the subject being in an equitable temperature, an upright posture and in a quiet relaxed state. To this end an interval of at least 1 h should be allowed after any meal or moderate exercise and 4 h after consuming alcohol. The subject should preferably not have smoked since the previous day (Table 20.2). However, if the subject is a very heavy smoker or has smoked within a few hours of the test the mixed venous carbon monoxide tension should be measured (Section 20.7.1). If the patient has reversible airflow limitation a bronchodilator aerosol should have been administered (see above).

To make the measurement of transfer factor the subject is seated upright in front of the apparatus; this is set so that the subject breathes air through the mouthpiece. A nose clip is worn. After a few normal breaths the subject breathes out to residual volume, then immediately and rapidly inhales the test gas to total lung capacity, holds the breath for approximately 8 s and finally breathes out at a moderately fast rate. After exhalation of 0.75 (range 0.7–1.0) l, a sample of 0.5 l to 1.0 l of alveolar gas is collected for analysis (see Footnote 20.1).

Footnote 20.1. In some laboratories the excursion of the kymograph is checked by having the subject take a full breath of air immediately prior to the test breath. This practice is inappropriate as it results in a spuriously high *Tl*.

Table 20.2 Preconditions for measurement of Tl,co.sb.

Aspect	Reason
Laboratory temperature – should be comfortable	A high or low temperature affects Vc (Table 20.11, page 253)
Analysers – should have been checked for linearity and accuracy (±1%)	Alinearity affects measurement of ratios of gas concentrations
Sample bag – deadspace should have been flushed with room air	Contamination from a previous test is an important source of error
Subject – should be rested, post-absorptive, seated, without reversible bronchoconstriction and not having smoked or taken alcohol that day	Activity and a supine posture increase Tl,co; the other items reduce it. After a recent cigarette the test should be postponed or co back pressure measured
Time should have been allowed after any previous test involving breathing O_2	Any additional oxygen in the alveolar gas reduces the uptake of co

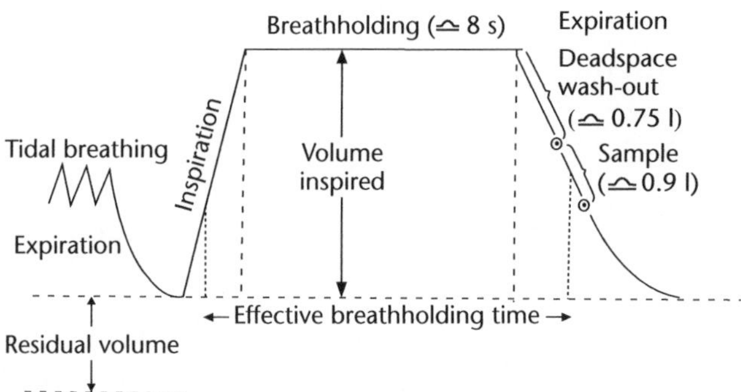

Fig. 20.3 Relationship of lung volume (l,BTPS) to time (s) during the breath-holding manoeuvre for determining the transfer factor (diffusing capacity) for the lung by the single-breath method. The subject breathes out to residual volume, inhales a vital capacity breath of the test gas, holds the breath for 8 s then exhales fully and moderately fast; after the exhalation of 750 ml a sample of 0.5 l or 1.0 l of alveolar gas is collected for analysis. Criteria for a technically satisfactory curve are illustrated in Fig 20.4 and given in Table 20.3. Provided these are met, the start of inspiration and of breath holding can be determined either by eye or by backward extrapolation from the linear part of the inspiratory limb of the curve [40] (cf. Fig. 12.7, page 139). By the method of Jones and Meade the effective duration of breath holding is taken to include two-thirds of the time of inspiration and the time of expiration up to half-way through the period of sample collection [34].

The spirogram, including the position of sampling, should be recorded and used to obtain the time of breath holding. The recommended method is that of Jones & Meade [34], Fig. 20.3 and also 'Time of breath holding' discussed above. Aspects of standardisation are summarised in Table 20.3.

Calculations. The transfer factor for carbon monoxide is for the lungs as a whole and is the rate constant for uptake of gas from the alveoli per minute per unit of alveolar tension in excess of the equilibrium back tension. In the SI system recommended by the European Respiratory Society the units for Tl,co are mmol min^{-1} and kPa^{-1}, whilst in the traditional system recommended by the American Thoracic Society they are ml min^{-1} mm Hg^{-1}. Conversion factors are given in Table 6.6 (page 56). Depending on the reader's preference either set of units can be inserted into the equations that follow. The starting point is eqn. 20.3 that describes the uptake per unit time. This can be rearranged as follows:

$$Tl\text{,co (in the chosen units)} = \frac{dF}{dt} \times V_A/22.4(F - F\bar{v})(P_B - P_{H_2O}) \quad (20.11)$$

where V_A is the alveolar volume in ml STPD, F is the instantaneous fractional concentration of carbon monoxide in the alveolar gas, t is time in minutes, and $F\bar{v}$ is the fractional concentration of carbon monoxide which would obtain in gas equilibrated with the mixed venous blood at the mean tension of oxygen in the alveolar capillaries. ($P_B - P_{H_2O}$) is the pressure of dry gas in the lung (kPa *or* mm Hg) and 22.4 is the volume in l STPD occupied by one mole of gas.

On rearrangement and integration this relationship becomes:

$$Tl\text{,co} = V_A/22.4(P_B - P_{H_2O}) \times 60/t \times \log_e[(F_o - F\bar{v})/(F_t - F\bar{v})] \quad (20.12)$$

where t is now the time of breath holding in seconds and Fo and Ft are the fractional concentrations of carbon monoxide in the alveolar gas at the beginning and end of this period.

In practice it is convenient to express the alveolar volume in l BTPS, to use logarithms to base 10 instead of to base e and to assume a constant barometric pressure. On substitution of the appropriate conversion factors the relationship becomes:

$$Tl\text{,co} = bV_A/t \times \log_{10}[(F_o - F\bar{v})/(F_t - F\bar{v})] \quad (20.13)$$

where V_A is now in l BTPS. The value of b in SI units is 53.6 ($b = (2.30 \times 60 \times 826)/(22.4 \times 0.133 \times (760 - 47))$ where 2.30 converts from $\log_e$ to $\log_{10}$, 60 from seconds to minutes, 826 from l BTPS to ml STPD and 0.133 between kPa and mm

Table 20.3 Summary of recommended procedures for measuring the *Tl*,co.sb. (See also Preconditions, Table 20.2).

$F_{I,CO}$	0.0025–0.003; if below this range the CO back tension should be allowed for
F_{I,O_2}	0.17–0.18 (but see page 240)
Inspired volume	>90% of largest measured vital capacity
Alveolar volume	The method should be stated. [$V_{A,eff}$ should always be calculated]
Washout volume	0.75 l–1.0 l (0.5 l if VC ≤ 2 l)
Sample volume	0.5 l–1.0 l collected over <3 s into bag of volume ≤1l
Time of inspiration	Normally <2.5 s; up to 4 s if there is airflow limitation
Breath holding	9 s–11 s (subject should relax against shutter)
Time of sample collection	<4 s [16]
Effective breath-holding time	Jones, Meade convention should be used
Number of tests	At least 2 that agree to within 10% and meet above criteria (the average $T1_{,CO}$ is used)
Interval between tests	At least 4 min with subject seated throughout
Gas analysis	Gas should be conditioned by absorbing CO_2 then water vapour, analysers should have been checked for linearity, the inspirate should be analysed as well as the 'alveolar' sample
Standardisation	Allowances may need to be made for back tension of carbon monoxide, carboxyhaemoglobin and haemoglobin concentrations and alveolar oxygen tension

Sources: [14–16, 30].

Hg. Alternatively, when it is intended to report the result in the traditional units ml min^{-1} $torr^{-1}$ the value of b is 160 (i.e. 53.6 × 22.4 × 0.133, see Table 6.6, page 56).

The fractional concentration of carbon monoxide in the alveolar gas at the start of breath holding (F_O) is obtained from the dilution of the helium by the following relationship:

$$F_O = F_{I,CO} \times F_{A,He}/F_{I,He} \qquad (20.14)$$

where F_O is the initial alveolar concentration and $F_{I,CO}$ is the concentration of carbon monoxide in the inspired gas. $F_{A,He}$ and $F_{I,He}$ are the concentrations of helium, respectively, in the alveolar and the inspired gas.

When breathing air, the back tension of carbon monoxide in the blood is usually small enough to be ignored. Equation 20.13 then simplifies to:

$$Tl_{,CO} \text{ (in the chosen units)} = bV_A/t \times \log_{10}\frac{(F_{I,CO} \times F_{A,He})}{(F_{A,CO} \times F_{I,He})} \qquad (20.15)$$

where $F_{A,CO}$ is the fractional concentration of carbon monoxide in the alveolar gas at the end of breath holding (i.e. Ft in eqn. 20.13) and the other symbols are as defined above.

VA measured by single-breath dilution of helium. The alveolar volume during breath holding (V_A) is best represented as the sum of the volume inspired and the residual volume obtained by an independent method (see above Which lung volume?). When the volume is that calculated from the dilution of the test inspirate [29] it is usually expressed as effective alveolar volume ($V_{A,eff}$) [14]. The following relationship is used:

$$V_{A,eff} = (V_{I ATPS} - V_{ID} - V_{DS}) \times F_{I,He}/F_{A,He} \times P_B/(P_B - P_{H_2O}) \times 310/(273 + T)\text{ l BTPS} \qquad (20.16)$$

where V_I is the volume of gas inspired in l ATPS, V_{ID} is the deadspace of the recording apparatus (l), V_{DS} is the anatomical deadspace (l), P_B is barometric pressure and ($P_B - P_{H_2O}$) is the pressure of dry gas in the lung in appropriate units (kPa or mm Hg), T is ambient temperature in °C; other symbols are as defined above. The term within the left hand bracket is the volume of inspired gas that enters the alveoli. The term $F_{I,He}/F_{A,He}$ is the ratio of the concentrations of helium in the inspired and the alveolar gas. The alveolar helium concentration should be corrected for any absorption of CO_2 prior to analysis (assumed to be 5% so the correction factor is 0.95) and for the deadspace of the sampling bag ($V_{ds,bag}$) using the correction factor $(V_s + V_{ds,bag})/V_s$ where V_s is the volume of the sample. A value is assumed for the anatomical deadspace; when expressed in ml it is approximately equal to the sum of the subject's age in years and body weight in pounds (kg × 2.2). Alternatively, in adults a value of 0.15 l can be used instead. The instrument deadspace is obtained from its dimensions or by water displacement and should include the volume of any filter fitted to the mouthpiece.

Nitrogen recovery method for measuring V_A. This method measures the dilution of nitrogen present in the residual volume of the lung. Compared with the helium method it can provide a better estimate of V_A in patients with airflow limitation [41]. An amended form of the eqn. 20.16 is used:

$$V_{A,eff(N_2)} = (V_{I\,ATPS} - V_{ID} - V_{DS}) \times [F_{A,N_2} - F_{I,N_2}]/[(F_{A,N_2} - F_{E,N_2}) \times 0.95]\ \text{l BTPS} \quad (20.17)$$

where $F_{,N_2}$ is fractional concentration of nitrogen, 0.95 corrects for the absorption of carbon dioxide (assumed to be 5%) and the other terms are as defined. The resident alveolar concentration of N_2 (F_{A,N_2}) is taken as that of dry gas after removal of CO_2 and is assumed to be 83.9% when breathing air. The expired nitrogen concentration can be measured directly. More often it is obtained by difference after absorbing carbon dioxide and analysing the other gases in the alveolar sample. Then:

$$F_{E,N_2} = [1 - F_{A,O_2} - F_{A,He} - F_{A,CO}] \quad (20.18)$$

The N_2 recovery technique depends on obtaining absolute concentrations of the other gases, including helium. This necessitates more careful calibration of the analysers compared with the single breath He dilution method, when only the ratio of the helium concentrations is required. The results have been reported as more variable than by the closed circuit helium dilution or plethysmograph methods [41]. The N_2 recovery method cannot be used with the Roughton–Forster method for measuring *D*m and *V*c as one of the test gas mixtures is then made up in oxygen (Section 20.8).

Allowance for absorption of water vapour. Removal of water vapour from the alveolar sample concentrates the other constituent gases by about 2% at 20°C [42]. The effect is small in relation to the assumptions made regarding the allowance for instrument and anatomical deadspace and the percentage of carbon dioxide removed during gas analysis (5%). Accordingly, adjustment for removal of water vapour is considered unnecessary during routine measurements. However, appropriate allowances may be required depending on how water and CO_2 affect the gas analysers and when precise adjustments are made including measuring the partial pressure of CO_2 [16].

Contamination of the sample bag deadspace. The deadspace of the sample bag may contain room air or alveolar gas from a previous test, either on the same or a different subject. The degree of contamination will alter with time as helium invariably escapes whilst carbon monoxide is retained. Such changes can lead to systematic error and inferior reproducibility. The difficulty can be overcome by routinely flushing the deadspace of the sample bag with room air from a cylinder of medical air or by using a pump. Alternatively, when the equipment is used with gas mixtures made up in oxygen for measurement of *D*m and *V*c the sample bag deadspace should be flushed with 100% oxygen to standardise the measurement conditions. An appropriate allowance is made for the contamination in the calculation.

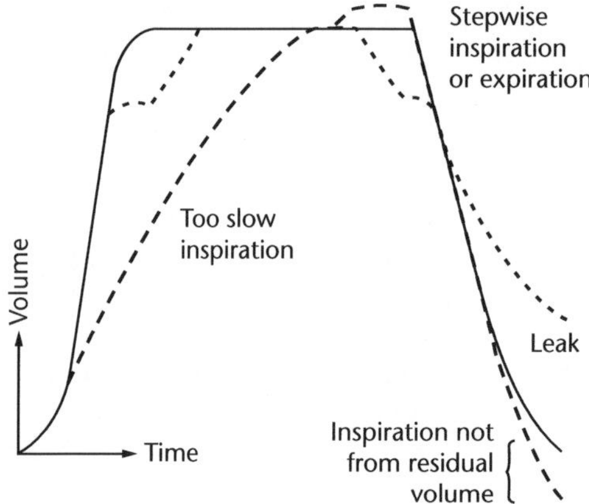

Fig. 20.4 Some faults in the breathing manoeuvre used for the measurement of *T*l,co.sb. The faults should be detected by scrutiny of the kymograph record; their occurrence should lead to the result being rejected.

Table 20.4 Common sources of error in gas analysis.

Gas	Method	Common fault	Feature*
Oxygen	Paramagnetic	cell mis-alligned	zero error
Helium	Katharometer	neglect of O_2 effect	proportional error
Carbon monoxide	Infrared	detector leaking	alinearity

* Illustrated in Fig. 7.13, page 78. The errors can be avoided using a three-point calibration when 1% accuracy is achievable.
Source: [43].

Quality control. Some procedural faults to be avoided when making the measurement are illustrated in Fig. 20.4 and common errors in gas analysis are given in Table 20.4 (see also Section 7.16). Alinearity of the helium or carbon monoxide analyser is particularly undesirable as it inevitably introduces bias into the ratios of gas concentrations. Provided the analysers are linear, absolute accuracy is mainly important where there is a need to adjust for back tension of CO and when using the nitrogen recovery method to estimate alveolar volume during the breath holding.

Other points that merit attention are summarised in Table 20.3. They include the possible need to standardise the result for the back tension of carbon monoxide and concentration of carboxyhaemoglobin in blood, the blood haemoglobin concentration, the alveolar oxygen tension and the lung volume (Section 20.7). These aspects are common to all techniques for measuring *T*l,co.

With proper attention to measurement techniques, the coefficient of variation of a single measurement of transfer factor or of *T*l/*V*A, including the within day and the between day variability (Section 25.6), is approximately 5%; that of the single-breath alveolar volume is approximately 3% [14]. The reproducibilities of *T*l within a session and over a year have been reported as, respectively, 3% and up to 9 % [44, 45]. Those for *D*m and *V*c are approximately 8% when analysed in the reciprocal form in which they are derived [46], see also Section 20.8. If the determination is made in duplicate this figure is reduced by the factor $1/\sqrt{2}$.

Given that a result is reproducible, its accuracy will depend on using valid parameters in all the calculations [47] and making appropriate allowances for the several physiological and biochemical variables that contribute to gas transfer. The order in which the allowances are made can also be important. Practices in all these respects still differ between laboratories so there is a need for awareness as to which allowances are made and which are left out.

20.4.1 Uncertainties and difficulties

Most technical problems in the measurement of *T*l,co.sb have been overcome. The improvements are due to attention to detail in gas analysis and use of standard procedural conventions in conjunction with the Jones–Meade method for defining breath-holding time and obtaining an alveolar sample for analysis. However early and late alveolar samples should be avoided [48]. Further consideration might be given to the choice of inert gas for the measurement of alveolar volume. Helium is widely used and is satisfactory on account of the relative ease with which it can be analysed accurately. However, the molecular weight is rather low. Methane is better in this respect and is convenient but the method has limitations and this is also the case for the resident gas (nitrogen recovery) method (see above). Some other topics where views diverge are indicated in Table 20.5.

The physical requirements of the test dictate the type of patients that can be assessed, in particular the need for a vital capacity of at least 1.5 l and ability to hold the breath for a minimum of 5 s. Patients with severe respiratory impairment cannot perform the test, but may be able to undertake a simplified rebreathing test instead (Section 20.5).

The test models the lungs as a single gas-exchanging vessel and this inevitably leads to difficulties when the lung function is uneven. In this circumstance the *T*l,co.sb should be interpreted in association with other tests, but steps can be taken to maximise the relevance of the result. For example *T*l,co measured using the single-breath lung volume (but not the multi-breath lung volume) is reduced by labile bronchoconstriction [30]. This creates uncertainty in interpretation that can be eliminated by prior bronchodilatation. Additional information is contained in the single-breath lung mixing index *V*A,eff/*V*A which should be obtained where this is practicable. The current recommendation is that *T*l,co.sb based on *V*A,eff should always be reported [16]; however, that based on *V*A (which also yields *V*A,eff/*V*A) is more informative.

From the nature of the model the alveolar volume during breath holding is an integral part of the measurement of *T*l,co.sb. In Forster's view it is no more than that [3]. Earlier measurements by Marie Krogh suggested otherwise [5], but her interpretation did not take into account regional differences in gas exchange. These alternative perspectives have practical implications that are considered subsequently (Section 20.9).

20.5 Measurement of *T*l,co.rb (rebreathing method)

By this method the subject rebreathes rapidly from a bag containing the test gas mixture [12]. The bag is emptied during each breath. To avoid error due to recirculation of blood that

Table 20.5 Controversies and former or current divergent practices.

Item		Comment
Terminology,	transfer factor (*T*l,co.sb)	Describes transfer process combining diffusion and chemical reaction
	diffusing capacity (*D*l,co.sb)	Is historic but potentially misleading descriptive term
	*K*co	Implies wrongly that the index is of fundamental importance
	*T*l/*V*A	Unpretentious but precise descriptive term
Units,	mmol min^{-1} kPa^{-1} (*T*l,co)	SI units (Recommended by UNESCO)
	ml min^{-1} mm Hg^{-1} (*D*l,co)	Traditional units (used in USA)
F_{I,O_2}	17%	Stabilises P_{A,O_2} at normal level (14.5 kPa, 108 mm Hg)*
	21%	Traditionally used in USA (provides sea level value at 1500 m). Sea level P_{A,O_2} 120 mm Hg (16 kPa)*
*V*A,	from dilution of gas inhaled (*V*A,eff)	Procedure is self-contained. Gives an unequivocal result that can be an underestimate, especially with labile bronchoconstriction
	from vol. of breath + RV (*V*A)	Yields upper limit for *T*l,co. Lower limit can then be calculable via *V*A,eff/*V*A
Prior bronchodilatation or not?		Bronchodilatation improves reproducibility and simplifies interpretation when *V*A,eff is used

* Provides the constant 'b' in Table 20.8 below.
Sources: [14–16, 30].

now contains some carbon monoxide, the period of rebreathing should be brief (ideally 10 s, cf. Section 17.3).

The procedure of rebreathing promotes mixing of gas in the lungs and on this account the method is increasingly being used for assessment of patients with uneven lung function. It is also used for those whose vital capacity is less than 1.5 l, so cannot be assessed by the single-breath method. The rebreathing bag can be disposable or capable of being sterilised, hence the procedure is suitable for patients who have or are particularly susceptible to respiratory infection, for example those with AIDS or cystic fibrosis [49].

20.5.1 Practical details

The procedure resembles the single-breath method in most respects except that rebreathing replaces breath holding. The rebreathing bag initially contains a volume of gas equal to the subject's forced expiratory volume (FEV_1). The subject is connected to it *after a forced expiration* and rebreathes for a period of up to 30 s at a frequency of 30 min^{-1}. The bag should empty with each inspiration. The contained gas is best sampled continuously by a pump that circulates the gas through analysers that have a rapid response. Alternatively, an early and a late sample can be taken from the bag over a timed period. Sampling should be at the end of expiration. The change in concentration of the carbon monoxide in the bag is plotted on a semi-log scale against the time from the start of the rebreathing. A linear relationship is to be expected and is used for the calculation. This is performed using a version of eqn. 20.13:

$$Tl,\text{co} = b(V\text{RV} + V\text{bag})/(t_2 - t_1) \times \log_{10}[(F_1,\text{co} - F\bar{v},\text{co})/(F_2,\text{co} - F\bar{v},\text{co})] \quad (20.19)$$

where VRV and V bag are the volumes of gas in l BTPS, respectively, in the residual volume of the lungs and in the bag at the start of the rebreathing procedure. The suffixes 1 and 2 refer to two points in time on the linear part of the exponential decay curve (cf. Fig. 20.1). The term in the left-hand bracket is the volume of gas from which carbon monoxide is absorbed during rebreathing; the assumption is made that it is also the effective alveolar volume. The volume is calculated from the dilution, in the lung, of helium present in the test gas mixture. This is done using a version of eqn. 20.16:

$$(V\text{RV} + V\text{bag}) = V\text{bag} \times F\text{I,He}/F\text{A,He} \text{ (l BTPS)} \quad (20.20)$$

where FI,He and FA,He are the fractional concentrations of helium in the bag before and at the end of the period of rebreathing; the latter is corrected for the absorption of carbon dioxide in the manner indicated on page 242. The method gives results that are significantly correlated with those by the single-breath method but are systematically lower. The reduction is mainly due to the measurement being made at a smaller average lung volume, but other factors, including the recirculation of blood through the lungs during rebreathing, can contribute to the difference.

20.5.2 Comment

Fast responding gas analysers are desirable, but not essential. The bag should be emptied during each breath and the breathing manoeuvre should be performed vigorously. These feats are beyond the ability of some patients. Feeble rebreathing can nonetheless yield a usable result. The method is subject to error if the alveolar oxygen tension is allowed to fall during the measurement. However, a raised oxygen tension can also cause error.

Several variants of the method are in current use, so there are no consistent reference values and results by the single-breath method cannot be used as they are not interchangeable. Thus, individual reference values should be compiled. In one study where the tidal volume was 80% of forced vital capacity rebreathed for 6 breaths, the following relationship was derived [49]:

Modified rebreathing

$$Tl,\text{co.rb} = -0.4 + 0.852\, Tl,\text{co.sb}\ (r = 0.97) \quad (20.21)$$

$$\text{Modified } V\text{A} = 0.3 + 1.070\, V\text{A,eff}\ (r = 0.96) \quad (20.22)$$

20.6 Measurement of *Tl*,co.ib (intra-breath method)

This method entails the subject inhaling a deep breath of test gas and then, following a short pause, exhaling at a constant, slow rate. Transfer factor is calculated from changes in composition of alveolar gas sampled during the exhalation [10, 50, 51]. The method is attractive for patients with a small vital capacity and those too breathless to sustain an adequate breath-holding period. In addition, as a research tool, the method might shed light on regional differences in gas transfer by comparing estimates of *Tl*,co.ib made early in expiration with those made late in expiration but before the onset of airway closure.

20.6.1 Practical details

In the intra-breath (constant exhalation) method the recommended test gas mixture comprises 0.3% carbon monoxide, 0.3% methane, 21% oxygen and the balance nitrogen [51]. The two carbon compounds are analysed using a rapid infrared two gas analyser. To make the measurement the subject inhales a vital capacity breath of the test gas then, after a pause of approximately 3 s, exhales to residual volume. The expiratory flow is maintained constant at 0.5 l s^{-1}. This is achieved by instructing the subject to follow a visual display. The process is assisted by having a resistance in the expired air line (e.g. an orifice of diameter 5 mm and length 13 mm). The resistance raises the proximal airway pressure to 2.6 cm H_2O at a flow of 0.5 l s^{-1}. During the exhalation, the methane concentration falls to a steady level, which is the alveolar concentration. The *Tl*,co.ib is proportional to the slope of the ln ($F_{A,CO}/F_{A_0,CO}$) on ln (V_A/V_{A_0}) before the onset of airway closure (closing volume). The slope of this relationship is dependent on the expiratory flow and the transfer factor is calculated from the following:

$$Tl_{,co.ib} = \dot{V}_E \frac{\ln F_{A,CO}/F_{A_0,CO}}{\ln V_A/V_{A_0}} \frac{60 \times 1000}{0.938 \times 101.3 \times 22.4} \quad (20.23)$$

where $\dot{V}_E$ is the mean expiratory flow (l s^{-1}), ln is the natural logarithm, $F_{A,CO}/F_{A_0,CO}$ is the ratio of carbon monoxide during exhalation to that at full inspiration, V_A/V_{A_0} is the ratio of alveolar volume during exhalation to that at full inspiration, 60 coverts time from s to min, 1000 converts volume from ml to l, 0.938 is the fraction of dry gas, 101.3 is standard barometric pressure (kPa) and 22.4 converts litres of CO to mol. Criteria for a satisfactory result include that the expiratory flow is within the range 0.3–0.7 l s^{-1} and the duration of expiration over which the relationship is linear is at least 1 s.

20.6.2 Limitations of intra-breath method

The value obtained for transfer factor differs depending on whether the respiratory manoeuvre is inspiratory, as in the single-breath method or expiratory as when constant exhalation is used [52]. The gas sampled early in expiration is subject to different influences from gas that is sampled later. First, the permeability of the alveolar membrane is greater because it is thinner. Second, the early samples tend to come from the lower rather than the upper zones of the lung (Fig. 16.2, page 184). The capillaries may have contained more blood in consequence. In addition, the residence time would have been shorter due to the test gas entering the lower zones after the upper zones. If the subject is a patient with airflow limitation the gradient in residence times may have been enhanced. There is a possibility that the method might shed light on regional differences in gas transfer, but ways of extracting the information and avoiding the various sources of bias appear not to have been worked out.

From the practical point of view, not all subjects can conform to a standardised procedure that entails breathing out at a constant, slow rate; variable expiratory flow can be a reason to reject a test. In addition, error may arise from the use of methane, either contamination of the gas sample by methane produced in the gut or difficulty with gas analysis. An alternative is to use helium and analyse the gas by mass spectrometry.

Reference values for the intra-breath method have been reported [53]. They resemble but are not identical with those for the single-breath and rebreathing methods and the limits of agreement can be wide. This is to be expected as the underlying assumptions and the technology are different and the measurements may not be made at the same lung volume [51, 54]. The latter difference can affect particularly the comparability of values for $Tl_{,co.ib}/V_A$ and $Tl_{,co.sb}/V_A$.

20.7 Contributions of haemoglobin and tensions of O_2 and CO

Introduction. Carbon monoxide in the fluid compartment of the lung combines with haemoglobin in the lung parenchyma in proportion to the total amount present (i.e. Hb concentration × V_c). The rate is influenced by the co-existing tensions of oxygen and carbon monoxide (the back tension) and the prevailing conditions of temperature and acid–base balance. The latter are assumed to be normal. An increased quantity of haemoglobin from any cause, or a reduced alveolar oxygen tension increases the rate and vice versa. Thus, the contributions of these features need to be characterised numerically.

20.7.1 Allowance for carboxyhaemoglobin

When a person inhales carbon monoxide the blood concentration of carboxyhaemoglobin rises by an amount that is determined by its dissociation curve (cf. Fig. 21.1, page 260). The compound and the gas quickly come into equilibrium, hence the tension of carbon monoxide in blood entering the alveolar capillaries reflects the dissociation of carboxyhaemoglobin. This back tension is a component of the transfer gradient for carbon monoxide as defined in eqn. 20.2. Through this relationship an increase in the blood concentration of carboxyhaemoglobin by 1% reduces the transfer factor by approximately 0.6% [55]. At the same time the additional coHb reduces the amount that is available to take up more carbon monoxide in the lungs [56]. This 'anaemia effect' reduces the transfer factor by an additional 0.4%, making a 1% reduction overall. Normally the blood of a non-smoker contains little carboxyhaemoglobin and the rise in blood concentration of coHb attributable to a single measurement of *Tl* is about 0.7% [57], so the back tension does not contribute materially to the result. When it does so an allowance should be made by inserting the back tension into eqn. 20.2 and subsequent equations. Some circumstances are listed in Table 20.6. The allowance is based on the back tension in mixed venous blood. Alternatively, the correction can be made in terms of the concentration of carboxyhaemoglobin [15].

Table 20.6 Circumstances when CO back tension may be important.

Increased catabolism of haemoglobin:
Haemolytic anaemia
Lead poisoning
Exposure to carbon monoxide:
Moderate or heavy smoking (>20 cigs or 1 pack per day)
Cigarette immediately prior to testing
Fumes from internal combustion engine in a confined space
Occupational exposure from welding, retorts, braziers etc (Section 37.4.1)
Carbon monoxide associated with test:
Repeated standard testing (e.g. >6 single-breath tests)
Test using low CO concentration (e.g. steady state or special procedure)

Measurement of CO back tension

Gasometric methods. By these methods the partial pressure of carbon monoxide in equilibrium with carboxyhaemoblobin is raised to a level where it becomes measurable. This is done by equilibrating the blood with oxygen.

The subject breathes oxygen for 5 min in order to raise the tension of oxygen in the alveolar gas. Equilibration is then achieved either by rebreathing oxygen from a closed circuit apparatus or a 5 l bag for 3 min [58], or breath holding for 25 s [59, 60]. One of the two former methods is preferable as the result is then independent of uneven lung function; in addition carbon dioxide can be absorbed by the rebreathing being conducted through a canister of soda lime.

By the end of the specified time almost complete gaseous equilibrium for carbon monoxide has been attained between the alveolar gas, the bag and carboxyhaemoglobin in the alveolar capillaries. The gas is then analysed for oxygen and carbon monoxide. This information is used to obtain the back tension of CO at the oxygen tension prevailing during the measurement of *Tl*,co via the following relationship:

$$P\text{CO} = P\text{O}_2 \times F\text{CO}/F\text{O}_2\,\text{kPa} \tag{20.24}$$

where Pco is the tension of carbon monoxide exerted by carboxyhaemoglobin at an oxygen tension of PO_2 in appropriate units. Fco and FO_2 are the fractional concentrations, respectively, of carbon monoxide and oxygen in the gas sample obtained after equilibration. This value is substituted for the term $P\bar{v}$,co in the equation used to calculate *Tl*,co.

Spectrophotometric method. By this method the venous blood saturations of haemoglobin with carbon monoxide and oxygen are measured by spectrophotometry. These values together with the alveolar oxygen tension are inserted into the Haldane equation (Footnote 19.3, page 231). The resulting value for back tension is used as described above.

Adjustment of Tl,co for [COHb]

The saturation of haemoglobin with carbon monoxide is measured using a CO oximeter and the resulting value substituted in the following empirical equation [55]:

$$Tl,\text{co, adjusted} = Tl,\text{co, observed}\,(1 + [\%\text{COHb}/100]) \tag{20.25}$$

This equation also adjusts for the effects of back tension, so should only be used if an overall correction is necessary but the back tension is not available.

20.7.2 Adjustment for haemoglobin concentration

Haemoglobin concentration influences the transfer factor via its effect on the reaction rate of carbon monoxide with oxyhaemoglobin, represented by θ in eqn. 19.13 (page 231). That equation (in either SI or traditional units) can be written in the form:

$$\frac{1}{Tl} = \frac{1}{Dm} + \frac{1}{\theta'[\text{Hb}]\,Vc} \tag{20.26}$$

where Dm is the diffusing capacity of the alveolar membrane, Vc is the volume of blood in the alveolar capillaries, θ' is the reaction rate at the average normal concentration for haemoglobin monomer in healthy men and women and [Hb] is the haemoglobin concentration as a fraction of normal. The units of the other variables are in Section 19.3.3. A material deviation of the haemoglobin concentration or of the oxygen tension from its normal level can lead to error in the interpretation of the transfer factor unless an appropriate allowance is made. This is best done by reporting the result adjusted to the reference haemoglobin concentration for the appropriate gender (Table 20.7) and to a standard oxygen tension. The recommended oxygen tensions are currently 16 kPa (120 mm Hg) in USA and elsewhere 14.6 kPa (110 mm Hg); the latter is more physiological (Table 20.5). Using these values, the corresponding value for $\theta(\theta s)$ can be obtained using eqn. 20.29 and Table 20.9. When Dm and Vc are measured in the manner that is described below the transfer factor under standard conditions (*Tl*,s) can be obtained using eqn. 20.26 by substituting θs for θ' [Hb]. Alternatively, when the transfer factor is measured at a normal oxygen tension but no data are available for Dm and Vc the correction is made using a version of the same equation:

$$Tl,\text{s} = Tl,\text{obs}\,(a + \theta\text{s}[\text{Hb}]) \div (a + \theta\text{s}) \times [\text{Hb}] \tag{20.27}$$

where *Tl*,obs is the transfer factor at the subject's own haemoglobin concentration, θs and [Hb] are defined above and a is the ratio Dm/Vc. This ratio is determined in part by the numerical values chosen for the reaction rate of carbon monoxide with oxyhaemoglobin; this is described below. A Dm/Vc ratio in SI units (mmol, kPa, min and l) of 230 and in traditional units (ml, min and torr) of 0.7 has been found to provide a valid correction [61, 62] (Table 20.7). An empirical correction can also be made provided there is a reasonable likelihood of it being

Table 20.7 Correction factors for standardising *Tl*,co to reference haemoglobin concentrations of 14.6 g dl^{-1} and 13.4 g dl^{-1} in men and women respectively (collectively eqns. 20.28).

Subjects	Relationship	Ref
Males, age >15 years	$Tls = Tlobs \times (10.22 + \text{Hb})/(1.7 \times \text{Hb})$	61
Females and males <15 years	$Tls = Tlobs \times (9.38 + \text{Hb})/(1.7 \times \text{Hb})$	15
Adult men and women	$Tls = Tlobs + 1.40\,([\text{Hb,ref}] - [\text{Hb,obs}])$ (SD 0.72)	63

Table 20.8 Factors for standardising Tl,co to a specified alveolar oxygen tension 'b'. For use with data at sea level when F_{I,O_2} is in the range 0.17 to 0.27.

Units	Factor = (Tl,co.st/Tl,co.obs)
SI	1.0 + 0.0262 (P_{A,O_2} – b) mmol min^{-1} kPa^{-1}
Traditional	1.0 + 0.0035 (P_{A,O_2} – b) ml min^{-1} mm Hg^{-1}

For 'b' see Table 20.5.
Source: [64].

applicable in the prevailing circumstances, e.g. [63]. Both the corrected and uncorrected values should be reported.

20.7.3 Empirical adjustment for oxygen tension

The relationship of Tl,co to oxygen tension is determined by the coefficient terms of the relationship that describes θco (eqn. 20.29). Unfortunately, the parameters of the equation are only known approximately. Therefore, there is a case for making any correction of transfer factor for oxygen tension on an empirical basis (Table 20.8). The reference oxygen tension should preferably be that normally present in the lungs during the breath-holding manoeuvre at sea level [14, 16] (also Table 20.5).

From Table 20.8 the difference in Tl,co.sb between measurements made using a test inspirate containing 17–18% oxygen and that using 21% oxygen is approximately 8%. The two concentrations reflect different measurement conventions in Europe and USA [14, 15] and should be taken into account when selecting reference values [16].

20.7.4 Reaction rate of carbon monoxide with oxyhaemoglobin (θCO)

In this and the following section the text can be read as relating to either SI or traditional units. For purposes of calculation the chosen units should be used consistently.

Numerical values for the reaction rate of carbon monoxide with partially oxygenated haemoglobin are needed for estimation of Dm and Vc by the Roughton–Forster method and to standardise Tl,co for haemoglobin concentration or alveolar oxygen tension. The values should preferably relate to *in vivo* conditions, including with respect to oxygen tension, and theoretically could be obtained from concurrent measurements of Tl,NO and Tl,co [65]. However, in practice the requisite assumptions cannot be relied on. Instead, values obtained *in vitro* are assumed to apply *in vivo* [66].

Aspects of the derivation. Carbon monoxide reacts with partially oxygenated blood according to the following reaction:

$$Hb_4(O_2)_3 + CO \xrightarrow{l'4} Hb_4(O_2)_3CO \qquad (20.28)$$

where the haemoglobin reactant has three of its four binding sites occupied by molecular oxygen, $l'4$ is the bimolecular reaction velocity constant for the binding of carbon monoxide to the fourth position on the haemoglobin molecule in the units mmol $l^{-1}s^{-1}$. The velocity constant is related to the reaction rate of carbon monoxide with blood (θco). The latter quantity was first reported by Roughton and Forster in the units ml/min/mm Hg/ml of blood containing haemoglobin at the average concentration of 14.6 g dl^{-1}. In SI units and making allowance for any haemoglobin which is already combined with carbon monoxide the reaction rate (θco) can be described by the following relationship:

$$\frac{1}{\theta co} = (\alpha + \beta P\bar{c},_{O_2}) \div [Hb] \times (1 - Sc,co/100) \qquad (20.29)$$

where $P\bar{c},O_2$ is the mean tension of oxygen in plasma in the alveolar capillaries in appropriate units, [Hb] is the concentration of haemoglobin in blood as a fraction of normal and Sc,co is the mean percentage saturation of haemoglobin with carbon monoxide; the latter term is only important after some carbon monoxide has been inhaled.

The reaction rate is influenced by the prevailing temperature and pH. It is also affected by the tension of carbon dioxide, which forms an intermediate complex with oxyhaemoglobin (CO_2,Hb_4O_6) [67]. Compared with Hb_4O_6 this complex reacts at different rates with oxygen and with carbon monoxide.

The parameters α and β, of eqn. 20.29 have been measured by a method that depends on the rapid mixing of suspensions of human red cells with plasma containing carbon monoxide in solution. The procedure is technically difficult so only a few determinations have been made. The results for four subjects reported in 1957 and for five that were confirmed in 1987 after being reported briefly in 1983, are given in Table 20.9. Both sets of values are in current use. The later determinations were made at physiological carbon monoxide tensions and appear to be more reliable (Table 20.9).

20.8 Measurement of *Dm* and *Vc* (Roughton–Forster method)

Outline. The recommended procedure for the measurement of the diffusing capacity of the alveolar membrane (Dm) and the volume of blood in the alveolar capillaries (Vc) entails solving the equation for transfer factor of Roughton and Forster that links the three variables (eqn. 19.13, page 231):

$$\frac{1}{Tl} = \frac{1}{Dm} + \frac{1}{\theta Vc} \qquad (19.13)$$

The transfer factor is measured at two levels of alveolar oxygen tension, the levels normally being near to those that obtain during breathing air and breathing oxygen. The corresponding values for the reaction rate (θco) are then obtained as described

Table 20.9 Parameters of eqn. 20.29 relating $1/\theta$ CO to $P\bar{c}$, O_2 for human blood at 37°C.

Parameter	α		β		
Units	SI	Traditional	SI	Traditional	Source
Roughton & Forster, 1957*	$(1–3) \times 10^{-3}$	0.34–1.0	0.134	6.1	[68]
Forster, 1987	3.9×10^{-3}	1.30	0.09	4.1	[69]

* the range for α reflects different assumptions about the permeability of the red cell membrane to CO from infinity down to 1.5 times that of the interior of the red cells. The lower values have been used in the present account.

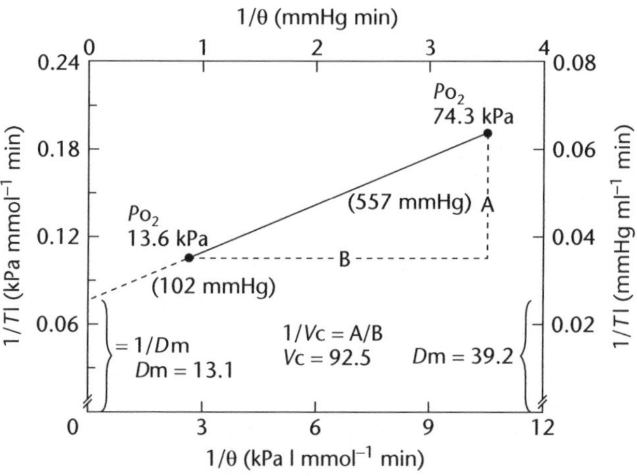

Fig. 20.5 Graphical solution to the eqn. 19.13 for determining the diffusing capacity of the alveolar capillary membrane and the volume of blood in the alveolar capillaries. The reciprocal of the transfer factor (diffusing capacity) for the lung ($1/Tl$) is plotted against the reciprocal of the reaction rate ($1/\theta$). The slope of the line is then the reciprocal of the volume of blood in the alveolar capillaries ($1/Vc$) and the intercept is the reciprocal of the diffusing capacity of the alveolar capillary membrane ($1/Dm$). Vc is here given in traditional units (ml). In SI units it is in l.

above. This procedure yields two values for Tl together with the corresponding values for θCO. The pairs of values are substituted in eqn. 19.13 to provide two simultaneous equations which are solved for Dm and Vc (see e.g. Fig. 20.5). The validity of the underlying assumptions is considered below.

Details of the Roughton–Forster procedure.

1 The back tension exerted by carboxyhaemoglobin present in mixed venous blood is measured by the rebreathing method (Section 20.7.1). For the present application, the method has the additional merit of raising the tension of oxygen in alveolar gas in preparation for the next stage in the procedure. However, this is not appropriate in all circumstances (see 'comment' below).

2 Immediately after the rebreathing and without the subject being taken off the apparatus, the transfer factor (Tl,CO) is determined using a test gas mixture that is made up in oxygen, not air. The alveolar sample that is collected is analysed for oxygen as well as for helium and carbon monoxide. The back tension of carbon monoxide exerted by carboxyhaemoglobin at this tension of oxygen is then calculated by the use of eqn. 20.24. The value so obtained is inserted into eqn. 20.13 for calculation of the transfer factor along with the other information obtained from the measurement.

3 The subject breathes air for 10 min to restore a normal alveolar oxygen tension. The measurement of the transfer factor is repeated using the normal gas mixture (Table 20.5). The resulting alveolar sample is similarly analysed for oxygen as well as other gases and the corresponding transfer factor is calculated by the use of eqn. 20.15.

4 The values for the transfer factor at the two tensions of oxygen are used to calculate Dm and Vc. This can be done graphically as in Fig. 20.5 or by use of the following relationships:

$$Vc = \frac{\beta(P_1 - P_2)}{[\mathrm{Hb}] \times (1/Tl_1 - 1/Tl_2)} \quad (20.30)$$

$$Dm = \frac{1/\theta_1 - 1/\theta_2}{(1/\theta_1 \times 1/Tl_2) - (1/\theta_2 \times 1/Tl_1)} \quad (20.31)$$

where, in SI or traditional units, Dm is the diffusing capacity of the alveolar capillary membrane, Vc is the volume of blood in the alveolar capillaries, [Hb] is the haemoglobin concentration as a fraction of normal and β is from Table 20.9. Tl_1 and Tl_2 are values for the transfer factor for carbon monoxide measured using the gas mixtures made up, respectively, of oxygen and air. P_1 and P_2 are the corresponding tensions of oxygen in plasma in the alveolar capillaries (Ppl,O_2). θ_1 and θ_2 are the reaction rates of carbon monoxide with oxyhaemoglobin that are obtained in these circumstances.

Values for Ppl,O_2. In the derivation of Vc the term ($P_1 - P_2$) can be approximated by the difference in the corresponding alveolar oxygen tensions, but for optimal accuracy the mean capillary oxygen tensions should be used. They are estimated using the basic equation for transfer factor (eqn. 20.1) in the form:

$$Dm,O_2 = O_2 \text{ uptake}/(P_{A},O_2 - P\bar{c},O_2) \quad (20.32)$$

where, in SI or traditional units, P_A,O_2 is the tension of oxygen in the alveolar gas, $P\bar{c}$,O_2 is the mean tension of oxygen in alveolar capillary plasma and Dm,O_2 is the resulting diffusing capacity of the alveolar capillary membrane for oxygen. The latter is linked to the Dm,CO through their respective diffusivities (Table 19.1, page 225). Then on rearrangement:

$$P\bar{c},O_2 = P\text{A},O_2 - 0.83\ O_2\ \text{uptake}/Dm,\text{CO} \quad (20.33)$$

where Dm,CO is the diffusing capacity of the alveolar capillary membrane for carbon monoxide in appropriate units. For the present application this quantity can be estimated with adequate accuracy from Tl breathing air using an appropriate multiplier. The Roughton–Forster values for α and β imply a multiplier of approximately 1.5, but a value in the range 3–5 is more likely to be correct (see above). A definitive value for Dm can now be calculated, either in two stages from eqns. 20.29 and 20.33 or using a combined equation. Then,

$$Dm,\text{CO} = \frac{Tl_1 \times Tl_2 \times (P_1 - P_2) - 0.83\ O_2\ \text{uptake}\ (Tl_2 - Tl_1)}{Tl_1 \times P_1 - Tl_2 \times P_2 - \alpha/\beta \times (Tl_2 - Tl_1)} \quad (20.34)$$

Comment. The Roughton–Forster method for partitioning $1/Tl$ has stood the test of time and yields intuitively sensible results. However, it is beset by uncertainties that have not been resolved.

1. Response of pulmonary vascular bed to oxygen. The method requires that the distribution of red blood cells in the pulmonary vascular bed is independent of oxygen tension. This condition appears to be met in normal circumstances. It is unlikely to be met when there is vasoconstriction that is ameliorated by breathing oxygen. However, the vasodilator response is not instantaneous, so the error can be minimised by confining the hyperoxia to the period of breath holding. This is done by using test gas that is made up with oxygen but having the subject breathe air prior to its inhalation. When this procedure is followed the reproducibility is likely to be reduced unless duplicate determinations are carried out.

2. Value for θ. The measurement of reaction rate is technically difficult [66]. This is reflected in the 1987 values for α and β differing from those obtained previously. The associated results for the volume of blood in the alveolar capillaries (Vc) are 1%–20% lower than when calculated using the 1957 values whilst the values for Dm are higher and more in line with morphological estimates. If the new parameters are correct the reference values for Dm in Chapter 26 and the values used to calculate Table 21.1 (page 259) and Fig. 21.2 (page 263) are too low. However, the reference values for Vc are not much affected. The findings reduce the impact of measurements of Dm and Vc in disease since they suggest that Vc is the main determinant of Tl. However, this in not in accord with the empirical evidence, in particular the dependence of Tl on lung volume, posture and haemoglobin concentration. There is a clear need to investigate these phenomena further by alternative methods. This has focussed attention on the possibility of estimating Dm and Vc from concurrent measurements of Tl,CO and Tl,NO at a single oxygen tension [65, 70], but at the time of writing the appropriate algorithm has not been established [71] and the relationship of Dm,NO to Tl,NO has not been established with confidence [2]. At postmortem Dm can be estimated anatomically [72, 73].

20.9 Interpretation of *Tl*,CO and related indices

Introduction. Transfer factor is the rate constant for the uptake of gas by the lungs as a whole, so is related to the size of the lungs. The size is related positively to stature and as a result stature is the principal reference variable for Tl,CO (Chapter 26). After allowing for stature, Tl,CO is related positively to alveolar volume standardised for stature [74]. This association is mediated through lung volume affecting the area and thickness of the alveolar capillary membrane (see below). Similarly in disease, Dm is reduced if the surface for gas exchange is reduced. It is also reduced if the diffusion pathway is lengthened by changes in the acinus or impeded by an increase in thickness of the alveolar capillary membrane. The rate factor for gas uptake by blood ($\theta\, Vc$) is also related to lung volume, but to a lesser extent (Fig. 20.6). It is very sensitive to changes in distribution of blood volume from any cause, for example to the increases that occur on adopting a supine position or as a result of exercise. Such variations appear not to have much effect on Dm.

20.9.1 Relationship of *Tl*,CO.sb to alveolar volume, including *Tl*/*V*A (*K*CO)

Underlying physiology. The lung volume between functional residual capacity and total lung capacity affects the transfer factor through its effects on the underlying processes and as a result of hysteresis [52]. Diffusion across the alveolar capillary membrane is enhanced when the lung is expanded, because the alveolar membrane increases in area and becomes thinner. As a consequence, Dm measured by the single-breath (breath holding) method is nearly proportional to lung volume (Fig. 20.6). By contrast, the volume of blood in lung capillaries (Vc) has an inverse relationship to lung volume; this is because capillaries in the walls of alveoli become flattened at near to total lung capacity (Fig. 11.2, page 119).

The respective relationships of Dm and Vc to lung volume determine the relationship for transfer factor; the relationship is curvilinear, but approximates to a linear relationship over the physiological range (Fig. 20.7).

Studies in healthy adults reported up to 1970, showed that the mean linear coefficient of transfer factor on alveolar volume was 0.86 mmol $\text{min}^{-1}\ \text{kPa}^{-1}\ \text{l}^{-1}$ (2.57 ml min^{-1} mm $\text{Hg}^{-1}\ \text{l}^{-1}$) and numerous similar relationships have been reported subsequently [46, 74]. All of them have a significant constant term. Thus, the

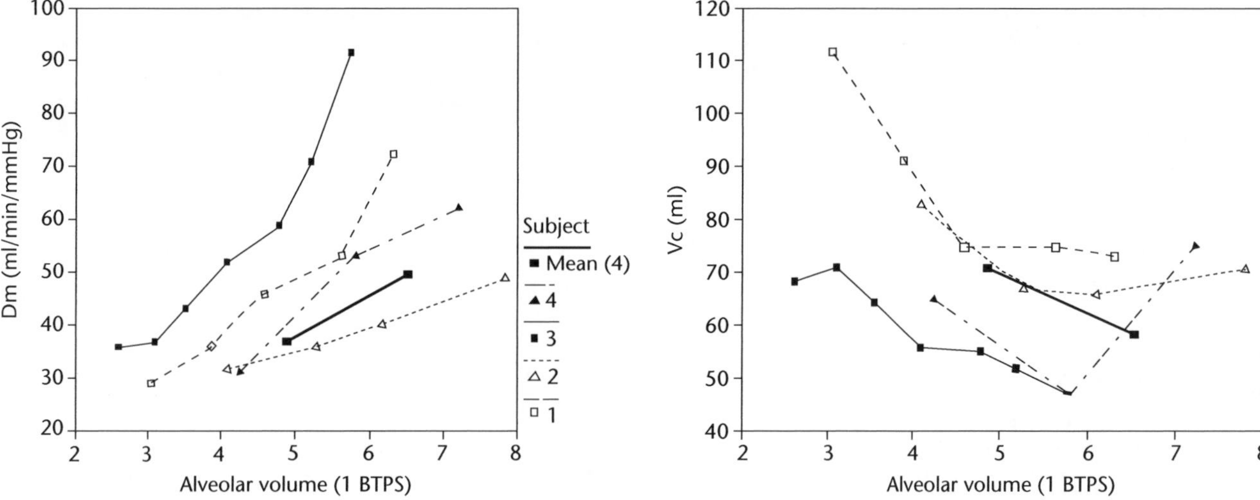

Fig. 20.6 Relationships of diffusing capacity of alveolar capillary membrane (Dm) and volume of blood in alveolar capillaries (Vc) to alveolar volume in healthy subjects. Sources: [75, 76]

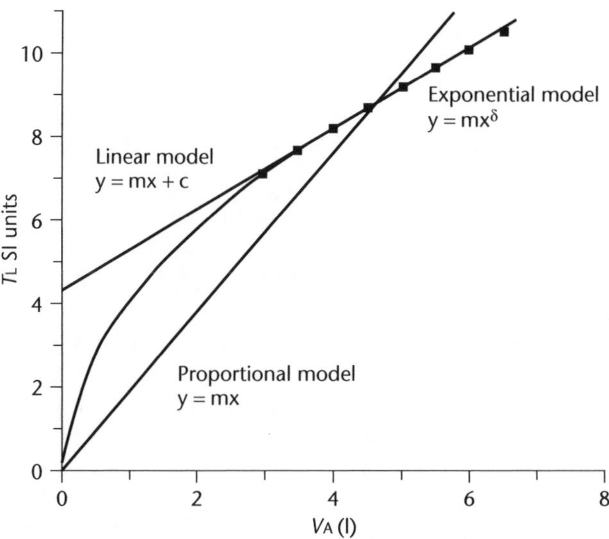

Fig. 20.7 Relationship of transfer factor to alveolar volume in one healthy subject. The data have been smoothed to illustrate alternative descriptive models. Source: [74]

relationship of transfer factor to alveolar volume can be described by a power function or linear equation (Footnote 20.2) but not by a proportionality. The implications of these observations are considered below.

Historical background. Marie Krogh pioneered the development of the single-breath (breath holding) method for measuring the transfer factor, then called diffusing capacity [5]. She observed that the index was greater at large than at small lung volumes, whilst for her data the ratio (Tl/V_A) was relatively constant. This suggested that the ratio provided a unique description of the gas-exchanging characteristics of the lungs. On this basis she introduced the terms 'permeability factor' or *diffusion constant* (kCO) with the units l (STPD) min^{-1} bar^{-1} per l (STPD) of alveolar volume (Footnote 20.3). The modern equivalent is Tl,co per litre of alveolar volume at BTPS (Tl/V_A) [14, 15, 16], alternatively designated KCO (or Dl/V_A).

Krogh made few observations, her method did not allow for regional inhomogenity or hysteresis and her conclusion was incorrect. Nonetheless her index endured. It has given rise to confusion because the model is unsound (see comment below) and aberrant units are sometimes used, either $k$co in the units of Krogh or Tl/V_A with alveolar volume in l ATP. The latter is unacceptable.

Footnote 20.2. Transfer factor of healthy white adults measured in a relaxed seated posture can be described in terms of age (year), height (m) and alveolar volume standardised for height $V_A.H^{-2}$. The equations are in SI units (mmol min^{-1} kPa^{-1}) and in traditional units (ml min^{-1} mm Hg^{-1}):

Adult men: Tl,co (SI units) $= 11.52 \times H - 0.051 \times Age + 2.72 \times V_A.H^{-2} - 12.35$ (RSD 1.17)

Dl,co (Trad units) $= 34.3 \times H - 0.15 \times Age + 8.11 \times V_A.H^{-2} - 36.8$ (RSD 3.49)

Adult women: Tl,co (SI units) $= 4.87 \times H - 0.019 \times Age + 2.29 \times V_A.H^{-2} - 3.03$ (RSD 0.92)

Dl,co (Trad units) $= 14.5 \times H - 0.06 \times Age + 6.82\ V_A.H^{-2} - 9.04$ (RSD 2.73)

RSD for these equations is narrower than for standard reference equations based on age and height.

Source: [74].

Footnote 20.3. Krogh's units are linked to the BTPS units of Tl/V_A by the relationship:

$$Tl/V_A\ (K\text{CO}) = k\text{CO}\ \frac{1000}{760} \times \frac{273}{310} \div 2.986\ \text{mmol min}^{-1}\ \text{kPa}^{-1} \qquad (20.35)$$

Table 20.10 Interpretation of *Tl*,co (normal, reduced or high with respect to Caucasian reference values) in circumstances likely to prevail in a clinic (see text). The information is amplified and referenced in Tables 20.11 and 20.12.

(A) Lung parenchyma is normal.

	Tl	*V*A	*Tl*/*V*A
Small *V*A e.g. ethnic,	N	↓	↑
submax inspiration	↓*		
restrictive defect (uncomplicated)	↓*		
Large *V*A e.g. some pts with asthma, acromegaly	↑*	↑	↓
Excision of normal lung tissue	↓	↓	↑
Exercise	↑	N	↑
Anaemia/polycythaemia with normal lungs	↓ / ↑	N	↓ / ↑

* normal after standardisation for *V*A [74].

(B) Lung parenchyma is abnormal (see text)

	Tl	*V*A	*Tl*/*V*A
Diffuse fibrosis	↓	↓	↑,N or ↓
Emphysema	↓	↑	↓↓
Pulmonary congestion*	↓	↓	↑,N or ↓
Lung haemorrhage	Varies with circumstances		↑

* Result variable (see Table 20.12).

Time constant for gas uptake (*tau*, CO). By analogy with electrical theory (Section 16.1.9) the *K*CO can be related to the time constant for the uptake of gas (τ CO); this is the time in seconds for the alveolar concentration of carbon monoxide (expressed as $\log_e F_{A,CO,t}$ as in eqn. 20.12) to fall exponentially to 37% of the initial value [77]. The τCO is numerically equal to 60/*K*CO. The index is mainly of theoretical interest.

20.9.2 Details of interpretation

*Interpretation of Tl/V*A. The *k*CO was introduced as a *primary* index of gas exchange having a proportional relationship to *Tl*,co [5] and this concept was transferred to *K*CO [2, 78]. For *Tl*,co.sb there is a proportional relationship in that the index (*Tl*,co.sb) is the volume of the gas exchanger (*V*A), multiplied by the terms that constitute *K*CO (eqn. 20.15). However, the relationship is merely a consequence of the method [3]. It does not exist for *Tl*,co.rb, where the volume of the gas exchanger is residual volume plus bag volume. In addition, the assumption of a proportional relationship does not obtain *in vivo*. Instead, the relationship of *Tl*,co to lung volume is nearly linear (Fig. 20.7). The primacy of *Tl* with respect to *K*CO is also supported by other evidence (Footnote 20.4).

The index describes the overall process of gas uptake in the prevailing circumstances. However, interpretation should take into account alveolar volume, evidence for uneven lung function and the underlying membrane and red cell conductances described by the Roughton–Forster relationship (eqn. 19.13 reproduced above).

The level of *K*CO (i.e. *Tl*/*V*A) is critically dependent on the lung volume [79]. As a result it is disproportionately high when lung volume is reduced and low when the lung size is increased (Table 20.10); thus it should not normally be interpreted in isolation. The index comes into its own in the unique circumstances of intra-alveolar haemorrhage when a reliable measurement of *Tl*,co may not be practicable, but a markedly raised *K*CO can be diagnostic [80, 81].

*Interpretation of Tl,*co, *Dm and Vc*. If alveolar volume is normal, the interpretation of *Tl*,co is likely to be unambiguous. If the alveolar volume is abnormal (either high or low) this must be taken into account when interpreting the *Tl*. When the abnormal *V*A is due to incomplete lung expansion or enlargement of the lungs with normal structure the allowance can be in terms of the linear model applied to *Tl* (Footnote 20.2). This can sometimes result in the salvaging of what was previously a technically

Footnote 20.4. Some additional reasons why *Tl*,co and not *K*CO is the primary measurement (and see text).

Aspect	Evidence
Reproducibility	On repeat measurements there is a negative relationship between *K*CO and *V*A. As a result *Tl*,co is relatively more reproducible than *K*CO [14]
Changes during growth	*Tl*,co increases progressively during growth but *K*CO declines, reflecting a disproportionate increase in lung volume (Chapter 26)
Ethnic variation	*Tl*,co is relatively independent of ethnic group, but *K*CO varies widely reflecting ethnic differences in lung size (Chapter 27)

Table 20.11 Circumstances that can affect the transfer factor (Tl,co) in subjects with healthy lungs (see text, also [84–89]).

Factors increasing Tl	Factors decreasing Tl	Principal variable
Exercise	Meals	Vc
Lying down	Standing up and other causes of peripheral blood pooling	Vc
Cold shower	Cutaneous vasodilatation	Vc
Increased sympathetic tone from other causes		Vc
(Müller manoeuvre)	Valsalva manoeuvre	Vc
	Night (cf. day)	Vc
	Smoking cigarettes	Vc
Growth (children) [Tl/VA ↓]	Age (adults)	Dm
Inhalation [Tl/VA ↓]	Exhalation [Tl/VA ↑]	Dm
Hypoxia	Breathing O_2 or CO	θco
Polycythaemia	Anaemia	θco

Table 20.12 Circumstances that can affect Tl,co in medical conditions. (see text, also [7, 90–96]). Tl/VA varies in the same direction as Tl except where indicated. Features in round brackets are somewhat variable.

Lung disorders	Dm	Vc	Tl	
Asthma	N or ↑	(N)	N or ↑	
Bronchitis	(N)	(N)	N or ↓	
Emphysema	↓	(↓)	N or ↓	[Kco ↓]
Diffuse infiltrations	↓	(↓)	↓	
Restrictive pleural disease	↓	(N)	(↓)	[Kco ↑]
Loss of lung tissue	↓	N or ↓	↓	
Cardiovascular disorders				
Hyperkinetic states	N	↑	↑	
Low cardiac output	N	↓	↓	
Raised pulmonary venous pressure:				
Minimal	N	↑	↑	
Intermediate	↓	↑	N	
Material (also other causes of pulmonary oedema)	↓	↓	↓	
Pulmonary embolism	↓	(–)	↓	
Good-pasture syndrome* (intrapulmonary haemorrhage, Tl/VA↑)		↑	↑	

* via effect on θco.

unsatisfactory measurement [74]. When the respiratory system is abnormal any of several processes may be involved and the existence of a linear relationship between Tl and VA cannot be assumed, but may obtain in some circumstances [82]. More data are needed. Meanwhile, awareness of the underlying relationships can assist in interpretation (Table 20.10). Errors that can be avoided by this approach include that, in interstitial fibrosis a normal Kco is a reassuring feature e.g. [83], and the use of Kco standardises Tl for variation in lung volume. Neither statement is correct!

Short-term variations in transfer factor are due to changes in pulmonary capillary blood volume (Vc). These occur over the cardiac cycle, with posture, exercise and secondary to changes in blood volume elsewhere in the body (Table 20.11). Vc decreases slightly with age.

In disease, the volume of blood in alveolar capillaries is increased by a rise in the pulmonary venous pressure such as occurs in mitral stenosis and left heart failure [90, 91]. It is also increased by the considerable augmentation to pulmonary blood flow that occurs in some forms of congenital heart disease (Section 41.18.2). The volume is usually normal in the early stages of chronic lung disease but declines in the later stages of this and other conditions when there is destruction of lung tissue and pulmonary hypertension (Table 20.12).

The membrane diffusing capacity (Dm) varies with the area of the alveolar capillary membrane and is subject to variation on this account, with respiratory manoeuvres, growth or as a result of respiratory and some systemic disorders (Table 20.12). The respiratory disorders include alveolitis, diffuse fibrosis, emphysema and conditions that can preferentially damage alveoli lining respiratory bronchioles (e.g. asbestosis) or limit lung expansion. Systemic disorders include those that give rise to lung infiltrates, interstitial or alveolar oedema, or cause damage to the capillary endothelium (e.g. non-insulin dependent diabetes [96]).

In most medical conditions in which *Tl* is reduced, the change reflects concordant reductions in *D*m and *V*c. However, when the changes in *D*m and θVc have opposite signs the effect on *Tl* is determined by their relative magnitudes. With changes in lung volume, the contribution of *D*m predominates (Fig. 20.6). By contrast when the pulmonary venous pressure is raised, as in mitral stenosis, the change in *Tl* can go either way [7, 90]. Initially, there is pulmonary congestion without transudation of fluid, hence *V*c is increased but *D*m is normal, so *Tl* is increased. Subsequently, as fluid accumulates in the interstitial tissue *D*m diminishes. This has an adverse effect on *Tl*, first returning it towards normal and later leading to it being reduced. The decline can then be aggravated by vascular thromboses and other changes.

In pulmonary embolism the changes include a redistribution of blood flow away from the obstructed and towards the non-obstructed parts of the pulmonary vascular bed. The changes reduce the area of surface available for gas exchange and hence *D*m. *V*c is reduced to a lesser extent on account of blood flow being diverted to those parts of the lung where gas exchange is taking place. In the obstructed regions the loss of perfusion can progress to closure of airways secondary to local hypocapnia [97] (see also Section 18.1.1). There is then the possibility that *D*m might decrease further.

Consequences for assessment of lung function. In most lung diseases lung diffusion is best monitored in terms of *Tl*. The principal reason for investigating the component terms is when *Tl* is increased or is normal despite clinical evidence for pulmonary congestion. However, the scope for specialist investigations may be enlarged as a consequence of studies into transfer factor for nitric oxide that are now in progress. Measurement of *D*m and *V*c can contribute to the assessment of gas exchange in a number of circumstances including lung trauma and the effects of drugs on the pulmonary circulation.

20.10 Measurement of *Tl*,NO (transfer factor for nitric oxide)

Some reasons for choosing to measure transfer factor for nitric oxide and an overview of the methods, with references, are given in Section 19.4.4. The methods are effectively those used to measure *Tl*,CO but with additional constraints. For example:

1 The concentrations used should be capable of being measured over a breathing manoeuvre that lasts up to 40 s, yet not such that oxidation to nitrogen dioxide poses a hazard.

2 Allowances need to be made for nitric oxide produced in the nose, airways and alveoli and for uptake during inspiration and expiration.

3 The slope of the alveolar plateau should be capable of interpretation in the presence of uneven lung function, despite being steep on account of the rapid uptake of NO.

Gas analysis. Nitric oxide is measured by a chemiluminescent method in which ozone is used to oxidise nitric oxide to nitrogen dioxide and photons of light; the latter are detected and quantified via a photomultiplier [98]. Early versions of the instrument had a slow response time so required static samples. More recent versions respond rapidly so studies during rebreathing and of single expirations can now be undertaken. Calibration can be with certified standard gas mixtures of nitric oxide in nitrogen. Alternatively, if the serial dilution method of calibration is used (Section 7.15.2) the diluent gas should be nitrogen. The zero point can be NO-free compressed air that has been passed through a filter packed with potassium permanganate.

Inspirate gas mixtures. Nitric oxide in multi-gas mixtures can oxidise to nitrogen dioxide, so mixtures for inhalation should be prepared immediately before use. This is done by adding an appropriate quantity from a stock cylinder containing 1000 ppm of NO in nitrogen to a bag that already contains the other constituents. The concentration that is used is in the range 5–40 parts per million, the lower concentration being appropriate for a 2-min period of steady state exercise and the higher for a single-breath (breath holding) test. A reasonable number of replicates can be carried out.

Back tension. Measurement of back tension is necessary because nitric oxide is excreted in material quantities from the nasal epithelium and in lesser amounts from the conducting airways. There is also some excretion from the lung parenchyma but the amount is small except when the peripheral tissues are inflamed or injured. The back tension is normally obtained by performing the test manoeuvre without, as well as with nitric oxide present in the test gas. During a single exhalation test the procedure for maintaining a constant expiratory flow usually entails breathing out through a resistance at a rate adjusted to keep the pressure in the mouth at a constant level. This has the additional advantage of preventing nasal contamination of the gas sample.

Derivation of Dm and Vc. Values for *Tl*,NO and *Tl*,CO obtained during the same breath-holding manoeuvre at a normal alveolar oxygen tension can be used to calculate *D*m and *V*c. To this end eqn. 19.13 is solved simultaneously for the two gases using appropriate values for *D*m,NO/*D*m,CO (approximately 2.0 from Table 19.2), θCO (from Table 20.9) and θNO; the latter has been given the value 1.5×10^3 mmol min^{-1} kPa^{-1}l^{-1} by Borland [99]. Then:

$$1/Tl{,}\mathrm{CO} = 1/Dm{,}\mathrm{CO} + 1/\theta\mathrm{CO}.Vc \qquad (19.13)$$

$$1/Tl{,}\mathrm{NO} = 1/2\ Dm{,}\mathrm{CO} + 1/\theta\mathrm{NO}.Vc \qquad (20.35)$$

from which it follows that:

$$Dm,\text{CO} = (\theta_{\text{NO}} - 2\theta_{\text{CO}})/(\theta_{\text{NO}}/Tl,\text{NO} - \theta_{\text{CO}}/Tl,\text{CO}) \quad (20.36)$$

$$Vc = 1/(\theta_{\text{CO}}/Tl,\text{CO} - \theta_{\text{CO}}/Dm,\text{CO}) \quad (20.37)$$

An alternative view is that θ_{NO} is effectively infinity, in which case $Dm,\text{CO} = 0.5 \times Dm,\text{NO} = 0.5\ Tl,\text{NO}$. This value for Dm,co can then be used in eqn. 20.37. To indicate the extent of the uncertainty both sets of values for Dm and Vc might be reported until such time as the matter has been resolved.

Comment. The transfer factor for nitric oxide differs from that for carbon monoxide in a number of respects (Table 19.3, page 229). As a result, the contribution of Dm to the transfer factor is larger for nitric oxide than for carbon monoxide; the respective ratios have been estimated as 40% and 17% [99]. Thus, even for nitric oxide the main constituent of the transfer factor is the diffusive resistance of the blood. The ratio $Tl,\text{NO}/Tl,\text{CO}$ has a wide range (approximately 3–5). In this it differs from $Tl,\text{O}_2/Tl,\text{CO}$ where the limits are narrow (Section 21.4.2), but whether the cause is technical or biological has still to be established.

Further development of the method could validate its use for estimation of Dm and Vc (e.g. [100]). This would represent a significant advance and be a means of avoiding the uncertainties associated with the Roughton–Forster method.

20.11 References

1. Cotes JE, Roughton FJW. Contributions to discussion. In: Dickens F, Neil E, eds. *Oxygen in the animal organism. Symposium of International Unions of Biochemistry and Physiological Sciences*, London 1–5 Sept 1963. Oxford: Pergamon 1964, 47–48.
2. Hughes JMB, Bates DV. Historical review: the carbon monoxide diffusing capacity (DL_{CO}) and its membrane (Dm) and red cell ($\theta.VC$) components. *Respir Physiol Neurobiol* 2003; **138**: 115–142.
3. Forster RE. The single-breath carbon monoxide transfer test 25 years on: a reappraisal. 1 Physiological considerations. *Thorax* 1983; **38**: 1–5.
4. Bartels H, Dejours P, Kellogg RH, Mead J. Glossary on respiration and gas exchange. *J Appl Physiol* 1973; **34**: 549–558.
5. Krogh M. The diffusion of gases through the lungs of man. *J Physiol* 1915; **49**: 271–296.
6. Filley GF, MacIntosh DJ, Wright GW. Carbon monoxide uptake and pulmonary diffusing capacity in normal subjects at rest and during exercise. *J Clin Invest* 1954; **33**: 530–539
7. Bates DV, Varvis CJ, Donevan RE, Christie RV. Variations in the pulmonary capillary blood volume and membrane diffusion component in health and disease. *J Clin Invest* 1960; **39**: 1401–1412.
8. Leathart GL. Steady-state diffusing capacity determined by a simplified method. *Thorax* 1962; **17**: 302–307.
9. Forster RE, Fowler WS, Bates DV, Van Lingen B. The absorption of carbon monoxide by the lungs during breathholding. *J Clin Invest* 1954; **33**: 1135–1145.
10. Newth CJL, Cotton DJ, Nadel JA. Pulmonary diffusing capacity measured at multiple intervals during a single exhalation in man. *J Appl Physiol* 1977; **43**: 617–625.
11. Gilson JC, Hugh-Jones P, Oldham PD, Meade F. Lung function in coal workers' pneumoconiosis. *Spec Rep Ser Med Res Counc (Lond)* 1955; **290**: 114–124 and 150–201.
12. Lewis BM, Lin T-H, Noe FE et al. The measurement of pulmonary diffusing capacity for carbon monoxide by a rebreathing method. *J Clin Invest* 1959; **38**: 2073–2086.
13. Kapitan KS, Wagner PD. Information content of multiple inert gas elimination measurements. *J Appl Physiol* 1987; **63**: 861–868.
14. Cotes JE, Chinn DJ, Quanjer PhH et al. Standardization of the measurement of transfer factor (diffusing capacity). Report of working party. Standardization of lung function tests, 1993 update. *Eur Respir J* 1993; **6**(Suppl 16): 41–53.
15. American Thoracic Society. Single breath carbon monoxide diffusing capacity (transfer factor). Recommendations for a standard technique – 1995 update. *Am J Respir Crit Care Med* 1996; **152**: 2185–2198.
16. MacIntyre N, Crapo RO, Viegi G et al. Standardisation of the single breath determination of carbon monoxide uptake in the lung – a joint official statement of ATS and ERS. *Eur Respir J* 2005; **26**: 720–735.
17. Kreukniet J. Relation between rebreathing CO-diffusing capacity of the lung and unequal ventilation. *Scand J Respir Dis* 1970; **51**: 49–54.
18. Cross CE, Gong H, Jr, Kurpershoeck CJ et al. Alterations in distribution of blood flow to the lung's diffusion surfaces during exercise. *J Clin Invest* 1973; **52**: 414–421.
19. Bouhuys A, Georg J, Jönsson R et al. The influence of histamine inhalation on the pulmonary diffusing capacity in man. *J Physiol (Lond)* 1960; **152**: 176–181.
20. Kreukniet J, Visser BF. The pulmonary CO diffusing capacity according to Bates and according to Filley in patients with unequal ventilation. *Pflügers Arch* 1964; **281**: 207–211.
21. Read J, Read DJC, Pain MCF. Influence of non-uniformity of the lungs on measurement of pulmonary diffusing capacity. *Clin Sci* 1965; **29**: 107–118.
22. Chinet A, Micheli JL, Haab P. Inhomogeneity effects on O_2 and CO pulmonary diffusing capacity estimates by steady-state methods. Theory. *Respir Physiol* 1971; **13**: 1–22.
23. Sundström G. Influence of body position on pulmonary diffusing capacity in young and old men. *J Appl Physiol* 1975; **38**: 418–423.
24. Kvale PA, Davis J, Schroter RC. Effect of gas density and ventilatory pattern on steady-state CO uptake by the lung. *Respir Physiol* 1975; **24**: 385–398.
25. Kindig NB, Hazlett DR. Temporal effects in the estimation of pulmonary diffusing capacity. *Q J Exp Physiol* 1977; **62**: 121–132.
26. Kety SS. The theory and applications of the exchange of inert gas at the lungs and tissues. *Pharmacol Rev* 1951; **3**: 1–41.
27. Forster RE. Exchange of gases between alveolar air and pulmonary capillary blood: pulmonary diffusing capacity. *Physiol Rev* 1957; **37**: 391–452.
28. Ogilvie CM, Forster RE, Blakemore WS, Morton JW. A standardized breathholding technique for the clinical measurement of the diffusing capacity of the lung for carbon monoxide. *J Clin Invest* 1957; **36**: 1–17.
29. Pelzar M, McGrath MW, Thompson ML. The effect of age, body size and lung volume change on alveolar-capillary permeability and diffusing capacity in man. *J Physiol (Lond)* 1959; **146**: 572–582.

30. Chinn DJ, Askew J, Rowley L, Cotes JE. Measurement technique influences the response of transfer factor (TlCO) to salbutamol in patients with airflow limitation. *Eur Respir J* 1988; **1**: 15–21.
31. Van Ganse W, Comhaire F, Van der Straeten M. Alveolar volume and transfer factor determined by single breath dilution of a test gas at various apnoea times. *Scand J Resp Dis* 1970; **51**: 82–92.
32. Leech JA, Martz L, Liben A, Becklake MR. Diffusing capacity for carbon monoxide. The effects of different derivations of breathhold time and alveolar volume and of carbon monoxide back pressure on calculated results. *Am Rev Respir Dis* 1985; **132**: 1127–1129.
33. Ferris BG Jr. Epidemiology standardisation project. *Amer Rev Respir Dis* 1978; **118**: 62–72.
34. Jones RS, Meade F. A theoretical and experimental analysis of anomalies in the estimation of pulmonary diffusing capacity by the single breath method. *Q J Exp Physiol* 1961; **46**: 131–143.
35. Graham BL, Dosman JA, Cotton DJ. A theoretical analysis of the single breath diffusing capacity for carbon monoxide. *IEEE Trans Biomed Eng* 1980; **27**: 221–227.
36. Graham BL, Mink JT, Cotton DJ. Improved accuracy and precision of single-breath CO diffusing capacity measurements. *J Appl Physiol* 1981; **51**: 1306–1313.
37. Graham BL, Mink JT, Cotton DJ. Overestimation of the single breath carbon monoxide diffusing capacity in patients with airflow obstruction. *Amer Rev Respir Dis* 1984; **129**: 403–408.
38. Graham BL, Mink JT, Cotton DJ. Effect of breath-hold time on Dlco(SB) in patients with airway obstruction. *J Appl Physiol* 1985; **58**: 1319–1325.
39. Meade F, Saunders MJ, Hyett F et al. Automatic measurement of lung function. *Lancet* 1965; **2**: 573–575.
40. Chinn DJ, Harkawat R, Cotes JE. Standardisation of single breath transfer factor (Tlco); derivation of breathholding time. *Eur Resp J* 1992;**5**: 492–496.
41. Cliff IJ, Evans AH, Pantin CAF, Baldwin DR. Comparison of two new methods for the measurement of lung volumes with two standard methods. *Thorax* 1999; **54**: 329–333.
42. Cotes, JE, Chinn DJ, Quanjer Ph et al. Standardisation of the measurement of transfer factor: allowance for water vapour in the analysis of helium concentration – reply. *Eur Resp J* 1995; **8**(10): 1814.
43. Chinn DJ, Naruse Y, Cotes JE. Accuracy of gas analysis in lung function laboratories. *Thorax* 1986; **41**: 133–137.
44. Punjabi NM, Shade D, Patel AM, Wise RA. Measurement variability in single breath diffusing capacity of the lung. *Chest* 2003; **123**: 1082–1089.
45. Hathaway EH, Tashkin DP, Simmons MS. Intra-individual variability in serial measurements of DLCO and alveolar volume over one year in eight healthy subjects using three independent measuring systems. *Am Rev Respir Dis* 1989; **140**: 1818–1822.
46. Cotes JE, Hall AM. The transfer factor for the lung; normal values in adults. In: Arcangeli E, ed. *Normal values for respiratory function in man.* Panminerva Medica 1970; 327–343.
47. Morris AH, Crapo, RO. Standardisation of computation of single breath transfer factor. *Bull Eur Physiopathol Respir* 1985; **21**: 183–189.
48. Tsoukias NM, Wilson AF, George SC. Effect of alveolar volume and sequential filling on the diffusing capacity of the lungs: 1. Theory. *Respir Physiol* 2000; **120**: 231–249.
49. Denison DM, Cramer DS, Hanson PJV. Lung function testing and AIDS. *Respir Med* 1989; **83**: 133–138.
50. Graham BL, Mink JT, Cotton DJ. Dynamic measurements of CO diffusing capacity using discrete samples of alveolar gas. *J Appl Physiol* 1983; **54**: 73–79.
51. Wilson AF, Hearne J, Brenner M, Alfonso R. Measurement of transfer factor during constant exhalation. *Thorax* 1994; **49**: 1121–1126.
52. Cassidy SS, Ramanathan M, Rose GL, Johnson RL Jr. Hysteresis in the relation between diffusing capacity of the lung and lung volume. *J Appl Physiol* 1980; **49**: 566–570.
53. Huang YC, Helms MJ, MacIntyre NR. Normal values for single exhalation diffusing capacity and pulmonary capillary blood flow in sitting, supine positions, and during mild exercise. *Chest* 1994; **105**: 501–508.
54. Felton C, Rose GL, Cassidy SS, Johnson RL. Comparison of lung diffusing capacity during rebreathing and during slow exhalation. *Resp Physiol* 1981; **43**: 13–22.
55. Mohsenifar Z, Tashkin DP. Effect of carboxyhemoglobin on the single breath diffusing capacity: an empirical correction factor. *Respiration* 1979; **37**: 185–191.
56. Frans A, Stanescu DC, Veriter T et al. Smoking and pulmonary diffusing capacity *Scand J Respir Dis* 1975; **56**: 165–183.
57. Frey TM, Crapo RL, Jensen RL, Elliott CG. Diurnal variation of the diffusing capacity of the lung: is it real? *Am Rev Respir Dis* 1987; **136**: 1381–1384.
58. Henderson M, Apthorp GH. Rapid method for estimation of carbon monoxide in blood. *Brit Med J* 1960; **2**: 1853–1854.
59. Jones RH, Ellicott MF, Cadigan JB, Gaensler EA. The relationship between alveolar and blood carbon monoxide concentrations during breathholding. *J Lab Clin Med* 1958; **51**: 553–564.
60. Kirkham AJT, Guyatt AR, Cumming G. Alveolar carbon monoxide: a comparison of methods of measurement and a study of the effect of change in body posture. *Clin Sci* 1988; **74**: 23–28.
61. Cotes JE, Dabbs JM, Elwood PC et al. Iron-deficiency anaemia: its effect on transfer factor for the lung (diffusing capacity) and ventilation and cardiac frequency during sub-maximal exercise. *Clin Sci* 1972; **42**: 325–335.
62. Clark EH, Woods RL, Hughes JMB. Effect of blood transfusion on the carbon monoxide transfer factor of the lung in man. *Clin Sci Mol Med* 1978; **54**: 627–631.
63. Marrades RM, Diaz O, Roca J et al. Adjustment of DLCO for hemoglobin concentration. *Am J Respir Crit Care Med* 1997; **155**: 234–241.
64. Kanner RE, Crapo RO. The relationship between alveolar oxygen tension and the single-breath carbon monoxide diffusing capacity. *Am Rev Respir Dis* 1986; **133**: 676–678.
65. Borland CDR, Cox Y. Effect of varying alveolar oxygen partial pressure on diffusing capacity for nitric oxide and carbon monoxide, membrane diffusing capacity and lung capillary blood volume. *Clin Sci* 1991; **81**: 759–765.
66. Holland RAB. O2 uptake kinetics of red blood cells. *Prog Respir Res* 1986; **21**: 1–4.
67. Sirs JA. The Bohr effect on the reaction of carbon monoxide with fully oxygenated haemoglobin. *J Physiol (Lond)* 1976; **263**: 475–488.
68. Roughton FJW, Forster RE, Cander L. Rate at which carbon monoxide replaces oxygen from combination with human haemoglobin in solution and in the red cell. *J Appl Physiol* 1957; **11**: 269–276.

69. Forster RE. Diffusion of gases across the alveolar membrane. In: Farhi LE, Tenney SM, eds. *Handbook of physiology, 4 gas exchange.* Bethesda, MD: American Physiological Society 1987; 71–88.
70. Guenard H, Vuene N, Vaida P. Determination of lung capillary blood volume and membrane diffusing capacity in man by the measurements of NO and CO transfer. *Respir Physiol* 1987; **70**: 113–120.
71. Borland C, Mist B, Zammit M, Vuylstreke A. Steady-state measurement of NO and CO lung diffusing capacity on moderate exercise in men. *J Appl Physiol* 2001, **90**: 538–544.
72. Weibel ER. Morphological basis of alveolar-capillary gas exchange. *Physiol Rev* 1973; **53**: 419–495.
73. Crapo JD, Crapo RO, Jensen RL et al. Evaluation of lung diffusing capacity by physiological and morphometric techniques. *J Appl Physiol* 1988: **64**: 2083–2091.
74. Chinn DJ, Cotes JE, Flowers R, et al. Transfer factor (diffusing capacity) standardised for alveolar volume; validation, reference values and applications of a new linear model to replace *K*co (*Tl*/*V*A). *Eur Respir J* 1996; **9**:1269–1277.
75. Hamer NAJ. Variations in the components of the diffusing capacity as the lung expands. *Clin Sci* 1963; **24**: 275–285.
76. Cotes JE, Meade F, Saunders MJ. Effect of volume inspired and manner of sampling the alveolar gas upon components of the transfer factor (diffusing capacity of the lung) by the single breath method. *J Physiol (Lond)* 1965; **181**: 73–75P.
77. Zamel N. Use of the RC time constant for CO in the measurement of diffusing capacity. *Am Rev Respir Dis* 1974; **110**: 683–684.
78. Hughes JMB, Pride NB. Perspective. In defence of the carbon monoxide transfer coefficient *K*co (*TL*/*V*A). *Eur Respir J* 2001; **17**: 168–174; *also Eur Respir J* 2001; **18**: 893–894.
79. Stam H, Kreuzer FJA, Versprille A. Effect of lung volume and positional changes on pulmonary diffusing capacity and its components. *J Appl Physiol* 1991; **71**: 1477–1488.
80. Ewan PW, Jones HA, Rhodes CG, Hughes JMB. Detection of intrapulmonary hemorrhage with carbon monoxide uptake. Application in Goodpasture's syndrome. *New Engl J Med* 1976; **295**: 1391–1396.
81. Greening AP, Hughes JMB. Serial estimations of carbon monoxide diffusing capacity in intrapulmonary haemorrhage. *Clin Sci* 1981; **60**: 507–512.
82. Stam H, Splinter TAW, Versprille A. Evaluation of pulmonary diffusing capacity in patients with a restrictive lung disease. *Chest* 2000; **117**: 752–757.
83. Wright PH, Hanson A, Kreel L, Capel LH. Respiratory function changes after asbestos pleurisy. *Thorax* 1980; **35**: 31–36.
84. Cotes JE, Snidal DP, Shepard RH. Effect of negative intra-alveolar pressure on pulmonary diffusing capacity. *J Appl Physiol* 1960; **15**: 372–376.
85. Ross JC, Ley GD, Coburn RF et al. Influence of pressure suit inflation on pulmonary diffusing capacity in man. *J Appl Physiol* 1962; **17**: 259–262.
86. Danzer LA, Cohn JE, Zechman FW. Relationship of Dm and Vc to pulmonary diffusing capacity during exercise. *Respir Physiol* 1968; **5**: 250–258.
87. Federspiel WJ. Pulmonary diffusing capacity: implications of two-phase blood flow in capillaries. *Respir Physiol* 1989; **77**: 119–134.
88. Kuwahira I, Ide M, Suzuki Y et al. Effect of cold pressor test on carbon monoxide diffusing capacity in normal subjects. *Respiration* 1989; **56**: 87–93.
89. Aftab N, Chinn DJ, Cotes JE, Smith SL. Effect of ambient temperature on small airway function. *J Physiol* 1987; **391**: 77P.
90. Gazioglu K, Yu PN. Pulmonary blood volume and pulmonary capillary blood volume in valvular heart disease. *Circulation* 1967; **35**: 701–709.
91. Guazzi M. Alveolar-capillary membrane dysfunction in chronic heart failure: pathophysiology and therapeutic implications *Clin Sci (Lond).* 2000; **98**: 633–641.
92. Bucci G, Cook CD, Hamann JF. Studies of respiratory physiology in children. VI Lung diffusing capacity, diffusing capacity of the pulmonary membrane and pulmonary capillary blood volume in congenital heart disease. *J Clin Invest* 1961; **40**: 1431–1441.
93. Pande JN, Gupta SP, Guleria JS. Clinical significance of the measurement of membrane diffusing capacity and pulmonary capillary blood volume. *Respiration* 1975; **32**: 317–324.
94. Puri S, Baker BL, Dutka DP et al. Reduced alveolar-capillary membrane diffusing capacity in chronic heart failure. Its pathophysiological relevance and relationship to exercise performance. *Circulation* 1995; **91**: 2769–2774.
95. Al-Rawas OA, Carter R, Stevenson RD et al. The alveolar-capillary membrane diffusing capacity and the pulmonary capillary blood volume in heart transplant candidates. *Heart* 2000; **83**: 156–160.
96. Guazzi M, Brambilla R, De Vita S, Guazzi MD. Diabetes worsens pulmonary diffusion in heart failure, and insulin counteracts this effect. *Am J Respir Crit Care Med* 2002; **166**: 978–982; *also Am J Respir Crit Care Med* 2003; **168**: 398–399.
97. Santolicandro A, Prediletto R, Fornai E et al. Mechanisms of hypoxaemia and hypocapnia in pulmonary embolism. *Am J Respir Crit Care Med.* 1995; **152**: 336–347.
98. Kharitonov S, Alving K, Barnes PJ. Exhaled and nasal nitric oxide measurements: recommendations. *Eur Respir J* 1997; **10**: 1683–1693.
99. Borland CDR, Cox Y. Effect of varying alveolar oxygen partial pressure on diffusing capacity for nitric oxide and carbon monoxide, membrane diffusing capacity and lung capillary blood volume. *Clin Sci* 1991; **81**: 759–765.
100. Tamhane RM, Johnson RL Jr, Hsia CCW. Pulmonary membrane diffusing capacity and capillary blood volume measured during exercise from nitric oxide uptake. *Chest* 2001; **120**: 1850–1856.

Further reading (see also Chapter 19)

Cadigan JB, Marks A, Ellicott MF et al. An analysis of factors affecting the measurement of pulmonary diffusing capacity by the single breath method. *J Clin Invest* 1961; **40**: 1495–1514.

Michaelson ED, Sackner MA, Johnson RL Jr. Vertical distributions of pulmonary diffusing capacity and capillary blood flow in man. *J Clin Invest* 1973; **52**: 359–369.

Scheid P, Piiper J. Blood gas equilibrium in lungs and pulmonary diffusing capacity. In: Chang HK, Paiva M, eds. *Respiratory physiology an analytical approach.* New York: Marcel Dekker, 1989: 453–497.

CHAPTER 21

The Oxygenation of Blood

The processes whereby the blood is oxygenated are reviewed in this chapter, including their dependence on the biochemical properties of haemoglobin and on the distributions of pulmonary ventilation, blood flow and gas transfer characteristics.

21.1 Overview

Achieving acceptable levels of oxygen and carbon dioxide in arterial blood depends on factors outside as well as within the lungs. The extrapulmonary determinants are the amounts and composition of the incoming air and mixed venous blood. The processes within the lungs are distribution, diffusion and chemical reactions. Of these the first two are considered as discrete entities in preceding chapters. The present chapter describes the chemical reactions and their interactions with the other processes. The final destination of oxygen is the mitochondria in muscle and other tissues (Section 28.9.1).

At each stage between inspired air and mitochondria the partial pressure of oxygen decreases compared with the previous stage so the flow of oxygen takes place as a series of cascades down a pressure gradient. The capacity of each stage can be expressed in terms of its conductance; this is the maximal quantity of oxygen per unit time that can be transferred per unit of pressure difference between the two ends of the stage under consideration. Some numerical values are given in Table 21.1.

The first stage reflects alveolar ventilation and is described by the term 'convective conductance'. At rest this conductance is low mainly because much of the minute volume is wasted in ventilating the physiological deadspace. On exercise the convective conductance rises because the alveolar ventilation increases to a greater extent than the deadspace ventilation. For the same reason the convective conductance increases with hypoxia. The alveolar oxygen tension provides the head of pressure for the second stage, which is diffusion of oxygen within the acini and its transfer across the alveolar capillary membrane into plasma in alveolar capillaries. This process occurs to different extents in the several parts of the lung, depending on the local anatomy and related circumstances. For the lungs as a whole the factors can be represented by the area and thickness of the alveolar capillary membrane and the volume and flow of blood in adjacent alveolar capillaries. The diffusive processes are the prelude to reversible combination of oxygen with haemoglobin. These aspects are considered, respectively, in Chapter 19 and the present chapter. The third and fourth stages are the transport of oxygen from the lungs to the tissue capillaries and the transfer from red blood cells into the tissues (Section 28.3). Here the oxygen is used as a hydrogen acceptor (Section 28.8.4) and for oxidation of substrate. The oxidative metabolism leads to the formation of carbon

Table 21.1 Representative mean oxygen tensions (Po_2) and conductances (G) for the several stages of oxygen transport in subjects assessed during rest and exercise at sea level and rest at an altitude of 5365 m (17,600 ft).

Conditions†	Rest				Exercise				Rest (Altitude)			
	Po_2		G		Po_2		G		Po_2		G	
Index units*	kPa	mm Hg	SI	trad	kPa	mm Hg	SI	trad	kPa	mm Hg	SI	trad
Inspired gas	20	150			20	150			9.4	71		
↓ convective (*airway*) G			2.2	0.3			15	2.0			3.9	0.52
Alveolar gas	13.3	100			13.3	100			5.6	42		
↓ alveolar capillary (*transfer*) G			7.5	1.0			22	2.9			19	2.50
Pulmonary capillaries	11.3	85			8.7	65			4.8	36		
↓ tissue capillary ($\dot{V}_A/\dot{Q}$) G			3.8	0.5			25	3.3			30	3.75
Tissue capillaries	7.3	55			4.7	35			4.3	32		
↓ tissue (*diffusive*) G			7.5	1.0			71	1.0			15	2.14
Tissue cells	5.3	40			3.3	25			3.3	25		
Overall conductance			1.0	0.14			6.0	0.8			2.4	0.33

†Oxygen uptakes are respectively rest 15 mmol min^{-1} (330 ml min^{-1}) and exercise 100 mmol min^{-1} (2.2 l min^{-1}).
*Units for G are in SI units mmol min^{-1}kPa^{-1} and in traditional units ml min^{-1} mm Hg^{-1}. Overall conductance was obtained from the sum of the reciprocals of the individual conductances; the reciprocals are the resistances to the flow of oxygen across the stages.
Source: adapted from [1].

dioxide; this returns along the same route to the atmosphere (Chapter 22).

21.2 Capacity of blood for oxygen

Blood carries oxygen in simple solution and combined with haemoglobin. The quantity in solution in plasma at 37°C is defined by the capacitance coefficient; this is approximately 0.01 mmol l^{-1} kPa^{-1}, equivalent to 0.03 ml/l/mm Hg (Table 19.1, page 225), hence for a subject breathing air at sea level the quantity of oxygen dissolved in arterial blood is approximately 0.13 mmol l^{-1} (0.3 ml/100 ml). When breathing 100% oxygen the concentration increases to approximately 0.9 mmol l^{-1} (2.0 ml/100 ml). These amounts are relatively small. The physiological requirement for oxygen is met by gas carried in combination with haemoglobin (see below, oxygen dissociation curve). The maximal quantity is then determined by the capacity of haemoglobin for oxygen, designated *Hufner's constant* [2]. In SI units this is 1 mmol of oxygen per mmol of haemoglobin; in traditional units 1.39 ml of oxygen per gram of haemoglobin. Hence, in a typical young man with a haemoglobin concentration of 9 mmol l^{-1} (14.6 g of haemoglobin per 100 ml) the oxygen capacity of the blood is 9 mmol l^{-1}, equivalent to 20 ml of oxygen per 100 ml of blood. The corresponding figures for women are 8.3 mmol l^{-1} (13.4 g of haemoglobin per 100 ml) and 18.6 ml of oxygen per 100 ml of blood. The oxygen capacity is reduced if some of the haemoglobin is combined with carbon monoxide (e.g. in smokers, Section 38.5), or present as methaemoglobin or other compound containing iron in the ferric state that does not transport oxygen.

Under normal conditions the quantity of oxygen in arterial blood is slightly less than the capacity, hence the blood is nearly fully saturated with oxygen (average saturation 97%). The saturation declines with age (Table 26.23, page 358) mainly due to a progressive deterioration in the matching of lung ventilation to perfusion. In some subjects this is aggravated by an increase in body fat.

21.2.1 Reaction of oxygen with haemoglobin

Reaction rate. Haemoglobin comprises four inter-linked polypeptide chains, each with a porphyrin ring containing an atom of iron attached to it. The iron is in the ferrous state and the chains are of two types (α and β, or in the foetus α and γ) with different composition and structure. The iron is capable of binding reversibly with oxygen, hence one molecule of haemoglobin can carry up to four molecules of oxygen. In the reduced state, due to the configuration of the polypeptide chains, the binding sites are relatively inaccessible to oxygen. They become more accessible after one of the four sites has been filled. Thereafter each reaction proceeds at a progressively increased rate. However, no one reaction is completed before the next one starts and as a result several compounds of oxygen combined to haemoglobin are present in the blood concurrently. This situation led Adair to develop his *intermediate compound hypothesis* [3]. He proposed that the reaction of oxygen with whole blood comprised four over-lapping stages, each with its own rate of forward and back reaction and intermediate compound:

$$Hb_4 + O_2 \leftrightharpoons Hb_4O_2 \quad (1)$$
$$Hb_4O_2 + O_2 \leftrightharpoons Hb_4O_4 \quad (2)$$
$$Hb_4O_4 + O_2 \leftrightharpoons Hb_4O_6 \quad (3)$$
$$Hb_4O_6 + O_2 \leftrightharpoons Hb_4O_8 \quad (4)$$

The equilibrium constant for each reaction is the ratio of the constants for the forward and backward reactions. Under physiological conditions the speed of the forward reactions increases by a factor of 500 between the first and fourth stages. The values for the intermediate stages have been estimated but not measured directly [4]. The physiological reaction rate for intact red cells is a weighted mean of the rates for the intermediate reactions and varies with circumstances including the prevailing temperature. In the blood, mixing of the plasma also contributes [5]. Other physiological variables are the prevailing oxygen tension and the change in blood pH caused by loss of carbon dioxide into the alveoli. The rate of loss depends on the speed of dissociation of carbamino-haemoglobin and the rate at which CO_2 is liberated from bicarbonate ions under the influence of carbonic anhydrase (Section 22.2.3). The effects of these factors are such that a single value for the reaction rate θO_2 is of limited usefulness [6]. However, a number of such determinations have been made. Early measurements have been reviewed by Roughton [7]. Subsequent measurements by different methods have yielded results in the range 0.9–8 mmol min^{-1} kPa^{-1} (2.7–26 vol/vol min^{-1} mm Hg^{-1}) [6, 8–10]. The wide range indicates that further clarification is necessary [11]. The rate is used in computations, for example for analysing gas exchange during exercise or at high altitude and for calculating the transfer factor for oxygen from that for carbon monoxide (Section 21.4.2).

21.2.2 Oxygen dissociation curve

The relationship of the oxygen content of haemoglobin to the prevailing oxygen tension under equilibrium conditions is portrayed by the haemoglobin dissociation curve for oxygen (Fig. 21.1). The S-shape of the curve was identified by Bohr [13] and its steep middle part was described mathematically by AV Hill [14]. Hill's equation is given by

$$\log y(1-y) = \log k + n(\log P_{O_2}) \quad (21.1)$$

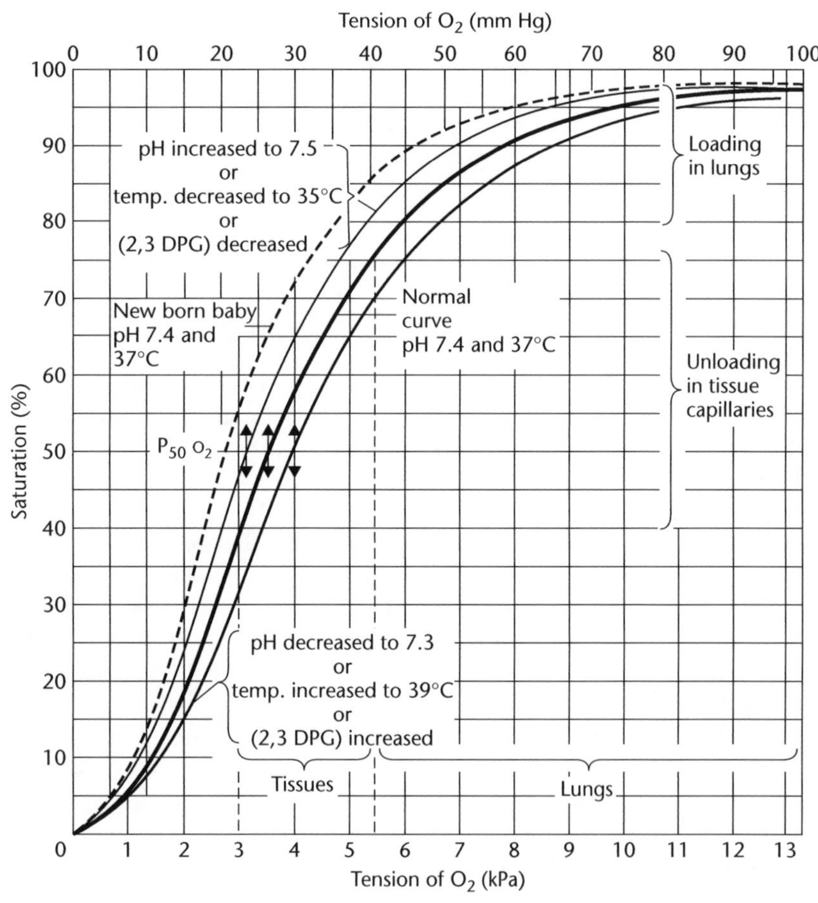

Fig. 21.1 Dissociation curves for oxyhaemoglobin compiled from data in the literature. The broad line is for pH 7.4 and 37°C (Table 21.2); the narrow lines show the effects of a change in pH or in body temperature.* The interrupted line is for a newborn baby. The brackets indicate the approximate saturations and tensions at which haemoglobin loads up with oxygen in the lungs and unloads in the tissue capillaries. The tension at which haemoglobin takes up oxygen is reduced when the subject is breathing a hypoxic gas mixture or the lungs are underventilated. The tension in the tissue capillaries is reduced by a low cardiac output such as occurs in patients with restrictive cardiac disease; low values also obtain during strenuous exercise.
*the following relationships were used in the construction of the curves:

$\log_{10}[P_{O_2}, 37°C / P_{O_2}, t°C] = 0.024\ (37 - t)$
$\log_{10}[P_{O_2}, \text{pH } 7.4 / P_{O_2}, \text{pHa}] = -0.48\ (7.4 - a)$

The curve for a newborn baby at pH 7.4 resembles that of an adult at pH 7.6. $P_{50}O_2$. (The two headed arrow is the tension of oxygen at which haemoglobin is 50% saturated.) Source: [12]

Table 21.2 Relationship of oxygen tension to saturation for normal blood at pH 7.4 and temperature 37°C.

Saturation	Oxygen tension		Saturation	Oxygen tension	
HbO_2 (%)	kPa	mm Hg	HbO_2 (%)	kPa	mm Hg
1	0.25	1.9	85	6.6	49.8
2	0.45	3.4	90	7.7	57.8
4	0.76	5.7	91	8.0	60.0
6	1.0	7.5	92	8.4	62.7
10	1.4	10.3	93	8.8	65.7
15	1.7	13.1	94	9.3	69.4
20	2.1	15.4	95	9.9	74.2
25	2.3	17.3	95.5	10.3	77.3
30	2.6	19.2	96	10.8	81.0
35	2.8	21.0	96.5	11.5	86.0
40	3.0	22.8	97	12.2	91.6
45	3.3	24.6	97.5	13.3	99.6
50*	3.55	26.6	98	14.8	111
55	3.8	28.7	98.5	17.2	129
60	4.2	31.2	99	21.2	159
65	4.5	34.0	99.5	30.0	225
70	4.9	36.9	99.8	46.7	350
75	5.4	40.4	99.9	66.7	500
80	5.9	44.5	99.95	93.3	700

*Corresponding O_2 tension is $P_{50}O_2$.
Source: [12].

where y is the fractional saturation of haemoglobin with oxygen, k is the dissociation constant and the exponent n is normally in the range 2.6–3.0. The equation can be used to obtain the $P_{50}O_2$ (see below, Role of 2,3 diphosphoglycerate). The data for the curve were collated by Severinghaus (Table 21.2) and represented as a continuous mathematical function by Kelman [15]. Minor changes have been made subsequently [16, 17]. The slopes of the lower and upper ends of the curve are due to reactions 1 and 4, respectively, whilst in the middle it is due mainly to reactions 2 and 3. The reaction rate approaches zero when the blood is fully saturated with oxygen.

The flat top to the curve stabilises the quantity of oxygen in the arterial blood (Section 21.3.2). It also contributes to the tension of oxygen in blood leaving the alveolar capillaries being nearly equal to that in the alveolar gas; how this is achieved is discussed below. The steep middle part of the curve ensures that a large proportion of the oxygen that is carried by the blood is delivered to the tissues at a relatively high tension. This attribute of haemoglobin is illustrated in the figure. Here the uptake of oxygen by haemoglobin is represented as taking place over a range of tensions of oxygen from 13.3 kPa (100 mm Hg), as is normally the case at sea level, to 6 kPa (45 mm Hg) which is the average tension at an altitude of 3300 m (11,000 ft). At sea level, the latter is equivalent to a subject breathing oxygen at a fractional concentration of 0.135 (13.5% O_2 in N_2); the corresponding saturations of haemoglobin with oxygen are 97% and 80%.

Unloading of oxygen occurs in the tissue capillaries at saturations that, near the venous ends of the capillaries, are less than those in the arterial blood by approximately 25% at rest and 50% during moderate exercise. Due to the shape of the dissociation curve the corresponding tensions of oxygen are in the range 5.3–2.9 kPa (40–22 mm Hg). Transport of oxygen is assisted by differences in pH, temperature and tension of carbon dioxide between the lungs and peripheral tissues. In the tissues the P_{CO_2} is relatively high, hence pH is low, on account of metabolism. This also raises the local temperature. These features are magnified by exercise in proportion to its intensity. Exercise can also lead to the formation of lactic acid (Section 28.9.2) and this further reduces the pH. The changes displace the dissociation curve to the right and have the effect of liberating oxygen from haemoglobin [18, 19]. The oxygen then passes by diffusion into the adjacent cells. This facilitating effect of P_{CO_2} (and hence of hydrogen ions) on delivery of oxygen to muscle and other tissues was described by Bohr (hence *Bohr effect*) [13]. It accounts for approximately 2% of the oxygen carried by blood.

In the lungs the temperature is lower than in the tissues and the pH is higher due to carbon dioxide passing out of the blood into the alveolar gas. These changes displace the dissociation curve to the left; they have the converse effect of increasing the uptake of oxygen by pulmonary capillary blood at the tension that obtains in the alveoli. The haemoglobin saturation rises in consequence and reduces the ability of the haemoglobin to retain carbon dioxide. The CO_2 is then unloaded into the plasma and thence into the alveolar gas. This feature is known as the *Haldane effect* [19]. It is the converse of the Bohr effect and reflects the interdependence of the transport of oxygen and carbon dioxide by blood [20, 21].

Role of 2,3 diphosphoglycerate. The substance 2,3 diphosphoglycerate (2,3 DPG) is present in red blood cells as a by-product of aerobic metabolism. It is formed from 1,3-diphosphoglycerate by the action of diphosphoglycerate synthase (Section 28.9.1). In most cells the reaction is quickly inhibited by accumulation of the end product. In red cells the inhibition is weak because 2,3 DPG is removed as it is formed. The molecules introduce themselves into spaces between the β polypeptide chains of the haemoglobin molecules [22]; this reduces the accessibility of the combining sites for oxygen. It also lowers the intracellular pH. As a result the dissociation curve in its lower part is displaced to the right by an amount which is proportional to the concentration present. 2,3 DPG is absent from purified haemoglobin solution and is present in reduced amounts in combination with foetal haemoglobin; these features lead to the dissociation curve being displaced to the left. The displacement is conveniently described in terms of the oxygen tension at which the haemoglobin is 50% saturated with oxygen ($P_{50}O_2$). The $P_{50}O_2$ can be obtained using eqn. 21.1 and is normally approximately 3.6 kPa (27 mm Hg) (Table 21.2); it is a function of the tension of carbon dioxide, the concentrations of hydrogen ions, chloride ions, 2,3 DPG and the prevailing temperature.

The effects of the chemical variables are interrelated because they combine at a limited number of locations on the haemoglobin molecule. Of these, the salt bridge between the imidazole group of β146 histidine and β94 aspartine is susceptible to pH changes in the physiological range and is believed to account for approximately half the normal Bohr effect. Half the remainder is due to oxygen linked binding of chloride ions. This linkage alters the ionisation at the NH_2-terminal α amino group on the α chain of the haemoglobin molecule. The corresponding terminal on the β chain of the molecule appears to be the main site of incorporation of carbon dioxide to form carbamic acid; this site also binds 2,3 DPG which then diminishes the carbamino reaction [23].

The reaction of 2,3 DPG with haemoglobin provides a means whereby the rate of metabolism, the supply of substrate and the level of tissue oxygenation can influence the extent to which oxygen is released from haemoglobin in the tissue capillaries. The metabolic pathway is illustrated by the central column in Table 21.3. The equilibrium between 1,3 and 2,3 DPG is influenced by a number of factors all of which contribute to the red cell concentration of the latter substance. Circumstances in which the level is altered are indicated in the table. When the haemoglobin is normal the $P_{50}O_2$ varies proportionately. However, with some haemoglobin variants the binding of 2,3 DPG is abnormal and the $P_{50}O_2$ is altered in consequence. The $P_{50}O_2$ concentration decreases when blood is stored. It also decreases with age [24]. The decline influences the level of tissue oxygenation and hence performance during exercise [e.g.25].

21.3 Transfer of oxygen across the alveolar capillary membrane

The quantity of oxygen that is transferred across the alveolar capillary membrane per unit time is the product of the transfer factor for oxygen and the transfer gradient (eqn. 20.1, page 235). The transfer factor depends on all the factors analysed in Chapter 19; they include diffusion and mixing within the alveolar capillary plasma (including the existence of possible boundary layer [5]), the permeability of the red cell membrane, combination of oxygen with haemoglobin and transport out of the lungs of the compound with haemoglobin. The reaction with haemoglobin has been described above. The transfer gradient and the way in which the dissociation curve maximises its effectiveness for oxygenating the blood are described next.

21.3.1 Some features of the transfer gradient

The transfer gradient is the amount by which the tension of oxygen in alveolar gas exceeds that in the pulmonary capillary blood. It is in effect the driving pressure for oxygenation of the blood. The tension in alveolar gas varies with ventilation minute volume and it is higher during inspiration than expiration (cf. Fig. 18.6, page 220). It is increased by breathing oxygen and is reduced by breathing gas in which the tension of oxygen is subnormal. The tension of oxygen in blood entering the gas-exchanging region of the lung is that in mixed venous blood. The tension is low during exercise (especially exercise performed under conditions

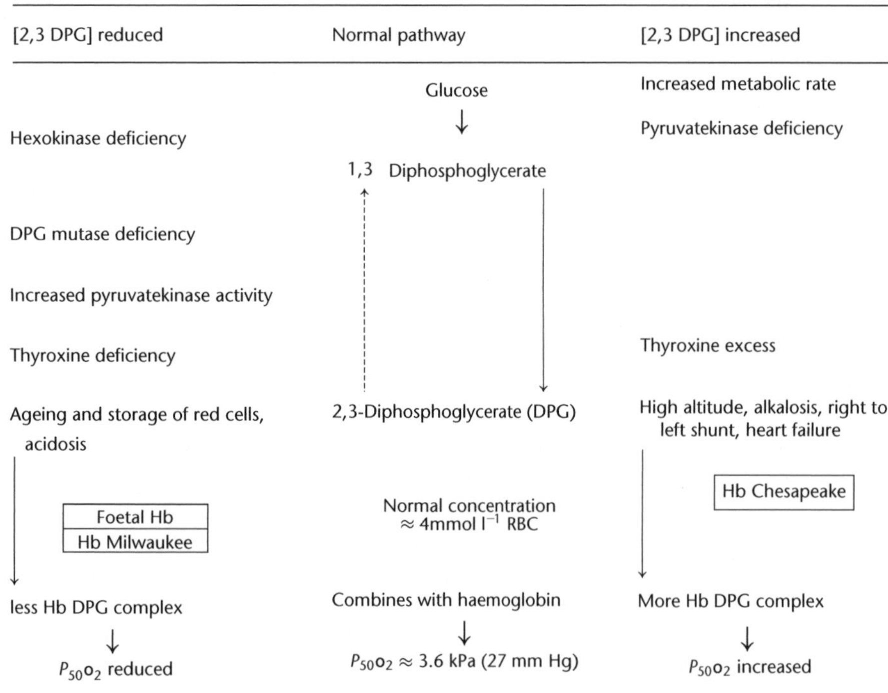

[2,3 DPG] reduced	Normal pathway	[2,3 DPG] increased
	Glucose	Increased metabolic rate
Hexokinase deficiency	↓	Pyruvatekinase deficiency
	1,3 Diphosphoglycerate	
DPG mutase deficiency		
Increased pyruvatekinase activity		
Thyroxine deficiency		Thyroxine excess
Ageing and storage of red cells, acidosis	2,3-Diphosphoglycerate (DPG)	High altitude, alkalosis, right to left shunt, heart failure
Foetal Hb Hb Milwaukee	Normal concentration $\approx$ 4mmol l^{-1} RBC	Hb Chesapeake
less Hb DPG complex	Combines with haemoglobin	More Hb DPG complex
↓	↓	↓
$P_{50}O_2$ reduced	$P_{50}O_2 \approx$ 3.6 kPa (27 mm Hg)	$P_{50}O_2$ increased

Table 21.3 Contribution of 2,3 diphosphoglycerate to shape of haemoglobin dissociation curve as described by $P_{50}O_2$ [23].

of hypoxia) and when cardiac output is reduced by shock or cardiac disease. The tension is relatively high if the cardiac output is increased without a coincident increase in the metabolism, for example with arteriovenous anastomosis or as a consequence of cutaneous vaso-dilatation due to a warm environment. The oxygen tension in blood as it *leaves* the capillary is usually that in the alveolar gas. This is the case for the majority of healthy persons breathing air at sea level when it is evidence for gas exchange being fully effective. However, in a small proportion of subjects during maximal exercise the end-capillary tension is less than in alveolar gas, indicating that in these instances the process of transfer cannot meet the demand for oxygen [26].

Gas transfer is also insufficient when the inspired oxygen tension is subnormal. In this circumstance the movement of oxygen molecules continues up to when the blood leaves the gas exchanging region and the end-capillary oxygen tension is invariably less than that in the alveoli. The end-capillary gradient is influenced by the shape of the dissociation curve and is discussed below. A gradient is more likely during exercise than at rest because the greater cardiac output leads to a more rapid flow of blood through the lungs; hence the time available for the exchange of gas (residence time) is reduced. In addition, there is a reduced O_2 tension in plasma entering the pulmonary capillaries during exercise and this increases the quantity of oxygen that must be transferred if the blood is to become fully oxygenated.

Role of blood flow. The flow of blood through the lungs contributes to the transfer factor for oxygen by replacing recently formed oxyhaemoglobin with partially reduced haemoglobin present in the mixed venous blood. This process lowers the tension of oxygen in the alveolar capillary plasma by the twin mechanisms of dilution and allowing less time for the dissociation of oxyhaemoglobin (i.e. it limits the back reaction). The effect is represented by the term $\beta\dot{Q}$ in eqn. 19.9 (page 230). It provides a mechanism whereby the process of transfer can adapt to an increase in metabolic demand such as occurs during exercise.

The flow of blood also makes a mechanical contribution to gas exchange (Section 19.3.3). The pulsations generated by cardiac systole promote mixing of fluid within the alveolar cells, the alveolar capillary plasma and the red cells. The flow itself influences the diameter and number of perfused capillaries that participate in gas exchange. The flow also influences the distances between the red cells [27]. During exercise these beneficial consequences of an increase in blood flow partially offset the deleterious effect on gas exchange of a concurrent reduction in residence time (see below, also Footnote 21.1).

Residence time. The residence time is also called transit time, but the latter term implies a continuous flow whereas in practice the flow exhibits pulsations. These have the effect that some or all of the blood in the gas exchanging vessels is replaced with each contraction of the heart. This blood is nearly stationary when gas exchange is taking place. Replacement is nearly complete when the capillary blood volume approximates to stroke volume as appears often to be the case.

The residence time defines the period available for gas exchange (Section 19.3.2). This is seldom a limiting factor in healthy subjects at sea level but becomes so if the alveolar oxygen tension is subnormal, if the surface for gas exchange is restricted or thickened as a result of disease, or if the residence time is reduced to a material extent (e.g. Footnote 19.4, page 231).

21.3.2 Gas transfer during normoxia, a worked example

The normal time course for exchange of oxygen along an alveolar capillary is illustrated in Fig. 21.2. Here the tension of oxygen in alveolar gas is 13.3 kPa (100 mm Hg) and the saturation of oxygen in mixed venous blood 70%. The corresponding oxygen tension at pH 7.4 is 4.9 kPa (37 mm Hg) (Fig. 21.1). The gradient for oxygen at the beginning of the alveolar capillary is then 8.4 kPa (i.e. 13.3 – 4.9) or 63 mm Hg. Since the subject has a normal transfer factor the considerable gradient leads to a large flow of oxygen by diffusion from the alveolar gas into the plasma entering the alveolar capillaries. As a result the tension of oxygen in the plasma and the saturation of haemoglobin with oxygen rise rapidly. Concurrently the tension of oxygen in the alveolar gas diminishes somewhat. These changes reduce the transfer

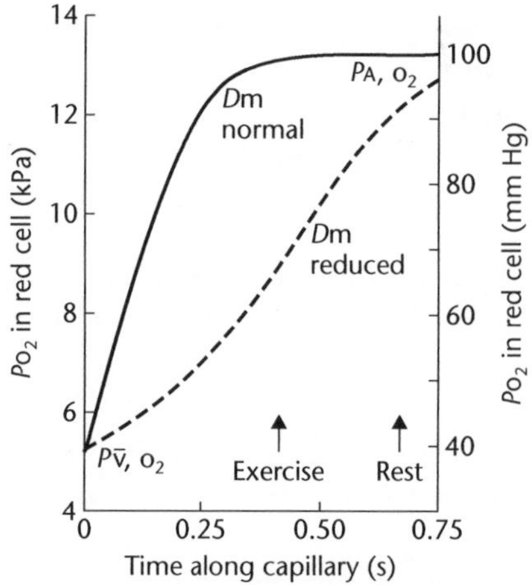

Fig. 21.2 Time course for the exchange of oxygen across the alveolar capillary membrane during breathing air. The curves were computed using the digital subroutines of Kelman [15]. The values assumed for Dm,o_2 were 13.3 and 3.3 mmol min^{-1}kPa^{-1} (40 and 10 ml min^{-1}mm Hg^{-1}). The time when the blood was assumed to leave the capillary is indicated by the arrows. When both Dm is reduced and the transit time is shortened by exercise the blood is incompletely oxygenated. The corresponding curves for CO_2 are shown in Fig. 22.2, page 278. Source: [28]

Footnote 21.1. In the case of carbon monoxide, gas transfer is facilitated by the physical processes outlined above. There is almost no contribution from blood flow (represented by the term $\beta\dot{Q}$) because dissociation of the compound with haemoglobin occurs slowly (Section 19.4.2).

gradient and hence the rate of flow of oxygen. But exchange of gas is now taking place on the flat part of the dissociation curve where the addition of a small volume of oxygen is sufficient to cause a large rise in the tension of oxygen in the blood. The volume of gas that must be transferred to attain equilibrium is now within the capacity for diffusion of the membrane and the rate of reaction with haemoglobin. On this account, in healthy subjects breathing air at sea level, the transfer gradient at the point where the blood leaves the alveolar capillaries is usually of negligible proportions [26]. The intermediate points can be calculated by the procedure of Bohr [29, 30].

21.3.3 Gas transfer during hypoxia, a worked example

In this example the alveolar oxygen tension is reduced to 6.9 kPa (52 mm Hg) as might occur when breathing a hypoxic gas mixture ($F\text{I}O_2 = 0.135$) or following ascent to an altitude of 3500 m (illustrated in Fig. 34.4, page 477). In this circumstance the saturation of oxygen in the mixed venous blood is about 60%, for which the corresponding tension at a pH of 7.4 is 4.1 kPa (31 mm Hg). The transfer gradient for oxygen at the beginning of the alveolar capillary is now 2.8 kPa (21 mm Hg) or approximately one-third of that obtained during breathing air at sea level. Consequently, the rate at which oxygen passes by diffusion from the alveolar gas into the blood entering the alveolar capillaries is much less and the rate of reaction with haemoglobin is also slower. In addition, at the end of the capillary the exchange of oxygen is still taking place on the steep linear part of the dissociation curve. The rate of transfer of oxygen that is necessary for the attainment of gaseous equilibrium then exceeds both the rate at which the oxygen can react with haemoglobin and the capacity for diffusion of the membrane. On this account, during hypoxia the tension of oxygen in the blood leaving the alveolar capillaries is lower than that in alveolar gas; the difference is small at rest but increases if the residence time is reduced by exercise when it may exceed 1.3 kPa (10 mm Hg). A similarly increased end-capillary gradient can occur when the gas-exchanging function of the lung is impaired by emphysema, diffuse interstitial fibrosis or other abnormality of the lung parenchyma (Fig. 21.2).

21.4 Measurement of transfer factor for oxygen ($T\text{l},O_2$)

21.4.1 Overview of methods

Measurement of $T\text{l},O_2$ is not as straightforward as for carbon monoxide because of the back tension generated by the dissociation of oxyhaemoglobin in alveolar capillaries. The back tension is allowed for in the classical steady state method of Riley and Lilienthal [31–33], described below. The method is of fundamental importance, but does not allow for uneven lung function and is not suitable for routine use. A simple alternative has been suggested [34]. The uncertainty associated with the back tension can be reduced by using an isotope of oxygen for which the initial back tension, but not that from subsequent dissociation of the compound with haemoglobin, is effectively zero. Both breath holding and rebreathing procedures have been used [35, 36, 11]; the latter minimises the effects of uneven lung function on the measurement.

As well as by direct measurement, $T\text{l},O_2$ can be obtained indirectly, for example by calculation following measurement of $T\text{l},\text{CO}$ [36]. A more accurate estimate can be obtained by comparison of the observed arterial oxygen saturation with that predicted from the distribution of ventilation–perfusion ratios obtained by the multiple inert gas elimination technique (MIGET) [37]. The method provides a standard against which results by other methods can be compared. The maximal values by this method come close to those predicted from morphometric measurements [38]. However, MIGET is a research procedure. For the present, the measurement of $T\text{l},O_2$ is mainly of theoretical interest.

21.4.2 Derivation of $T\text{l},O_2$ from $T\text{l},\text{CO}$

The term $D\text{m}$ for oxygen exceeds that for carbon monoxide because the gases differ in their solubility and diffusivity in lung tissue (Table 19.2, page 228). The difference can be allowed for by substitution into eqn. 19.13 of the appropriate conversion factor. Then:

$$\frac{1}{T\text{l},O_2} = \frac{1}{1.23D\text{m,CO}} + \frac{1}{\theta O_2 V\text{C}} \qquad (21.2)$$

where 1.23 is the rate of diffusion of oxygen relative to that for carbon monoxide. The reaction rate for oxygen with reduced haemoglobin (θO_2, see Section 21.2.1) cannot be specified with similar certainty as published values differ and vary with circumstances. A value of 0.9 mmol $\text{min}^{-1}\text{ml}^{-1}$ (2.73 vol/vol min^{-1} mm Hg^{-1}) can be used [8, 36]. Alternatively an overall conversion factor of 1.2 can be applied to the measured value for $T\text{l},\text{CO}$. This approach has been validated for persons with normal lungs [36]; it is unlikely to be as accurate if the lung function is uneven [36]. In addition, the value calculated for $T\text{l},O_2$ relates to the conditions prevailing during the measurement of $T\text{l},\text{CO}$. Hence, the conditions should be appropriate. For example, if oxygen exchange in the steady state is of interest the $T\text{l},\text{CO}$ should be measured by a steady state method.

21.4.3 $\dot{V}\text{A}/\dot{Q}$ method for $T\text{l},O_2$ (Summary)

The $\dot{V}\text{A}/\dot{Q}$ method for $T\text{l},O_2$ weights the diffusing characteristics of the different compartments according to their blood flow, assuming that the ratio $D/\dot{Q}\beta$ is constant for all compartments, where D is diffusing capacity, $\dot{Q}$ is blood flow and β is the whole blood capacitance coefficient for oxygen (Section 19.2.2). In hypoxia β is assumed to be constant. β for oxygen is given by $(C\text{a},O_2 - C\bar{\text{v}},O_2)/(P\text{a},O_2 - P\bar{\text{v}},O_2)$ which is the slope of the oxygen dissociation curve (Fig. 21.1). The quantity is different from that for plasma, which is given in Table 19.2 (page 228).

For any compartment (j) the end-capillary oxygen tension gradient can be calculated making the assumption that the process of equilibration is exponential, then:

$$(P\text{A}j - Pc'j) = (P\text{A}j - P\bar{v})\, e^{-(D/\dot{Q}\beta)} \qquad (21.3)$$

where the terms within the brackets are, on the left the end-capillary oxygen tension gradient and on the right the transfer gradient [39].

21.4.4 Method of Riley and Lilienthal [31–33].

By this method the lungs are regarded as an idealised single phase mixing chamber. The transfer factor (diffusing capacity of the lung for oxygen) is obtained using a version of eqn. 20.2 (page 235):

$$Tl,O_2 = O_2 \text{ uptake per min}/(P\text{A},O_2 - P\bar{c},O_2) \qquad (21.4)$$

where Tl,O_2 is the transfer factor for the lungs for oxygen in appropriate units, $P\text{A},O_2$ is the tension of oxygen in the alveolar gas, as defined by the alveolar air equation (Section 18.4.3) and $P\bar{c},O_2$ is the mean capillary oxygen tension. It is the tension associated with the mean concentration of oxyhaemoglobin in alveolar capillaries and relates to conditions of gaseous equilibrium.

Procedure. The data required for the calculations are obtained during two periods of steady state exercise performed with the subject breathing, respectively, air and a hypoxic gas mixture ($F\text{I},O_2$ is usually 0.12). Mixed expired gas is collected during the 4th to 6th min, the minute volume and the concentrations of O_2 and CO_2 are obtained by analysis and these quantities are used to calculate the consumption of oxygen and respiratory exchange ratio (Section 7.8.2). Arterial blood is sampled and analysed for Pa,O_2 and Pa,CO_2. Respiratory exchange ratio and Pa,CO_2 are inserted into the alveolar air equation for calculation of mean alveolar oxygen tension. Alternatively, at the cost of some loss of accuracy the Pa,O_2 can be obtained by analysis of end tidal gas using a respiratory mass spectrometer or other rapid analyser for oxygen. When this is done the arterial oxygen tension is obtained via the oxygen dissociation curve from the arterial oxygen saturation measured by pulse oximetry (Section 7.8.1).

Calculations. The consumption of oxygen and the tension of oxygen in alveolar gas are obtained in the manner described above. The mean tension of oxygen in the alveolar capillaries cannot be determined directly. Instead it is obtained by integration in the manner first described by Bohr [29, 30]. For this purpose, values are calculated for the tension of oxygen down the length of the capillary from estimates of tension at the two ends; a mean value is then obtained by integration. The measurement is made over a range of oxygen tensions that lie on the linear part of the oxygen dissociation curve; this is usually achieved using a hypoxic gas mixture ($F\text{I}O_2 = 0.12$). Alternatively, to avoid a need for integration, the following equation can be used:

$$Tl,O_2 = \frac{\dot{n}O_2 \text{ or } \dot{V}O_2}{(Pc',O_2 - P\bar{v},O_2)} \log_e \frac{(P\text{A},O_2 - P\bar{v},O_2)}{(P\text{A},O_2 - Pc',O_2)} \qquad (21.5)$$

where $P\bar{v},O_2$, Pc',O_2 and $P\text{A},O_2$ are, respectively, the tensions of oxygen in the blood entering and leaving the alveolar capillaries and in the alveolar gas [40]. The tension of oxygen in the blood entering the alveolar capillaries is that of the mixed venous blood; the tension at the end of the capillary is obtained by a process of trial and error that was developed by Lilienthal and Riley. The method entails measurement of the difference in the tension of oxygen between the alveolar gas and the arterial blood during normoxia and during hypoxia. The difference is partitioned into two compartments as follows:

$$(P\text{A},O_2 - Pa,O_2) = (P\text{A},O_2 - Pc',O_2) + (Pc',O_2 - Pa,O_2) \qquad (21.6)$$

where Pc',O_2 and Pa,O_2 are, respectively, the tensions of oxygen in the blood leaving the alveolar capillaries and the left ventricle. The left-hand term is then the A-a difference, the middle term is the diffusion gradient between the alveolar gas and the blood leaving the alveolar capillaries and the right-hand term is the component due to the venous admixture effect.

The partitioning is done first for data obtained when the subject is breathing air, by assuming a value (usually 0.1 kPa or 1 mm Hg) for the diffusion gradient; this permits calculation of Pc',O_2 by subtraction and hence of the venous admixture effect by use of eqn. 18.20, page 217. The same venous admixture is then applied to calculate the end-capillary oxygen tension (Pc',O_2) during hypoxaemia. The end-capillary tension so obtained is fed into the integration procedure for calculating the mean tension of oxygen in the pulmonary capillary blood; this, in turn, is substituted in eqn. 21.4 in order to calculate the diffusing capacity of the lungs for oxygen. The value assumed for the diffusion gradient at the point where the blood leaves the alveolar capillaries when the subject is breathing air is next examined to find out if it is consistent with the diffusing capacity that is calculated from it. If this is not the case an alternative value is assumed and the process is repeated, until by trial and error, values are obtained which are mutually consistent.

Comment. The reproducibility of the method is surprisingly good considering the complexity of the procedure. This is a consequence of the shape of the dissociation curve by which, when breathing air, the greater part of the tension difference for oxygen between the alveolar gas and the arterial blood can be attributed to uneven distribution of lung ventilation and perfusion. The part attributable to the transfer gradient is relatively small. The reverse is the case when breathing gas deficient in oxygen. Most of the A-a difference is now due to the transfer gradient rather than to venous admixture.

The accuracy of the method depends on the extent to which the lung can be treated as a single mixing chamber and on other assumptions that are to some extent incorrect. They are:

1 The alveolar air equation provides a reasonable estimate of the alveolar oxygen tension (not true where there is $\dot{V}_A/\dot{Q}$ inequality).

2 The venous admixture effect does not differ to a material extent between breathing air and breathing gas deficient in oxygen (not true where there is labile hypoxic pulmonary vasoconstriction, Section 17.2.2).

3 Blood flows along alveolar capillaries at a uniform rate; this is assumed for the Bohr integration.

4 The haematocrit of alveolar capillary blood is the same as that in the blood sample taken for analysis [41].

5 The reaction rate θO_2 is relatively constant along the length of the alveolar capillaries. This is likely to be correct when the arterial oxygen saturation is lower than 90%. It may not hold for breathing air.

When Tl,O_2 is measured during exercise the results are only slightly less than those by other methods. This is due to the errors largely cancelling out. However, at rest the values obtained using the single compartment model are materially lower. This is due to uneven lung function.

21.4.5 Effects on Tl,O_2 of uneven lung function

In many disorders the mechanisms that regulate the distributions of pulmonary ventilation and blood flow are impaired (Section 18.1.1). This affects the distribution of ventilation with respect to perfusion ($\dot{V}_A/\dot{Q}$ ratios) and results in hypoxaemia. The mechanism is illustrated by a worked example below. There are similar variations in the transfer characteristics with respect to ventilation (Tl/V_A ratios) and to perfusion within those parts of the lungs where gas exchange takes place ($Tl/\dot{Q}c$ ratios). The effects of these types of uneven lung function have been studied using models [42].

The error in the measurement of Tl,O_2 introduced by uneven lung function is reduced by exercise because alveolar ventilation and pulmonary blood flow are both increased. An increase in alveolar ventilation increases the transfer gradient for oxygen and hence the accuracy with which the mean alveolar oxygen tension can be estimated. An increase in blood flow improves its distribution; this reduces the dispersion of $Tl/\dot{Q}c$ ratios and stabilises the contribution of the term $\beta\dot{Q}$ in the gas exchange equation (eqn. 19.8, page 230). Hence, Tl,O_2 should be measured during exercise where this is practicable.

Abnormal conditions of the lung parenchyma including emphysema, interstitial fibrosis, alveolitis and interstitial oedema reduce the transfer factor for oxygen. These conditions also give rise to uneven lung function; hence, in circumstances when the level of Tl,O_2 might be informative the accuracy of the measurement is most compromised. The error is much less for carbon monoxide (Section 19.4.2).

21.5 Respiratory determinants of arterial oxygen tension and saturation: some worked examples

The tensions of oxygen and carbon dioxide and the saturation of haemoglobin in arterial blood are determined by the composition of inspired gas, barometric pressure, lung function and the composition of blood in pulmonary arteries, including the effects of any shunts. In this section the respired gas is air at sea level.

21.5.1 Alveolar ventilation

For this overview, the alveolar ventilation is defined for the lungs as a whole as that part of the minute volume that participates in gas exchange. Its mean composition lies somewhere between that of inspired gas and gas in equilibrium with mixed venous blood. Within these limits the composition of alveolar gas is determined by the rates at which oxygen and carbon dioxide in the alveoli exchange with the environment (i.e. alveolar ventilation) and, across the alveolar capillary membrane, with plasma in the alveolar capillaries (i.e. diffusion and combination with haemoglobin). When alveolar ventilation is high relative to perfusion, the gas tensions in the alveoli move towards those in inspired air; when it is low, the tensions approach those of mixed venous blood.

The relationships between alveolar ventilation and gas tensions and the consequences for arterial oxygen saturation can be explored using models. In the present instance these relate to a healthy subject at rest breathing air at sea level. The overall respiratory exchange ratio is 0.8.

In the simplest case the respiratory exchange ratio is independent of the level of alveolar ventilation and the lungs behave as an ideal mixing chamber in which the tension of oxygen in mixed end-capillary blood is equal to that in alveolar gas. Under these conditions the tensions of oxygen and carbon dioxide are sensitive to small changes in alveolar ventilation (Fig. 21.3). By contrast, because the upper part of the dissociation curve is relatively flat, the *saturation* of haemoglobin with oxygen is nearly independent of the level of alveolar ventilation until this is greatly reduced. On account of these differences, a progressive reduction in alveolar ventilation causes hypercapnia before it gives rise to hypoxaemia.

The consequences for gas exchange of the model lung comprising not one but two gas-exchanging units that are differently ventilated and perfused are described next.

21.5.2 Two-compartment model of normal gas exchange

Tensions of oxygen and carbon dioxide: contribution of uneven distribution ($\dot{V}_A/\dot{Q}$). In each gas-exchanging unit of healthy lungs the exchanges across the alveolar capillary membrane proceeds nearly to equilibrium. As a result the tension of oxygen in any

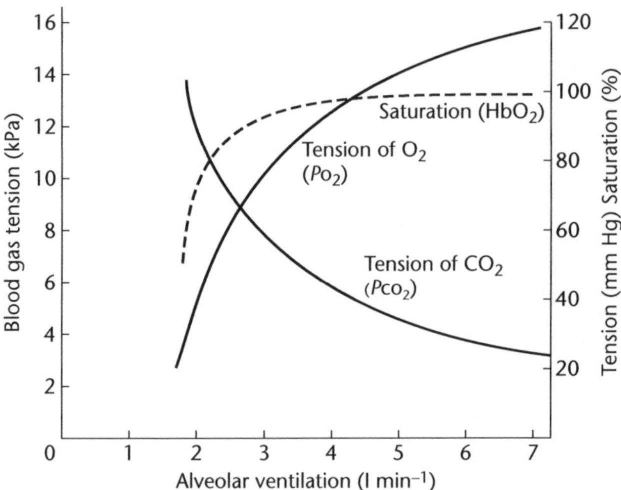

Fig. 21.3 Relationship of the composition of blood leaving the alveolar capillaries to the level of alveolar ventilation (for derivation see Footnote 21.2). The tensions of oxygen and carbon dioxide are sensitive to small changes in alveolar ventilation. By contrast, on account of the shape of the dissociation curve, the oxygen saturation is relatively independent of the level of ventilation until this is greatly reduced.

alveolus is effectively the same as that in blood leaving the corresponding alveolar capillary. Heterogeneity is introduced because ventilation and perfusion are not uniformly matched throughout the lungs. This leads to differences in gas tension between acini. The differences occur both within and between regions, with the largest difference between the apex and base of the lungs (Fig. 21.4).

Overall gas exchange is the resultant of gas from all the alveoli merging to form mixed alveolar gas and blood from all the capillaries merging to form pulmonary venous blood. However, the amalgamations occur in different proportions in the gas phase compared with the blood phase. The composition of the mixed alveolar gas is unduly influenced by gas from acini whose ventilation is excessive for their perfusion. This circumstance is associated with a relatively high tension of oxygen and low tensions of carbon dioxide and nitrogen. Similarly, the composition of the pulmonary venous blood is unduly influenced by blood from acini whose perfusion exceeds their ventilation. This circumstance is associated with a relatively high tension of carbon dioxide and low tension of oxygen. Thus, as a result of $\dot{V}_A/\dot{Q}$ inequality the tension of O_2 in systemic arterial blood is invariably lower and the tension of CO_2 is higher than in mixed alveolar gas. This *distribution effect* is illustrated by a numerical example in Table 21.4 where the calculations are based on a model comprising two compartments. The related changes in the tension of nitrogen are given below.

Shape of the dissociation curves for O_2 and CO_2. A second factor that increases the alveolar–arterial gas tension difference for oxygen is that the oxygen dissociation curve is asymptotic (i.e. has a flat top). As a result, a normal average alveolar oxygen tension of 15 kPa (110 mm Hg) is sufficient to almost fully saturate blood with oxygen. Well-ventilated alveoli that have an oxygen tension greater than this cannot raise their haemoglobin saturation further, so the additional ventilation is not used effectively. By contrast the saturation of blood from acini having a low $\dot{V}_A/\dot{Q}$ ratio is inevitably reduced. When mixing occurs between blood from poorly ventilated and well-ventilated alveoli the quantity of oxygen in blood from alveoli with a high ventilation–perfusion ratio does not make up for the diminished quantity in the blood from poorly ventilated alveoli. The content and saturation of oxygen in the mixed blood is reduced in consequence. This *dissociation curve effect* is relatively unimportant for carbon dioxide because the CO_2 dissociation curve, unlike for oxygen, is essentially linear over the physiological range (Fig. 21.5).

Alveolar–arterial tension difference for nitrogen. The alveolar partial pressures of oxygen and carbon dioxide are determined in part by the intrapulmonary processes that have been described. These give rise to compensatory changes in the tension of nitrogen; the changes are local to each part of the lungs and reflect that, in the absence of respiratory movements, the pressure throughout the lungs is atmospheric. Where the $\dot{V}_A/\dot{Q}$ ratio is above the average, as at the apices of the lungs, the alveolar oxygen tension is relatively high; the alveolar nitrogen tension is low in consequence and nitrogen moves from the mixed venous blood into the gas phase. Contrary changes occur in regions of low $\dot{V}_A/\dot{Q}$. When summed for the lungs as a whole, the nitrogen tension of pulmonary blood (and hence systemic arterial blood) exceeds that in mixed alveolar gas (Fig. 21.4). The a-A D_{N_2} varies inversely with the extent of $\dot{V}_A/\dot{Q}$ inequality from approximately 0.4 kPa (3 mm Hg) in healthy subjects to 3 kPa (20 mm Hg) in patients with uneven lung function. The difference reflects mainly the contribution of blood from poorly ventilated alveoli (low $\dot{V}_A/\dot{Q}$). The information provided by the measurement

---

Footnote 21.2. Derivation of Fig. 21.3. For the lungs as a whole the product of alveolar ventilation and alveolar concentration of carbon dioxide is the rate at which carbon dioxide leaves the body in the expired gas. When the subject is in a steady state this is the same as the rate of evolution of carbon dioxide into the alveoli. Then for CO_2:

$$F_{A,CO_2} = P_{A,CO_2}/(P_B - P_{H_2O}) = f\,[\dot{n}_{CO_2} \text{ (or } \dot{V}_{CO_2})/\dot{V}_A] \quad (21.7)$$

$$P_{A,CO_2} = f(\dot{n}_{CO_2} \text{ or } \dot{V}_{CO_2})/\dot{V}_A = f\,[(\dot{n}_{O_2} \text{ or } \dot{V}_{O_2})R/\dot{V}_A] \quad (21.8)$$

where F_{A,CO_2} is the concentration of carbon dioxide in the alveolar gas and P_{A,CO_2} is the corresponding CO_2 tension (kPa or mm Hg); $\dot{n}$ and $\dot{V}$ are the rates of exchange of the relevant gases in mmol min^{-1} and ml STPD min^{-1}, and R is the respiratory exchange ratio. $\dot{V}_A$ is the alveolar ventilation (l BTPS min^{-1}). The factors f are required to bring the disparate units into forms that are mutually compatible (Sections 6.4 and 6.6). The corresponding relationships for oxygen were obtained by substitution in the alveolar air equation (Section 18.4.3) then obtaining the equivalent saturations by reference to the haemoglobin dissociation curve for oxygen (Fig. 21.1).

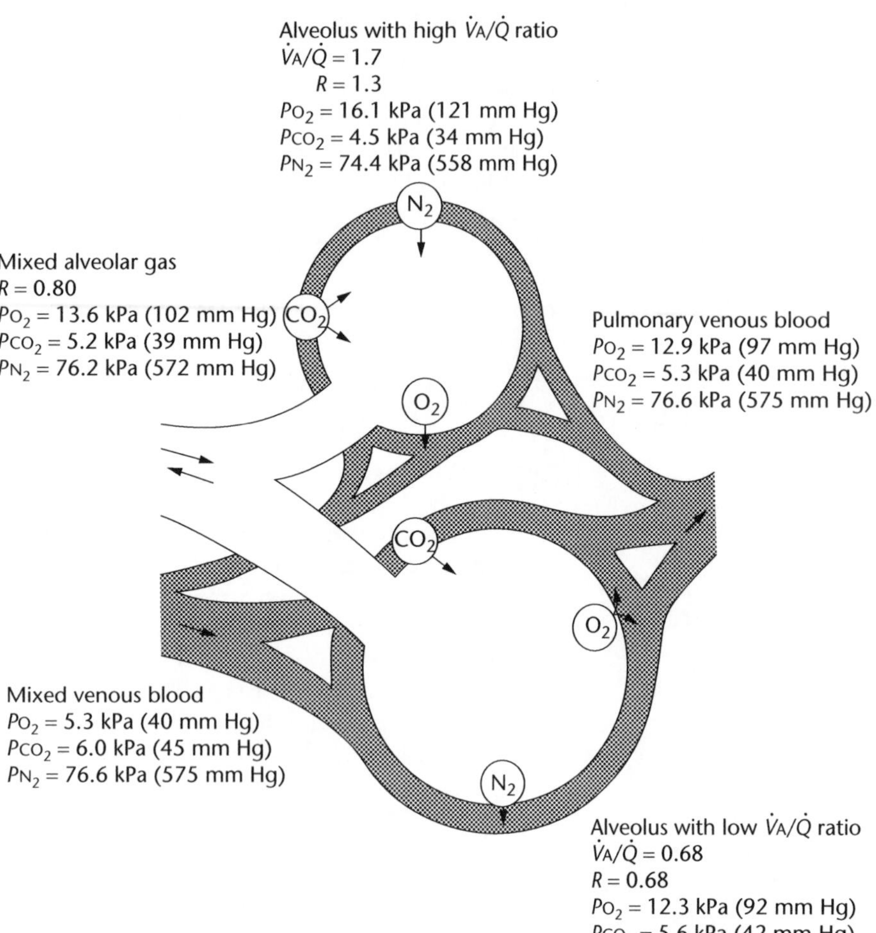

Fig. 21.4 Two-compartment model to illustrate the consequences for gas exchange of uneven lung function. In this instance the inequality is due to the vertical gradient of lung function, for which the mechanical basis is given in Chapter 16 (Fig. 16.2, page 184). The upper alveolus has a relatively high $\dot{V}_A/\dot{Q}$ ratio. Due to the dissociation curve effect it has a higher respiratory exchange ratio and lower nitrogen tension compared with the lower alveolus. Due to the distribution effect this inequality leads to differences in tension for oxygen, carbon dioxide and nitrogen between mixed alveolar gas and pulmonary venous, hence mixed arterial blood. Source: [43]

Table 21.4 Consequences for gas exchange of $\dot{V}_A/\dot{Q}$ inequality: a numerical example based on a hypothetical two-compartment model.

		Compartment			
		C1	C2	Combined	A-a difference
Gas phase					
Ventilation ($\dot{V}_A$)	l min^{-1}	4	1	5	
O_2 tension (P_{A,O_2})	kPa (mm Hg)	16.7 (125)	9.3 (70)	15.2 (114)	
CO_2 tension (P_{A,CO_2})	kPa (mm Hg)	4.5 (34)	6.7 (50)	4.9 (37)	
N_2 tension (P_{A,N_2})	kPa (mm Hg)	74 (554)	79 (593)	75 (562)	
Blood phase					
Blood flow ($\dot{Q}$)	l min^{-1}	2.5	2.5	5	
O_2 tension (P_{a,O_2})	kPa (mm Hg)	16.7 (125)	9.3 (70)	13.0 (97.5)*	
Saturation (S_{a,O_2})	%	98.5	92	95	
P_{a,O_2} (from dissociation curve)	kPa (mm Hg)			11.3 (85)	3.9 (29)
CO_2 tension (P_{a,CO_2})	kPa (mm Hg)	4.5 (34)	6.7 (50)	5.6 (42)*	0.7 (5)
N_2 tension (P_{a,N_2})	kPa (mm Hg)	74 (554)	79 (593)	76.5 (573)	1.5 (11)
$\dot{V}_A/\dot{Q}$	–	1.6	0.4	1.0	

Note: Alveolar ventilation and pulmonary blood flow are both 5 l/min but are distributed differently. The ventilation of the compartments is in the ratio 4 : 1 but the blood flow is uniform. On the assumption that there is gaseous equilibrium across the alveolar capillary membrane, the a-A difference for O_2 due to the distribution effect is 15.2 – 13.0 = 2.2 kPa (16.5 mm Hg). The additional difference due to the dissociation curve effect is 13.0 – 11.3 = 1.7 kPa (12.5 mm Hg). The a-A difference for CO_2 (5.6 – 4.9 = 0.7 kPa or 5 mm Hg) is due solely to the distribution effect. It has been calculated assuming a linear CO_2 dissociation curve. (cf. Fig. 21.5).

* average of values for the two compartments.

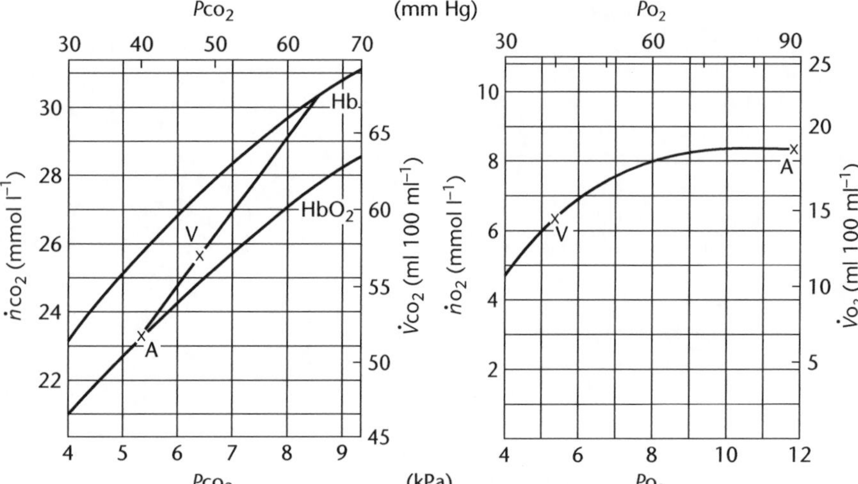

Fig. 21.5 Whole blood dissociation curves for carbon dioxide and oxygen over the physiological range in a healthy subject at rest. The points A and V are, respectively, for arterial and mixed venous blood. Between A and V the relationship for CO_2 is effectively linear but not that for O_2 Sources: [19, 44]

complements that from the a-A difference for carbon dioxide which is mainly due to alveoli having a high $\dot{V}A/\dot{Q}$ ratio (Table 21.5). The nitrogen difference is independent of any intrapulmonary shunt. This is because the gas is neither produced nor metabolised so the tension it exerts is the same throughout the systemic circulation, including in the arterial and mixed venous blood. The a-A D_{N_2} was formerly used as an index of uneven lung function [45].

21.6 Investigation of hypoxaemia, including use of models

21.6.1 Introduction

The cause of hypoxaemia can be environmental, for example that due to hypoxia, or can arise from inadequate gas transfer (as occurs in some people during maximal exercise), from insufficient respiratory drive (as with hypoventilation), or from pathological changes in the lungs, as occur in many diseases of the lungs and cardiovascular system (Table 21.6). Multiple causes are common.

In clinical practice hypoxaemia due to defective gas transfer occurs mainly on exercise (e.g. Fig. 21.2). In addition, the transfer factor for carbon monoxide is reduced. Defective gas transfer is a feature of emphysema and of alveolar congestion, alveolitis and interstitial fibrosis. Hypoxaemia at rest is usually due to impaired distribution ($\dot{V}A/\dot{Q}$ effect) except during anaesthesia when it is often due to a shunt (Sections 42.3.5 and 42.3.6). Uneven lung function causes hypoxaemia in patients with narrowing of peripheral airways, including many of those who have chronic obstructive lung disease (COPD, Section 40.3). Hypoxaemia from this cause varies inversely with the level of cardiac output and is a conspicuous feature of left heart failure where the output is low, but not of asthma associated with a raised output [46].

If the transfer factor is normal, hypoxaemia that is secondary to uneven lung function can be diagnosed by administration of oxygen in low dosage. This corrects hypoxaemia from this cause, but not that due to a shunt. When both abnormalities may be present, their relative contributions can be assessed in terms of the five-compartment model; this subdivides the physiological

Table 21.5 The levels of oxygen and carbon dioxide associated with the five-compartment model of ventilation–perfusion relationships illustrated in Fig. 18.1, page 211.

		Alveolar tension		Blood content	
Site	$\dot{V}A/\dot{Q}$ ratio	Oxygen	Carbon dioxide	Oxygen	Carbon dioxide
Anatomical shunt and non-ventilated alveoli	0	–	–	As mixed venous blood	
Anatomic deadspace and non-perfused alveoli	∞	As inspired gas*		–	–
Underventilated or overperfused alveoli	0–0.9	Low	High	Low*	High*
Ideal alveoli	0.9	Normal	Normal	Normal	Normal
Overventilated or under-perfused alveoli	0.9–∞	High*	Low*	*Not raised*	Low
Principal consequences		$\dot{V}A$ increased		SaO_2 reduced	

Note: The dominant effects on mixed alveolar gas and pulmonary venous blood are indicated by *. They are due solely to the distribution effect except in the case of oxygen in blood where the contribution of the dissociation curve is indicated by italics.

Table 21.6 Some cardio-respiratory causes of hypoxaemia.

Airway obstruction (acute or chronic)
Uneven lung function ($\dot{V}A/\dot{Q}$)
Diseases of lung parenchyma (transfer defect)
Pulmonary congestion of cardiac origin
Respiratory distress syndrome (neonatal and subsequently)
Shunt from any cause (intrapulmonary, cardiovascular or portal-pulmonary)
Pulmonary embolism
Circumstances associated with anaesthesia and thoracic surgery

shunt into an anatomical shunt and alveolar blood shunt compartment (Table 21.5). The methods are described in Chapter 18.

The multiple inert gas elimination technique (Section 18.2) provides more detailed information, but is seldom a realistic option. In some circumstances a perfusion scan will be appropriate (Section 18.6). Alternatively, the approach can be semi-quantitative in terms of an O_2–CO_2 diagram or chart that relates oxygen saturation measured by pulse oximetry to inspired oxygen tension. The latter is technically undemanding yet can provide semi-quantitative information on the relative contributions to hypoxaemia of the shunt and $\dot{V}A/\dot{Q}$ compartments.

21.6.2 Graphical analysis of gas exchange. Oxygen–carbon dioxide diagram

The oxygen–carbon dioxide diagram (Fig. 21.6) describes gas exchange under steady state conditions in ideal lungs, in which ventilation and perfusion are distributed uniformly and the arterial and alveolar tensions of carbon dioxide are equal. The alveolar oxygen tension is that which is consistent with the levels of the other variables; it is calculated using the alveolar air equation (Section 18.4.3).

The diagram is complicated because the relationships of blood gas concentration to partial pressure for oxygen and carbon dioxide are both curvilinear and inter-dependent (Sections 21.2.1 and 22.2.2). Nevertheless the diagram provides mutually compatible values for the ventilation–perfusion and respiratory exchange

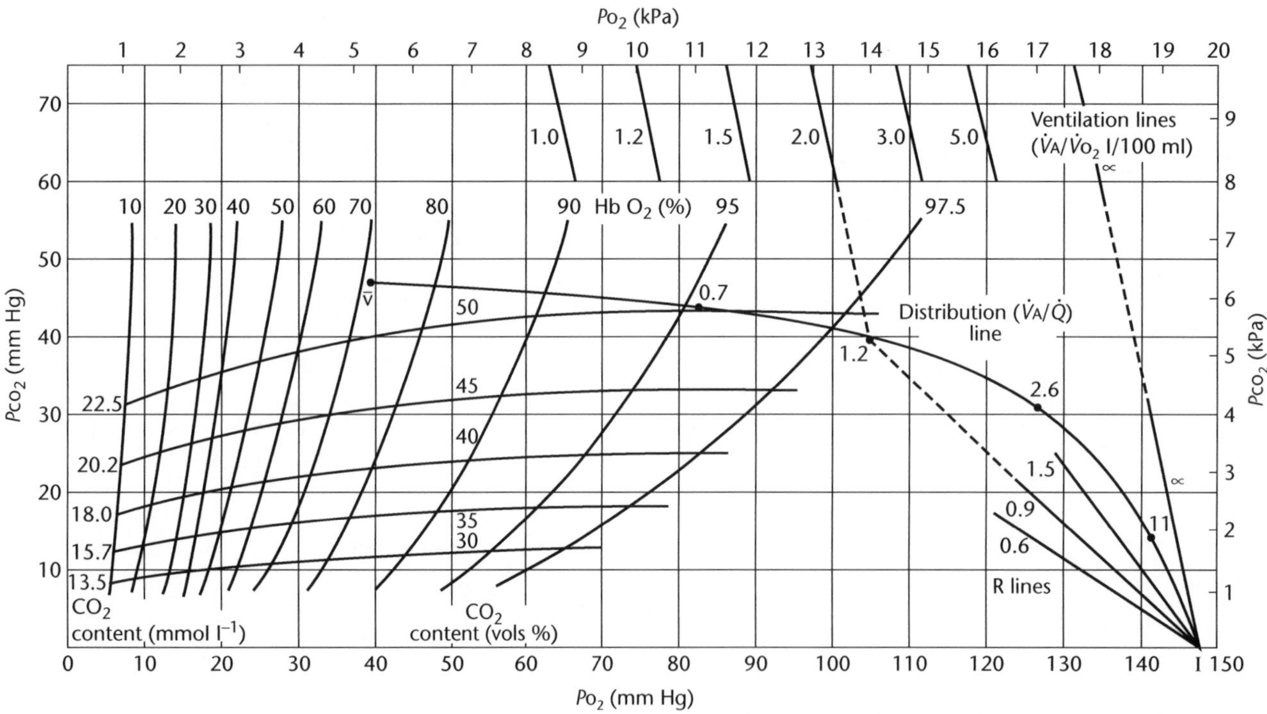

Fig. 21.6 O_2–CO_2 diagram of Rahn and Fenn. The grid of curved lines illustrates the normal relationships of the tensions of oxygen and carbon dioxide to the haemoglobin saturation and the content of carbon dioxide in blood. The lines for respiratory exchange ratio (*R* lines) radiate from a point (I) which describes the inspired gas (in this case air). Alveolar ventilation (units l/min per 100 ml/min of oxygen uptake) is represented by parallel lines of which that for infinite ventilation has an *R* value of infinity. The curved distribution line illustrates the combinations of oxygen and carbon dioxide tension associated with different ventilation-perfusion ratios: its limits are inspired gas ($\dot{V}A/\dot{Q} = \infty$) and mixed venous blood ($\dot{V}A/\dot{Q} = 0$). The dashed lines converge on a point on the distribution line where the $\dot{V}A/\dot{Q}$ ratio is 1.2. For an alveolus having this ratio of ventilation to perfusion the alveolar ventilation would be expected to be 2.0 l/100 ml, the respiratory exchange ratio 0.9 and the tensions of oxygen and carbon dioxide respectively 13.9 and 5.2 kPa (104 and 39 torr). The corresponding values for oxygen saturation and carbon dioxide content of blood can also be read off the diagram. Source: [47].

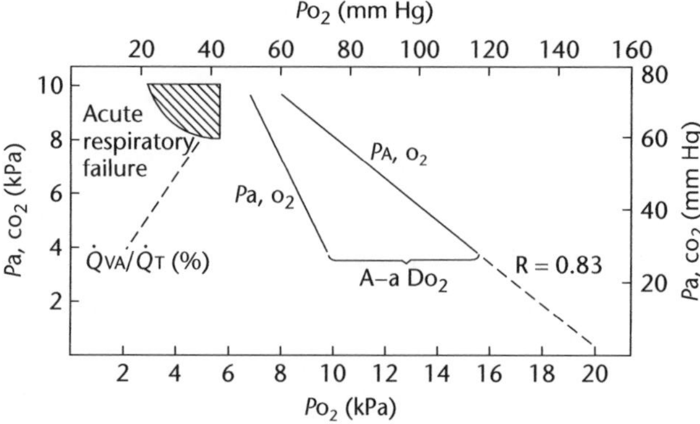

Fig. 21.7 O_2–CO_2 diagram for patients in respiratory failure. The lines describe the inter-relationships between alveolar and arterial blood gas tensions, and venous admixture effect for 487 patients with lung disease. The alveolar oxygen tensions (PA,O_2), calculated using the alveolar air equation (Section 18.4.3), lie on the line for $R = 0.83$ (cf. Fig. 21.6). The diagram shows that patients with a *high* arterial tension of carbon dioxide can have a smaller alveolar-arterial oxygen tension difference (A-aDo$_2$) but a larger venous admixture ($\dot{Q}$VA/$\dot{Q}$T) than patients with a *low* tension of carbon dioxide; the difference reflects the level of alveolar ventilation and hence the alveolar oxygen tension. Thus the two indices of uneven distribution are not interchangeable. The shaded area indicates the arterial blood gas tensions before treatment with oxygen in 81 patients with acute respiratory failure. The lowest recorded A-a, O_2 was 2.5 kPa (19 mm Hg) and the highest Pa,co$_2$ 11.7 kPa (88 mm Hg). Sources: [48, 49].

ratios and the compositions of inspired gas and mixed venous blood; when three of these quantities are known or assumed the fourth can be read off the diagram.

Historically the diagram was a remarkable achievement and it led to the concept that the gas-exchanging characteristics of the lung could be described using inert gases in which the relationships of concentration to partial pressure are linear (Section 18.2.1). For patients with lung disease the diagram indicates the limits for mutually compatible levels of the different variables and also the levels that are compatible with life (Fig. 21.7). Where there is a wide range of ventilation–perfusion ratios the increased A-a difference for oxygen is mainly due to lung units that have a high $\dot{V}$A/$\dot{Q}$ ratio. Such differences reflect uneven lung function but not the extent of hypoxaemia. The latter is determined mainly by the amount and composition of blood that perfuses poorly ventilated alveoli and by the blood shunt compartment (Section 18.4.6).

In practice the O_2–CO_2 diagram is of limited usefulness. This is because the principal outcome, the difference in oxygen tension between ideal alveolar air and arterial blood, is not specific to uneven lung function, but can also be due to impaired gas transfer or shunt. In addition, use of the diagram entails direct measurement of the tensions of oxygen and carbon dioxide in arterial blood. These limitations are overcome in the PIo$_2$ vs Spo$_2$ diagram that is described next.

21.6.3 *P*Io$_2$ vs *S*po$_2$ oxygen diagram

This model relates the arterial oxygen saturation measured by pulse oximetry (Spo$_2$) to the inspired oxygen partial pressure (PI,o$_2$). It describes observations made under steady state conditions during which the saturation is varied by changing the tension of oxygen in inspired gas. The model that is used is one of several alternatives to the classical five-compartment model of gas exchange in the lungs (Section 18.1.3) [50, 51]. In this instance two compartments are used; the first describes the transfer of oxygen from inspired gas to blood leaving the alveolar capillaries. The second is from this stage onwards. The oxygen tension at the demarcation point is that in equilibrium with mixed oxygenated blood leaving the alveolar capillaries (i.e. mixed end-capillary oxygen tension Pc′,o$_2$). This quantity is less than the alveolar oxygen tension calculated from the alveolar air equation by an amount that reflects the imbalance between ventilation and perfusion. It exceeds the systemic arterial oxygen tension on account of the anatomical shunt.

The Pc′,o$_2$ cannot be measured directly. In the model it is inferred from the relationship of arterial oxygen saturation obtained by pulse oximetry to inspired oxygen tension. The relationship is obtained by having the subject breathe some 7–10 gas mixtures chosen to produce saturations in the range 85%–99%. Each gas mixture is breathed for 3–5 min. The method uses assumed values for the arterio-venous oxygen difference and the oxygen capacity of haemoglobin (Section 21.2.1). The haemoglobin concentration is assumed unless the measured value is available. The derivation depends on the property of a raised alveolar oxygen tension to reduce and, at high tensions, to

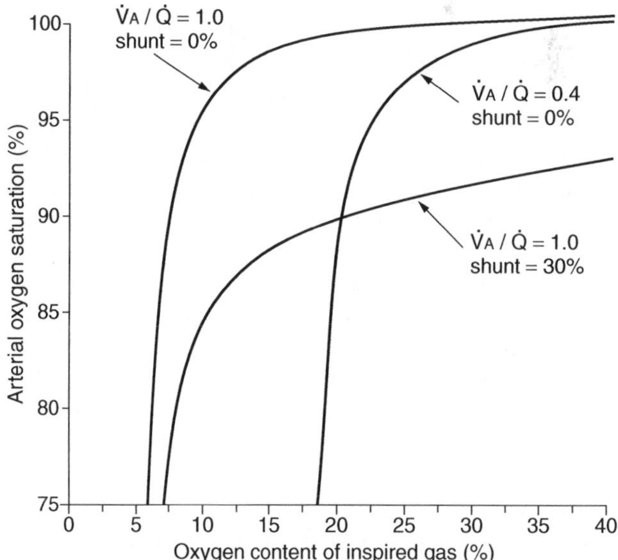

Fig. 21.8 The relationships between Sa o$_2$, $\dot{V}$A/$\dot{Q}$ and Shunt % in a model lung comprising two differently ventilated compartments of which one was normal and the other had either a reduced $\dot{V}$A/$\dot{Q}$ ratio or a large shunt. Source: [53, 54].

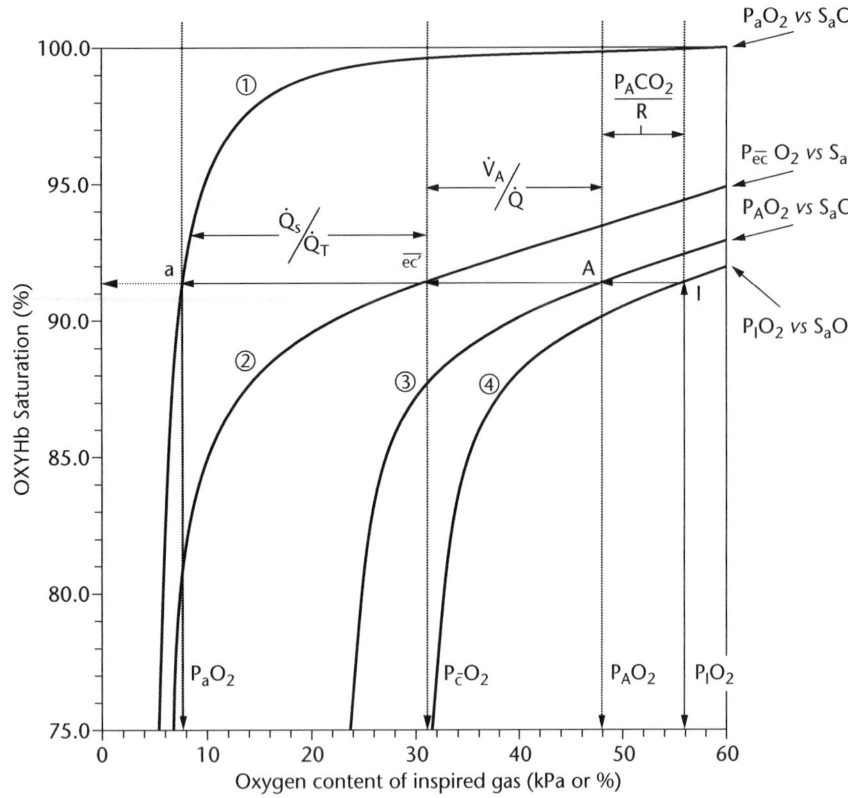

Fig. 21.9 Model to show the effects of a 30% shunt and uneven lung function on oxygen saturation (So_2) at different stages in the movement of oxygen from inspired gas to arterial blood. Curve 1: relationship of So_2 to oxygen tension for arterial blood. This is a standard dissociation curve (cf. Fig. 21.1). Curve 2: relationship of So_2 to mean end-capillary oxygen tension (Pc',o_2). The curve is displaced downwards. Curve 4: corresponding relationship for inspired oxygen tension (i.e. Spo_2 vs $P\text{I}o_2$ diagram). The curve is displaced to the right without change in shape. The displacement is on account of both uneven lung function ($\dot{V}\text{A}/\dot{Q}$, Curve 2 – Curve 3) and dilution of ideal alveolar air by deadspace gas (designated $Pa,co_2/R$, Curve 3 – Curve 4). Source: [51].

eliminate hypoxaemia due to ventilation–perfusion inequality, whilst not affecting that due to the anatomical shunt (Sections 18.4.5 and 18.4.6). Successive approximations are used to obtain values for the mean virtual shunt that is compatible with the other quantities.

In nine normal subjects the mean virtual shunt was reported as 8.1 (SD 1.49)% and the mean drop in oxygen tension over the first compartment (mean $P\text{I}o_2 - Pc',o_2$) was 6.0 (SD 0.47) kPa (45 mm Hg). The analysis was reported as accounting for 88% of the variance in the data [51]. In healthy subjects, the shunt by this method appears to be larger than by the traditional method. If this is a real difference, possible reasons might be the action of oxygen in relaxing smooth muscle in the walls of pulmonary arterioles and the maximal concentration of oxygen in the inspired gas being limited to 60%. In patients with disturbed lung function the mean virtual shunt appears to reflect the real shunt, with values in the range 12%–33% being reported during thoracotomy [52]. An enlarged oxygen tension difference ($P\text{I},o_2 - Pc',o_2$) reflects a reduced relationship of pulmonary ventilation to perfusion together with any effect due to impaired gas transfer.

In graphical terms, a reduction in Spo_2 due to a shunt displaces the graph relating saturation to Pc',o_2 in a downward direction (i.e. a given inspired oxygen tension is associated with a lower saturation). Converting Pc',o_2 to inspired oxygen tension ($P\text{I},o_2$) then shifts the displaced curve to the right (i.e. a given saturation is achieved at a higher oxygen tension, Fig. 21.8). In healthy lungs the shift is a result of alveolar gas being diluted with gas from the physiological deadspace and on account of the R effect (Fig. 21.6). With uneven lung function a further shift occurs due to the low $\dot{V}\text{A}/\dot{Q}$ ratio reducing the mixed end-capillary oxygen tension with respect to that in ideal alveolar air. These two causes of lateral displacement of the curve can be separated if the arterial partial pressure of carbon dioxide (Pa,co_2) is known. The result can be interpreted visually in terms of the downward and lateral displacements of the $P\text{I}o_2$ vs Spo_2 graph (Fig. 21.9).

When the haemoglobin concentration is within normal limits, the Spo_2 vs $P\text{I}o_2$ diagram provides a visual indication of the mechanism of hypoxaemia (e.g. Fig. 42.5, page 601). However, if the haemoglobin concentration is atypical a computational interpretation should be used. The model is suitable for large-scale clinical use [55].

21.7 References

1. Otis AB., In: Fishman AP, ed. *Handbook of Physiology* (Section 3). IV: 1–11. Bethesda, MD: American Physiological Society, 1987.
2. Edsall JT. Hemoglobin and the origins of the concept of allosterism. *Fed Proc* 1980; **39**: 226–235.
3. Adair GS. The hemoglobin system. The oxygen dissociation curve of hemoglobin. *J Biol Chem* 1925; **63**: 529–545.

4. Gill SJ, Di Cera E, Doyle ML et al. Oxygen binding constants for human hemoglobin tetramers. *Biochemistry* 1987; **26**: 3995–4002.
5. Huxley VH, Kutchai H. Effect of diffusion boundary layers on the initial uptake of O_2 by red cells. Theory versus experiment. *Microvasc Res* 1983; **26**: 89–107.
6. Heidelberger E, Reeves RB. Factors affecting whole blood O_2 transfer kinetics: implications for $\theta(O2)$. *J Appl Physiol* 1990; **68**: 1865–1874.
7. Roughton FJW. Kinetics of gas transport in blood. *Br Med Bull* 1963; **19**: 80–89.
8. Staub N, Bishop JM, Forster RE. Importance of diffusion and chemical reaction rates in O_2 uptake in the lung. *J Appl Physiol* 1962; **17**: 21–27.
9. Holland RAB, Shibata H, Scheid P, Piiper J. Kinetics of O_2 uptake and release by red cells in stopped-flow apparatus: effects of unstirred layer. *Respir Physiol* 1985; **59**: 71–91.
10. Yamaguchi K, Glahn J, Scheid P, Piiper J. Oxygen transfer conductance of human red blood cells at varied pH and temperature. *Respir Physiol* 1987; **67**: 209–223.
11. Piiper J. Alveolar-capillary gas transfer in lungs: development of concepts and current status. *Adv Exp Med Biol* 1994; **345**: 7–14.
12. Severinghaus JW. Blood gas calculator. *J Appl Physiol* 1966; **21**: 1108–1116.
13. Bohr C, Hasselbalch KA, Krogh A. Ueber einen in biologischer Beziehung wichtigen ubr die Kohlensaurespannung des Blutes auf desen Sauerstoffbindung ubt. *Scand Arch Physiol* 1904; **16**: 402–412.
14. Hill AV. The possible effects of the aggregation of the molecules of haemoglobin on its dissociation curves. *J Physiol (Lond)* 1910; **40**: P IV–VII.
15. Kelman GR. Digital computer subroutine for the conversion of oxygen tension into saturation. *J Appl Physiol* 1966; **21**: 1375–1376.
16. Olszowka AJ, Wagner PD. Numerical analysis of gas exchange. In: West JB, ed. *Pulmonary gas exchange.* Vol 1. Ventilation, blood flow and diffusion. New York: Academic Press, 1980; 263–306.
17. Winslow RM, Samaja M, Winslow NJ et al. Simulation of continuous blood O_2 equilibrium curve over physiological pH, DBG and PCO_2 range. *J Appl Physiol* 1983; **54**: 524–529.
18. Lapennas GN. The magnitude of the Bohr coefficient: optimal for oxygen delivery. *Respir Physiol* 1983; **54**: 161–172.
19. Christiansen J, Douglas CG, Haldane JS. The absorption and dissociation of carbon dioxide by human blood. *J Physiol (Lond)* 1914; **48**: 244–271.
20. Hlastala MP. Significance of the Bohr and Haldane effects in the pulmonary capillary. *Respir Physiol* 1973; **17**: 81–92.
21. Grant BJB. Influence of Bohr–Haldane effect on steady-state gas exchange. *J Appl Physiol* 1982; **52**: 1330–1337.
22. Bunn HF, Jandl JH. Control of hemoglobin function within the red cell. *N Eng J Med* 1970; **282**: 1414–1421.
23. Kilmartin JV, Rossi-Bernardi L. Interaction of hemoglobin with hydrogen ions, carbon dioxide, and organic phosphates. *Physiol Rev* 1973; **53**: 836–890.
24. Purcell Y, Brozovic B. Red cell 2.3-diphosphoglycerate concentration in man decreases with age. *Nature (Lond)* 1974; **251**: 511–512.
25. Oski FA, Gottlieb AJ, Miller WW, Delivoria-Papadopoulos M. The effects of deoxygenation of adult and fetal hemoglobin on the synthesis of red cell 2,3-diphosphoglycerate and its in vivo consequences. *J Clin Invest* 1970; **49**: 400–407.
26. Dempsey JA, Wagner PD. Exercise-induced arterial hypoxemia. *J Appl Physiol* 1999; **87**: 1997–2006.
27. Federspiel WJ. Pulmonary diffusing capacity: implications for two-phase blood flow in capillaries. *Respir Physiol* 1989; **77**: 119–134.
28. Wagner PD, West JB. Effects of diffusion impairment on O_2 and CO_2 time courses in pulmonary capillaries. *J Appl Physiol* 1972; **33**: 62–71.
29. Bohr C. Uber die spezifische Tatigkeit der Lungen bei der respiratorischen Gasaufnahme. *Scand Arch Physiol* 1909; **22**: 221–280.
30. Briehl RW, Fishman AP. Principles of the Bohr integration procedure and their application to measurement of diffusing capacity of the lung for oxygen. *J Appl Physiol* 1960; **15**: 337–348.
31. Lilienthal J Jr, Riley RL, Proemmel DD, Franke RE. An experimental analysis in man of the oxygen pressure gradient from alveolar air to arterial blood during rest and exercise at sea level and at altitude. *Am J Physiol* 1946; **147**: 199–216.
32. Riley RL, Cournand A, Donald KW. Analysis of factors affecting partial pressure of oxygen and carbon dioxide in gas and blood of lungs: methods. *J Appl Physiol* 1951; **4**: 102–120.
33. Riley RL, Shepard RH, Cohn JE et al. Maximal diffusing capacity of the lungs. *J Appl Physiol* 1954; **6**: 573–587.
34. Rosenhamer GJ, Friesen WO, McIlroy MB. A bloodless method for measurement of diffusing capacity of the lungs for oxygen. *J Appl Physiol* 1971; **30**: 603–610.
35. Hyde RW, Forster RE, Power GG et al. Measurement of O_2 diffusing capacity of the lungs with a stable O_2 isotope. *J Clin Invest* 1966; **45**: 1178–1193.
36. Meyer M, Scheid P, Riepl G et al. Pulmonary diffusing capacities for O_2 and CO measured by a rebreathing technique. *J Appl Physiol* 1981; **51**: 1643–1650.
37. Hammond MD, Hempleman SC. Oxygen diffusing capacity estimates derived from measured $\dot{V}A/\dot{Q}$ distributions in man. *Respir Physiol* 1987; **69**: 129–147.
38. Weibel ER. Morphometric model for pulmonary diffusing capacity. 1. Membrane diffusing capacity. *Respir Physiol* 1993; **93**: 125–149.
39. Piiper J, Scheid P. Model for alveolar-capillary equilibration with special reference to O_2 uptake in hypoxia. *Respir Physiol* 1981; **46**: 193–208.
40. Scheid P, Piiper J. Blood gas equilibrium in lungs and pulmonary diffusing capacity. In: Chang HK, Paiva M, eds. *Respiratory physiology an analytical approach.* New York: Marcel Dekker, 1989: 453–497.
41. Staub NC. The interdependence of pulmonary structure and function. *Anesthesiology* 1963; **24**: 831–854.
42. Cross CE, Gong H Jr, Kurpershoek CJ et al. Alterations in distribution of blood flow to the lung's diffusion surfaces during exercise. *J Clin Invest* 1973; **52**: 414–421.
43. West JB. *Ventilation/blood flow and gas exchange.* Oxford: Blackwell Scientific Publications, 1965.
44. Dill DB. *Handbook of respiratory data in aviation.* Washington DC: Office of Scientific Research and Development. 1944.
45. Kloche FJ, Rahn H. The arterial–alveolar inert gas ('N_2') difference in normal and emphysematous subjects, as indicated by the analysis of urine. *J Clin Invest* 1961; **40**: 286–294.
46. West JB, Wagner PD. Pulmonary gas exchange. *Am J Respir Crit Care Med* 1998; **157**: S82–S87.
47. Rahn H, Fenn WO. *A graphical analysis of the respiratory gas exchange.* Washington DC: *American Physiological Society,* 1955.

48. Refsum HE, Kim BM. The alveolo-arterial oxygen tension difference at varying alveolar ventilation in patients with pulmonary disease breathing air. *Clin Sci* 1967; **33**: 569–576.
49. McNicol MW, Campbell EJM. Severity of respiratory failure. Arterial blood-gases in untreated patients. *Lancet* 1965; **1**: 336–338.
50. Thews G, Schmidt W. Partitioning the alveolar–arterial O_2 pressure difference under normal, hypoxic and hyperoxic conditions. *Respiration* 1976; **33**: 245–255.
51. Sapsford DJ, Jones JG. The PIO_2 vs SpO_2 diagram: a non-invasive measure of pulmonary oxygen exchange. *Eur J Anaesthesiol* 1995; **12**: 375–386.
52. Gray L de, Rush EM, Jones JG. A noninvasive method for evaluating the effect of thoracotomy on shunt and ventilation perfusion inequality. *Anaesthesia* 1997; **52**: 630–635.
53. Sapsford DJ, Jones JG. Derivation of V_A/Q from the position of the P_{IO_2} vs. SpO_2 curve. *Br J Anaes* 1992; **69**: 541p.
54. Jones JG, Jones SE. Discriminating between the effect of shunt and reduced V_A/Q on arterial oxygen saturation is particularly useful in clinical practice. *J Clin Monit* 2000; **16**: 337–350.
55. Kjaergaard S, Rees S, Malczynshi J et al. Non-invasive estimation of shunt and ventilation-perfusion mismatch. *Intensive Care Med.* 2003; **29**: 727–734.

Further reading

Barcroft J. *The respiratory function of the blood. Haemoglobin, Part 11.* London: Cambridge University Press, 1928.

Finley TN, Swenson EW, Comroe JH Jr. The cause of arterial hypoxaemia at rest in patients with 'alveolar-capillary block syndrome'. *J Clin Invest* 1962; **41**: 618–622.

Hsia CCW. Respiratory function of hemoglobin. *New Eng J Med* 1998; **338**: 239–247.

Perutz MF. Molecular anatomy, physiology, and pathology of hemoglobin. In: Stamatoyannopoulos G, Nienhuis AW, Leder P, Majerus PW, eds. *The molecular basis of blood disease.* Philadelphia: WB Saunders, 1987: 127–178.

Rørth M, Astrup P, eds. *Oxygen affinity of hemoglobin and red cell acid base status.* Copenhagen: Munksgaard, 1972. See especially article by F.J.W. Roughton et al.

West JB, ed. *Pulmonary gas exchange. Vol 1. Ventilation, blood flow and diffusion.* New York: Academic Press, 1980.

Zetterstrom H. Assessment of the efficiency of pulmonary oxygenation. The choice of oxygenation index. *Acta Anaesthesiol Scand* 1988; **32**: 579–584.

CHAPTER 22

Gas Exchange for Carbon Dioxide and Acid–Base Balance

Gas exchange for CO_2 disposes of a waste product and is a means of preserving the body's internal acid–base environment. This chapter summarises present views.

22.1 Introduction

The oxidation (or more accurately the dehydrogenation) of carbohydrate, fat and, to a lesser extent, protein provide the energy for most bodily functions. The principal end product is carbon dioxide. This gas is produced by all tissues, especially muscles during exercise when the quantity reflects the level of activity and the type of fuel (Section 28.9.1). The CO_2 is disposed of by being transported in blood returning to the lungs, and then excreted in the alveolar fraction of expired gas. Throughout this journey the gas is in equilibrium with water with which it combines to form carbonic acid that then dissociates into hydrogen ions and bicarbonate ions. The hydrogen ions are neutralised by buffer systems within the blood including bicarbonate salts and compounds with proteins, especially haemoglobin. The level at which the systems operate is set by the kidneys through the selective excretion or retention of sodium and other substances. The settings can be modified by some medical disorders and also by altered respiratory drive associated with acclimatisation to high altitude.

The processes that contribute to the carriage and disposal of carbon dioxide also provide immediate and some longer term protection against other acidic substances that enter the blood. The substances include lactic acid (formed during strenuous exercise or as a result of hypoxia), keto-acids in diabetes mellitus and other acid (or alkali) residues as may be formed during metabolism or enter the body by ingestion. The protection is by storage in tissues, including muscle, and by changes in alveolar ventilation that increase or decrease the pulmonary excretion of CO_2 as the circumstances require.

In patients with damaged lungs the level of ventilation that is needed to maintain the blood gases at their normal level can become unsustainable. When this happens the P_{CO_2} rises so the blood becomes more acid (see Footnote 22.1).

The pH of the blood is usually preserved by the excretion of an acid urine. If this mechanism is inadequate for any reason the pH falls and the patient can then be in serious difficulties. The condition may be treatable, but first the biochemical abnormalities should be identified. In most respiratory patients this can be achieved in terms of base excess and P_{CO_2} as represented by the Siggaard-Anderson nomogram [1]. However, for some complex abnormalities there may be a need to make allowances for additional variables (see e.g. SID, below).

Footnote 22.1. The relative acidity of the blood reflects the concentration of free hydrogen ions $[H^+]$. This quantity is usually represented by its reciprocal, pH (i.e. $\log_{10}(1/[H^+])$), cf. Section 7.11.1).

22.2 Gas exchange for CO_2

22.2.1 Overview

Carbon dioxide is a highly diffusible gas that is produced by all cells during metabolism. The gas is in solution in the cell cytoplasm and from there passes by diffusion into plasma perfusing the adjacent capillaries [2]. It then moves into red cells where about 90% becomes hydrated under the influence of the enzyme carbonic anhydrase. The CO_2 subsequently reenters the plasma where it is present as bicarbonate ions buffered by plasma proteins. Of the remaining 10%, approximately half is transported in solution, whilst the other 5% can be accounted for by CO_2 attached to protein as carbamate compound. Almost all of this is carbamino-haemoglobin as the quantity that combines with plasma proteins is too small to contribute to gas exchange [3, 4].

Carbon dioxide in the blood is conveyed to the lungs where the changes associated with gas uptake in the tissue capillaries are reversed. This leads to carbon dioxide passing into the alveoli as a gas that is then voided to atmospheric air by ventilation of the lungs.

Carbon dioxide is normally present in arterial blood in a concentration and at a tension of approximately 22 mmol l^{-1} (50 ml/100 ml) and 5.3 kPa (40 mm Hg). Under resting conditions the corresponding values for mixed venous blood are 24 mmol l^{-1} (54 ml/100 ml) and 6.1 kPa (46 mm Hg). The corresponding values during moderate exercise might be, respectively, 26 mmol l^{-1} (58 ml/100 ml) and 7.3 kPa (55 mm Hg). In these examples the transfer gradient at rest is of the order of 0.8 kPa (6 mm Hg) and on moderate exercise 2.0 kPa (15 mm Hg). A small gradient is an important feature of homeostasis whereby the pH throughout the body is maintained at a nearly constant level. This stability depends on the chemical properties of blood and the mechanisms that regulate acid–base balance throughout the body. The chemical properties determine the shape of the dissociation curve for carbon dioxide. The mechanisms include those that determine the level of alveolar ventilation (Chapter 23) and the excretory activity of renal tubules (Section 22.3.5).

22.2.2 Whole blood dissociation curve for carbon dioxide

The transport system for carbon dioxide operates over a very small range of partial pressures. This is due to the steep slope of the blood dissociation curve whereby a small change in gas tension is associated with a relatively large change in gas content (Fig. 21.5, page 269, also [5]). This feature has the effect of minimising the difference in pH between tissues and lungs. The relevant curve (the *in vivo* dissociation curve) is for conditions prevailing in the alveolar capillaries; these can be simulated using freshly drawn arterial whole blood as the concentrations of 2,3-diphosphoglycerate are the same in both. The physiological curve differs from those of mixed venous and arterial blood due to the processes of gas exchange leading to progressive changes in pH, oxygen saturation and other variables along the length of the alveolar capillaries. The curve has been described mathematically [6, 7]:

$$C\text{CO}_2\cdot\text{blood} = C\text{CO}_2\cdot\text{plasma} \times \left[1 - \frac{0.0289 \times [\text{Hb}]}{(3.352 - 0.456 \times S\text{O}_2) \times (8.142 - \text{pH})}\right] \qquad (22.1)$$

where $C\text{CO}_2\cdot\text{plasma} = 2.226 \times s \times \text{plasma } P\text{CO}_2 \times (1 + 10^{\text{pH}-\text{p}K'})$, $C\text{CO}_2$ is CO_2 content, $S\text{O}_2$ is O_2 saturation, s is the plasma CO_2 solubility coefficient, and pK' is the apparent pK from the equations of Kelman [8].

The *in vivo* dissociation curve connects at its lower and upper ends with the curves for oxygenated and partially reduced haemoglobin. The latter are separated by a distance that represents the difference in content of carbon dioxide between oxygenated and venous blood at the same $P\text{CO}_2$. This quantity of carbon dioxide is transported between the tissues to the lungs in association with reduced haemoglobin. In the tissues the take up of CO_2 is facilitated by the unloading of oxygen from haemoglobin, whilst in the lungs the influx of oxygen facilitates the efflux of CO_2. This oxylabile component of CO_2 exchange was identified by Christiansen, Douglas and Haldane and is known as the *CDH or Haldane effect* [5]. It is due to reduced haemoglobin being a better buffer of hydrogen ions and binding more carbon dioxide as carbamate than is the case for oxygenated haemoglobin. The size of the effect is related to the gas tensions, the blood pH and the concentration of 2,3-diphosphoglycerate.

The *in vivo* dissociation curve for CO_2, unlike that for oxygen, is effectively linear over the physiological range (Fig. 21.5, page 269). This is an advantage when there is a wide range of ventilation–perfusion ratios throughout the lung, as gas exchange in acini with a high $\dot{V}\text{A}/\dot{Q}$ ratio can compensate for those where the $\dot{V}\text{A}/\dot{Q}$ ratio is lower (Section 21.5.2). In addition, modest changes in alveolar ventilation have an immediate effect on CO_2 excretion and hence provide a physiological mechanism for regulating blood $P\text{CO}_2$ and pH. But the relative linearity of the dissociation curve renders the attainment of gaseous equilibrium across the alveolar capillary membrane more difficult. This is because there is no tailing off of the volume flow of gas as equilibrium approaches, as is the case for oxygen (Section 21.3.2).

The slope of the CO_2 dissociation curve is used in the O_2–CO_2 diagram (Fig. 21.6, page 270) and in the several carbon dioxide methods for measuring cardiac output (Section 17.3.2). For the latter application, the information that is summarised in eqn. 22.1 can also be obtained from a nomogram (Fig. 17.6, page 203, [9]).

22.2.3 Uptake of carbon dioxide by blood

Carbon dioxide that is formed in the tissues passes rapidly by diffusion into the plasma of the adjacent capillaries. Here some of the gas hydrates slowly to form carbonic acid; this dissociates into bicarbonate ions and hydrogen ions. The latter displace sodium from combination with phosphate and protein in the plasma. The hydration reaction is mediated via a low energy form of the enzyme carbonic anhydrase (carbonic anhydrase I) that is present in the capillary endothelium. However, most of the dissolved carbon dioxide passes from the plasma into the red cells; here the greater part is hydrated through the mediation of the high energy form of carbonic anhydrase (carbonic anhydrase II):

$$CO_2 + H_2O \underset{}{\overset{\text{carbonic anhydrase}}{\leftrightharpoons}} HCO_3^- + H^+ \qquad (22.2)$$

Understanding the role of this enzyme in gas exchange was advanced by Roughton and his successive collaborators [10, 11]. The enzyme contains zinc. The structure and chemistry of the enzyme have been the subject of recent dramatic advances [12].

In the red cells the hydration of carbon dioxide to form carbonic acid is the start of a series of reactions and migrations of ions for which the traditional model is shown in Fig. 22.1. The carbonic acid dissociates into bicarbonate ions and hydrogen ions; the hydrogen ions displace potassium ions from combination with haemoglobin in the interior of the red cell. This process is assisted by the dissociation of oxyhaemoglobin. The oxygen passes into the tissues and by doing so liberates haemoglobin that takes up hydrogen ions more readily in its reduced than in its oxidized form. Subsequently, according to the model the bicarbonate ions diffuse out of the red cells, where their concentration is high, into the plasma and the extracellular fluid where their concentration is lower. The apparent migration is now known to reflect a reduction in $[HCO_3^-]$ in the red cells and rise in concentration in the plasma as a consequence of diffusion of CO_2, without a migration of ions taking place. The bicarbonate ions in the cells are replaced by chloride ions. This exchange is called the chloride shift, or the Hamburger shift after its discoverer. It is an active process mediated by a carrier protein in the cell membrane and can be inhibited by drugs including salicylates and frusemide [13]. The anion exchange leads to the uptake of carbon dioxide by blood in the tissue capillaries being shared between red cells and plasma, although the red cells contain the bulk of the protein upon which the process depends. The participation of the extracellular fluid leads to the dissociation curve for carbon dioxide in the body differing from that in the blood [14].

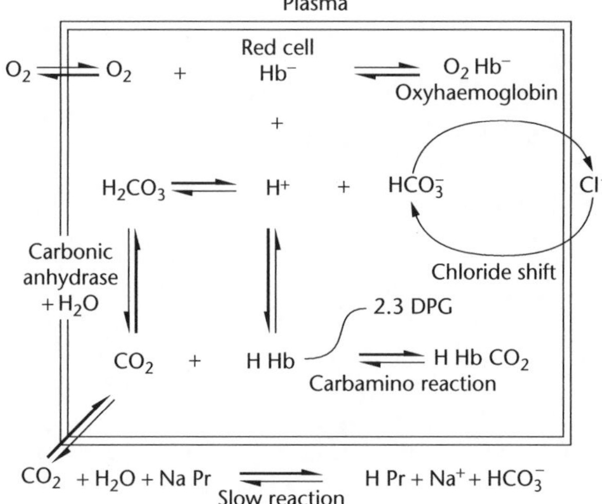

Fig. 22.1 Role of haemoglobin in the transport of carbon dioxide. The directions of the reactions are indicated by the width of the arrows; these are broad for the tissue capillaries and narrow for the alveolar capillaries. In the tissue capillaries the oxygen is liberated from oxyhaemoglobin (O_2Hb^-) that then reverts to the ionic form Hb^-; these ions are reduced to haemoglobin (HHb) by hydrogen ions (H^+) formed by dissociation of carbonic acid (H_2CO_3). The reduced haemoglobin accepts carbon dioxide to form carbamino-haemoglobin. The reduced haemoglobin also combines with 2,3 DPG and this reaction reduces the extent of the carbamino reaction. In the tissues, bicarbonate formed by the dissociation of carbonic acid exchanges with chloride ions in the extracellular fluid. Source: [11]

22.2.4 Carbamino-haemoglobin

As well as the reactions with water some carbon dioxide combines with reduced haemoglobin to form a compound of a carbamino type:

$$\text{HbNH}_2 + CO_2 \leftrightharpoons \text{HbNHCOOH} \leftrightharpoons \text{HbNHCOO}^- + H^+ \qquad (22.3)$$

In the tissue capillaries the forward reaction is facilitated by the quantity of reduced haemoglobin rising as the oxyhaemoglobin gives up its oxygen. The process is reversed in the lungs; hence the reaction contributes to the CDH effect whereby the extent of oxygenation of haemoglobin influences the transport of carbon dioxide. The mechanism is believed to explain approximately 10% of the total transport in normal circumstances and up to 19% in the foetus, but these figures are subject to revision [3]. The effect is represented in the O_2–CO_2 diagram by the curvature of the isopleths for the carbon dioxide content of blood (Fig. 21.6, page 270).

The formation of carbamate occurs at terminal amino groups on the β chains of deoxygenated haemoglobin molecules and, to a lesser extent, on the α chains. However, the former reaction is diminished by 2,3 DPG which competes for the same sites (Section 21.2.2); the organic phosphates do not compete for the sites on the α chains which in practice contribute equally with the β chains to the oxylabile carbamate transport of carbon dioxide [15].

22.2.5 Release of CO_2 in the lungs

In the lungs the chemical changes are the reverse of those that occur in the tissues. They are initiated and sustained by the reciprocal changes that take place in the tensions of carbon dioxide and oxygen. The fall in the tension of carbon dioxide alters the position of equilibrium between dissolved carbon dioxide and carbonic acid. The rise in the tension of oxygen increases the concentration of oxyhaemoglobin; this reduces the quantity of carbamino-haemoglobin and also liberates hydrogen ions from reduced haemoglobin. The hydrogen ions in turn contribute to the release of carbon dioxide from bicarbonate. The temperature in the lungs is lower than that in the tissues by, on average, 0.5°C; this also contributes to the release of carbon dioxide. The CO_2 that is released diffuses rapidly in the aqueous phase of the lung tissue and thence into the alveoli. However, in addition to being a conduit for CO_2, the lung water smoothes the fluctuations in CO_2 exchange that occur during the respiratory cycle. The fluctuations exceed those for oxygen on account of the dissociation curve being steeper [16] and are transmitted to the blood where they contribute to control of breathing (Section 23.5.3).

22.2.6 Rate of equilibration

Carbon dioxide is a very soluble gas; hence, from eqn. 19.4 (page 227) the rate of diffusion across the alveolar capillary membrane (Dm,CO_2) might be expected to be high, exceeding that for oxygen by a factor of 20.3 (Table 19.1, page 225). Studies using radioisotope-labelled gases including $^{13}CO_2$, $C^{16}O^{18}O$ and $C^{18}O_2$, suggest that the hypothesis is correct [17, 18]. On this basis West and Wagner have computed the likely time course for exchange of carbon dioxide along the length of a representative alveolar capillary (Fig. 22.2). The analysis shows that, assuming a standard dissociation curve, the diffusivity of carbon dioxide is adequate for the attainment of gaseous equilibrium before the blood leaves the alveolar capillary. This appears not to be the case in practice.

The paradox of a relatively slow overall equilibration time for carbon dioxide despite its high diffusivity is due to the chemical processes. These are slower than those for oxygen [20], partly because the oxygenation of haemoglobin needs to be completed before carbon dioxide can achieve equilibrium between red cells and plasma. In addition, the red cell membrane is permeable to chloride ions but relatively impermeable to hydrogen ions. As a result the anions and carbon dioxide molecules migrate between red cells and plasma in the manner described above. The half-time for completion of the exchanges is approximately 15 s [21]. This exceeds the sampling time for measurements made during exercise; hence, the tension of carbon dioxide in arterial blood can be less than that in the alveolar gas [22]. In this circumstance an empirical correction factor can be used (eqn. 17.6. page 202). An end capillary gradient can also occur if carbonic anhydrase is inhibited by acetazolamide, or if anion transport is depressed by salicylates, or the lung parenchyma is damaged by disease.

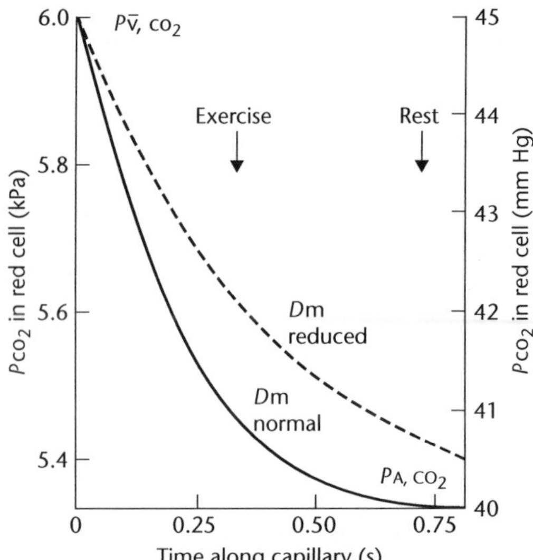

Fig. 22.2 Time course for the diffusion of carbon dioxide across the alveolar capillary membrane during breathing air. The curves were computed using the digital subroutines of Kelman [8]. The value assigned to Dm,CO_2 was 20 times Dm,O_2.(cf. Fig. 21.2, page 263). The times when the blood was assumed to leave the capillary is indicated by arrows. When both Dm is reduced and the transit time is shortened by exercise the diffusion of CO_2 is incomplete. In this event, the associated tendency towards hypercapnia is corrected by an increase in ventilation. Source: [19]

22.3 Acid–base balance

22.3.1 Overview

The relative steepness and the linearity of the *in vivo* CO_2 dissociation curve have the consequence that the carbon dioxide content of arterial blood is exquisitely sensitive to the amount of alveolar ventilation. In health this is regulated to maintain the P_{CO_2} at its normal level for most of the time. During sleep the respiratory drive diminishes and the P_{CO_2} rises (Section 32.4). During exercise of moderate or high intensity, the respiratory drive is increased by a rise in the level of lactate in the blood (Section 28.9.2). There is then an increase in alveolar ventilation, additional carbon dioxide is exhaled, the arterial P_{CO_2} falls and the blood pH is restored to near to its previous level. Subsequently the lactate is disposed of and a normal blood P_{CO_2} is restored. In this instance the acid–base disturbance is of short duration. Converse changes that can be of much longer duration occur following ascent to altitude. Here the hypoxia drives respiration to increase the level of alveolar ventilation. This maximises the tension of oxygen in alveolar gas and hence in arterial blood, but at the expense of lowering the tension of carbon dioxide. The hyperventilation raises the blood pH and leads to compensatory changes by the kidneys that modify the buffering capacity of the blood (Section 34.2). In this way the blood pH is restored but the alveolar hyperventilation and hence the hypocapnia persist or are enhanced (Section 34.4).

These examples indicate that achieving an adequate arterial oxygen tension has priority over maintaining a normal blood pH. Both have priority over the level of blood $P\text{CO}_2$ that can vary within wide limits. This sequence was apparent on a larger scale during the emergence of terrestrial life from the sea. The arterial oxygen tension increased a little whilst the $P\text{CO}_2$ increased approximately fourfold (Section 1.2). Regulation of blood pH is a means of preserving the working environment of the cells in the brain and other tissues, especially the extent of dissociation of imidazole-NH groups in proteins [23]. The primacy or alpha status of this reaction led to the systems that regulate it being designated the *alphastat* [24]. The mechanisms entail adjustments to alveolar ventilation and to the balance between acidic and basic (i.e. alkali) constituents of blood and cerebrospinal fluid (acid–base balance). The ventilatory mechanism is important as it has a shorter time constant than the other mechanisms. As a result, traditional acid–base physiology was primarily in terms of the level of plasma bicarbonate with respect to that expected for the prevailing level of $P\text{CO}_2$, as calculated using the Henderson–Hasselbalch equation (eqn. 7.16, page 70). By this approach the difference between the calculated and observed values for $[HCO_3^-]$ was the *base excess* [25]. The terminology associated with this traditional approach to acid–base physiology is included in Table 6.1 (page 53) and examples of its use are given in Figs 22.3 and 22.4.

22.3.2 Indices: base excess, strong ion difference, anion gap

The concentration of hydrogen ions is influenced by the concentrations of other ions, especially those that are 'strong' i.e. fully dissociated. The principal strong ions are the cations Na^+ and K^+ and the anion Cl^-. The difference between their respective molar concentrations is traditionally described as *buffer base* [35]. It can also be referred to as *strong ion difference* (SID [36]), where in normal circumstances $SID = [Na^+] + [K^+] - [Cl^-]$. However, SID also takes note of other strong ions where these are present, for example lactic acid during strenuous exercise, hyperventilation or circulatory failure and keto-acids in uncontrolled diabetes. The quantity normally has a value of approximately 40 mEq/l and is exactly balanced by contributions from weak ions (i.e. those that are not fully dissociated). The principal ions in this category are bicarbonate ions $[HCO_3^-]$ and ionised proteins $[A^-]$. Hence, from the law of electrical neutrality:

$$[SID] - [HCO_3^-] - [A^-] - [CO_3^{2-}] + [H^+] - [OH^-] = 0 \qquad (22.4)$$

In this equation the first three left-hand terms are defined above, the fourth is carbonate from dissociation of bicarbonate and the last two are from dissociation of water. SID is derived from this equation by inserting measured or calculated values for the other variables.

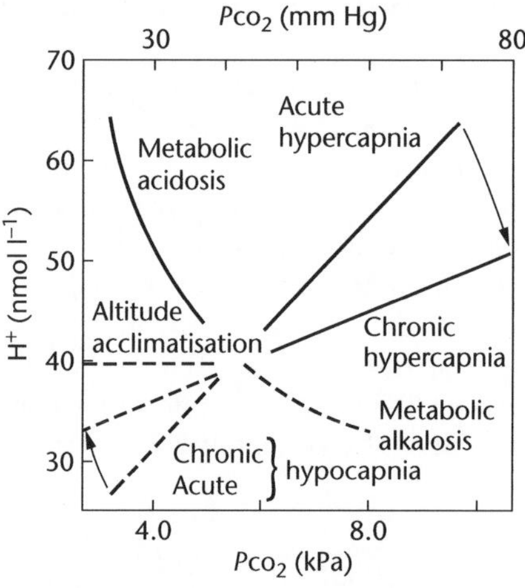

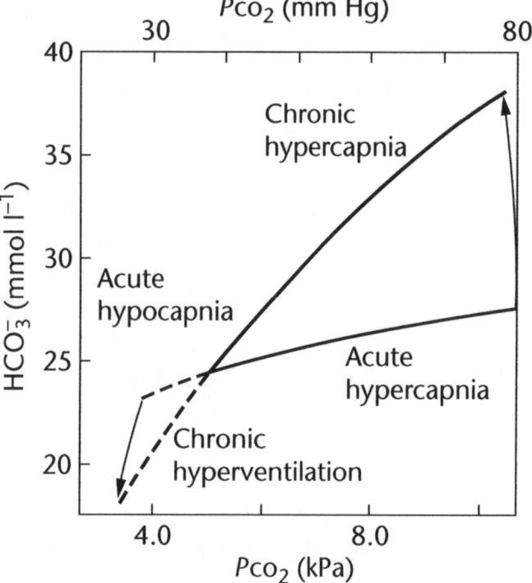

Fig. 22.3 Adaptation of the buffering capacity of the blood to a change in the tension of carbon dioxide. The diagrams show steady-state values for the blood hydrogen ion concentration and plasma bicarbonate at a range of tensions of carbon dioxide produced by breathing mixtures of CO_2 in air. In SI units, the following relationships were used:
acute hypercapnia in healthy subjects [26]:
$H^+ = 0.77 \times 7.5\ P\text{CO}_2 + 8.0$
$HCO_3^- = 24.7 \times 7.5\ P\text{CO}_2 \div (0.77 \times 7.5\ P\text{CO}_2 + 8.0)$.
Chronic hypercapnia in patients with chronic lung disease [27]:
$H^+ = 0.3 \times 7.5\ P\text{CO}_2 + 26.8$
$HCO_3^- = 24.7 \times 7.5\ P\text{CO}_2 \div (0.3 \times 7.5\ P\text{CO}_2 + 26.8)$.
Primary metabolic acidosis [28]: $P\text{CO}_2 = 962 \div (7.5 \times ([H^+] - 12))$.
For $P\text{CO}_2$ in mm Hg the factor 7.5 was omitted.
Additional sources: [29, 30]

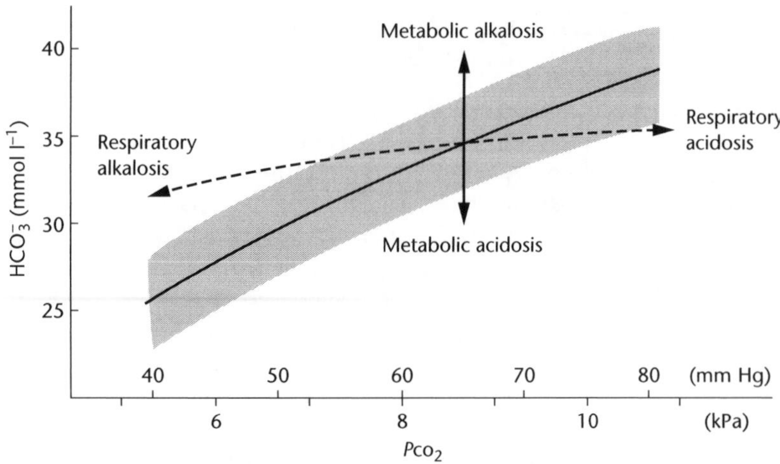

Fig. 22.4 Changes effected by disturbed acid–base on the relationship of plasma bicarbonate to PCO$_2$ (from Fig. 22.3, right): the shaded area shows estimated 95% confidence limits. The interrupted line shows the effect of a recent change in alveolar ventilation and is based on the relationship for acute hypercapnia in the right-hand half of Fig. 22.3. The corresponding blood hydrogen ion concentrations can be obtained by reference to the left-hand half of that figure. Source: [31], see also [32–34]

In biochemical analysis of plasma the commonly measured substances are sodium, chloride and bicarbonate, whilst the contributions of $[K^+]$ and the last three substances in eqn. 22.4 are very small. Hence, the relationship that includes SID can be simplified to:

$$\text{Anion gap} - [A^-] - [etc] = 0 \qquad (22.5)$$

where *anion gap* is $[Na^+] - [Cl^-] - [HCO_3^-]$, whilst $[etc]$ refers to other variables [37, 38]. Their contribution is normally very small, in which case the anion gap is filled by anions from dissociated proteins, particularly albumen. In practice, the mass of ionised protein $[A^-]$ is not readily established but it can be represented by the total protein mass since more than 90% of the protein is normally in an ionised form and the mass of the H^+ ions is negligible. Hence, the term in eqn. 22.5 can be replaced by *total weak acid* (Atot) with which it is in equilibrium (i.e. $[\text{Atot}] = [A^-] + [H^+]$). [Atot] is normally in the range 8–16 mmol l^{-1} and is proportional to the quantity of protein. The coefficient of proportionality is 0.24, so $[\text{Atot}] = 0.24\,[\text{Pr}]$, where [Pr] is the concentration of plasma proteins ([Pr] in the units g l^{-1}). The measured concentration of albumin can also be used for the calculation [39].

Consideration of the ionic balance exemplified by the indices SID, anion gap and Atot has increased understanding of the mechanisms of acid–base disturbance in different circumstances [40–43]. Some of these are indicated below.

22.3.3 Respiratory alkalosis and acidosis

An alteration to respiratory drive changes the alveolar ventilation and causes immediate *converse* changes in blood carbon dioxide tension and hydrogen ion concentration (PCO$_2$ and $[H^+]$). Such changes are of respiratory origin and this is recognised in the terminology that relates to trends in hydrogen ion concentration over time, not to the actual levels [44]. *Respiratory alkalosis* is when an increase in ventilation raises the pH in the direction of alkalosis, and *respiratory acidosis* is when a decrease in ventilation reduces the pH in the direction of acidosis. Some causes are given below (Table 22.1).

The terminology also extends to respiratory compensation for changes in $[H^+]$ brought about by metabolic processes. *Compensatory respiratory alkalosis* is when a rise in blood $[H^+]$ (metabolic acidosis) triggers an increase in alveolar ventilation. The change compensates for the acidaemia by promoting the excretion of carbonic acid as carbon dioxide. It does not extend fully to the cerebro-spinal fluid (see below). The situation needs to be distinguished from the compensated respiratory alkalosis that can be obtained as a result of acclimatisation to high altitude (Section 34.2).

Similarly, *compensatory respiratory acidosis* is a response to a low blood $[H^+]$ of metabolic origin (metabolic alkalaemia). This reduces the drive to respiration and leads to compensatory hypercapnia which, when it occurs, can restore the $[H^+]$ towards normal.

The dissociation curve that describes the relationship of blood hydrogen ion concentration to the content of CO_2 in blood is relatively steep (Fig. 22.3). As a result, changes in $[H^+]$ of respiratory origin are small in relation to the quantities of carbon dioxide that are retained or expired. Thus, in the absence of complicating factors, a change in ventilation that alters the pH by 0.1 units can represent an increase in PCO$_2$ of approximately 2.6 kPa (20 mm Hg) or a reduction in PCO$_2$ of 1.3 kPa (10 mm Hg), see also Footnote 22.2. The immediate buffering mechanisms that are responsible are indicated above (Fig. 22.1). The mechanisms

Footnote 22.2. PCO$_2$ in arterial plasma varies inversely with level of alveolar ventilation as in eqn. 21.7 (see Footnote 21.2, page 267). In traditional units the eqn. has the form:

$$P\text{aCO}_2 = 0.863\,\dot{V}\text{CO}_2/\dot{V}\text{A}$$

where $\dot{V}$CO$_2$ is CO_2 output in ml STPD min^{-1} and $\dot{V}$A is alveolar ventilation in l BTPS min^{-1}. 0.863 is 713/(1000 × 0.826) and converts fractional concentration to partial pressure, ml to l and volume from BTPS to STPD conditions (Section 6.6).

Table 22.1 Respiratory causes of acid–base disturbance.

Mechanism	Respiratory acidosis	Respiratory alkalosis
Intrapulmonary	Increased work of breathing, weakness of respiratory muscles from any cause	Transfer defect†, pulmonary vascular disease or embolism. Pneumothorax
Altered hypoxic drive	In patients with hypoxaemia drive reduced by O_2 therapy (can result in CO_2 narcosis)	Drive increased by hypoxic gas mixture, altitude
Stimulation of C fibre receptors (J receptors)	-	Raised pulmonary capillary pressure, interstitial oedema (e.g. secondary to cardiac abnormality)
Brain stem	Structural damage	Localised lesions, Cheyne–Stokes breathing, hyperthermia
Voluntary or psychogenic	Breathing gas enriched with CO_2 [40]	Over-breathing*, ventilator therapy
Drugs	Respiratory depressants	Salicylates, methylxanthines, β-adrenergic agonists
Hormones	-	Progesterone, thyroxine

† especially in absence of restrictive ventilatory defect and if J receptor stimulation coexists.
* can be complicated by tetany due to formation of calcium carbonate (from $CO_3{}^{2-}$) reducing the plasma concentration of Ca^{2+}.
Sources: [41, 45].

and hence the dissociation curve are modified substantially if a metabolic disturbance coexists (Fig. 22.3). They are also modified by compensatory mechanisms of which the most important reside in the renal tubules (see below).

22.3.4 Changes in cerebrospinal fluid

A change in the tension of carbon dioxide in the jugular venous blood leads to an equivalent movement of the gas into or out of the cerebrospinal fluid (CSF). The initial response is rapid, but the time to equilibrium is prolonged because the area of choroid plexus across which the exchange takes place is relatively small. Buffering in the cerebrospinal fluid is dependent on electrolytes, not proteins as is the case for blood [46]. As a result, the equilibrium tension of carbon dioxide is, on an average, higher in CSF than that in arterial blood. The mean difference is approximately 1 kPa (8 torr) and the pH is lower in consequence (mean value approximately 7.33). In addition a change in the tension of carbon dioxide produces a somewhat larger change in pH in CSF than in blood. However, the deviation from the normal pH is reduced over a period of days. This is a result of active transport of ions across the blood-to-CSF barrier. Before the process is complete, the brain is particularly vulnerable to a change in the tension of carbon dioxide. For this reason, the condition of carbon dioxide narcosis is more likely to occur following a rise in $P\text{CO}_2$ that is of moderate size but rapid onset, than a larger rise that occurs more slowly.

22.3.5 Renal mechanisms

The renal tubules receive a filtrate of plasma and condition it before the residue is passed on to the bladder. Regulation is achieved by varying the proportions and amounts in which constituents of tubular fluid are reabsorbed into the blood [47]. The kidneys respond to uncomplicated respiratory alkalaemia by reducing the reabsorbtion of sodium. The response is rapid, the effect is detectable within a few hours, and by the second or third day the pH is usually restored to very near the initial value. The principal exception is prolonged exposure to high altitude; here renal adaptation is delayed by interaction with other effects of hypoxaemia (Section 34.2). In this circumstance the blood pH returns to normal over about a month. Respiratory alkalosis occurring as a result of medical conditions (Table 22.1) is seldom completely compensated.

The kidneys respond to acidaemia by retaining sodium and excreting more chloride ions. Alternatively, where the acidaemia is due to lactate or ketones these ions are excreted in preference to Cl^-. In this circumstance the keto-acidosis or lactacidosis may be complicated by hyperchloraemic acidosis. In addition, some hydrogen ions enter the urine as ammonium salts and acid phosphates via the following reactions:

$$NH_3 + H^+ = NH_4{}^+ \quad (22.6)$$

$$HPO_4{}^{2-} + H^+ = H_2PO_4{}^- \quad (22.7)$$

The resulting increase in the concentration of sodium in plasma represents an increase in SID and is associated with an increase in the plasma concentration of bicarbonate. Other tissues also contribute to the changes; these come into effect rapidly at first and subsequently more slowly, until the blood hydrogen ion concentration is restored to near to its initial value. However, in respiratory acidosis, unlike respiratory alkalosis occurring at high altitude, the compensation for a change in $[H^+]$ is seldom complete (Fig. 22.3).

Table 22.2 Some causes of metabolic acidosis and alkalosis.

System	Metabolic acidosis (SID reduced)	Metabolic alkalosis (SID elevated)
Gastro-intestinal tract	Diarrhoea (loss of Na^+) Utero-sigmoidostomy (gain in Cl^-)	Vomiting, gastric aspiration (loss of Cl^-)
Ingestion	NH_4Cl (gain in Cl^-), salicylates, ethylene glycol (glycolate), methanol (formate)	Ant-acids (including $NaHCO_3$), sodium penicillin (gain in Na^+). Licorice , carbenoxalone (mineralocorticoids)
Metabolic	Lactic acidosis from exercise or hypoxaemia, diabetic keto-acidosis (i.e. with C=O groups)	Dehydration with loss of Cl^-
Renal	Tubular acidosis (loss of Na^+), renal failure (retention of SO_4^{2-})	Diuretic therapy with K^+ depletion
Endocrine		Aldosteronism

Source: adapted from [41].

Table 22.3 Acid–base disturbances of multiple aetiology.

Type	Conditions
Double metabolic acidosis	Diabetic + renal acidosis or lactacidosis
Respiratory and metabolic acidosis	Respiratory acidosis + hypoxaemic lactacidosis
Respiratory acidosis and metabolic alkalosis	Respiratory failure + diuretic and steroid therapy Metabolic hypokalaemia + weak respiratory muscles
Metabolic alkalosis and respiratory alkalosis	Post-op. nasogastric aspiration + mechanical ventilation
Metabolic acidosis and alkalosis	Severe vomiting + metabolic acidosis
Metabolic acidosis + respiratory alkalosis [Pa,CO_2 > expected for metabolic abnormality]	Additional respiratory stimulation [see Table 22.1].

Source: adapted from [41].

22.3.6 Metabolic acidosis and alkalosis

Acidic and basic substances that pass into the blood as a consequence of normal or abnormal metabolism have effects on the blood hydrogen ion concentration that are analogous to those of CO_2. Their origins are metabolic, hence *metabolic acidosis* and *metabolic alkalosis*, but again these descriptive terms relate to the direction of change and not to the actual hydrogen ion concentration. The terms compensatory metabolic acidosis and alkalosis are also used. Some circumstances associated with metabolic acid–base disturbances are given in Table 22.2.

Many seriously ill patients have metabolic acidosis [48]. The cause is usually a reduced supply of oxygen to the tissues; either there is hypoxaemia from acute respiratory failure or the blood supply is reduced by shock [49]. The lactic acid is then produced by all cells except those in the brain. This *Type A lactacidaemia* can also occur transiently during heavy exercise (Chapter 28). In *Type B lactacidaemia* the source of the lactic acid is the liver. It is due to this organ changing from being a net consumer of lactic acid, converting it to carbohydrate, to being a producer. The condition can occur in diabetes mellitus, liver disease, acute alcoholic intoxication and treatment with oral hypoglycaemic biguanides such as phenformin.

22.3.7 Acid–base disturbances of multiple aetiology

An acid–base disturbance often has more than one cause. Some examples are given in Table 22.3. Diagnosis is often difficult in these circumstances [48–50].

22.4 References

1. Siggaard-Anderson O. The acid-base status of the blood. *Scand J Clin Lab Invest* 1963; **15**(Suppl 70): 1–134.
2. Hyde RW, Puy RJM, Raub WF, Forster RE. Rate of disappearance of labelled carbon dioxide from the lungs of humans during breath holding: a method for studying the dynamics of pulmonary CO_2 exchange. *J Clin Invest* 1968; **47**: 1535–1552.

3. Klocke RA. Carbon dioxide transport. In: Crystal RG et al, eds. *The lung, scientific foundations.* 2nd ed. Philadelphia: Lippencott-Raven, 1997: 1633–1642.
4. Geers C, Gros G. Carbon dioxide transport and carbonic anhydrase in blood and muscle. *Physiol Rev* 2000; **80**: 681–715.
5. Christiansen J, Douglas CG, Haldane JS. The absorption and dissociation of carbon dioxide by human blood. *J Physiol (Lond)* 1914; **48**: 244–271.
6. Visser BF. Pulmonary diffusion of CO_2. *Phys Med Biol* 1960; **5**: 155–166.
7. Douglas AR, Jones NL, Reed JW. Calculation of whole blood CO_2 content. *J Appl Physiol* 1988; **65**: 473–477.
8. Kelman GR. Digital computer procedure for the conversion of P_{CO_2} into blood CO_2 content. *Respir Physiol* 1967; **3**: 111–116.
9. McHardy GJR. The relationship between the differences in pressure and content of carbon dioxide in arterial and venous blood. *Clin Sci* 1967; **32**: 299–309.
10. Meldrum NU, Roughton FJW. Carbonic anhydrase. Its preparation and properties. *J Physiol (Lond)* 1933; **80**: 113–142.
11. Roughton FJW. Transport of oxygen and carbon dioxide. In: Fenn WO, Rahn H., eds. *Handbook of physiology, Vol 1: Respiration* (Section 3). Bethesda, MD: American Physiological Society, 1964: 767–825.
12. Tripp BC, Smith K, Ferry JG. Carbonic anhydrase: new insights for an ancient enzyme *J Biol Chem* 2001: **276**: 48615–48618.
13. Kloche RA. Velocity of CO_2 exchanges in blood. *Ann Rev Physiol* 1988; **50**: 625–637.
14. Michel CC. The *in vivo* carbon dioxide dissociation curve of true plasma. *Respir Physiol* 1966; **1**: 121–137.
15. Kilmartin JV, Rossi-Bernardi L. Interaction of hemoglobin with hydrogen ions, carbon dioxide, and organic phosphates. *Physiol Rev* 1973; **53**: 836–890.
16. Lin KM, Cumming G. A model of time-varying gas exchange in the human lung during a respiratory cycle at rest. *Respir Physiol* 1973; **17**: 93–112.
17. Schuster KD. Kinetics of pulmonary CO_2 transfer studied by using labelled carbon dioxide $C^{16}O^{18}O$. *Respir Physiol* 1985; **60**: 21–37.
18. Heller H, Fuchs G, Schuster KD. Single-breath diffusing capacities for NO, CO and $C^{18}O_2$ in rabbits. *Pflugers Arch* 1988; **435**: 254–258, erratum 581.
19. Wagner PD, West JB. Effects of diffusion impairment on O_2 and CO_2 time courses in pulmonary capillaries. *J Appl Physiol* l972; **33**: 62–71.
20. Mochizuki M, Kagawa T. Numerical solutions of partial differential equations describing the simultaneous O_2 and CO_2 diffusions in the red blood cell. *Jpn J Physiol* 1986; **36**: 43–63.
21. Forster RE, Crandall ED. Time course of exchanges between red cells and extracellular fluid during CO_2 uptake. *J Appl Physiol* 1975; **38**: 710–718.
22. Piiper J, Meyer M, Marconi C, Scheid P. Alveolar-capillary equilibration kinetics of $^{13}CO_2$ in human lungs studied by rebreathing. *Respir Physiol* 1980; **42**: 29–41.
23. Rahn H, Reeves RB, Howell BJ. Hydrogen ion regulation, temperature and evolution. *Am Rev Respir Dis* 1975; **112**: 165–172.
24. Reeves RB. An imidazole alphastat hypothesis for vertebrate acid-base regulation; tissue carbon dioxide content and body temperature in bullfrogs. *Respir Physiol* 1972; **14**: 219–236.
25. Astrup P, Severinghaus JW. *History of acid–base physiology.* Stockholm: Munksgaard, 1986.
26. Brackett NC Jr, Cohen JJ, Schwartz WB. Carbon dioxide titration curve of normal man. *New Engl J Med* 1965; **272**: 6–12.
27. Van Ypersele de Strihou C, Brasseur L, de Coninck J. The 'carbon dioxide response curve' for chronic hypercapnia in man. *New Engl J Med* 1966; **275**: 117–122.
28. Bone JM, Cowie J, Lambie AT, Robson JS. The relationship between arterial P_{CO_2} and hydrogen ion concentration in chronic metabolic acidosis and alkalosis. *Clin Sci* 1974; **46**: 113–123.
29. Flenley DC. Another non-logarithmic acid–base diagram? *Lancet* 1971; **1**: 961–965; **2**, 160–161.
30. Dulfano MJ, Ishikawa S. Quantitative acid-base relationships in chronic pulmonary patients during the stable state. *Am Rev Respir Dis* 1966; **93**: 251–256.
31. Cohen JJ, Schwartz WB. Evaluation of acid–base equilibrium in pulmonary insufficiency. *Am J Med* 1966; **41**: 163–167.
32. Arbus GA, Herbert LA, Levesque PR et al. Characterization and clinical application of the 'significance band' for acute respiratory alkalosis. *New Engl J Med* 1969; **280**: 117–123.
33. Goldstein MB, Gennari FJ, Schwartz WB. The influence of graded degrees of chronic hypercapnia on the acute carbon dioxide titration curve. *J Clin Invest* 1971; **50**: 208–216.
34. Ingram RH, Miller RB, Tate LA. Acid-base response to acute carbon dioxide changes in chronic obstructive pulmonary disease. *Am Rev Respir Dis* 1973; **108**: 225–231.
35. Jorgensen K, Astrup P. Standard bicarbonate, its clinical significance, and a new method for its determination. *Scand J Clin Lab Invest* 1957; **9**:122–132.
36. Stewart P. Modern quantitative acid-base chemistry. *Can J Physiol Pharmacol* 1983; **61**: 1444–1461.
37. Narins RG, Jones ER, Stom MC et al. Diagnostic strategies in disorders of fluid, electrolyte and acid–base homeostasis. *Am J Med* 1982; **72**: 496–520.
38. Ishihara K, Szerlip HM. Anion gap acidosis. *Semin Nephrol* 1998; **18**: 83–97.
39. Kowalchuk JM, Scheuermann BW. Acid–base regulation: a comparison of quantitative methods. *Can J Physiol Pharmacol* 1994; **72**: 818–826.
40. Pingree BJW. Acid–base and respiratory changes after prolonged exposure to 1% carbon dioxide. *Clin Sci* 1977; **52**: 67–74.
41. Jones NL. Acid–base physiology. In: Crystal RG et al, eds. *The lung, scientific foundations.* 2nd ed. Philadelphia: Lippioncott-Raven, 1997.
42. Corey HE. Stewart and beyond: New models of acid-base balance. *Kidney Int* 2003; **64**: 777–787; *also Kidney Int* 2004; **65**: 1112–1113.
43. Story DA. Bench-to-bedside review: a brief history of clinical acid-base. *Crit Care* 2004; **8**: 253–258.
44. van Ypersele de Strihou C, Frans A. The respiratory response to chronic metabolic alkalosis and acidosis in disease. *Clin Sci Mol Med* 1973; **45**: 439–448.
45. Epstein SK, Singh N. Respiratory acidosis. *Respir Care* 2001; **46**: 366–383.
46. Nattie EE. Ionic mechanisms of cerebrospinal fluid acid-base regulation. *J Appl Physiol* 1983; **54**: 3–12.
47. Koeppen BM, Steinmetz PR. Basic mechanisms of urinary acidification. *Med Clin North Am* 1983; **67**: 753–770.
48. van der Beek A, de Meijer PH, Meinders AE. Lactic acidosis: pathophysiology, diagnosis and treatment. *Neth J Med* 2001; **58**: 128–136.

49. Galley HF, Webster NR. Acidosis and tissue hypoxia in the critically ill: how to measure it and what does it mean. *Crit Rev Clin Lab Sci* 1999; **36**: 35–60.

50. Battle DC, Hizon M, Cohen E et al. The use of the urinary anion gap in the diagnosis of hyperchloremic metabolic acidosis. *New Eng J Med* 1988; **318**: 594–599.

Further reading

Henderson LJ. *Blood: a study in general physiology.* New Haven: Yale University Press, 1928.

Hill EP, Power GG, Longo LD. Mathematical simulation of pulmonary O_2 and CO_2 exchange. *Am J Physiol* 1973; **224**: 904–917.

Peters JP, Van Slyke DD. *Quantitative clinical chemistry,* vol 1, *Interpretations.* Baltimore: Williams & Wilkins, 1931.

Piiper J. Carbon dioxide-oxygen relationships in gas exchange of animals. In memory of Hermann Rahn. *Boll Soc It Biol Sper* 1991; **67**: 635–658.

Rahn H, Prakash O, eds. *Acid–base regulation and body temperature.* Boston: Martinus Nijhoff, 1985.

Rørth M, Astrup P, eds. *Oxygen affinity of hemoglobin and red cell acid base status.* Copenhagen: Munksgaard, 1972. See in particular article by Roughton F.J.W. et al.

Siggaard Andersen O. The acid–base status of the blood. *Scand J Clin Lab Invest* 1963; **15**(Suppl 70): 1–134.

Stewart PA. *How to understand acid–base: a quantitative acid-base primer for biology and medicine.* New York: Elsevier, 1981.

CHAPTER 23

Control of Respiration

An ability to regulate the exchange of gases between the lungs and surrounding air (external respiration) is necessary for homeostasis. This chapter describes the control mechanisms and the means whereby their effectiveness can be assessed.

23.1 Introduction

Breathing is regulated such that the tensions of oxygen and carbon dioxide and the concentration of hydrogen ions in arterial blood and cerebral extracellular fluid are maintained at nearly constant levels. The regulatory mechanisms operate over a wide range of levels of metabolism and altered acid–base balance, and also during speaking, eating, drinking and other activities. Controlled changes in breathing form part of the homeostatic responses to many circumstances including hypoxaemia, hypercapnia, hyperthermia and pregnancy, as well as diseases of the lungs and the cardiovascular system.

23.2 Central respiratory activity

23.2.1 Functional anatomy

Breathing is controlled by the activity of networks of neurones in the medulla and pons. These networks are involved in the rhythmic contractions of the respiratory muscles, coordinate the responses to speech and swallowing, and respond to sensory information from receptors in the lungs, carotid bodies and other parts of the brain. The motor pathway is via the spinal cord, the phrenic nerves (that innervate the diaphragm) and the nerves that supply the intercostal, abdominal and other respiratory muscles. Their action is influenced by the elastic recoil, resistance to movement and inertance of the lung and chest wall, all of which are monitored by receptors in the thorax. The activity of these networks can be overridden by spinal cord reflexes in response to local sensory inputs and by voluntary action emanating from higher centres in the brain.

The respiratory neurones are organised into three principal collections; the pontine respiratory group (previously known as the pneumotaxic centre) in the pons, and the dorsal respiratory group and ventral respiratory group in the medulla.

Pontine respiratory group. The PRG is organised around the nucleus parabrachialis medialis (*n*PBM), the nucleus parabrachialis lateralis (*n*PBL) and the Kölliker–Fuse nucleus (KFN). These areas contain both expiration-related and inspiration-related neurones, as well as those that are active during the transition phase between inspiration and expiration (known as *phase spanning*).

The function of the PRG is not precisely known, but is thought to play a role in the regulation of respiratory phase switching.

Dorsal respiratory group. The DRG is in the dorsomedial part of the medulla and is associated with the nucleus tractus solitarius (*n*TS). It receives afferent fibres from the lungs and extrathoracic airways via the vagus nerves and is rich in inspiration-related neurones. These neurones can be divided into two main types depending upon their response to inflation [1]. The Iα (Rα) neurones have a discharge pattern resembling that of phrenic motor neurones; they are actively inhibited by lung inflation, hence are inhibited by lung volume related afferents, the so-called inspiratory off-switch mechanism. Activity in the Iβ (Rβ) neurones is excited by inflation, possibly via stimuli from stretch receptors. The DRG receives afferent information from respiratory related mechano- and chemoreceptors.

Ventral respiratory group. The VRG lies in a ventral column which, in an approximate order from above downwards, is formed from the Bötzinger complex (within the nucleus retrofacialis), the nucleus paraambigualis (*n*PA) and the parallel-sited nucleus ambiguus (*n*A), the nucleus retroambigualis (*n*RA), the nucleus retrofacialis (*n*RF) and the Aoki group of inspiration-related relay neurones in the first and second segments of the spinal cord. Both inspiratory and expiratory neurones are present, the former found predominately in the middle segment (around the *n*PA and *n*A) whilst the latter are in proportionately larger numbers at the rostral and caudal ends (Bötzinger complex and *n*RA, see Fig. 23.1).

The Bötzinger complex has widespread expiratory functions and activates, via expiration-related (E-R) neurones, the bulbar (E-R) neurones, primarily towards the end of prolonged expiration. Other neurones inhibit the inspiration-related activity of the *n*A. The *n*A itself contributes motor neurones that supply the laryngeal muscles via the vagi.

The *n*PA contains mainly inspiration-related (I-R) premotor neurones. The majority of fibres cross to the contralateral side of the brain stem and activate the motor neurones of the phrenic nerve and inspiratory intercostal muscles. In the case of the intercostal motor neurones the activation is via direct bulbo-spinal pathways but in the case of the phrenics some of the premotor neurones are relayed in the Aoki centres. The discharge of most I-R premotor neurones increases progressively throughout inspiration.

The *n*RA contains mainly premotor (expiratory) neurones that make synaptic contacts with motor neurones in the spinal cord; the latter supply expiratory internal intercostal muscles.

Just caudal to the nucleus retrofacialis in the ventral respiratory group is the pre-Bötzinger complex that has been postulated to be the site of rhythm generation. Neurones in this area possess pacemaker-like properties, with periodic membrane potential depolarization adequate for rhythmogenesis [2].

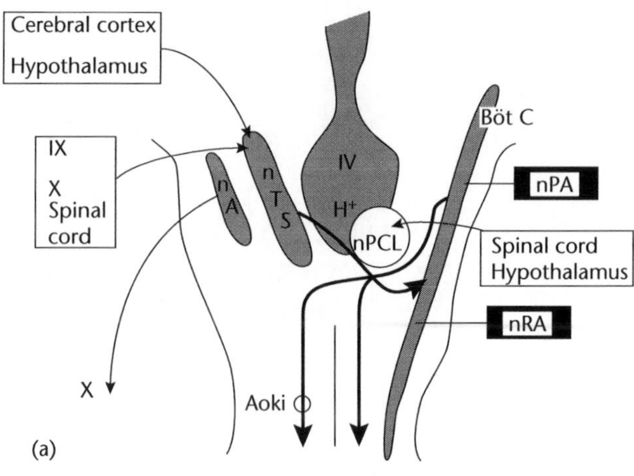

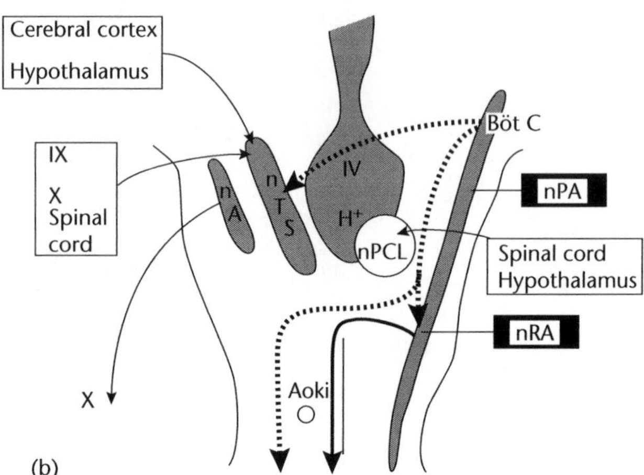

Fig. 23.1 Some ventral respiratory nuclei in the medulla and spinal cord with their most readily identifiable connections. The nuclei exist as pairs on each side of the mid line but for convenience only one of each pair is shown. Broad arrows indicate pathways that are particularly active (a) during inspiration and (b) during expiration. *n*A = nucleus ambiguus; *n*TS = nucleus of tractus solitarius; *n*PCL = nucleus paragiganto cellularis lateralis; Böt C = Bötzinger complex;
*n*RA = nucleus retroambigualis; *n*PA = nucleus paraambigualis;
IV = fourth ventricle

23.2.2 Rhythm generation

Inspiration. Central inspiratory activity increases in intensity with time during each inspiration then stops at the onset of expiration. The time profile, as reflected by activity in the phrenic nerve, resembles that of the volume change. Both have a relatively linear profile but variable duration. Inspiratory activity is influenced by the level of central excitation; this is reduced by sleep, anaesthesia, sedative drugs and appropriate hypnotic suggestion. It is also reduced by hypoxia acting on the central nervous system. Central excitation is increased by exercise and by stimulant drugs. The latter differ in their specificity, from convulsant drugs, which are non-specific, to progesterone that appears to affect only the drive to inspiration. The intensity of inspiratory activity is also influenced by stimuli from chemoreceptors and sensory nerve endings. The strength of the stimulus influences the total phrenic discharge per unit time; the half-time for the resulting inspiration is similar following stimulation from hypoxia (via the peripheral chemoreceptors), hypercapnia and exercise. The half-time is reduced when the stimulus is hyperthermia, which also changes the pattern of breathing. Inspiration is terminated by inhibition of the discharges from the inspiratory premotor neurones. The inhibition arises within the brain stem but is modulated by afferent information of which the most important is that from the lungs and carotid body. The excitability of this inspiratory off-switch (see below) is influenced by the rate and volume of inspiration; these features are reflected in the activity of the Iβ (Rβ) neurones of the dorsomedial group referred to above. The cutoff itself could similarly be effected by late-onset inspiration-related neurones such as are present in the dorsomedial and ventricle groups of respiratory neurones. However, the evidence appears to be mainly circumstantial.

Expiration. Inspiratory muscle activity continues into the early part of expiration when it opposes the expiratory effect of lung elasticity and slows the rate of expiration. The contraction is a positive feature of breathing and not a mere tailing off of the previous inspiration because it is associated with a switch in activity of premotor neurones; there is inhibition of neurones that fire during inspiration and activation of others that fire during early expiration. Expiratory muscles do not normally contract during this period but will do so if the drive to ventilation is increased. The contraction is accompanied by firing of expiratory premotor neurones in the *n*RA but the linkage is less strong than is the case for inspiration. The expiration related neuronal activity is increased in response to hypercapnia.

The duration of expiration (tE) is influenced by the Hering–Breuer mechanism (Section 23.3.2); it appears to vary with the integral of expired volume with respect to time during expiration. Expiratory time is therefore influenced by expiratory flow; the latter is a function of end inspiratory volume, the tailing off of inspiratory muscle activity and laryngeal calibre. The calibre in turn is under reflex control from pulmonary stretch receptors.

Respiratory rhythmicity. The mechanism of rhythm generation remains largely unknown. The best starting point is the model of von Euler [3] although it is no longer considered to be complete. In this model the drive to breathe is a continuous phenomenon which is inhibited periodically to allow expiration to take place in a mainly passive manner. The inhibition is by what has been termed an *inspiratory off-switch.* The inspiration is driven by a central inspiratory excitation that is determined by an inspiratory ramp generator. There is no equivalent expiratory drive so the system is asymmetrical. In this model the inspiratory activity originates in local neuronal circuits within the medulla. The circuits do not give rise to peaks of electrical activity so are not readily identifiable. Their location is not known but it probably includes the nucleus paragiganto cellularis lateralis (*n*PCL) which is near to the nucleus retrofacialis in the VRG. The *n*PCL adjoins the CO_2-sensitive region of the floor of the fourth ventricle and is connected to the *n*TS which in turn receives brainstem inputs from peripheral chemoreceptors. It also has rich connections with other brainstem nuclei and with the spinal cord. Some of the neurones contain serotonin, catecholamines, and other pharmacologically active substances. Inactivation of the nucleus by local cooling has been shown to cause apnoea.

The original von Euler model has been progressively elaborated so that there are now two main models of respiratory rhythmicity. The first is based upon cell network interactions i.e. neural networks. This model has two potential forms; the *bistable oscillator*, composed of two populations of inspiratory and expiratory neurones in which dominant activity periodically passes from one group to the other, and *inhibitory phasing,* in which rhythm is generated by inhibitory interneurones interacting with inspiratory neurones. This latter version is of interest because it does not entail active inhibition by expiratory neurones. The second model is based upon endogenously active pacemaker cells with an intrinsic respiratory pattern. Until recently this model has been considered to be attractive but virtually impossible to prove. However, an area close to the nucleus retrofacialis has been found to be necessary in the genesis and maintenance of respiratory rhythm; Smith and colleagues [2] demonstrated that in the neonatal rat rhythmic breathing ceased when the brainstem was sectioned immediately below the pre-Bötzinger complex, very near to the nucleus retrofacialis. Since then further studies have confirmed the pre-Bötzinger complex as a site of respiratory rhythm in the neonatal rat and cat, whether this area is as important in man remains unproven.

23.3 Peripheral neural inputs

23.3.1 Upper respiratory tract

Sensory information from the epithelium and mucosa of the nose, pharynx and larynx is supplied to the nuclei of the Bötzinger complex via the trigeminal and glossopharyngeal nerves and the nucleus of the tractus solitarius [4], (see also Table 3.2, page 29). The information provides the basis for sneezing, coughing and other reflexes, many of which have a protective role (Section 37.2.1).

23.3.2 Slowly adapting receptors

In most laboratory animals the principal inspiratory off-switch mechanism (see above) is the Hering–Breuer inflation reflex. The stimulus is lung inflation, primarily an increase in tension of the airway wall, which is detected by the slowly adapting stretch receptors (SARs, originally known as pulmonary stretch receptors). These are located close to smooth muscle cells in both the extra- and intrathoracic lower airways. The information is transmitted up the vagi and leads to a reflex inhibition of inspiratory motor output and prolongation of the subsequent expiration. It also influences the calibre of the larynx and trachea. The response is modified by the action of pulmonary C-fibre receptors (also called J receptors; see below).

The Hering–Breuer reflex is well developed in many mammals and in newborn babies. In adults the inhibition has a high threshold and is normally only demonstrable at tidal volumes in excess of 1 l [5], despite the receptors themselves responding to all levels of volume change. In some mammalian species vagotomy results in greater tidal volumes and a slower respiratory rate. In man, denervation of the lungs as occurs during heart-lung transplantation is not associated with any apparent deviation from the normal pattern of resting ventilation either when the subject is awake or during the several stages of sleep [6]. These latter observations weaken the von Euler hypothesis for respiratory regulation as applied to man. However, the major role which the hypothesis attributes to the stretch receptors might be shared with tendon organs and other non-pulmonary afferents; if so, this has still to be demonstrated. The threshold for activation of the reflex may not hold for the calibres of the larynx and trachea which have been shown to be regulated by the Hering–Breuer mechanism at all levels of tidal volume [7].

The Hering–Breuer inflation reflex is inactivated by inhalation of local anaesthetic aerosol or carbon dioxide in high concentration. It is facilitated by an increase in the rate of rise in central inspiratory activity such as occurs with hyperthermia, and also by vibration applied to the chest wall, presumably via activation of intercostal muscle spindles. The response to vibration can also include a reduction in ventilation minute volume [8]. Both types of stimuli increase the frequency of breathing by reducing the duration of inspiration. A similar reduction does not occur with hypoxia, hypercapnia or exercise; instead an increase in central inspiratory activity from these causes appears to raise the threshold volume at which the inflation reflex operates.

23.3.3 Rapidly adapting receptors

These receptors were originally described as mechanoreceptors excited by lung hyperinflation [9]. They were subsequently shown to be stimulated by rapid deflation, pneumothorax, and particularly by lung irritants [10], hence they became known as lung irritant receptors. However, these rapidly adapting receptors (RARs) are probably mechanoreceptors like the SARs, with the two groups being at opposite ends of one continuum [11].

The RARs are found in the airway epithelium from the trachea to the respiratory bronchioles, and the reflex responses depend to some degree on their location. When stimulated the receptors fire rapidly and then quickly accommodate. Stimulation of those in the trachea and upper airways produces bronchoconstriction, increased mucus production and possibly coughing. Stimulation of those in the more distal airways reduces the duration of the respiratory cycle but may increase ventilation by an increase in phrenic nerve activity and an increase in deadspace ventilation resulting from the shallow, rapid breathing (tachypnœa).

23.3.4 C-fibre endings

Receptors served by small non-myelinated nerve fibres in the vagi also contribute to the control of breathing. Evidence for their presence in the lung parenchyma was obtained by Paintal who called them juxta-pulmonary capillary or J-receptors [11], but receptors with similar innervation and function also occur in the airways; they have been respectively designated as either pulmonary or bronchial C-fibre receptors [12] depending upon position and accessibility. The receptors contribute afferent information to the central pattern generator but the response is to some extent masked by that to the slowly adapting stretch receptors; it becomes apparent when the latter are blocked by cooling the vagi to 4–8°C. Vagal cooling leads to a shortening of the time of expiration and an increase in minute volume. This response was first observed but misinterpreted by Head who, in 1889 [13] described a paradoxical inspiratory response to lung inflation after cooling the vagi; some of the effects formerly attributed to slowly adapting pulmonary stretch receptors (SAR) are in fact due to C-fibre receptors. The SARs contribute to tachypnoea by shortening the time of inspiration, the C-fibre receptors do so by shortening the time of expiration.

Pulmonary C-fibres (J-receptors) are stimulated by pulmonary congestion, embolism and infection and by a number of chemical substances (Table 23.1). The response is an inspiratory

Table 23.1 Conditions that can activate bronchial and/or pulmonary C-fibre receptors.

*Intrapulmonary condition**	*Lung autocoids*†
Diffuse pulmonary infiltration	Bradykinin
Increased pulmonary blood flow	Histamine‡
Lung inflation	Prostaglandins‡ ($F_2\alpha$, E_1, E_2, I_2 etc)
Pulmonary anaphylaxis	Serotonin
Pulmonary embolism‡	
Pulmonary inflammation	*Other substances*
Pulmonary oedema	Ammonia‡
Raised pulmonary venous pressure‡	Capsicum‡
	Carbon dioxide
*Anaesthetic agents**	Chlorine
Chloroform	Ozone*
Ether	Phenyl diguanide‡¶
Halothane	Sodium dithionite
Trichlorethylene	Sulphur dioxide†‡
	Tobacco smoke†‡

* Mainly pulmonary receptors (J receptors).
† Mainly bronchial receptors.
‡ Irritant receptors also active.
¶ Effect not demonstrable in man.
Source: [12].

apnoea followed by rapid shallow breathing; in addition there is usually bradycardia and hypotension. Bronchoconstriction, somatic motor inhibition and increased airway secretion can also occur. The initial apnoea is due to generalised inhibition of respiratory activity involving the inspiratory and expiratory premotor neurones in the *n*TS and motor neurones supplying the intercostal muscles. The mechanism of the subsequent shortening of the time of expiration appears not to have been established. Stimulation of C-fibre receptors causes the shallow rapid breathing, in many abnormal conditions of the lung parenchyma (e.g. Figs 28.11 and 28.12, pages 397 and 398) and in left heart failure.

During breathing carbon dioxide C-fibre receptors contribute to the increase in frequency of breathing. The frequency is therefore increased by cooling the vagi to block afferent fibres from pulmonary stretch receptors, and decreased only when all vagal afferents are interrupted. However, the mechanism whereby carbon dioxide activates the C-fibre receptors is not known. By contrast during exercise there is evidence for the C-fibre activity being increased by the increase in pulmonary blood flow; even so, there appears to be only inferential evidence that C-fibre receptors contribute to exercise tachypnoea secondary to pulmonary congestion.

23.3.5 Spinal mechanisms

The efferent nerve impulses from the respiratory reticular formation converge upon the respiratory motor neurones in the spinal cord; here they summate with excitatory impulses from other sources including Golgi tendon organs and muscle spindles in the intercostal muscles and diaphragm. The tendon organs are tension receptors. They provide a safety mechanism whereby an undue increase in tension in an intercostal muscle can inhibit the α motor neurone that is causing the muscle to contract. The tendon organs also supply information to higher centres in the brain stem. By this route they may contribute to the inspiratory off-switch mechanism.

The muscle spindles, abundant in the intercostals, are effectively length receptors; they consist of sensory nerve endings joined to small muscle fibres enclosed in a fusiform sheath

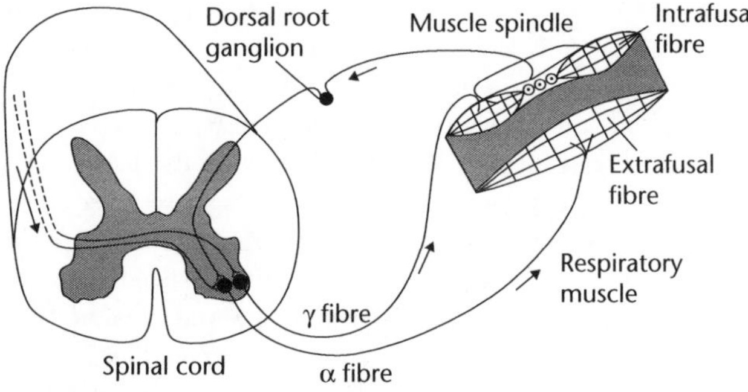

Fig. 23.2 Diagram illustrating the role of muscle spindles in regulating the contraction of respiratory muscles. See text for details.

(Fig. 23.2). The endings respond to stretching of the central portion of the spindle. The intrafusal muscle fibres are innervated from the spinal cord by unmyelinated fibres from γ motor neurones. The sensory endings communicate through afferent nerves with the α motor neurones in the spinal cord that supply the respiratory muscles. This arrangement provides the basis for a local control mechanism whereby the intensity of contraction of the respiratory muscles is tightly regulated with respect to local events in the lungs and thorax [14].

At the start of inspiration nerve impulses from the respiratory reticular formation activate both γ and α motor neurones. The discharge of the γ motor neurones leads to contraction of the intrafusal muscle fibres; this causes traction on the sensory endings in the spindles. Concurrently the discharge of the α motor neurones contracts the extrafusal fibres of the respiratory muscles. When the contraction is accompanied by shortening of the muscle, the length of the spindle, and hence the traction which is exerted on the sensory ending, is reduced. The discharge from the ending reflects the balance between the two forces. When the shortening of the extrafusal fibres lags behind that of the spindles the discharge from the sensory endings stimulates the α motor neurones to increase the strength of contraction of the respiratory muscles.

When the respiratory muscles shorten at a greater rate than the spindles the stimulation of the α motor neurones is reduced. In this way the strength of the contraction of the respiratory muscles is modified by the extent to which it causes the required chest wall movement. In man these responses have a latency of 33 ms to 85 ms [15], which is shorter than the minimum voluntary reaction time; their effect is to stabilize the lung volume or the rate of change of lung volume against the mechanical load which is applied. The muscle spindles can also be stimulated by vibration applied to the chest wall; by this means they can contribute to the inspiratory off-switch mechanism (Section 23.3.4).

23.4 Central chemoreceptors

Structural aspects. The central inspiratory activity is augmented by tonic stimulation from chemosensitive areas present on the ventrolateral surface of the medulla [16]. These areas, the extent of which is still in some doubt [17, 18], appear to be organised into three chemoresponsive regions. One is located rostrally and another more caudally; the third, intermediate region, on the basis of experiments involving suppression of activity by cooling, has been argued to be either part of a signal pathway [19, 20] or a site close to the principle areas of respiratory activity [21].

Central response to hypercapnia. The gross chemosensitive areas have been identified, but the actual chemosensitive cells have not; indeed, even the mechanism by which the signal is developed remains in doubt. Both hydrogen ion concentration and tension of CO_2 appear to be effective stimuli, although it is generally accepted that the hydrogen ion is the actual agent and the action of CO_2 is through the production of H^+ via carbonic acid. The response is transmitted via cholinergic nerves that are stimulated by acetyl choline. The response to hydrogen ions is blocked by atropine. It is also blocked by cooling or applying local anaesthetic to the adjacent surface of the medulla, this projects to the nucleus paragiganto cellularis (*n*PGC), the retrofacial nucleus (*n*RF) and the nucleus of the tractus solitarius (*n*TS). The signal here summates with afferent information from other sources including the skeletal muscles [21]. The action of the central chemoreceptors has the effect of protecting the central nervous system from changes in hydrogen ion concentration including those that result from strenuous exercise (Section 28.4.6). The chemoreceptors themselves are not in direct contact with the arterial blood but are surrounded by brain extracellular fluid (ECF) that is in direct contact with cerebrospinal fluid (CSF). The arterial blood is kept separate by the blood–brain barrier. The barrier is readily permeable to CO_2 but effectively impermeable to bicarbonate, lactic acid and other fixed acids. Stimulation of the central chemoreceptors depends therefore upon the H^+ concentration of brain ECF; this is determined by the Henderson-Hasselbalch equation via CO_2 and HCO_3^- since there is little other buffering (eqn. 7.16, page 70). The importance of the CSF and hence the ECF was demonstrated by Leusen [22]. This work lead to the concept of a relatively superficial chemoreceptor, not one deeply situated in the medulla as are the respiratory centres.

Central effects of hypoxia. After inactivation of the peripheral (carotid) chemoreceptors, hypoxia depresses central inspiratory activity, reduces tidal volume and can cause a tachypnoea resembling that associated with hyperthermia (Section 36.1). The respiratory depression is not as a result of a direct action on specific oxygen chemoreceptors, but has been postulated to be due to hyperpolarisation of respiratory neurones caused by changes in concentration of neurotransmitter substances. Hypoxia reduces the concentrations of excitatory neurotransmitters, including monoamines and acetylcholine, whilst the concentrations of the inhibitory substances such as γ aminobutyric acid (GABA), adenosine and endogenous opioids are increased. The importance of substances such as GABA in this role [23] have been questioned, and the magnitude of the hypoxic respiratory depression ascribed to washout of CO_2 at the site of the central chemoreceptors due to an increase in cerebral blood flow [24].

The actions of the inhibitory neurotransmitters can be reduced by antagonists that block the relevant receptors (Table 23.2). These blocking agents have each been shown to partially

Table 23.2 Some mediators of hypoxic respiratory depression.

Mediator	Antagonist
γ-Aminobutyric acid (GABA)*	Bicuculline
Adenosine	Theophylline
Endogenous opioids	Naloxone

* synthesis is enhanced and degradation impeded by lactacidosis.

reverse the hypoxic depression, which is therefore presumably due to more than one inhibitor. The site of this hypoxic depression overlies the central chemoreceptors. However, whilst the depression affects the level of inspiratory activity, there is a normal increase in response to a rise in P_{CO_2} or H^+; the sensitivity of the central receptors to hypercapnia is not affected by hypoxia.

In adults central hypoxic depression of respiration occurs only with severe hypoxia and is normally more than compensated for by the drive from the peripheral chemoreceptors. By contrast, in the newborn respiratory depression can occur with lesser degrees of hypoxaemia; the depression can be alleviated by naloxone, which is evidence for it being due in part to endogenous opioids. The production of these opioids is stimulated by some anaesthetic agents, and by high tensions of carbon dioxide. For this reason naloxone can alleviate carbon dioxide narcosis (Section 35.7.2). Endorphines also contribute to the respiratory depression observed in patients with a very high airway resistance (Section 40.3), but endogenous opioids do not contribute to the control of breathing in normal circumstances.

23.5 Peripheral chemoreceptors (carotid and aortic bodies)

23.5.1 Physiology

The partial pressures of oxygen, carbon dioxide and/or hydrogen ion concentration in arterial blood are monitored by the carotid and the aortic bodies. These are small nodes that are closely related to the carotid bulb and to the arch of the aorta from which they obtain a rich blood supply. The function of the aortic bodies is similar to that of the carotid bodies, but they contribute very little to respiratory control; the following therefore relates to the carotid body whose function was suggested by de Castro [25] in 1926 and confirmed by Heymans four years later [26].

Functional anatomy. Information on arterial P_{CO_2}, P_{O_2} and pH is transmitted via the carotid sinus nerves to the *n*TS and other centres in the brain (Fig. 23.1). By this means the carotid bodies contribute a chemoreceptor drive to respiration; this has been investigated in depth and is described below. The mechanism of chemoreception, however, is poorly understood. The node diameter is normally 1–2 mm but it is increased by chronic hypoxia such as occurs as a result of residence at high altitude (Section 34.2) or chronic lung disease. The nodes have a glomerular structure with a connective tissue casing containing clusters of cells surrounded and invaded by large glomerular capillaries. The capillaries can be bypassed by arterio-venous anastomoses. The glomerular cells are of two types. The type I cells are relatively large (diameter 8–12 μm), have vesicles containing many types of neurotransmitters in their cytoplasm, make contact with other type I cells and have a rich covering of nerve endings; a single nerve fibre may innervate several cell clusters, some type I cells may have terminals from different fibres. Most of the nerve endings arise from sensory neurones with cell bodies located in the petrosal ganglion of the glossopharyngeal nerve (9th cranial nerve). The type II cells have long thin cytoplasmic processes that envelop and insinuate between type I cells; they resemble the Schwann cells that protect and nourish nerve axons. Blood flow is high, as is oxygen consumption. This is generally taken to be indicative of intense metabolic activity. The blood vessels are innervated from the superior cervical ganglion of the sympathetic nervous system and local parasympathetic ganglion cells that are supplied by the carotid sinus branch of the glossopharyngeal nerve [27].

Role of glomus cells. The glomus cells have a high metabolic rate and require a high ambient oxygen tension for the full oxygenation of their contained cytochrome. Therefore, they become short of oxygen when the tension in the arterial blood is reduced or the flow of blood to the capillary network is decreased. Either event leads to non-aerobic metabolism in the node and local production of metabolites that stimulate the adjacent nerve endings. The release of these transmitter substances is Ca_2^+ dependent [27].

A number of transmitter substances appear to contribute to the response. Dopamine is released from the glomus cells in response to hypoxia but has a mainly inhibitory effect on chemoreceptor activity. [28, 29]. By contrast the effects of released noradrenaline and adenosine [30] are mainly excitatory. The noradrenaline probably acts by altering the distribution of blood flow within the glomeruli. This increases the sensitivity to hypoxia and hypercapnia and contributes to the increase in ventilation that occurs during exercise (see also [31]).

The glomus cells also contain catecholamines, encephalins, vasoactive intestinal peptides and substance P that are released by hypoxia; the encephalins reduce and the latter two substances enhance the ventilatory response to hypoxia. Recent studies have suggested that nitric oxide (NO) and carbon monoxide (CO) may also have a role in chemoreception and be produced within the carotid body [32, 33]. Thus, the glomus cells contain many potential transmitter substances and some or all of them are likely to contribute to signal transduction and/or transmission.

Role of carotid sinus nerves. The type I cells or the adjacent nerve endings respond to hypoxia, hypercapnia and pH, but are considered to be effective O_2 receptors in that the primary response to CO_2 and pH is centrally mediated (see Section 23.4). Lack of oxygen increases the rate of firing of afferent nerve fibres in the carotid sinus nerves. Most of the fibres are myelinated but non-myelinated fibres also respond. The association between the nerve discharge and oxygen tension is weak at tensions in excess of approximately 13 kPa (100 mm Hg). Below this level the rate of firing varies inversely with oxygen tension. The rate is also influenced by the coexisting arterial tension of carbon dioxide and/or concentration of hydrogen ions. When these are increased the response to hypoxia is augmented in a multiplicative fashion; when they are reduced the response to hypoxia is diminished or absent. The response to hypoxia is therefore markedly affected by the prevailing level of CO_2 and pH [27]. However, for the response to hypoxia to be suppressed the carbon dioxide tension must be very low. It should be noted that the receptors are responsive to the partial pressure (tension) of the gases, not the concentration.

The response latency is of the order of 0.3 s and the time to peak nerve discharge in the range 1 s–3 s. The pattern of firing is mainly random but exhibits a periodicity at the frequency of breathing up to a maximum of 20 min^{-1} for oxygen and 70 min^{-1} for carbon dioxide and/or hydrogen ion concentration [34]. The oscillations contribute to the regulation of breathing (see below). As well as hypoxic hypoxia the chemoreceptors respond to stagnant hypoxia associated with a reduction in systemic blood pressure and histotoxic hypoxia such as follows the administration of cyanide. There is little response to a reduction in delivery of oxygen caused by anaemia or inhalation of carbon monoxide (Section 37.4.1).

23.5.2 Chemoreceptor drive to respiration: introduction

Lack of oxygen in the arterial blood depresses the central nervous system; at the same time it increases the flow of sensory information from the chemoreceptors. Hyperoxia has the opposite effect. Abrupt changes in the concentration of oxygen in the inspired gas are followed within a few seconds by changes in ventilation; the latter initially mirror the changes in chemoreceptor activity (Fig. 23.3).

The immediate changes in ventilation that follow a step change in the $P\text{I}O_2$ are subsequently diminished, or even reversed, by changes in the tension of carbon dioxide that are secondary to the change in ventilation. The secondary adjustments are most marked at rest when they lead to the steady-state ventilation during moderate hypoxaemia not being materially changed compared with breathing air, whilst during oxygen breathing the ventilation is usually increased. The changes that underlie this paradoxical behaviour are illustrated in Fig. 23.4.

Inhalation of gas low in oxygen causes an immediate increase in ventilation; this then increases the excretion of carbon dioxide from the lung and reduces the tension of carbon dioxide in arterial blood. As a result the stimulus to inspiration from carbon dioxide decreases, and the ventilation declines towards that obtained when breathing air. Converse changes occur during the inhalation of 100% oxygen; there is then an immediate decrease in ventilation minute volume, resulting in less carbon dioxide being excreted and a rise in the tension of carbon dioxide in the arterial blood, stimulating breathing. The rise in the tension of carbon dioxide also dilates cerebral arterioles and increases the flow of blood to the brain. This change causes a rise in cerebral PO_2, which is in addition to that due to the initial enrichment of the inspired gas with oxygen. The two processes combine to increase the concentration of oxyhaemoglobin in the blood in the cerebral capillaries; less reduced haemoglobin is then available to take up and transport carbon dioxide from the brain in the

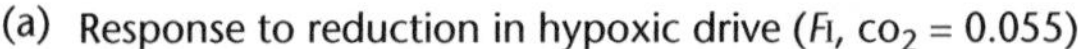

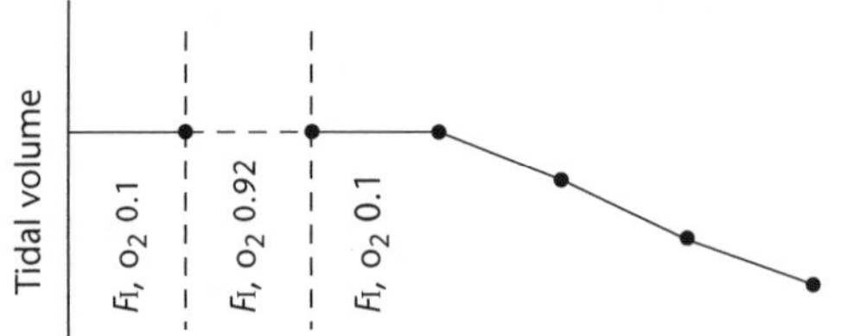

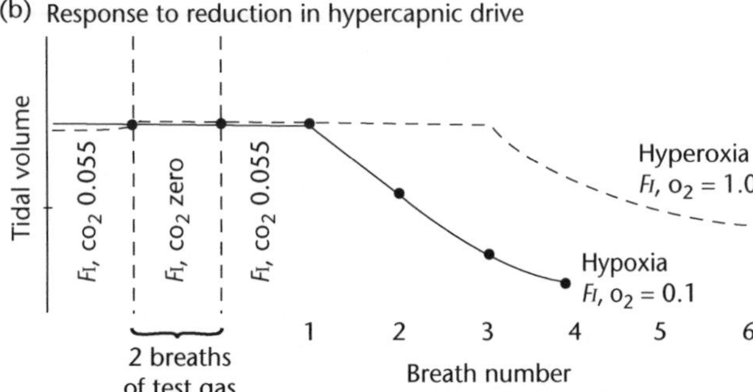

Fig. 23.3 Response of ventilation to a brief change in the concentration of oxygen or carbon dioxide in inspired gas. In (a) the carbon dioxide is held constant whilst the oxygen is increased sufficiently to greatly reduce the peripheral chemoreceptor drive. The reduction in ventilation is detectable two breaths later. In (b) the oxygen is held constant whilst the carbon dioxide is reduced. During hypoxia, when the chemoreceptor drive is intact, the reduction in ventilation is again detectable two breaths later: when the peripheral chemoreceptor drive is eliminated by breathing oxygen, the reduction is only detectable after four breaths. The delay represents the additional time needed for the blood to reach the central chemoreceptors. Source: [35].

form of carbamino-haemoglobin. The tension of carbon dioxide in the medulla rises in consequence and this further increases the hypercapnoeic drive to respiration. At rest, the increase more than compensates for the reduction in peripheral chemoreceptor drive caused by the hyperoxia; as a result, the steady-state ventilation at rest when breathing oxygen exceeds that when breathing air by about 2 l min^{-1}.

During exercise the factors that contribute to transport of carbon dioxide are similar to those at rest. However, the chemoreceptor drive is increased by a rise in blood noradrenaline and other factors (see above). When oxygen is administered during exercise, the reduction in chemoreceptor drive exceeds the gain in hypercapnoeic drive so ventilation decreases and the tension of carbon dioxide rises. The rise can be material, of the order of 1.3 kPa (10 torr), and occurs in patients with lung disease as well as healthy subjects. The hypercapnia is therefore evidence for the material role of chemoreceptor drive in regulating the respiration during exercise.

The signal from the chemoreceptors is in the form of afferent discharges in the carotid sinus nerves. These reflect the mean gas tensions in the arterial blood and the fluctuations that occur between inspiration and expiration (Fig. 23.5). Changes in the mean level of discharge are responsible for much of the chemoreceptor drive to respiration, but it has also been suggested that oscillations in the partial pressures of the gas can contribute materially [34, 37].

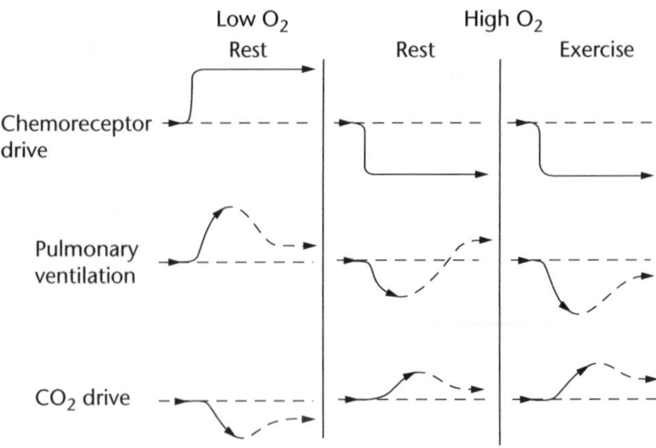

Fig. 23.4 The sequence of events following a change in the chemoreceptor drive to respiration. Inspiration of gas deficient in oxygen increases the drive; this stimulates respiration, washes out carbon dioxide and decreases the overall stimulus to breathing. The ventilation then declines to a new equilibrium value where the increased chemoreceptor drive is nearly offset by the reduced drive from carbon dioxide. When breathing oxygen converse changes take place. However, they are partly offset by a concurrent increase in the carbon dioxide drive due to a reduction in the buffering capacity of blood perfusing the brain. At rest this change causes an increase in the ventilation above that when breathing air. On exercise the effect is concealed by the relatively greater importance of the chemoreceptor drive.

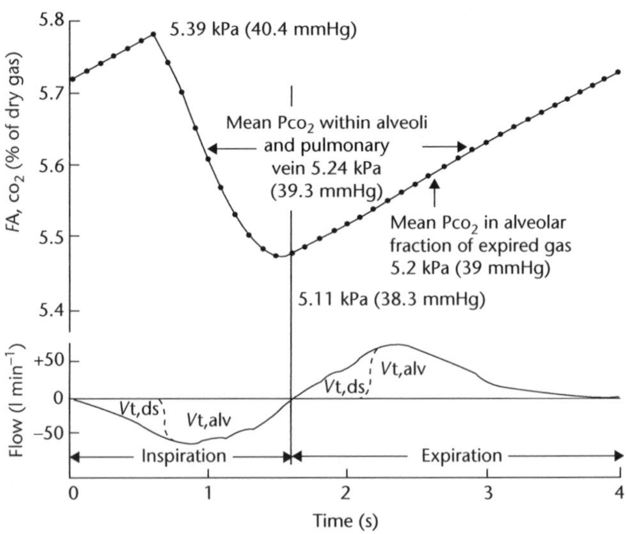

Fig. 23.5 Alveolar carbon dioxide tension (P_{A,CO_2}) over one respiratory cycle showing a linear rise during the expiratory phase. The lower tracing shows that to obtain the mean P_{A,CO_2} the optimal time for sampling the alveolar gas is shortly after mid expiration. $V_{t,ds}$ and $V_{t,alv}$ are respectively the deadspace and alveolar fractions of the tidal volume. Source: [36].

It has been shown that the timing of the peak discharge in relation to the breathing cycle can influence respiration. Peaks in late expiration or early inspiration prolong the relevant inspiration whilst peaks at other times prolong the next post-expiratory pause. The mechanism may contribute to control of breathing during sleep and when the rhythm of breathing is disturbed by speech or coughing. The frequency of discharge increases during the upstroke of the $P\text{a},CO_2$ oscillation seen during exercise and this could contribute to the increase in ventilation (cf. Table 28.4, page 396). Chemoreceptor drive is also important when the central drive to respiration is reduced or the ability of the respiratory apparatus to increase ventilation is impaired. In such circumstances respiration may depend solely upon the chemoreceptor drive; if this is removed by administration of oxygen the breathing becomes reduced and may cease altogether (Section 35.7.2).

23.5.3 Hypercapnoeic drive

The hypercapnoeic drive to respiration is mediated via the carotid and central chemoreceptors (Fig. 23.3). There may also be receptors that monitor the tension of carbon dioxide in pulmonary venous blood. Similar receptors exist in birds and their presence in mammals has been deduced from the discharge pattern of selected single fibres in the vagus nerve. However, no pulmonary chemoreceptors have yet been found in man and study of patients following heart lung transplantation does not suggest a role for such receptors in the control of breathing. The effective stimulus to the known receptors is either $P\text{CO}_2$ or hydrogen ion concentration at the receptor site, and the response is critically influenced by the coexisting $P\text{O}_2$. For peripheral chemoreceptors either CO_2 tension or hydrogen ion concentration is an effective stimulus; the response is dependent on and interacts with that of oxygen. This is discussed below. For central chemoreceptors the usual stimulus is $P\text{CO}_2$ because the CO_2 readily diffuses to the receptor site; it is independent of oxygen tension except to the extent that hypoxaemia depresses central nervous activity. However, the response is modulated by concurrent changes in blood flow to the central medulla which appears to be more sensitive to hypoxia and hypercapnia (both of which cause vasodilatation) than blood flow to other parts of the brain.

Study of the ventilation responses to carbon dioxide is complicated by the responses being influenced by the way in which the gas is administered. Rebreathing from a bag containing high oxygen levels produces progressively increasing hypercapnia with hyperoxia. The peripheral chemoreceptors are suppressed by the hyperoxia and therefore do not contribute.

The response is that to $P\text{CO}_2$ levels at the central chemoreceptors (Section 23.4). It relates to conditions of hyperoxia when the buffering of carbon dioxide by haemoglobin is reduced (Section 22.2.3). In contrast, breathing mixtures of carbon dioxide in air stimulates both central and peripheral chemoreceptors; however, the resulting increase in ventilation raises the alveolar oxygen tension and hence reduces the hypoxic drive unless the inspired oxygen tension is adjusted concurrently. In addition, the increase in ventilation proportionally increases the carbon dioxide delivered to the lungs, which delays the attainment of a steady state for up to 20 min. During this time the renal excretion of bicarbonate is increased; as a consequence if several gas mixtures are used consecutively the resulting acid–base changes can modify the ventilatory response. A few decades ago Cummin and colleagues [38] reintroduced an alternative technique in which the quantity of additional CO_2 (the CO_2 mass load) was constant and independent of the ventilatory response. This technique appears capable of further application.

Hypercapnoeic drive extends over a wide range of tensions of carbon dioxide from an upper limit when carbon dioxide depresses central nervous activity to a lower limit when the ventilation is apparently independent of the carbon dioxide tension. Respiratory depression occurs as a result of inhaling high concentrations of carbon dioxide ($F\text{I},CO_2 > 0.08$). Dissociation of ventilation from carbon dioxide tension occurs following voluntary over-breathing which increases the elimination of CO_2 and lowers the alveolar carbon dioxide tension. In between these limits the ventilatory response to hypercapnia can be described by a linear equation:

$$\dot{V}\text{A} = S(P_\text{A}, \text{CO}_2 - B) \tag{23.1}$$

where A is alveolar ventilation (l min^{-1}), $P\text{A},CO_2$ is alveolar carbon dioxide tension (kPa or torr) and S and B are constants. Whilst breathing air, the sensitivity to carbon dioxide (S) is normally in the range 7.5–52 $\text{l min}^{-1}\ \text{kPa}^{-1}$ (1.0–7.0 $\text{l min}^{-1}\ \text{mm Hg}^{-1}$). The constant term B is approximately 4.7 kPa (35 mm Hg). The respiratory sensitivity to carbon dioxide varies inversely with the tension of oxygen (Fig. 23.6).

The respiratory sensitivity to CO_2 (S) is also affected by other circumstances of which some are shown in Fig. 23.7, for example the sensitivity (top left panel) is increased in response to noradrenaline, progesterone, almetrine, persistent hyperventilation, a reduction in carotid blood flow and following administration of neurotransmitter substances (see above Role of glomus cells). Reductions in sensitivity occur during sleep and anaesthesia and with propranolol, dopamine, encephalins and other substances. It is also reduced when the work of ventilating the lung is increased as a result of disease of the lung or the chest wall. However, if the disease process affects only the mechanical functions of the lung and not the control system, the response will be within normal limits when expressed in terms of the work that is performed on the lung (Fig. 23.8, also Section 9.7.1).

The intercept B is related to the concentration of bicarbonate in blood plasma (Fig. 23.7, top right panel); it is reduced when bicarbonate is decreased by metabolic acidosis or by persistent over-breathing such as occurs at high altitude, in pregnancy and with some diseases of the lung parenchyma. It is also reduced by exercise. The threshold is increased by the ingestion of bicarbonate or by a depression of respiration sufficient to cause the retention of carbon dioxide in the arterial blood such as occurs,

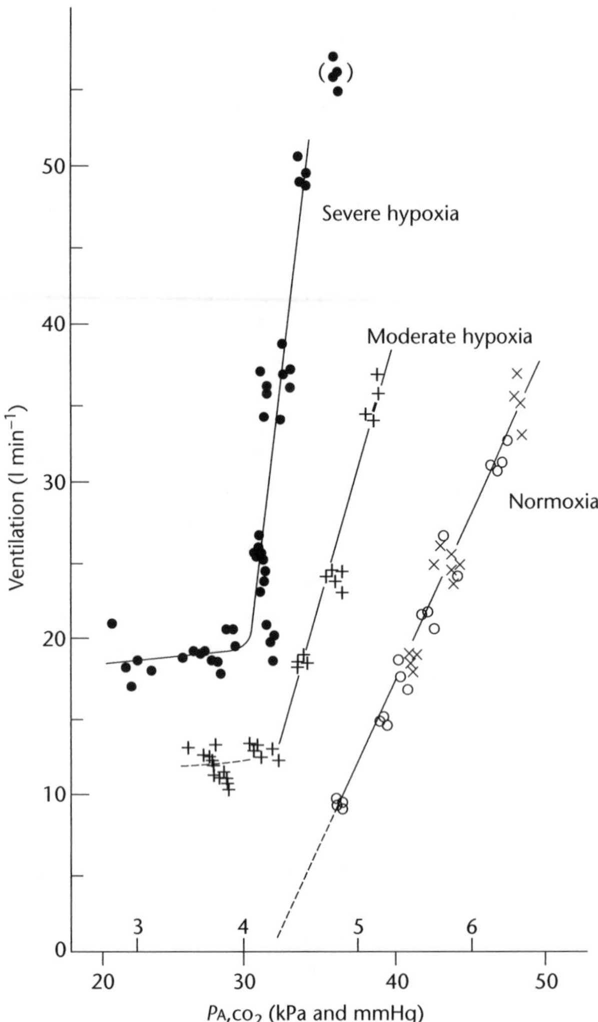

Fig. 23.6 Relationship of ventilation to alveolar tension of carbon dioxide (P_{A,CO_2}) under steady state conditions of severe hypoxia (P_{A,O_2}, 4.9 kPa, 37 torr), moderate hypoxia (P_{A,O_2}, 6.3 kPa, 47 torr) and normoxia. During hypocapnoeic hypoxia the ventilation is nearly independent of P_{A,CO_2}. Source: [39]

for example, in some patients with an obstructive type of ventilatory defect. The threshold is increased during sleep as a result of the administration of sedative drugs, including morphine and codeine. It is also affected by changes in the concentration of hydrogen ions in arterial blood. The intercept is independent of oxygen tension and many of the other factors that influence respiratory sensitivity.

23.5.4 Hypoxic drive

The response of ventilation to hypoxic drive from peripheral chemoreceptors can be described in terms of the factors A and C of Lloyd and Cunningham that are illustrated in Fig. 23.7; their measurement is given in Section 23.9. The factors have values that are usually of the order of 2.7 to 6.7 kPa (20–50 torr). A reduced response is a feature of the people who are born and grow up at high altitude, subjects with mountain sickness and patients with cyanotic congenital heart disease (Sections 34.2 to 34.5). An intermediate response is observed in some athletes. The response to hypoxia is less labile than that to hypercapnia, e.g. it is not affected by an alteration in the acid–base balance of the blood and is relatively less affected by partial obstruction to the lung airways. At the onset of isocapnœic hypoxia there is a brisk ventilatory response that declines after a few minutes to an intermediate level. The initial decline appears to be due to adenosine exerting a central inhibitory action; the inhibition can be reversed by aminophylline acting as an adenosine antagonist. The residual response appears not to adapt with time, consequently the chemoreceptor drive continues to operate when the activity of the respiratory centre is depressed by narcotic agents or cerebral hypoxia to the extent that carbon dioxide no longer exerts its central stimulant effect. In these unfavourable circumstances the maintenance of spontaneous respiration depends entirely upon the chemoreceptor drive.

23.6 Unifying theories of chemical control

The increase in ventilation produced by an increase in CO_2, the injection of acids and the production of lactate all have in common an increase in H^+. The demonstration of areas in the central nervous system responsive to H^+ stimuli led to the view that H^+ was the origin of chemical drive [42]. This was later modified to account for the ventilatory response to altitude and eventually for the discovery by Heymans of the peripheral chemoreceptors [43, 44]. This Reaction Theory, as it was termed, was effectively ignored as efforts were made to describe the interactions of CO_2, oxygen and H^+ upon ventilation [45]. Thus, Gray introduced the Multiple Factor Theory [46] that described ventilation in the steady state as being the resultant of an additive interaction, viz:

$$\text{Ventilation} = 0.22[H^+] + 2.62 P_{CO_2} - 18 + 2.118 \times 10^{-8}(104 - P_{O_2})^{4.9} \quad (23.2)$$

Lloyd and Cunningham have subsequently used the following empirical, hyperbolic equation, by which ventilation is the resultant of a multiplicative interaction:

$$\text{Ventilation} = D[A/(Pa, o_2 - C) + f](Pa, co_2 - B) \quad (23.3)$$

where the ventilation minute volume in l BTPS min^{-1}, P_{a,O_2} and P_{a,CO_2}, in kPa (or mm Hg) are the tensions of oxygen and carbon dioxide in arterial blood and B is the intercept for carbon dioxide (see above). D is the ventilatory response to carbon dioxide in oxygen and has the units litres BTPS min^{-1} kPa^{-1} (or mm Hg^{-1}), A is the tension of oxygen at which the response to carbon dioxide is twice that which obtains when breathing 100% oxygen and C is the tension of oxygen at which the stimulant effect of hypoxaemia

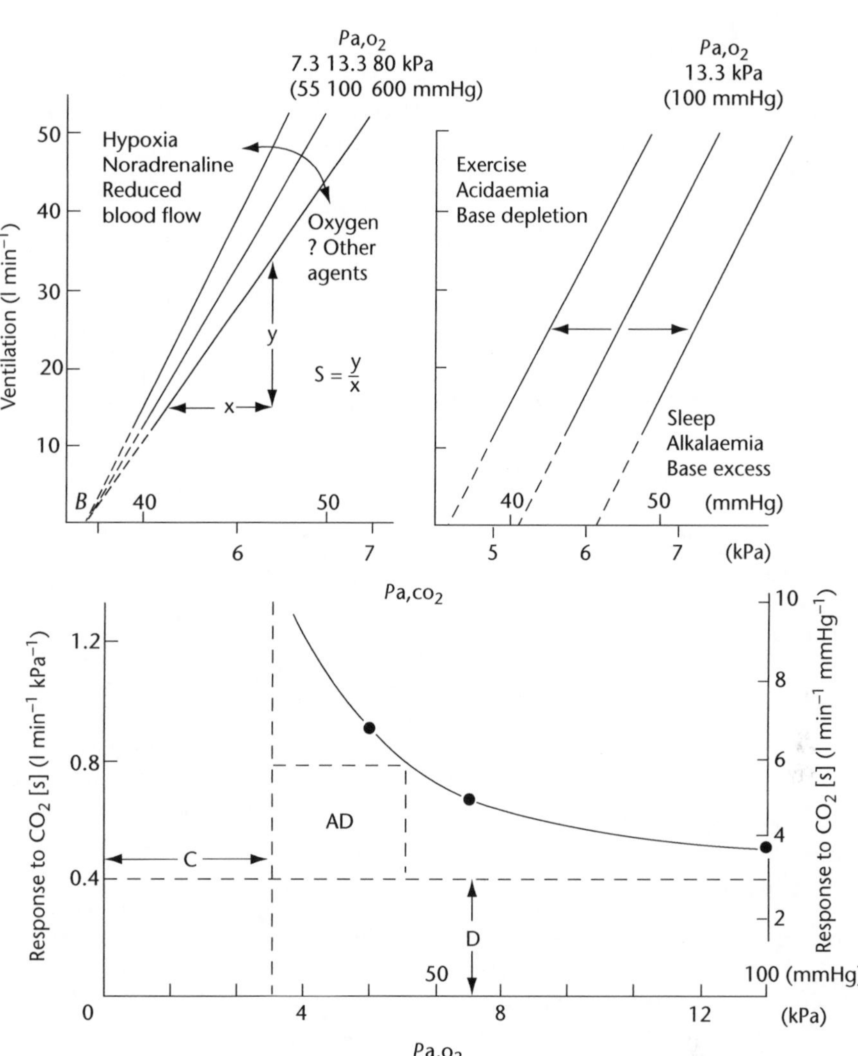

Fig. 23.7 Top: The relationship of the ventilation minute volume to the end-tidal or arterial tension of carbon dioxide for a subject breathing mixtures of CO_2 and O_2 in nitrogen. On the left the regression lines for different tensions of oxygen converge on the point B. The response to carbon dioxide (S) at any tension of oxygen is calculated in the manner indicated. On the right are some factors that determine the value for B under steady state conditions. Somewhat higher values obtain during rebreathing. Bottom: The relationship of the response to carbon dioxide (S) to the tension of oxygen. D is the response of ventilation to carbon dioxide when the subject is breathing gas containing oxygen in a fractional concentration of approximately 0.95. C is the oxygen tension at which the response to carbon dioxide is infinite and A is another factor that describes the response of ventilation to hypoxaemia. Source: [40].

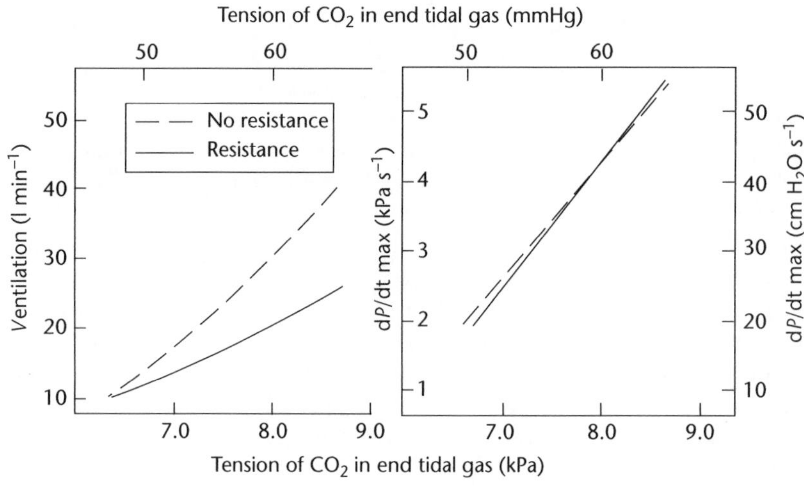

Fig. 23.8 Effect of respiratory resistance upon the ventilation minute volume and the (dP/dt)max during rebreathing carbon dioxide in oxygen. Source: [41].

reaches its maximal value. The tension C is believed to be that at which there is a zero tension of oxygen in the chemoreceptor cells. The constant f is 7.5 in SI units and 1.0 in traditional units. The term within the right-hand bracket is the effective stimulus to respiration by carbon dioxide. The remaining terms (illustrated in the lower part of Fig. 23.7) describe the response of the subject to this stimulus under the conditions of measurement.

The factor D, which is the ventilatory response to hyperoxic hypercapnia, is usually in the range 5–22.5 $\mathrm{l\,min^{-1}\,kPa^{-1}}$ (0.7–3.0 $\mathrm{l\,min^{-1}\,mm\,Hg^{-1}}$). The response is related to the vital capacity of the subject and for men and women of European descent may, on average, be described by the following relationship:

$$D = 7.5[0.89 + 0.35\,\mathrm{VC}\ \mathrm{SD}\,0.58]\,\mathrm{l\,min^{-1}\,kPa^{-1}} \qquad (23.4)$$

where VC is the vital capacity in litres and 7.5 converts between SI and traditional units. For people of some other ethnic groups the value for D is reduced (Section 27.1.6).

The central role of H^+ as the principal if not the sole determinant of central chemoreceptor stimulation is now widely accepted, but the position with regard to the peripheral chemoreceptors is still controversial.

23.7 Behavioural control

23.7.1 Volitional breathing

Breathing is generated, and ultimately controlled, through activities in the brainstem, but it is modulated volitionally, e.g. to subserve speech, for defaecation, in emotive circumstances and during breath holding. Some of these activities entail higher centre control by the motor cortex.

The representation of respiratory muscles in the primary motor cortex in humans was suggested in 1936 by Foerster [47]. More recent studies using percutaneous electrical and transcranial magnetic stimulation have identified a fast conduction pathway from the motor cortex to the diaphragm [48–50]. In addition, studies of brain activity using positron emission tomography (PET) and functional magnetic resonance imaging (fMRI) have highlighted areas of the motor cortex, thalamus and cerebellum that are associated with volitional breathing [51–54].

Patients with congenital hypoventilation syndrome (CCHS) apparently lack the medullo-spinal pathways that facilitate reflexogenic breathing [55]. These patients rely on volitional breathing at all times, suggesting that cortical control is not completely integrated with the brainstem respiratory control centre. However, evidence suggests that the volitional control of breathing acts via corticobulbar pathways that are known to directly innervate the medullary respiratory centres [56, 57]. Thus, the motor cortex has the neuronal apparatus to act directly on the respiratory apparatus and to modulate activity in the medullary respiratory control centre. The available evidence does not delineate the precise form the integration takes or the extent to which it is used.

23.7.2 Learned responses

It has recently become apparent that in addition to the control of breathing being subject to volitional influences, there is a degree of modulation or plasticity within the system with several reports of a form of respiratory memory. This respiratory memory may be of short duration, i.e. lasting several minutes, termed short-term potentiation (STP), or may last for hours or days when it is known as long-term modulation (LTM). An example of the former has been demonstrated in cats [58] and more recently in humans [59, 60].

The magnitude and development of STP are similar to the slow changes in ventilation that occur at the beginning and end of exercise, so it is possible that STP contributes to the ventilatory responses [61]. The dynamics of STP development and after-discharge may also contribute to the ventilatory chemoflex dynamics during hypoxic and hypercapnoeic challenge [62].

Evidence for LTM is less well documented. An enhanced ventilatory response to steady-state exercise, with a disproportionate increase in breathing frequency and corresponding decrease in tidal volume, has been observed following repeated short exposures to hypercapnoeic exercise in goats. This finding is evidence for LTM in an animal model [61, 63–65]. The role of LTM in the ventilatory response to exercise in humans is less clear; there are few studies extant and their conclusions are conflicting [66–69]. It has also been reported that the enhanced exercise ventilatory response is not dependant upon either exercise conditioning or CO_2, but can be achieved by targeted breathing at rest; this suggests that LTM of ventilation may be induced by repetitive reinforcement learning without the need for a specific exercise or hypercapnoeic stimulus [70]. The stimulus in this latter study was applied intermittently over a period of 4 weeks, substantially longer than the other studies. A possible explanation is that LTM, like any other response to training, is critically related to the intensity or the time course of the stimulus.

LTM could reflect an increase in activity in the neural pathways involved in the ventilatory response to exercise; if so a possible mechanism is that it facilitates synaptic transmission by mobilising activity in related neural pathways, a process described as synaptic plasticity [71].

Short- and long-term modulations of ventilation are a means for adapting the ventilatory response so they remain appropriate under changing conditions. Thus, the present findings, if confirmed, have wide ranging implications for ventilatory control in a variety of circumstances, including during early development, exposure to abnormal environments, ageing and in the presence of lung disease.

23.8 Pattern of breathing

The respiratory control system determines the pattern of breathing and the lung volume from which it starts (i.e. functional residual capacity). The pattern embraces the volume–time profile of the entire breath of which the principal dimensions are the tidal volume and the separate durations of inspiration and expiration. These attributes exhibit slight variation from breath to breath, with the principal variable being the duration of inspiration; at any level of ventilation the mean inspiratory flow rate is relatively constant. This is illustrated in Fig. 28.7 (page 393) where flow is described by the slopes of the lines relating tidal volume to time of inspiration or expiration. The range of normal variation is represented by the thickened portions of the lines. An increase in minute volume is achieved by an increase in inspiratory and expiratory flows and by shortening of the time of expiration, the time of inspiration (t_I) is much less affected. During moderate exercise or hypoxia, t_I is at the resting level. However, t_I diminishes when tidal volume exceeds about half the vital capacity. The reduction is due to the Hering–Breuer inflation reflex. The duration of inspiration is also reduced during hyperthermia (Section 23.2.2). With this exception, the pattern of breathing during increased ventilation under steady state conditions is independent of the stimulus. The pattern can be summarized for the whole breath by the relationship of ventilation to tidal volume (Fig. 23.9).

The constancy of the pattern is evidence for the different respiratory drives converging before they influence the central pattern generator. However, the constant pattern is not achieved immediately; instead the initial response varies depending on the stimulus. When this acts via the carotid chemoreceptors the first response is usually a shortening of the time of expiration (t_E) and hence an increase in respiratory frequency. When the stimulus acts via central chemoreceptors, for example while breathing carbon dioxide in oxygen, the initial response is an increase in tidal volume without much change in respiratory frequency. In this event the apparent constancy of breath duration is due to converse changes in its components: t_E decreases as might be expected but t_I increases. The latter change is responsible for the initial increase in tidal volume [73].

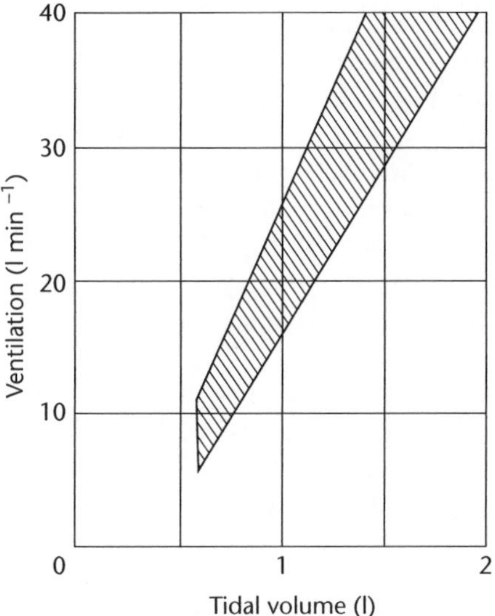

Fig. 23.9 Relationship of exercise ventilation to tidal volume in healthy adults of European descent. The form of the relationship is y = mx + c. For steady state conditions Hey and colleagues found the average values of m and c to be, respectively, 28.3 (SD 5.7) and 0.32 (SD 0.13) [72]. The tidal volume is also related to vital capacity (Fig. 29.10, page 434) and to ethnic group (Table 27.3, page 368).

Inspiration is by contraction of inspiratory muscles; any increase in flow is due to more rapid contractions. Expiration is normally passive and results from the elastic recoil of the lung overcoming the thoracic resistance. The volume–time relationship during passive expiration has been described as follows [74]:

$$Vt_x = Vt_o\ e^{-t_x(RC)^{-1}} \quad (23.5)$$

where Vt_x is volume at time t_x, Vt_o is volume at the start of expiration and RC is the product of compliance and resistance which is the time constant of the lung (Section 16.1.9). In a normal adult at rest the time constant is approximately 0.4 s (compliance 2.0 l kPa^{-1}, thoracic resistance 0.2 kPa l^{-1}s). A complete expiration will occupy approximately four time constants, which is approximately 1.6 s; this is somewhat less than is normally observed at rest. The difference is due to expiration being slowed by contraction of the inspiratory muscles. Progressive shortening of the duration of expiration as tidal volume increases is due to airway resistance decreasing as inspired volume increases and due to progressive removal of constraints on expiration. For example, the calibre of the larynx is increased by (1) contraction of the posterior cricoarytenoid muscle, (2) activity of the inspiratory muscles in early expiration and (3) the subject changing from nose to mouth breathing. During nearly maximal breathing the former two changes are partly reversed in conjunction with increased activity of the accessory muscles of expiration. Diseases of the heart or lungs that change the lung compliance and resistance alter the time constant and hence the pattern of breathing in the expected directions (Section 28.4.7).

23.9 Assessment of respiratory control

23.9.1 Introduction

The respiratory control system maintains normal, and virtually constant, tensions of oxygen and carbon dioxide, and concentration of hydrogen ions in arterial blood and cerebral extracellular fluid in a wide range of circumstances (Section 23.1). The system is robust, but can be overloaded. The subject is then in respiratory failure. Faulty respiratory control leads to inappropriate levels of ventilation or an abnormal pattern of breathing; the changes alter the levels of the arterial blood gases which in turn can have consequences for all bodily organs and systems, particularly the central nervous system (see Footnote 23.1).

In patients with lung disease disturbance to respiratory control usually occurs in association with hypoxaemia, hyper- or hypocapnia, breathlessness or somnolence. There may also be evidence for secondary changes, for example acid–base changes that correct a respiratory acidosis or alkalosis, pulmonary hypertension that may progress to right heart failure or polycythaemia that may be complicated by intravascular thromboses.

The principle of testing is to alter a component of the drive to breathe and measure the response. The alteration can be a modification of the existing stimulus or the introduction of a new one, the response can be the change in ventilation or in respiratory work or a related variable (see Fig. 23.9, also below, Mouth occlusion pressure). The relationship of the response to the change in respiratory drive should be linearised by an appropriate transformation if it is not linear to start with (Section 5.3); the respiratory sensitivity is then described by one of the parameters of the resulting regression equation (e.g. eqn. 23.1).

23.9.2 Conditions of measurement

In everyday life the respiratory drive varies from breath to breath in response to the many factors that influence it; this is reflected in cyclical variations in the pattern of breathing (e.g. Fig. 28.7, page 393). The drive diminishes on closing the eyes and increases momentarily with every external stimulus. Thus, to obtain a representative result the findings for a number of breaths should be averaged and the conditions of measurement should be standardised. This is particularly important at rest when steady state measurements tend to be unreliable because some subjects hyperventilate if they become aware that interest is being taken in their breathing. Such hyperventilation is less likely when the subject's attention is occupied by reading a bland book or by performing an exercise test. In addition, since the drive to respiration is normally increased during exercise, an assessment under these conditions may reveal an abnormality that is not detectable at rest. Precautions need to be taken when making a steady state assessment, e.g. the subject should be in a post-absorptive state and not stimulated by caffeine, alcohol, or extraneous sights or sounds [75]. Before the test the subject should empty the bladder, adopt a comfortable posture, take trouble over the adjustment of the mouthpiece, nose clip and other respiratory apparatus, then relax for 30 min. During the test the subjects should preferably not think about their breathing and not consciously try to influence it. When the test entails switching between gas mixtures, this should be done in such a way that the subject is not aware of its occurrence; the gases should be of the same temperature and humidity and not taste differently.

Footnote 23.1 The brain is especially vulnerable on account of its high metabolic rate and inability to accumulate an oxygen debt. As a result it is totally dependent on the current delivery of oxygen by the circulation.

23.9.3 Ventilation and arterial blood gases

Before proceeding to specific tests there is much to be learnt from observing the patient and noting the respiratory frequency. Depending on circumstances the next step is likely to be the measurement of arterial oxygen and carbon dioxide tensions and blood pH. Complementary information can be obtained from measurement of the volume and composition of expired gas.

Arterial blood gases. The subject should be at rest, relaxed and in a post-absorptive state. The blood should preferably be sampled via an indwelling arterial cannula and a period of approximately 30 min allowed for the subject's breathing to stabilise before the blood is taken. It should be handled and analysed appropriately (see Sections 7.9 to 7.11). Interpretation of the blood gas tensions and $[H^+]$ depends on knowledge of the normal levels (Table 26.23, page 358). Usually only minor changes occur during moderate steady state exercise.

The arterial oxygen tension is low in newborn babies (Section 24.5). It rises to a steady level at about the third week of extrauterine life and thereafter remains fairly constant into adulthood. Subsequently, the tension declines with age due to the lung function becoming progressively more uneven (Section 25.9). The tension of oxygen usually varies inversely with body mass and is reduced by uneven lung ventilation–perfusion ratios such as are caused by smoking, chronic bronchitis or emphysema. Other relatively common causes of hypoxaemia are hypoventilation and a vascular shunt of blood across the lungs. Pa,o_2 exhibits circadian variation, being less during sleep than in the waking state (Section 25.6). There is also a small monthly oscillation in women, with relatively high values in the luteal phase of the menstrual cycle when progesterone stimulates respiration (Section 25.8.1).

The tension of carbon dioxide in arterial blood resembles that of oxygen in being relatively low in newborn babies. Subsequently, when the subject is awake, it stabilises at around 5.3 kPa (40 mm Hg) increasing somewhat during sleep (Section 32.4.1). The level falls if respiratory drive is increased (e.g. at altitude or in women when the blood concentration of progesterone is elevated). During moderate steady state exercise the arterial CO_2 tension can deviate upwards or downwards, reflecting alterations in respiratory control and in the tension of CO_2 in mixed venous blood (including a contribution from the exercising muscles). These and other circumstances need to be taken into account when deciding whether or not the arterial blood gases are abnormal.

Normal values at rest exclude gross abnormalities but not changes that occur during sleep or progressive exercise. Hence, measurement in these circumstances can be appropriate.

Ventilation minute volume. The information is likely to be obtained as part of another investigation, usually a progressive exercise test, which in a respiratory patient should ideally be performed on a treadmill (Section 29.4.1). Information on respiratory control is obtained at near to the point of discontinuing the exercise and also, in patients who are not grossly disabled, from the relationships of ventilation to uptake of oxygen and tidal volume, and the respiratory exchange ratio (see Section 29.8).

23.9.4 Ventilatory response to CO_2

The response is the increase in ventilation per unit increase in tension of carbon dioxide (Fig. 23.7). The derivation requires measurements of ventilation at a minimum of two levels of carbon dioxide tension. Under these circumstances:

$$S = \frac{\dot{V}_{E(1)} - \dot{V}_{E(2)}}{Pa,CO_{2(2)} - Pa,CO_{2(1)}} = \frac{\Delta \dot{V}_E}{\Delta Pa,CO_2} \quad 1\ \text{min}^{-1}\ \text{kPa}^{-1}(\text{or mm Hg}^{-1}) \qquad (23.6)$$

where S is the response of ventilation to carbon dioxide, $\dot{V}_E$ is the ventilation minute volume in $1\ \text{min}^{-1}$ and Pa,CO_2 is the tension of carbon dioxide in the arterial blood in kPa or mm Hg. The subscripts (1) and (2) refer, respectively, to measurements made at low and high tensions of carbon dioxide. When the range of ventilation–perfusion ratios is within normal limits the tension of carbon dioxide may be obtained by rapid analysis of the respired gas (Fig. 18.6, page 220); formerly an end-tidal gas sampler might have been used (Fig. 1.3, page 10). Where pulmonary gas exchange is uneven the arterial or arterialised venous blood should be measured (Section 7.11).

The end-tidal gas tensions can also be measured by the rebreathing method of Read [76]. The subject rebreathes from a bag that initially contains between 3 and 5 l of gas comprising approximately 5% CO_2 with the remainder being oxygen. The duration of rebreathing is 4 min or until the concentration of CO_2 has risen to approximately 70–80 mm Hg. The bag is usually contained in a box with a separate outlet that is connected to a dry gas meter, spirometer or pneumotachograph for measurement of ventilation. After 3 or 4 breaths the P_{CO_2} in the end-tidal gas is assumed to be the same as that in the bag; the latter is measured with an analyser having a response time of less than 0.2 s. The ventilatory response to carbon dioxide is the slope of the relationship of ventilation to P_{CO_2} over the range where this is linear; alinearity is often apparent at low tensions of carbon dioxide and either these points or the first 45 s of rebreathing should be excluded from the analysis. Reproducibility is influenced by the number and accuracy of the measurements of ventilation minute volume; these should be made over finite numbers of whole breaths where it is practicable. Alternatively, timed intervals of 30 s (or 15 s) can be used. Repeating the test after an interval of 10 min will improve the accuracy, but some subjects develop a headache, so the use of duplicates may be inadvisable, especially where there is a need for serial measurements. Values for the index in healthy subjects are influenced by the size of the lung and by ethnic group (Section 27.2.6, Papua New Guinea); reference values are given above (Section 23.5.3). The procedure also yields the response time for the increase in ventilation and the tension of carbon dioxide in the mixed venous blood (Section 17.3.2).

When the steady-state method is used the subject breathes one of two appropriate concentrations, usually 3% and 6% of CO_2 in oxygen for 20 min. On each occasion the ventilation is measured over the last 5 min and if arterial blood is to be collected it is sampled over 2 min.

For the constant inflow method [38], carbon dioxide in the dosage 0–0.8 $1\ \text{min}^{-1}$ is added to the inhaled air whilst the subject is breathing through a mouthpiece (or close fitting mask). The CO_2 is delivered into wide bore tubing 3 cm proximal to the inspiratory valve. The concentrations of oxygen and carbon dioxide at the mouth and in the mixed expired gas are monitored using a respiratory mass spectrometer. The oral CO_2 concentrations are used to estimate the arterial carbon dioxide tension (Fig. 23.5).

23.9.5 Chemoreceptor drive

Hypoxic drive. The response to hypoxic drive can be obtained by an isocapnoeic technique in which the ventilation is related to the alveolar oxygen tension during hypoxia of increasing intensity [77]. The tension of carbon dioxide in the alveolar gas is kept constant using an approach similar to that for the isocapnoeic technique described below. The hypoxic response is obtained from the following relationship:

$$\dot{V}_E = \dot{V}_{E,0} + 7.5A(w)/(P_{A,O_2} - 32)1\ \text{min}^{-1} \qquad (23.7)$$

where P_{A,O_2} is the tension of oxygen in the alveolar gas in mm Hg and 7.5 converts to kilopascals. $\dot{V}_E$ is ventilation ($l_{STPD}\ \text{min}^{-1}$) and $\dot{V}_{E,0}$ is ventilation extrapolated back to zero P_{A,O_2}. The response term A(w) is similar to the product term AD of Lloyd and Cunningham (eqn. 23.3).

The ventilatory response to hypoxia can also be expressed in logarithmic form or in terms of the extent of desaturation of the arterial blood measured by oximetry. For the latter [78] the oxygen saturation is used rather than P_{O_2} because the relationship between ventilation and saturation is linear. The test can be performed using pulse oximetry.

Technique of Lloyd and Cunningham. The drive from carotid chemoreceptors varies inversely with oxygen tension starting from a tension of approximately 25 kPa (200 mm Hg). Below this upper limit the chemoreceptors also respond to carbon dioxide, and the response interacts with that to oxygen. The interaction can be described using the relationship of Lloyd and Cunningham (eqn. 23.3 and Fig. 23.7). The constants A, B, C and D together describe the ventilatory responses to hypoxia and hypercapnia. In subjects with a normal range of ventilation–perfusion ratios the test may be done by an isocapnoeic technique. The subject breathes oxygen to which controlled quantities of carbon dioxide are added through rotameters. The flow is adjusted to maintain the ventilation minute volume at a predetermined level in the range 20 l min^{-1} to 60 l min^{-1}. The test is continued until a steady level has been established. The hypercapnoeic drive is then reduced and the hypoxic drive increased by the addition of nitrogen at a rate which is determined by trial and error to keep the level of ventilation constant. During this procedure five determinations are made of the tensions of oxygen and carbon dioxide in the end-tidal gas or the arterial blood; one determination is also made at a lower level of ventilation. These data are used to calculate the indices A, B, C and D. Some results are in Section 23.5.3.

23.9.6 Other methods

Mouth occlusion pressure. The strength of the inspiratory drive can be assessed from the rate of change of pressure that develops in the airway when it is occluded suddenly whilst the subject is breathing in. The measurement is made 0.1 s from the start of inspiration, hence the term $P_{0.1}$. This index has the advantage of requiring only relatively simple equipment, but the disadvantage of interrupting breathing and hence being applicable to only a small proportion of breaths. An alternative is the dP/d$t$max, which is the maximal rate of rise of pressure at the start of the inspiration, when a small resistance is interposed in the external airway [79]. The dP/d$t$max does not disturb ventilation and can be measured at each breath so is more reproducible than $P_{0.1}$ (Fig. 23.8). The pressure that is developed varies with the initial length of the muscle fibres, and hence with FRC. This variable should be taken into account when interpreting the result (e.g. with respiratory muscle abnormalities, in emphysema or during exercise).

Transcranial magnetic stimulation. The technique of magnetic stimulation of bulbospinal pathways in the neck can be used to investigate diaphragmatic weakness (Section 9.9.3). It has recently been extended by using stimulation of the cranium to initiate diaphragmatic contraction via corticospinal pathways as well. The former pathway is direct and virtually automatic. The latter includes a component that is at least partly under voluntary control. Comparison of the two responses is providing new information about the contribution to respiratory control of higher centres in the brain [80, 81].

Work of breathing. The non-elastic work done on the lungs during inspiration provides a measure of respiratory drive which, like the $P_{0.1}$ (see above) is nearly independent of the functional condition of the lung. The work can be obtained from measurements of oesophageal pressure throughout inspiration; the instantaneous pressures together with the corresponding volumes above functional residual capacity are used to delineate a volume–pressure curve. The inspiratory work is given by the area of the inspiratory part of the curve (Fig. 9.3, page 103). The method provides a means for validating other simpler procedures; it is seldom used for assessment on account of entailing intubation of the oesophagus.

Oxygen cost of breathing. The consumption of oxygen by the respiratory muscles reflects the respiratory drive. The consumption can be estimated from measurements of the uptake of oxygen made using a closed circuit spirometer [82]. The spirometer is fitted with an absorber for CO_2 and filled with 100% oxygen. The ventilation is varied by arranging that the subject rebreathes from a length of wide-bore tubing introduced between the mouthpiece and the spirometer circuit. In terms of ventilation the oxygen cost (in SI or traditional units) is given by:

$$\text{Oxygen cost} = \frac{O_{2\,\text{uptake}(2)} - O_{2\,\text{uptake}(1)}}{\dot{V}\mathrm{E}_{(2)} - \dot{V}\mathrm{E}_{(1)}}\ \text{mmol l}^{-1} \qquad (23.8)$$

where O_2 uptake is in SI or traditional units, $\dot{V}\mathrm{E}$ is the ventilation minute volume in l min^{-1} and (1) and (2) refer, respectively, to measurements made when breathing 100% oxygen and mixtures of CO_2 in oxygen obtained by rebreathing. The oxygen cost bears a curvilinear relationship to ventilation (Fig. 9.4, page 104). The work and the oxygen cost of breathing are increased by disease of the lung or the chest wall that increase the work of breathing. By contrast, the oxygen cost is within normal limits if the hypoventilation is due to reduced activity of the respiratory centre but the lungs are normal. In such cases the result should be expressed in terms of the hypercapnoeic drive to respiration:

$$O_2\ \text{cost} = \frac{[O_{2\,\text{uptake}(2)} - O_{2\,\text{uptake}(1)}]}{[Pa,\mathrm{CO}_{2(2)} - Pa,\mathrm{CO}_{2(1)}]}\ \text{mmol min}^{-1}\ \text{kPa}^{-1} \qquad (23.9)$$

where Pa,CO_2 is the tension of carbon dioxide in arterial blood in kPa and the other terms are as defined above. This index provides a measure of the activity of the respiratory centre that is independent of the structural integrity of the lungs and thoracic cage.

23.10 Overview

New techniques and concepts, including brain imaging, transcranial magnetic stimulation and investigations into behavioural control of breathing are rendering obsolete the traditional views of respiratory control. Now it is apparent that most parts of the brain contribute, the system is flexible and responds to changing circumstances to a greater extent than was at one time thought. The implications of these findings are still being worked out. Meanwhile, the simple traditional tests of respiratory control still have a place in assessment; they may have more to offer in the future, for example in the assessment of bronchodilatation for relief of breathlessness on exertion.

23.11 References

1. von Baumgarten R, Kanzow E. The interaction of two types of inspiratory neurons in the region of the tractus solitarius of the cat. *Arch Ital Biol* 1958; **96**: 361–373.
2. Smith JC, Ellenberger HH, Ballanyi K et al. Pre-Botzinger complex: a brain stem region that may generate respiratory rhythm in mammals. *Science* 1991; **254**: 726–729.
3. von Euler C. Brainstem mechanisms for generation and control of breathing pattern. In: Cherniack NS, Widdicombe JG, eds. *Handbook of physiology. The respiratory system 2: control of breathing.* Bethesda, MD: American Physiological Society, 1986: 1–67.
4. Widdicombe JG. Airway receptors. *Resp Physiol* 2001; **125**: 3–15.
5. Hamilton RD, Winning AJ, Horner RL, Guz A. The effect of lung inflation on breathing in man during wakefulness and sleep. *Respir Physiol.* 1988; **73**: 145–54.
6. Shea SA, Horner RL, Banner NR et al The effect of human heart-lung transplantation upon breathing at rest and during sleep. *Respir Physiol* 1988; **72**: 131–149.
7. Cohen MI. Phrenic and recurrent laryngeal discharge patterns and the Hering-Breuer reflex. *Am J Physiol* 1975; **228**: 1489–1496.
8. Colebatch JG, Gandevia SC, McCloskey DI. Reduction in inspiratory activity in response to sternal vibration. *Respir Physiol* 1977; **29**: 327–338.
9. Larrabee MG, Knowlton GC. Excitation and inhibition of phrenic motoneurones by inflation of the lungs. *Am J Physiol* 1946; **147**: 90–99.
10. Widdicombe JG. Respiratory reflexes in man and other mammalian species. *Clin Sci* 1961; **21**: 163–170.
11. Paintal AS. Vagal sensory receptors and their reflex effects. *Physiol Rev* 1973; **53**: 159–227.
12. Coleridge JCG, Coleridge HM. Afferent C-fibre innervation of the lungs and airways and its functional significance. *Rev Physiol Biochem Pharmacol* 1984; **99**: 1–110.
13. Head H. On the regulation of respiration. *J Physiol (Lond)* 1889; **10**: 1–71.
14. Sears TE. Efferent discharges in alpha and fusimotor fibres of intercostal nerves of the cat. *J Physiol (Lond)* 1964; **174**: 295–315.
15. Newsom Davis J, Sears TA. The effects of sudden alterations in load on human intercostal muscles during voluntary activation. *J Physiol (Lond)* 1967; **190**: 36P–38P.
16. Loeschcke HH. Review lecture: central chemosensitivity and the reaction theory. *J Physiol (Lond)* 1982; **332**: 1–24.
17. Coates EL, Li A, Nattie E. Widespread sites of brainstem ventilatory chemoreceptors. *J Applied Physiol* 1993; **75**: 5–14.
18. Severinghaus JW. Invited editorial on "Widespread sites of brainstem ventilatory chemoreceptors". *J Appl Physiol* 1993; **75**: 3–4.
19. Schlaefker ME, See WR, Loeschcke HH. Ventilatory response to alterations of H^+ ion concentration in small areas of the ventral medullary surface. *Respir Physiol* 1970; **10**: 198–212.
20. Schlaefker ME. Central chemosensitivity: a respiratory drive. *Rev Physiol Biochem Pharmacol* 1981; **90**: 171–244.
21. Nattie HH. Central chemoreception. In: Demsey JA, Pack AI, eds. *Regulation of Breathing.* 2nd ed. New York: Marcell Dekker, 1995: 493–510.
22. Leusen IR. Chemosensitivity of the respiratory centre. Influence of CO_2 in the cerebral ventricles on respiration. *Am J Physiol* 1954; **176**: 39-44.
23. Melton JE, Neubauer JA, Edelman NH. GABA antagonism reverses hypoxic respiratory depression in the cat. *J Appl Physiol* 1990; **69**: 1296–1301.
24. Berkenbosch A, Olievier CN, DeGoede J. Respiratory responses to hypoxia. Peripheral and central effects. In Semple SJG, Adams L, Whipp BJ, eds. *Modelling and control of ventilation.* New York: Plenum, 1995: 251–256.
25. De Castro F. Sur la structure et l'innervation de la glande carotidienne (glomus caroticum) de l'homme et des mammiferes, et sur un nouveau système d'innervation autonome du neuf glossopharyngien. *Trab Lab Invest Biol Univ Madrid* 1926; **24**: 365-432.
26. Heymans C, Bouchaert JJ, Dautrebande L. Sinus carotidien et reflexes respiratoire II. *Arch Intern Pharmacodyn* 1930; **39**: 400–408.
27. Fidone SJ, Gonzalez C. Initiation and control of chemoreceptor activity in the carotid body. In: Fishman AP, Cherniack NS, Widdicombe JG, Geiger SR, eds. *Handbook of physiology III, The respiratory system* vol 2 part 1. Bethesda, MD: American Physiologiy Society, 1986: 247–312.
28. Ward DS, Bellville JW. Reduction of hypoxic ventilatory drive by dopamine. *Anaesth Analg* 1982; **61**: 333–337.
29. Delpierre S, Fornaris M, Guillot C, Grimaud C. Increased ventilatory chemosensitivity induced by domperidone, a dopamine antagonist, in healthy humans. *Bull Eur Physiopathol Respir* 1987; **23**: 31–35.
30. Yamamoto M, Nishimura M, Kobayashi S et al. Role of endogenous adenosine in hypoxic ventilatory response in humans: a study with dipyridamole *J Appl Physiol* 1994; **76**: 196–203.
31. Foo IT, Warren PM, Drummond GB. Influence of oral clonidine on the ventilatory response to acute and sustained isocapnic hypoxia in human males. *Br J Anaesth* 1996; **76**: 214—220.
32. Prabhakar NR. Dinerman JL, Agani FH, Snyder SH. Carbon monoxide: A role in carotid body chemoreception. *Proc Natl Acad Sci USA* 1995; **92**: 1994–1997.
33. Wang ZZ, Stensas LJ, Berdt DS et al. Mechanisms of carotid body inhibition. *Arterial chemoreceptors: cell to system.* New York: Plenum, 1994: 229–235.
34. Cross BA, Davey A, Guz A et al. The pH oscillations in arterial blood during exercise: a potential signal for the ventilatory response in the dog. *J Physiol (Lond)* 1982; **329**: 57–73.
35. Cunningham DJC, Lloyd BB, Miller JP, Young JM. The time course of human ventilation after transient changes in P_{A,CO_2} at two values of P_{A,O_2}. *J Physiol (Lond)* 1965; **179**: 68P–70P.

36. DuBois AB, Britt AG, Fenn WO. Alveolar CO_2 during the respiratory cycle. *J Appl Physiol.* 1952; **4**: 535–548.
37. Black AMS, Goodman NW, Nail BS et al. The significance of the timing of chemoreceptor impulses for their effect upon respiration. *Acta Nerobiol Exp* 1973; **33**: 139–147.
38. Cummin ARC, Alison J, Jacobi MS et al. Ventilatory sensitivity to inhaled carbon dioxide around the control point during exercise. *Clin Sci* 1986; **71**: 17–22.
39. Nielsen M, Smith M. Studies on the regulation of respiration in acute hypoxia. *Acta Physiol Scand* 1951; **24**: 293–313.
40. Lloyd BB, Cunningham DJC. A quantitative approach to the regulation of human respiration. In Cunningham DJC, Lloyd BB, eds. *The regulation of human respiration.* Oxford: Blackwell Scientific Publications, 1963: 331–349.
41. Matthews AW, Howell JBL. Assessment of the responsiveness to carbon dioxide in patients with chronic airways obstruction by rate of inspiratory pressure development. *Clin Sci* 1976; **50**: 199–205.
42. Astrup P, Severinghaus JW. *History of acid—base physiology.* Stockholm: Munksgaard, 1986.
43. Winterstein H. Die regulierung der atmung dursch das blut. *Pfluger's Arch Gasemte Physiol* 1911; **138**: 167–184.
44. Winterstein H. Die reaktionstheorie rer atmungsregulation. *Pfluger's Arch Gasemte Physiol* 1921; **187**: 293–298.
45. Winterstein H, Gokhan N. Ammoniumchlorid-acidosis und reaktiontheorie der atmungsregulation *Arch Intern Pharmacodyn* 1953; **93**: 212–282.
46. Gray JS. *Pulmonary ventilation and its physiological regulation.* Springfield: Thomas, 1950.
47. Foerster O, Motorische F u B: In: Bumke O, Foerster O, eds. *Handbook der Neurologie* Berlin: Springer-Verlag, 1936: 50–51.
48. Gandevia SC, Rothwell JC. Activation of human diaphragm from the motor cortex. *J Physiol (Lond)* 1987; **384**: 109—118.
49. Murphy K, Mier L, Adams L, Guz A. Putative cerebral cortical involvement in the ventilatory response to inhaled CO2 in conscious man. *J Physiol (Lond)* 1990; **420**: 1–18.
50. Corfield DR, Murphy K, Guz A. Does the motor cortical control of the diaphragm 'bypass' the brain stem respiratory centres in man? *Respir Physiol* 1998; **114**: 109–117.
51. Colebatch JG, Adams L, Murphy K et al. Regional cerebral blood flow during volitional breathing in man. *J Physiol (Lond)* 1991; **443**: 91–103.
52. Ramsay SC, Adams L, Murphy K et al. Regional cerebral blood flow during volitional expiration in man: a comparison with volitional inspiration. *J Physiol (Lond)* 1993; **461**: 85–101.
53. Fink GR, Adams L, Watson JD et al. Hyperpnoea during and immediately after exercise in man: evidence of motor cortical involvement *J Physiol (Lond)* 1995; **489**: 663–675. Erratum, *J Physiol (Lond)* 1996; **494**.
54. Evans KC, Shea SA, Saykin AJ. Functional MRI localisation of central nervous system regions associated with volitional inspiration in humans. *J Physiol (Lond)* 1999; **520**: 383–392.
55. Gozal D. Congenital central hypoventilation syndrome: an update. *Pediat Pulmonol* 1998; **26**: 273–282.
56. Rikard-Bell GC, Bystrzycka EK, Nail BS. The identification of brainstem neurones projecting to thoracic respiratory motoneurones in the cat as demonstrated by retrograde transport of HRP. *Brain Res Bull* 1985; **14**: 25–37.
57. Rikard-Bell GC, Bystrzycka EK, Nail BS. Cells of origin of corticospinal projections to phrenic and thoracic respiratory motoneurones in the cat as shown by retograde transport of HRP. *Brain Res Bull* 1985; **14**: 39–47.
58. Eldridge FL, Gill-Kumar P. Central neural respiratory drive and afterdischarge. *Respir Physiol* 1980; **40**: 49–63.
59. Swanson GD, Ward DS, Bellville JW. Posthyperventilation isocapnic hyperpnoea. *J Appl Physiol* 1976; **40**: 592–596.
60. Fregosi FF. Short-term potentiation of breathing in humans. *J Appl Physiol* 1991; **73**: 892–899.
61. Eldridge FL, Waldrop TG. Neural control of breathing during exercise. In: Whipp BJ, Wasserman K, eds. *Exercise, pulmonary physiology and pathophysiology.* New York: Dekker, 1991: 309–370.
62. Poon CS. Synaptic plasticity and respiratory control. In: Khoo MCK, ed. *Bioengineering approaches to pulmonary physiology and medicine.* Los Angeles: Plenum, 1999: 93–113.
63. Mitchell GS, Foley KT, McGuirk S et al. Effects of chronic thoracic dorsal rhizotomy (TDR) on ventilatory control during mild exercise in goats. *FASEB J* 1988; **2**: A1508.
64. Mitchell GS, Douse MA, Foley KT. Receptor interactions in modulating ventilatory activity. *Am J Physiol* 1990; **259**: 911–920.
65. Martin PA, Mitchell GS. Long-term modulation of the exercise ventilatory response in goats. *J Physiol (Lond)* 1993; **470**: 601–617.
66. Turner DL, Bach KB, Martin PA et al. Modulation of ventilatory control during exercise. *Respir Physiol* 1997; **110**: 277–285.
67. Moosavi SH, Guz A, Adams L. Repeated exercise paired with "imperceptible" deadspace loading does not alter VE of subsequent exercise in humans. *J Appl Physiol* 2002; **92**: 1159–1168.
68. Cathcart AJ, Herrold N, Turner AP et al. Absence of long-term modulation of ventilation by dead-space loading during moderate exercise in humans. *Eur J Appl Physiol* 2005; **93**: 411–420.
69. Wood HE, Fatemian M, Robbins PA. A learned component of the ventilatory response to exercise in man. *J Physiol (Lond)* 2003; **553**: 967–974.
70. Reed JW, Coates JC. Induction of long-term modulation of the exercise ventilatory response in man. *Adv Exp Med Biol* 2001; **499**: 221–224.
71. Paulsen O, Sejnowski TJ. Natural patterns of activity and long-term synaptic plasticity. *Curr Opin Neurobiol* 2000; **10**: 172–179.
72. Hey EN, Lloyd BB, Cunningham DJC et al. Effects of various respiratory stimuli on the depth and frequency of breathing in man. *Respir Physiol* 1966; **1**: 193–205.
73. Gardner WN. The pattern of breathing following step changes of alveolar partial pressure of carbon dioxide and oxygen in man. *J Physiol (Lond)* 1980; **300**: 55–73.
74. Brody AW, Wander HJ, O'Halloran PS et al. Correlations, normal standard, and interdependence in tests of ventilatory strength and mechanics. *Am Rev Respir Dis* 1964; **89**: 214–235.
75. Severinghaus JW. A proposed standard determination of ventilatory responses to hypoxia and hypercapnia *Chest* 1976; **70**: 129–131.
76. Read DJC. A clinical method for assessing the ventilatory response to carbon dioxide. *Aust Ann Med* 1967; **16**: 20–32.
77. Weil JV, Byrnne-Quinn E, Sodal ID et al. Hypoxic ventilatory drive in normal man. *J Clin Invest* 1970; **49**: 1061–1072.

78. Rebuck AS, Campbell EJM. A clinical method for assessing the ventilatory response to hypoxia. *Am Rev Respir Dis* 1974; **109**: 345–350.
79. Milic-Emili, J. Recent advances in clinical assessment of control of breathing. *Lung* 1982; **160**: 1–17.
80. Straus C, Locher C, Zelter M et al. Facilitation of the diaphragmatic response to transcranial magnetic stimulation by increases in human respiratory drive. *J Appl Physiol* 2004; **97**: 902–912.
81. Demoule A, Verin E, Ross E et al. Intracortical inhibition and facilitation of the response of the diaphragm to transcranial magnetic stimulation. *J Clin Neurophysiol* 2003; **20**: 59–64.
82. Campbell EJM, Westlake EK, Cherniack RM. The oxygen consumption and efficiency of the respiratory muscles of young male subjects. *Clin Sci* 1958; **18**: 55–64.

CHAPTER 24

Newborn Babies, Infants and Young Children (Ages 0–6 Years)

Infant lung function testing is a relatively new subject. This chapter describes the methods and underlying neonatal physiology. Lung function and exercise in older children are reviewed in Chapters 25, 26 and 31.

24.1 Introduction

Most babies develop normally during intrauterine life and are successful in changing from placental to pulmonary gas exchange (see below). In a few babies the normal progression is deranged. The resulting abnormalities include developmental disorders such as bronchial dysplasia, lung hypoplasia, sequestration of parenchymal tissue and congenital diaphragmatic hernia, prematurity, placental insufficiency and atelectasis. Subsequently, some infants will develop an acute or subacute infection, cystic fibrosis [1] or a disorder arising from maternal smoking or atopy (Sections 37.3 and 15.3, also [2,3]). The management of these conditions and their complications will be helped in many instances by measurement of arterial blood gases and limited or detailed assessment of lung function.

The assessment of lung function can be undertaken at any age from birth onwards. In neonates and young infants, specialist equipment, staff and procedures are necessary, the latter being based on best current practices. These have been reviewed on behalf of ATS and ERS by Stocks and others [4–6] and further reviews are likely in future. The success rate for the assessments is high. In the age range 2–5 years the forced oscillation technique can be relied upon to provide useful information. The application of other measurements is limited by the ability of the child to cooperate and the patience and persuasiveness of the operator. Scaled down versions of adult equipment can be used. From the age of 6 onwards the lung function can usually be assessed by standard methods if the approach is made at the child's level and ample time is allowed for the measurements.

24.2 Summary of neonatal respiratory physiology

Airway dynamics. The bronchial architecture of the lungs are fully formed by the 16th week of gestation (Section 3.3.3) and the airways are normally fully patent at birth. The patency is achieved by a combination of anatomical features and lung elasticity, but unlike in adults the elastic recoil at small lung volumes is not reinforced by the elastic recoil of the chest wall, which is still conspicuously weak. Possibly on this account the resistance to flow in peripheral airways represents a relatively large proportion of total airway resistance. As a result airways often close during tidal breathing and airway obstruction is relatively common [7], also below 'Consequences for external respiration'. However, from studies based on models the diameters of these airways appear to be larger than might be expected for a scaled down version of adult lungs [8]. Further development of this approach is to be expected.

Gas exchange. By the time of birth the main structures of the lungs are normally fully formed and ready to function (Section 3.3). In utero gas exchange is via the placental circulation. It is assisted by the haemoglobin dissociation curve for oxygen of the foetus being to the left of that in the adult (Fig. 21.1, page 260) and the haemoglobin concentration being somewhat higher. The positions of the curves reflect the respective concentrations of blood electrolytes and the structure of foetal haemoglobin; this leads to it taking up less 2,3-diphosphoglycerate than is the case for adult haemoglobin (Section 21.2.2) [9]. The displacement of the curve facilitates the absorption by the foetus of oxygen from the maternal blood. The process is assisted by the passage of acid substances across the placenta in the reverse direction (Bohr effect, Section 21.2.2). Transfer of oxygen is facilitated by cytochrome P450 in the placental cells. The function of this substance is impaired by carbon monoxide from tobacco smoke and by barbiturates, diphenhydramine and some other drugs.

Changes at birth. The changes initiated by the onset of uterine contractions include clearance of secretions from the airways and alveolar ducts, onset of ventilation and exposure to conditions outside the uterus. These changes are followed by reduction in pulmonary vascular resistance and a redistribution of blood flow from the placental to pulmonary circulation.

Fluid is cleared mainly by absorption; this is enhanced by increases in the blood levels of adrenaline and arginine that are stimulated by the uterine contractions. Additional fluid is expelled from the lungs by compression of the thorax during the second stage of labour. Breathing is initiated by the deluge of sensory stimuli to which the baby is subjected at birth; the stimuli augment the drive to breathe and cause the baby to take its first breath. The resulting expansion of the lung exerts traction on blood vessels from interstitial lung tissue and this lowers the pulmonary vascular resistance. The onset of breathing raises the alveolar oxygen tension and leads to the release of prostacyclin into the blood; both these factors contribute to vasodilatation. At the same time the ventilation lowers the tension of carbon dioxide and this together with release of nitric oxide promotes vasodilatation and inhibits vasoconstriction (Section 17.2). Concurrently, the interruption of blood flow to the placenta raises the resistance in the systemic circulation. The changes create a pressure gradient between the left and right atria and lead to closure of the foramen ovale. At about the same time the muscle of the ductus arteriosus contracts to occlude the lumen. This diverts the entire right ventricular output through the lungs.

Consequences for external respiration. Following the onset of respiration the functional residual capacity becomes stabilized within a few breaths; thereafter the ventilation minute volume, the alveolar ventilation and the work of breathing are comparable to those in adults when allowance is made for the difference in metabolic rate. The nasal resistance is relatively high, accounting for approximately half the total airway resistance (Footnote 24.1).

At the same time the chest wall is very compliant. Hence, any undue narrowing of airways leads to inward movement of intercostal spaces during inspiration. Such narrowing is more common in infant boys than girls. The difference has implications for reference values (Section 24.5) and consequences that extend into adult life (Sections 25.2 and 25.3).

The elastic recoil of the chest wall is low so it does not expand the lung as much as in older subjects. As a result, tidal breathing takes place from a small lung volume. The time of expiration is correspondingly brief, giving more time for inspiration. The tidal volume per unit of body mass is not dissimilar to that in older children and adults. The small FRC is associated with closure of some airways at the end of expiration and to the ventilation being distributed preferentially towards the upper zones. There is no similar bias in perfusion. As a result, compared with older children and adults there is more $\dot{V}_A/\dot{Q}$ inequality and a relatively large intrapulmonary shunt of blood. The arterial blood oxygen tension is rather low in consequence. As if to accommodate to this situation, the chemoreceptors in the carotid body contribute little to the control of breathing until a few days after birth [10].

Ventilation and consumption of oxygen are related to the body mass of the infant. Oxygen consumption also varies with age, being relatively less on the day of birth than on subsequent days; it diminishes when the baby is hypoxaemic and varies with the ambient and the deep body temperatures.

Reference values for lung function in newborn infants are given in Section 24.5.

24.3 Some problems at birth

24.3.1 Asphyxia neonatorum

In normal circumstances ventilation starts promptly at birth, but occasionally the baby remains apnoeic or the ventilation is slow and feeble. This is most likely to happen following a protracted or difficult delivery. If it persists for more than 2 min from the time of birth active steps need to be taken to secure the ventilation of the lung. The measures can include gentle inflation of the chest via a mask and resuscitation bag or, when personnel with the necessary skills are in attendance, an endotracheal catheter.

24.3.2 Respiratory distress syndrome (RDS)

Adaptation to breathing air usually occurs very rapidly. However, a very few babies (about 1%) have difficulty in breathing either at birth or within the first 2 h thereafter. The condition, known

Footnote 24.1. The high nasal resistance needs to be borne in mind when interpreting measurements of intrapulmonary resistance in this age group (see Forced oscillation method below, also Section 14.3.5).

as respiratory distress syndrome of the newborn (RDS) is due to prematurity leading to the baby's lungs not producing sufficient surfactant [11]. Aggravating factors include delivery by Caesarian section before onset of labour and asphyxia at birth. RDS is often transient but can progress.

Course if untreated. In progressive respiratory distress syndrome the respiratory rate rises to between 60 and 100 breaths per min; the chest wall appears to be drawn in during inspiration and the infant makes a grunting noise during expiration. Cyanosis develops and, in the absence of ventilatory support, often is not corrected by the administration of oxygen; the hypoxaemia is associated with hypercapnia. Death is from respiratory failure. At postmortem some respiratory bronchioles, alveolar ducts and atria are found to be lined with hyaline eosinophilic material and many air sacs and alveoli contain no air; there may be numerous haemorrhages.

Lung physiology. The condition is due to the fluid in the alveoli not having the normal property of lowering the surface tension at an air-to-water interface. This important observation arose from the work of Avery and Mead and of Pattle (Section 11.3). The deficiency is due mainly to immaturity affecting the synthesis of surface-active material by the type II alveolar pneumonocytes (Section 3.3.6). The high surface tension reduces the lung compliance; hence the tidal volume and functional residual capacity are smaller than they normally are. The shallow breathing leads to unequal expansion of alveoli and atelectases. The resulting ventilation–perfusion inequality causes hypoxaemia (Section 21.5.2).

The hypoxaemia raises the pulmonary arterial pressure and hence alters the pressure gradient between the right and left atria. Mixed venous blood then passes through the foramen ovale and ductus arteriosus into the systemic arterial circulation. In this way the hypoxaemia aggravates the condition, since the secondary vascular changes further lower the tension of oxygen and raise the tension of carbon dioxide in the arterial blood. The hypoxaemia also depresses the activity of the respiratory reticular formation since the response to chemoreceptor drive is not well developed at birth (Section 24.2).

Outcome. RDS is usually caused by insufficient surfactant that is a consequence of prematurity. Thus, prevention is often possible by taking measures to ensure that the pregnancy continues to term and by stimulating production of surfactant both before and immediately after birth.

Once developed, RDS usually resolves spontaneously through the reversal of the lung pathology on the third to fifth day. The long-term prognosis is usually excellent. However, a few children have continuing difficulties; these are associated with inflammatory changes throughout the lung parenchyma. The condition may progress to chronic lung disease that is then difficult to treat. Possible causes include pre- or postnatal infection, protracted positive pressure ventilation, excessive administration of oxygen and the steroid therapy affecting the development of alveoli (Section 41.12). Another complication can be retrolental fibroplasia due to high partial pressure of oxygen affecting the development of the retina (Section 35.7.2).

Initial treatment is directed to securing time for the type II alveolar cells to start producing surface-active material. This can usually be achieved by administration of bovine or synthetic surfactant within a few minutes of birth. The availability of these substances is one of the great success stories of respiratory medical science [12, also see, e.g.13, 14]. The treatment may entail use of an incubator and negative pressure ventilation tuned to the spontaneous respiratory cycle (Section 42.5). In addition, the systemic arterial blood is likely to require monitoring by ear lobe oximetry or sampling the blood directly from a cranial or upper limb artery (Section 7.9).

24.4 Assessment of lung function in neonates and infants (ages 0–2 years)

24.4.1 Introduction

In the neonatal lung function laboratory the mechanical and bellows function of the lungs and thoracic cage can now be assessed with acceptable accuracy [4–6]. The measurements are of airway and thoracic resistance, lung and chest wall compliance, lung volumes and flows, including timed flows and forced expiratory flow–volume curves. In addition, the transfer factor can be measured using a steady state method but the index is of limited usefulness in infancy. The methods are scaled down versions of those described in previous chapters, with modifications to compensate for infants not being able to perform respiratory manoeuvres. The findings are revealing the normal functional evolution of the lungs (Section 24.5) and the short- and long-term features of lung diseases in children.

General considerations. The proposed measurements should be appropriate to the condition of the infant and the reason for the assessment. These features should be discussed with the parent or a responsible person and consent obtained. The laboratory should be warm (23–25 °C) and equipped with appropriately miniaturised apparatus that can be sterilised. The characteristics of the analysers should be adequate with respect to linearity, frequency response and stability [6, No.1], also Sections 7.3, 7.4, 7.5 and 7.15). The measurements should be made by a minimum of two persons with the appropriate training.

Conditions of measurement. The assessment procedures are usually applied during quiet non-REM sleep, as occurs after a feed. An appropriate sedative is usually required at beyond 1-month postnatal age. It is invariably needed from 3 months. Chloral hydrate in the dose 50–100 mg/kg is unlikely to affect lung function. The infant is studied in a supine position. The oxygen saturation is usually monitored by a probe applied to the lateral border of the foot or to the toe. Connection with the respiratory equipment is usually made via an oro-nasal mask. The mask should fit snugly and not leak at the line of contact with the face. To achieve this, more than one face piece and a supply of silicone putty or petroleum jelly should be available. The seal should be tested for leaks by occluding the external airway. For measurements that require forced expiration the infant is wrapped in an inflatable jacket; this should fit snugly but not constrict the chest and should be removed before other measurements are made [15, 16].

Measurement of mass and length. The principal reference variables for indices of lung function in neonates and infants are body mass and body length (stature). The mass is usually obtained before a feed, by weighing the baby wearing a dry nappy. Length in the supine position is measured with an infant stadiometer. Two helpers are needed, one to position and hold the head and the other to position the trunk and depress the knees against the table.

24.4.2 Measurement of ventilation and tidal volume

Pneumotachography. Ventilation minute volume and its subdivisions respiratory frequency and tidal volume are best measured using either a pneumotachograph connected to a face mask or a respiratory inductance plethysmograph. A mask is usually simple to apply, well tolerated and accurate within the limits of the calibration, provided the seal with the face is intact. The seal should be checked frequently. The method has the disadvantage that the presence of the mask may alter the pattern of breathing.

Respiratory inductance plethysmography (RIP). An inductance plethysmograph senses and interprets changes in the circumferences of the thorax and abdomen throughout the respiratory cycle. The device is arranged to fit snugly, but without restricting the respiratory movements. Its main use is for monitoring the pattern of breathing. Where the pattern is stable the device can be calibrated and then used to measure ventilation minute volume. Calibration entails measuring the redistribution of air between thorax and abdomen that occurs when the airway is occluded. The procedure has been called qualitative diagnostic calibration (QDC) [17]. It can be performed automatically during the first 5 min of use. The calibration is relative to the ventilation at the time. Absolute calibration is achieved by measuring tidal volume during the procedure. Reliable measurements can then be made for as long as the balance between the respiratory and abdominal components of breathing are maintained. The procedure can be combined with electrocardiography when it is used for monitoring for hypopnoea, apnoea and related acute life threatening events (designated ALTE).

Monitoring temperature of expired air. The times of inspiration and expiration, including the time taken to achieve peak expiratory flow, can be measured using temperature sensitive probes placed at the external nares and the lips. The accuracy is limited by the response time of the probe. The signal can mislead if the probe is dislodged or the external temperature changes abruptly.

24.4.3 Measurement of forced expiratory flow (forced compression techniques)

Partial expiratory flow–volume curves. Spontaneous forced expiration can be measured during crying but the flows are not reproducible. As a result the use of crying has been replaced by the rapid thoraco-abdominal compression technique in which pressure is applied to the trunk via an inflatable jacket. In an infant who is breathing spontaneously the pressure is usually applied at the end of inspiration when the lung volume is the functional residual capacity plus tidal volume. The procedure then yields a partial expiratory flow–volume curve. It can be used for infants to identify the presence of obstruction to airflow (Fig. 24.1). The equipment is illustrated in Fig. 24.2.

In pre-term infants the volume axis can be unstable, in which case the reproducibility of the flow is unsatisfactory. It can be improved by using the elastic equilibrium point as a volume landmark. This is done by preceding the forced expiration with inflations to briefly inhibit spontaneous breathing [20]. Alternatively, where the subject is intubated and deeply sedated or anaesthetised, the reproducibility can be improved by combining the compression with tracheal suction.

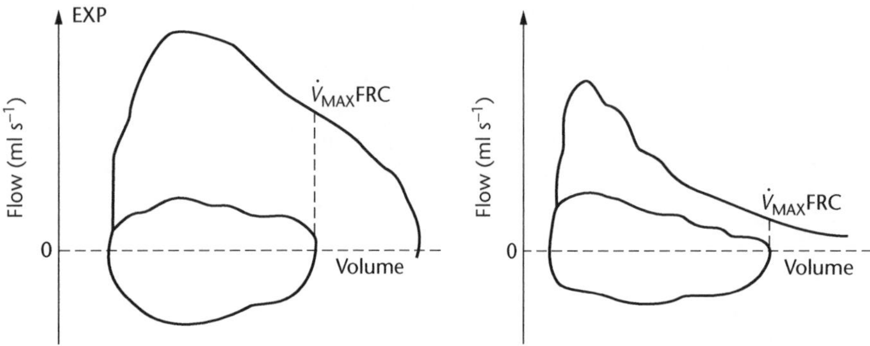

Fig. 24.1 Forced partial expiratory flow-volume curves superimposed on those for tidal breathing. *Left* Result for a healthy infant. *Right* Curve showing airflow limitation. Source: [18].

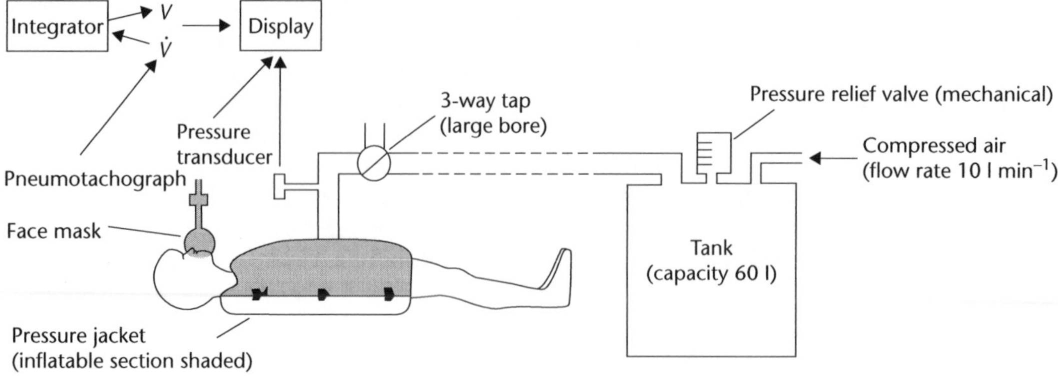

Fig. 24.2 Equipment for measuring forced expiratory flows in infants. The equipment comprises a pneumotachograph with integrator, an oronasal mask, a compression jacket, a gas reservoir with pressure relief value (range 0–10 kPa, 0–100 cm H_2O), and a three-way tap with wide bore connections. Source: [19].

Table 24.1 Representative values for functional residual capacity measured by helium dilution in healthy infants.

Length, cm	50	60	70	80	90
FRC_{He}, ml	72	114	168	236	318
95% limits	51–102	81–161	119–237	166–333	226–448

Source: [21].

Lung inflation followed by compression. The raised volume rapid thoraco-abdominal compression technique (RVRTC) can be used to obtain indices of forced expiratory flow and volume that approximate to those for older subjects (Sections 12.4 and 12.5). The conditions of measurement are described above. Inflation towards total lung capacity is made in a series of 3–5 steps using air from a reservoir or pump at a pressure of up to 3 kPa (30 cm H_2O). Higher pressures can lead to air being forced into the oesophagus. The inflations activate the Hering–Breuer reflex to cause relaxation of the respiratory muscles. After the inflation the thorax is compressed using the method described above.

The flow data are integrated over a timed period to obtain forced expiratory volume in a timed period. In infants aged less than 3 months a time of 0.4 s (i.e. $FEV_{0.4}$) is recommended [22]. The $FEV_{0.5}$ can be used subsequently up to the preschool period when a change can be made for a longer time (Fig. 24.6). The data over a complete exhalation yield forced vital capacity and indices from the forced expiratory flow–volume curve including the forced expiratory flow at functional residual capacity ($\dot{V}max_{FRC}$) and when 75% of forced vital capacity has been expired ($FEF_{75\%FVC}$). The former is more reproducible [22]. The indices can be used to measure airflow limitation [23], monitor bronchodilator therapy [24] and investigate bronchial responsiveness [25], see also Sections 15.7.2 and 15.8. The flow–volume curves can throw light on obstruction to airflow [26].

Forced inflation followed by tracheal suction. Infants can be assessed under fully controlled conditions if they are relaxed and ventilated via a tracheal catheter. The criteria for the investigation are necessarily strict, but for those who meet them the findings can be informative. This is because the volume history is readily standardised, the attainment of total lung capacity is achieved by applying a more negative pressure to the thorax than is practicable in the absence of intubation and complete exhalation down to residual volume is ensured by suction applied to the endotracheal tube. The volume history is standardised by making three initial inflations each followed by passive deflation before the full manoeuvre. In these circumstances the reproducibility of the flow and volume indices is of a high order. The interpretation is as for the previous method.

A variant of this procedure, involving negative expiratory pressure (NEP) is now sometimes used in adults (Section 12.5.1). It can be used in young children to establish whether they have achieved flow limitation during forced expiratory manoeuvres [27].

24.4.4 Measurement of lung volumes

Gas dilution methods. In infants who are breathing spontaneously, functional residual capacity (FRC) is readily obtained by the closed circuit helium dilution method or by the open circuit nitrogen washout method. Both methods can be applied during normal sleep or sedation using essentially the same procedures as for older subjects (Section 10.3). With proper attention to detail the results by the two methods are interchangeable. A washin/washout procedure with sulphur hexafluoride as the indicator gas analysed by an ultrasonic flow meter can also be used [28]. Results for all these methods are less than those for the plethysmograph method (see Table 24.1, cf. Fig. 24.4). The procedure can be extended to include total lung capacity by combining it with the inflation technique described above. Residual volume can also be obtained by combining it with compression [29]. The ratios FRC/TLC and RV/TLC provide estimates, respectively, of pulmonary hyperinflation and air trapping [30].

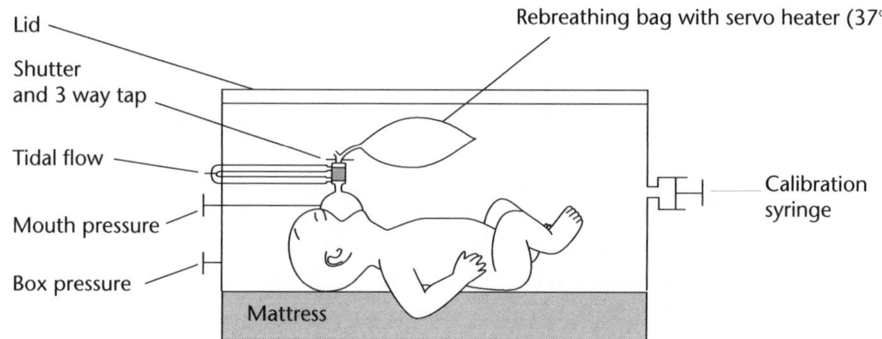

Fig. 24.3 Whole body plethysmograph for the measurement of lung volumes and airway resistance in babies. Source: [31].

Plethysmograph method. Thoracic gas volume (TGV) can be measured by whole body plethysmography in the way described for older subjects (Section 14.6, also Fig. 24.3). However, accurate results are dependent on having a minimal deadspace and making proper allowance for the deadspace that remains. Neglect of these precautions in the past has led to results by this method being unduly high both in absolute terms (Fig. 24.4) and in comparison with gas dilution methods [32]. The measurement can be combined with that of airway resistance and used for assessment of change in airway calibre. The measurement can also be used to obtain flow–volume curves that are without error from dynamic compression of intrathoracic gas (Section 12.5.1).

Other methods. In sick infants the lung volume can be estimated from chest radiographs [33] but the method has not been refined to the extent that it has in adults (Section 10.3.4).

24.4.5 Measurement of compliance and resistance

Lung and chest wall compliance

The stiffness of the lungs is increased in respiratory distress syndrome (Section 24.3.2) so the measurement of lung compliance can contribute to the management of that condition. The measurement is made in several ways.

Classical method. The tidal breathing method of Mead and Whittenberger measures the dynamic lung compliance. This can be applied to infants using essentially the same procedure as for adults (Section 11.8.4). The compliance is then the tidal volume divided by the difference in pleural pressure between the start and end of inspiration. The pleural pressure is measured via a catheter placed in the oesophagus (Section 11.8.1). However, the measurement may not be representative when a supine posture is adopted (Fig. 24.3). In addition, increased gradients of pleural pressure may occur on account of paradoxical chest movements,

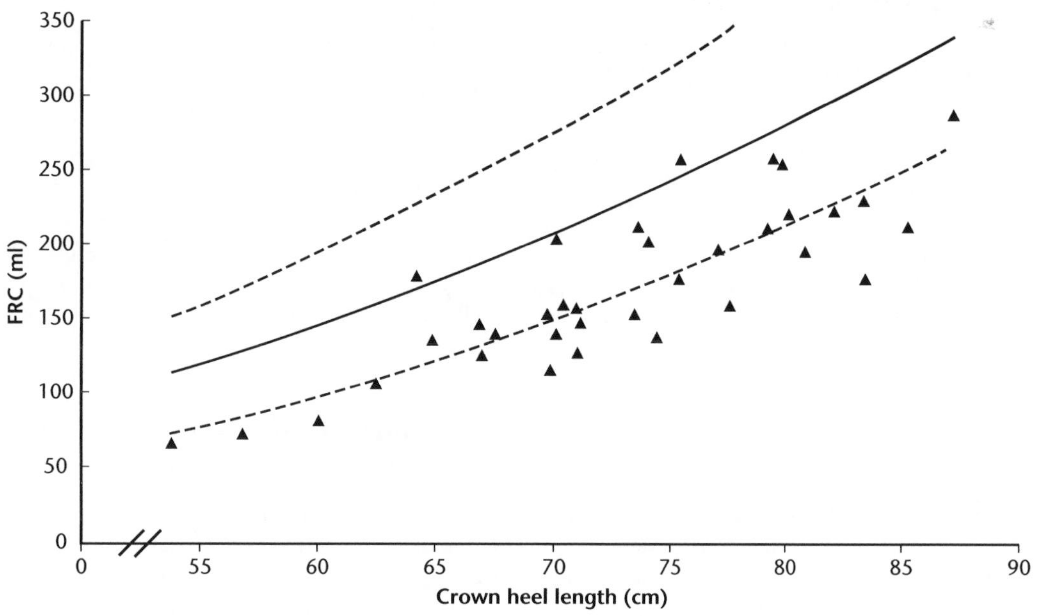

Fig. 24.4 Relationship of FRC measured by whole-body plethysmography to length in infants of both sexes. Continuous line with 95% limits are from [21]. The closed symbols are recent plethysmographic data; they lie below the mean line and more nearly resemble results obtained by the helium dilution method (Table 24.2). Source: [32].

rapid breathing (f_R > 60/min) or airflow obstruction. The reliability of the oesophageal pressure should be checked by comparing it over two or three breaths with that measured in a closed face mask. The two should agree to within 10%.

Spirometric method. The total respiratory compliance can be measured during closed circuit spirometry, with weights applied to the spirometer bell. The compliance is then the volume change divided by the mean increase in pressure within the circuit. In young infants the compliance measured in this way is effectively that of the lungs since the compliance of the thoracic cage is relatively high. The chest wall compliance decreases as the infant gets older and after the age of 6 months it makes a material contribution to the total respiratory compliance. The method is only suitable before this age. Subsequently, the occlusion technique can be used.

Occlusion technique. Static lung compliance can be obtained from measurements of volume and of pressure in the mouth during brief occlusion of the airway. The measurement is made during tidal breathing and is suitable throughout the first year of life. It depends on the Hering–Breuer inflation reflex causing the respiratory muscles to relax during the occlusion, hence mouth pressure becomes equal to alveolar pressure. The linear part of the relationship of mouth pressure to lung volume is then the total respiratory compliance [34]. The method depends on the accuracy of the measurement of alveolar pressure; this can be under-estimated if there is airway narrowing or over-estimated as a consequence of adduction of the larynx. The latter error can be overcome by use of a tracheal catheter.

Airway and chest wall resistance (including nasal resistance)

Combined with measurement of compliance. The occlusion technique for measuring compliance can be extended to also measure the resistance. For this purpose a passive expiratory flow–volume curve is recorded following release of the occlusion. Then, provided the respiratory muscles remain relaxed, the slope of the linear part of the curve is the time constant of the respiratory system. The time constant is the product of total thoracic resistance and compliance (Section 16.1.9); hence, as the compliance is measured by the procedure the resistance can be calculated. In practice, in the presence of airway obstruction, pressures may not equilibrate rapidly enough to measure elastic recoil at the airway opening. It is then not possible to represent the respiratory system by a single time constant.

Plethysmograph method. Airflow limitation in babies can be assessed by measurement of airway resistance using whole body plethysmography (Section 14.6.3). In adults this usually entails panting. In infants the alternative is to supply the pneumotachograph with air at body temperature saturated with water vapour. The equipment is illustrated above (Fig. 24.3); its use requires a high level of technical competence [6, No.9]. Where this is available the procedure works well in most babies, especially those with a raised airway resistance. The result (expressed as specific airway conductance) can be used to discriminate between upper and lower airway disease.

Forced oscillation technique (FOT). The impedance of the respiratory system is measured by applying forced oscillations to the contained air (Section 14.4.4). The method is widely used on account of not requiring much cooperation from the subject, but has the disadvantage for infants that much of the resistance is in the nose. In addition, when the oscillations are applied at the mouth, part of the resulting flow is absorbed in moving the wall of the upper airway. The movement can be reduced by applying the oscillations to the nose as well as to the mouth. This is done by enclosing the head in a box. However, the procedure is difficult to apply to infants [35].

24.4.6 Measurement of transfer factor (diffusing capacity)

In newborn infants the transfer factor is measured by the steady state carbon monoxide method ($Tl_{co,ss}$) [36]. The method is modified from that for adults (Section 20.3).

24.5 Reference values (infants and young children)

Information on lung function in healthy neonates and infants is available from many laboratories. However, in most instances few subjects have been studied and the measurements have not always been made by exactly the same methods or to the same technical standards. Hence, there are as yet no agreed reference values and more studies using standard methods are needed. In addition, the ethnic origin and environmental factors, including exposure to tobacco smoke, should be taken into account. Gender affects forced expiratory flows, which are greater in girls, but not the static lung volumes; the latter are independent of gender after crown-heel length has been allowed for. Some results that appear to meet present day criteria are summarised here (Tables 24.1 and 24.2, also Figs 24.4–24.6). The values are comparable to those for adults when allowance is made for the difference in body size.

24.6 Indications for testing lung function in infancy

Modern infant lung function testing originated in 1949 in an academic department of physiology [39] and much subsequent effort has been devoted to perfecting the methods for application to patients. There are still relatively few reports of successful use, but as a result of intensive development work the number can be expected to increase. However, the procedures are expensive to deploy and some are invasive, so if they are to be used on a regular

Table 24.2 Average lung function in healthy infants born at term.

	Units	Mean values and ranges (±2 SD)	
Details of subjects:			
Postnatal age*	weeks	6.2	3.4–10
Body mass	kg	4.5	2.9–6.1
Crown-heel length (l)	cm	55.4	49–61
Measurements during spontaneous breathing:			
Tidal volume (Vt)	ml kg^{-1}	8.6	6.4–10.8
Respiratory frequency (fR)	per min	45.1	27.7–62.5
Duration of inspiration (tI)	s	0.58	0.4–0.76
Duration of expiration (tE)	s	0.80	0.44–1.16
Pa,O_2	kPa and mm Hg	9.0 and 68	–
$\dot{Q}_s/\dot{Q}_t$	%	10	–
FRC	ml	see Fig. 24.4	
Measurements entailing augmented breathing and/or thoraco-abdominal compression:			
Total respiratory resistance (Rrs)	kPa l^{-1}s	3.98	1.7–6.3
Total respiratory compliance (Crs)	ml $kPa^{-1}kg^{-1}$	9.0	5.9–12.1
Inflation volume (Vinf)	ml kg^{-1}	23.4	15.6–31.2
$\dot{V}\,max_{FRC}\,^{0.5}$(ml s^{-1}) (Fig. 24.5)	Boys 4.22 + 0.0021 1^2 RSD 3.01, R^2 0.48		
	Girls –1.23 + 0.242 1 RSD 2.72, R^2 0.49		
$\ln FEV_{0.5}$ (ml s^{-1}) boys and girls	−3.88 + 2.113 ln (length) + 0.139 ln (age) ± 14%†		
lnFVC (ml) (Fig. 24.6)	−5.804 + 2.614 ln (length) + 0.144 ln (age) ±15%†		

* Corrected for gestational age.
† Age in weeks.
Sources: [21 and 32–39].

basis the benefits must clearly outweigh the disadvantages. This aspect has recently been reviewed (Table 24.3).

24.7 Lung function in children aged 2–6 years

The lung function of children between the ages of approximately 2 and 6 years was formerly a closed subject that is now in process of rapid development. As a result a success rate of 70% to 80% can now be achieved for most of the techniques listed in Table 24.4. The essential ingredients for a successful outcome include an appropriate setting and approach to the child (see Section 31.2), also [41], ample time and application of charm and guile. If not too ill, the child usually finds the experience fun! The subject is reviewed by Stocks [46].

Table 24.3 Situations for which infant lung function testing should be recommended.

Unexplained tachypnoea, hypoxia, cough or respiratory distress not diagnosed by clinical means.
Continuous chronic airways obstruction not responding to standard treatment (Section 15.7).
Circumstances where there is a need for evidence to assist in formulating clinical policy.
Research and development.

Source: Adapted from [40].

24.8 Older children

Lung function, body dimensions, body composition and exercise in older children can be assessed by the methods used for adults.

Table 24.4 Measurements usually tolerated by young children.

Aspect	Indices	
Anthropometry	Stature (standing height), body mass	Section 4.3.2
Ventilatory capacity	Forced ventilatory flows and volumes, e.g. PEF, $FEV_{0.5}$ [41].	Sections 12.3, 12.4 and 12.5
Airway resistance	Whole body plethysmography [42], interrupter technique [43], forced oscillation technique [44].	Section 14.6 Section 14.4.6 Section 14.4.4
Ventilation inhomogenity	Lung clearance index [45].	Section 16.2.7
Transcutaneous Po_2	For evaluating bronchodilatation [43].	Sections 7.10 and 15.7.2
Bronchial provocation	Atopy, presence of exercise-induced asthma	Sections 15.3 and 15.8

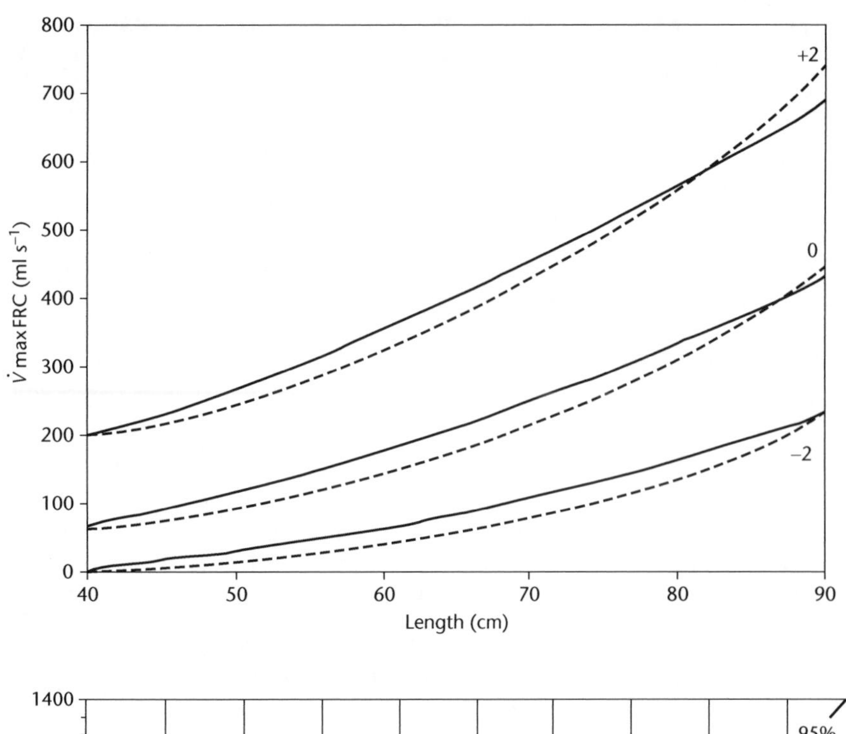

Fig. 24.5 Relationships of $\dot{V}max_{FRC}$ to length in 459 infants aged 3–15 weeks. The pairs of lines are 98th, 50th and 2nd percentiles (continuous for girls and interrupted for boys). The gender difference is significant. Source: [37]

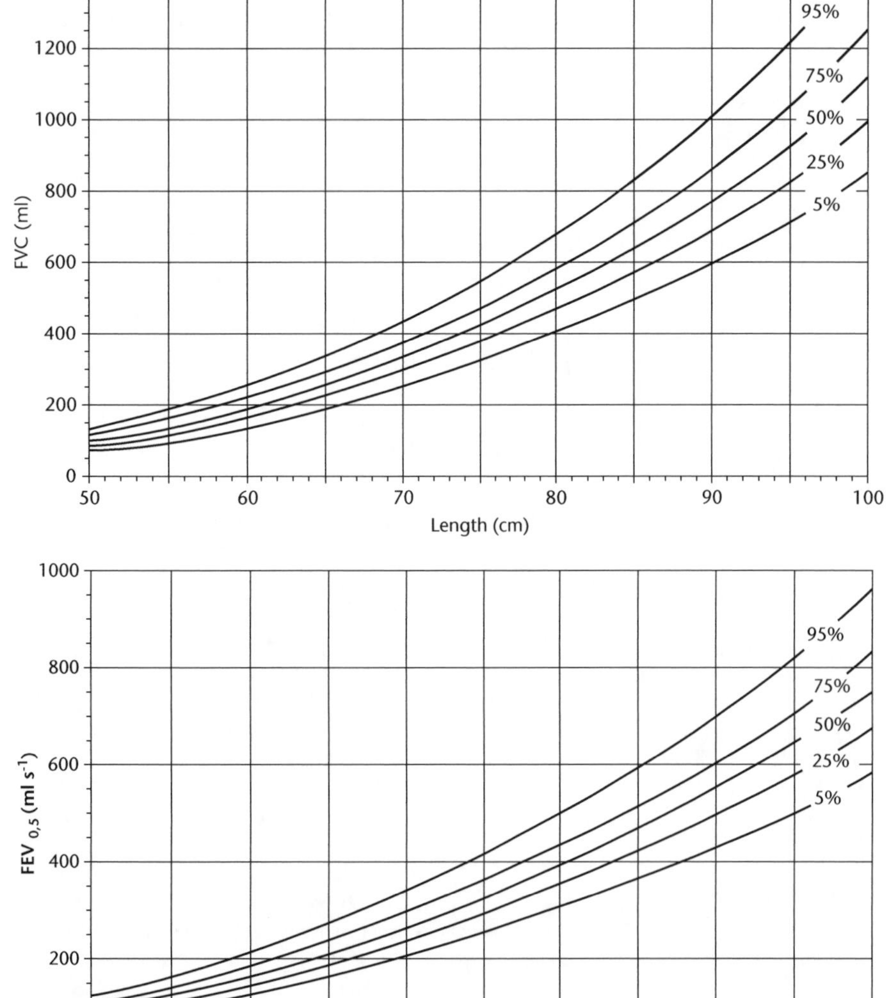

Fig. 24.6 Relationships of $FEV_{0.5}$ and FVC (ml) to length in 155 infants of both sexes aged 3–149 weeks, showing percentiles. The inflation pressure was 30 cm H_2O and the compression up to 120 cm H_2O. In these figures no separate allowance is made for age (cf. Table 24.1). Source: [38]

The assessment should be conducted in an ambience and with a style appropriate to the age group (see Chapter 31, Exercise in Children). Reference values are discussed in Chapters 26 and 31.

24.9 References

1. Ranganathan SC, Stocks J, Dezateux C et al. The evolution of airway function in early childhood following clinical diagnosis of cystic fibrosis. *Am J Respir Crit Care Med* 2004; **169**: 928–933.
2. Stocks J, Dezateux C. The effect of parental smoking on lung function and development during infancy. *Respirology* 2003; **8**: 266–285.
3. Frey U, Kuehni C, Roiha H et al. Maternal atopic disease modifies effects of prenatal risk factors on exhaled nitric oxide in infants. *Am J Respir Crit Care Med* 2004; **170**: 260–265.
4. Stocks J, Sly PD, Tepper RS, Morgan E, eds. *Infant respiratory function testing*. New York: Wiley-Liss, 1996.
5. Stocks J, Sly P, Morris MG, Frey U. Standards for infant respiratory function testing: what(ever) next? *Eur Respir J* 2000; **16**: 581–584.
6. Stocks J, Gerritsen J, eds. *Standards for infant respiratory function testing*: ERS/ATS Task Force.
   No. 1. Frey U, Stocks J, Coates A, Sly P, Bates J. Specifications for equipment used for infant pulmonary function testing. *Eur Respir J* 2000; **16**: 731–740.
   No. 2. Sly PD, Tepper R, Henschen M et al. Tidal forced expirations. *Eur Respir J* 2000; **16**: 741–748.
   No. 3. Frey U, Stocks J, Sly, P, Bates J. Specifications for signal processing and data handling used for infant pulmonary function testing. *Eur Respir J* 2000; **16**: 1016–1022.
   No. 4. Bates JHT, Schmalisch D, Filbrun D, Stocks J. Tidal breathing analysis for infant pulmonary function testing. *Eur Respir J* 2000; **16**: 1180–1192.
   No. 5. Gappa M, Colin AA, Goetz I, Stocks J. Passive respiratory mechanics: the occlusion techniques. *Eur Respir J* 2001; **17**: 141–148.
   No. 6. Stocks J, Godfrey S, Beardsmore C et al. Plethysmographic measurements of lung volume and airway resistance. *Eur Respir J* 2001; **17**: 302–312.
   No. 7. Morris MG, Gustafsson P, Tepper R et al. The bias flow nitrogen washout technique for measuring functional residual capacity in infants. *Eur Respir J* 2001; **17**: 529–536.
   No. 8. Frey U, Reinmann B, Stocks J. The infant lung function model: a mechanical analogue for testing infant lung function equipment. *Eur Respir J* 2001; **17**: 755–764
   No. 9. Reinmann B, Stocks J, Frey U. Assessment of an infant whole body plethysmograph using an infant lung function model. *Eur Respir J* 2001; 17: 765–772.
7. Stocks J, Hislop AA. Structure and function of the respiratory system: Development aspects and their relevance for aerosol therapy. In Bisgaard H, O'Callaghan C, Smaldon GC eds. Drug delivery to the lung: clinical aspects. Marcel Dekker, New York 2002; 47–104.
8. Lambert RK, Castile RG, Tepper RS. Model of forced expiratory flows and airway geometry in infants. *J Appl Physiol* 2004; **96**: 688–692.
9. Lucius H, Gahlenbeck H, Kleine H-O et al. Respiratory functions, buffer system and electrolyte concentrations of blood during human pregnancy. *Respir Physiol* 1970; **9**: 311–317.
10. Hertzberg T, Lagercrantz H. Postnatal sensitivity of the peripheral chemoreceptors in newborn infants. *Arch Dis Child* 1987; **62**: 1238–1241.
11. Copland IB, Post M. Understanding the mechanisms of infant respiratory distress and chronic lung disease. *Am J Respir Cell Mol Biol* 2002; **26**: 261–265.
12. Lenfant C. Lung research: government and community. The 1982 Burns Anderson Lecture. *Am Rev Respir Dis* 1982; **126**: 753–757.
13. Sweet DG, Halliday HL. Current perspectives on the drug treatment of neonatal respiratory distress syndrome. *Paediatr Drugs* 1999; **1**: 19–30.
14. Suresh GK, Soll RF. Current surfactant use in premature infants. *Clin Perinatol* 2001; **28**: 671–694.
15. Lum S, Hoo AF, Stocks J. Influence of jacket tightness and pressure on raised lung volume forced expiratory maneuvers in infants. *Pediatr Pulmonol* 2002; **34**: 361–368.
16. Lum S, Hulskamp G, Hoo AF et al. Effect of raised lung volume technique on subsequent measures of V'maxFRC in infants. *Pediatr Pulmonol* 2004; **38**: 146–154.
17. Sackner MA, Watson H, Belsto AS et al. Calibration of respiratory inductive plethysmography. *J Appl Physiol* 1989; **66**: 410–420.
18. Tepper RS, Morgan WJ, Cota K, Taussig LM. Expiratory flow limitation in infants with bronchopulmonary dysplasia *J Pediat* 1986; **109**: 1040–1046.
19. Beardsmore CS, Godfrey S, Silverman M. Forced expiratory flow-volume curves in infants and young children. *Eur Resp J* 1989; **2**(Suppl. 4): 154S–159S.
20. Henschen M, Stocks J, Hoo Ah-F, Dixon P. Analysis of forced expiratory maneuvers from raised lung volumes in preterm infants. *J Appl Physiol* 1998; **85**: 1989–1997.
21. Stocks J, Quanjer Ph H. Reference values for residual volume, functional residual capacity and total lung capacity. *Eur Respir J* 1995; **8**: 492–506.
22. Ranganathan SC, Hoo AF, Lum SY et al. Exploring the relationship between forced maximal flow at functional residual capacity and parameters of forced expiration from raised lung volumes in healthy infants. *Pediatr Pulmonol* 2002; **33**: 419–428.
23. Hanrahan JP, Tager IB, Castle RG et al. Pulmonary function measures in healthy infants. Variability and size corrections. *Am Rev Respir Dis* 1990; **141**: 1127–1135.
24. Sheikh S, Castile R, Hayes J et al. Assessing bronchodilator responsiveness in infants using partial expiratory flow-volume curves. *Pediatr Pulmonol* 2003; **36**: 196–201.
25. Maxwell DL, Prendiville A, Rose A, Silverman M. Lung volume changes during histamine-induced bronchoconstriction in recurrently wheezy infants. *Pediatr Pulmonol* 1988; **5**: 145–151.
26. LeSouef PN, Hughes DM, Landau LI. Shape of forced expiratory flow-volume curves in infancy. *Am Rev Respir Dis* 1988; **138**: 590–597.
27. Jones MH, Davis SD, Kisling JA et al. Flow limitation in infants assessed by negative expiratory pressure. *Am J Respir Crit Care Med* 2000; **161**: 713–717.
28. Schibler A, Hall GL, Businger F et al. Measurement of lung volume and ventilatory distribution with an ultrasonic flow meter in healthy infants. *Eur Respir J* 2002; **20**: 912–918.
29. Morris MG. A novel non-invasive technique for measuring the residual lung volume by nitrogen washout with rapid thoracoabdominal compression in infants. *Thorax* 1999; **54**: 874–883
30. Hammer J, Numa A, Newth CJL. Total lung capacity by N_2 washout from high and low lung volumes in ventilated infants and children. *Am J Respir Crit Care Med* 1998; **158**: 526–531.

31. Milner AD. Lung function testing in infancy. *Arch Dis Child* 1990; **65**: 548–552.
32. Hulskamp G, Hoo AF, Ljungberg H et al Progressive decline in plethysmographic lung volumes in infants: physiology or technology? *Am J Respir Crit Care Med* 2003; **168**: 1003–1009.
33. Fumey MH. Nickerson BG, Birch M. et al. A radiographic method for estimating lung volumes in sick infants. *Pediat Pulmonol* 1992; **13**: 42–47.
34. Fletcher ME, Dezateux CA, Stocks J. Respiratory compliance in infants – a preliminary evaluation of the multiple interrupter technique. *Pediatr Pulmonol* 1992; **14**: 118–125.
35. Desager KN, Cauberghs M, Naudts J, Van de Woestijne KP. Influence of upper airway shunt on total respiratory impedance in infants. *J Appl Physiol* 1999; **87**: 902–909.
36. Jongste JC, Mercus PJFM, Stam H. Lung diffusion capacity. In: Eber E, Hammer J, eds. *Pediatric pulmonary function testing.* Basel: Karger 2005.
37. Hoo AF, Dezateux C, Hanrahan JP et al. Sex-specific prediction equations for Vmax(FRC) in infancy: a multicenter collaborative study. *Am J Respir Crit Care Med* 2002; **165**: 1084–1092.
38. Jones M, Castile R, Davis S et al. Forced expiratory flows and volumes in infants: normative data and lung growth. *Am J Respir Crit Care Med* 2000; **161**: 353–359.
39. Cross KW. The respiratory rate and ventilation in the newborn baby. *J Physiol (Lond)* 1949; **109**: 459–474.
40. Godfrey S, Bar-Yishay E, Avital A, Springer C. What is the role of tests of lung function in the management of infants with lung disease? *Pediatr Pulmonol* 2003; **36**: 1–9.
41. Aurora P, Stocks J, Oliver C et al. Quality control of spirometry in preschool children with and without lung disease. *Am J Respir Crit Care Med* 2004; **169**: 1152–1159.
42. Bisgaard H, Nielsen KG. Plethysmographic measurements of specific airway resistance in young children. *Chest* 2005; **128**: 355–362.
43. Beydon N, Trang-Pham H, Bernard A, Gaultier C. Measurement of resistance by the interrupter technique and of transcutaneous partial pressure of oxygen in young children during methacholine challenge. *Pediatr Pulmonol* 2001; **31**: 238–246.
44. Wilson NM, Bridge P, Phagoo SB, Silverman M. The measurement of methacholine responsiveness in 5 year old children: three methods compared. *Eur Respir J* 1995; **8**: 135–140.
45. Aurora P, Bush A, Gustafsson P et al. Multibreath washout as a marker of lung disease in preschool children with cystic fibrosis. *Am J Respir Crit Care Med* 2005; **171**: 249–256.
46. Stocks J. Pulmonary function tests in infants and young children. In: Cherniack V. et al, eds. *Kendig's disorders of the respiratory tract in children.* 7th ed. Philadelphia, Elsevier, 2006; 129–167.

PART 3
Normal Variation in Lung Function

CHAPTER 25

Normal Lung Function from Childhood to Old Age

The progression of lung function mirrors that of life itself. This chapter provides an overview from the age of approximately three years through to the end. The section on ageing includes its effects on the circulation and performance during exercise. Models of the changes and reference values are in Chapter 26. Genetic variation is in Chapter 27.

25.1 Introduction

The lungs develop as gland-like structures during intrauterine life. They become organs of gas exchange with the admission of the first breath, grow steadily during childhood, participate in the adolescent growth spurt and attain optimal performance early in adult life. The function remains at this level, usually with only minor fluctuations, for up to 20 years then starts to decline. The decline reflects the ageing of the lungs and progresses at an increasing rate as time passes. The level of function at any point in the sequence and the rate of decline are influenced by environmental factors and by parallel changes in other components of the body (Fig. 25.1).

25.2 Childhood and adolescence

25.2.1 Early changes

The structures of the lungs have nearly attained their adult form by age 4 years (Section 3.3) and soon after this the arterial oxygen tension stabilises at its adult levels [2]. By age 6 years effective mechanisms are in place for controlling respiration and the distribution of lung ventilation and perfusion. Concurrently there is a progressive increase in the elastic recoil of the lungs. This increases the traction on small airways and hence the forced expiratory flow relative to lung volume [3–6]. The point of closure of airways occurs at a progressively smaller lung volume, so the closing capacity is reduced. There are concurrent increases in the outward recoil of the thoracic cage and the strength of the respiratory muscles (Sections 24.2). Both changes increase the total lung capacity. The calibre of the trachea and other large airways also increase, but not always in proportion to the size of the lungs. The dissociation between the two has been described as *dysanapsis* (unequal growth) [7], see also Section 25.3.1. The different aspects of growth during childhood are summarised in Table 25.1.

25.2.2 Factors that influence development

The principal cause for differences in lung function between children seen at one point in time or longitudinally is that they

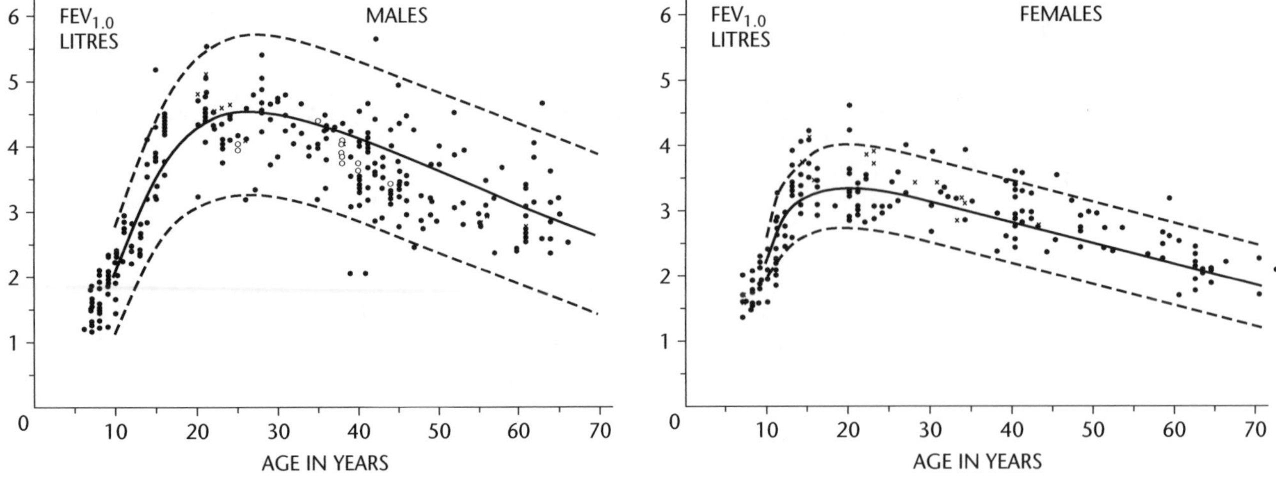

Fig. 25.1 Cross-sectional relationship of forced expiratory volume to age for healthy persons. Source: [1].

differ in size. This is the outcome of a number of factors of which some are considered below (see also Table 25.2).

Skeletal dimensions. In children the largest single determinant of body size and hence of lung size is stature. This variable accounts for approximately 80% of the explained variance between subjects for most indices of lung function (Table 25.3). Sitting height reflects trunk size and also describes much of the variance, but rather less than does stature. However, this situation may change as young people in many countries are currently becoming taller mainly due to their legs continuing to grow in late adolescence, but without much change in trunk length [11]. It is not known at present if the factors that are responsible [12] also influence the lungs. Some additional variation is explained by differences in thoracic dimension, expressed either as sternal length and chest width and depth [13] or as their product which is thoracic volume index [10]. The contribution of the dimensions can also be demonstrated cross-sectionally (Table 25.3). The usefulness of chest dimensions for describing the lung function of young people appears not to extend into adult life.

Body fat and muscle. After allowing for stature some 10% of the remaining variability in lung function between children can be explained by differences in body composition expressed as fat free mass index (FFM/stature^2) and body fat as percentage of body mass [14]. Additional muscle is associated with physical activity and above average production of growth hormone. At the local level it also increases the inspiratory capacity. Additional fat in the thorax and abdomen reduce the lung volumes by occupying space locally and by raising the diaphragm. The fat can also affect the movement of the chest wall.

Variations in the amounts and distribution of muscle and fat occur within each gender group and also between them as in general, boys have more muscle and girls more fat. However, unlike for most indices in adults, an allowance for body muscle does not eliminate altogether the differences between the genders (Table 25.4 cf. Section 25.7). The distribution of any excess

Table 25.1 Effects of somatic growth on lung function in children.

Aspect of growth	Response	Effect on lung function
Thoracic cage elongates and becomes wider and deeper.	Thoracic cavity expands	lung volumes ↑ ventilatory capacity ↑ transfer factor ↑
Quantity of lung tissue increases	Elastic recoil increases	closing capacity ↓ maximal expiratory flows ↑
Chest wall alters in shape	Outward recoil increases	total lung capacity ↑
Muscles, including respiratory muscles enlarge	Muscle strength increases	Inspiratory capacity is increased; this affects total lung capacity, vital capacity and FEV_1
Quantity of fat increases, especially in some girls.	Fat can accumulate in thoracic cavity, abdomen and bosom	Lung volumes and exercise tidal volume (Vt_{30}) can be diminished
Large airways increase in length and diameter	Dysanaptic/isotropic growth	See text

Table 25.2 Circumstances that can affect the size and function of apparently healthy lungs.

Circumstance	Feature	Effect
Genetic factors	Gender	Sections 25.3 and 25.7
	Ethnic group	Chapter 27
	Shared genes	Family resemblance in lung function (especially between identical twins)
Nutrition (*in utero* and childhood)	Adequate nutrition and some dietary factors are necessary. A surplus leads to fat. Insufficiency stunts growth and reduces muscle strength	Deficiencies (or obesity) lead to the lungs being small*
Muscle strength and training	Respiratory muscles are developed by swimming, rowing, underwater diving, high levels of ventilation (e.g. with exercise or at high altitude) and increased respiratory work (some childhood asthmatics)†. Inactivity or muscle weakness from any cause is a disadvantage	Strength of respiratory muscles affects inspiratory capacity and probably also exercise tidal volume (Vt_{30}). ‡
Onset of puberty	The pubertal growth spurt is associated with increased production of growth hormone	Thoracic cavity is enlarged and muscle strength increased, particularly in boys
Raised growth hormone level	Hormone production is increased during puberty and by physical exercise (see above). Some pituitary tumours also produce it	TLC and *Tl* are increased
Domestic circumstances	Potential for physical activity e.g. living in apartment with lift or on a hillside [8]. Walking or going by vehicle to school	As for muscle strength
Polluted air	Tobacco fume (personal or environmental), also cannabis. Fume from gas or solid fuel appliances	Airways are narrowed

* Starvation can increase the lung size both absolutely due to loss of body fat and relative to stature. The latter effect is sometimes observed in asthmatic children taking oral steroids; it is then a consequence of the reduction in height upon which the reference value is based.
† This effect is confined to children and is not observed in adults [9].
‡ Singing or playing a wind instrument may have a similar effect.

Table 25.3 The contribution of stature and individual chest dimensions to the explained variance in lung function of healthy white children aged 8–17 years. In this analysis chest dimensions did not contribute significantly to the description of FRC or RV.

				Additional explained variance after allowance for stature (%)				
Sex	Index	N	Explained variance due to Stature (%)	Chest width	Chest depth	Sternal length	TVI*	Bi-acromial width
Boys	ln FEV_1	98	84.3	1.5	1.0	1.3	2.8	2.0
	ln FVC	98	88.9	1.8	1.5	0.8	2.8	2.4
	ln TLC	73	88.5	1.3	1.1	0.5†	1.9	2.4
	ln IC	73	79.2	2.0	2.0	0.7†	3.7	3.4
	ln *Tl*	73	86.4	0.7†	0.1†	0†	0.2†	1.9
Girls	ln FEV_1	129	86.0	2.0	2.4	0.1†	2.3	1.3
	ln FVC	129	86.2	1.9	3.0	0.1†	2.4	0.8
	ln TLC	85	72.8	2.6	2.1	0.3†	3.0	2.3
	ln IC	85	51.8	3.0	3.2	0.8†	4.3	2.9
	ln *Tl*	87	64.0	2.6	0.2†	0.2†	0.9†	2.1

* Thoracic volume index (chest width × chest depth × sternal length) [10].
† Non-significant contribution ($p > 0.05$).
Source: Chinn DJ, Cotes JE, Martin AJ, Hey E. unpublished.

Table 25.4 Average percentage differences in indices of lung function between boys and girls aged 8–16 years.

Index	Reference variable (the figures are percentages)		
	Stature	Sitting height	Stature, Fat% & FFMI
FEV_1	−5	−8	−4
FVC	−9	−11	−7
TLC	−7	−10	−6
IC	−11	−13	−8
FRC	ns	−6	ns
Tl	−9	−11	−7

Notes: The table shows the differences that remain after allowing for different anthropometric features. FFMI is fat-free mass index.
ns = not significant. There were no gender differences for RV, *K*co (*T*l/*V*A) and PEF.
Source: [14].

Table 25.5 Air pollutants that can damage the lungs.*

Type	Source
Domestic	Parental smoking Fumes from stoves, open fires and cookers Contributors to sick building syndrome
Personal	Smoking tobacco or cannabis
Environmental	Smoke from domestic and industrial chimneys (aggravated by geographical features and temperature inversions) Fumes and small airborne particles from motor vehicles and aircraft engines Oxidation products (ozone and oxides of nitrogen) Agricultural fungicides and insecticides Public health and crowd control agents Other toxic agents

* These topics are reviewed in Chapter 37.

fat as between the thorax and abdomen on the one hand and the hips on the other is also important. The distribution can be influenced by ethnic group. The effect of allowing for body composition is greatest for those children who have more or less fat and/or muscle compared with the average child. Body mass index, because it combines information on both fat and muscle, does not provide similar information (Section 4.6, also [15]).

Environmental factors including level of habitual activity. Sustained activity influences the production of growth hormone and this affects the lungs. As a result the lungs are relatively large in children who grow up amongst hills or in mountainous regions or who are exposed to the rigors of a cold climate. The lungs are relatively small among those who live in high-rise flats with lifts and have few opportunities for recreation [8].

At high altitude the effect on the lungs of physical activity can be facilitated by a direct contribution from hypoxia. In children who regularly experience exercise-induced airflow obstruction the additional respiratory work might also be expected to affect the lungs.

The amount and composition of the diet, including the content of vitamins and related factors, influences the growth of the lungs. This effect is both direct and by providing some protection against infections and the effects of breathing polluted air (Table 25.5). Additional factors can influence the degree of protection that is provided. They include atopic status, other genetic features and exposure to sunlight. The latter determines the intrinsic production of vitamin D.

Role of developmental age. The development of the lungs does not take place at a uniform rate with respect to somatic growth [16, 17] or the passage of time [18]. Instead, the different features have their own characteristic patterns that exhibit perturbations depending on the environmental exposures and in relation to puberty. The age of onset of puberty differs between the sexes (see below). As a result the different lung function indices need individual consideration, both biologically and in terms of the models that are used to describe them (Section 26.1.4). A model for lung function in childhood can include a term for age (e.g. Section 26.3.3) but here age is a surrogate for a biological variable, not a primary determinant of lung function.

25.3 Puberty and transition to adult lung function

See Footnote 25.1

25.3.1 Contribution of gender

Before puberty the lung function indices that include inspiratory capacity are on average some 7% larger in boys than in girls of the same stature [14, 19] (also Table 25.4). This is due to boys having larger inspiratory capacities relative to stature because of their greater muscle strength. The residual and expiratory reserve volumes are similar in boys and girls, as are the forced expiratory flows (PEF, FEF_{50} and FEF_{75}). However, when related to lung volume the flows are, on average, larger in girls, suggesting that their airways are shorter and wider [20]. This dissociation between the dimensions of the lungs and airways is a consequence of unequal growth (*dysanapsis* [7]). The inequality originates in early childhood [21].

In the UK puberty usually occurs at a mean age of approximately 12 years in girls and 14 years in boys, but with wide individual variation. Its duration is approximately 3 years. Before puberty and also after puberty the relationships of lung function to stature are relatively linear. At puberty the growth in stature

Footnote 25.1. Reference values that span puberty are in Sections 26.3.2 and 26.3.3.

exhibits a temporary increase, the adolescent growth spurt. There is an even more marked increase in growth of the lungs. This reveals itself as a discontinuity in the relationship of lung function to stature and is initially due to growth in length of the thoracic cavity. Subsequently, in young men, after longitudinal growth has ceased the lateral and antero-posterior dimensions of the thoracic cage continue to increase (see skeletal dimensions above). There may be some flattening of the diaphragm. The strength of the respiratory muscles also increases, particularly in boys. The growth in thoracic length leads to the step increase being less conspicuous when related to trunk length than to stature [19].

25.3.2 Girls and young women

The earlier onset of puberty in girls leads to their lungs growing rapidly at a time when the lungs of boys are growing relatively slowly. As a result, the size of the lungs of girls catches up with and temporarily exceeds that of boys of the same age, though this may not be the case for forced vital capacity on account of the greater muscle strength of boys. The step increase in lung function in girls in the UK currently occurs at an average stature of 1526 mm, but with some individual variation [19]. For the indices FEV_1, FVC and PEF the increase amounts to some 10%. It is much less or absent for the other indices. This is due in part to growth being terminated abruptly by fusion of epiphyses at a relatively young age (see also skeletal dimensions above). Thereafter, FEV_1 may increase by a small amount (e.g. 10 ml $year^{-1}$), whilst FVC can decline on account of accumulation of fat. The latter trend is frequently reversed in early adult life.

25.3.3 Boys and young men

In boys the step increase in lung function associated with puberty currently occurs in the UK at an average stature of 1625 mm and age 14 year [19]. It is on average 16%, which is larger than in girls and affects most indices of lung function. The changes are associated with proportional growth of the airways and lung parenchyma, so the lungs exhibit *isotropic* growth [22]. As a result the step increase affects indices of flow as well as of volume and gas exchange. Thereafter, FEV_1 and FVC continue to increase until about 25 years of age. Up to about 17 years of age the growth is linked to that of stature, with an additional component from enhanced strength of the respiratory muscles (e.g. Fig. 9.1, page 101). At approximately age 18 years growth in stature ceases but the thoracic cavity continues to enlarge, mainly as a result of the thorax becoming wider. Other thoracic dimensions also increase, but to a lesser extent (Table 25.3), and enhance the lung function of young men compared with young women. The resulting differences continue into and throughout adult life.

This third stage in the development of the lungs of young men possibly differs from the others in that the increases in total mass of the lungs and the quantity of collagen appear to lag behind the increase in lung volume. This could be a factor in the lungs of men being more susceptible to wear and tear later in life compared with the lungs of women (Section 25.7, see also Section 37.3). However, the final mass relative to body size and the mechanical properties of the lungs of men and women are similar [23, 24].

25.4 Lung function in early adulthood

After the impressive improvement in lung function that occurs during adolescence a plateau is reached. However, this is an average response and it conceals individual differences, with the majority of people showing small changes, either up or down, over the next decade [25]. The changes have been explored for FEV_1 and FVC, where there are ample data. The fluctuations are mainly due to environmental factors, including those listed in Table 25.5 and to changes in body composition [26], but not all the factors that contribute to variation around the plateau have been identified. During the plateau phase the lungs start to be affected by a progressive loss of lung tissue, including elastic tissue, that is part of the process of ageing. The changes can begin in adolescence. They occur earlier in smokers than in non-smokers and affect all aspects of lung function (Section 25.9). For descriptive purposes the ageing process is under way when the partial regression coefficient of lung function on age changes sign (from positive to negative or vice versa). The age at the transition occurs earlier for indices that are mainly determined by lung elasticity than for those to which muscle strength or structural changes in the lungs make a material contribution (e.g. Table 25.6.). The points of transition differ between men and women (Table 26.28, page 361). Reference values are in Section 26.4.

25.5 Variation in lung function between adults

25.5.1 Roles of body fat and muscle

Fat can be laid down in the mediastinum, around the heart, in the pleural space and above the diaphragm. In any of these positions it occupies space that would otherwise be available for alveolar air. Similarly, in the abdomen, fat can accumulate round the kidneys, other organs and in the mesentery. Additional

Table 25.6 Mean age at the start of lung function decline in 488 shipyard workers.

	Age at start of decline (year)	
	Smokers *	non-smokers
FEV_1	18.5	25.1
FVC	25.8	35.6
PEF	35.0	45.2

Notes: For interpretation see text
* Smoked at some time during period of follow up (7.2 years). For each index the decline started earlier in the smokers ($p < 0.05$).
Source: Chinn DJ, Cotes JE. Unpublished.

fat reduces the functional residual capacity both directly by its presence in the thorax and indirectly by raising the diaphragm. Thus, a high level of body fat reduces the static lung volumes whilst a low level enhances them. On this account fat located mainly in the abdomen, as in men with a 'beer belly', can restrict the vital capacity (Fig. 4.4, page 35). Fat in the bosom can also have a dynamic effect by causing rapid, shallow breathing during exercise (Section 28.4.3).

The quantity of fat is best expressed as a percentage of body mass (Fat%, Section 4.7.1) and this index describes some of the gender difference in lung function [27]. Abdominal fat can be represented by the ratio of the waist to hip circumferences which is larger in men than women [28, 29]; the reverse is the case for body fat generally (Section 4.7).

Body mass index. Fat constitutes an important component of body mass index, but this index also includes the fat free mass, of which the largest component is muscle (see below). For most indices of lung function the contributions of fat and muscle are in opposition and such indices are independent of BMI. The principal exception is expiratory reserve volume (ERV) where the effects of the two components are synergistic in reducing ERV. Thus, for cross-sectional studies BMI can be a reference variable for this index and hence also for functional residual capacity [27].

The situation is different for longitudinal studies since body fat is relatively labile whilst in most people who are free from active disease the quantity of muscle usually only declines by a small amount between early adult life and late middle age. As a result a *change* in BMI (ΔBMI) usually represents a change in body fat. In longitudinal studies ΔBMI has been found to be a useful guide to change in lung function [26, 30, 31].

25.5.2 Roles of habitual activity and athletic training

Accessory muscles of respiration. The accessory muscles of respiration act by raising and expanding the rib cage (Section 9.4). As a result their strength contributes to the inspiratory capacity. The increase can be linearly related to maximal inspiratory pressure [32] and to fat-free body mass (FFM), with which it is correlated positively. The change is often not accompanied by a corresponding increase in the forced expiratory volume, so $FEV_1\%$ (FEV_1/FVC) can be relatively low [33]. The increase in vital capacity is then associated with a reduction in forced expiratory flow at small lung volumes ($FEF_{75\%FVC}$, [34]); the mechanism is unclear.

Habitual activity. Physical activity develops the relevant skeletal muscles; it also gives rise to high levels of ventilation that exert a training effect on the respiratory muscles. In addition, concern for physical fitness may also lead to a person eating a 'healthy' diet and having a low body fat in consequence. Thus, the effects of activity and physical training are multidimensional.

A high level of habitual physical activity contributes to the lung function of people living at high altitude or in hilly terrain, many agriculturists, nomads and those who participate in gymnastics, ball games, athletics and active outdoor recreations. In some circumstances the high level of activity is mandatory from an early age, whilst in others it is acquired during adolescence or subsequently. The former activities, in particular, are associated with an increase in the size of the lung and its capacity to transfer gas (Table 25.7). The changes are partly due to the release of growth hormone which activates several insulin growth factors, including IGF-1 and 2, to stimulate tissue growth (Section 28.12). On this account habitual activity during childhood can influence respiratory function in adult life.

Athletic training

Overview. Athletes do not comprise a homogenous group. Middle-distance runners have long legs, often are lightly built and have high aerobic capacities whereas sprinters and weight lifters have greater muscle strength and different overall physical dimensions. A well-developed shoulder girdle is a feature of weight lifters, rowers and canoeists, archers, deep-sea divers and other swimmers. Long distance swimmers usually have a thick layer of subcutaneous fat that provides buoyancy as well as insulation. In all sportsmen and women the quantity of the

Table 25.7 Habitual activity and transfer factor. The transfer factor, standardised for age, stature and haemoglobin concentration (Tls,st) is here related to physical condition as reflected by exercise cardiac frequency, standardised for oxygen uptake and body muscle ($fC_{45,st}$).

Activity level	Group	$fC_{45,st}$ (per min)	Tls,st (SI units)*
High	New Guinea highlands	122†	11.0†
Medium	New Guinea coastal	135	9.6
	UK housewives	134	9.4
Low	Jamaican housewives	145†	7.7†

Notes: The data are for young women studied during the International Biological Programme. The association between the variables is consistent with the transfer factor (which is nearly independent of ethnic group) being influenced by previous habitual activity (*see* also Section 28.6).

* For conversion to traditional units see Table 6.6 (page 56).

† Significant difference compared with UK housewives ($p < 0.05$).

Source: [35].

Table 25.8 Lung volume and the response to exercise in 35 amateur racing cyclists compared with the average for healthy young men of the same age and stature (respectively, 22 years and 1.75 m).

Indices	Cyclists*	Controls
Forced expiratory volume (FEV_1) (l)	4.60	4.38
Inspiratory capacity (l)	3.75	3.40
Expiratory reserve volume (l)	1.37	1.54
Transfer factor (mmol min^{-1} kPa^{-1} and ml min^{-1} mm Hg^{-1})	13.4 (39.9)	12.3 (36.6)
Kco (Tl l^{-1})	2.01 (5.99)	1.83 (5.46)
Exercise cardiac frequency† (min^{-1})	109	122
Maximal O_2 uptake (mmol min^{-1} and l min^{-1})	196 (4.39)	158 (3.53)
Maximal exercise ventilation (l min^{-1})	161	127

* All values for cyclists are significantly different from those for control subjects ($p < 0.05$).
† At oxygen uptake = 67 mmol min^{-1} (1.5 l min^{-1}).
Source: [36].

relevant muscle is increased, there is usually an increase in respiratory muscle strength and, for most sports, the quantity of body fat is below average. In addition, an athlete may have another anatomical feature that confers a respiratory advantage, for example a long trunk length in a swimmer. As a result, participants in many sports, including middle distance running, cycling or swimming events, usually have above average levels of lung function compared with a general population (Table 25.8). However, such persons often have a more active lifestyle than most of their peers, so the association between extent of regular exercise and lung function is partly causal [37, 38]. A diminution in the level of activity reverses most of the effects of training, particularly those that were acquired in the recent past. For example, in a study of divers after a deep dive, the half time for restoration of vital capacity to its pre-dive level was approximately 4 weeks [39] (also Fig. 35.2, page 490). Similarly, an increase in maximal breathing capacity measured at constant air density resulting from participation in a mountaineering expedition to high altitude, diminishes after return to sea level. By contrast, changes acquired over a long period of time tend to persist. For this reason the level of previous activity should be taken into account when interpreting lung function in an individual (e.g. Table 25.2).

Lung volumes and ventilatory capacity. Development of the accessory muscles of respiration increases inspiratory capacity, whilst a below average amount of body fat enlarges expiratory reserve volume. Both effects increase total lung capacity, vital capacity and indices dependent on them. Forced expiratory volume, because it is dependent on lung elasticity is relatively independent of physical activity and as a consequence the training can reduce the ratio of FEV_1 to vital capacity. It can also reduce maximal flows at small lung volumes (see 'Accessory muscles of respiration' above). Peak expiratory flow and maximal breathing capacity can be increased.

Transfer factor. Physically active persons tend to have a high transfer factor. This is due in part to their usually having relatively large lungs, hence a large surface area for exchange of gas. When the activity starts in childhood there is also suggestive evidence for an increase in density of alveolar capillaries. Thus, transfer factor can be increased by exercise during the period of growth but not during adult life [9]. A possible mechanism could be that prolonged activity increases the production of growth hormone and this promotes the growth of the lungs. Activity also affects total body haemoglobin and other variables but the changes are transient.

Ventilatory response to carbon dioxide. In divers, underwater swimmers and persons who undertake periods of breathing against a resistance the ventilatory response to carbon dioxide is often reduced; the tolerance to carbon dioxide of such subjects can be increased [40]. The phenomenon appears to be an adaptation to an increase in the work of breathing. It can also occur with athletic training. In the swimmers it may be due in part to their having a high proportion of body fat, sufficient to increase the work of breathing. Obese individuals exhibit a similar response.

25.6 Cyclical variation in lung function

The function of the lungs exhibits seasonal and diurnal variations about a mean which itself changes with age. In women additional changes occur in phase with the menstrual cycle. The variations relate to the pattern of sleep, posture, meals, ambient temperature and, in females, levels of hormone production. Hours of daylight can also contribute.

Central drive to respiration is reduced by normal sleep, though not by rapid eye movement sleep (REM sleep). The sequence of sleep and wakefulness leads to a diurnal variation in alveolar ventilation which is lower at night. The reduction raises the tension of carbon dioxide and lowers the tension of oxygen in arterial blood. The variation is linked to sleep and has not been observed if the subject remains awake (Section 32.4.2). Other variations are linked to the change in posture that accompanies sleep. The act of lying down raises the diaphragm and alters the position of equilibrium of the thorax. Inspiratory capacity is then increased and ERV reduced. Concurrently, the vital capacity is reduced by influx of blood into the lungs from elsewhere in the body. This, and other causes of redistribution of blood affect the transfer factor (Table 20.11, page 253).

The ambient temperature contributes to the regulation of respiration and the inhalation of cold air causes bronchoconstriction in subjects with reactive airways. These and other factors interact with cyclical changes in blood cortisol and adrenaline levels to cause diurnal variations in lung function [41]. The increase in airway resistance can summate with that due to latent asthma to cause nocturnal wheeze [42]. The raised resistance reduces forced expiratory volume and peak expiratory flow, increases functional residual capacity and contributes to less uniform distribution of inspired gas [43], cf. Fig. 15.1, page 168. The changes can overflow into daytime; for example, airway resistance declines between morning and afternoon by approximately 2.5% per hour [44]. A suggestion that there are similar oscillations in transfer factor [45] has not been confirmed [46].

Seasonal variation in airway resistance and FEV_1 is relatively common and can be associated with any of several environmental factors. These include ambient temperature, hours of daylight, particulate air pollutants, ozone levels, airborne spores, pollen or mites, and other variables. The amplitude of the variation in FEV_1 is small, approximately 0.1 l [47–50].

Implications for measuring lung function. The time of day and the season are important for longitudinal studies of groups of subjects amongst whom a cyclical variation can be of similar magnitude to that due to age, air pollution or other factor. Such variations can summate with others including those due to ingestion of food. Representative results are likely to be obtained when the measurements are made in a controlled environment during office hours, preferably during the morning or mid afternoon, but not after a heavy meal [51, 52]. The time of day should also be standardised when undertaking trials into the action of drugs that can affect airway calibre (Section 15.7.2).

25.7 Differences in function between men and women

Relevance of body composition and age. Compared with men, women usually have smaller lungs and lower ventilatory capacity and transfer factor. Part of the difference is due to women on average being smaller and the discrepancies are less when size is taken into account. But, how this is done greatly influences the outcome [53, 54]. In two studies where stature was allowed for using a linear model the average gender differences in vital capacity were, respectively, approximately 900 ml and 720 ml [55, 27]. In the latter study the difference was the same at all ages. It was mainly due to the men having a larger inspiratory capacity and this in turn was due to them being more muscular and having less body fat than the women. Hence, the gender differences in FVC and IC did not reside in the lungs but in the anatomical features of the thorax.

For FEV_1, FRC, RV and *Tl* the gender difference varied depending on the age of the subjects. The age dependency was eliminated when the lung function was expressed on a proportional basis by using logarithms. In the case of FRC this transformation also eliminated the gender difference itself. For transfer factor and FEV_1 the gender difference remained, but for transfer factor it was eliminated when allowance was made for fat free mass. The mechanism for this was unclear, but it could have reflected an association between FFM and total body haemoglobin. Thus, taking aspects of body composition into account can eliminate the difference between men and women for some indices of lung function.

Gender and ventilatory capacity. The greater size of the lungs of young men compared with young women appears to extend to all its component parts, including the air sacs, the alveoli and the air passages from respiratory bronchioles to trachea. The airway resistance of men is somewhat less in consequence. This factor contributes to the men having the larger FEV_1. However, the proportion of the forced vital capacity that can be expired in the first second (FEV%) is less for men than for women. The lower ratio is partly due to the denominator in men, but not in women, continuing to enlarge during early adulthood when the forced expiratory volume is already declining. In addition, the tracheal cross-sectional area appears to be more closely related to lung volume in women than that in men, possibly on account of the women not having a third phase of lung growth (Section 25.3.2).

Gender and lung elasticity. The lungs of men are more compliant than the lungs of women, mainly because they are larger. This difference reflects the respective respiratory muscle strength in the two sexes. However, the sex difference in compliance disappears when the volume–pressure curves are expressed in terms of a theoretical maximal volume that is independent of muscle strength [24]. When this is done the results suggest that the bulk elastic properties of the lungs of young men and women are identical.

Gender and blood gases. The distribution of ventilation–perfusion ratios and the tension of oxygen in the arterial blood are similar in men and women. However, the tension of carbon dioxide is somewhat lower in women as a result of the rise in blood concentration of progesterone that occurs during the second half of the menstrual cycle (Section 25.8.1). The progesterone increases the respiratory drive and this in turns lowers the constant term *B* of the ventilatory response to carbon dioxide (Section 23.5.3). The drive and the value for *B* change further during pregnancy (Section 25.8.2).

Gender and exercise. During submaximal exercise, standardised for consumption of oxygen, the ventilation and cardiac frequency are on average higher in women compared with men. For a given alveolar ventilation, women have a smaller tidal volume and greater frequency of breathing. As a result a larger volume of air per minute is used to flush the anatomical deadspace. In addition, women experience additional respiratory drive from progesterone during the luteal phase of the menstrual cycle (*q.v.*). The shallower, more rapid breathing pattern of women may contribute to their being more likely than men to experience arterial hypoxaemia during nearly maximal exercise [56].

Women on average have smaller hearts than men and the contractions are likely to be less powerful owing to women usually taking less exercise. As a result, stroke volumes are smaller in women than in men. However, relative to uptake of oxygen the requirement for blood flow is no less, so the smaller stroke volume is compensated for by a higher cardiac frequency; the cardiac frequency at a given uptake of oxygen is greater in consequence. In young adults, the gender difference in exercise cardiac frequency can be eliminated by making allowance for fat-free mass (Fig. 29.11, page 434). The gender-related differences in the ventilatory responses to exercise emerge during adolescence; the circulatory differences are related to body size and appear to be intrinsic (Section 31.1).

The effects of size extend to maximal exercise where the smaller tidal volume and stroke volume lead to the maximal levels of ventilation, cardiac output and oxygen uptake usually being less in women than in men. For comparable levels of habitual activity and haemoglobin concentration the lower exercise capacity of women can be explained by their lesser muscularity [57].

Gender and ageing. With advancing years the lung function of men deteriorates to a greater extent than that of women, so the initial male superiority diminishes. The deterioration is accentuated by exposure to tobacco smoke and other atmospheric pollution to which men are usually exposed to a greater extent than women. However, the causes of deterioration are primarily biological. Intrinsic causes are considered subsequently (Section 25.9.1). One extrinsic cause in middle age is an accumulation of body fat. Women usually accumulate more fat than men but the effect on the lungs is greater in men. This is due to the distribution of fat differing between the sexes (Section 4.7.1). The additional fat aggravates the increase in breathlessness on exertion that is a normal feature of ageing (Section 25.10.2).

Summary. On average, the lung function of women is less than that of men. The difference reflects gender-related differences in body size and composition, the age at which growth ceases and the somewhat different lifestyles of the two sexes.

25.8 Menstrual cycle and pregnancy

25.8.1 Menstrual cycle

Physiological responses. In adult women the blood concentration of progesterone is higher during the later luteal phase of the menstrual cycle than during the earlier follicular phase. The additional progesterone raises the basal metabolism and increases the body temperature by approximately 0.5°C. There are comparable increases in the temperature thresholds for cutaneous vasodilatation, shivering and chest sweating [58]. The consequent redistribution of blood volume leads to more blood being present in the lung capillaries and hence to a rise in transfer factor. The central respiratory drive is increased [59]; this increases the ventilation and tidal volume at rest, during exercise and in response to hypoxia and hypercapnia [60]. As a result, the arterial carbon dioxide tension is lower at the end than at the start of the menstrual cycle. However, the endurance performance of the inspiratory muscles is improved. There is little change in the cardiovascular responses to exercise or maximal oxygen uptake [61].

Lung airways. Women with asthma may experience an exacerbation in the pre-menstrual period. The symptoms can be accompanied by a reduction in peak expiratory flow, but no changes have been observed in FEV_1 or airway reactivity [62]. The mechanism appears not to be related to progesterone. By contrast, progesterone can ameliorate inflammation of the airways from ozone when the exposure occurs during the luteal phase of the menstrual cycle [63].

25.8.2 Pregnancy

Pregnancy affects the lungs and cardiovascular system through the presence of the pregnant uterus and as a consequence of changes in blood concentration of sex hormones. The physiological consequences are progressive into the third trimester. They are somewhat ameliorated when the head of the foetus descends into the pelvis and this process is accelerated after birth. However, full restoration to the pre-pregnant lung function takes several months.

The presence of the uterus in the abdomen raises the diaphragm (Fig. 4.4, page 35); this reduces the expiratory reserve volume and hence the functional residual capacity (FRC) [64]. The reduction is approximately 25% at the 36th week of pregnancy, but it has relatively little effect on other aspects of lung function on account of increased excursion of the ribs. As a result the inspiratory capacity is increased. The total lung capacity, FEV_1 and other indices of ventilatory capacity are usually unaffected by pregnancy.

There is similarly no change in closing capacity which can therefore exceed FRC in some women. When this occurs, a proportion of airways are closed throughout the respiratory cycle. The blood that perfuses them is not oxygenated, so it causes hypoxaemia. This venous admixture effect is greater in a supine than upright posture [65]. It can be enhanced by obesity. Some pregnant women experience snoring at night, particularly those with pre-eclampsia. The condition is associated with narrowing of the upper airway at the level of the oropharyngeal junction [66].

The mass of the uterus contributes to an increase in body mass and this exerts a proportional effect on the energy cost of activities that entail work against gravity (e.g. walking). As a result the oxygen uptake is increased. Additional energy is expended because the metabolic rate is increased [67].

Another factor raising the body mass is additional fluid, including that in the blood where it reduces the haemoglobin concentration. The extra fluid plus the increased uptake of oxygen increase the cardiac output and its components, the cardiac frequency and stroke volume. At 26 weeks of pregnancy the blood flow to the uterus has been reported as approximately $2.5\,l\,min^{-1}$. The additional blood flow needed for exercise is that to be expected for the increase in uptake of oxygen [68]. In most women in whom the measurement has been made the maximal oxygen uptake is relatively normal. However, where rapid glycolysis occurs (Section 28.4.6) its consequences are enhanced because the buffering of lactic acid is reduced [69].

Ventilation minute volume at rest and on exercise is increased during pregnancy [70, 71]. This is a consequence of both an increase in metabolism and respiratory drive from progesterone. The latter increases the $P_{0.1}$ (Section 23.9.6). The hyperventilation increases progressively throughout pregnancy and causes a nearly linear decline in the tension of carbon dioxide in the arterial blood. The tension is on average 4.0 kPa (30 torr) at the 8th week and 3.7 kPa (28 torr) at term, but with wide individual variations [70]. The change has the effect of enhancing the excretion of carbon dioxide by the foetus at the cost of increasing the mother's breathlessness on exertion. The extra ventilation is achieved mainly by an increase in tidal volume; inspection of published data [71] suggests that $\dot{V}_{E45}$ and Vt_{30} (Section 28.4.3) are both increased.

The transfer factor (diffusing capacity) is affected by many of the features of pregnancy, including haemodilution, transfer of iron from mother to foetus and an increase in cardiac output. The effects of the changes are most apparent early in pregnancy when *Tl*,co is increased. Subsequently, the index reverts towards its normal level [72, 73].

25.9 Effects of age on the lungs

25.9.1 Underlying considerations

Methodology. Conclusions about change in lung function with increasing age can be unreliable. This is because most studies are cross-sectional. The subjects are all survivors from amongst their birth cohort, but the comparison group of younger persons is diluted by many who will not survive to a comparable age. This source of error can be reduced by longitudinal study. Ideally the study should start at or before birth [e.g. 74] and be continued through to postmortem examinations. Despite the obvious difficulties such studies are now being undertaken by institutions. In addition, useful information can be obtained from short-term follow-up of cohorts (Section 8.2.2).

For investigating ageing, the mathematical model should include as many as possible of the relevant formative variables and their interactions, adjustments for co-linearity and terms to allow for the rate of deterioration with age being curvilinear (Section 5.6). This rigour is necessary because of the apparently large contributions to the ageing process of lifestyle and environmental factors. For making comparisons between the lung function of men and women a proportional model can be appropriate (Section 5.3, also Section 25.7, *Relevance of body composition and age*).

Mechanisms. During adult life the function of the lung declines. The principal cause is deterioration in the tissues of which the lungs are composed. In addition, the strength of the respiratory muscles is reduced (Fig. 9.1, page 101) and the stiffness of the thoracic cage is increased. Analogy with other tissues suggests that the intrapulmonary changes are due in part to an impaired nutrient blood supply from the bronchial arteries. An additional factor is internal destruction by superoxides and proteolytic enzymes, including those from macrophages attracted to the alveoli in response to adverse circumstances [e.g. 75]. The resulting changes can include digestion of alveolar walls, reduced permeability of cell membranes and alterations to the structure of collagen and elastin. The lungs then become more rigid. The tensile strength of the parenchyma is reduced, as is the ability of epithelial cells to recover after injury. The changes impair all aspects of lung function, but their extent varies between individuals [76]. The average changes for the principal indices of lung function are detailed in Sections 26.5 and 26.6.

The features of ageing can be ameliorated by an appropriate diet [77] and aggravated by exposure to polluted atmospheres, including particulates and tobacco smoke (Chapter 37) [78, 79]. Single episodes of acute chest illness do not have a deleterious effect unless recovery is incomplete [47, 80].

Structural changes. The ageing process is associated with progressive fibrosis of the internal linings of pulmonary arteries and venules. In lungs inflated to a standard pressure the air sacs are enlarged, there are fewer of them and there are more holes (fenestrations) in alveolar wall [81–83], also Section 3.3.5. As a result the surface for gas exchange is decreased [84]. The calibre of the respiratory bronchioles can be increased. This change is a step towards the development of centrilobular or focal emphysema (Section 40.3, *Pathology*). However, the calibre of non-respiratory bronchioles is independent of age. The quantities of elastin and collagen in the lung parenchyma are reported as unchanged or somewhat reduced, but there is an increased quantity of elastin in the vessels, airways and pleura [85]. The production of surfactant may be impaired [86].

25.9.2 Lung function

Lung elasticity. In men who are non-smokers and, to a lesser extent in women, the elastic recoil pressure of the lung decreases with age (in other words the compliance increases) [87, 88]. The reduction in recoil is not apparent when the lungs are filled with saline [89]. Hence, it is due to a reduction in surface forces. This is a consequence of the decrease in alveolar surface area referred to above. The change has the important effect of reducing the traction on the walls of bronchioles [90, 91]. This leads to these airways narrowing and closing prematurely during expiration. As a result, the closing volume, closing capacity [92] and residual volume increase with age. The changes contribute to increased ventilation–perfusion inequality (*q.v.*).

Lung volumes. Total lung capacity is usually reported as being independent of age. This is because the reduction in lung elastic recoil (described above) is nearly matched by the combined effects of the respiratory muscles being weaker and the thoracic cage being stiffer. However, the model does not apply to excised lungs [93]. It also neglects body fat that, on average, increases with age from early adulthood to late middle age. The additional fat can reduce the lung volumes (Section 25.5.1). The effect can be allowed for by standardising the volumes to a constant Fat%. In one study where this was done the sign of the partial regression coefficient of TLC on age was increased from negative to zero in women and from zero to positive in men [27]. This suggested that the lungs expand with age, as might be expected from the observed increase in lung compliance (see above). The apparent gender difference could reflect a greater tendency for women to gain fat and for men to lose lung elasticity as they grow older. The same features appear to be a factor in men, who are at a greater risk than women of developing emphysema and chronic non-specific lung disease (Section 37.5).

Residual volume increases with age as a direct consequence of the reduction in elastic recoil (see above). The increase is larger than the change in total lung capacity, so vital capacity decreases with age (Sections 26.5 and 26.6). This consequence of diminished recoil is supplemented by accumulation of fat and reduced strength in the respiratory muscles, so the reduction in vital capacity with age has several causes. Ageing further reduces forced vital capacity because the loss of recoil leads to dynamic compression of lung airways during forced expiration (Section 12.5.1).

Of the other subdivisions of total lung capacity, after allowance for changes in body composition inspiratory capacity is independent of age, whilst the effects of age on functional residual capacity and expiratory reserve volume are relatively small [27].

Ventilatory capacity. All the indices of ventilatory capacity decline with age. The decline is greater in men than in women (Sections 26.5 and 26.6). For both sexes it begins in early adult life and starts at a younger age for indices that depend solely on lung elasticity compared with those such as peak flow that are to some extent effort dependent. The onset of the decline is brought forward by smoking (Table 25.6). The subsequent rate of decline is mainly a manifestation of reduced lung recoil pressure and predominantly affects flow in small airways. Thus, from Table 26.16 (page 347) the percentage reductions between the ages of 25 and 65 years in men are on average 85% for $FEF_{75\%FVC}$ and 54% for $FEF_{50\%FVC}$ compared with 18% for PEF (reductions expressed as recommended in Section 5.4.3). In reality the rate of decline accelerates with age, so it is correlated with the initial size of the lung [53]. The decline also speeds up when there are respiratory symptoms.

The decline in ventilatory capacity with age is independent of the airway resistance which, at a lung volume of about 1 l in excess of the functional residual capacity, shows no significant upward trend with age. The change with age in the resistance to movement of the chest wall is also poorly documented. It is probably increased as both the total pulmonary resistance and the oxygen cost of breathing rise with age. Concurrently, the strength of the respiratory muscles declines, but the contribution of this factor to the reduction in ventilatory capacity is unclear.

Comment. Knowledge of the mechanics of ageing is still incomplete. The subject merits more research.

Ventilation–perfusion inequality. With increasing age, the range of expansion ratios of alveoli widens and the indices of uneven ventilation show deterioration in consequence. For example, the physiological deadspace as percentage of tidal volume doubles between the ages of 20 and 60 years. This is due to an increase in the number of alveoli with a high ventilation–perfusion ratio, hence they are poorly perfused in relation to their ventilation. The wider range of expansion ratios also leads to an increase in the single-breath nitrogen index of uneven ventilation; in one study of men between the ages of 33 and 66 years the index increased from 1.34% to 2.3% [94]. The closing volume (Section 16.2.5) increases as well.

In the pulmonary vascular bed, the walls of small pulmonary arteries become stiffer and autonomic regulation is impaired [95, 96, 97]. The changes lead to blood flow becoming more pulsatile and to loss of the vertical gradient of perfusion whereby lower regions are better perfused that upper ones [98]. At the same time, there is an increase in the proportion of alveoli that have a low ventilation–perfusion ratio, for example those that constitute the closing volume; this increases the mean alveolar to arterial tension difference for oxygen and reduces the arterial oxygen tension by about 1 kPa (6 mm Hg) [99]. There is a concurrent reduction in the arterial oxygen saturation from about 97% to 94% (Table 26.23, page 358).

Gas exchange. The rate of diffusion of gas across the alveolar capillary membrane declines with age. This is mainly because the increase in mean diameter of alveoli lengthens the average distance that gas molecules must travel to reach the alveolar membrane. The change reduces the transfer factor (diffusing capacity) and *D*m, the diffusing capacity of the alveolar capillary membrane. A contributory factor might be the associated loss of alveolar surface. However, whether this represents alveolar capillaries or inter-capillary spaces is unclear as the density of alveolar capillaries and the volume of blood that participates in gas exchange (*V*c) have both been reported as being independent of age [100], also Table 26.16, page 347.

25.10 Effects of age on responses to exercise

25.10.1 Interaction with ageing of the lungs

Ageing of the lungs begins in the third decade of life and thereafter progresses at an increasing rate. The deterioration is more marked in men than women. The features are reviewed in the preceding section. One of the most important features is increasing fenestration of alveolar walls leading to loss of alveoli. This process reduces the total alveolar surface area and hence the lung elastic recoil; it is aggravated by smoking. The resulting decrease in lung recoil reduces forced expiratory flow at small lung volumes and increases residual volume. The loss of elasticity is associated with an increase in mean alveolar diameter. This impairs gas exchange. Other primary changes include a reduction in strength of respiratory muscles and increased rigidity of the chest cage. All these features of ageing along with others, including changes in body fat, affect the physiological responses to exercise.

They interact with similar changes in the cardiovascular system to increase breathlessness and reduce capacity for exercise in elderly people (Fig. 25.2).

However, whilst the pulmonary changes are conspicuous and have immense clinical implications for patients with lung diseases, it is the reduction in maximal cardiac output that normally limits performance [101, 102].

25.10.2 Oxygen consumption, ventilation and breathlessness

At rest, the requirement for oxygen decreases with age, reflecting a reduction in the number of metabolically active cells. The ventilation to alveoli participating in gas exchanging declines as a result. However, gas exchange is impaired by $\dot{V}_A/\dot{Q}$ inequality, so ventilation is wasted on parts of the lungs that are poorly perfused with blood. The two changes are of nearly equal magnitude. As a result, the ventilation under quiet resting conditions shows no significant change with age despite a material change in its effectiveness.

During exercise the requirement for oxygen increases because motor co-ordination deteriorates. This leads to older people expending additional energy in overcoming friction in muscles and joints and in preserving the balance. Hence, for a given quantity of external work, the consumption of oxygen increases with age. The ventilation for a given task increases in consequence. The ventilation is further increased by it being unevenly distributed with respect to perfusion [103]. This has the effect that, below Owles point (Section 28.4.3), the ventilation standardised for uptake of oxygen shows a material increase (Fig. 25.3). The increase is not due to hyperventilation, since the arterial carbon dioxide tension remains at a normal level. This is evidence that, during exercise, the respiratory sensitivity to carbon dioxide does not change with age [105]. However, the rate of increase in ventilation at the start of exercise is reduced (see below). In addition, Owles point occurs at a progressively lower oxygen uptake as age increases (see below); this raises the ventilation further.

The increased ventilatory cost of exercise in elderly people contributes to their experiencing breathlessness when performing tasks that went without comment when they were younger. The breathlessness is aggravated by the associated decline in ventilatory capacity with age. The two effects can summate (Fig. 25.4).

25.10.3 Contribution of cardiovascular system

The relationship of cardiac output to uptake of oxygen is independent of age until quite late in life. This is due to an increase in

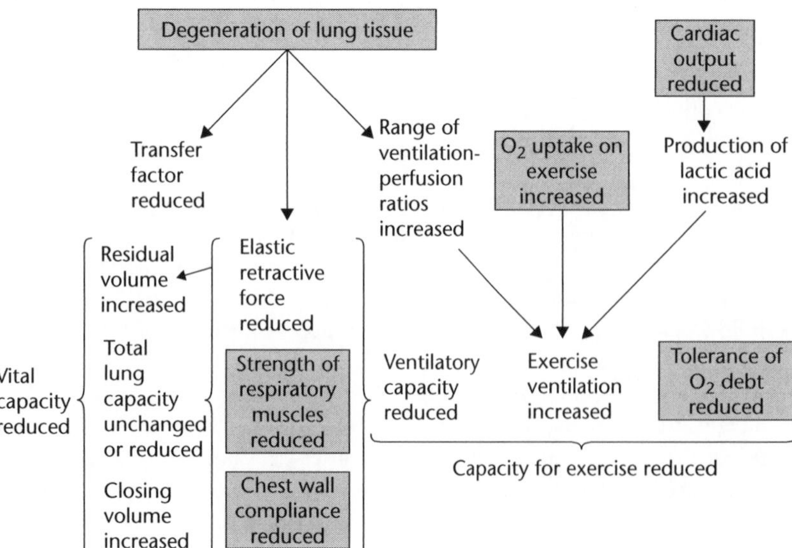

Fig. 25.2 Effects of age upon lung function and the capacity for exercise.

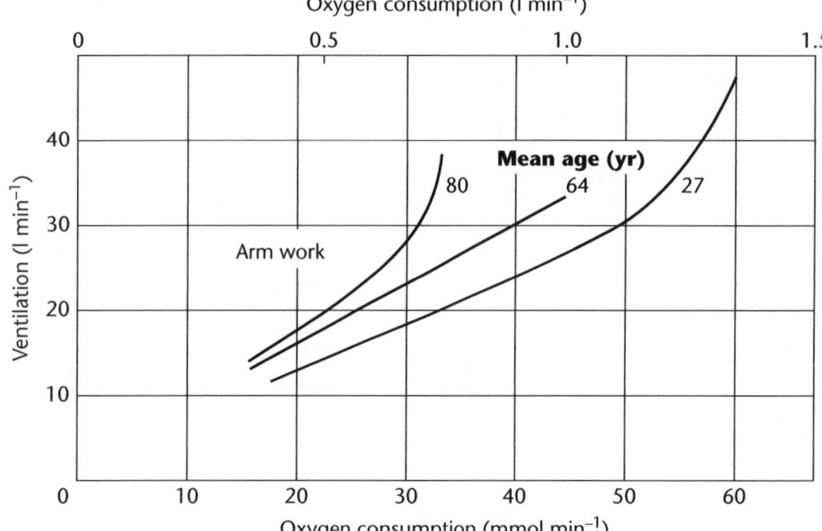

Fig. 25.3 Effect of age (expressed as the mean for each group of subjects) on the relationship of ventilation to consumption of oxygen for men performing work with the arms. The ventilation is higher and the onset of curvilinearity in the relationship occurs earlier in the older subjects. Source: [104].

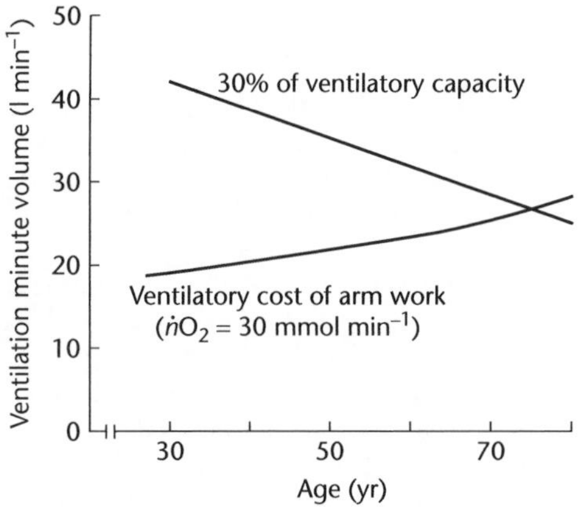

Fig. 25.4 Concurrent changes with age in the ventilatory cost of a task entailing an oxygen uptake of 30 mmol min^{-1} (0.67 l min^{-1}) from Fig. 25.3 and in an index of maximal ventilation calculated from FEV_1. According to the model the task might be expected to give rise to breathlessness beyond 75 years of age. Source: [106].

stroke volume with age compensating for a reduction in cardiac frequency (Sections 28.5 and 28.6). The reduction is more consistent for maximal than for submaximal exercise. It reflects an alteration in the balance between sympathetic and parasympathetic tone. The reduction in maximal frequency begins in early adulthood and is the main cause for the maximal cardiac output and the capacity for exercise decreasing with age. When the lungs are healthy the principal associated symptom is as much fatigue as breathlessness (Section 28.8.3).

In the systemic circulation the distensibility of arteries and arterioles diminish with age, so the systolic blood pressure and pulse wave velocity usually increase. The peripheral vascular bed tends to shrink and there is an increase in the response of the blood pressure to isometric work. In addition, the circulatory adaptations at the start of exercise occur relatively slowly in older people (Section 28.6.1). This retards the increase in ventilation at the start of exercise and extends the time constants for the responses of gas exchange to sinusoidal work [107].

The overall effect of the vascular changes with age is to reduce the delivery of oxygen to muscles that are active. The muscles then resort to rapid glycolysis with production of lactic acid at lower levels of energy expenditure than in younger subjects (Section 28.4.6). The changes lead to the increase in ventilation associated with strenuous exercise occurring at a progressively lower level of exercise as age advances. This sequence can be described as a reduction with age in the anaerobic threshold, but the terminology is imprecise. The changes are greatly influenced by any reduction in habitual activity as normally occurs with advancing age (Section 28.12). This effect is reversible, as old people respond well to physical training within their competence.

25.11 References

1. Berglund E, Birath G, Bjure J et al. Spirometric studies of normal subjects. 1. Forced expirograms in subjects between 7 and 70 years of age. *Acta Med Scand* 1963; **173**: 185–192.
2. Gaultier C, Boule M, Allaire Y et al. Determination of capillary oxygen tension in infants and children. *Bull Eur Physiopathol Respir* 1978; **14**: 287–297.
3. Cook CD, Helliesen PJ, Agathon S. Relation between mechanics of respiration, lung size and body size from birth to young adulthood. *J Appl Physiol* 1958; **13**: 349–352.
4. Mansell AL, Bryan AC, Levison H. Relationship of lung recoil to lung volume and maximum expiratory flow in normal children. *J Appl Physiol* 1977; **42**: 813–823.
5. Zapletal A, Paul T, Samanek M. Pulmonary elasticity in children and adolescents. *J Appl Physiol* 1976; **40**: 953–961.
6. Knudson RJ, Slatin RC, Lebowitz MD. The maximal expiratory flow-volume curve. *Amer Rev Respir Dis* 1976; **113**: 587–600.

7. Green M, Mead J, Turner JM. Variability of maximum expiratory flow-volume curves. *J Appl Physiol* 1974; **37**: 67–74.
8. Jones PRM, Baber FM, Heywood C, Cotes JE. Ventilatory capacity in healthy Chinese children: relation to habitual activity. *Ann Hum Biol* 1977; **4**: 155–161.
9. Reuschlein PS, Reddan WG, Burpee J et al. Effect of physical training on the pulmonary diffusing capacity during submaximal work. *J Appl Physiol* 1968; **24**: 152–158.
10. Neve V, Girard F, Flahault A, Boule M. Lung and thorax development during adolescence: relationship with pubertal status. *Eur Resp J* 2002; **20**: 1292–1298.
11. Dangour AD, Schilg S, Hulse JA. Cole TJ. Sitting height and subischial leg length centile curves for boys and girls from southeast England. *Ann Hum Biol* 2002; **29**: 290–305.
12. Gasser T, Sheehy A, Molinari L, Largo RH. Growth processes leading to a large or small adult size. *Ann Hum Biol* 2001; **28**: 319–327.
13. DeGroodt EG, van Pelt W, Borsboom GJJM et al. Growth of lung and thorax dimensions during the pubertal growth spurt. *Eur Respir J* 1988; **1**: 102–108.
14. Cotes JE, Dabbs JM, Hall AM, *et al.* Sitting height, fat free mass and body fat as reference variables for lung function in healthy British children: comparison with stature. *Ann Hum Biol* 1979; **6**: 307–314.
15. Bedogni G, Iughetti L, Ferrari M et al. Sensitivity and specificity of body mass index and skinfold thicknesses in detecting excess adiposity in children aged 8–12 years. *Ann Hum Biol* 2003; **30**: 132–139.
16. Sherrill DL, Camilli A, Lebowitz MD. On the temporal relationship between lung function and somatic growth. *Am Rev Respir Dis* 1989; **140**: 638–644
17. Hopper JL, Hibbert ME, Macaskill GT et al. Longitudinal analysis of lung function growth in healthy children and adolescents. *J Appl Physiol* 1991; **70**: 770–777.
18. Hurwitz S, Allen J, Liben A, Becklake MR. Lung function in young adults: evidence for differences in the chronological age at which various functions start to decline. *Thorax* 1980; **35**: 615–619.
19. Rosenthal M, Bain SH, Cramer D et al. Lung function in white children aged 4 to 19 years: 1-spirometry. *Thorax* 1993; **48**: 704–802.
20. Hibbert M, Couriel JM, Landau LI. Changes in lung, airway and chest wall function in boys and girls between 8 and 12 years. *J Appl Physiol* 1984; **57**: 304–308.
21. Martin TR, Feldman HA, Fredberg JJ et al. Relationship between maximal expiratory flows and lung volumes in growing humans. *J Appl Physiol* 1988; **65**: 822–828.
22. Martin TR, Castile RG, Fredberg JJ et al. Airway size is related to sex but not lung size in normal adults. *J Appl Physiol* 1987; **63**: 2042–2047.
23. Whimster WF, Macfarlane AL. Normal lung weights in a white population. *Am Rev Respir Dis* 1974; **110**: 478–483.
24. Gibson GJ, Pride NB, O'Cain C, Quagliato R. Sex and age differences in pulmonary mechanics in normal nonsmoking subjects. *J Appl Physiol* 1976; **41**: 20–25.
25. Robbins DR, Enright PL. Sherrill DL Lung function development in young adults: is there a plateau phase? *Eur Respir J* 1995; **8**: 768–772.
26. Chinn DJ, Cotes JE, Reed JW. Changes in body mass can affect interpretation of longitudinal measurements of ventilatory capacity (FEV_1 & FVC). *Thorax* 1996; **51**: 699–704.
27. Cotes JE, Chinn DJ, Reed JW. Body fat, fat percentage, and fat free mass as reference variables for lung function: effects on terms for age and sex. *Thorax* 2001; **56**: 839–844.
28. Ashwell M, Cole TJ, Dixon AK. Obesity: new insight into the anthropometric classification of fat distribution shown by computed tomography. *BMJ* 1985; **290**: 1692–1694.
29. Lazarus R, Gore CJ, Booth M et al. Effects of body composition and fat distribution on ventilatory function in adults. *Am J Clin Nutr* 1998; **68**: 35–41.
30. Cotes JE, Gilson JC. Effects of inactivity, weight gain and antitubercular chemotherapy upon lung function in working coal-miners. *Ann Occup Hyg* 1967; **10**: 327–335.
31. Chen Y, Horne SL, Doseman JA. Body weight and weight gain related to pulmonary function decline in adults: a six year follow up study. *Thorax* 1993; **48**: 375–380.
32. Fisher AB, DuBois AB, Hyde RW et al. Effect of 2 months' undersea exposure to N_2-O_2 at 2.2 Ata on lung function. *J Appl Physiol* 1970; **28**: 70–74.
33. Bouhuys A, Beck GJ. Large lungs in divers? *J Appl Physiol* 1979; **47**: 1136–1137.
34. Davey IS, Cotes JE, Reed JW. Relationship of ventilatory capacity to hyperbaric exposure in divers. *J Appl Physiol* 1984; **56**:1655–1658.
35. Cotes JE, Anderson HR, Patrick JM. Lung function and the response to exercise in New Guineans: role of genetic and environmental factors. *Phil Trans R Soc B.* 1974; **268**: 349–361.
36. Cotes JE, Dabbs JM, Daley C *et al.* Above-average exercise capacity in competition cyclists: relationship to body muscle. *J Physiol* (Lond) 1971; **218**: 63–64P.
37. Andrew GM, Becklake MR, Guleria JS, Bates DV. Heart and lung functions in swimmers and non-athletes during growth. *J Appl Physiol* 1972; **32**: 245–251.
38. Eriksson BO, Lundin A, Saltir B. Cardiopulmonary function in former girl swimmers and the effects of physical training. *Scand J Clin Lab Invest* 1975; **35**: 135–145.
39. Cotes JE, Davey IS, Reed JW, Rooks M. Respiratory effects of a single saturation dive to 300 m. *Br J Ind Med* 1987; **44**: 76–82.
40. Florio JT, Morrison JB, Butt WS. Breathing pattern and ventilatory response to carbon dioxide in divers. *J Appl Physiol* 1979; **46**: 1076–1080.
41. Spengler CM, Shea SA. Endogenous circadian rhythm of pulmonary function in healthy humans. *Am J Respir Crit Care Med* 2000; **162**: 1038–1046; also *Am J Respir Crit Care Med* 2002; **166**: 1005.
42. Calhoun WJ. Nocturnal asthma (Review) *Chest* 2003; **123**(suppl): 399S–405S
43. Kerr HD. Diurnal variation of respiratory function independent of air quality. *Arch Environ Health* 1973; **26**: 144–152.
44. McDermott M. Diurnal and weekly cyclical changes in lung airways resistance. *J Physiol (Lond)* 1966; **186**; 90P–92P.
45. Cinkotai FF, Thomsen ML. Diurnal variation in pulmonary diffusing capacity for carbon monoxide. *J Appl Physiol* 1966; **21**: 539–542
46. Frey TM, Crapo RO, Jensen RL, Elliott CG. Diurnal variation of the diffusing capacity of the lung: is it real? *Am Rev Respir Dis* 1987; **136**: 1381–1384.

47. McKerrow CB, Rossiter CE. An annual cycle in the ventilatory capacity of men with pneumoconiosis and of normal subjects. *Thorax* 1968; **23**: 340–349.
48. Scarlett JF, Abbott KJ, Peacock JL et al. Acute effects of summer air pollution on respiratory function in primary school children in southern England *Thorax* 1996; **51**: 1109–1114.
49. Senthilselvan A, Dosman JA, Semchuk KM et al. Seasonal changes in lung function in a farming population. *Can Respir J* 2000: **7**: 320–325.
50. Kopp MV, Bohnet W, Frischer T et al. Effects of ambient ozone on lung function in children over a two summer period. *Eur Respir J* 2000; **16**: 893–900.
51. Borsboom GJ, van Pelt W, van Houwelingen HC et al. Diurnal variation in lung function in subgroups from two Dutch populations: consequences for longitudinal analysis. *Am J Respir Crit Care Med* 1999; **159**: 1163–1171.
52. Teramoto S, Suzuki M, Matsui H et al. Influence of age on diurnal variability in measurements of spirometric indices and respiratory pressures. *J Asthma* 1999; **36**: 487–492.
53. Cole TJ. Linear and proportional regression models in the prediction of ventilatory function *J R Stat Soc* 1975; **138**: 297–328.
54. Dirksen A, Groth S. Calculation of reference values for lung function tests. *Bull Eur Physiopathol Respir* 1986; **22**: 231–37.
55. Amrein R, Keller R, Joos H, Herzog H. Valeurs theoriques nouvelles de l'exploration de la fonction ventilatoire du poumon. *Bull Eur Physiopathol Respir* 1970; **6**: 317–349.
56. Harms CA, McClaran SR, Nickele GA et al. Exercise-induced arterial hypoxaemia in healthy young women. *J Physiol (Lond)* 1998; **507**: 619–628.
57. Von Dobeln W. Human standard and maximal metabolic rate in relation to fat-free body mass *Acta Physiol Scand* 1956; **37**(Suppl 126).
58. Hessemer V, Bruck K. Influence of menstrual cycle on shivering, skin blood flow, and sweating responses at night. *J Appl Physiol* 1985; **59**: 1902–1910.
59. Bayliss DA, Millhorn DE. Central neural mechanisms of progesterone action: application to the respiratory system. *J Appl Physiol* 1992; **73**: 393–404.
60. Schoene RB, Robertson HT, Pierson DJ, Peterson AP. Respiratory drives and exercise in menstrual cycles of athletic and nonathletic women. *J Appl Physiol* 1981; **50**: 1300–1305.
61. Marsh SA, Jenkins DG. Physiological responses to the menstrual cycle: implications for the development of heat illness in female athletes. *Sports Med* 2002; **32**: 601–614.
62. Pauli BD, Reid RL, Munt PW et al. Influence of the menstrual cycle on airway function in asthmatics and normal subjects. *Am Rev Respir Dis* 1989; **140**: 258–262.
63. Fox SD, Adams WC, Brookes KA, Lasley BL. Enhanced response to ozone exposure during the follicular phase of the menstrual cycle. *Environ Health Perspect* 1993; **101**: 242–244.
64. Contreras G, Gutierrez M, Beroiza T *et al.* Ventilatory drive and respiratory muscle function in pregnancy. *Am Rev Respir Dis* 1991; **144**: 837–841.
65. Craig DB, Toole MA. Airway closure in pregnancy. *Can Anaesth Soc J* 1975; **22**: 665–672.
66. Izci B, Riha RL, Martin SE et al. The upper airway in pregnancy and pre-eclampsia. *Am J Respir Crit Care Med* 2003; **167**: 137–140.
67. Carpenter MW, Sady SP, Sady MA et al. Effect of maternal weight gain during pregnancy on exercise performance. *J Appl Physiol* 1990; **68**: 1173–1176.
68. Sady SP, Carpenter MW, Thompson PD et al. Cardiovascular response to cycle exercise during and after pregnancy. *J Appl Physiol* 1989; **66**: 336–341.
69. Lotgering FK, Struijk PC, van Doorn MB et al. Anaerobic threshold and respiratory compensation in pregnant women. *J Appl Physiol* 1995; **78**: 1772–1777.
70. Spatling L, Fallenstein F, Hutch A *et al.* The variability of cardiopulmonary adaptation to pregnancy at rest and during exercise. *Br J Obstet Gynaecol* 1992; **99**(Suppl 8): 1–40.
71. Field SK, Bell SG, Cenaiko DF, Whitelaw WA. Relationship between inspiratory effort and breathlessness in pregnancy. *J Appl Physiol* 1991; **71**: 1897–1902.
72. Milne JA, Mills RJ, Coutts JR et al. The effect of human pregnancy on the pulmonary transfer factor for carbon monoxide as measured by the single breath method. *Clin Sci Mol Med* 1977; **53**: 271–276.
73. McAuliffe F, Kametas N. Rafferty GF et al. Pulmonary diffusing capacity in pregnancy at sea level and at high altitude. *Respir Physiol Neurobiol* 2003; **134**: 85–92.
74. Lamont DW, Parker L, Cohen MA et al. Early life and later determinants of adult disease: a fifty year follow-up study of the Newcastle thousand families cohort. *Public Health* 1998; **112**: 85–93.
75. Bowler RP, Crapo JD. Oxidative stress in allergic respiratory diseases. *J Allergy Clin Immunol* 2002: **110**: 349–356.
76. Zeleznik J. Normative ageing of the respiratory system. *Clin Geriatr Med* 2003; **19**: 1–18.
77. Butland BK, Fehily AM, Elwood PC. Diet, lung function, and lung function decline in a cohort of 2512 middle aged men. *Thorax* 2000; **55**: 102–108.
78. Zhu S, Manuel M, Tanaka S *et al* Contribution of reactive oxygen and nitrogen species to particulate-induced lung injury. *Environ Health Perspect* 1998; **106**: 1157–1163.
79. Wright JL. The importance of ultramicroscopic emphysema in cigarette smoke-induced lung disease. *Lung* 2001; **179**: 71–81.
80. Fletcher C, Peto R, Tinker C, Speizer FE. *The natural history of chronic bronchitis and emphysema.* Oxford: Oxford University Press, 1976.
81. Verbeken EK, Cauberghs M Mertens I et al. The senile lung. Comparison with normal and emphysematous lungs. 2. Functional aspects. *Chest* 1992; **101**: 800–809.
82. Gillooly M, Lamb D. Airspace size in lungs of lifelong non-smokers: effect of age and sex. *Thorax* 1993; **48**: 39–43.
83. Pump K. Emphysema and its relation to age. *Am Rev Respir Dis* 1976; **114**: 5–13.
84. Thurlbeck WM. The internal surface area of non-emphysematous lungs. *Am Rev Respir Dis* 1967; **95**: 765–773.
85. Pierce JA, Ebert RV. Fibrous network of the lung and its change with age. *Thorax* 1965; **20**: 469–476.
86. Shimura S, Boatman ES, Martin CJ. Effects of ageing on the alveolar pores of Kohn and on the cytoplasmic components of alveolar type II cells in monkey lungs. *J Pathol* 1986; **148**: 1–11.
87. Niewoehner DE, Kleinerman J, Liotta I. Elastic behavour of postmortem human lungs: effects of ageing and mild emphysema. *J Appl Physiol* 1975; **39**: 943–949.
88. Colebatch HJH, Ng CKY. A longitudinal study of pulmonary distensibility in healthy adults. *Respir Physiol* 1986; **65**: 1–11.

89. Haber PS, Colebatch HJH, Ng CKY, Greaves IA. Alveolar size as a determinant of pulmonary distensibility in mammalian lungs. *J Appl Physiol* 1983; **54**: 837–845.
90. Turner JM, Mead J, Wohl ME. Elasticity of human lungs in relation to age. *J Appl Physiol* 1968; **25**: 664–671.
91. Knudson RJ, Clark DF, Kennedy TC, Knudson DE. Effect of ageing alone on mechanical properties of the normal adult human lung. *J Appl Physiol* 1977; **43**: 1054–1062.
92. Bode FR, Dosman J, Martin RR *et al.* Age and sex differences in lung elasticity and closing capacity in nonsmokers. *J Appl Physiol* 1976; **41**: 129–135.
93. Berend N, Skoog C, Waszkiewicz L, Thurlbeck WM. Maximum volumes in excised human lungs: effects of age, emphysema and formalin fixation. *Thorax* 1980; **35**: 859–864.
94. Cohn JE, Donoso HD. Mechanical properties of lung in normal men over 60 years old. *J Clin Invest* 1963; **42**: 1406–1410.
95. Dice FH. Cellular and molecular mechanisms of ageing. *Physiol Rev* 1993; **73**: 149–159
96. Lakatta EG. Cardiovascular regulatory mechanisms in advanced age. *Physiol Rev* 1993; **73**: 413–467.
97. Folkow B, Svanborg A. Physiology of cardiovascular ageing. *Physiol Rev* 1993; **73**: 725–764.
98. Holland J, Milic-Emili J, Macklem PT, Bates DV. Regional distribution of pulmonary ventilation and perfusion in elderly subjects. *J Clin Invest* 1968; **47**: 81–92.
99. Cardus J, Burgos F, Diaz O et al. Increase in pulmonary ventilation-perfusion inequality with age in healthy individuals. *Am J Respir Crit Care Med* 1997; **156**: 648–653.
100. Butler C, Kleinerman J. Capillary density: alveolar diameter, a morphometric approach to ventilation and perfusion. *Am Rev Respir Dis* 1970; **102**: 886–894.
101. Åstrand P-O, Rodahl K. *Textbook of work physiology.* 3rd ed. London: McGraw-Hill, 1986.
102. Higginbotham MB, Morris KG, Williams RS et al. Physiologic basis for the age-related decline in aerobic work capacity. *Am J Cardiol* 1986; **57**: 1374–1379.
103. Poulin MJ, Cunningham DA, Paterson DH *et al.* Ventilatory response to exercise and carbon dioxide in men and women 55 to 86 years of age. *Am J Respir Crit Care Med* 1994; **149**: 408–415.
104. Norris AH, Shock NW, Yiengst MJ. Age differences in ventilatory and gas exchange responses to graded exercise in males. *J Gerontol* 1955; **10**: 145–155.
105. McConnell AK, Semple ESG, Davies CTM. Ventilatory responses to exercise and carbon dioxide in elderly and young subjects. *Eur J Appl Physiol* 1993; **91**: 43–56.
106. Cotes JE. Assessment of disablement due to impaired respiratory function. *Bull Eur Physiopathol Respir* 1975; **11**: 210P–217P.
107. Cunningham DA, Himann JE, Paterson DH, Dickinson JR. Gas exchange dynamics with sinusoidal work in young and elderly women. *Respir Physiol* 1993; **91**: 43–56.

Further reading

Growth of the lungs

Lebowitz MD, Holberg CJ, Knudson RJ, Burrows B. Longitudinal study of pulmonary function development in childhood, adolescence, and early adulthood. *Am Rev Respir Dis* 1987; **136**: 69–75.

Schrader PC, Quanjer PhH, Olievier ICW. Respiratory muscle force and ventilatory function in adolescents. *Eur Respir J* 1988; **1**: 368–375.

Effects of age

Bode FR, Dosman J, Martin RR *et al* Age and sex differences in lung elasticity, and in closing capacity in nonsmokers. *J Appl Physiol* 1976; **41**: 129–135.

Frank NR, Mead J, Ferris BG Jr. The mechanical behaviour of the lungs in healthy elderly persons. *J Clin Invest* 1957; **36**: 1680–1687.

Holland J, Milic-Emili J, Macklem PT, Bates DV. Regional distribution of pulmonary ventilation and perfusion in elderly subjects. *J Clin Invest* 1968; **47**: 81–92.

Janssens JP, Pache JC, Nicod LP. Physiological changes in respiratory function associated with ageing. *Eur Respir J* 1999; **13**: 197–205.

Knudson RJ, Clark DF, Kennedy TC, Knudson DE. Effect of ageing alone on mechanical properties of the normal adult human lung. *J Appl Physiol* 1977; **43**: 1054–1062.

Kronenberg RS, Drage CW. Attenuation of the ventilatory and heart rate responses to hypoxia and hypercapnia with aging in normal men. *J Clin Invest* 1973; **52**: 1812–1819.

Mittman C, Edelman NH, Norris AH, Shock NW. Relationship between chest wall and pulmonary compliance and age. *J Appl Physiol* 1965; **20**: 1211–1216.

Ranga V, Kleinerman J, Ip MPC, Sorensen J. Age-related changes in elastic fibers and elastin of lung. *Am Rev Respir Dis* 1979; **119**: 369–381.

Sorbini CA, Grassi V, Solinas E, Muiesan G. Arterial oxygen tension in relation to age in healthy subjects. *Respiration* 1968; **25**: 3–13.

CHAPTER 26

Reference Values for Lung Function in White (Caucasian) Children and Adults

This chapter describes the derivation and use of reference values and identifies equations for white children and adults (Caucasians).

26.1 Basic considerations

26.1.1 Definitions

A measurement of lung function is only useful after it has been interpreted, for example a result may be judged normal or abnormal for a particular subject. Alternatively, the measurement may be unsound or the comparison not appropriate. The first conclusion depends on having a result with which the new measurement can be compared. It can be a previous result for the same subject or an estimate based on experience of other people with similar characteristics. These alternative standards are, respectively, internal and external reference values. They estimate the lung function at one point in time, so are cross-sectional.

An *internal reference value* is a result obtained before the event that led to the new measurement. The event might be an illness, active intervention (e.g. inhalation of a broncho-active drug) or passage of time since the last assessment. The time interval is usually short, so no external reference is necessary. However, if the interval is in years, rather than days or months, an estimate of the change to be expected over the period might assist in interpretation. That estimate is a *longitudinal reference value.* It is used for monitoring a population, but has wide confidence limits so is not accurate when applied to an individual subject. For a subject seen in an occupational context, the inaccuracy can sometimes be reduced by reference to the result of a lung function assessment performed as part of a pre-employment examination. This requires that the result should have been preserved [1].

An *external reference value* describes the level of an index for a group of healthy persons, i.e. the *reference population,* in terms of defining variables, known as *reference variables.* Commonly used reference variables are ethnic group, age, gender and one or more indices of body size. Thus, the reference value is generated from an equation and the result for an individual subject is obtained by inserting values for his or her features into the equation. For the purposes of this chapter the person is white, i.e. of European descent, so the ethnic group is Caucasian.

The appropriateness of a reference value depends on all its features matching those of the person being assessed (Table 26.1).

Where reference values are obtained and used locally their appropriateness is seldom in doubt, but in other circumstances the match between local circumstances and published reference values requires that both should conform to the same standards. Inevitably these standards need to be of the highest,

Table 26.1 Features to be considered when choosing a reference value.

Category	Feature
Genetic attributes	Ethnic group Gender (atopic status)
Environmental exposures	Altitude Climate Air pollution Smoking history
Biological attributes	Age Nutrition, hence body fat Customary activity, hence muscle strength Absence of disease (i.e. subjects are healthy) Cohort is appropriate [2]
Technical attributes	Measurement protocol Equipment (including calibration and method of use) Definition (and mode of calculation) of the index

since anything less may have unpredictable consequences. These considerations require that reference values should be reviewed periodically and, where necessary, modified to accommodate new technical developments.

26.1.2 Reference subjects

Criteria

(i) Obligatory criteria. Reference subjects need to have healthy lungs contained in reasonably healthy bodies. They should also conform to appropriate criteria from amongst those listed in Table 26.1. The need for respiratory health requires that subjects are without respiratory symptoms, especially regular cough, phlegm production, wheeze or undue breathlessness on exertion, have no history of chest disease and have not had an acute respiratory illness within the last 6 weeks [3, 4]. Thus, normality is defined in terms of what can be established during a population survey, without reference to chest radiography or other investigations. In the past an additional criterion was that subjects were free from airways obstruction as indicated by the ratio FEV_1/FVC (FEV%) exceeding 70%. However, this criterion should not be used as it does not take into account that FEV% normally declines with age [5].

(ii) Conditional criteria. Many reference values describe biologically healthy subjects for whom an important criterion is that they should never have smoked tobacco (or cannabis) [6]. Such subjects are described as 'never smoked' (Section 37.3). Alternatively, the reference subjects can include asymptomatic smokers. The former values are appropriate for purposes of life assurance, whilst the latter may be preferable for assessing the effect of an occupational exposure.

Role for local subjects. The choice of reference values is likely to be based on authoritative recommendations, but should be confirmed locally. This is particularly important for a laboratory that has recently been set up, where the staff or equipment have changed or the local population or local methodology for assessment has unusual features. In any of these circumstances the recommended reference values should be calibrated against those for an appropriate group of subjects recruited and assessed locally. This can lead to an informed choice being made. Alternatively, the usual reference values can be adapted to local circumstances [7]. This can be done using fewer data than are required for obtaining local reference values, but the latter are preferable where they are available.

Recruitment. Community reference values are representative if they are based on subjects selected at random from the relevant population. This is practicable for most indices of lung function. The sampling may need to be stratified in order to ensure adequate representation of subjects who have a feature that is uncommon, for example great age or an usual stature (Section 8.2.4).

The newer or laboratory based tests often rely on subjects recruited casually, for example hospital staff and visitors, and members of local organisations. This type of recruitment usually yields representative values, except for exercise studies where a sample recruited casually is often biased in favour of persons who are physically active.

Recruitment for longitudinal studies is discussed in Section 26.7.

26.1.3 Quality control

Reference values are the standards for interpreting lung function in individual subjects, so their reliability must be above any dispute. To this end, the methods used for obtaining them should be appropriate and the equipment should meet the relevant criteria for overall characteristics, response time and accuracy. The observer should have been trained and the circumstances of the test should minimise biological variation. The procedure and performance of the test, including the intermediate results, should be technically satisfactory and the results should be calculated in the recommended manner. The choices in all these respects are reviewed throughout this book; quality control is addressed specifically in Sections 2.5 and 7.16.

26.1.4 Models (mathematical equations) that form the basis for reference values

Reference values are equations that describe indices of lung function in terms of one or more reference variables (Table 26.2). The choice of which reference values to use is influenced by the index being described and the category of person, for example

Table 26.2 Some reference variables for indices of lung function.

Type	Variable
Categorical variables (yes or no)	Ethnic group (cf. Chapter 27)*
	Gender*
	Smoking status (Section 37.3)
Anthropometric variables	Stature (standing height)*
	Sitting height
	Thoracic dimensions (Sections 4.4 and 4.5)
	Body composition (fat and FFM)†
Biological variables	Age*‡
	Activity grade
	Stage of puberty (children)

* Standard for most indices.
† Recommended.
‡ Age should be in decimal years (Table 5.1, page 43) for longitudinal studies and where a term for age is applied to data for children.

children, adolescents, adults or the elderly. Inclusion of a variable in the model implies that it can account for a useful part of the variation in the index for persons in the relevant category. The association need not be causal. The number of variables depends on the index, for example, it is more for primary indices such as FEV_1 and FVC, to which both body size and age contribute, than for their ratio (FEV%) where the size term is largely eliminated on account of appearing to nearly the same relative extent in both numerator and denominator of the relationship. However, the dependence of FEV_1 and FVC on size is only nearly equal, so in order to describe FEV% with maximal accuracy there may be a need for a size term as well (e.g. Table 26.20, page 355). The reference variables should, so far as is possible be independent of each other (Section 5.6.2).

Types of model. The majority of reference values are for subgroups of subjects classified by age group (children, adolescents, adults and the elderly). The models (Table 26.3) are relatively simple; their accuracy is greatest for subjects in the middle of the respective age ranges. Continuous models that make allowance for the transitions between the several age groups are inevitably more complicated (Section 26.7). The different models are described below in relation to the subjects for whom they are appropriate. Their accuracy is expressed in terms of a residual standard deviation, 95% confidence limits or coefficient of variation about the relationship. The appropriate expression to use depends on the distribution of the data and this in turn determines the type of relationship that is appropriate (Section 5.3).

Table 26.3 Some models used for reference values.

Model	Relationship
Simple linear	$y = mx + c$
Multiple linear	$y = m_1x + m_2z + c$
Logarithmic*	$\ln y = m\ln(x) + c$
Proportional*	$y = cx^m$
Exponential	$y = ae^{kx}$
Hyperbolic	$y = x(k + \text{stature})/(k - \text{stature})$
Polynomial	$y = c + m_1x + m_2x^2 + m_3x^3 + m_4x^4 \ldots$ etc
Hybrid	$\ln y = a + [b + c\ \text{Age}]\ \text{Stature}$
Splined or continuous piecewise linear	See Section 26.7

* See Footnote 26.1.

26.1.5 Strategies for selecting reference values

The reference values that are adopted should describe accurately the lung function of healthy members of the communities served by the laboratory. The first step is to ensure that the definitions and methods for the proposed reference values are compatible with those used locally. This should be the case but in practice may not be. For example, in respect of transfer factor (diffusing capacity), the European and US protocols for alveolar oxygen tension are different. This might be expected to result in small systematic differences in the results (Section 20.4.1).

The second step is to make measurements on local subjects, usually groups of 20 to 40 in each relevant category, and compare the results with those predicted by commonly used reference values, e.g. [7]. A good approach is to calculate the standardised residuals (Section 5.6.4) and check their distribution against age and height for the two sexes separately. The mean Z-score should be around zero and the SD of the residuals should be about 1.

Each class of index should be assessed individually. It is an advantage if the reference equations have all been obtained from the same group of subjects as the results are then internally consistent. Alternatively, individual equations from different published sets can be selected. In practice, there is little to choose between the commonly used equations. Reference values should be changed infrequently as experience in interpretation is gained through the consistent use of a single set.

26.2 Pre-school children (ages 3–6 years)

Assessment of lung function of young children has been improved by use of the interrupter technique for measurement of respiratory resistance (Rint) [8, 9] and of incentive spirometry and animation programmes for measurement of spirometric indices [10–13]. For spirometry the success rate is now approximately 85%, with most of the failures in the younger children. However, the technique is demanding on both clinical scientist and child (Section 24.7). Reference values for the age range 2–7 years are in Table 26.4. Values for infants including the younger end of this age range are in Section 24.5.

26.3 Children of school age

26.3.1 Models based on stature

Stature contributes more to the variance of lung function in children than any other single variable and the relationships on

Table 26.4 Reference values for respiratory resistance by the interruptor method (Rint) and spirometric indices in pre-school aged children. Stature in cm.

Index	n	Range		Equation	RSD or CoV*	Source
		Age	Stature			
Rint (insp) kPa l^{-1}s	54	2–7	90–127	2.59 – 0.017 St	0.12	[8]
Rint (insp) kPa l^{-1}s	284	3–6.4	94–130	2.276 – 0.0137 St	0.19	[9]
Rint (exp) kPa l^{-1}s	54	2–7	90–127	2.61 – 0.016 St	0.13	[8]
Rint (exp) kPa l^{-1}s	284	3–6.4	94–130	2.127 – 0.0125 St	0.20	[9]
FEV_1 (ml)	184	3–7	87–127	0.004737 $St^{2.63}$	11.2%	[10]
FVC (ml)	184	3–7	87–127	0.001204 $St^{2.95}$	11.7%	[10]
PEF (l s^{-1})	184	3–7	87–127	(1.687×10^{-5}) $St^{2.54}$	15.1%	[10]

* RSD is residual standard deviation and CoV is coefficient of variation (%).

stature provide reference values for most lung function indices. The majority of the relationships are proportional ones [14]. They can be expressed either in this form (Table 26.5) or in the logarithmic form used to derive them (Footnote 26.1).

Alternatively, when expressed in terms of residual standard deviations the model provides percentiles that describe the lung function relative to that of the children in the reference population (Section 26.3.5).

The accuracy of the simple model can be improved if allowance is also made for body composition (Fat% and fat-free mass) and/or thoracic dimensions (Table 26.2 and Table 25.3, page 319). In the case of transfer factor (Tlco,sb) the accuracy in a number of circumstances is also improved when allowance is made for alveolar volume standardised for stature [16] (also Table 26.11, page 341).

The simple model does not take into account the accelerated growth of lung function that occurs at adolescence. As a result, the process of averaging (e.g. Fig. 26.3) tends to over-estimate some indices of lung function before puberty and under-estimate them afterwards.

26.3.2 Models that allow for puberty

Puberty in boys is accompanied by an increase in the rate of growth of the whole body. The lungs are particularly affected because, as well as an increase in thoracic dimensions, the respiratory muscles become stronger. In girls the changes are smaller because growth ceases sooner and the increase in muscle strength is less marked.

Footnote 26.1. The proportional model (Table 26.3) can be derived from the logarithmic model as ln FEV = m ln(Stature) + c (± RSD); then FEV = antilog $c\times$ Stature^m (±CoV%), where ln is natural logarithm and CoV (coefficient of variation) is residual standard deviation as a percentage of the mean value.
Example: ln FEV = 3.09 × ln (Stature, m) – 0.283 (RSD = 0.12); hence, FEV = 0.753 × Stature$^{3.09}$ (CoV 12%)

Table 26.5 Simple reference equations for lung function in healthy boys and girls of European descent, ages 8–16 years. Stature (St) is in metres. Gas volumes are in l BTPS. The equations are displayed graphically in Figs 26.1 and 26.2.

Index	Gender	Relationship on stature (m)	CoV %
TLC (l)	M	1.227 $St^{2.80}$	9
	F	1.189 $St^{2.64}$	10
VC and FVC (l)	M	1.004 $St^{2.72}$	11
	F	0.946 $St^{2.61}$	10
IC (l)	M	0.720 $St^{2.55}$	15
	F	0.657 $St^{2.47}$	14
ERV (l)	M	0.264 $St^{3.37}$	24
	F	0.283 $St^{2.90}$	19
FRC (l)	M	0.500 $St^{3.12}$	17
	F	0.528 $St^{2.81}$	17
RV (l)	M + F	0.237 $St^{2.77}$	27
$FEV_{0.75}$ (l)	M	0.780 $St^{2.67}$	11
	F	0.744 $St^{2.66}$	11
FEV_1 (l)*	M	0.812 $St^{2.77}$	10
	F	0.788 $St^{2.73}$	10
PEF (l s^{-1})	M + F	7.59St – 5.53	13†
Tl (SI)‡	M	2.695 $St^{2.46}$	14
	F	2.536 $St^{2.33}$	13
Dm (SI)‡¶	M	5.161 $St^{2.07}$	21
	F	4.023 $St^{2.41}$	21
Vc (l)	M	0.0177 $St^{2.91}$	22
	F	0.0199 $St^{2.40}$	24
Tl/V_A‡	M + F	2.359 $St^{-0.4}$	12

* Measured without backward extrapolation: if this practice is adopted add 2.5% (Section 12.6.2).
† RSD: residual standard deviation (but expressed here as a percentage of the predicted value).
‡ mmol min^{-1} kPa^{-1} and (in the case of Tl/V_A) l^{-1}; to convert to ml min^{-1} mm Hg^{-1} multiply by 2.99.
¶ The values for Dm are influenced by assumptions made about the reaction rate θ (Section 20.7.4).
Source: [15]

The effects of the pubertal growth spurt can be allowed for by expanding the simple model with additional terms. The terms can be anatomical, developmental or empirical.

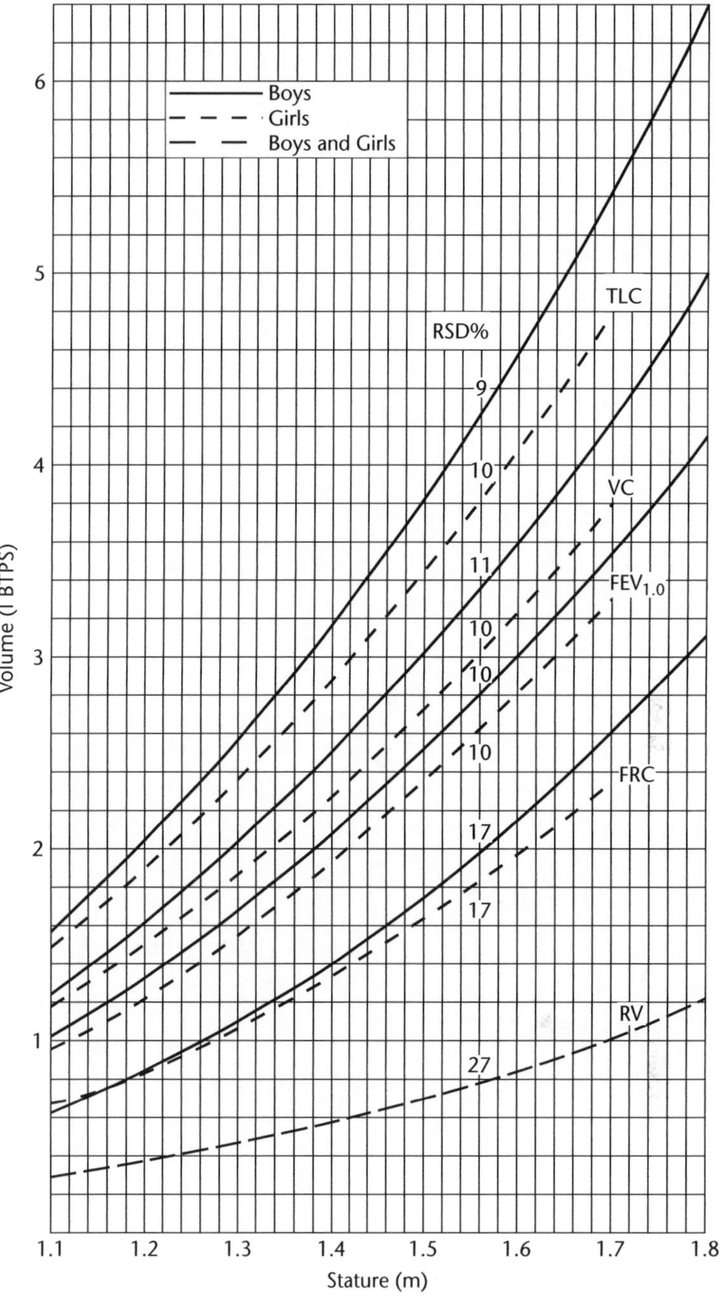

Fig. 26.1 Relationship of total lung capacity (TLC), vital capacity (VC) and forced vital capacity (FVC), forced expiratory volume (FEV_1), functional residual capacity (FRC) and residual volume (RV) to stature in healthy boys and girls of European descent. Source: [15].

Anatomical model. The model includes terms for thoracic dimensions and fat-free mass, all of which enlarge at puberty (Tables 25.3 and 25.4, pages 319 and 320). The enlargement keeps pace with the increase in lung function [17, 18].

Developmental model. The model uses stage of puberty as an additional reference variable [17, 18]. There are three linear terms, with different regression coefficients on stature for before puberty, during puberty, when allowance is made for stage of puberty [19], and after puberty. The model can be appropriate for indices that are markedly affected by puberty, including most indices of lung function in boys and FEV_1, FVC and PEF in girls. For other indices in girls a polynomial equation can be used instead (Table 26.8).

The developmental model adds a new dimension to reference values for adolescents and yields values that merge into those for adults. It is recommended for circumstances when it can be applied. However, the model has the disadvantage of requiring a dedicated staff member who can guide the subject into making a self-assessment of his or her stage of puberty as illustrated in photographs. This is beyond the scope of most laboratories, so in practice the middle term of the model can seldom

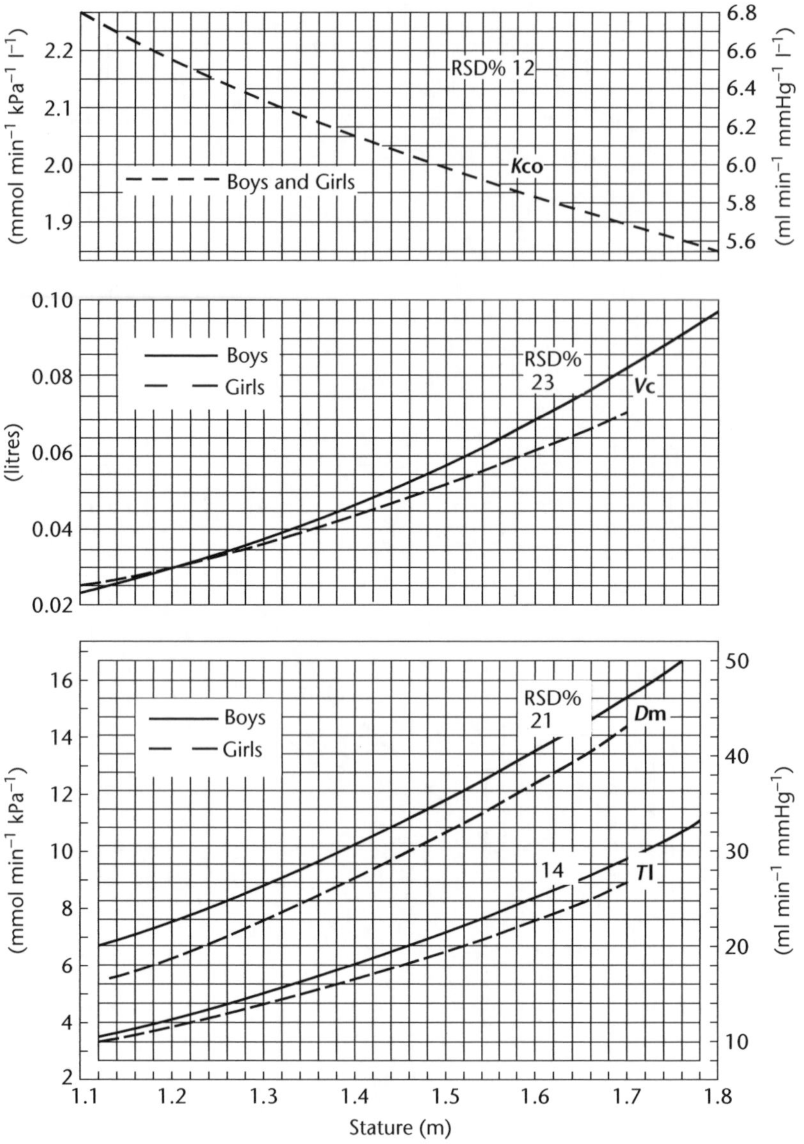

Fig. 26.2 Relationship of transfer factor (diffusing capacity) for the lungs (*T*l), its subdivisions (*D*m and *V*c), and the diffusion constant (*K*co, i.e. *T*l/*V*A) to stature in healthy boys and girls of European descent. The values for *D*m are influenced by assumptions made about the reaction rate θ. Source: [15].

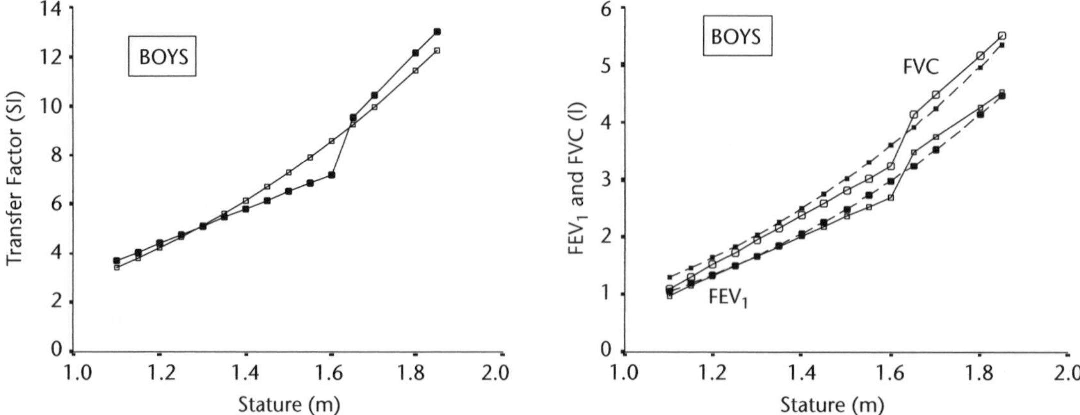

Fig. 26.3 Transfer factor for carbon monoxide, FEV_1 and FVC relative to stature in boys. Comparison of simple reference equations on stature [15] with those incorporating a step change at puberty [17, 18].

be defined quantitatively. In this event, either the term for stage of puberty can be replaced by a step increase (simplified developmental model discussed below) or an empirical model used instead.

Simplified developmental model. For this model, the middle term that spans the 5 stages of puberty is replaced by a step increase located at its midpoint (Tables 26.6 and 26.7). For Caucasian boys and girls living in the UK at the end of the 20th century the corresponding statures were, respectively, 1625 mm and 1526 mm [17, 18]. This approximation has the advantages of simplicity and of retaining optimal relationships of lung function to stature over most of the range of statures covered by the model. However, a step change in the relationship at puberty of up to 16% is not physiological and its location may not be appropriate for some children, including those who experience enhanced or retarded growth, those whose nutrition is inadequate and members of other ethnic groups. These considerations suggest that the modified model should be used with circumspection.

Table 26.6 Equations for indices of lung function relative to stature (m) in healthy white boys aged 4–19 years. Over the five stages of puberty (average stature 1.625 m) there is a step increase of approximately 16%.

	Stature (m)	Equation (y = m St + c) m	c	Coefficient of variation (%)
FEV_1 (l)	<1.626	3.425	−2.78	13
	>1.625	5.21	−5.108	
FVC (l)	<1.626	4.29	−3.619	12
	>1.625	6.78	−7.038	
FEV_1/FVC (%)		−10.0	100	1.2 + 5.0 St
PEF (l s^{-1})	<1.626	7.3	−5.98	18
	>1.625	12.5	−13.14	
FEF_{50} (l s^{-1})*	<1.626	4.0	−2.91	24
	>1.625	4.8	−3.38	
PIF (l s^{-1})	<1.626	5.4	−4.31	38 − 12 St
	>1.625	8.5	−7.96	
TLC (l)	<1.626	4.976	−3.828	12
	>1.625	9.586	−10.648	
FRC (l)	<1.626	2.394	−1.716	34.1 − 12 St
	>1.625	5.918	−7.036	
RV (l)	<1.626	0.818	−0.283	28
	>1.625	3.095	−3.905	
*Tl*co (SI)†	<1.626	7.0	−3.99	4.3 + 8 St
	>1.625	17.3	−19.0	
*V*A (l)	<1.626	4.357	−3.49	11
	>1.625	8.67	−9.785	
*K*co (SI)†	<1.626	−1.3	4.13	11
	>1.625	0	2.1	
*R*aw (kPa l^{-1}s)	<1.626	−0.26	0.634	65
	>1.625	−0.12	0.36	

* This source also gives equations for FEF_{75} but the confidence limits are very wide.

† Units for *Tl* and *K*co (*Tl*/*V*A) mmol min^{-1} kPa^{-1} and l^{-1}. For traditional units (ml min^{-1} mm Hg^{-1}) multiply by 2.99.

Source: [17, 18].

Table 26.7 Equations for indices of ventilatory capacity relative to stature (m) in healthy white girls aged 4–19 years. Over the five stages of puberty (average stature 1.525 m) there are step increases for FEV_1, FVC and PEF of approximately 10%.

	Stature (m)	Equation (y = m St + c) m	c	Coefficient of variation
FEV_1 (l)	<1.526	3.316	−2.734	13.6
	>1.525	4.112	−3.68	
FVC (l)	<1.526	3.918	−3.311	13.9
	>1.525	4.512	−3.881	
FEV_1/FVC (%)		−9.8	104	8
PEF (l s^{-1})	<1.526	7.9	−6.79	20
	>1.525	6.4	−3.94	
FEF_{50} (l s^{-1})	<1.526	4.1	−3.03	24
	>1.525	2.3	0.49	
FEF_{75} (l s^{-1})	<1.526	1.5	−0.807	56 − 18 St
	>1.525	2.7	−2.12	
PIF (l s^{-1})	<1.526	6.1	−5.14	47 − 19 St
	>1.525	3.26	−0.379	

Source: [18].

26.3.3 Empirical models

Hybrid model of Quanjer and colleagues. [20] This model uses the association of growth in stature at puberty with age to improve significantly the simple proportional model relating lung function to stature (Table 26.3). That relationship now becomes:

$$\ln y = a \ln \text{St} + b\,(\text{Age} \times \text{St}) + c \qquad (26.1)$$

where y is an index of lung function

The model is illustrated in Tables 26.9 and 26.10. It can be recommended for circumstances when the reference variables are limited to gender, stature and age (decimal years). However, where the data include thoracic dimensions the model can be refined further (e.g. Table 25.3, page 319). In the case of transfer factor additional considerations apply (see below).

Hybrid model for transfer factor. The hybrid model can be used for transfer factor (*Tl*co,sb) as for other indices of lung function. However, where alveolar volume is available, this variable can replace the A × St interaction term in the reference equation (Table 26.11). The new term has the form (V_A/St^3) because it is then independent of stature in children and adolescents (age range 7.9–20 years). The equivalent term in adults is (V_A/St^2) (see Footnote 20.2, page 251). The circumstances when the use of the model is appropriate are in Section 20.9.2.

Table 26.8 Equations for lung volumes, transfer factor and *Raw* based on a fifth degree polynomial model using stature (m) in healthy white girls aged 4–19 years. The equations are appropriate for a height range of 1.1–1.75 m. The coefficients must not be rounded.

	Intercept	Regression coefficients on stature (m) St	St^2	St^3	St^4	St^5	Coefficient of variation (%)
FRC (l)	−33.928	114.78	−136.745	69.82277567	−12.725216	0	17
TLC (l)	−234.078	703.067	−780.2979	381.00528	−68.597971	0	12
RV (l)	610.323	−2091.427	2858.6128	−1945.88828	659.4203	−88.899	28
*Tl*co (SI)*	−577.13	1678.1	−1811.017	863.6953	−152.87	0	11
*V*A (l)	−289.408	843.755	−912.67633	435.1045553	−76.69615	0	11
*K*co (SI)*	4.14	−1.3	0	0	0	0	0.68 + 7.3 St
Raw (kPa l^{-1}s)	0.7	−0.31	0	0	0	0	55

* Units for *Tl* and *K*co (*Tl* /*V*A) mmol min^{-1} kPa^{-1} and l^{-1}. For traditional units (ml min^{-1} mm Hg^{-1}) multiply by 2.99.
Source: [17].

Table 26.9 Reference equations for FEV_1 and FVC using stature (m) and an age–stature interaction (A × St, where age is in decimal years) in healthy children and adolescents of European descent.

Index	Sex	Equation	RSD%
ln FVC	M	−1.2782 + [1.3731 + 0.0164 Age] St	10.3
	F	−1.4507 + [1.4800 + 0.0127 Age] St	10.6
ln FEV_1	M	−1.2933 + [1.2669 + 0.0174 Age] St	10.9
	F	−1.5974 + [1.5016 + 0.0119 Age] St	10.6

RSD: residual standard deviation.
FVC (litres) = $antilog_e$ (ln FVC). Hence, FVC = $e^{ln(FVC)} = 2.71828^{ln(FVC)}$.
Source: [20].

Multiple quadratic model. The model comprises linear and quadratic terms on age and a quadratic term on stature [22]. It has been used for reference values of dynamic spirometry obtained from a representative sample of the US general population; this included 878 young Caucasians aged 8–20 years. Examination of mean data suggests that for male young persons the values are similar to those reported above, whilst for females the values given by this model are slightly higher. The equations are included in Table 26.21 (page 357).

26.3.4 Reference values independent of body size

Reference values for indices that are independent of size can mostly be described by a mean value with its standard deviation. The indices include those for gas exchange and some ratios that describe a volume or resistance per litre of lung volume (Table 26.12). Such indices are nearly constant throughout childhood. Thus, as a first approximation the specific conductance, i.e. (airway resistance × lung volume)$^{-1}$, can be described by a single number as can, over most of its range, the specific compliance, i.e. compliance ÷ lung volume. The static recoil pressure, for example that at 90% of total lung capacity, is related to stature but the retraction coefficient, which is the maximal recoil pressure ÷ total lung capacity, is independent of it. The constancy of these indices throughout childhood is due to the airway conductance and the static compliance both increases as the lung gets larger.

Table 26.10 Reference equations for TLC and subdivisions using stature (m) and an age–stature interaction (Age × St, where age is in decimal years) in healthy children and adolescents of European descent.

Index*	Sex	Equation	RSD%†
ln TLC	M	−1.115 + [1.442 + 0.0137 Age] St	10.5
	F	−1.254 + [1.530 + 0.0108 Age] St	9.8
ln IC	M	−1.627 + [1.412 + 0.0104 Age] St	15.3
	F	−1.858 + [1.543 + 0.0062 Age] St	13.3
ln FRC	M	−2.078 + [1.522 + 0.0163 Age] St	18.1
	F	−2.059 + [1.518 + 0.0156 Age] St	15.4
ln ERV	M	−2.772 + [1.600 + 0.0172 Age] St	23.6
	F	−3.306 + 2.177 St	19.1
ln RV	M	−2.853 + [1.470 + 0.0148 Age] St	26.6
	F	−2.450 + [1.069 + 0.0260 Age] St	26.6
ln VC	M	−1.331 + [1.451 + 0.0131 Age] St	11.0
	F	−1.597 + [1.655 + 0.0066 Age] St	10.3
RV/TLC %	M	Mean (SD) = 19.4 (4.4)	–
	F	Mean (SD) = 21.3 (4.8)	–

* TLC: total lung capacity, IC: inspiratory capacity, FRC: functional residual capacity, ERV: expiratory reserve volume RV: residual volume, VC: vital capacity.
† RSD: residual standard deviation.
TLC (litres) = $antilog_e$ (ln TLC). Hence, TLC = $e^{ln(TLC)} = 2.71828^{ln(TLC)}$.
Source: [21].

Reference values not given elsewhere. Relationships which describe some indices of forced expiratory flow, lung mechanics, closing volume and respiratory muscle strength are given in Table 26.13. Some of these relationships are illustrated in Figs 26.4 and

Table 26.11 Reference equations for single breath carbon monoxide transfer factor (*Tl*, SI units) using stature (m) and an age–stature interaction (A × St, where age is in years) and alveolar volume (*V*A, litres) in healthy children and adolescents of European descent.

Index	Sex	Equation	RSD%
ln V_A	M	$-1.174 + [1.452 + 0.0126 \text{ Age}]$ St	10.9
	F	$-1.262 + [1.453 + 0.0134 \text{ Age}]$ St	11.0
ln *Tl*	M	$-0.326 + [1.387 + 0.0117 \text{ Age}]$ St	12.6
	M	$-1.365 + 1.824$ St $+ 0.582$ (V_A/St^3)*	10.8
	F	$-0.237 + [1.299 + 0.00786 \text{ Age}]$ St	12.0
	F	$-1.177 + 1.646$ St $+ 0.584$ (V_A/St^3)*	10.2
Tl/*V*A	M	$2.402 - 0.203$ St	0.24
	F	$3.117 - 0.750$ St	0.22

Data for 455 boys of mean age 15.2 (SD 2.9, range 7.9–19.9) years and 266 girls of mean age 13.6 (SD 3.0, range 7.9–19.8) years.
RSD: residual standard deviation.
Tl (mmol min^{-1}kPa^{-1}) = antilog$_e$ (ln *Tl*). Hence, $Tl = e^{\ln(Tl)} = 2.71828^{\ln(Tl)}$.
For traditional units (ml min^{-1} mm Hg^{-1}) multiply by 2.99.
Source: [21] also unpublished*.

26.5. The peak expiratory flows for very young children (Stature <1.1 m, Fig. 26.5) were obtained by voluntary effort after a full inspiration.

26.3.5 Longitudinal growth charts (percentiles)

Derivation. A reference equation describes the overall relationship of a lung function test in terms of the reference variables. When applied to a reference population the results for half the individuals will fall on or below the regression line and half above it. Thus, the regression is the 50th percentile. The spread of results about the regression equation is given by the residual standard deviation (RSD), which for the proportional model used in Table 26.5 is related to the level of lung function, so is a percentage (the coefficient of variation). Five per cent of results are more than 1.64 RSD below the mean line; hence the mean minus 1.64 RSD is described as the 5th percentile. Other percentiles are given in Table 5.7 (page 50). For the proportional model the percentiles are constructed using the form

$$\ln y(a) = (m \ln x + c) \pm \text{Za,RSD} \qquad (26.2)$$

where $y(a)$ is the value of y at the percentile a and Za,RSD is the standardised deviate associated with that percentile (Table 5.7). Percentiles are not normally used for adults, because most data are described better by a linear than by a proportional relationship (Section 26.5).

Relevance. Expressing a lung function result as a percentile indicates its likely normality and provides a basis for possible action.

Table 26.12 Lung function in healthy children (male (M), female (F) or both sexes); indices that are effectively independent of age and body size.

	Mean values				Source
Lung volumes and ventilatory capacity					
$FEV_{0.75}$ % ($FEV_{0.75}$/FVC)	81 F		78 M	RSD 5	[15]
FEV_1 % (FEV_1/FVC)	88 F		84 M		[23]
$FEV_{0.75}$ %/FEV_1(%)		93		RSD 2.7	[15]
RV % (RV/TLC)		24		RSD 2.4	[24]
FRC % (FRC/TLC)		47		RSD 5	[15]
$FEF_{50\%VC}$/TLC (s^{-1})		0.95		RSD 0.15	[25]
$FEF_{40\%TLC}$/TLC (s^{-1})		0.91		RSD 0.14	[25]
PEF / TLC (s^{-1})		1.32		RSD 0.22	[25]
Lung mechanics					
sGaw (Gaw/TGV) ($s^{-1}kPa^{-1}$)		2.0		1.4–4.6	[26]
(s^{-1}cm H_2O^{-1})		0.2		0.14–0.46	
sC (Cstat/FRC) (kPa^{-1})		0.57		–	[27]
(cm H_2O^{-1})		0.057		–	
Indices of gas distribution					
Vd/*Vt* (rest) (%)		26		RSD 7	[28]
Lung clearance index		7.8		RSD 0.9	[29]
Indices of gas exchange (boys and girls)					
	kPa		mm Hg		
P_{A,O_2}	14.0, RSD 0.2		104.9, RSD 1.7		[30]
$Pa,_{O_2}$	12.7, RSD 0.5		95.5, RSD 3.7		[30]
A-aD_{O_2}	1.3, RSD 0.6		9.4, RSD 4.8		[30]
$Pa,_{CO_2}$	4.9, RSD 0.2		37.1, RSD 1.6		[30]
PH		7.39, RSD 0.01			[30]

Table 26.13 Regression relationships describing aspects of lung function not included elsewhere. Most are for boys and girls of stature >1.1 m. Stature (St) is in m (or cm where indicated) and body mass (BM) in kg. The abbreviations are explained in Table 6.2, page 53.

Index		Units	Relationship	RSD% (or units)	Figure	Source
Cstat		$l\ kPa^{-1}$*	$0.418\ St^{2.18}$	32%	26.4	[24]
Gaw		$l\ s^{-1} kPa^{-1}$*	1.63 TGV + 0.71	27%	26.4	[26]
CV/VC		%	26.12 – 1.25 Age	30%	26.4	[27]
R total		$kPa\ l^{-1} s$*	7.39/antilog(0.89 St)	21%	26.5	[31]
R total		$kPa\ l^{-1} s$*	$1.81\ St^{-7.39}$	35%	26.5	[‡]
PEF ($St \leq 1.1$ m)		$l\ s^{-1}$	4.93 St – 2.9	14%	26.5	[‡]
*P*stat 90% TLC		kPa	$2.04\ St - 0.0018\ St^2$	78.6%	–	[32]
$FEF_{50\%FVC}$						
	M	$l\ s^{-1}$	5.43 St – 4.58	0.47†	26.5	[25]
	F	$l\ s^{-1}$	4.48 St – 3.37	0.49†	26.5	[25]
$FEF_{75\%FVC}$						
	M	$l\ s^{-1}$	2.82 St – 2.31	0.40†	26.5	[25]
	F	$l\ s^{-1}$	2.48 St–1.86	0.40†	26.5	[25]
*P*Emax						
	M	(cm H_2O)	5.5 Age + 35	18.4	–	[33]
	F	(cm H_2O)	4.8 Age + 24	17.0	–	[33]
*P*Imax						
	M	(cm H_2O)	0.75BM + 44.5	21.1	–	[33]
	F	(cm H_2O)	0.57BM + 40	19.8	–	[33]
Log ($R_{f0,\ 8Hz}$)			10.990 – 2.370 log St (cm)	–	–	[34]
Log ($R_{f0,\ 12Hz}$)			10.357 – 2.259 log St (cm)	–	–	[34]
Log ($R_{f0,\ 16Hz}$)			8.705 – 1.945 log St (cm)	–	–	[34]

* For conversion to traditional units see Table 6.6 (page 56).

† at stature 1.5 m.

‡ Unpublished data of Robinson M (1973).

For example, children in the top and bottom 5% may merit special consideration. In addition, each child's lung normally grows along his or her own percentile [35]. As a consequence, percentiles can be used to monitor progress and identify trends in response to treatment or progression of disease. Indices that behave in this way include TLC, VC, FEV_1 and respiratory pressures but not RV.

The model is inevitably an approximation because it is based on the one variable, i.e. stature, and does not take account of puberty. However, where there are sufficient data this difficulty can be minimised by reporting values for each year of age [36]. Average values are displayed in Fig. 26.6.

26.4 Young persons aged 16–25 years

The lung function of young persons aged 16–25 years can be described in terms of stature using relationships developed for children of school age (see previous sections). Alternatively, in healthy males the lung function can be described in terms of thoracic dimensions, for which age is a surrogate measure. Hence, the partial regression coefficients on stature and age are both positive (Table 26.14). In healthy females skeletal growth ceases at about 16 years of age, and for most indices the term for age is not significant. However, some teenage girls increase their body mass by accumulating additional fat. When this change is represented by a term for body mass index (i.e. mass independent of stature) in a multiple regression equation the *average* partial regression coefficient is negative (Table 26.15). However, the coefficient is positive for the minority of young women who increase their BMI by accumulating additional muscle (Section 4.7.1).

26.5 Adults aged 25–65 years

Introduction. The lung function of adults is traditionally represented as a linear decline from a peak or high plateau at ages 20–25 years through to death. The model that is used is a multiple regression (Table 26.3) with a constant term and linear terms on stature and age, see eqn. 5.12, terms *a*, *b* and *c* (page 49). In subjects with spinal curvature the stature can be replaced by a function of arm span (Section 4.3.2).

The model can accommodate additional terms, for example indices of body composition such as Fat% and fat-free mass [37]. Body mass index can also be included, but is of limited usefulness for describing the level of lung function as it does not distinguish between the sometimes contrary effects of the component terms for fat and muscle. In most studies the basic model accounts for some 60% of the variance in the population data. It is convenient because it is simple, the principal reference variables (stature

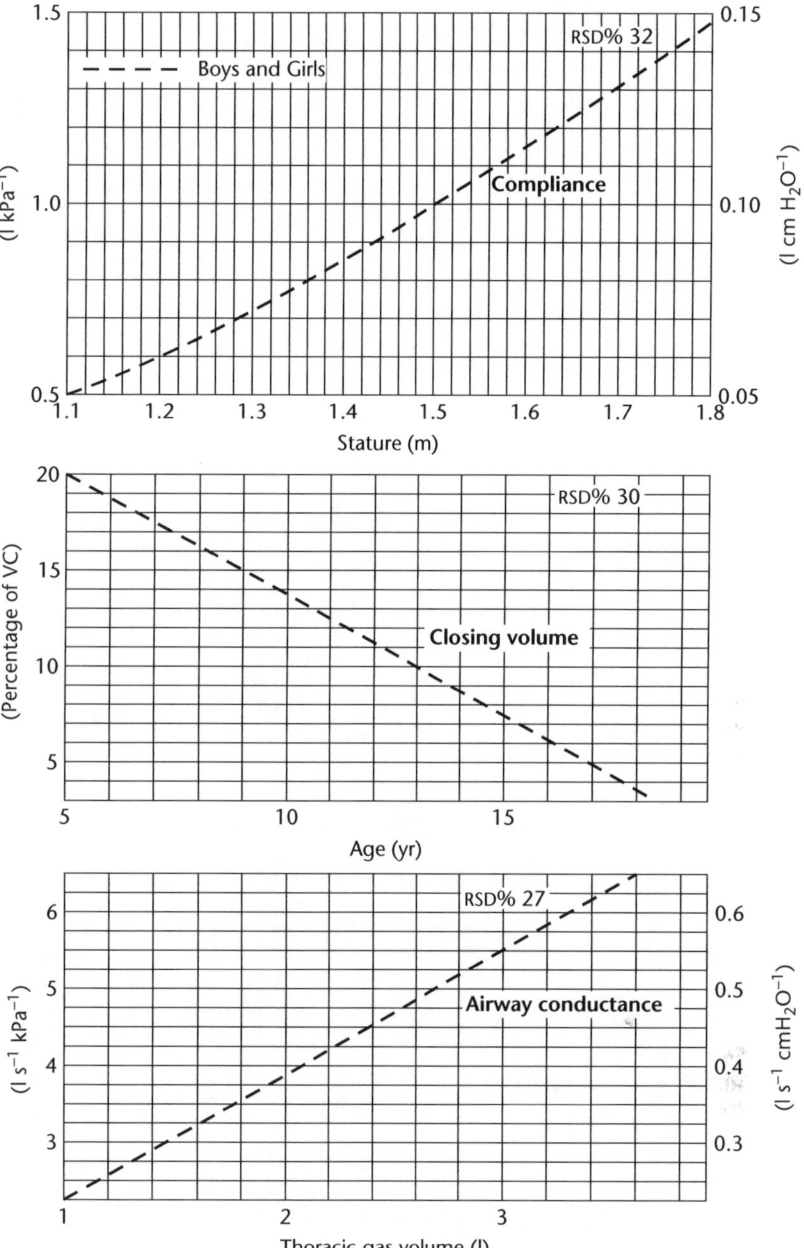

Fig. 26.4 Relationship of compliance to stature, closing volume to age, and airway conductance to thoracic gas volume in healthy boys and girls of European descent (for sources see Table 26.13).

and age) are usually available, the partial regression coefficients (parameters) of the equations have been obtained and cross-checked in numerous studies and most people who use the equations have extensive experience of their features and limitations.

Comments on the model. The model is simplistic because the lung function of the adult emerges out of that of the child, so the plateau has been subject to numerous influences, including those listed in Table 26.2, not all of which can be allowed for by using a term for stature. Allowance is normally made for the principal *categorical* variables in that table, but not for the other variables. Similarly, the decline that occurs throughout adult life depends on many factors in addition to age. Neglect of them leads to the model slightly over predicting the lung function of young and old adults.

The form of the model implies that the increment of lung function per unit of stature is the same for short and tall people; at the present time this appears to be the case. The model also implies that the decline in lung function throughout adult life is the same at all ages and is independent of stature and smoking habits. This is incorrect. The decline with age increases with age [38, 39]; in absolute units it is also greater for tall than for short people and it can be represented as occurring at a greater rate in smokers than in non-smokers. Allowances for these aspects

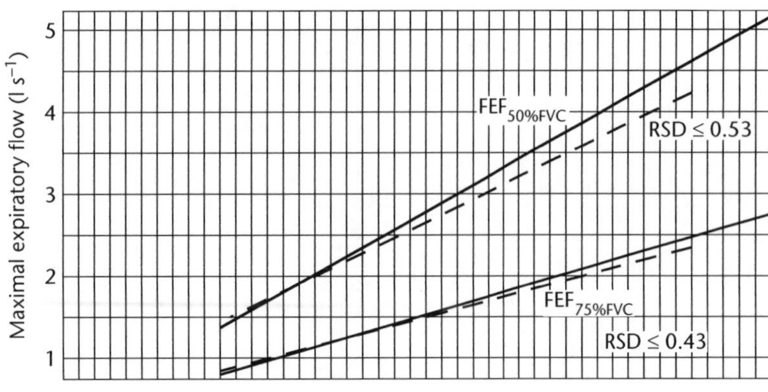

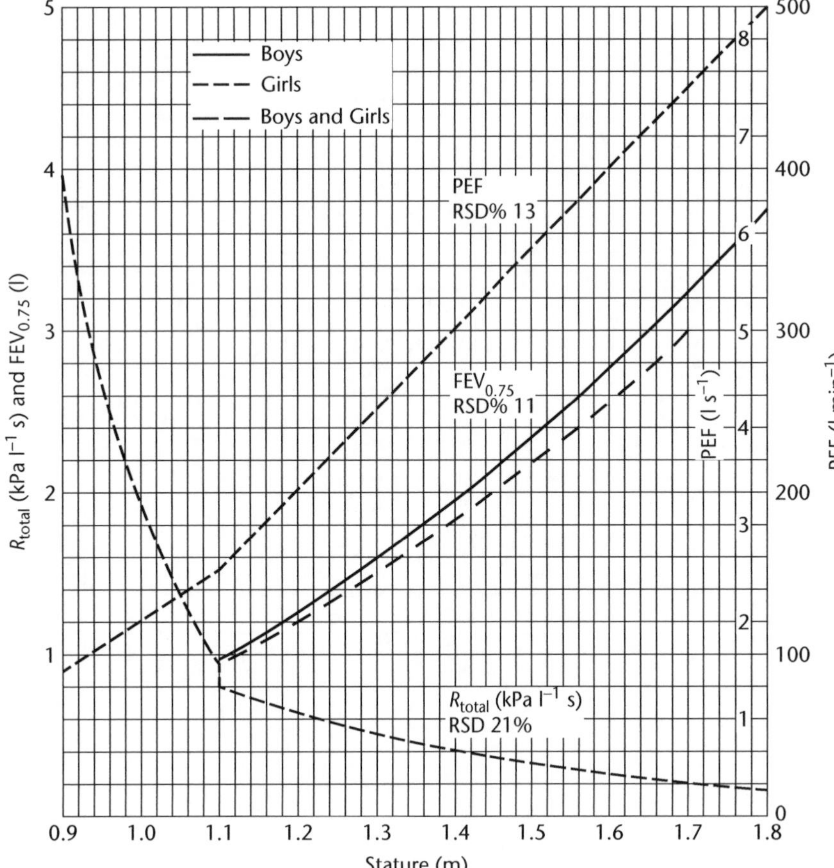

Fig. 26.5 Forced expiratory flow when 50% and 75% of forced vital capacity have been expired ($FEF_{50\%\,FVC}$ and $FEF_{75\%\,FVC}$), total thoracic resistance (R total), peak expiratory flow (PEF) and forced expiratory volume ($FEV_{0.75}$) in healthy boys and girls of European descent (for sources see Tables 26.5 and 26.13).

can be made by adopting a more complex model that includes quadratic and interaction terms, for example

$$\begin{aligned} y = {} & (a \times \text{stature}) + (b \times \text{age}) + (c \times \text{stature}^2) + (d \times \text{age}^2) \\ & +(e \times \text{if smoker}) + (f \times \text{age} \times \text{smoking}) \\ & +(g \times \text{age} \times \text{stature}) + \cdots + Z(\pm \text{RSD}) \end{aligned} \quad (26.3)$$

An alternative model proposed by Cole [40] has the form

$$y\ \text{st}^{-2} = k_1 k_2 \exp(a + b \times \text{age}) \quad (26.4)$$

where k_1 and k_2 are coefficient terms for gender and for ethnic group. Versions of this model have now been used in a number of investigations but mostly in single ethnic groups (see Section 26.7). For example

$$y = \exp^{(b0 + b1\text{Age} + b2\text{Age}^2 + b3 \ln \text{stature})}. \quad (26.5)$$

The full potential of the multiplicative model has still to be established.

Reference equations for white adults. Most laboratories use and come to feel at ease with a single set of reference equations for

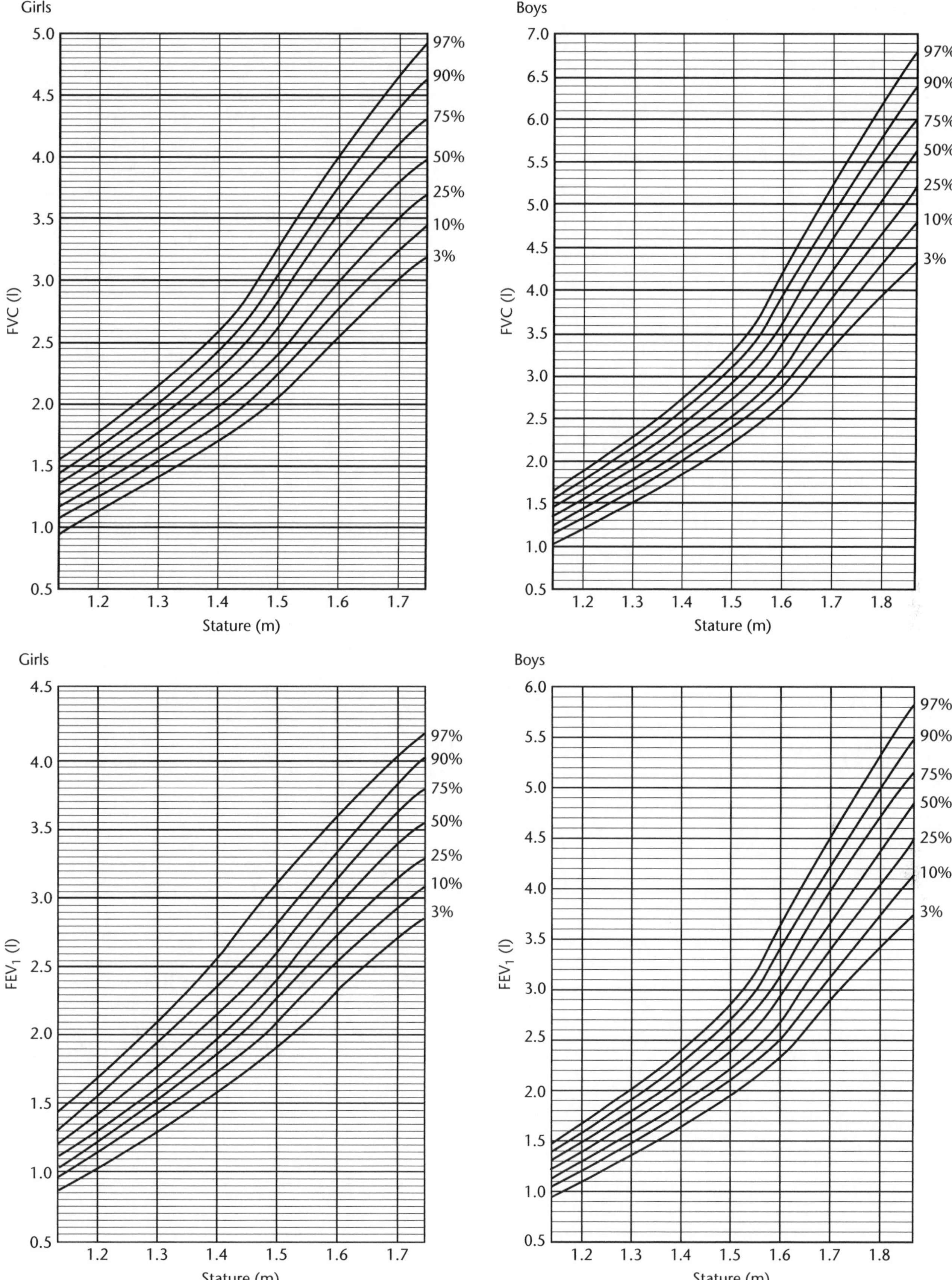

Fig. 26.6 Percentiles describing the development of forced expiratory volume and vital capacity in white children aged 6–18 years in six US cities. Source: [36].

Table 26.14 Regression equations describing the lung function of 701 asymptomatic young men aged 16–25 years studied cross-sectionally.

	Regression coefficients			
	Age (years)	Stature (m)	Constant	RSD
Forced expiratory volume (l)	–	5.03	−4.48	0.48
Forced vital capacity (l)	0.024	6.72	−6.96	0.51
FEV_1% (of FVC)	−0.61	−7.41	107.2	6.3
Peak expiratory flow (l s^{-1})	0.044	7.90	−5.17	1.37
Total lung capacity (l)	0.098	8.83	−10.91	0.65
Inspiratory vital capacity (l)	0.060	6.90	−8.02	0.55
Residual volume (l)	0.032	1.96	−2.97	0.30
RV% (of TLC)	0.25	6.65	0.28	4.0
Transfer factor (SI units)	0.13	12.7	−13.1	1.58
*K*co (*T*l/*V*A)	−0.006*	−0.59	3.00	0.23

*In asymptomatic smokers. Smoking did not affect the other indices.
Source: Chinn DJ, Bridges N, Cotes JE, unpublished.

all commonly used indices of lung function. The set is usually for men and women of working age. Lung function in old age is considered subsequently (Section 26.6). The core indices are for ventilatory capacity by dynamic spirometry, static lung volumes by helium dilution or plethysmography and transfer factor (diffusing capacity) with related variables. One set, that included a wide range of indices, was compiled for the first edition of this book (1965) and revised subsequently. The present version is given in Table 26.16. Additional relationships for PEF on age and stature (cm) and for indices with allowances for body composition are given in Tables 26.17 and 26.18. Some of the relationships, also those for closing volume, are displayed in Figs 26.7–26.10. The series compiled by Quanjer for the European Coal and Steel Community is also widely used, despite there being difficulty with *K*co and FEV% (see 'Features of the different series' below). The equations are listed in Table 26.19 and illustrated in Figs 26.11 and 26.12. In the USA the principal equations include those of Crapo, based on experience at Salt Lake City in the foothills of the Utah mountains, Morris reflecting the lung function of the state of Michigan and for dynamic spirometry Hankinson whose subjects were a sample of the general US population. Where they can be compared the three series yield similar results, except for transfer factor. For this index the results from Salt Lake City are higher than those from Michigan due to the lower oxygen tension associated with the altitude (1400 m). Reference equations from the US are given in Tables 26.20 and 26.21, also Figs 26.13 and 26.14 (pages 355 to 357). The average levels of function for the three recommended series are compared in Table 26.22 and associated text (see also Footnote 26.2). Reference values for other indices of lung function are in Tables 26.23 and 26.24.

Usually one of the recommended sets of reference values (lung function, ECSC or US) will meet local circumstances (Sections 26.1 and 26.2).

Features of the different series of reference values. The lung function of white adults is inevitably influenced by environmental factors (Table 25.2, page 319), but not by country of residence. Yet the three series of reference values given above show notable differences for some indices (Table 26.22). These are at least partly due to the criteria used for selecting the subjects. In the lung function series and that for the European Coal and Steel Community the subjects were asymptomatic (Section 26.1.2). Potential subjects were not excluded if they were asymptomatic smokers. The subjects for the US studies were non-smokers. In addition, the lung function and US equations were each the

Footnote 26.2. Notable omissions are where some of the methods have been superceded (e.g. [67, 68, 69]). In addition, the equations for FEV_1 have been increased by a factor of 1.025 to allow for the protocols in the original studies not including backward extrapolation.

Table 26.15 Regression equations describing the lung function of 84 asymptomatic young women aged 16–25 years studied cross-sectionally.

	Regression coefficients				
	Age (years)	Stature (m)	BMI (kg m^{-2})	Constant	RSD
Forced expiratory volume (l)	−0.034	4.49	–	−3.48	0.31
Forced expiratory volume (l)	–	4.71	−0.246	−3.97	0.31
Forced vital capacity (l)	–	5.03	–	−4.52	0.39
FEV_1% (of FVC)	–	–	−0.49	96.9	5.3
Peak expiratory flow (l s^{-1})	–	9.43	–	−8.44	0.90
Total lung capacity (l)	–	6.18	−0.044	−4.14	0.47
Inspiratory vital capacity (l)	–	4.51	–	−3.81	0.42
Residual volume (l)	–	1.33	−0.054	0.23	0.30
RV% (of TLC)	–	–	−0.88	44.0	5.1
Transfer factor (SI units)	–	11.07	–	−9.09	1.56
*K*co (*T*l/*V*A)	–	–	–	1.90	0.29

Source: Cotes JE, Chinn DJ, Ashton I, unpublished

Table 26.16 Reference values for white adults revised from those in previous editions of this book. Regression relationships for the prediction of indices of lung function from age (year), stature (st, m) and in some instances body mass (BM, kg) or body mass index (BMI, kg m^{-2}) in asymptomatic adult male and female subjects of European descent. Gas volumes are expressed at BTPS. Equations for gas exchange have been converted from traditional to SI units.

		Regression coefficients						
	Sex	Stature	Age	BM or BMI	Constant	RSD	Figure	Source
Total lung capacity (TLC, l)*	M	8.67	–	–	–8.49	0.91	26.7	[41]
	F	7.46	–0.013	–	–6.42	0.51	26.8	[42]
Expiratory and forced vital capacity (FVC, l)*	M	5.20	–0.022	–	–3.60	0.58	26.7	[43]
	F	4.66	–0.029	–	–2.88	0.44	26.8	[42]
Residual volume (RV, l)*	M	2.7	+0.017	–	–3.45	0.39	26.7	[44]
	F	2.8	+0.016	–	–3.54	0.31	26.8	[42]
Functional residual capacity (FRC, l)	M	5.95	+0.019	–0.086 (BMI)	–5.53	0.59	–	[37]
	F	4.06	–	–0.09 (BMI)	–1.46	0.46	–	[37]
Inspiratory capacity (IC, l)*	M	2.35	–0.020	+0.017 (BM)	–1.40	0.47	–	[46]
	F	2.88	–	+0.014 (BM)	–3.09	0.40	–	[41]
Expiratory reserve volume (ERV, l)*	M	3.50	–0.012	–0.018 (BM)	–2.84	0.38	–	[46]
	F	3.35	–0.018	–0.019 (BM)	–2.12	0.33	–	[41]
(RV/TLC%)	M	–	+0.343	–	+16.7	4.8	26.7	[44]
	F	–	+0.43	–	+14.33	5.7	26.8	[42]
Forced expiratory volume(FEV_1 l)*†	M	3.71	–0.032	–	–1.44	≈0.5	26.7	[47]
	F	3.37	–0.030	–	–1.46	0.37	26.8	[42]
FEV_1/FVC (%)†	M	–	–0.382	–	+94.1	7.37	26.7	[48]
	F	–	–0.228	–	+88.7	6.4	26.8	[42]
Maximal voluntary ventilation (MVV, l min^{-1})	M	134	–1.26	–	–21.4	29.0	–	[43]
	F	81	–0.57	–	–5.5	10.7	–	[49]
Peak expiratory flow (PEF, l s^{-1})§	M	St x	(–0.025	–	+6.58)	1.0	26.7§	[50]
	F	6.23	–0.035	–	–1.88	1.1	26.8	[51]
Forced mid-expiratory flow (FEF_{25-75} l s^{-1})	M	–	–0.057	–	+6.38	1.09	–	[52]
	F	–	–0.063	–	+6.14	0.77	–	[52]
Forced expiratory flow ($FEF_{50\% FVC}$ l s^{-1})	M	2.72	–0.061	+0.04 (BMI)	+1.52	1.38	–	¶
	F	3.28	–0.049	+0.04 (BMI)	–0.17	1.04	–	¶
Forced expiratory flow ($FEF_{75\% FVC}$ l s^{-1})	M	1.00	–0.033	–	+1.28	0.55	–	¶
	F	1.11	–0.032	–	+0.94	0.49	–	¶
Combined obstruction index (page 190)	M (? and F)	–	0.312	–0.221 (BMI)	17.2	4.1	–	¶
Compliance. (10^2.exp k $pressure^{-1}$)	M and F		0.0929		+9.71	2.84	–	[53]
Transfer factor (*T*l,co sb)‡	M	10.9	–0.067	–	–5.89	1.71	26.7	[41]
	F	7.1	–0.054	–	–0.89	1.20	26.8	[54]
*K*co (*T*l / *V*A)†	M	–	–0.013	–	2.20	0.27	26.9	[55]
	F	–	–0.007	–	2.07	0.20	26.9	[55]
1/*D*m‡	M and F	–0.054	+0.00036	–	+0.135	0.006	26.9	[41]
l/*V*c (ml^{-1})	M	–0.0201	–	–	+0.047	0.003	26.9	[56]
	F	–0.0274	–	–	+0.061	0.006	26.9	[41]

* The accuracy is improved by the additional inclusion of terms for Fat% and/or fat-free mass index (see Table 26.18).

† Increased by 2.5% to allow for original measurement not including backward extrapolation. (Section 12.6.2).

‡ Equations in SI units (i.e. mmol min^{-1} kPa^{-1} and their reciprocal). To convert to traditional units (ml, min and torr) multiply throughout by 2.99, see Table 6.6 (page 56). An extended version that allows for alveolar volume is in Footnote 20.2, page 251.

§ Figure 26.7 includes the linear form of the curvilinear equation (PEF = 5.455 St – 0.0437 Age + 1.9687); the two equations give very similar results but these are now subject to revision following efforts to linearise the instrument scales (see Section 12.3.2). Equations for the Wright peak flow meter are in Table 26.17.

¶ Chinn DJ, Cotes JE. Unpublished.

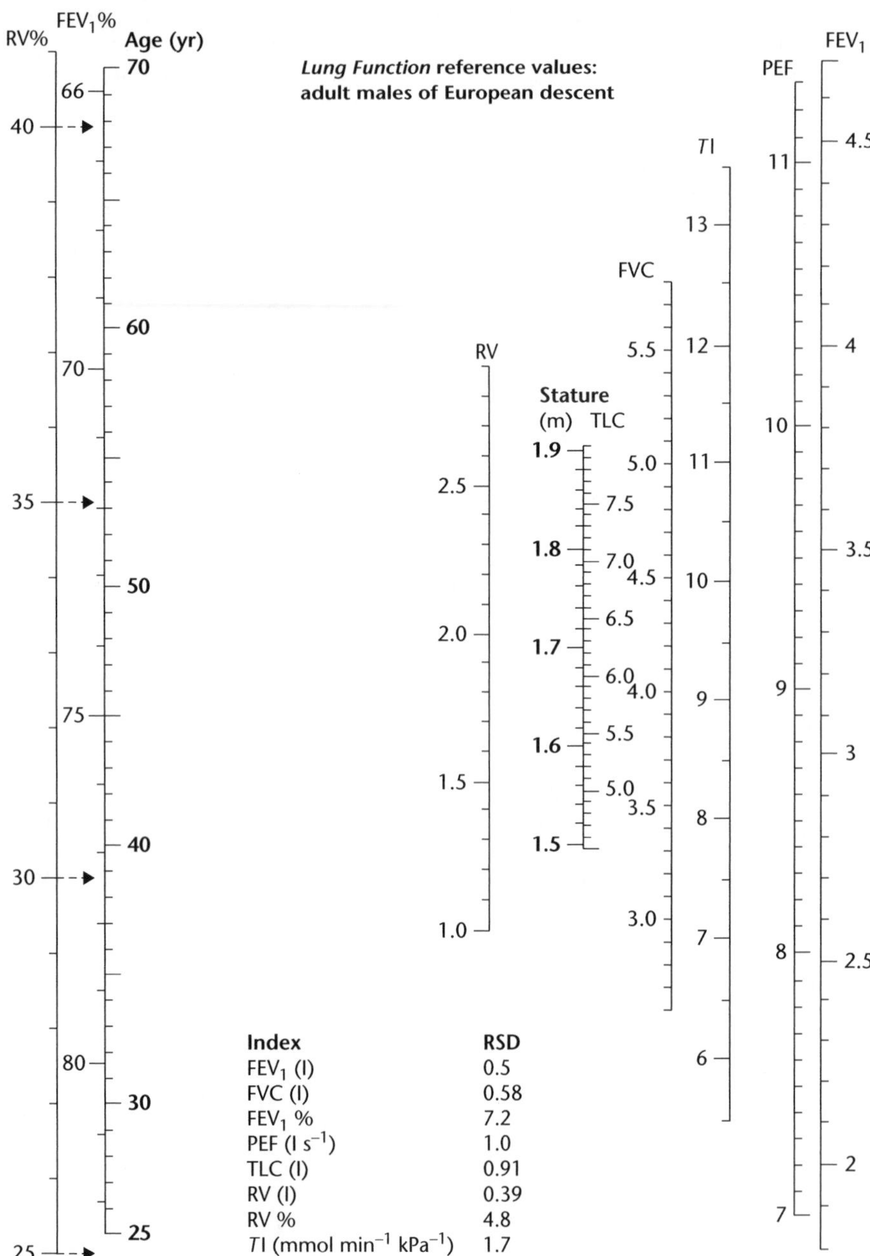

Index	RSD
FEV_1 (l)	0.5
FVC (l)	0.58
FEV_1 %	7.2
PEF (l s^{-1})	1.0
TLC (l)	0.91
RV (l)	0.39
RV %	4.8
Tl (mmol min^{-1} kPa^{-1})	1.7

Fig. 26.7 Nomogram relating indices of lung function to stature and age for healthy adult males of European descent (from Table 26.16). To use the nomogram a ruler is placed to overlie the age and stature of the subject, the lung function is then given by the intersections with the vertical lines. However, RV% and the FEV% are related only to age and TLC only to stature so these indices should be read directly from the respective columns. When stature is measured in inches these should be converted to metres by dividing by 39.4. Values for FEV_1 and FEV_1% should be increased by 2.5% to allow for original measurement not including backward extrapolation (Section 12.6.2). The data for PEF should be adjusted for the non-linearity of the original scale: PEFcorrected = 53.2 + 0.585 PEFobs + 0.00075 $(PEFobs)^2$ (see Table 12.3, page 133)

outcome of single investigations, so the subjects and methods were known. For the present compilation published studies were reviewed and representative equations selected. The summary equations in the ECSC series were each calculated using values culled systematically from a number of primary sources. As a result some equations included data obtained by more than one method; this was the case for *K*co (*Tl*/*V*A) where *V*A was not defined in a consistent manner (Section 20.9.1), and for FEV_1 where the measurement technique appears not to have been standardised for backward extrapolation. After allowing for this, the ECSC values of FEV% are rather high for asymptomatic smokers; the cause appears not to have been identified. In other respects, results for the lung function and ECSC series are comparable and either series is suitable for circumstances where smoking history is not an issue, including most occupational and many clinical applications. The US equation for TLC in males is unusual in that the partial regression coefficient on age is positive. This probably reflects the biological relationship but in the present instance may have been influenced by the reference population including some relatively young subjects [62]. The US equations are widely used and are especially suitable for when the early effects of smoking are being investigated. The quadratic equations (Table 26.21 page 357) extend into an older age group than the other series.

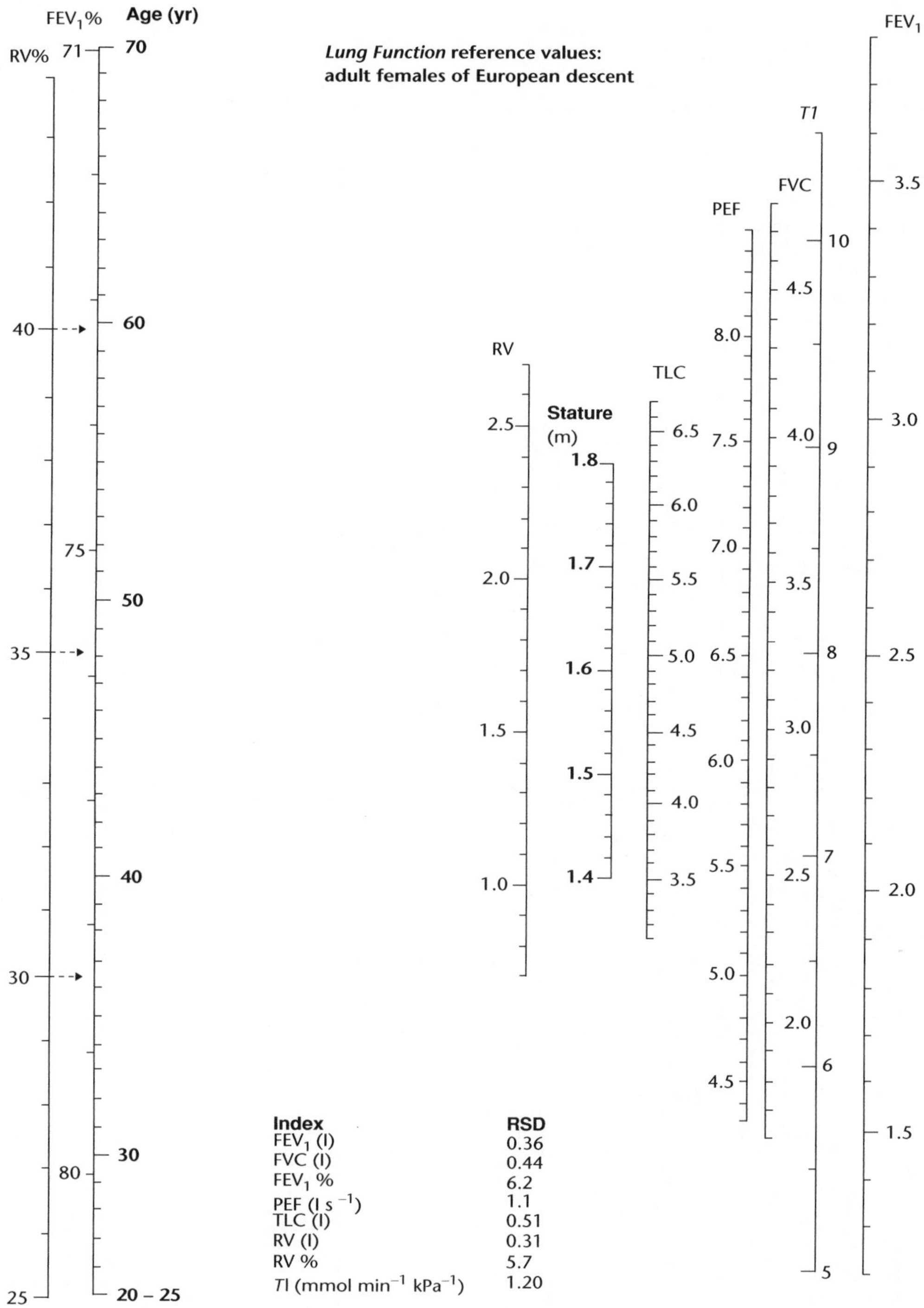

Fig. 26.8 Nomogram relating indices of lung function to stature and age for healthy adult females of European descent (from Table 26.16; see also caption to Fig. 26.7).

Other reference values. Reference values for lung function indices not given in Tables 26.16 to 26.20 are in Tables 26.23 to 26.25 (pages 358 to 360). Reference equations which describe the physiological response to exercise, including ventilation, tidal volume and cardiac frequency are given in Section 29.5 (page 434).

26.6 Adults aged 65 years onwards

Adult reference values are usually derived from subjects that can be studied in sufficient numbers to obtain representative results. Hence, they are appropriate for similar persons who are able-bodied. The very old tend to be less accessible for study.

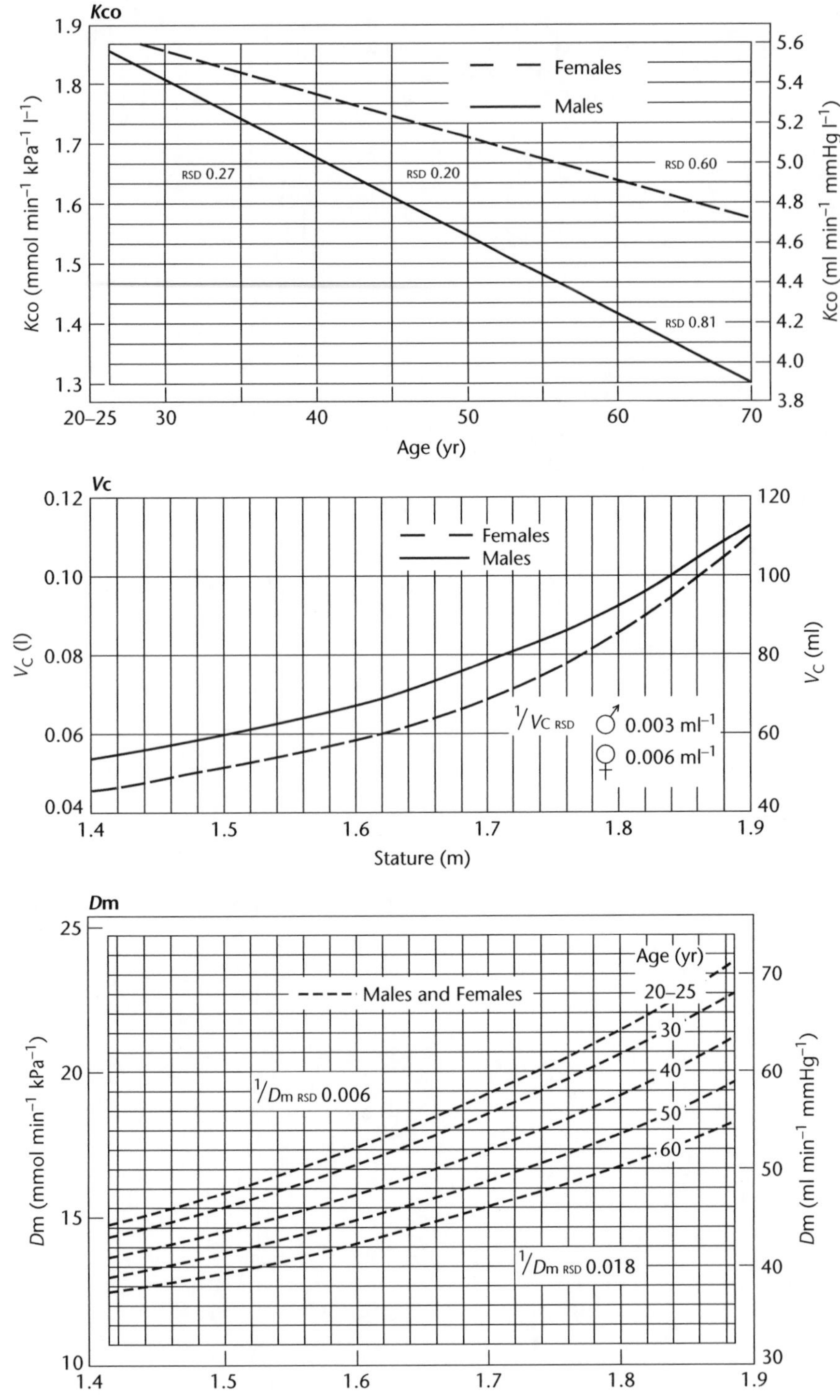

Fig. 26.9 Diffusion constant (*k*co or [*T*l/*V*A]), volume of blood in the alveolar capillaries (*V*c) and the diffusing capacity of the alveolar capillary membrane (*D*m) in healthy adults of European descent. Sources: see Table 26.16 (page 347).

They also vary in their ability to perform measurements to the required technical standard. They are survivors of a larger cohort amongst whom relatively impaired lung function may have been a factor associated with early demise [77]. The association need not have been causal. These features point to the lung function of elderly subjects being above the average for their cohort. In practice, the values are usually consistent with those given by reference equations for adults of working age, despite the extrapolation that this entails [78, 79]. Thus, for white adults, either the equations given in Tables 26.16–26.21 or dedicated

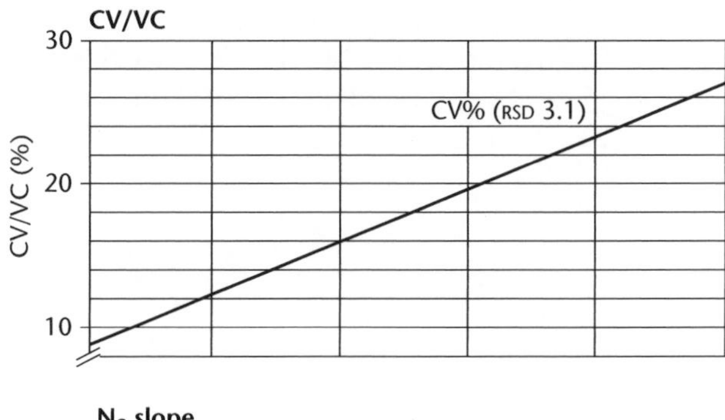

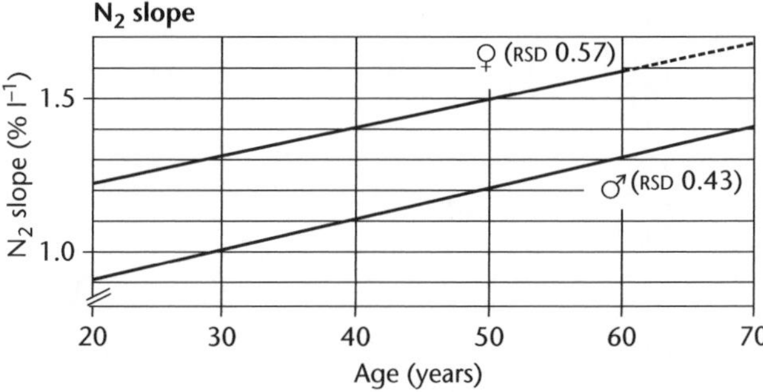

Fig. 26.10 Closing volume as a percentage of vital capacity and nitrogen slope for non-smokers. The values for smokers are on average twice those for non-smokers but with a wide scatter. Sources: [57, 58]. Note that the line for N_2 slope in women should stop at age 60 (equations: N_2 slope (M) = 0.71 + 0.10 age, (F) = 1.036 + 0.009 age).

Table 26.17 Reference equations for $\log_e$ peak expiratory flow (l min^{-1}) measured using a correctly calibrated Wright peak flow meter in male and female non-smokers aged 15 – 85 years. The original equations [59] have been recalculated following revision of the scales [60] (see Section 12.3.2).

			RSD
Men:	ln (PEF) =	$0.755 \log_e A - 0.021 A - 104.1 St^{-1} + 5.16$	46 l.min^{-1}
Women:	ln (PEF) =	$0.486 \log_e A - 0.016 A - 76.8 St^{-1} + 5.43$	

A is age in years and St is stature in cm.

equations (e.g. Tables 26.26 and 26.27, pages 360 and 361) can be used. Where available the equations should be for the local population [22, 80–85]. However, external reference values are of limited usefulness for elderly subjects. For clinical management, the aim should be to obtain serial measurements that provide internal reference values and to assess the amount of function that remains.

26.7 Comprehensive cross-sectional and longitudinal models

For historical reasons the lung function of children including adolescents is usually considered separately from that of adults and geriatric patients. This is appropriate for most applications, but not for medical care of young people with respiratory problems that accompany them into adult life, including chronic infections, cystic fibrosis and asthma. At the other end of life the present linear models are also inadequate as the decline with age is curvilinear. These considerations have led to a search for a comprehensive alternative. An early example is given in Fig. 25.1 (page 318), where part of the curve and associated limits were drawn by hand. Recent work has been directed to finding a mathematical alternative. This may need to be specific to individual indices of lung function as the pattern of change is not the same for all of them [86].

On account of convenience and availability of the information the comprehensive models have been in terms of age and stature and confined to data for subjects who have never smoked. However, this convention has led to neglect of physique (e.g. Table 26.18), habitual activity and other factors that contribute to variation between individuals at one point in time. It also cannot explain the *cohort effect* whereby there are systematic differences in lung function between those born in different decades. The evidence for this extends back to 1846 (Section 1.4.1). Data for a relatively large number of subjects are needed to construct the new models and up to the present this has led to the analyses being confined to indices of ventilatory capacity.

26.7.1 Cross-sectional models

Cross-sectional models now have the flexibility to provide a good empirical description of indices of lung function from childhood to old age. They are based on versions of eqn. 26.4, for example Table 26.21 on page 357. A more recent model that has been used in several studies is given in Table 26.27 (page 361).

Such equations have been found to provide concordant descriptions of FEV_1 and FVC for healthy Caucasian men and women who have never smoked, independent of the country in which they live, e.g. [22, 80–84]. The equations can include a realistic lower limit of normal that allows for the dispersion of the results increasing as people grow older [80]. These relationships can be recommended where the main requirement is for cross-sectional reference values for FEV_1 and FVC. They are less satisfactory for FEV_1/FVC on account of the two indices having different determinants; this can lead to the mean levels of FEV% differing systematically between communities [80]. The relationships do not describe longitudinal changes in individuals. This is because the determinants of cross-sectional and longitudinal relationships are different. For example, in a longitudinal study of shipyard workers the principal correlate with a decline in lung function was an increase in body mass [87], a term that only appears rarely in current relationships [88], see also Fig. 4.3, page 35. For this and similar reasons the partial regression coefficient on age from a cross-sectional reference equation is not a good guide to the longitudinal decline [89].

Table 26.18 Reference equations for white adults that include significant terms for body composition*.

Index*	Sex	Stature	Age	Fat%	FFMI†	Constant	RSD
		Partial regression coefficients					
TLC	M	9.64	0.025	−0.051	0.058	−11.1	0.64
	F	7.82	ns	−0.038	ns	−5.92	0.52
	M and F	8.42	ns	−0.024	ns	−7.42	0.62
IC	M	3.44	ns	ns	0.13	−5.16	0.48
	F	3.84	ns	ns	0.084	−5.06	0.36
	M and F	3.54	ns	ns	0.114	−5.04	0.44
ERV*	M and F	2.82	−0.007	−0.033	−0.069	−0.77	0.42
RV	M	2.57	0.033	−0.017	ns	−3.81	0.33
	F	2.56	0.024‡	−0.025	ns	−2.63	0.30
FVC	M	6.76	−0.011¶	−0.047	0.069	−6.70	0.52
	F	4.84	−0.018	−0.030	ns	−2.57	0.46
	M and F	6.21	−0.012	−0.040	0.046	−5.38	0.50
FEV_1	M	4.80	−0.026¶	−0.031	0.041	−3.61	0.48
	F	3.05	−0.022	−0.022	ns	−0.47	0.35

ns: not significant ($p > 0.05$).
* See Table 26.16 for more information, including relationships for describing FRC and ERV that include BMI. For these indices, after allowing for BMI the term for gender was still significant.
† Fat free mass index (FFM × St^{-2}).
‡ The apparent increase with age in women was significantly less than in men.
¶ Allowing for body composition significantly reduced the partial regression coefficient on age.
Source: [37].

Table 26.19 Summary equations (reference values) of European Coal and Steel Community. These equations are for asymptomatic subjects and calculated using representative values from other equations. St is stature in metres, Age is in years, RSD is in brackets. Abbreviations are as given in Table 26.16. The equations are given as nomograms in Figs 26.11 and 26.12.

	Men	Women
TLC (l)	7.99 St − 7.08 (0.7)	6.60 St − 5.79 (0.60)
FVC (l)	5.76 St − 0.026 Age − 4.34 (0.61)	4.43 St − 0.026 Age − 2.89 (0.43)
RV (l)	1.31 St + 0.022 Age − 1.23 (0.41)	1.81 St + 0.016 Age − 2.00 (0.35)
FRC (l)	2.34 St + 0.009 Age − 1.09 (0.60)	2.24 St + 0.001 Age − 1.00 (0.50)
RV/TLC (%)	0.39 Age + 13.96 (5.46)	0.34 Age + 18.96 (5.83)
FEV_1 (l)	4.30 St − 0.029 Age − 2.49 (0.51)	3.95 St − 0.025 Age − 2.60 (0.38)
FEV_1/FVC (%)*	87.21 − 0.18 Age (7.17)	89.10 − 0.19 Age (6.51)
PEF ($l\ s^{-1}$)†	6.14 St − 0.043 Age + 0.15 (1.21)	5.50 St − 0.030 Age − 1.11 (0.90)
FEF_{25-75} ($l\ s^{-1}$)	1.94 St − 0.043Age + 2.70 (1.04)	1.25 St − 0.034 Age + 2.92 (0.85)
*T*lco (SI)	11.11 St − 0.066 Age − 6.03 (1.41)	8.18 St − 0.049 Age − 2.74 (1.17)
*K*co (SI)*‡	–	–

* See footnotes to Table 26.16.
† The data for PEF should be adjusted for the non-linearity of the original scale:
PEFcorrected = 53.2 + 0.585 PEFobs + 0.00075 $(PEFobs)^2$ (see Table 12.3, page 133)
‡ Use instead *T*lco / TLC [61].
Source: [5].

26.7.2 Progression of lung function throughout life

The principal difficulty confronting the model maker is that for subjects assembled at one point in time, the older and younger members will have experienced different environmental exposures and selection factors [90–93]. As a result they cannot be represented as the same individuals at different stages of life. The short-term progression of present day subjects can be constructed prospectively from serial measurements made at intervals of between 5 and 10 years on a population consisting of subjects of all ages. The interval is long enough to obtain an estimate of the current decline with age (Section 8.2.3), but short enough that the same observers and equipment can be used for the measurements. However, this degree of technical standardisation is difficult to achieve in practice [94]. Data from well-planned long-term investigations can also be used, but even here technical mishaps and unexplained perturbations cannot

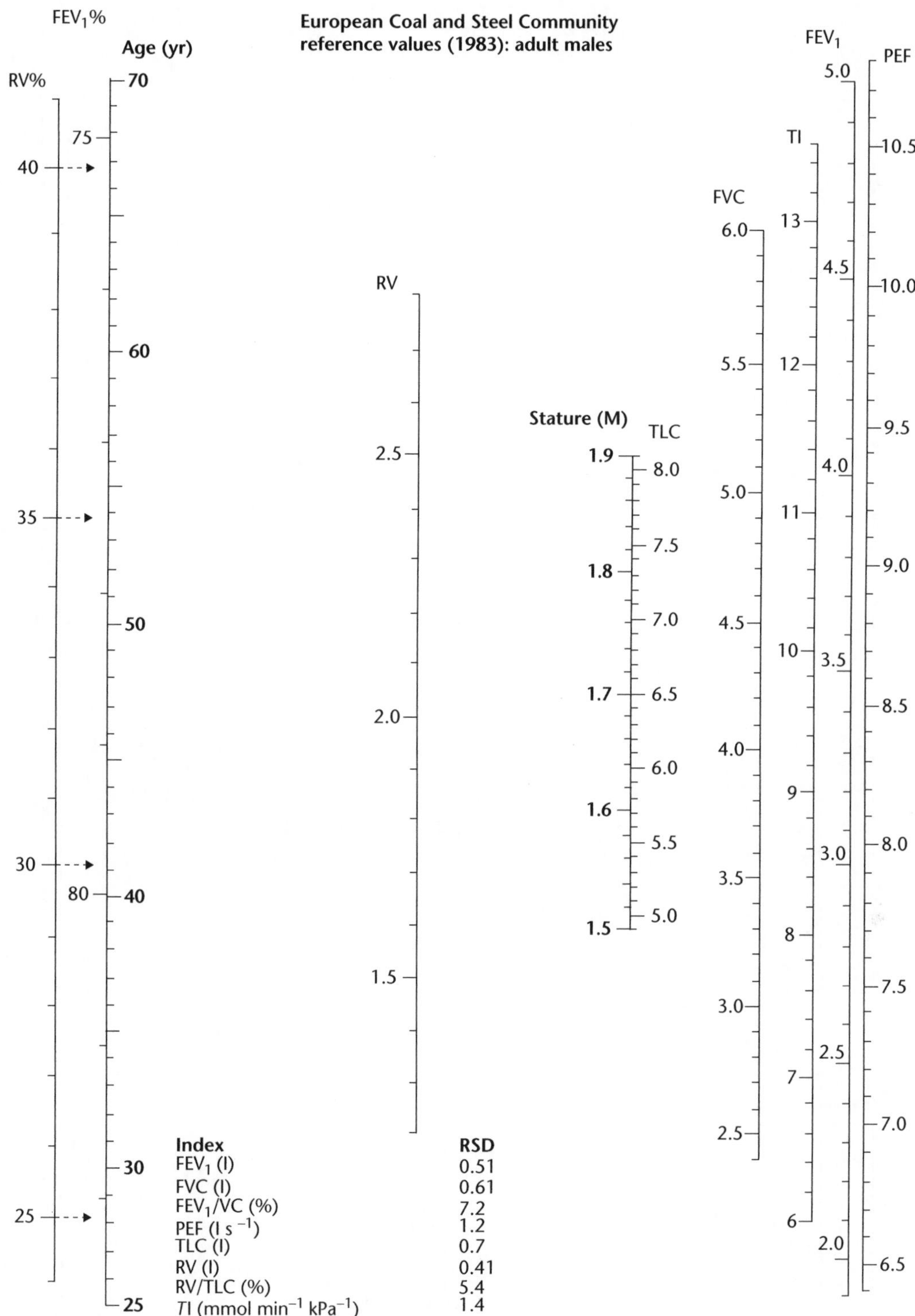

Fig. 26.11 Nomogram relating the lung function of adult males to age and stature using the summary equations of the European Coal and Steel Community (Table 26.19). To use the nomogram a ruler is placed to overlie the age and stature of the subject; the lung function is then given by the intersections with the vertical lines. However, RV% and the FEV% are related only to age and TLC only to stature so these indices should be read directly from the respective columns. When stature is measured in inches these should be converted to metres by dividing by 39.4. The data for PEF should be adjusted for the non-linearity of the original scale (see footnote to Table 26.19).

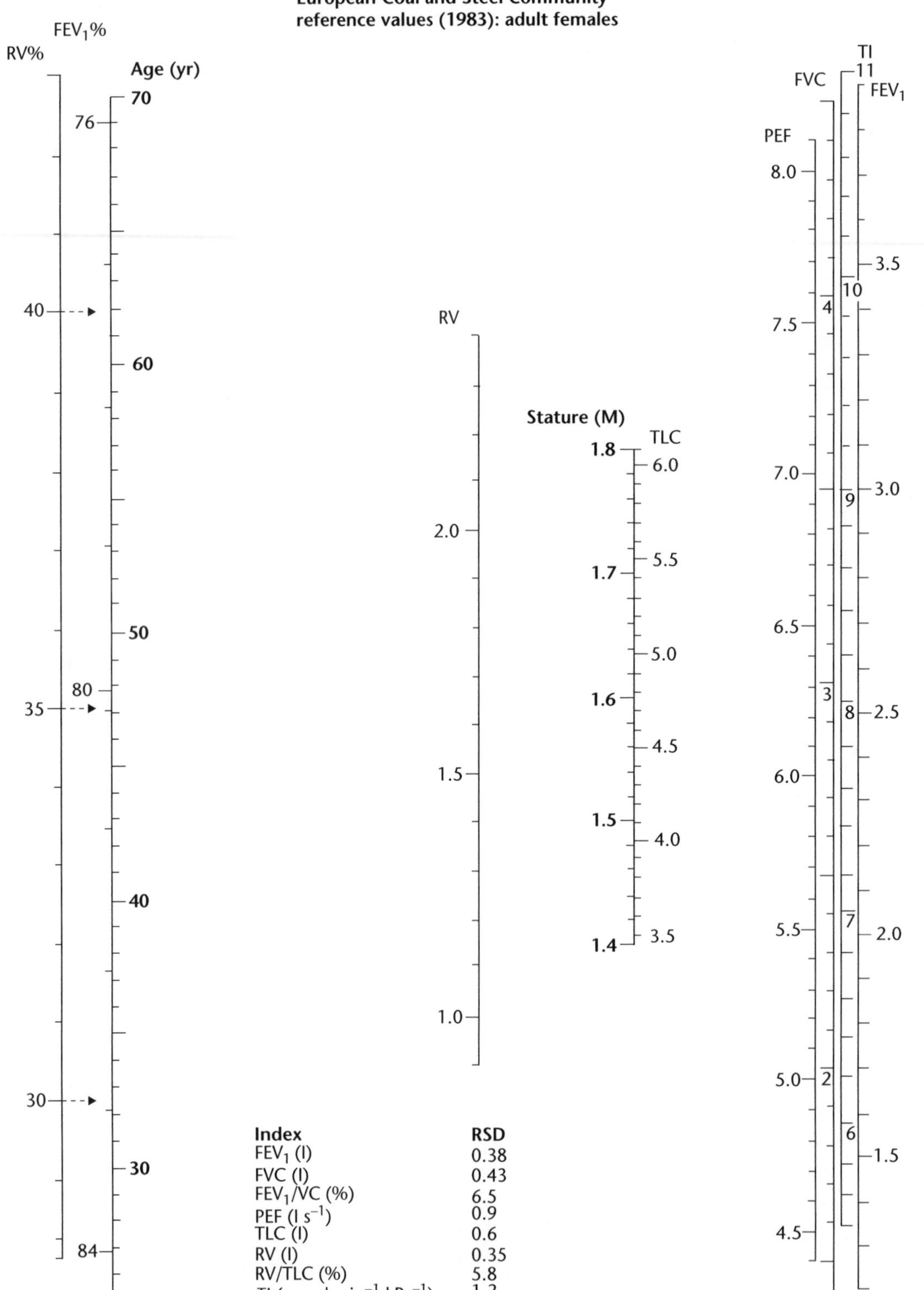

Fig. 26.12 Nomogram relating the lung function of adult females to age and stature using the summary equations of the European Coal and Steel Community (Table 26.19, see also caption to Fig. 26.11).

Table 26.20 Linear regression equations that describe the lung function of white adults (non-smokers) in USA., selected from [3]. Stature (St) is in metres, Age is in years, RSD is in brackets. Abbreviations are as in Table 26.16. The equations are given as nomograms in Figs 26.13 and 26.14.

	Men	Women	Source
TLC (l)	7.95 St + 0.003 Age − 7.33 (0.79)	5.90 St − 4.54 (0.54)	[62]
FVC (l)*	7.74 St − 0.021A − 7.75 (0.51)	4.14 St − 0.023A − 2.20 (0.44)	[63]
RV (l)*	2.16 St + 0.021 Age − 2.84 (0.37)	1.97 St + 0.020 Age − 2.42 (0.38)	[62]
FRC (l)	4.72 St + 0.009 Age − 5.29 (0.72)	3.60 St + 0.003 Age − 3.18 (0.52)	[62]
RV/TLC (%)	0.309 Age + 14.1 (4.38)	0.416 Age + 14.35 (5.46)	[62]
FEV_1 (l)*	5.66 St − 0.023 Age − 4.91 (0.41)	2.68 St − 0.025 Age − 0.38 (0.33)	[63]†
FEV_1/FVC (%)	110.2 − 13.1 St‡ − 0.15 A (5.58)	124.4 − 21.4 St − 0.15 Age (6.75)	[63]†
FEF_{25-75} (l s^{-1})*	5.79 St − 0.036 Age − 4.52 (1.08)	3.00 St − 0.031 Age − 0.41 (0.85)	[64]
$FEF_{50\%FVC}$ (l s^{-1})	6.84 St − 0.037 Age − 5.54 (1.29)	3.21 St − 0.024 Age − 0.44 (0.98)	[64]
$FEF_{75\%FVC}$ (l s^{-1})	3.10 St − 0.023 Age − 2.48 (0.69)	1.74 St − 0.025 Age − 0.18 (0.66)	[64]
Dl (ml min^{-1}mm Hg^{-1})	16.4 St − 0.229 Age + 12.9 (4.84)	16.0 St − 0.111 Age + 2.24 (3.95)	[65]
*K*co (*Dl*/*V*A)	10.09 − 2.24 St − 0.031 Age (0.73)	8.33 − 1.81 St − 0.016 Age (0.80)	[65]

* For these indices marginally greater accuracy (up to age 80 years) is achieved by using a quadratic model (Table 26. 21).

† The regression equations of Crapo et al. are identical for practical purposes [66].

‡ Coefficient on stature is not significant.

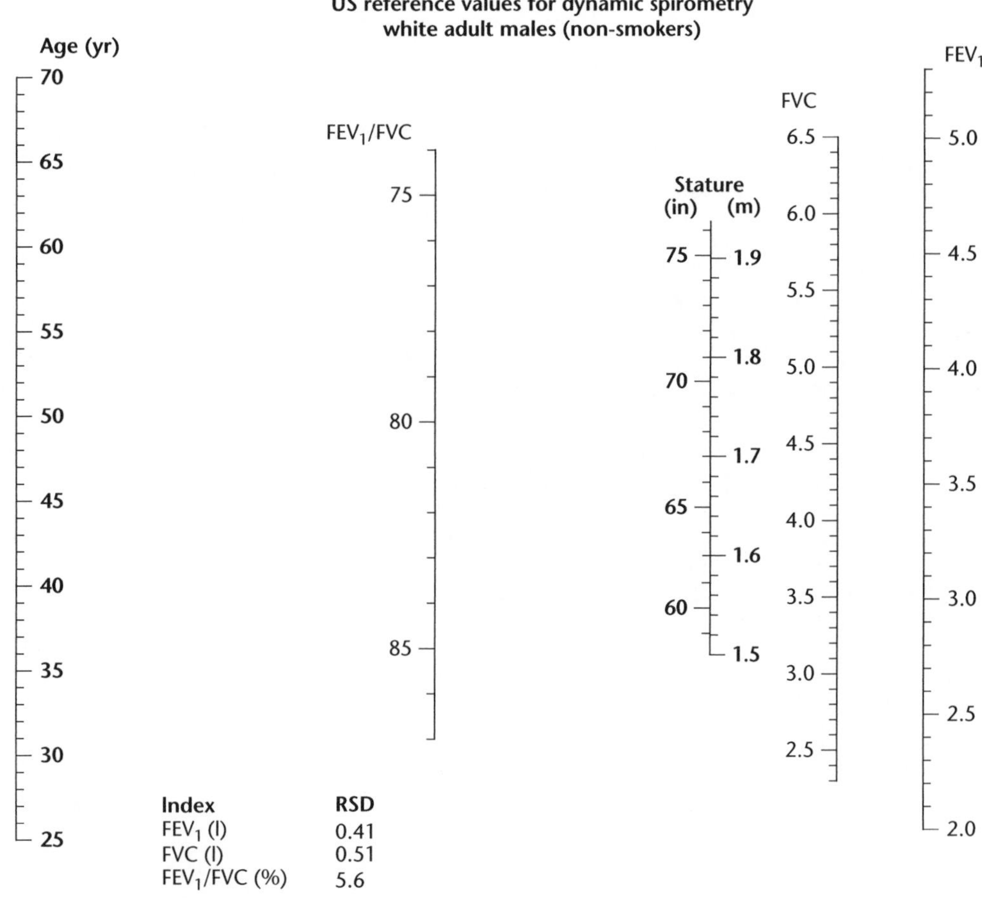

Fig. 26.13a Two part nomogram relating the lung function of adult US white males to age and stature (part 2 is overleaf) . The regression equations are given in Table 26.20 and the use of the nomogram is in the caption to Fig. 26.7.

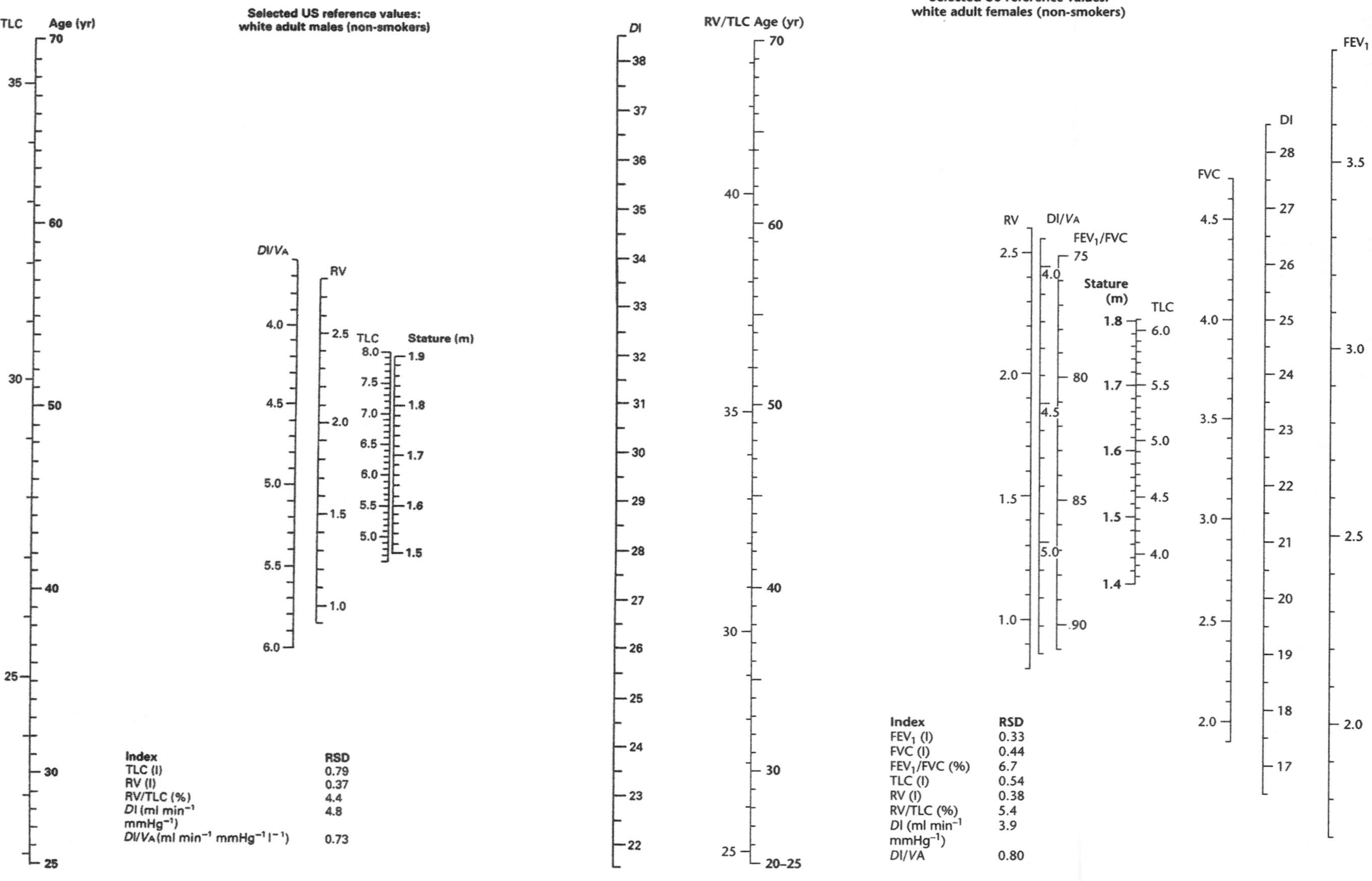

Fig. 26.13b (*Continued*)

Fig. 26.14 Nomogram relating the lung function of adult US white females to age and stature, see caption to Fig. 26.13 part 1 for practical details.

Table 26.21 Multiple quadratic equations for dynamic spirometry in Caucasians aged 8 – 80 years. (data of Hankinson and colleagues for subjects living in USA who have never smoked). The equations are of the form $y = a + b\ \text{age} + c\ \text{age}^2 + d\ \text{St}^2$, where age is in years and stature is in metres. The lower limit of normal is given by $e\ \text{St}^2$ in the same units.

Index		a	b	c	d	e
Males aged 8–19 years	FEV_1 (l)	−0.745	−0.0411	0.00448	1.410	1.161
	FVC (l)	−0.258	−0.2041	0.0101	1.864	1.569
Females aged 8–17 years	FEV_1 (l)	−0.871	0.0654		1.150	0.928
	FVC (l)	−1.208	0.0592		1.481	1.220
Males aged 20–80 years	FEV_1 (l)	0.554	−0.0130	−0.000172	1.410	1.161
	FVC (l)	−0.193	0.00064	−0.000269	1.864	1.569
Females aged 18–80 years	FEV_1 (l)	0.433	−0.00361	−0.000194	1.150	0.928
	FVC (l)	−0.356	0.0187	−0.000382	1.481	1.220
Males aged 8–80 years	FEV%	88.07	−0.207			78.4*
Females aged 8–80 years	FEV%	90.81	−0.212			81.0*

* Lower limit of normal for FEV% (FEV_1/FVC).
Source: [22].

Table 26.22 Average lung function at age 45 years given by reference equations from *Lung Function* (LF, Table 26.16), European Coal and Steel Community (ECSC, Table 26.19), and USA.

	Men (mean stature 1.75 m)				Women (mean stature 1.65 m)			
	LF	ECSC	USA [a]	USA [b]	LF	ECSC	USA [a]	USA [b]
FEV_1 (l)	3.62*	3.73	3.94	3.94	2.77*	2.79	2.91	3.01
FVC (l)	4.51	4.57	4.84	5.00	3.50	3.24	3.59	3.74
FEV_1/FVC (%)	76.9*	79.1†	80.5	78.8	78.4*	80.5†	82.3	81.2
TLC (l)	6.68	6.90	6.72	–	5.30	5.10	5.20	–
RV (l)	2.04	2.05	1.87	–	1.80	1.71	1.73	–
RV/TLC (%)	32.1	31.5	28.0	–	33.7	34.3	33.1	–
*T*lco (SI)	10.2	10.4	10.5	–	8.39	8.55	7.93	–
(trad.)	30.3	31.1	31.4	–	25.1	25.6	23.7	–
*K*co (SI)	1.61	(1.51)‡	1.60	–	1.75	(1.68)‡	1.54	–
(trad.)	4.83	(4.51)‡	4.77	–	5.23	(5.01)‡	4.62	–
PEF ($l\ s^{-1}$)	9.54	8.96	NA	9.78	6.82	6.61	NA	7.03
$FEF_{50\%FVC}$ ($l\ s^{-1}$)	4.51	4.89†	4.78	–	3.99	4.08†	3.78	–
$FEF_{75\%FVC}$ ($l\ s^{-1}$)	1.55	2.06†	1.91	–	1.33	1.72†	1.56	–
FEF_{25-75} ($l\ s^{-1}$)	3.81	4.16†	3.98	3.62	3.30	3.45†	3.15	3.01

[a]: Table 26.20.
[b]: Table 26.21.
SI: Units are mmol min^{-1} kPa^{-1} (and l^{-1}); traditional units are ml min^{-1} mm Hg^{-1} (and l^{-1}).
* Adjusted for backward extrapolation (Table 26.16).
† Other evidence suggests that the equation gives results which may be too high.
‡ From *T*lco/TLC (see Table 26.19).

altogether be avoided (Fig. 7.10, page 76) also [64]. In addition, where measurement practices have subsequently been shown to be sub-optimal it is not always practicable to make a correction (e.g. Footnote 26.2).

An impressively complete data set for longitudinal studies is that established in Arizona by Burrows and colleagues, and this has been the starting point for numerous analyses. In consideration of this task several mathematical difficulties have been identified and overcome [95, 96]. One approach has been to create smooth curves by splining; this entails inserting additional variables at empirically chosen ages to match the data [97, 98]. Another has been to construct a series of joined up linear relationships; hence, creating a continuous piecewise linear model [22, 99]. When this is done the ages at the break points coincide with biological features, namely the start and finish of the adolescent growth spurt and end of the plateau of lung function in early adult life (Table 26.28, page 361). The break points are not the same in men and women.

Table 26.23 Approximate values in healthy men at rest for some indices of pulmonary function which are not included in Tables 26.16–26.20; in most instances they also apply to women. SI units are given first; traditional units are in brackets.

Index	Units	Age 20		Age 60
Ventilation and metabolism				
$\dot{V}_E$	$l\ min^{-1}$		6.0–10.0	
$\dot{V}_A$	$l\ min^{-1}$		4.0–7.5	
f_R	min^{-1}		12–20	
V_d	ml	100		200
$\dot{n}_{O_2}$ ($\dot{V}_{O_2}$)	$mmol\ min^{-1}$ ($ml\ min^{-1}$)		11–13 (250–300)	
$\dot{n}_{CO_2}$($\dot{V}_{CO_2}$)	$mmol\ min^{-1}$ ($ml\ min^{-1}$)		9–11 (200–240)	
R	–		0.8 (0.7–0.9)	
Gas exchange				
P_{A,CO_2}	kPa (torr)		4.7–6.1 (35-46)	
P_{a,CO_2}	kPa (torr)		4.8–6.3 (36-47)	
C_{CO_2}	$mmol\ l^{-1}$		24–34	
P_{A,O_2}	kPa (torr)		13–15 (100–110)	
P_{a,O_2}*	kPa (torr)	13.2 (99)		11.9 (89)
S_{a,O_2}	%	95–97.5		93–96
pH (arterial blood)	$-\log_{10}$ cH		7.45–7.35	
cH	$nmol\ l^{-1}$		36–44	
$\dot{V}_A/\dot{Q}$ relationships				
N_2 index (s.b.)	% N_2 per 500 ml		see Fig. 26.10	
Closing volume	% of VC		see Fig. 26.10	
F_{A,N_2} after 7 min of O_2	%	1.5		2.5
Lung clearance index	–		5–10	
V_A eff/V_A	–	0.9–1.0		0.85–0.95
$\dot{Q}va/\dot{Q}t$	%	2		4
$\dot{Q}s/\dot{Q}t$	%	1		2
Lung mechanics				
R total (Table 14.1)†	$kPa\ l^{-1}\ s$ ($cm\ H_2O\ l^{-1}\ s$)		0.12–0.44 (1.3–4.4)	
Raw‡	$kPa\ l^{-1}\ s$ ($cm\ H_2O\ l^{-1}\ s$)		0.05–0.2 (0.5–2.0)	
sGaw	$s^{-1}\ kPa^{-1}$ ($s^{-1}\ cm\ H_2O^{-1}$)		1.3–3.5 (0.13–0.35)	
Cstat¶	$l\ kPa^{-1}$ ($l\ cm\ H_2O^{-1}$)		0.9–4.0 (0.09–0.40)	
sC	kPa^{-1} ($cm\ H_2O^{-1}$)		0.3–1.4 (0.03–0.14)	
Recoil pr. (max)	kPa (cm H_2O)		1.2–3.7 (12–37)	
(TLC-20% VC)§		1.4 (14)		0.9 (9)
Cth	$l\ kPa^{-1}$ ($l\ cm\ H_2O^{-1}$)		1.0–3.5 (0.1–0.35)	

* P_{a,O_2} (SI) = 0.133 [104 – 0.24 Age, RSD 7.9]. [70]
† [71], The ECSC [5] gives R total in SI units as <0.3 and sGaw >0.85 and >1.04 in men and women, respectively.
‡ Raw (SI) = [4.2/TGV: range (2.9–7.7)/TGV] ÷ 9.8 [72]
¶ Cstat (SI) = 9.8 [0.353 St (m) – 0.347, RSD 0.081]. [Bevan C, McKerrow CB. unpublished], see also [73–75].
§ Pstat (TLC-20% VC) (SI) = [16.67 – 0.13 Age, RSD 2.13] ÷ 9.8.
To convert the equations to traditional units the term outside the bracket should be omitted.

The information content of the relationships might be increased by the inclusion of additional reference variables. But the first attempt at this using body mass index raised hopes that have still to be fulfilled [100]. There is a better prospect of success with more focussed indices of body dimensions and composition, also possibly the level of habitual activity and environmental exposure. The inclusion of such reference variables in a joined up linear model merits further consideration.

26.8 Interpreting reference values

Non-random presentation for assessment. Reference equations describe the test results of groups of people with apparently healthy lungs. Their application to an individual subject depends on that subject being a member of the group and selected *at random* from it. This condition is almost never met! Instead, the subject selects himself or herself for assessment because of symptoms that may be contributed to by below average lung

Table 26.24 Reference values for maximal respiratory pressures in healthy men and women based on age (year) and stature (m).

Index	Units	Gender	Equation	RSD
PEmax (from TLC)	cm H_2O	M	180 − (0.91 × Age)	31
	cm H_2O	F	3.5 + (55 × St)	16
PImax (from RV)	cm H_2O	M	142 − (1.03 × Age)	28
	cm H_2O	F	−43 + (71 × St)	21

Source: [33].

function. This is the case for most patients with chronic respiratory disorders, e.g. [38]. As a result, the selection of subjects does not meet an essential condition for statistical interpretation of data. Instead, the calculated significance of any deviation from the mean for the population is inevitably an over-estimate and a rogue result cannot be ruled out. The main justification for the method is that the information it provides has been found to be of practical use.

Estimates of variability. A reference value is usually described in terms of an equation containing one or more continuous variables, for example age and/or stature. The scatter about the relationship depends on its form (e.g. proportional or linear etc. as given in Table 26.3 and Section 5.6), and on the technical and biological factors that contribute. In children before puberty the most commonly used reference equations represent the lung function indices as being proportional to stature (Table 26.3). Any deviation from the expected level can then be expressed on a proportional basis. The same principle applies to complex cross-sectional relationships (Section 26.7.1). However, in this instance the scatter is not uniform throughout life and this needs to be taken into account when constructing a lower limit of normal [80]. In adults, against expectations, the scatter about the regression relationship is seldom very different for the high and low levels of a variable. Instead, it is usually relatively constant over the range of the observations [101]. As a consequence the practice of expressing the scatter as a coefficient of variation (Footnote 26.3) is rarely appropriate; it is similarly inappropriate to express an observed result as a percentage of its reference value [3, 5].

The extent of the error from using a percentage depends on the range of the principal reference variable. Where this is small and remote from zero, as in the case of an index that is related mainly to stature (e.g. inspiratory capacity) the error from using a percentage is small. It is also small for comparisons between levels of function in men and women. The error is large and not acceptable for indices to which age makes an important contribution.

Footnote 26.3. The coefficient of variation is the standard deviation as a percentage of the mean value (i.e. 100. SD/mean).

The disadvantage of not being able to use proportional relationships can be overcome by use of alternative units, for example expressing the lung function per unit of stature squared (eqn. 26.4) or stature cubed [38]. These techniques can be useful for statistical analyses.

Standard deviation units. For most indices of lung function, the relative constancy of the scatter in adults has the important consequence that, as a first approximation, a single residual standard deviation can be used to describe it. Greater precision is possible by allowing for the increase in scatter that is apparent at the extremes of the age distribution, but the improvement is usually small. As a result, a comparison between an observed and predicted result should normally be in terms of the standardised residual [3, 5, 102]. It is calculated as:

$$\text{Standardised residual} = (\text{observed value-predicted value})/\text{RSD} \quad (26.6)$$

where RSD is the residual standard deviation about the regression equation. Where the relationship conforms to accepted statistical criteria, a result that deviates by more than 1 SD units from the mean in the direction of abnormality may merit critical attention. When the deviation exceeds 1.64 SD units the result has a less than one in twenty chance of being normal (Table 5.7, page 50). In clinical practice the criterion is not met for the reason given above.

Which reference values should be used? External reference values are appropriate for interpreting the lung function of a subject who is being assessed for the first time, so no previous internal reference value is available for comparison. For such a person the choice is likely to be between a value obtained on subjects who have never smoked and one for persons who are asymptomatic, including asymptomatic smokers. In the present context it is between the reference values based on those originally compiled for Lung Function (Table 26.16) or the ECSC series (Table 26.19) and the majority of series that were obtained subsequently. In most circumstances the choice is less important than that the operator should be familiar with and know the limitations of the series they use. Reference values obtained from lifetime non-smokers are appropriate for purposes of life insurance and where the pulmonary condition may have been caused mainly by smoking, for example COPD (Sections 37.3 and 40.3). However, for assessing another condition in a subject who smokes or is exposed to tobacco fume in the course of his/her work, or domestic and leisure activities the values for asymptomatic subjects are more appropriate. The number of circumstances where the latter conditions apply is still considerable, though it is diminishing.

Possibly, of greater relevance is the variety of reference variables that are included in the regression equation (Table 26.2). The commonly used variables are gender, ethnic group, age and stature, of which stature is normally the most important. The term for gender is in some circumstances a surrogate for body composition, yet the latter indices do not appear in any ATS/ERS

Table 26.25 Reference values for indices derived from moments analysis of the forced expiratory spirogram in healthy men and women. Age in year and stature (St) in metres.

Index*	Truncation†	Units	Gender	Equation	RSD
ln MTT	75%	s	M	−3.46 + 0.0048 Age + 1.15 St	0.21
	90%	s	M	−3.14 + 0.0099 Age + 1.10 St	0.23
	100%	s	M	−2.18 + 0.0143 Age + 0.72 St	0.27
ln MTT	75%	s	F	−2.62 + 0.0036 Age + 0.72 St	0.18
	90%	s	F	−2.41 + 0.0097 Age + 0.70 St	0.21
	100%	s	F	−1.65 + 0.0169 Age + 0.32 St	0.25
MR	75%	–	M	1.189 + 0.0020 Age	0.036
	90%	–	M	1.195 + 0.0049 Age	0.066
	100%	–	M	2.324 + 0.0063 Age − 0.54 St	0.144
MR	75%	–	F	1.171 + 0.0018 Age	0.042
	90%	–	F	1.129 + 0.0058 Age	0.068
	100%	–	F	2.055 + 0.0104 − 0.55 St	0.132

* MTT: mean transit time (also first moment, M1), MR: moment ratio, = ($\sqrt{M2}$)/M1
† Percentage of FVC expired
Source: [76]

Table 26.26 Reference equations for indices that relate to ventilatory capacity in white adults aged 65–85 years*.

Index	Gender	Partial regression coefficient on Stature (m)	Partial regression coefficient on Age (year)	Constant	RSD
FEV_1 (l)	M	2.60	−0.037	1.05	0.44
	F	2.44	−0.028	0.12	0.29
FVC (l)	M	4.33	−0.034	−0.99	0.52
	F	4.09	−0.034	−1.39	0.32
FEF_{25-75} (l s^{-1})	M	0.74	−0.054	4.56	0.60
	F	0.47	−0.034	3.18	0.42
PEF (l s^{-1})	M	2.20	−0.134	16.0	2.13
	F	0.67	−0.019	6.6	0.85
		Body mass (kg)			
P_{Imax}	M	0.22	−1.0	149	25.6
(suction, cm H_2O)	F	0.22	−0.90	118	23.2
P_{Emax}	M	0.61	−2.27	278	31.7
(pressure, cm H_2O)	F	0.79	−1.68	179	45.7

* Mean data:
Men: n = 112, St 1.71 (1.60–1.82) m, Age 72.4 (66–83) years, BM 79.7 (62–97) kg.
Women: n = 176, St 1.57 (1.47–1.67) m, Age 75.2 (66–87) years, BM 65.7 (49–86) kg.
(39% of these volunteer subjects were excluded on health grounds and about 10 % on technical grounds).
Source: [78, see also 79].

recommendations. The indices of body fat and muscle can contribute more to the explained variance than some recommended indices [37], so there is still scope for improvement.

A consideration of physique (e.g. thoracic width) and body composition (fat and muscle) can help to position a subject's lung function within the normal range. Another pointer is a subject's previous measurement since people tend to track along their percentile (Section 26.3.5). Thus, old results from another hospital or a pre-employment examination [1] should be looked for. A further approach might be to use the position of one index as a guide to the position of another. Unfortunately, this assumption is false, since if an individual is described in terms of a number of indices these will inevitably be scattered over their normal ranges [103]. As a result, it is virtually impossible for a subject to be average with respect to all indices at the same time! For this reason the accuracy of prediction is greatest when the mean value for a group of subjects is required. For individual subjects the accuracy of prediction is inevitably much less. It is

Table 26.27 Example of a parsimonious model used to describe the FEV_1 and FVC of Caucasians aged 16–90 living in the UK [80]. The model is $y = e^{(b_1+b_2A+b_3A^2+b_4 \ln St)}$. The parameters of equations for calculating reference values and the corresponding lower limits of normal are in the table.

Gender	Index*	Predicted†	Regression coefficients			
			Intercept (b_1)	Age (b_2)	Age^2 (b_3)	ln stature (cm) (b_4)
Male, aged 16–25 years	ln FEV_1	Mean	−10.41186	0.09569	−0.00221	2.10839
		LLN	−10.75820	0.10320	−0.00231	2.10839
Male, aged 16–25 years	ln FVC	Mean	−11.45146	0.09895	−0.00216	2.32222
		LLN	−11.63230	0.09795	−0.00217	2.32222
Male, aged >25 years	ln FEV_1	Mean	−9.37674	0.00183	−0.00011	2.10839
		LLN	−9.72308	0.00933	−0.00021	2.10839
Male, aged >25 years	ln FVC	Mean	−10.36706	0.00434	−0.00011	2.32222
		LLN	−10.54790	0.00334	−0.00012	2.32222
Female, aged ≥16 years	ln FEV_1	Mean	−8.49717	0.00422	−0.00015	1.90019
		LLN	−8.68467	0.00495	−0.00018	1.90019
Female, aged ≥16 years	ln FVC	Mean	−9.66999	0.00837	−0.00017	2.14118
		LLN	−9.84941	0.00772	−0.00018	2.14118

* Example: Predicted FVC (litres) = antilog$_e$ (lnFVC). Hence, FVC = $e^{\ln(FVC)} = 2.71828^{\ln(FVC)}$.
Worked example: Expected FVC for a man aged 30 years, stature 180 cm is $y = e^{(-10.36706+0.00434\times30-0.00011\times30^2+2.3222\times\ln 180)} = 5.60$ l (LLN = 4.50 l).
† LLN: lower limit of normal (5th percentile).

Table 26.28 Age at breakpoints in non-smokers.

Lung function index	Males		Females	
	Breakpoint (years)	95% CI	Breakpoint (years)	95% CI
FEV_1	12.4	11.7, 13.9	9.6*	9.0, 10.2
	17.4	16.6, 19.2	15.5*	14.9, 16.2
	25.9	23.2, 30.9	27.4	24.8, 29.6
FVC	12.4	11.2, 13.4	10.1*	9.9, 10.4
	18.0	16.6, 19.2	18.0	17.2, 19.2
	25.8	23.2, 30.8	46.4*	41.7, 50.1

* $p < 0.05$
Source: [98].

least for subjects whose reference values lie at the lower end of the physiological range [101]. There are two reasons for this. First, the reference population will have contained relatively few of such subjects. Second, an RSD that is nearly independent of age will represent a relatively high proportion of the mean for subjects with the lower values. Thus, for many reasons only limited importance should be attached to a single comparison of an observed with an expected result.

Making sense of the results

Results at one point in time. An isolated abnormal finding can be difficult to interpret, so the best strategy is to look for features that characterise a syndrome of lung function, for example normal function, a transfer defect or obstructive ventilatory defect (Chapter 39). To this end, each index can be considered in terms of three categories, probably normal (within 1 SD), borderline or probably abnormal (between 1 SD and 2 SD) and definitely abnormal (2 SD or beyond). For the reason given above this last category can only be defined with certainty if the result is outside the normal range. In a person of normal physique a difference from the mean in excess of 2 SD is likely to be abnormal. However, where the physique is abnormal, neglect of this factor can itself lead to the lungs being considered abnormal when in fact the abnormality lies in the surrounding structures [37].

These considerations have important practical implications. They include that the subject's lung function should be given in absolute units and the reference values should preferably include the normal range. Where the deviation is in SD units the reference variables should be stated. If, as is likely to be the case, these are age and stature, a statement should be made on body

Table 26.29 Some reasons for two results not being identical.

Mechanism	Comment
Technical	Instrument failure
	Calibration error
	Measurement variation
Biological	Biological variation
	Alteration in environment
	Ageing
	Change in health
	Result of an intervention

composition. In addition, any conclusion or recommendation for action based solely upon the use of predicted values should, so far as possible, be confirmed by clinical, radiographic or other means. This applies particularly to major medical or surgical treatment for which an abnormal lung function result should be a confirmatory and not the principal reason for taking action.

Repeat measurements. When a measurement is repeated the reference value is usually the previous measurement. The new result will usually be different by an amount that varies with circumstances, so the reason should be established (Table 26.29).

Where the change is relevant its magnitude should be established. This can be indicated by the confidence limits of the measurement. If the change can be represented as a proportional one the calculation should make allowance for regression to the mean. This is best done in the form Δx (%) $= 100(x_1 - x_2)/[0.5(x_1 + x_2)]$ (Section 15.7.2). Where the interval between measurements is a period of years the longitudinal reference value should be consulted, but is likely to be of limited usefulness unless changes in body composition have been taken into account [87]. Even when this is done the interpretation is difficult since smoking, atopic status and related variables have a material influence on the outcome [99, 104]. Thus, interpretation is a difficult subject and whilst aspects can be automated there is still need to utilise experience and to undertake more research.

26.9 References

1. Chinn DJ, Cotes JE, Fechner M, Elliott C. Pre-employment lung function at age 16 years as a guide to that in adult life. *Br J Industr Med* 1993; **50**: 422–427.
2. Van Pelt W, Borsboom GJ, Rijken B et al. Discrepancies between longitudinal and cross-sectional change in ventilatory function in 12 years of follow-up. *Am J Respir Crit Care Med* 1994; **149**: 1218–1226.
3. American Thoracic Society. Lung function testing; selection of reference values and interpretative strategies. *Am Rev Respir Dis* 1992; **145**: 1202–1218.
4. Stocks J, Quanjer PhH. Reference values for residual volume, functional residual capacity and total lung capacity. ATS workshop on lung volume measurements. Official statement of the European Respiratory Society. *Eur Respir J* 1995; **8**: 492–506.
5. Quanjer PhH, ed. Standardized lung function testing. *Bull Eur Physiopathol Respir* 1983; **19**(Suppl 5): 1–95.
6. Crapo RO, Morris AH. Standardized single breath normal values for carbon monoxide diffusing capacity. *Am Rev Respir Dis* 1981; **123**: 185–189.
7. Nysom K, Ulrik CS, Hesse B, Dirksen A. Published models and local data can bridge the gap between reference values of lung function for children and adults. *Eur Respir J* 1997; **10**: 1
8. Merkus PJ, Mijnsbergen JY, Hop WC, de Jongste JC. Interrupter resistance in preschool children: measurement characteristics and reference values. *Am J Respir Crit Care Med* 2001; **163**: 1350–1355.
9. Lombardi E, Sly PD, Concutelli G et al. Reference values of interrupter respiratory resistance in healthy preschool white children. *Thorax* 2001; **56**: 691–695.
10. Eigen H, Bieler H, Grant D et al. Spirometric pulmonary function in healthy preschool children. *Am J Respir Crit Care Med* 2001; **163**: 619–623.
11. Vilozni D, Barker M, Jellouschek H et al. An interactive computer-animated system (Spirogame) facilitates spirometry in preschool children. *Am J Respir Crit Care Med* 2001; **164**: 2200–2205.
12. Crenesse D, Berlioz M, Bourrier T, Albertini M. Spirometry in children aged 3 to 5 years: reliability of forced expiratory manoeuvres. *Paediatr Pulmonol* 2001; **32**: 56–61.
13. Nystad W, Samuelsen SO, Nafstad P et al. Feasibility of measuring lung function in preschool children. *Thorax* 2002; **57**: 1021–1027.
14. Quanjer PH, Stocks J, Polgar G et al. Compilation of reference values for lung function measurements in children. *Eur Respir J* 1989; **2**(Suppl 4): 184S–261S.
15. Cotes JE, Dabbs JM, Hall AM et al. Lung volumes, ventilatory capacity and transfer factor in healthy British boy and girl twins. *Thorax* 1973; **28**: 709–715.
16. Chinn DJ, Cotes JE, Flowers R et al. Transfer factor (diffusing capacity) standardised for alveolar volume; validation, reference values and applications of a new linear model to replace *K*co (*T*l/*V*A). *Eur Respir J* 1996; **9**: 1269–77.
17. Rosenthal M, Cramer D, Bain SH et al. Lung function in white children aged 4 to 19 years: 2. Single breath analysis and plethysmography. *Thorax* 1993; **48**: 803–808.
18. Rosenthal M, Bain SH, Cramer D et al. Lung function in white children aged 4 to 19 years: 1. Spirometry. *Thorax* 1993; **48**: 794–808.
19. Tanner JM. Growth at adolescence. 2nd ed. Oxford: Blackwell Scientific Publications, 1962.
20. Quanjer PhH, Borsboom GJJM, Brunekreef B et al. Spirometric reference values for white European children and adolescents: Polgar revisited. *Pediatr Pulmonol* 1995; **19**: 135–142.
21. Chinn DJ, Cotes JE, Martin AJ. Modelling the lung function of Caucasians during adolescence as basis for reference values. *Ann Hum Biol*, 2006; **33**: 64–77.
22. Hankinson JL, Odencrantz JR, Fedan KB. Spirometric reference values from a sample of the general US population. *Am J Respir Crit Care Med* 1999; **159**: 179–187.
23. Strang LB. The ventilatory capacity of normal children. *Thorax* 1959; **14**: 305–310.
24. Helliesen PJ, Cook CD, Friedlander L, Agathon S. Studies of respiratory physiology in children. I. Mechanics of respiration and lung volumes in 85 normal children 5 to 17 years of age. *Pediatrics* 1958; **22**: 80–93.

25. Zapletal A, Motoyama EK, van de Woestijne KP et al. Maximum expiratory flow-volume curves and airway conductance in children and adolescents. *J Appl Physiol* 1969; **26**: 308–316.
26. Zapletal A, Samanek M, Tuma S et al. Assessment of airway function in children. *Bull Physiopathol Respir* 1972; **8**: 535–544.
27. Mansell A, Bryan C, Levison H. Airway closure in children. *J Appl Physiol* 1972; **33**: 711–714.
28. Beaudry PH, Wise MB, Seely JE. Respiratory gas exchange at rest and during exercise in normal and asthmatic children. *Am Rev Respir Dis* 1967; **95**: 248–254.
29. Kjellman B. Ventilatory efficiency, capacity and lung volumes in healthy children. *Scand J Clin Lab Invest* 1969; **23**: 19–29.
30. Levison H, Featherby EA, Weng TR. Arterial blood gases, alveolar-arterial oxygen difference and physiologic deadspace in children and young adults. *Am Rev Respir Dis* 1970; **101**: 972–974.
31. Mansell A, Levison H, Kruger K, Tripp TL. Measurement of respiratory resistance in children by forced oscillations. *Am Rev Respir Dis* 1972; **106**: 710–714.
32. Zapletal A, Paul T, Samanek M. Pulmonary elasticity in children and adolescents. *J Appl Physiol* 1976; **40**: 953–961.
33. Wilson SH, Cooke NT, Edwards RHT, Spiro SG. Predicted normal values for maximal respiratory pressures in caucasian adults and children. *Thorax* 1984; **39**: 535–538.
34. Ducharme FM, Davis GM, Ducharme GR. Pediatric reference values for respiratory resistance measured by forced oscillation. *Chest* 1998; **113**: 1322–1328.
35. Hibbert ME, Hudson IL, Lanigan A et al. Tracking of lung function in healthy children and adolescents. *Pediatr Pulmonol* 1990; **8**: 172–177.
36. Wang X, Dockery DW, Wypij D et al. Pulmonary function between 6 to 18 years of age. *Pediatr Pulmonol* 1993; **15**: 75–88.
37. Cotes JE, Chinn DJ, Reed JW. Body fat, fat percentage, and fat free mass as reference variables for lung function: effects on terms for age and sex. *Thorax* 2001; **56**: 839–844.
38. Fletcher C, Peto R, Tinker C, Speizer FE. The natural history of chronic bronchitis and emphysema. Oxford: Oxford University Press, 1976.
39. Burrows B, Lebowitz MD, Camilli AE, Knudson RJ. Longitudinal changes in forced expiratory volume in one second in adults. Methodologic considerations and findings in healthy nonsmokers. *Am Rev Respir Dis* 1986; **133**: 974–980.
40. Cole TJ. The influence of height on the decline in ventilatory function. *Int J Epidemiol* 1974; **3**: 145–I52.
41. Cotes JE, Meade F, Saunders MJ, Hall AM. Equation computed for earlier editions of this book from measurements made in the laboratory and on respiratory surveys.
42. Hall AM, Heywood C, Cotes JE. Lung function in healthy British women. *Thorax* 1979; **34**: 359–365.
43. Kory RC, Callahan R, Boren HG, Syner JC. The veterans administration—army cooperative study of pulmonary function. 1. Clinical spirometry in normal men. *Am J Med* 1961; **30**: 243–258.
44. Goldman HI, Becklake MR. Respiratory function tests. Normal values at median altitudes and the prediction of normal results. *Am Rev Tuberc* 1959; **79**: 457–467.
45. Grimby G, Soderholm B. Spirometric studies in normal subjects. III. Static lung volumes and maximum voluntary ventilation in adults with a note on physical fitness. *Acta Med Scand* 1963; **173**: 199–206.
46. Becklake MR, Fournier-Massey G, McDonald JC et al. Lung function in relation to chest radiographic changes in Quebec asbestos workers. I. Methods, results and conclusions. *Bull Physiopathol Respir* 1970; **6**: 637–659.
47. Cotes JE, Rossiter CE, Higgins ITT, Gilson JC. Average normal values for the forced expiratory volume in white Caucasian males. *Br Med J* 1966; **1**: 1016–1019.
48. Berglund E, Birath G, Bjure J et al. Spirometric studies of normal subjects. 1. Forced expirograms in subjects between 7 and 70 years of age. *Acta Med Scand* 1963; **173**: 185–192.
49. Lindall A, Medina A, Grismer JT. A re-evaluation of normal pulmonary function measurements in the adult female. *Am Rev Respir Dis* 1967; **95**: 1061–1064.
50. Leiner GC, Abramowitz S, Small MJ et al. Expiratory peak flow rate. Standard values for normal subjects. *Am Rev Respir Dis* 1963; **88**: 644–651.
51. Pelzer AM, Thomson ML. Expiratory peak flow. *Br Med J* 1964; **2**: 123.
52. Birath G, Kjellmer I, Sandqvist L. Spirometric studies in normal subjects. 2. Ventilatory capacity tests in adults. *Acta Med Scand* 1963; **173**: 193–198.
53. Colebatch HJH, Greaves IA, Ng CKY. Exponential analysis of elastic recoil and aging in healthy males and females. *J Appl Physiol* 1979; **47**: 683–691.
54. Billiet L, Baiser W, Naedts JP. Effet de la taille, du sexe et de l'age sur la capacité de diffusion pulmonaire de l'adult normal. *J Physiol (Paris)* 1963; **55**: 199–200.
55. Cotes JE, Hall AM. The transfer factor for the lung; normal values in adults. In: Arcangeli P, ed. *Normal values for respiratory function in man.* Torino: Panminerva Medica, 1970: 327–343.
56. Frans A. Les valeurs normales du volume capillaire pulmonaire (Vc) et de la capacite de diffusion de la membrane alveolo-capillaire (DM). In: Arcangeli P, ed. *Normal values for respiratory function in man.* Torino: Panminerva Medica, 1970: 352–363.
57. McCarthy DS, Spencer R, Greene R, Milic-Emili J. Measurement of 'closing volume' as a simple and sensitive test for early detection of small airway disease. *Am J Med* 1972; **52**: 747–753.
58. Buist AS, Ross BB. Quantitative analysis of the alveolar plateau in the diagnosis of early airway obstruction. *Am Rev Respir Dis* 1973; **108**: 1078–1087.
59. Nunn AJ, Gregg I. New regression equations for predicting peak expiratory flow in adults. *BMJ* 1989; **298**:1068–1070.
60. Miller MR. Peak expiratory flow meter scale changes: implications for patients and health professionals. *Airways J* 2004; **2**: 80–82.
61. Love RG, Seaton A, also Quanjer PhH. About the ECCS summary equations (Letters to the Editor). *Eur Respir J* 1990; **3**: 489–490.
62. Crapo RO, Morris AH, Clayton PD, Nixon CR. Lung volumes in healthy nonsmoking adults. *Bull Eur Physiopathol Respir* 1982; **18**: 419–425.
63. Miller A, Thornton JC, Warshaw R et al. Mean and instantaneous expiratory flows, FVC and FEV_1: prediction equations from a probability sample of Michigan, a large industrial state. *Bull Eur Physiopathol Respir* 1986; **22**: 589–597.
64. Knudson RJ, Lebowitz MD, Holberg CJ, Burrows B. Changes in the normal maximal expiratory flow-volume curve with growth and aging. *Am Rev Respir Dis* 1983; **127**: 725–734.
65. Miller A, Thornton JC, Warshaw R et al. Single breath diffusing capacity in a representative sample of the population of Michigan, a large industrial state. *Am Rev Respir Dis* 1983; **127**: 270–277.

66. Crapo RO, Morris AH, Gardner RM. Reference spirometric values using techniques and equipment that meet ATS recommendations. *Am Rev Respir Dis* 1981; **123**: 659–664.
67. Knudson RJ, Slatin RC, Lebowitz MD, Burrows B. The maximal expiratory flow volume curve. Normal standards, variability and effects of age. *Am Rev Respir Dis* 1976; **113**: 587–600.
68. Knudson RJ, Kaltenborn WT, Knudson DE, Burrows B. The single-breath carbon monoxide diffusing capacity. Reference equations derived from a healthy nonsmoking population and effects of hematocrit. *Am Rev Respir Dis* 1987; **135**: 805–811.
69. Paoletti P, Viegi G, Pistelli G et al. Reference equations for the single-breath diffusing capacity. A cross-sectional analysis and effect of body size and age. *Am Rev Respir Dis* 1985; **132**: 806–813.
70. Raine JM, Bishop JM. A-a difference in O_2 tension and physiological dead space in normal man. *J Appl Physiol* 1963; **18**: 284–288.
71. Pride NB. The assessment of airflow obstruction. Role of measurements of airways resistance and tests of forced expiration. *Brit J Dis Chest* 1971; **65**: 135–169.
72. Briscoe WA, DuBois AB. The relationship between airway resistance, airway conductance and lung volume in subjects of different age and body size. *J Clin Invest* 1958; **37**: 1279–1285.
73. Frank NR, Mead J, Ferris BG Jr. The mechanical behaviour of the lungs in healthy elderly persons. *J Clin Invest* 1957; **36**: 1680–1687.
74. Frank NR, Mead J, Siebens AA, Storey CF. Measurements of pulmonary compliance in seventy healthy young adults. *J Appl Physiol* 1956; **9**: 38–42.
75. Gibson GJ, Pride NB, O'Cain C, Quagliato R. Sex and age differences in pulmonary mechanics in normal nonsmoking subjects. *J Appl Physiol* 1976; **41**: 20–25.
76. Miller MR, Grove DM, Pincock AC. Time domain spirogram indices. Their variability and reference values in nonsmokers. *Am Rev Respir Dis* 1985; **132**: 1041–1048.
77. Friedman GD, Klatsky AL, Siegelaub AB. Lung function and risk of myocardial infarction and sudden cardiac death. *New Engl J Med* 1976; **294**: 1071–1075.
78. Enright PL, Adams AB, Boyle PJ, Sherrill DL. Spirometry and maximal respiratory pressure references from healthy Minnesota 65-to 85-year-old women and men. *Chest* 1995; **108**: 663–669; erratum, Ibid page 1776.
79. Enright PL, Kronmal RA, Higgins M et al. Spirometric reference values for women and men ages 65–85: cardiovascular health study. *Am Rev Respir Dis* 1993; **147**: 125–133.
80. Falaschetti E, Laiho J, Primatesta P, Purdon S. Prediction equations for normal and low lung function from the Health Survey for England. *Eur Respir J* 2004: **23**: 456–463.
81. Gore CJ, Crockett AJ, Pederson DG et al. Spirometric standards for healthy adult lifetime nonsmokers in Australia. *Eur Respir J* 1995; **8**: 773–782.
82. Brandli O, Schindler CH, Kuenzli N et al. Lung function in never smoking adults: reference values and lower limits of normal of a Swiss population. *Thorax* 1995; **51**: 277–283.
83. Langhammer A, Johnsen R, Gulsvik A et al. Forced spirometry reference values for Norwegian adults: the bronchial obstruction in Nord-Trondelag study. *Eur Respir J* 2001; **18**: 770–779.
84. Garcia-Rio F, Pino JM, Dorgham A et al. Spirometric reference equations for European females and males aged 65–85 years. *Eur Respir J* 2004; **24**: 397–405.
85. Hardie JA, Vollmer WM, Buist AS *et al.* Reference values for arterial blood gases in the elderly. *Chest* 2004; **125**: 2053–2060.
86. Hurwitz S, Allen J, Liben A, Becklake MR. Lung function in young adults: evidence for differences in the chronological age at which various functions start to decline. *Thorax* 1980; **35**: 615—619.
87. Chinn DJ, Cotes JE, Reed JW. Longitudinal effects of change in body mass on measurements of ventilatory capacity. *Thorax* 1996; **51**: 699–704.
88. Nevill AM, Holder RL. Identifying population differences in lung function: results from the Allied Dunbar national fitness survey. *Ann Hum Biol* 1999; **26**: 267–285.
89. Ware JH, Dockery DW, Louis TA et al. Longitudinal and cross-sectional estimates of pulmonary function decline in never-smoking adults. *Am J Epidemiol* 1990; **132**: 685–700.
90. Kannel WB, Lew EA. Vital capacity as a predictor of cardiovascular disease: the Framingham study. *Am Heart J* 1983; **105**: 311–315.
91. Carpenter L, Beral V, Strachan D et al. Respiratory symptoms as predictors of 27 year mortality in a representative sample of British adults. *BMJ* 1989; **299**: 357–361.
92. Ebi-Kryston KL, Hawthorne VM, Rose G et al. Breathlessness, chronic bronchitis and reduced pulmonary function as predictors of cardiovascular disease mortality among men in England, Scotland and the United States. *Internat J Epidemiol* 1989; **18**: 84–88.
93. Grievink L, Smit HA, Ocke MC et al. Dietary intake of antioxidant (pro)-vitamins, respiratory symptoms and pulmonary function: the Morgen study. *Thorax* 1998; **53**: 166–171.
94. Graham WGB, O'Grady RV, Dubuc B. Pulmonary function loss in Vermont granite workers. *Am Rev Respir Dis* 1981; **123**: 25–28.
95. Lefante JL. The power to detect differences in average rates of change in longitudinal studies. *Stat Med* 1990; **9**: 437–446.
96. Rijcken B, Schouten JP, Weiss ST, Ware JH. ERS/ATS workshop on longitudinal analysis of pulmonary function data, Barcelona, September 1995. *Eur Respir J* 1997; **10**: 758–763.
97. Sherrill DL, Lebowitz MD, Knudson RJ, Burrows B. Methodology for generating continuous prediction equations for pulmonary function measures. *Comput Biomed Res* 1991; **24**: 249–260.
98. Sherrill DL, Lebowitz MD, Knudson RJ, Burrows B. Continuous longitudinal regression equations for pulmonary function measures. *Eur Respir J* 1992; **5**: 452–462.
99. Sherrill DL, Enright PL, Kaltenborn WT, Lebowitz MD. Predictors of longitudinal change in diffusing capacity over 8 years. *Am J Respir Crit Care Med* 1999; **160**: 1883–1887.
100. Pistelli F, Bottai M, Viegi G *et al.* Smooth reference equations for slow vital capacity and flow-volume curve indices. *Am J Respir Crit Care Med* 2000; **161**: 899–905.
101. Sobol BJ, Weinheimer B. Assessment of ventilatory abnormality in the asymptomatic subject: an exercise in futility. *Thorax* 1966; **21**: 445–449.
102. Guidelines for the measurement of respiratory function; recommendations of the British Thoracic Society and the Association of Respiratory Technicians and Physiologists. *Respir Med* 1994; **88**: 165–194.
103. Williams RJ. Standard human beings versus standard values. *Science* 1957; **126**: 453–454.
104. Burrows B, Knudson RJ, Cline MG, Lebowitz MD. Reexamination of the risk factors for ventilatory impairment. *Am Rev Respir Dis* 1988; **138**: 829–836.

Further reading

Bachofen H, Hobi HJ, Scherrer M. Alveolar-arterial N_2 gradients at rest and during exercise in healthy men of different ages. *J Appl Physiol* 1973; **34**: 137–142.

*de Kroon JPM, Joosting PE, Visser BF. Les valeurs normales de la capacité vitale et du volume expiratoire maximum seconde. *Arch Mal Prof* 1964; **25**: 17–30.

Drouet D, Kauffman F, Brille D, Lellouch J. Valeurs spirographiques de référence: Modèles mathématiques et utilisation pratique. *Bull Eur Physiopathol Respir* 1980; **16**: 747–767.

Georges R, Saumon G, Loiseau A. The relationship of age to pulmonary membrane conductance and capillary blood volume. *Am Rev Respir Dis* 1978; **117**: 1069–1078.

Gulsvik A, Bakke P, Humerfelt S et al. Single breath transfer factor for carbon monoxide in an asymptomatic population of never smokers. *Thorax* 1992; **47**: 167–173.

Hertle FH, George R, Lange HJ. Die arteriellen blutgaspartialdrucke und ih re Beziehungen zu Alter und Anthropometrischen Grössen. *Rev Inst Hyg Mines* 1971; **28**: 1–30.

Higgins MW, Keller JB. Seven measures of ventilatory lung function. Population values and a comparison of their ability to discriminate between persons with and without chronic respiratory symptoms and disease, Tecumseh, Michigan. *Am Rev Respir Dis* 1973; **108**: 258–272.

*Lawther PJ, Brooks AGF, Waller RE. Respiratory function measurements in a cohort of medical students: a ten-year follow-up. *Thorax* 1978; **33**: 773–778.

*Lundsgaard C, Van Slyke DD. Studies of lung volumes: 1. Relation between thorax size and lung volume in normal adults. *J Exp Med* 1916; **27**: 65–86.

Paoletti P, Pistelli G, Fazzi P, Viegi G, Di Pede F, Guiliano G et al. Reference values for vital capacity and flow-volume curves from a general population study. *Bull Eur Physiopathol Respir* 1986; **22**: 451–459.

Pistelli R, Brancato G, Forastiere F, Michelozzi P, Corbo GM, Agabiti N et al. Population values of lung volumes and flows in children: effect of sex, body mass and respiratory conditions. *Eur Respir J* 1992; **5**: 463–470.

*Ringqvist T, Ringqvist I. Respiratory forces and variations of static lung volumes in healthy subjects. *Scand J Clin Lab Invest* 1974; **33**: 269–276.

Roberts CM, MacRae KD, Winning AJ et al. Reference values and prediction equations for normal lung function in a non-smoking white urban population. *Thorax* 1991; **46**: 643–650.

Roca J, Sanchis J, Agusti-Vidal A et al. Spirometric reference values from a Mediterranean population. *Bull Eur Physiopathol Respir* 1986; **22**: 217–224.

Vooren PH, van Zomeren BC. Reference values of total respiratory resistance, determined with the "opening" interruption technique. *Eur Respir J* 1989; **2**: 966–971.

*Reference of historical interest.

CHAPTER 27

Genetic Diversity: Reference Values in Non-Caucasians

Ethnic differences in lung function are of increasing importance as a result of the population of the world becoming more mobile. This chapter reviews the present situation.

27.1 Overview

27.1.1 Relevance of race

The genus *Homo sapiens* emerged by a combination of genetic mutation and natural selection from within the primate family. It became subdivided into three principal racial groups (Table 27.1) each with distinguishing features reflecting a shared genetic inheritance. The features were perpetuated by inbreeding; this occurred as a result of proximity, cultural preference and geographical separation.

The identifying features of the races were initially those that could be seen at a glance including the appearance of the skin, hair and face. However, the genetic differences also include body proportions, fat distribution, predisposition to diseases (e.g. diabetes) and the size and function of the lungs. Groupings of these features may have arisen by accident, but more probably they were combinations that permitted a few individuals to survive in previously unfavourable habitats; this is consistent with recent evidence from mitochondrial DNA on the growth of populations [1]. The large lungs and fair skins of Caucasians could have sustained an aquatic phase in their migration from Africa [2] and contributed to their subsequent survival in northern regions where the atmosphere absorbed some ultraviolet light from the sun. By contrast, the long legs, lightly built bodies and dark skins of the Black Africans probably contributed to their survival amongst the wild animals and hot sun of sub-Saharan Africa. If these speculations have substance, the racial differences had a purpose that arose outside the lungs. Now they can contribute to reference values for lung function in individual subjects. The contribution is less than that of genetic variables within racial groups. In addition, to an increasing extent a person's race is becoming obscured by interbreeding arising from migration, war and individual circumstances. Finally, the term has acquired disagreeable overtones and this has led to it being replaced by 'ethnic group'.

27.1.2 Ethnic factor in lung function

Ethnic group describes a person's cultural identity. Historically it was based on race, but the description is strongly influenced by geographical and other factors including the social group to which the person belongs. Initially the groups were large, for example all Afro Americans comprised one ethnic group, currently described as 'blacks'. However, such large groups have a

Table 27.1 Principal ethnic groups.

Group	Origin	Other regions
Caucasian*	Europe	worldwide (Whites)
Indian †	South Asia	plantations worldwide
Hispanic ‡	Central and South America	N. America
Mongoloid*	East Asia	Eskimo, Indians of North and South America
Black African*	Sub-Saharan Africa	North America (Blacks)
Oceanian (see text)	Australia	Indonesia
	Pacific islands	New Zealand

* Primary racial group, now widely dispersed.

† Subdivided by locality (including north, south and east India, Pakistan, Bangladesh, Sri Lanka).

‡ Formerly Spanish or Portuguese, now with Black African and South American Indian admixture.

Table 27.2 Examples of genetic abnormalities with ethnic affiliations.

Abnormality	Condition	Affiliation
HbS formation	Sickle cell anaemia	W. Africa, Arabia
HbA deficiency	β-Thalassaemia	E. Mediterranean
Hb α chain abnormal	α-Thalassaemia	Southeast Asia
G6PD deficiency	Haemolytic anaemia	Black African people
Cystic fibrosis	Dysfunction of exocrine glands	North Europeans
Retrovirus HTLV-1	Spastic paraparesis	Afro-Caribbeans, Japanese
HLA BW 46	Antigenic variant	Cantonese
HLA BW 42	Antigenic variant	Black African people

Hb, haemoglobin; G6PD, glucose 6 phosphate dehydrogenase; HLA, human leucocyte antigen. Source: [4]

progressive tendency to subdivide and the physical component become diluted. As a result the concept of an ethnic factor in lung function is less useful than it was a few years ago and a more precise description is desirable [3]. This might embrace the racial group, countries of origin and present residence. For example, studies have been conducted of people who migrated from sub-Saharan Africa or south India to work in plantations in other countries. Currently, some of them still live in rural communities, but many have moved elsewhere. As a result the lung function of the succeeding generations have been subject to numerous influences and a single 'ethnic factor' cannot be assumed. The principal ethnic groups are listed in Table 27.1. They mostly have a genetic (racial) component, modified by environmental influences that include previous geographical location and cultural practices, including diet and prevalence of smoking.

As a result of these changes the genetic component to the lung function may no longer be identifiable. However, the ethnic ancestry can still be relevant for health in other ways (Table 27.2).

An association between ethnic group and lung function was observed in the 1960s, first from casual observations [5–7], then after standardising for age, stature and level of activity [8]. The magnitude and extent of ethnic differences in lung function were explored during the International Biological Programme. Representative groups of subjects were used and the results appeared to be unequivocal; the lung size relative to stature of Asian Indians, sub-Saharan Africans and Australian Aboriginals was smaller than that of Europeans. The lung function of mongoloid peoples was intermediate (e.g. Fig. 27.1).

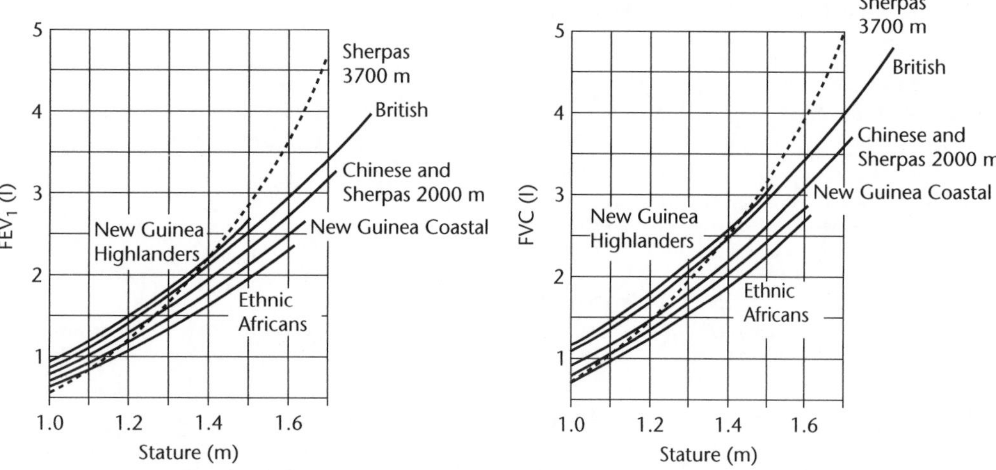

Fig. 27.1 Forced expiratory volume and forced vital capacity as a function of stature in boys of various ethnic groups studied in their traditional environments during the International Biological Programme. Values for girls are on average lower by approximately 10% (Table 25.4, page 320). Compared with native British children the values for rural Jamaicans of African origin, Chinese and New Guinean coastal and highland children differed, respectively, by approximately −23%, −9%, −16% and +5%. The lung function of children from many parts of South Asia is similar to that of the Jamaicans. The large lungs of the Sherpa children is of environmental origin. Sources: [9–14], also text.

The observed differences were of such magnitude that to neglect them could lead to errors in diagnosis and medical treatment, and to some people with healthy lungs failing a pre-employment medical examination or being turned down for life insurance. Clearly the ethnic factor was important. However, the association with ethnic group has turned out to be less simple than at first appeared.

27.1.3 Variables sometimes linked to ethnic group

Geographical location. Traditional ethnic groups had strong geographical associations. This led to their being identified with particular terrains, sources of food, climate, parasites and other features that can influence the level of habitual activity. A high level of activity during childhood stimulates the lungs to grow and enhances the ability to transfer gas. An associated increase in muscle strength enlarges the vital capacity. The effect of exercise is prominent for people living in temperate rather than tropical climates and where the terrain is mountainous (Table 27.3).

The geographical influence is most apparent for high altitude populations when hypoxia provides an additional stimulus to lung growth (Section 25.2.2). However, lower altitudes also have an effect. Thus, in a review of lung function in Africans, the altitude at which the people lived was the largest single cause of variation between studies. For FVC in men the altitude effect was approximately 0.2 l/1000 m [15].

Diet. Insufficient calories or a low protein diet can restrain the physical development of the body including the lungs. The cause can be a traditional diet, religious preference, or unfavourable geographic and economic circumstances. Any of these can be associated with ethnic group. In the case of Japanese people a traditional diet contributed to their having small lungs. Changing to a western style, higher protein diet led to a material increase in stature and also in the size of the lungs relative to stature [16]. Thus, the extent of acculturation related to ethnic group can influence lung function. Other than Japan this factor appears to operate for some people in New Guinea, other pacific islands and parts of the Indian subcontinent, but the reasons for the small lungs are multi-factorial. If diet was the only consideration a change to a western diet would increase the lung size relative to stature to the level of Caucasians but this has not been observed.

27.1.4 Biases introduced by migration

In historical times migration was a hazardous procedure, involving dangers on the journey, conflict on arrival and hardship during the process of becoming established. Death was common at each stage, so those who succeeded were typically robust, resourceful and lucky. These considerations still apply in the usually less stressful conditions of today. They contribute to the migrants often having superior lung function compared with persons of similar age and stature who remain at home [17]. Formerly, this was particularly the case with people attracted or moved forcibly to undertake physically demanding jobs as mercenaries or workers in plantations or mines. The principal requirements were then a robust physique and ability to undertake physical work; both factors that can be associated with relatively large lungs. As a result, the lung function of a parent community can under-represent that of a daughter community in another location.

27.1.5 Miscegenation: evidence for autosomal inheritance of lung function

Terminology. Ethnic terminology is often inaccurate on account of lagging behind the demographic reality. This is because migration is usually followed by intermarriage into an indigenous population. Its extent varies depending on the strength of

Table 27.3 Relation of lung function and the cardiorespiratory response to exercise to ethnic group and level of habitual activity in young women. The lung function has been standardised for age, stature and, where appropriate, haemoglobin concentration. The exercise ventilation has been standardised to an oxygen uptake of 45 mmol l^{-1}, (1.0 l min^{-1}, V_{E45}) and the cardiac frequency to a fat-free mass of 40 kg (fc_{45} ,st). The data suggest that the transfer factor is influenced by previous habitual activity and the exercise tidal volume standardised for vital capacity (V_{t30}, ex. st) by ethnic group. The lung volume and probably the exercise ventilation are influenced by both factors.

Activity:	High	Medium		Low
Subjects:	New Guinea highlanders	New Guinea coastal people	UK housewives	Jamaican housewives
fc_{45}, st (min^{-1})	122*	135	134	145*
Tl s,st (mmol min^{-1} kPa^{-1}) †	11.0*	9.6	9.4	7.7*
Vt_{30}, ex. st (l)	1.07*	1.01*	1.34	1.11*
TLC st (l)	4.82	4.12*	4.97	4.22*
V_{E45}(l min^{-1})	24.6*	27.6	26.9	29.5*

* Significant difference compared with UK housewives ($p < 0.05$).

† For conversion to traditional units see Table 6.6 (page 56)

Source: [13].

cultural identity within the respective groups and on demographic and economic pressures. In some circumstances the mixing is minimal. In others it is extensive, as in the USA were people of African origin are described as Black Americans, yet as long ago as 1969, the Caucasian admixture in the average black urban American was in excess of 22% [18]. The proportion is likely to have risen subsequently.

Inheritance. For people of mixed Black African and white ancestry, the lung volume has been found to be intermediate between those of the parents and capable of being described on a four-point scale reflecting the ethnicity of the four grandparents [9]. Hence, lung function, like stature, is inherited equally from both parents (autosomal). In the study cited, the score for ethnicity could be replaced by a score for skin colour. Australian Aboriginals show a similar pattern (*q.v.*).

Magnitude of the ethnic factor. For any single pair of ethnic groups an estimate of the size of the ethnic factor will vary depending on the allowances made for co-related variables. Differences of up to 30% have been observed (Fig. 27.1) but more than one variable may have contributed. The ethnic factor is being reduced progressively by miscegenation and will eventually be eliminated. Until this happens, the factor to be quoted should be that for ethnically pure communities. In individuals the factor may need to be modified to allow for interbreeding, when the allowance should be the mean of those appropriate for the ethnic group of each of the four grandparents.

27.1.6 Ethnic factor in ventilatory responses to exercise and breathing CO_2

A person's exercise capacity (maximal oxygen uptake) is greatly influenced by his or her genetic constitution; this determines the limits within which environmental factors can operate (Section 28.3). The ethnic component of the constitution contributes to the *type* of exercise that can be performed best. Long limbs, as in Black Africans, facilitate running and boxing whereas large lungs, as in Caucasians, facilitate swimming. Other related features, including the length and mass of the trunk, may contribute to these associations.

The lung function is influenced by the extent to which an activity, including one with an ethnic component, develops the accessory muscles of respiration. Through this association the ethnic group can have a secondary effect on the lung function. However, this is smaller than the primary effect of ethnic group in influencing the total lung capacity and subdivisions. The latter contribute to exercise tidal volume, but except in relation to swimming this does not appear to affect performance. The relationship of submaximal exercise tidal volume to vital capacity appears to be independent of ethnic group [9, 13]. This is also the case for the submaximal cardiac frequency standardised for oxygen uptake, habitual activity and quantity of body muscle (e.g. Table 27.3).

The respiratory sensitivity to carbon dioxide has been found to be reduced amongst people in New Guinea [19] but not in people from Nigeria [20]. The cause for the different responses is unclear. Recent work on the control of breathing suggests that a cultural explanation is possible (Section 23.7.1). Thus, in these respects as in others, the full relevance of the ethnic connection has still to be worked out.

27.1.7 Inheritance of lung function within ethnic groups

In racially mixed communities the possibility of ethnic differences in lung function has attracted attention because of the association with physical appearance. In ethnically homogeneous communities there are comparable differences between and within families; this has become apparent through study of twins. In this situation, within pair differences in lung function standardised for stature are consistently smaller for identical than for non-identical pairs. The differences are largely due to anatomical factors and those that affect patterns of growth and the dimensions of the large airways [21, 22]. Other contributory factors include the level of habitual activity [23, 11, 24], susceptibility to tobacco smoke and liability to respiratory infections [25]. These features can have a genetic component. However, information on a possible familial factor in lung function is not yet in a form where it can be used to improve the accuracy of reference values.

27.1.8 Reference variables

The reference variables now used for study of ethnic variation are stature in children and stature and age in adults. These variables appear to account for the greater part of the variance. Another variable might be sitting height or trunk length since the relatively short trunks of Black African people contribute to their small lungs. However, even within that community sitting height is a less good predictor than stature [9, 26]. Amongst Mongoloid people an allowance for sitting height *enhances* the ethnic factor since, compared with Caucasians their trunks are relatively long whereas their lungs are usually smaller. Thus, the case for using trunk length as a reference variable for describing ethnic differences in lung function is not strong. There is a better case for using thoracic dimensions [5] and/or distribution of body fat (Section 4.6), but these options appear not to have been explored in detail.

Additional variables that influence indices of lung size are specific lung compliance and maximal respiratory pressures. If one of these indices varied between ethnic groups it might be eligible for use as a reference variable. However, both indices appear to be independent of ethnic group [27, 28, 29]. In the case of maximal respiratory pressures, the absence of ethnic variation is consistent with the common experience that peak expiratory flow is independent of ethnic group. Thus, in this as in other respects the case for additional or specific reference variables has still to be made.

Table 27.4 Contribution of ethnicity to reference values for lung function and indices of standardised submaximal exercise.

Present	Probable	Absent
FEV_1 and FVC	Vt_{30}	PEF
TLC, IC and ERV	Sco_2	*Tl*
Tl/*VA*		MEP and MIP
		CI
		fC_{45} and VE_{45}

27.1.9 Technical factors in interpretation

Recent studies confirm that forced expiratory volume, vital capacity and total lung capacity exhibit systematic differences between ethnic groups. Other indices may be subject to ethnic variation but in most instances the differences appear to be small and of similar magnitude to those associated with environmental factors (Table 27.4). Ethnic differences are apparent in young children [30], but have not been observed in neonates.

Estimates of any possible ethnic effects are subject to error from sub-optimal sampling strategies especially with respect to environmental factors, variations in the definition of what constitutes a healthy person, use of equipment having different performance characteristics, imperfect measurement of stature and variation in experience of statistics [31]; Chapter 5 provides examples of these. In addition, the lung function is subject to secular trends and there can be biological quirks, e.g. when the lung function of smokers is found to be superior to that of non-smokers. The optimal biological models can also differ between groups, as for Sherpa children compared with others in Fig. 27.1. Amongst the latter a proportional model can be fitted to the data, so the ethnic differences can be represented by percentages. Where a proportional or additive model does not fit the data, any single ethnic factor is inevitably an approximation. It may, nonetheless be useful.

Against this background the present selection of reference values and commentary should be regarded as a guide at one point in time. Any lung function laboratory should check their reference values against groups of healthy volunteers selected for this purpose. Such checks are particularly important where the techniques or the subjects do not match exactly those used for the reference values that are available locally.

27.2 Lung function analysed by ethnic group and geographical location

27.2.1 South Asia, including Indian subcontinent

The lung function reported from India and other parts of South Asia exhibits considerable diversity (e.g. Table 27.5).

Contributory factors are racial differences, use of a wide variety of equipment and numerous environmental influences including nutrition, climate, terrain and prevalence of disease. Many aspects are in the process of change, so recent local reference values should be used where these are available. They are needed especially for ventilatory capacity, total lung capacity and functional residual capacity. Transfer factor and residual volume are less subject to racial variation. Consequently, where *Tl* is well maintained but alveolar volume is low (as in South Indians) the *K*co (*Tl*/*V*a) is correspondingly increased. *Tl* can be reduced on account of anaemia, particularly in women [38], so standardisation to a normal haemoglobin concentration is recommended.

Table 27.5 Mean ventilatory capacity at age 35 years, height 1.65 m for men from different parts of the Indian subcontinent: comparison with other ethnic groups.

Origin	Domicile	FEV_1 (l)	FVC (l)	Source
Kolkata†	India	3.03	3.68	[32]
W. Pakistan	UK	3.20	3.72	[33]
Delhi	India	3.24	4.03	[34]
Uttar Pradesh	Guyana	2.79	3.42	[35]
Chennai (city)*	India	2.66	3.34	[36]
Chennai (rural)	India	2.51	3.15	[37]
Black African	Guiana	2.95	3.59	[35]
Caucasians	Various	3.48	4.21	Table 26.16

* Formerly Madras
† Formerly Calcutta

North India and Pakistan. These lands have been subject to numerous invasions including that of Macedonians under Alexander the Great, Moguls and others. As a result the predominant racial group is Caucasian. The population includes the former martial races of India; their lung function can resemble that of Caucasians [39]. Compared with these people the lung volumes and ventilatory capacity of Pakistanis [40] and North Indians, including from Delhi and Haryana, are usually reported as being somewhat lower, but higher than in South Indians [32, 34, 41, 42]. Rural people and those living in the hills often have superior lung function to urban dwellers [43].

North Indian migrants to UK appear to have similar lung function to that of their parent communities (see also Section 27.1.4). By contrast the lung function of migrants to UK from Pakistan is only slightly less than, or matches, that of Caucasians. Thus, depending on circumstances either local values (Fig. 27.2) or Caucasian reference values should be used.

Children up to age 16 years. Amongst boys up to age 16 years the relationship of FEV_1 to height appears to be well established [44–48], there is reasonable agreement for FVC and some diversity for PEF; the last possibly reflecting differences in muscle strength. Amongst girls there are also some unexpected results including relatively low values for urban children in Delhi [46]. In several studies, values for FVC are not materially larger than those for FEV_1. As a result, high values are reported for FEV% ($100 \times FEV_1/FVC$). In addition, some comparisons between lung function in boys and girls do not show the expected differences.

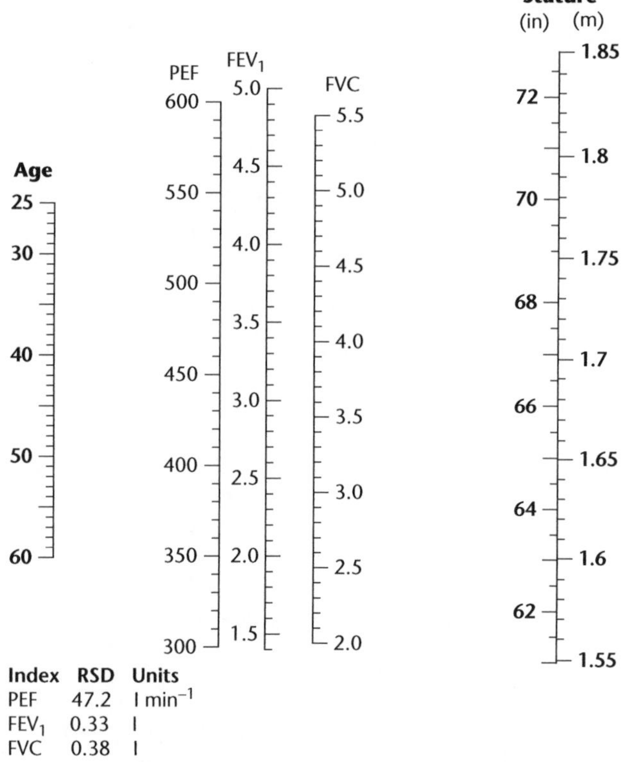

Fig. 27.2 Nomogram relating FEV_1, FVC and PEF (Wright peak flow meter) to age and stature for men from Pakistan working in the UK. Source: [33]. In the case of PEF an adjustment should be made for alinearity in the scale of the meter (Section 12.3.2).

The explanations of these findings are at present unclear. Some consistent features and results that appear common to many parts of India are illustrated in Figs 27.3 and 27.4. Additional values for children from the Punjab are overleaf in Table 27.6.

South India. The people of South India and Bangladesh do not have the physique or levels of activity of those in the north and their standardised lung function is lower [35, 36, 38, 49]. The main cause appears to be genetic, but standard of living also contributes via its effects on growth and physique [50], onset of puberty and amount of chest illness. A rural or deprived urban environment is disadvantageous [e.g. 37]. The lung function of South Indians is shared with daughter communities comprising present and past former plantation workers throughout the world (Table 27.1). Some reference values for adults are given in Table 27.6; those for ventilatory capacity are illustrated in Figs 27.5 and 27.6. The lung function of South Indian children appears not to have been reviewed recently and more data are needed. Meanwhile, use may be made of the factor given in the caption to Fig. 27.1.

The levels of lung function in all these populations are systematically lower than in Caucasians. Similar relatively low values (on average 16–28% lower) have been observed for non-smoking Asian Indians living in the USA [51] (also Table 27.6).

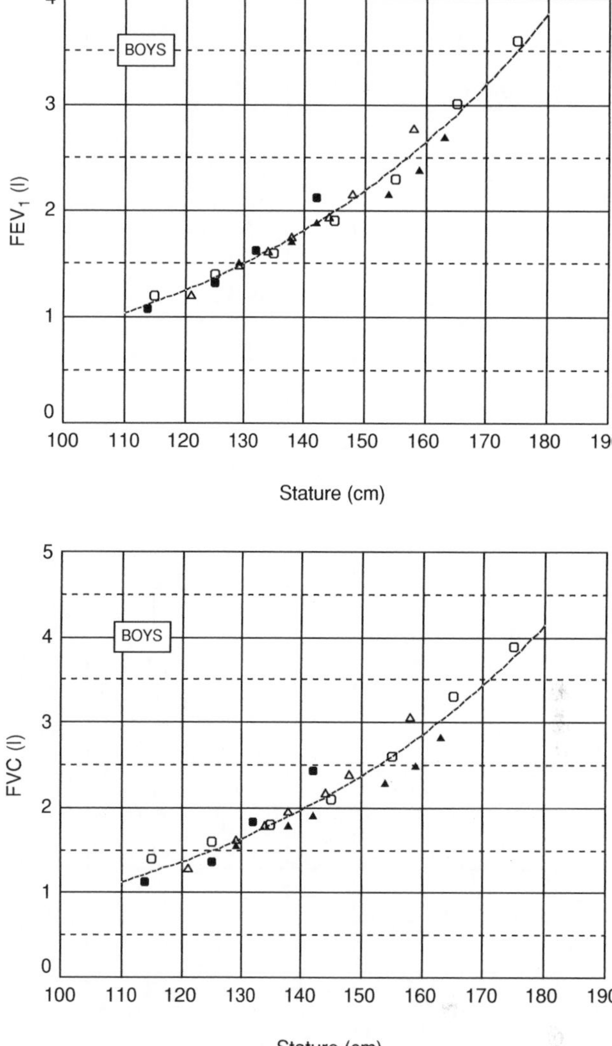

Fig. 27.3 Representative values for FEV_1 and FVC in boys aged up to 16 years from mainly northern India. The relationships were obtained by fitting exponential models to mean data; these were from [44] –open triangles, [45] – open circles, [46] – closed triangles, [47] – closed circles. The equations were: $FEV_1 = 0.1306 \times e^{(0.0188\,\text{Stature,cm})}$ ($R^2 = 0.973$) and $FVC = 0.1457 \times e^{(0.0186\,\text{Stature,cm})}$ ($R^2 = 0.938$). The coefficients of variation about the relationships are likely to be of the order of 11% [14]. Comparable relationships in girls are in Fig. 27.4 (overleaf).

Malay people. The indigenous people of Malaya are related to those of South India and they have similar lung function [52, 53]. The lung function of Malay migrants to Singapore has been reported as being less than that of the local Chinese by a factor between 5% and 10%. Migrants to Singapore from India on average recorded values that were slightly but not significantly lower [54, 55].

Sinhalese. The ventilatory capacity and lung volumes of the people of Sri Lanka resemble those of South Indians. However, the

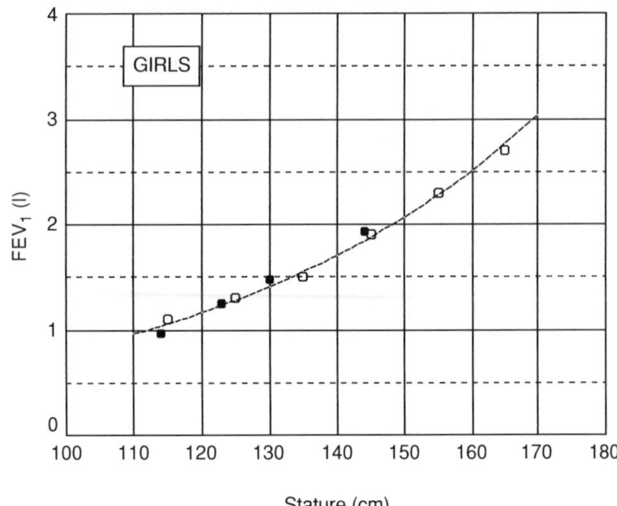

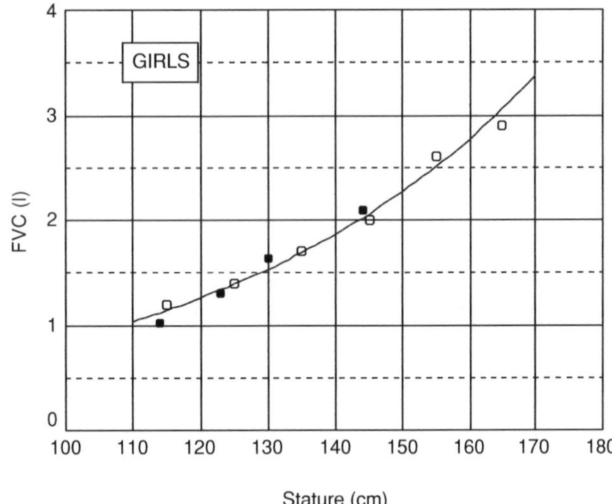

Fig. 27.4 Representative values for FEV_1 and FVC in girls aged up to 16 years mainly from northern India. The relationships were obtained by fitting exponential models to mean data; these were from [45] – open circles, [47] – closed circles. The data of Sharma et al [46] yielded systematically lower values. The equations were: $FEV_1 = 0.1162 \times e^{(0.0192\,\mathrm{Stature,cm})}$ ($R^2 = 0.988$) and $FVC = 0.1184 \times e^{(0.0197\,\mathrm{Stature,cm})}$ ($R^2 = 0.978$). By analogy with similar studies of Caucasian girls [14] the coefficients of variation about the relationships are likely to be of the order of 10%.

function of young persons may be improving relative to that of older generations. The transfer factor is similar to that of Caucasians and other ethnic groups [56].

27.2.2 Mexicans and Hispanic Americans

The people of Mexico are Spanish speaking but many of them have African and Mongoloid people amongst their ancestors. Their lung function has been studied locally [57] and in the USA where Hispanic Americans now comprise an increasing proportion of the local population. They are often of stocky physique with a relatively short trunk. The standardised lung function does not differ significantly from that of Caucasians [58, 59].

Table 27.6 Reference values for South Indian men and women.

Index	Gender	Regression equation (significant terms only)	RSD	Figure	Source
FEV_1(l)	M	3.96 St – 0.021 A –3.13	0.37‡	27.5	[36]
	M	3.5 St – 0.026 A –1.94	0.39	–	[51]*
FEV_1(l)	F	2.74 St – 0.010 A –2.0	0.31‡	27.6	[36]
	F	2.1 St – 0.021 A –0.40	0.28	–	[51]*
FVC (l)	M	5.03 St – 0.014 A –4.49	0.46‡	27.5	[36]
	M	4.3 St – 0.024 A –2.75	0.48	–	[51]*
FVC (l)	F	3.70 St – 0.007 A –3.19	0.38‡	27.6	[36]
	F	2.7 St – 0.020 A –0.84	0.35	–	[51]*
TLC (l)	M	7.6 St + 0.0006 A^2–8.27	0.564	–	[38]†
	M	6.4 St – 0.017 A –5.15	0.828	–	[51]*
TLC (l)	F	3.6 St + 0.00024 A^2–2.31	0.404	–	[38]†
FRC (l)	M	4.7 St + 0.00035 A^2–5.34	0.470	–	[38]†
	F	2.6 St + 0.00022 A^2–2.12	0.340	–	[38]†
RV (l)	M	2.8 St + 0.00043 A^2–3.60	0.399	–	[38]†
	F	NS (mean value 1.06)	0.26	–	[38]†
*T*l,st (SI)‡	M	11 St –0.00009 A^2–8.67	1.519	–	[38]†
	F	4.9 St –0.00113 A^2+0.83	1.127	–	[38]†

Stature (St) is in metres, age (A) is in years
* Asian Indians resident in US.
‡ RSD not reported. Value cited is from another study that yielded a similar result [35].
† Ages 15 – 40 years. Due to the inclusion of adolescents some coefficients on age are positive.
Units mmol $min^{-1}kPa^{-1}$; standardised to [Hb] = 14.6 g dl^{-1}. See also [38].

27.2.3 Middle East and North Africa

The people of these lands are predominantly Semitic, mainly Arabs (Fellahin and Bedouin) from the Arabian Peninsula whose language is Arabic. The principal exceptions are Iran where the majority are Persians, and Israel where the population is now cosmopolitan. These are considerable admixtures of other groups including Kurds (Iraq and Iran), Berbers (North Africa), Copts (Egypt) and Druze (Lebanon and adjacent countries); the last have a cultural affinity with Iran. The *Persians* came originally from the Caucasus and adjacent parts of Central Asia and at one time occupied Northern India. Thus, the lung function of the region might be expected to resemble that of Caucasians in Europe and elsewhere. For Iran this appears to be the case [60], with any small differences probably having a technical explanation.

The ventilatory function of adult *Jordanians* in Amman is also similar to that of Caucasians and this finding could reflect the lung function of Arab people generally [61]. However,

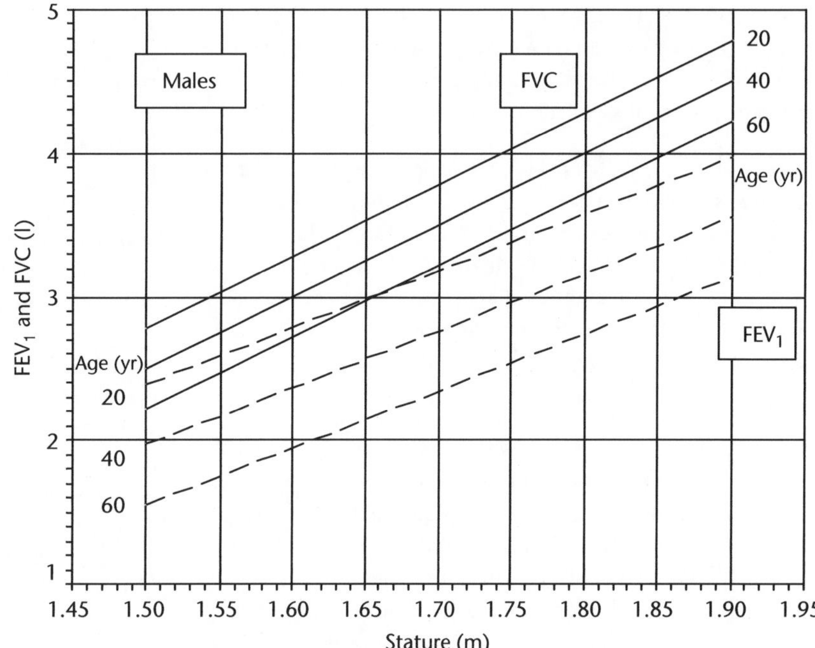

Fig. 27.5 FEV_1 and FVC related to age (year) and stature (m) in adult males from South India. Equations are given in Table 27.6. Source: [36]

Amman is set in mountains, where the altitude is 774 m above sea level and the associated physical activity might contribute to an above average lung function. Lower levels of lung function have been reported for children and adults living at sea level in Benghazi, *Libya* [62,63]. The mean difference was approximately 19%. This is larger than might be expected from the difference in altitude [15], so other factors probably contributed as well.

27.2.4 Mongoloid people

These people came from what is now East Asia. The largest group is the *Chinese* who whilst centred in East Asia are now found throughout the world. On average, they have a high trunk length to leg length ratio. Despite this the ventilatory capacity of Chinese adults is usually somewhat less than that of Caucasians; a difference of 7% is probably representative [54, 64]. In children the difference for FEV_1 is less or non-existent [55, 65, 66]. However,

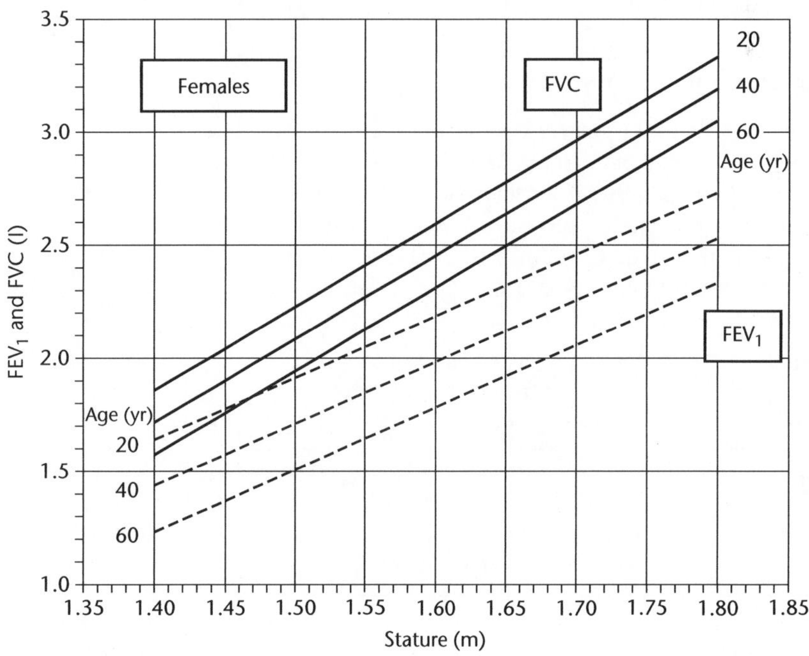

Fig. 27.6 FEV_1 and FVC related to age (year) and stature (m) in adult females from South India. Equations are given in Table 27.6. Source: [36]

in some cities the population density is high, the air is polluted and the children take little exercise. These factors appear to be having an adverse effect on the lung function of children and increasingly of adults as well.

American Indians. These are Mongoloid people who walked from Asia into what is now Alaska, at a time when the continents were joined up; they have features in common with the Chinese. The standardised lung function of Indians now living in the USA is not significantly different from that of white Americans [67, 68]. The lung function of Indians in Central and South America appears not to have been reported.

Inuit. (*Eskimos*). The Inuit are a Mongoloid people of stocky physique, many of whom live within the Arctic Circle. Acculturation has improved the health of young people and increased life expectancy, but physical fitness has deteriorated and body fat has increased. As a result of these changes the height-standardised FEV_1 and FVC at age 20 years has improved significantly over the 20 years up to 1990. By contrast, amongst adults the longitudinal decline with age has accelerated, particularly amongst men. Smoking is not a significant contributory factor [69]. The recent lung function of Canadian Inuits is similar to or slightly better than that of Caucasians (Table 27.7).

Similarly, Greenlandic Inuit children have superior lung function to their Danish counterparts despite the Greenlanders having much respiratory illness in early childhood. The difference affects both sexes and is more apparent in the older than younger children. It has been attributed in part to environmental factors, possibly a diet rich in fish oil, and much physical activity [70]. The results of further investigations will be of interest.

Mongolians. The lung function of adults in the People's Republic of Mongolia is within 1–2% of that of Caucasians [71].

27.2.5 Sub-Saharan Africans

The dark skinned people of Central and Southern Africa have long legs, lightly built trunks and pigmented skin. Formerly, these features could have contributed to survival (Section 27.1.1). Some groups including those from West Africa, also had small lungs relative to the size of their bodies [15]. This observation was first made on the descendants of people who were taken as slaves to work in the plantations of the New World, including USA, West Indies and Central America, e.g. [35]. The studies led to the prevailing view that the lung volumes and related indices of people of West African descent standardised for age and height are on average 87% of those of Caucasians [72–76]. This factor is appropriate for use in children (Fig. 27.1, also Section 26.3.5). However, in adults studied cross-sectionally the difference is mainly in the constant term of the regression equations, not the coefficients on age and stature. As a result, the racial difference from Caucasian lung function can be expressed in absolute units, for example in men and women, respectively, for FEV_1 –0.45 l and –0.4 l, and for FVC –0.7 l and –0.61 l. However, compared with men and women from South India living and working in the same environment the FEV_1 and FVC are slightly greater in the West Africans (mean difference 0.14 l) [35]. Reference values for adults of West African descent are given in Table 27.8 and Figs 27.7 and 27.8. Reference values for non-white children living in the UK are given in Table 27.9 (page 378) and percentile charts (Section 26.3.5) for FEV_1 and FVC in black children living in the United States are given in Fig. 27.9 (page 377).

The above factors can be used in conjunction with reference values for Caucasians to describe the ventilatory capacity of some but not all people from sub-Saharan Africa. Other circumstances that influence the level of the result include altitude during childhood and the cohort defined by the year of study [15, 78, 79]. In addition, the pattern of results is complicated by technical factors that can introduce bias and by some of the populations for study comprising people of mixed ethnic origin. However, within populations the result is likely to be independent of chronic airways obstruction as the prevalence of that condition is relatively low amongst black people [80, 81]. A complete map of African lung function has still to be compiled.

Table 27.7 Lung function in adult Inuit (1990).

Gender	Indices	Equation	RSD
Men ($n = 70$)	FVC (l)	4.20 St − 0.044 Age − 0.34	NA
	FEV_1(l)	3.27 St − 0.040 Age − 0.53	NA
Women ($n = 55$)	FVC (l)	6.18 St − 0.029 Age − 4.87	NA
	FEV_1 (l)	5.56 St − 0.031 Age − 4.43	NA

NA: not available.
Source: [69].

27.2.6 Oceanians, including Australian aboriginals

Oceania comprises the islands in the Pacific Ocean, Australia and New Zealand. They were originally inhabited by Melanesians and

Table 27.8 Reference equations for ventilatory capacity and total lung capacity in adults of West African descent. The reference variables are stature (St), in meters, and age, (A) in years.

Index	Equation	RSD
FEV_1(l) M	3.40 St − 0.024 A − 1.82	0.37
F	2.45 St − 0.018 A − 1.04	0.31
FVC (l) M	4.44 St − 0.024 A − 2.90	0.46
F	3.15 St − 0.020 A − 1.55	0.38
TLC (l) M	9.04 St − 9.58	0.68
F	6.03 St − 5.31	0.46
VC (l) M	6.47 St − 0.019 A − 6.24	0.50
F	4.78 St − 0.004 A − 4.63	0.44

Residual volume and transfer factor were as for Caucasians (Chapter 26).
Source: [9, 35].

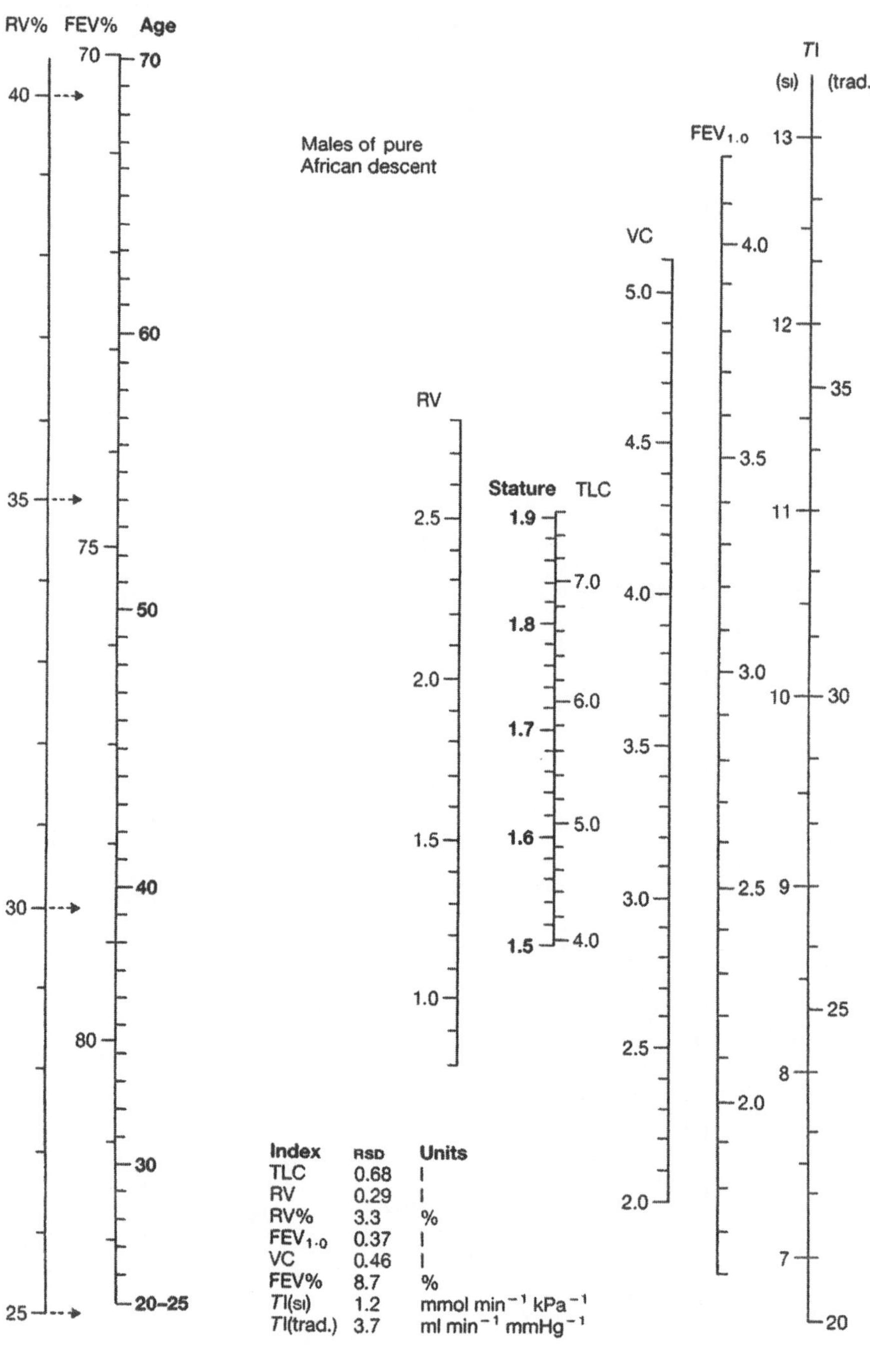

Fig. 27.7 Nomogram relating indices of lung function to stature and age for healthy adult men of African descent. The RV% and FEV% are related only to age and the TLC only to stature. Source: [9].

Micronesians who migrated from southeast Asia to Australia, and by Polynesians who went from China to New Zealand via the Philippines. These movements will have influenced the lung function of the respective populations.

Australian Aboriginals. Australia was first populated some 50,000 years ago by small groups of people who had sailed from Timor or walked from New Guinea across the bed of what is now the Arafura sea. Other groups followed. They spread out thinly across the continent, so were subject to geographical separation that perpetuated any initial differences in genetic constitution. Recently, this diversity has been enhanced by mixed marriages (miscegenation). The consequences for lung function are not known.

Aboriginal people usually have broad nostrils and many have learnt to play musical instruments that necessitate control of the soft palate, including nasal pipes and the aerophone or drone pipe. The latter entails simultaneous inspiration into the lungs and expiration of air stored in the buccal cavity. Thus, when measuring lung function the use of a nose clip is essential.

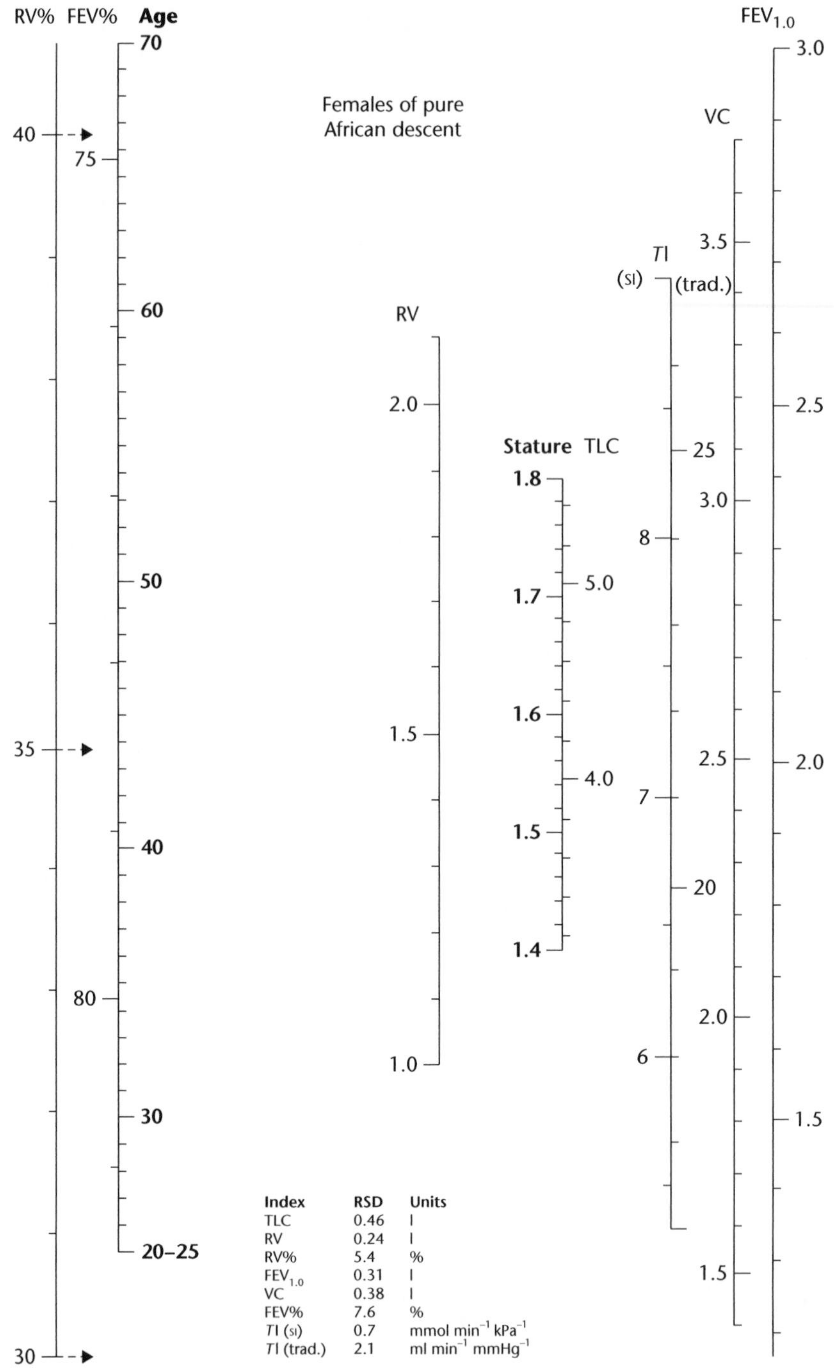

Index	RSD	Units
TLC	0.46	l
RV	0.24	l
RV%	5.4	%
$FEV_{1.0}$	0.31	l
VC	0.38	l
FEV%	7.6	%
Tl (SI)	0.7	mmol min^{-1} kPa^{-1}
Tl (trad.)	2.1	ml min^{-1} $mmHg^{-1}$

Fig. 27.8 Nomogram relating indices of lung function to stature and age for healthy adult women of African descent. The RV% and FEV% are related only to age and the TLC only to stature. Source: [9].

The lung function standardised for age and stature of asymptomatic Aboriginals is reported as 75% of that of Caucasians [82]. In this they resemble some of the present inhabitants of southeast Asia. Contributory factors in some subjects can include clinically silent lung airway disease, the possession of a short trunk relative to stature and/or central obesity. People of mixed race (usually Aboriginal mother and Caucasian father) have intermediate values.

New Zealand Maoris. The Maoris are Mongoloid people who reached New Zealand by boat from the Philippines some 1000 years ago. Their lung function is reported as being less than that of Caucasians. In adults the difference is of the order of 10% [83], similar to that of some other Mongoloid people (*q.v.*). In children the ethnic difference varies linearly with stature [84], so it cannot be represented by a single number. The association with stature may reflect an early onset of puberty.

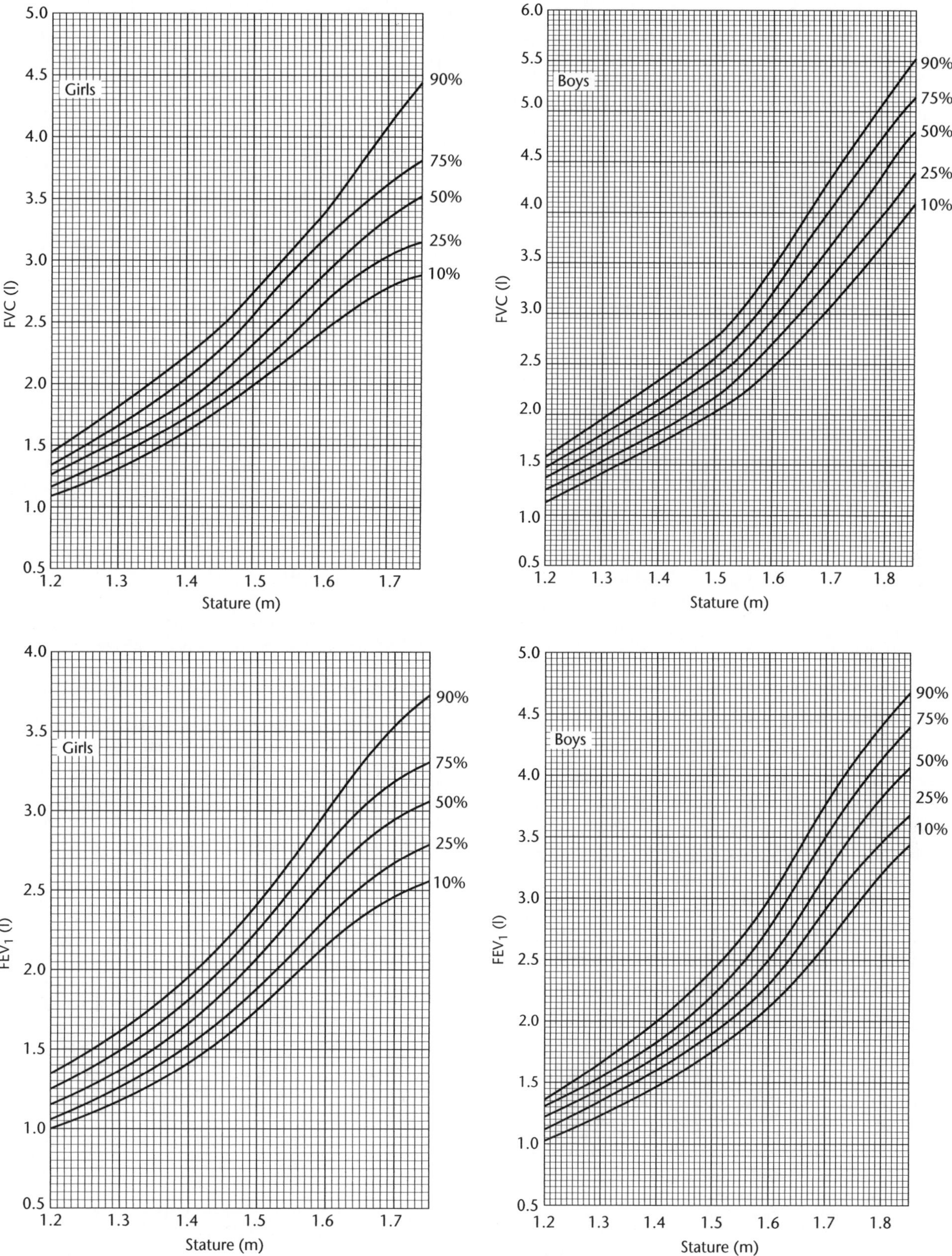

Fig. 27.9 Percentiles describing the development of forced expiratory volume and vital capacity in black children aged 6–18 years in six US cities. Source: [77].

Table 27.9 Reference values for ventilatory capacity of children in Nottingham, UK some of whose parents came from West Africa or the Punjab.

Index	Eqn for Caucasians	Factors for other children	Coefficient of variation
FEV_1 (l)	$0.731 \times St^{2.95}$	−12% if male −15% if female,	12%
FVC (l)	$0.837 \times St^{3.00}$	−13% if male −20% if female,	12%
PEF (l min^{-1})*	$2.26 \times St^{2.33}$	None	14%

* An adjustment should be made for alinearity in the scale of the meter (Section 12.3.2). Source: [76].

Papua New Guinea. The lung function of people in Papua-New Guinea was investigated in the early 1970s as part of the International Biological Programme. At that time, compared with Caucasians, the standardised lung volumes and FEV_1 of people on the coast were smaller by a factor of approximately 10% in men and 12 % in women. There was no difference in transfer factor (Table 27.3). The lung function of highlanders more nearly resembled that of Caucasians [85]. The standardised ventilation and cardiac frequency during submaximal exercise reflected the levels of habitual activity, but standardised tidal volume was smaller and ventilatory response to carbon dioxide less than in Caucasians [13, 19].

27.3 Perspective

A person's genetic constitution influences the size of the lungs relative to indices of body length. Some of the variation on this account is associated with racial group. Additional variation is contributed by selective migration, nutrition, habitual activity and other environmental factors. Together these features give rise to ethnic differences in lung volumes and related indices between peoples. The variations are of sufficient size so neglect of them can lead to the lung function being interpreted incorrectly. In some situations this can have serious consequences. For example, in sickle cell disease the use of inappropriate reference values can lead to a misdiagnosis of restrictive lung disease.

The magnitude of the ethnic factor can be up to 25%, but is usually less. It is also diminishing as a result of miscegenation, improvements in nutrition and hygiene and improvements in the quality of the measurements. In the future it could be further reduced by extending the range of anthropometric reference variables by which the lung function is described. Meanwhile, the best available allowance should be made; to this end, where there is uncertainty the need to establish an ethnic identity should be explained to the subject and, if necessary, the ethnic pedigree established. This can be used to interpolate between reference values for the parent populations. Local reference values or those given in the text should be used where appropriate. The use of standard factors without reference to local environmental and cultural circumstances can mislead [40]; they should only be used where there is no locally derived alternative (Table 27.10).

Table 27.10 Approximate factors for converting reference values for FEV_1 and FVC in Caucasian men to reflect the average lung function of other ethnic groups. For women a larger adjustment is usually needed.

Group	Factor*
North Indians and Pakistanis	1.0–0.87
South Indians, other southeast Asians	0.87–0.75
Hispanics	1.0
Orientals (men and women), from:	
Hong Kong, Inuit, Mongolians, North American Indians	1.0
Others	0.9
Sub-Saharan Africans	0.87 †
Polynesians and New Guineans	0.9
Australian Aboriginals	0.75–0.87‡

* The factor can be increased by 0.1 for persons who were physically very active in their youth or reared at altitude.
† Alternatively, for FEV_1 in men and women use −0.45 and −0.41, for FVC use −0.7 and −0.61.
‡ If mixed descent.
Notes: Factors for children are in the caption to Fig. 27.1. Locally determined reference values should be used where these are available. For details see text.

Future compilations of reference values should focus on the definition of the populations being investigated and the quality of the physiological and anthropometric measurements. The environmental conditions should be recorded. Consideration should be given to making additional anthropometric measurements, including thoracic dimensions and indices of body fat and fat-free mass; these should be analysed in a form that is independent of stature (Chapter 4 and Section 5.6.2).

27.4 References

1. Sykes B. *The seven daughters of Eve.* London: Bantam Press, 2001.
2. Hardy A, Tobias P. Cited in Douglas K. Taking the plunge. *New Sci* 2000; **2266**: 29–33.
3. Bhopal R. Glossary of terms relating to ethnicity and race: for reflection and debate. *J Epidemiol Comm Health* 2004; **58**: 441–445.
4. Cruickshank K, Beevers, DG eds. *Ethnic factors in health and disease.* London: Wright, 1989.
5. Paul R, Fletcher GH, Addison G. A comparative study between Europeans and Africans in the mining industry of Northern Rhodesia. *Med Proc* 1960; **6**: 69–77.
6. Glass WI. Ventilatory function differences between Polynesian and European rope workers. *N Z Med J* 1962; **61**: 433–444.
7. Abramowitz S, Lewis GC, Lewis WA et al. Vital capacity in the Negro. *Am Rev Respir Dis* 1965; **92**: 287–292.
8. Cotes JE, Malhotra MS. Differences in lung function between Indians and Europeans. *J Physiol (Lond)* 1965; **177**: 17P–18P.

9. Miller GJ, Cotes JE, Hall AM et al.Lung function and exercise performance of healthy Caribbean men and women of African ethnic origin. *Q J Exp Physiol* 1972; **57**: 325–341.
10. Anderson HR, Anderson JA, Cotes JE. Lung function values in healthy children and adults from highland and coastal areas of Papua New Guinea. *Papua New Guinea Med J* 1974; **17**: 165–167.
11. Jones PRM, Baber FM, Heywood C, Cotes JE. Ventilatory capacity in healthy Chinese children: relation to habitual activity. *Ann Hum Biol* 1977; **4**: 155–161.
12. Bangham CRM, Veale KEA. Ventilatory capacity in healthy Nepalese. *J Physiol (Lond)* 1977; **265**: 31P–32P.
13. Cotes JE, Anderson HR, Patrick JM. Lung function and the response to exercise in New Guineans; role of genetic and environmental factors. *Phil Trans R Soc B*. 1974; **268:** 349–361.
14. Cotes JE, Dabbs JM, Hall AM et al. Lung volumes, ventilatory capacity and transfer factor in healthy British boy and girl twins. *Thorax* 1973; **28**; 709–715.
15. White NW, Hanley JH, Lalloo UG, Becklake MR. Review and analysis of variation between spirometric values reported in 29 studies of healthy African adults. *Am J Respir Crit Care Med* 1994; **150**: 348–355.
16. Massey DG, Fournier-Massey G. Japanese-American pulmonary reference values - influence of environment on anthropology and physiology. *Environ Rec* 1986; **39**: 418–433.
17. Miall WE, Ashcroft MT. Lovell HG, Moore FA. Longitudinal study of the decline in adult height in two Welsh communities. *Human Biol* 1967; **39**: 445–454.
18. Reed TE. Caucasian genes in American negroes. *Science* 1969; **165**: 762–768
19. Patrick JM, Cotes JE. Anthropometric and other factors affecting respiratory responses to CO_2 in New Guineans *Phil Trans R Soc Lond (Biol)* 1974; **268**: 363–373.
20. Patrick JM. Respiratory responses to CO_2-rebreathing in Nigerian men. *Q J Exp Physiol Cogn Med Sci* 1976; **61**: 85–93.
21. Cotes JE, Heywood C, Laurence KM. Determinants of respiratory function in boy and girl twins. In: Weiner JS, ed.*Physiological variation and its genetic basis.* Vol. 17. *Symposia of Society for the Study of Human Biology*, London: Taylor and Francis, 1977: 77–85.
22. Schwartz J, Katz SA, Fegley RW, Tockman MS. Sex and race differences in the development of lung function. *Am Rev Respir Dis* 1988; **138**: 1415-1421; also Brooks LE et al. Sex and race differences in the development of lung function. *Am Rev Respir Dis* 1989; **140**: 855.
23. Miller GJ, Saunders MJ, Gilson RJ, Ashcroft MT. Superior lung function and exercise performance of Jamaican children belonging to a hill farming community as compared with their urban copatriots. *Thorax* 1976; **31**: 481–482.
24. Kagamimori S, Robson JM, Heywood C, Cotes JE. Genetic and environmental determinants of the cardio-respiratory response to submaximal exercise – a six year follow-up study of twins. *Ann Hum Biol* 1984; **11**: 29–38.
25. Lung and Asthma Information Agency. *Ethnic variation in lower respiratory disease.* London. Public Health Science Dept. St George's Hospital, Factsheet 2000/1
26. Harik-Khan RI, Fleg JL, Muller DC, Wise RA. The effect of anthropometric and socioeconomic factors on the racial difference in lung function. *Am J Respir Crit Care Med* 2001; **164**: 1647–1654.
27. Chan C-C, Cheong T-H, Poh S-C, Wang Y-T. Lung elastic recoil in normal young adult Chinese compared with Caucasians. *Eur Respir J* 1995; **8**: 446–449.
28. Donnelly PM, Yang T-S, Peat JK, Woolcock AJ. What factors explain racial differences in lung volumes? *Eur Respir J* 1991; **4**: 829–838.
29. Johan A, Chan CC, Chia HP et al. Maximal respiratory pressures in adult Chinese, Malays and Indians. *Eur Respir J* 1997, **10**: 2825–2828.
30. Pool JB, Greenough A. Ethnic variation in respiratory function in young children *Respir Med* 1989; **83**: 123–125.
31. Chinn S, Rona RJ. Height and age adjustments for cross sectional studies of lung function in children aged 6–11 years. *Thorax* 1992; **47**: 707–714.
32. Chatterjee S, Saha D, Chatterjee BP. Pulmonary function studies in healthy non-smoking men of Calcutta. *Ann Hum Biol* 1988; **15**: 365–374.
33. Malik MA, Moss E, Lee WR. Prediction values for the ventilatory capacity in male West Pakistani workers in the United Kingdom. *Thorax* 1972; **27**: 611–619.
34. Jain SK, Ramiah TJ. Normal standards of pulmonary function tests for healthy Indian men 15–40 years old: comparison of different regression equations (prediction formulae). *Indian J Med Res* 1969; **57**: 1453–1466.
35. Miller GJ, Ashcroft MT, Swan AV, Beadnell HMSG. Ethnic variation in forced expiratory volume and forced vital capacity of African and Indian adults in Guyana. *Am Rev Respir Dis* 1970; **102**: 979–981.
36. Kamat SR, Tyahi NK, Rashid SSA. Lung function in Indian adult subjects. *Lung India.* 1982; **1**: 11–21.
37. Milledge JS. Vital capacity and forced expiratory volume one second in South Indian men. *Ind J Chest Dis* 1965; **2**: 97–103.
38. Vijayan VK, Kuppurao KV, Venkatesan P et al. Pulmonary function in healthy young adult Indians in Madras. *Thorax* 1990; **45**: 611–615.
39. Cotes JE, Dabbs JM, Hall AM et al. Lung function of healthy young men in India: contributory roles of genetic and environmental factors. *Proc R Soc Lond (Biol)* 1975; **191**: 413–425.
40. Nadeem MA, Raza SN, Malik MA. Ventilatory function of healthy, urban, non-smoking, Pakistani young adults aged 18–24 years. *Respir Med* 1999; **93**: 546–551.
41. Jain SK, Gupta CK. Lung function studies in healthy men and women over forty. *Indian J Med Res* 1967; **55**: 612–619.
42. Mahajan KK, Mahajan A, Mishra N. Pulmonary functions in healthy females of Haryana. *Indian J Chest Dis Allied Sci* 1997; **39**: 163–171.
43. Patel RK, Bhagat GR, Kaji BC et al. Study of pulmonary function tests in 2000 healthy persons in Gujarat *J Assoc Physicians India* 1998; **46**: 689–694.
44. Chatterjee S, Mandal A. Pulmonary function studies in healthy schoolboys of West Bengal. *Japanese J Physiol* 1991; **41**: 797–808.
45. Chowgule RV, Shetye VM, Parmar JR. Lung function tests in normal Indian children. *Indian Pediatr* 1995; **32**: 185–191.
46. Sharma PP, Gupta P, Deshpande R, Gupta P. Lung function values in healthy children (10–15 years). *Indian J Pediatr* 1997; **64**: 85–91.
47. Mahajan RKK, Mahajan A. Ventilatory function tests in school children of 6—13 years. *Indian J Chest Dis Allied Sci* 1997; **39**: 97–105.
48. Vijayan VK, Reetha AM, Kuppurao KV et al. Pulmonary function in normal south Indian children aged 7 to 19 years. *Indian J Chest Dis Allied Sci* 2000; **42**: 147–156.
49. Mathur N, Rastogi SK, Husain T, Gupta BN. Lung function norms in healthy working women. *Indian J Physiol Pharmacol* 1998; **42**: 245–251.
50. Mukhopadhvay S, Macleod KA, Ong TJ, Ogston SA. "Ethnic" variation in childhood lung function may relate to preventable nutritional deficiency *Acta Pediatr* 2001; **90**: 1299–1303.

51. Fulambarker A, Copur AS, Javeri A et al. Reference values for pulmonary function in Asian Indians living in the United States. *Chest* 2004; **126**: 1225–1233.
52. Ismail Y, Azmi NN, Zurkurnain Y. Lung function in Malay children *Med J Malaysia* 1993; **48**: 171–174.
53. Singh R, Singh HJ, Sirisinghe RG. Spirometric studies in Malaysians between 13 and 69 years of age. *Med J Malaysia* 1993; **48**: 175–184.
54. Chia SE, Wang YT, Chan OY, Poh SC. Pulmonary function in healthy Chinese, Malay and Indian adults in Singapore. *Ann Acad Med* 1993; **22**: 878–884.
55. Connett GJ, Quak SH, Wong ML et al. Lung function reference values in Singaporean children aged 6–18 years. *Thorax* 1994; **49**: 901–905.
56. Editorial. Respiratory function tests: reference norms for the Sinhalese. *Ceylon Med J* 1995; **40**: 53–58.
57. Perez-Padilla R, Regalado-Pineda J, Rojas M et al. Spirometric function in children of Mexico City compared with Mexican–American children. *Pediat Pulmonol* 2003; **35**: 177–183.
58. Crapo RO, Jensen RL, Lockey JE et al. Normal spirometric values in healthy Hispanic Americans. *Chest* 1990; **98**: 1435–1439
59. Hankinson JL, Odencrantz JR, Fedan KB. Spirometric reference values from a sample of the general U.S. population. *Am J Respir Crit Care Med* 1999; **159**: 179–187.
60. Golshan M, Nematbakhsh M, Amra B, Crapo RO. Spirometric reference values in a large Middle Eastern population. *Eur Respir J* 2003; **22**: 529–534.
61. Sliman NA, Dajani BM, Dajani HM. Ventilatory function test values of healthy adult Jordanians. *Thorax* 1981; **36**: 546–549.
62. Shamssain MH, Thompson J, Ogston SA. Forced expiratory volume in normal Libyan children aged 6–19 years. *Thorax* 1988; **43**: 467–470.
63. Shamssain MH. Forced expiratory indices in normal Libyan men. *Thorax* 1988; **43**: 923–925.
64. Korotzer B, Ong S, Hansen JE. Ethnic differences in pulmonary function in healthy nonsmoking Asian-Americans and European-Americans. *Am J Respir Crit Care Med* 2000; **161**: 1101–1108.
65. Ip MSM, Karlberg EM, Karlberg JPE et al.Lung function reference values in Chinese children and adolescents in Hong Kong. 1. Spirometric values and comparison with other populations. *Am J Respir Crit Care Med* 2000; **162**: 424–429.
66. Ip MSM, Karlberg EM, Chan K-N. et al. Lung function reference values in Chinese children and adolescents in Hong Kong. 2.Prediction equations for plethysmographic lung volumes. *Am J Respir Crit Care Med* 2000; **162**: 430–435.
67. Wall MA, Olson D, Bonn BA et al. Lung function in North American Indian Children: reference standards for spirometry, maximal expiratory flow volume curves and peak expiratory flow. *Am Rev Respir Dis* 1982; **125**: 158–162.
68. Crapo RO, Lockey J, Aldrich V et al. Normal spirometric values in healthy American Indians. *J Occup Med* 1988; **30**: 556–560.
69. Rode A, Shephard RJ. The ageing of lung function: cross-sectional and longitudinal studies of an Inuit community. *Eur Respir J* 1994; **7**: 1653–1659.
70. Krause TG, Pedersen BV, Thomsen SF et al. Lung function in Greenlandic and Danish children and adolescents. *Resp Med* 2005; **99**: 363–371.
71. Crapo RO, Jensen RL, Oyunchimeg M et al. Differences in spirometric reference values: a statistical comparison of a Mongolian and a Caucasian study. *Eur Respir J* 1999; **13**: 606–609.
72. Rossiter CE, Weill H. Ethnic difference in lung function; evidence for proportional differences. *Int J Epidemiol* 1974; **3**: 55–61.
73. Binder RE, Mitchell CSA, Schoenberg JB, Bouhuys A. Lung function among black and white children. *Amer Rev Respir Dis* 1976; **114** 955–959.
74. Patrick JM, Femi-Pearse D. Reference values for $FEV_{1.0}$ and FVC in Nigerian men and women: a graphical summary. *Niger Med J* 1976; **6**: 380–385.
75. Dockery DW, Berkey CS, Ware JH et al. Distribution of forced vital capacity and forced expiratory volume in one second in children 6 to 11 years of age. *Am Rev Respir Dis* 1983; **128**: 405–412.
76. Patrick JM, Patel A. Ethnic differences in the growth of lung function in children: a cross-sectional study in inner-city Nottingham. *Ann Hum Biol* 1986; **13**: 307–315.
77. Wang X, Dockery DW, Wypij D et al. Pulmonary function between 6 to 18 years of age. *Pediatr Pulmonol* 1993; **15**: 75–88.
78. Mengesha YA, Mekonnen Y. Spirometric lung function tests in normal non-smoking Ethiopian men and women. *Thorax* 1985; **40**: 465–468, *erratum Thorax* 1986; **41**: 223
79. Orie NN. Comparison of normal respiratory function values in young Kenyans with those of other Africans and Caucasians. *East Afr Med J* 1999; **76**: 321–334.
80. Miller GJ, Ashcroft MT. A community survey of respiratory disease among East Indian and African adults in Guyana. *Thorax* 1971; **26**: 331–338.
81. Cookson JB, Mataka G. Prevalence of chronic bronchitis in Rhodesian Africans. *Thorax* 1978; **33**: 328–334.
82. Thompson JE, Sleigh A, Passey ME et al. Ventilatory standards for clinically well Aboriginal adults *Med J Aust* 1992; **156**: 566–569.
83. De Hamel FA, Welford B. Lung function in Maoris and Samoans working in New Zealand. *NZ Med J* 1983; **96**: 560–562.
84. Asher MI, Douglas C, Stewart AW et al. Lung volumes in Polynesian children. *Am Rev Respir Dis* 1987; **136**: 1360–1365.
85. Cotes JE, Saunders MJ, Adam JER et al. Lung function in coastal and highland New Guineans: comparison with Europeans. *Thorax* 1973; **28**: 320–330.

Further reading

Bhattacharya AK, Banerjee S. Vital capacity in children and young adults of India. *Indian J Med Res* 1966; **54**: 62–71.

Bhopal R. Is research into ethnicity and health racist, unsound or important science? *BMJ* 1997; **314**: 1751.

Boyce AJ, Haight JS, Rimmer DB, Harrison GA. Respiratory function in Peruvian Quechua Indians. *Ann Hum Biol* 1974; **1**: 137–148.

Da Costa JL. Pulmonary function studies in healthy Chinese adults in Singapore. *Am Rev Respir Dis* 1971; **104**: 128–131.

Edwards RHT, Miller GJ, Hearn CED, Cotes JE. Pulmonary function and exercise responses in relation to body composition and ethnic origin in Trinidadian males. *Proc R Soc Lond (Biol)* 1972; **181**: 407–420.

Enright PL, Arnold A, ManolioTA, Kuller LH. Spirographic reference values for healthy elderly Blacks. *Chest* 1996; **110**: 1416–1424.

Lam K-K, Pang S-C, Allan WGL et al. A survey of ventilatory capacity in Chinese subjects in Hong Kong. *Ann Hum Biol* 1982; **9**: 459–472.

Malik SK, Jindal SK, Jindal V, Bausal S. Peak expiratory flow rate in healthy adults. *Ind J Chest Dis* 1975; **17**: 166–171.

Marcus EB, Maclean CJ, Curb JD et al. Reference values for FEV in Japanese-American men from 45 to 68 years of age. *Am Rev Respir Dis* 1988; **138**: 1393–1397.

Schwartz J, Katz SA, Fegley RW, Tockman MS. Sex and race differences in the development of lung function. *Am J Respir Dis* 1988; **138**: 1415–1421.

Smolej-Narancic N, Pavlovic M, Rudan P. Ventilatory parameters in healthy nonsmoking adults of Adriatic island (Yugoslavia). *Eur Respir J* 1991; **4**: 955–964.

Yang T-S, Peat J, Keena V et al. Review of the racial differences in the lung function of normal Caucasian, Chinese and Indian subjects. *Eur Respir J* 1991; **4**: 872–880.

Yokoyama T, Mitsufuji M. Statistical representation of the ventilatory capacity of 2247 healthy Japanese adults. *Chest* 1972; **61**: 655–661.

PART 4
Exercise

CHAPTER 28

Physiology of Exercise and Changes Resulting from Lung Disease

During exercise the role of the lungs is to sustain the required ventilation without undue breathlessness. This role is compromised by lung diseases. The normal and clinical physiology of exercise is described in this chapter. Details of clinical exercise testing, including reference values and interpretation are given in Chapter 29, exercise capacity and disability are in Chapter 30 and exercise in children is in Chapter 31.

28.1 Some basic concepts

What is exercise? Exercise entails contraction and relaxation of voluntary muscles. The contraction can be short-lived (a kick), sustained (carrying an object), or repetitive (walking), and can be isometric (tug-of-war) or isotonic (standing erect from squatting, or lifting a weight) but in most normal activities it is a combination of all of these. The exercise usually involves many muscle groups, most of which are performing physical work. This is done when the force produced by a muscle in a particular direction results in a movement in the same direction. The work is the product of the force and the distance. If there is no movement (as when straining against a stationary object) no work is done; thus the term static work is a misnomer.

The work done in effecting a particular movement is strictly independent of the time the movement takes, but the time determines the rate of work; this is the power output and has the units: force × distance ÷ time. Examples are kg m min^{-1} and watts that are used to describe power output during cycle ergometry (Section 29.4.3). Some components of work are in Table 28.1. This table also lists other calls on a person's metabolism when they perform work. The need to meet them has the consequence

Table 28.1 Components of the energy cost of exercise.

Component		Example or comment
Anticipation of exercise		Increased metabolism produces heat
Work done against:	An ergometer	Treadmill, cycle, ladder mill etc
	Gravity	Lifting the trunk, as in walking
		Lifting the limbs, as in cycling
	Wind resistance	Running
	Body mass	Alternating acceleration and deceleration as when walking
External friction		Heat in bearings of ergometer, tyre in contact with road etc.
Internal friction		Work of breathing – increased by hyperbaria and lung diseases, reduced at high altitude
		Movement of joints
		Circulation of blood
Generation of heat		Warm up, shivering

that measurable external work only accounts for about a quarter of the total energy expended during exercise. The rest is dissipated in other ways (Table 28.1).

The main source of energy is aerobic catabolism (combustion) of food, including glycogen that is present in muscle fibres and glucose and fatty acids that are transported there by circulating blood. During exercise of moderate intensity the supply of these substances (the substrates) usually keeps up with the demand, hence the designation *steady state exercise.* The metabolic processes are facilitated by enzymes present in mitochondria. The concentrations of the relevant enzymes are highest in *Type 1 muscle fibres* (slow twitch); these fibres have a high oxidative potential (Section 28.9.1). In addition, at the start of exercise or when the demand is further increased, extra energy can be obtained almost immediately by non-oxidative metabolism of glucose and glycogen, hence the designation rapid glycolysis (Section 28.9.2). The process was formerly incorrectly called anaerobic metabolism. Rapid glycolysis is conducted by enzymes present in the cytoplasm of muscle fibres, particularly that of *Type 2 fibres* (fast twitch). It carries the penalty that the immediate end product is lactic acid. Small quantities can be metabolised or reconverted to glycogen, but lactic acid that accumulates in the blood causes acidaemia and stimulates breathing. The resulting breathlessness and fatigue progressively discourage further exertion. During recovery after such exercise additional oxygen (the so called *oxygen debt*) is used to dispose of the lactic acid, rebuild the stores of adenosine tri-phosphate (ATP) and phosphocreatine in the muscles and reoxygenate myoglobin; the latter is an oxygen-binding protein found in muscle. These aspects are described subsequently. The oxygen cost of heavy exercise is the sum of the oxygen consumed during the exercise and the oxygen debt. During exercise of nearly maximal intensity the metabolic need is met by a combination of aerobic and rapid glycolysis, but a point comes when the aerobic mechanism is making a maximal contribution and the subject has attained his or her *aerobic capacity.* The corresponding oxygen uptake is the *maximal oxygen uptake.* This is designated $\dot{V}O_2max$ and $\dot{n}O_2max$, respectively, in the traditional and SI systems.

Terminology for maximal exercise. In most circumstances, the maximal oxygen uptake is a capacity measurement in that it is not increased by a further increase in the external work. Hence, aerobic capacity and maximal oxygen uptake are synonymous. The associated work level is actually submaximal as, given the motivation, a further increase can be achieved using energy obtained by rapid glycolysis. A different situation obtains at high altitude or with many medical conditions, including respiratory disorders. Here, exercise of increasing intensity is limited by breathlessness or another symptom before the oxygen uptake has reached a plateau value. As a result the aerobic capacity cannot be measured. In this circumstance (but not otherwise) the maximal oxygen uptake is a peak value that corresponds to the limiting work rate and is designated $\dot{V}O_2peak$ or *symptom limited maximal oxygen uptake* (e.g. $\dot{V}O_2max,s\,l$). The distinction is important for those respiratory patients where there is a need to establish if he or she has exercised maximally within the constraint imposed by respiratory impairment (Section 28.8.1). The exercise protocol is summarised in Section 29.3.

Units of maximal oxygen uptake. Maximal oxygen uptake (aerobic capacity) is best reported as oxygen uptake in mmol min^{-1} or l STPD min^{-1}. This figure is then interpreted for the individual subject by making allowance for age, body size and expected power output. The latter depends mainly on the quantity of muscle and the intensity of its use. When these variables are allowed for, aerobic capacity is nearly independent of gender (Section 28.10). Hence, maximal O_2 uptake is usually best described by a linear regression that includes terms for fat free mass and, the rating for habitual activity (Table 29.15, page 433). If fat-free mass is not available, it can be replaced in the regression by terms for age, body mass and stature. The traditional alternative of expressing $\dot{V}o_2$max per kg body mass, although widely used is not acceptable because the relationship of uptake to mass is not a proportionality [1] (also Section 5.3.1). Use of $\dot{V}o_2$max per kg can lead to the erroneous conclusion that small persons, by virtue of their size, are necessarily fitter than larger ones!

28.2 Oxygen cost of exercise

Most sustainable activities depend on aerobic glycolysis, hence the activities can be quantified in terms of the associated consumption of oxygen. The average oxygen costs of a range of activities are indicated in Fig. 28.1.

In almost all instances the cost is related positively to body mass; the dependence is high for exercise done against gravity as in walking up an incline or performing stepping exercise, and low for cycle ergometry, where most of the work is done against the ergometer. Any of these forms of exercise can be used in the assessment of the physiological responses, so the different relationships of oxygen cost to rate of work and body mass need to be taken into account when interpreting the results (e.g. Table 29.3 cf. Table 29.5, also Table 29.5, pages 420–423).

For any activity the oxygen cost is reduced by familiarity and by training through better coordination and economy of movement. These attributes are affected negatively by increasing age and by ill health. The oxygen cost is increased in obesity. The

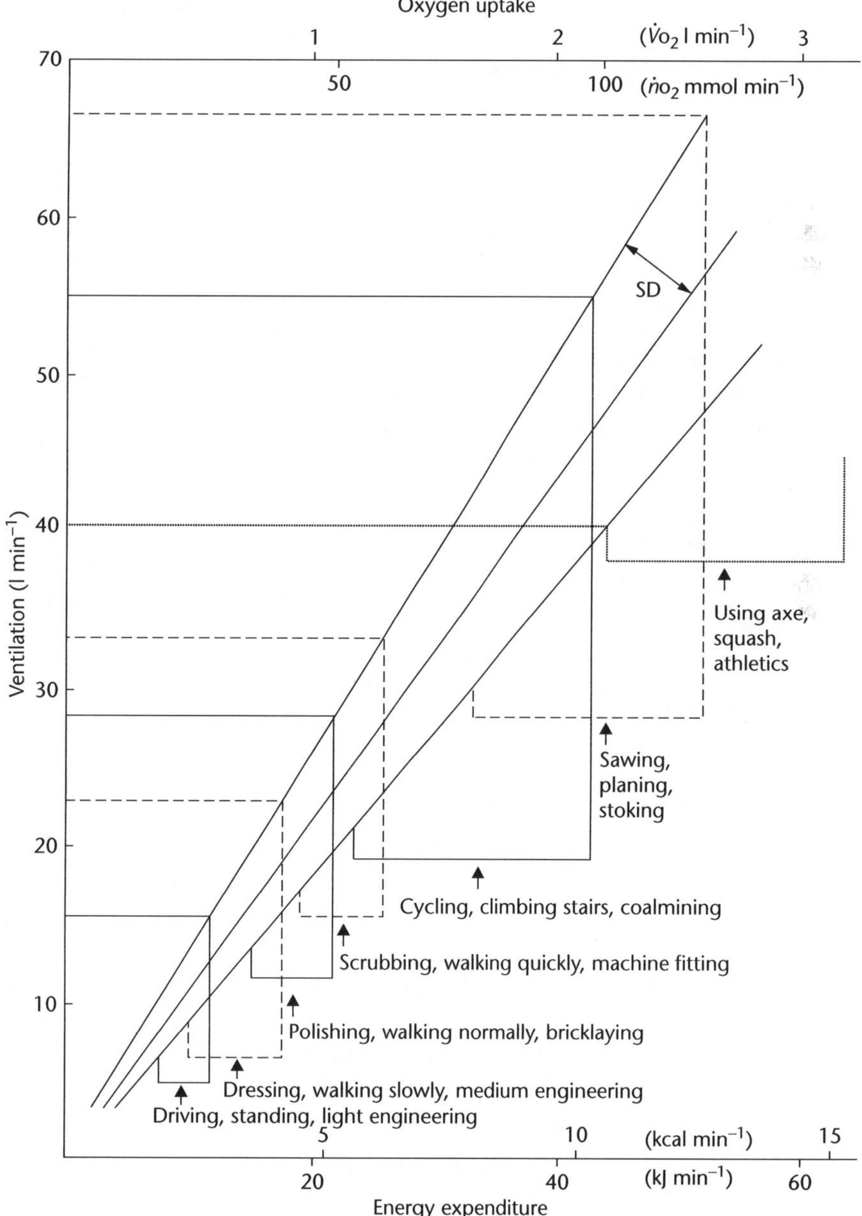

Fig. 28.1 Average energy and ventilatory costs of activities for healthy men with an indication of the between-subject variation (given by the vertical and horizontal lines). In women the ventilatory costs are similar but the energy costs are approximately 10% lower. Ventilation is increased by age, smoking, respiratory symptoms and other factors; it is below average in persons who are physically fit. Source: [2]

extra mass of fat exerts a training effect, but this is more than offset by the additional energy cost of movement (Table 28.1). Energy costs are increased in hyperthyroidism [3].

The measurement of oxygen cost is an integral part of any assessment where there is an interest in physical performance. However, during a routine exercise test the measurement is useful mainly as providing a reference variable for interpreting the ventilatory and cardiovascular responses. The component of oxygen uptake that is attributable to the oxygen cost of breathing can be a factor limiting exercise in some circumstances (Section 9.7.2).

28.3 Determinants of exercise capacity: an overview

During the course of man's evolution the capacity for exercise has been a key factor in survival in competition with the animal kingdom, fellow humans and the constraints imposed by the environment. These aspects are brought together in Fig. 28.2.

The principal *anatomical* determinant of exercise capacity is body size. This influences the dimensions of the oxygen transport system, the mass of muscle that can be brought into use, and the mechanical conditions under which the muscle operates. Body size is influenced by both genetic and environmental factors. A person's genes determine his or her potential for exercise. Environmental factors, including diet and habitual activity determine the extent to which the potential is realised. Growth hormone and anabolic steroids are intermediaries, particularly during adolescence. Gender and age are also important.

The principal *physiological* determinants of exercise capacity are those of the respective aerobic and glycolytic pathways, particularly the oxygen transport chain; these comprise ventilation of the lungs (also called external respiration), diffusion of oxygen from lungs to blood, circulation of blood transporting oxygen attached to haemoglobin, diffusion of oxygen across the capillary muscle membrane and within the muscle, and manipulation of oxygen by enzymes within mitochondria (Chapter 21). A similar transport chain conveys carbon dioxide in the reverse direction (Chapter 22). The capacities of the different components of the chain for oxygen are approximately matched. Thus, in one study, differences in aerobic power between groups of subjects were associated with similar differences in lung function, total body haemoglobin, cardiac interval (hence stroke volume) during standard exercise, total body potassium (hence body cell mass) and muscle size [5] (see also Fig. 4.1, page 32). The matching can be disturbed by a number of factors such as, for the lungs, having asthma in childhood or, for the muscles, the techniques of body building. The matching is never perfect so the stages do not contribute equally to exercise limitation. Instead, the principal limiting factor in normal circumstances is now believed to be diffusion of oxygen across the capillary muscle membrane (Sections 28.8.3 and 28.8.4). The resulting flow of oxygen is greatly influenced by the mean capillary oxygen tension and hence the ability of the circulation to deliver blood to the muscle capillaries. This implies that the limit is set by the circulation. By contrast the lungs normally have spare capacity; this is called upon at high altitude and is used up in the early stages of many lung diseases. The principal factors that contribute to limitation are summarised in Table 28.2. Some details, including the role

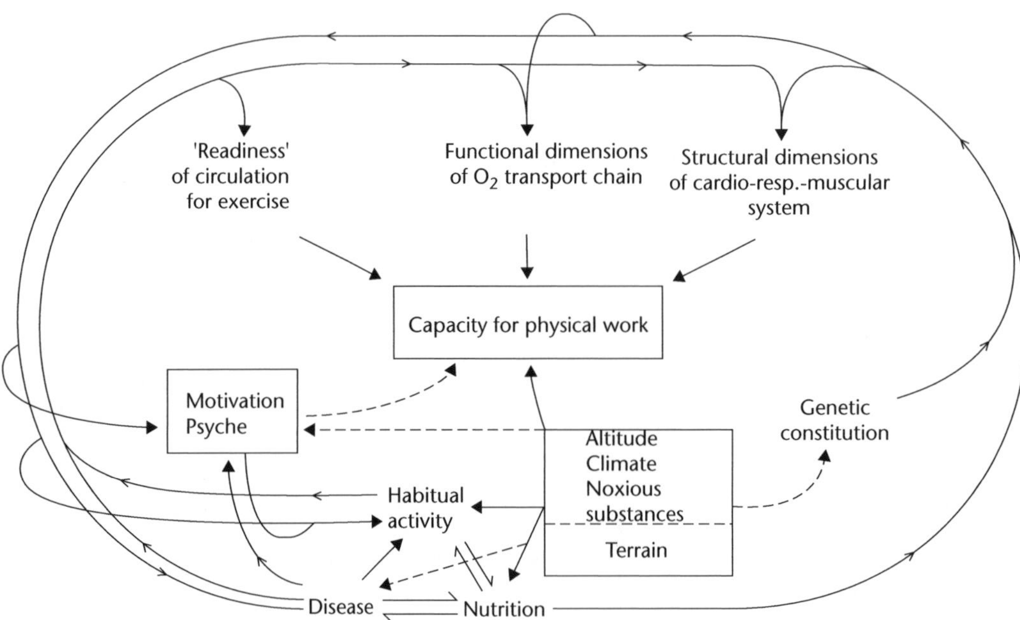

Fig. 28.2 Determinants of capacity for physical work. Source: [4]

Table 28.2 Causes of a reduced exercise capacity.

Mechanism	Conditions that can render it critical
Oxygen cost increased	Obesity, hyperthyroidism
Exercise ventilation approaches limiting value	Ventilatory capacity reduced or respiratory drive increased (e.g. by hypoxia, over-breathing etc)
Ventilation wasted by: shallow, rapid breathing. $\dot{V}A/\dot{Q}$ imbalance	Lung diseases, pulmonary congestion.
Gas transfer inadequate	At altitude, hypoxia at sea level Diseases/disorders of lung parenchyma
Insufficient oxyhaemoglobin	Anaemia (converse is polycythaemia), vascular shunt, haemoglobin inactivated by CO or other substance
Cardiac output insufficient	Especially if sedentary lifestyle, cardiac disorder, insufficient blood volume (Section 28.8.3) or requirement increased by hyperthermia
Reduced muscle blood flow	Lack of use. Unfavourable distribution of cardiac output
Insufficient O_2 transfer from muscle capillaries	A high requirement for oxygen
Tissue hypoxia	Rarely a limiting factor, except with poisoning, e.g. by cyanide
Altered metabolism	Myopathy, increased rapid glycolysis (from any cause)
Disagreeable sensation (usually breathlessness)	Secondary to lung disease or other factor Low tolerance of discomfort Aggravating psychological factor

of gas exchange and the differences between what are essentially circulatory and ventilatory causes of limitation are considered in Section 28.8.

28.4 Respiratory response to exercise

28.4.1 Introduction

The level of ventilation is controlled by the respiratory reticular formation in the medulla. This has an intrinsic rhythmicity that is continuously modified by positive and negative stimuli from a number of sources. They include the cerebral cortex, hypothalamus, other parts of the brain, central and peripheral chemoreceptors and mechanoreceptors in the airways, lung parenchyma and muscles, including the respiratory muscles (Chapter 23). An increase in ventilation occurs on exercise and can give rise to breathlessness on exertion. This symptom is an inevitable accompaniment of heavy exercise and is the commonest symptom experienced by patients with lung disease. Hence, the level of ventilation is an appropriate starting point for consideration of the physiological response to exercise.

28.4.2 Ventilation during exercise of constant intensity

At the start of exercise of constant intensity the ventilation typically increases abruptly (Fig. 28.3). The increase is accompanied by and probably contributes to a rise in cardiac output [7]. It appears to be due in part to an increased central drive to breathe [8], also known as central command [9], but other factors also contribute [10]. The initial increase in ventilation (phase 1) is followed by a slower progressive rise (phase 2). This leads into a ventilatory plateau, at which the level reflects the rate of work. If the rise is assumed to be exponential, it can be described by the time constant (*tau*, Section 20.9.1, also Section 29.3.2: 'Submaximal steady state protocol'). The time constants for the on- and off-transients at the start and end of exercise vary with age, physical condition and the intensity of the exercise. During moderate exercise the half times are of the order of 30 s [11]. During phase 2 the ventilation lags behind the metabolic changes with the result that arterial oxygen tension falls temporarily and carbon dioxide tension rises. The subsequent equilibrium occurs earlier for oxygen than for carbon dioxide (Fig. 28.4).

During exercise that can be sustained the plateau of ventilation (phase 3) is relatively stable and the subject is in a steady state. However, the ventilation may drift upwards after some 10–20 min as the body temperature rises [13]. During more strenuous exercise the plateau is replaced by a progressive rise. This is associated with a metabolic acidosis from lactic acid and leads to the exercise no longer being sustainable (Section 28.4.6).

At the end of exercise the changes in ventilation are the opposite of those at the start. Initially there is a precipitate reduction as central respiratory drive is withdrawn (phase 4). The arterial tension of carbon dioxide rises transiently in consequence (Fig. 28.4). Subsequently, the ventilation declines to the resting level (phase 5). The recovery takes approximately 5 min following steady state exercise, but longer if there has been a metabolic acidosis; the time is needed to pay off the oxygen debt including that associated with lactic acid (see 'What is exercise' above, also Section 28.9.2).

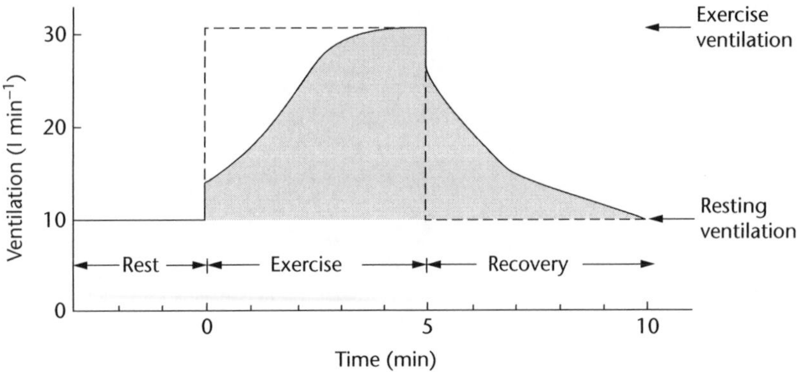

Fig. 28.3 Diagram showing the features of the ventilatory response to moderate exercise. The phases are described in the text. The area that is shaded represents the excess exercise ventilation (EEV) [6]. The part of the EEV that is incurred during recovery is normally equal to the ventilation deficit at the start of exercise; hence the two areas bounded by the curve and the interrupted lines are normally of equal size. The recovery area is larger when there is an oxygen debt.

Steady state exercise is used when it is proposed to study gas exchange, respiratory control and the circulatory adaptations to exercise (Section 29.3.2). Most routine exercise testing now entails progressive exercise (see below).

28.4.3 Ventilation during progressive exercise

For progressive exercise that is sustainable by aerobic glycolysis the ventilation is linearly related to uptake of oxygen. However, when the range of work levels include those that entail rapid glycolysis, the ventilation increases disproportionately, so the relationship of ventilation on O_2 uptake becomes curvilinear (Fig. 28.5). The onset of curvilinearity is designated *Owles point* [15]. Similar points on related graphs have other names; they include anaerobic threshold, lactic acid threshold and ventilatory threshold (Section 28.4.6). The ventilation can also be related to output of carbon dioxide (see below 'Carbon dioxide output').

How should ventilation be standardised?

Ventilation during progressive exercise can be related to time of exercise, rate of external work, carbon dioxide output or oxygen uptake. Of these, all but oxygen uptake has serious limitations as a means of standardising the ventilation.

Time during exercise implies the existence of a standard protocol of which currently there appears to be little prospect.

Rate of external work against an ergometer can be used to standardise ventilation and other variables within one type of ergometry (e.g. walking, cycling, stepping, climbing). It has the limitation that the rate may be in terms of arbitrary units such as when the subject attains a specified combination of treadmill speed and slope. Also the energy expenditure can be influenced by the length or mass of the subject's legs (Section 29.3.2). However, for some applications this is acceptable (provided the ergometer has been calibrated (Section 29.3). The use of percentage of maximal attained work level can be meaningful if the factor limiting exercise is the same for all the subjects.

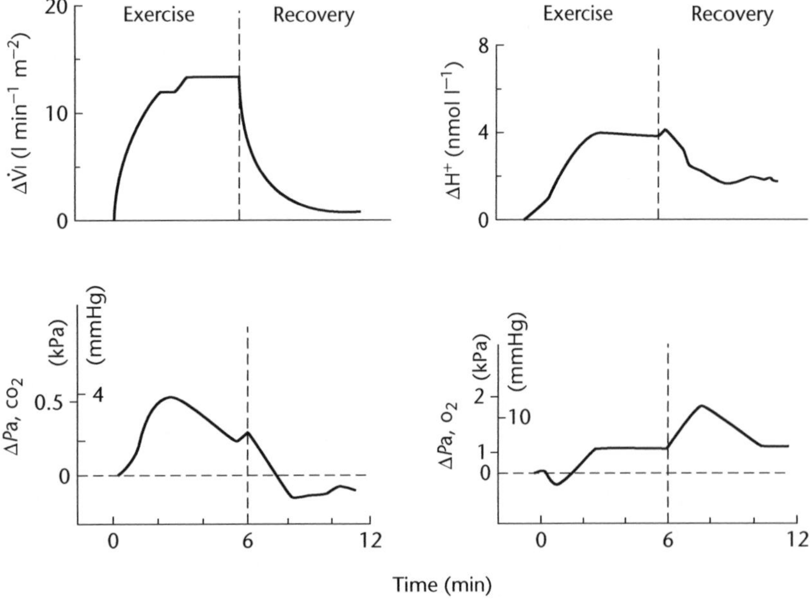

Fig. 28.4 Mean time course of deviations from resting values for ventilation ($\dot{V}_I$), hydrogen ion concentration $[H^+]$ and arterial tensions of carbon dioxide and oxygen (Pa,CO_2 and Pa,O_2) during and after moderate exercise in 5 healthy subjects. Source: [12]

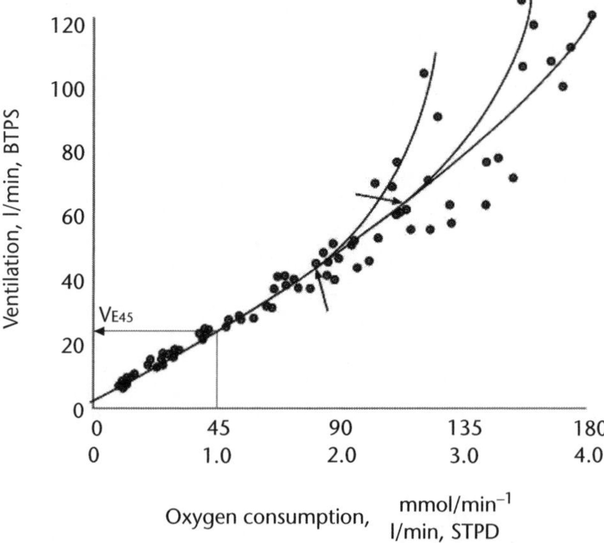

Fig. 28.5 Relationship of ventilation to uptake of oxygen during exercise in representative healthy subjects. Redrawn from [14]. The regression line has been fitted to the data points to the left of the lower arrow and does not go through the origin. The subsequent extrapolations are arbitrary to illustrate possible positions of Owles point (e.g. right hand arrow) but do not reflect the responses of individual subjects; (cf. Fig. 28.10). The figure also shows the derivation of the ventilation index $\dot{V}_{E45}$ (SI units), $\dot{V}_{E1.0}$ in traditional units.

Carbon dioxide output has the apparent advantage that its relation to ventilation, unlike that of oxygen, does not show an inflection point (Fig. 28.6b, also [16]). However, this is because the increase in ventilation at the inflection point for oxygen itself increases the elimination of carbon dioxide. Thus, CO_2 output is determined partly by the level of ventilation so, on its own, should not be used to describe it. Where standardisation is primarily in terms of O_2 uptake, additional standardisation in terms of CO_2 output or respiratory exchange ratio can sometimes be informative (Section 29.8.1).

Oxygen uptake during exercise reflects all components of the energy cost (see Table 28.1) and is only influenced by ventilation to the extent that the latter contributes to the oxygen cost of breathing – a second order effect. Thus, O_2 uptake is a suitable reference variable for defining ventilation. In the case of exercise below Owles point, a ventilation that is high relative to O_2 uptake is due to non-metabolic factors, for example an increase in respiratory drive from another cause, an alveolar deadspace or shallow breathing. Any of these factors can contribute to increased exercise ventilation in respiratory patients.

Indices of ventilation relative to O_2 uptake

Ventilation equivalent. Traditionally ventilation ($\dot{V}_E$) was considered to be proportional to oxygen uptake ($\dot{V}_{O_2}$) [14]. On this basis, the slope of the relationship ($\dot{V}_E/\dot{V}_{O_2}$) at oxygen uptakes below Owles point was a constant, designated ventilation equivalent (VE). Unfortunately, this convenient hypothesis ignored that the relationship is not a proportionality but has a significant constant term (Figs 28.5 and 28.6b, also Section 5.3.1). On this account, the ratio $\dot{V}_E/\dot{V}_{O_2}$ varies depending on the oxygen uptake (Fig. 28.6c). In descriptive terms, the ventilation equivalent decreases between rest and Owles point and then increases progressively. One implication is that every value for ventilation equivalent above Owles point has its duplicate below it. Thus, ventilation equivalent is an ambiguous index that is not independent of oxygen uptake. It should not be used to describe the level of ventilation during exercise.

Indices based on a linear model. The relationship of $\dot{V}_E$ to $\dot{V}_{O_2}$ is normally linear between rest and Owles point, so can be described by the parameters *m* and *c* of a linear equation (e.g. Table 29.15, page 433). Unpublished data suggest that in healthy young adults the parameters exhibit relatively little variation between individuals of the same sex. The slope is increased if the breathing is very shallow (airway deadspace effect), lung function is uneven ($\dot{V}_A/\dot{Q}$ effect), the respiratory drive is increased (RER increased) or Owles point is not identified correctly. The intercept reflects the ventilation of the deadspace per minute; it is not entirely independent of the slope.

For purposes of interpreting the ventilatory response to exercise, the use of the two parameters *m* and *c* of the linear equation (i.e. $y = mx + c$) can be inconvenient. Alternatively, the information they provide can be pooled and any ambiguity as to the appropriate work level avoided by using as an index the ventilation at a designated uptake of oxygen, for example 1.0 l min^{-1} or its SI equivalent 45 mmol min^{-1}, hence $\dot{V}_{E1.0}$ and $\dot{V}_{E45}$ [18]. This index has the merits that it is unambiguous, reflects the ventilation during normal daily activities (Fig. 28.1) and is increased if there is uneven lung function caused by smoking or any of several disease processes. However, a raised value may also be due to Owles point occurring at below the designated oxygen uptake (e.g. 45 mmol min^{-1} or 1.0 l min^{-1}). To allow for this, the interpretation should include noting the respiratory exchange ratio (see below) and inspecting the $\dot{V}_E/\dot{V}_{O_2}$ curve.

In population studies the $\dot{V}_{E45}$ is increased if there is a history of wheeze occasionally or other apparently trivial respiratory symptom, so the definition of the population is important [19]. Amongst asymptomatic adults (non-smokers) who agreed to perform an exercise test, mean values for $\dot{V}_{E45}$ in men and women, respectively, were in one study 23.1 and 26.0 l min^{-1} ($n = 373$ and 201) and in another 22.4 and 26.7 ± 3.68 l min^{-1} [20, 21]. In both studies the $\dot{V}_{E45}$ varied directly with the response to respiratory drive as reflected in the respiratory exchange ratio (RER) or position of Owles point. It varied inversely with tidal volume. Allowance for these variables can greatly increase the accuracy of the reference values (e.g. residual standard deviation about the regression for men can be reduced to 2.0 l min^{-1}, Table 29.15, page 433). Ventilation in medical conditions is considered in Section 28.4.7

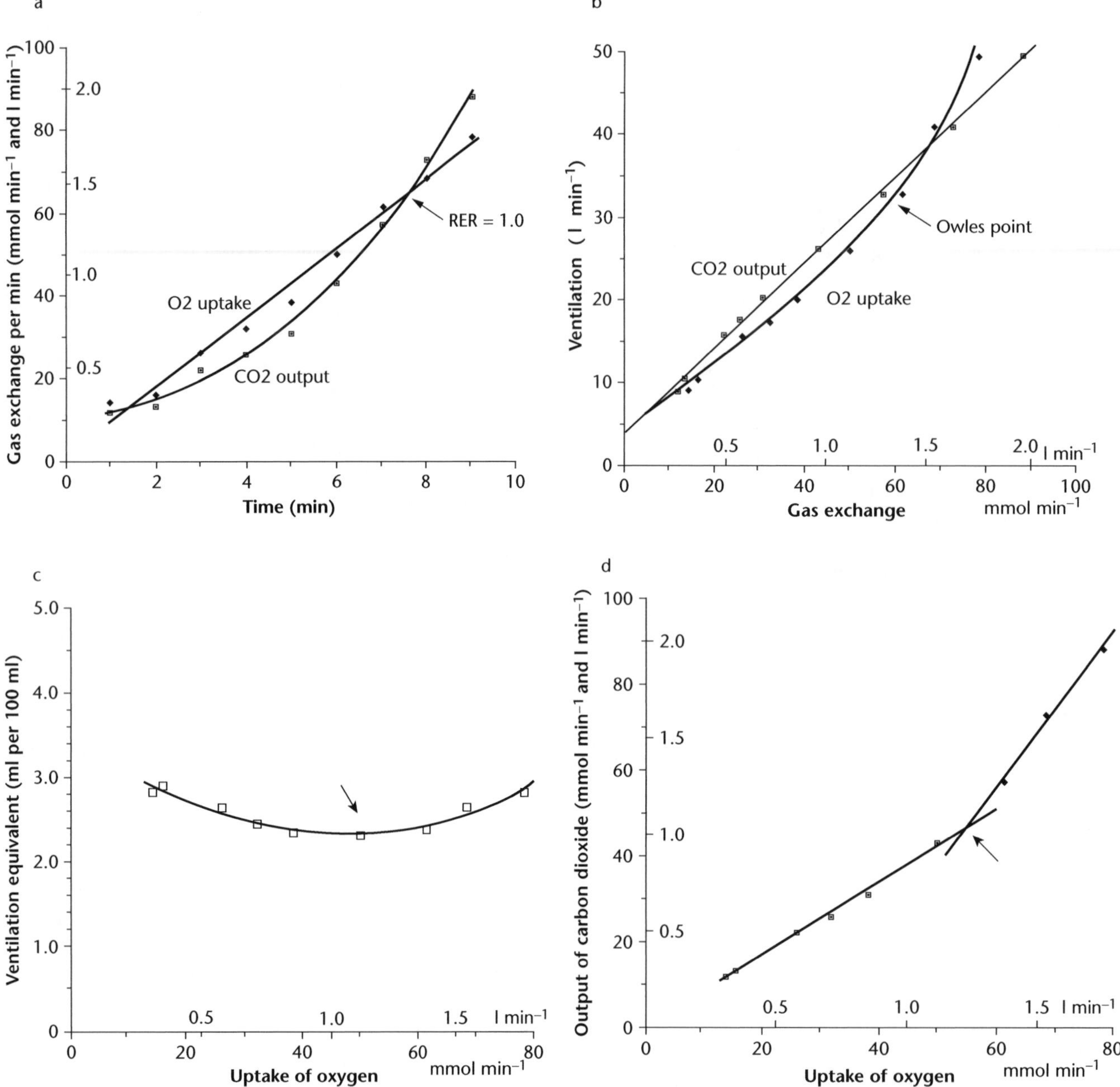

Fig. 28.6 Ventilation and gas exchange during progressive exercise on a cycle ergometer in a healthy subject breathing air. (a) *Oxygen uptake and CO_2 output versus time during exercise.* The relationship for oxygen is linear reflecting the progressively increasing rate of work. That for CO_2 is initially lower reflecting the metabolism of carbohydrate (Respiratory quotient 0.8, Section 28.4.4). Subsequently CO_2 output increases disproportionately in association with increases in ventilation and in blood concentration of lactic acid (Section 28.4.6). As a result, the respiratory exchange ratio (CO_2 output / O_2 uptake) rises. Where the two lines cross the RER is unity. (b) *Ventilation versus gas exchange.* The relationship for oxygen is linear up to Owles point. (The intercept on the ventilation axis represents ventilation of the physiological deadspace.) Beyond Owles point, due to lactic acid and related factors, the ventilation increases disproportionately (Fig. 28.5). The extra ventilation increases the output of CO_2; this linearises the relationship for CO_2 as displayed here. (The extra CO_2 is shown as a rising curve in Panel a.) The present relationship for CO_2 starts above that for O_2 because of the RQ effect. (c) *Ventilation equivalent (ventilation/O_2 uptake) versus O_2 uptake.* The initial decline reflects a progressive increase in tidal volume, hence a decrease in deadspace ventilation relative to minute volume (see Section 28.4.5). The subsequent rise in the curve starts at Owles point (shown by arrow). (d) *CO_2 output versus O_2 uptake.* This relationship can be used to obtain anaerobic threshold (AT) by the V-slope method [17], also Section 28.4.6. The method applies a minimal standard deviation procedure (MSD) to construct two lines that converge on the AT. The paper should be consulted for details.

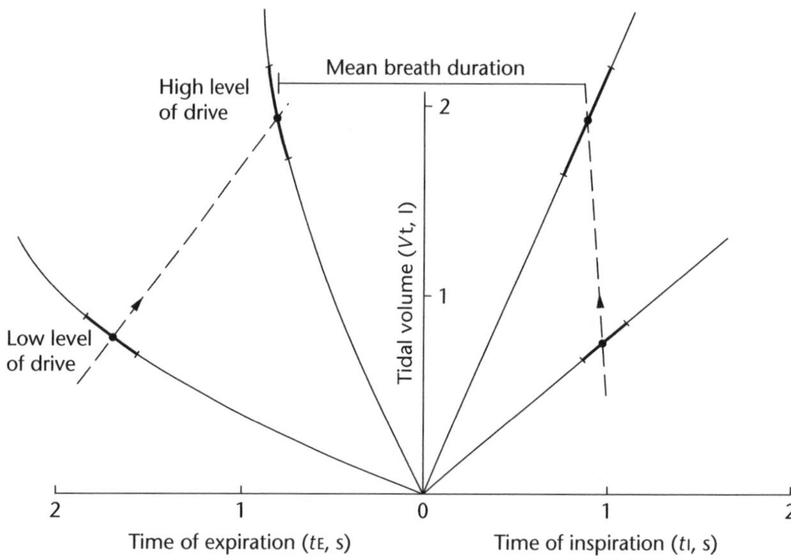

Fig. 28.7 Idealised relationship of the durations of inspiration and expiration to tidal volume during exercise and breathing air enriched with carbon dioxide. The two pairs of continuous lines are for low and high levels of respiratory drive, with the thickened portions showing the mean values and the variation between breaths under steady state conditions. The arrows show the direction of change as the level of drive is increased; there is an increase in tidal volume and a reduction in the mean duration of each breath that is due mainly to shortening of expiration. In the circumstances indicated the time of inspiration is relatively constant; it is reduced during heavy exercise, hyperthermia and stimulation of pulmonary J receptors. Source: [22]

28.4.4 Respiratory exchange ratio (RER)

This index is the ratio of carbon dioxide output to oxygen uptake under the dynamic conditions of exercise. It is considered here because it can illuminate the level of ventilation during exercise. The RER is superimposed on an underlying ratio, the respiratory quotient (RQ), that is determined by the average carbon and oxygen contents of the diet (see Footnote 28.1).

The variations in RER above or below the RQ reflect changes in the level of ventilation relative to the production of carbon dioxide by metabolic activity after allowance has been made for changes in the quantity of carbon dioxide stored in the body. Thus, at the start of exercise the increased central drive to respiration eliminates some carbon dioxide before there is much increase in uptake of oxygen, hence the respiratory exchange ratio rises (Fig. 29.1. page 418). Subsequently, the increase in uptake of oxygen is reflected in the alveolar gas, whilst part of the corresponding output of carbon dioxide is taken up by body stores. Hence, the RER falls, then settles at a level that is appropriate for the metabolic demand. During progressive exercise the demand rises and the additional energy is supplied by modifications to the on-going metabolic processes in the muscle; this can entail liberation of lactic acid in the blood (Section 28.9.2). The acid stimulates ventilation and causes a progressive increase in RER. The transition usually takes place at an oxygen uptake in excess of 45 mmol min^{-1} ($\dot{V}O_2 = 1.0$ l min^{-1}) in healthy men (e.g. Fig. 28.5), but at a lower uptake in many women and respiratory patients. In some circumstances RER at the same work level (i.e. RER_{45}) can be a reference variable for ventilation during submaximal exercise (Table 29.15, page 433).

28.4.5 Respiratory frequency and tidal volume

The increase in ventilation that occurs on exercise is achieved by increases in both tidal volume and respiratory frequency. As a result the breathing cycle becomes shorter and the ventilatory flows increase. The shortening is due mainly to a shorter time of expiration (t_E), whilst the time of inspiration (t_I) is only reduced to a notable extent once tidal volume has attained its maximal value (Fig. 28.7). The increase in tidal volume is achieved by encroaching on both the inspiratory and the expiratory reserve volumes; the resting respiratory level is lower in consequence [23]. The attainment of maximal ventilation entails the mutual adjustment of all these variables [24].

The relationship between ventilation ($\dot{V}_E$) and tidal volume (Vt) is curvilinear. Traditionally it has been described by a linear equation up to a limiting value (Vtmax) that is approximately 60% of vital capacity (VC) (Fig. 28.8), also [25, 26]. Over this range the relationship can be described by the slope and intercept of a linear equation. Alternatively, a curvilinear model can be used.

In healthy individuals when ventilation is driven by hypercapnia or hypoxia the Hey plot resembles that during exercise. The slope is increased by hyperthermia and when pulmonary J receptors are activated (see Section 28.7.3). However, as with ventilation and oxygen uptake, description of the relationship between ventilation and tidal volume requires a minimum of two parameters (slope and intercept) and this reduces the ease with which data can be manipulated. The difficulty can be overcome, and uncertainty as to the best form of the relationship avoided, by using as an index a point near the middle of the relationship, for example the tidal volume at a minute volume of 30 l min^{-1} (Vt_{30} [18]). The Vt_{30} is usually unambiguous. Once obtained, it

Footnote 28.1. For a person on a normal diet the mean RQ is approximately 0.8. This is a weighted average for all foodstuffs. The range is from 1.0 for carbohydrate for which combustion involves equal quantities of oxygen and carbon dioxide (i.e. $C_6H_{12}O_6 + O_2 = 6CO_2 + 6H_2O$) to 0.7 for fat where the requirement for oxygen is higher.

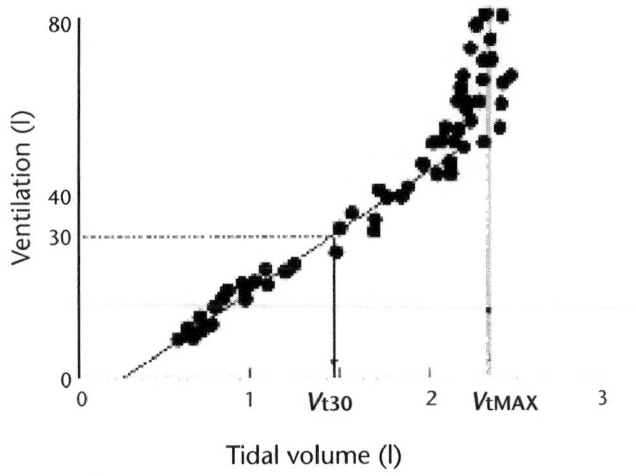

Fig. 28.8 Relationship of ventilation to tidal volume (Hey plot). The derivation of the index Vt_{30} is superimposed. [Redrawn from 25]

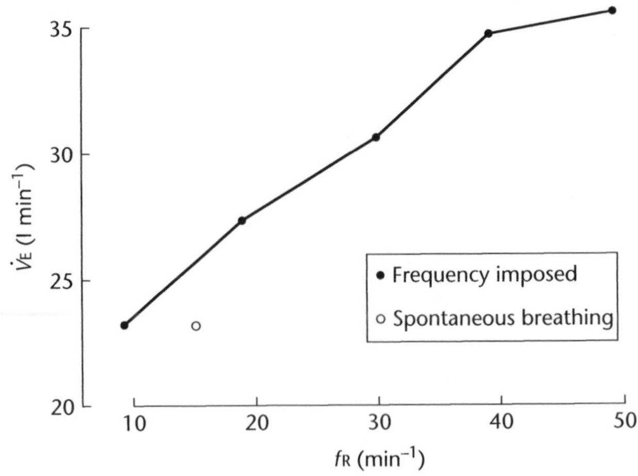

Fig. 28.9 Ventilation during steady state cycling in a healthy subject to show the effect of a voluntary increase in respiratory frequency. This increased the deadspace ventilation per minute and hence the overall ventilation. The respiratory exchange ratio was constant throughout.

can be used to calculate the corresponding respiratory frequency (fR_{30} in breaths per minute $= 30/Vt_{30}$). The two indices can be used interchangeably. However, their associations are different.

The tidal volume, both maximal and as Vt_{30}, has a dimensional relationship to VC ([25, 26],also Table 29.15, page 433). Expressed in these terms the Vt_{30} is similar between adults and children of the same gender, but female subjects often breathe more shallowly and rapidly than males [27] (see also Fig. 31.1, page 446). On theoretical grounds inspiratory capacity might be expected to be a better reference variable [28], but this appears not to be the case.

Respiratory frequency is best considered independent from tidal volume because it is subject to its own control mechanisms, including those associated with thermal panting. In addition, it contributes to the volume of air used per minute to ventilate the anatomical deadspace (i.e. $\dot{V}$E.anat.ds $= f$R $\times$ deadspace) and hence to the ventilation per minute (Fig. 28.9). The frequency/tidal volume relationship in medical conditions is discussed in Section 28.4.7.

28.4.6 Anaerobic threshold: useful index or dangerous fallacy?

The inflection on the relationship between ventilation and uptake of oxygen (see Figs 28.5 and 28.6b) marks an increase in respiratory drive. Owles observed that the increase nearly coincided with a notable rise in the blood concentration of lactic acid and attributed it to anaerobic metabolism (rapid glycolysis) in the exercising muscles [15]. The metabolic process is described in Section 28.9.1. The rise in blood lactate is progressive but in some circumstances can appear to be sudden as though marking a transition from aerobic glycolysis to one that involves lactic acid; hence, the terms *anaerobic threshold* (AT), *gas exchange threshold* ($\dot{V}O_2$,AT) and *lactic acid threshold*, though the latter should only apply in circumstances when blood lactic acid concentration has been measured directly. The corresponding oxygen uptake is near to that at which the subject can no longer achieve a steady state during sustained exercise. Hence, the AT is widely considered to be a fundamental yet accessible index of exercise limitation [29]. However, the evidence does not support this interpretation:

(1) During rapid glycolysis the muscle oxygen tension remains above the critical level needed for electron transport and oxidative phosphorylation even at the breaking point of exercise [30]. Thus, the muscle metabolism is not anaerobic (see also [31]).

(2) There is no discontinuity in the relationship of blood lactate to oxygen consumption, so there is no threshold. Instead, in subjects who have fasted overnight the lactate concentration falls during light exercise, reflecting an increase in utilisation relative to production [32–34]. With more intense exercise the balance is reversed. Overall, the relationship of lactate concentration to oxygen consumption is exponential (Fig. 28.10).

(3) The derivation of AT depends on internal consistency between, on one hand Owles point and similar discontinuities on related graphs (Table 28.3) and, on the other the concentration of blood lactate. This is not observed; instead, the ventilatory threshold can differ from the gas exchange threshold and both can precede the level at which the lactate concentration in blood rises above its level prior to exercise [35] also Fig. 28.5. In addition, the discontinuity in the graph relating ventilation to oxygen uptake (Owles point) can occur without lactacidaemia in McArdle's disease, a condition in which the muscles do not produce lactic acid (Section 28.9.3). Hence, the concept of a *metabolic* threshold is not correct.

(4) An alternative mechanism for Owles point has been identified. The ventilatory response depends on the integrity of the carotid chemoreceptors [36], so the stimulus is a humoral agent linked to muscle metabolism. For the reasons given, the mediator appears not to be lactic acid. A material factor is potassium, for which the blood concentration mirrors the ventilation quite closely in a range of circumstances [37]. However, the match is not perfect [38], so other mediators may contribute as well.

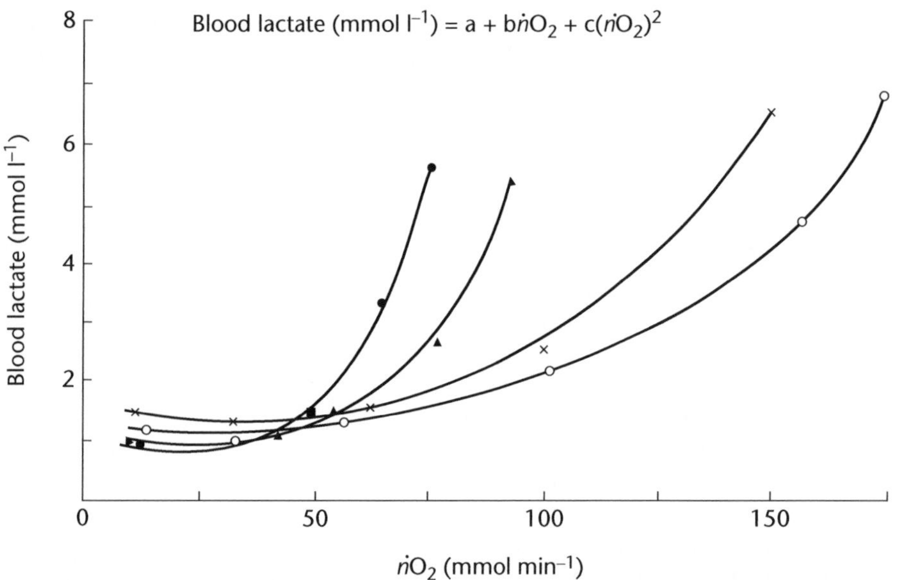

Fig. 28.10 Curves relating blood lactate concentration to oxygen uptake during periods of steady state exercise of successively increased intensity in four healthy subjects who had fasted for 12 h. There was no threshold. However, the oxygen uptake at a specified lactate concentration (e.g. 4 mmol l^{-1}) was negatively correlated with and could be used to estimate the aerobic capacity ($\dot{V}O_2max$). Source: [33]

Features of AT. The oxygen uptake at Owles point ($\dot{V}O_2$,AT) marks a discontinuity in the ventilatory response to progressive exercise that is apparent in healthy persons and others whose capacity for exercise is limited by circulatory factors (Section 30.5.1). Below Owles point the exercise can be sustained, whilst at higher levels of uptake the ventilation can rise exponentially. This has implications for employment (Section 30.6). The $\dot{V}O_2$,AT is correlated with, and can be used to estimate the maximal oxygen uptake where this is determined by circulatory factors, but for this purpose the oxygen uptake at an RER of 1.0 or at a blood lactate concentration of 4 mmol l^{-1} appear to be better guides [19, 33].

In line with these other indices, $\dot{V}O_2$,AT is reduced by inactivity and enhanced by physical training; thus, where these topics are of interest the measurement may be of practical use. However, the index may mislead if the subject's cooperation is suboptimal or the exercise is limited by non-circulatory factors, including a raised ambient temperature [39], anaemia or respiratory disease [40].

In healthy subjects the $\dot{V}O_2$,AT varies with the type of exercise (hand cranking, cycling or work on a treadmill) because this determines the size of the muscle groups that are involved. For exercise with large muscle groups it is approximately 50–60% of aerobic capacity (range 40–80%).

Measurement of AT. The several methods are indicated in Table 28.3. They are usually applied concurrently and the results averaged. Alternatively, if the lactate threshold is of interest it can be estimated during successive periods of steady state exercise of increasing intensity. Time should be allowed for full recovery between periods as otherwise the result may be influenced by a warm-up effect. The lactate concentration can be estimated using peripheral venous blood sampled 2 min after the end of exercise. The observed level should be compared with the level before exercise which is likely to be in the range 0.5–1.0 mmol l^{-1} (cf. Fig. 28.10).

28.4.7 Exercise ventilation in medical conditions

Submaximal exercise ventilation. The main adaptive response to impaired lung function is an increase in ventilation relative to uptake of oxygen during exercise. This can cause breathlessness that reduces the subject's ability to take exercise. Hence, the detection and interpretation of an unduly high exercise ventilation can contribute to medical management. The usual cause is that ventilation is wasted as a result of $\dot{V}A/\dot{Q}$ imbalance (alveolar deadspace effect, Section 18.4.1). In the absence of an exercise test this can escape notice, especially if the arterial oxygen saturation and transfer factor are relatively normal. Augmented respiratory drive can increase the ventilation in patients whose arterial oxygen tension falls on exercise or who are anxious and hyperventilate on this account. In both instances RER is increased. Functional over-breathing is seldom deliberate. Another important cause of increased ventilation is shallow rapid breathing. This increases the ventilation per minute of the anatomical deadspace. The tachypnoea can be evident at all times or only on exercise. The causes include progressive pulmonary congestion and structural abnormalities of the lungs whose effects may not be apparent at rest (see 'Tidal volume and respiratory frequency in medical conditions' below). Some causes are listed in Table 28.4 and some clinical examples are given in Tables 29.11 and 29.12 (pages 429 and 430).

Table 28.3 Graphical identification of ventilatory threshold (AT).

Graph				
y-axis	*x*-axis	Example	Identifier	Ref
CO_2 output	O_2 uptake	Fig. 28.6d	Intersection point of 2 regression lines if data are of this form (V-slope method).	40, 41
Ventilation equivalent (VE)	O_2 uptake	Fig. 28.6c	VO_2 where VE is minimal (Plot of VE versus VCO_2 remains linear)	29
PO_2 (end tidal) (dual criteria)	O_2 uptake	–	VO_2 where PO_2(end tidal) is minimal (Plot of VCO_2 versus PO_2 (end tidal) remains linear)	29
Ventilation	O_2 uptake	Figs 28.5 and 28.6b	Onset of curvilinearity	15

Amongst men working in a shipyard, the average increase in $\dot{V}_{E45}$ (ventilation at O_2 uptake 1.0 l min^{-1}) associated with moderate asbestosis (mean score for small opacities 5.63 ILO units) was 6.0 l min^{-1} [42]. Amongst women with pulmonary congestion due to mitral stenosis, the $\dot{V}_{E33}$ (ventilation at O_2 uptake 0.75 l min^{-1}) was increased by an average of 13.5 l min^{-1} [43]. Similar changes have been observed in patients with alveolitis due to beryllium disease [44]. In both instances contributory factors were hypoxaemia from alveolitis, and shallow breathing from activation of pulmonary receptors (Section 23.3.4). The changes were reversed by treatment (Table 28.5 and Fig. 28.11).

In emphysema and in interstitial fibrosis an increase in $\dot{V}_{E45}$ can be due to an enlarged alveolar deadspace ($\dot{V}_A/\dot{Q}$ effect) reflecting uneven lung function, an enlarged anatomical deadspace from centrilobular emphysema or loss of alveoli from respiratory bronchioles, or to progressive hypoxaemia. This is partly a consequence of the uneven lung function but, unlike in patients with primary disease of the airways, the increased $\dot{V}_E$ is mainly due to hypoxaemia secondary to defective gas transfer [45]. If the resulting hypoxaemia is corrected by administration of oxygen the excess exercise ventilation immediately reverts towards normal. However, where the previously increased ventilation had caused hypocapnia leading to compensatory acid–base changes, the full recovery of ventilation occurs gradually (cf. Sections 22.3.3 and 34.2). Conversely, in patients in whom the work of breathing is greatly increased the ventilatory response

Table 28.4 Some causes for an increased ventilation during submaximal exercise.

Mechanism	Example	
Increased ventilation of airway or alveolar deadspaces.	Shallow, rapid breathing: (RER can be normal)	Functional (e.g. anxiety) Mechanical (e.g. fibrosis of lung or pleura, obesity) Reflex (central or pulmonary) Thermal panting
	Uneven lung function: ($\dot{V}_A/\dot{Q}$ imbalance, RER often somewhat increased)	Diseases of airways or lung parenchyma Occlusions of pulmonary arteries
Increased alveolar ventilation (RER increased).	Lactacidaemia:	Heavy or unaccustomed exercise
	Hypoxia:	High altitude, aviation
	Hypoxaemia:	$\dot{V}_A/\dot{Q}$ imbalance Transfer defect Pulmonary shunt
	Central respiratory drive increased:	Hyperthermia Brain stem lesion
	Humoral agent:	Progesterone Noradrenaline
	Voluntary hyperventilation:	Apprehension Malingering

RER is respiratory exchange ratio (CO_2 output/O_2 uptake).

to exercise may be subnormal. Hypoxaemia is also a component of the increases in ventilation associated with multiple small pulmonary emboli and with cyanotic congenital heart disease (Sections 41.5.1 and 41.18.2). In the latter instance any effect of administering oxygen is usually small.

Tidal volume and respiratory frequency in medical conditions. The exercise tidal volume is below normal and the respiratory frequency is increased in patients in whom lung expansion is restricted (for example by diffuse interstitial fibrosis). This feature contributes to breathlessness by increasing the ventilation per minute that is wasted in flushing the anatomical and alveolar deadspaces, e.g. [46]. Shallow breathing also occurs during nearly maximal exercise in some patients with COPD or asthma when the change is a component of ventilatory limitation of exercise (Section 28.7.2). It is then associated with a rise in end expiratory lung volume and reduction in inspiratory capacity [47, 48], see Section 29.8.2. Shallow breathing can also limit exercise in other conditions but the mechanisms and consequences are less well documented. Interpretation can be assisted by expressing exercise tidal volume and respiratory frequency at a ventilation minute volume of 30 l min^{-1} (Vt_{30} and fR_{30}, Section 28.4.5). The indices have the merit of being related to the maximal tidal excursion of the lung (and hence the forced vital capacity (FVC)), so by taking this dimension into account the contribution of reflex and other factors can be identified.

Expressed in these terms an abnormal pattern of breathing can take several forms [49]. These are illustrated in Tables 29.11, 29.12 and 30.6, respectively, on pages 429, 430 and 442.

1 Vt_{30} is above or below the average for healthy persons, but is nearly normal after standardising for VC. This appears to be the case for patients with acromegaly, interstitial fibrosis (without much pleural thickening) and in the early or intermediate stages of chronic airways obstruction (e.g. Table 29.11).

2 Vt_{30} is increased relative to VC. This is observed in some asthmatics in whom the relatively deep breathing maximises the airway calibre (e.g. Table 29.11). The change reduces the ventilation per minute of the airway deadspace relative to alveolar ventilation and hence reduces the standardised ventilation during submaximal exercise ($\dot{V}E_{45}$).

3 Vt_{30} is reduced relative to VC. The cause of this dynamic limitation to lung expansion can be mechanical as in some patients with pleural thickening or obesity (Tables 29.11, 29.12 and 30.6). Alternatively, it can reflect a change in respiratory control. The causes include stimulation of pulmonary receptors by acute alveolitis or pulmonary congestion (Figs 28.11 and 28.12) [50, 51], increased central nervous activity as with some focal brain lesions, hyperthermia or voluntary rapid breathing (Fig. 28.9).

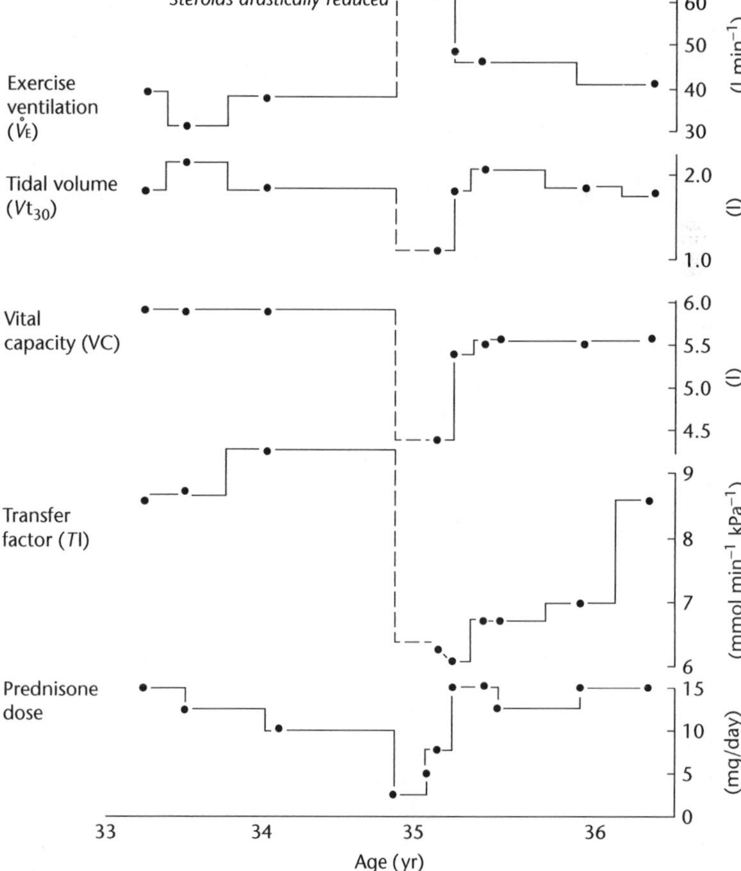

Fig. 28.11 Tachypnoea associated with acute alveolitis in a patient with beryllium disease. The episode was precipitated by a reduction in the dosage of prednisone. This exacerbated the transfer defect (very low transfer factor with gross exercise hypoxaemia); it also caused rapid shallow breathing with a reduced Vt_{30} (and hence raised fR_{30}) relative to the values expected for VC; the reductions were: observed 0.7 l, expected from ΔFVC 0.26 l. The exercise ventilation standardised for oxygen uptake (in this instance 67 mmol min^{-1}, equal to 1.5 l min^{-1}) was increased in consequence. Source: [44]

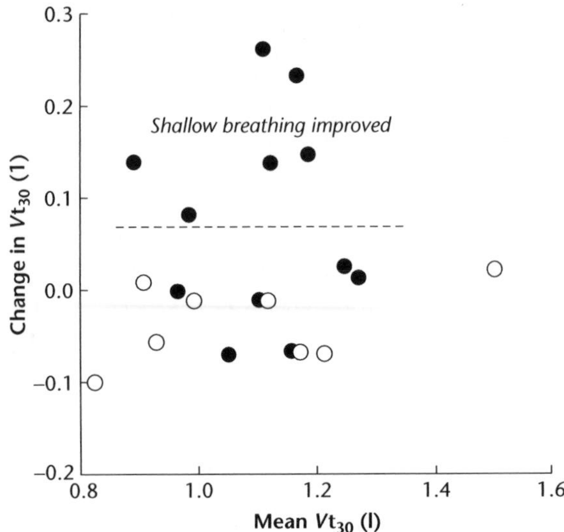

Fig. 28.12 Partial correction of shallow breathing (tachypnoea) following relief of pulmonary congestion in women with mitral stenosis. The figure shows the change in Vt_{30} subsequent to an operation on the mitral valve. In the 12 women in whom the operation was successful the Vt_{30} increased ($p < 0.02$) (closed circles), whereas there was no change in Vt_{30} in the 8 women in whom the operation was not successful (open circles) [43]. (*See also* Table 28.5 on page 402).

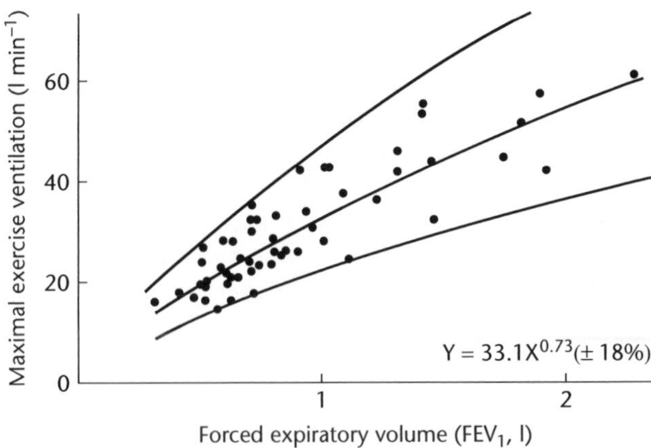

Fig. 28.13 Relationship of maximal exercise ventilation to forced expiratory volume for well-motivated patients with chronic lung disease. In patients not limited by breathlessness or in whom motivation is suspect the maximal ventilation is often below the lower confidence limit. Source: [53]

The ventilation minute volume is influenced by the pattern of breathing that is adopted.

The maximal tidal volume during progressive exercise in most respiratory patients resembles that in healthy subjects, being approximately 60% of FVC e.g. [26]. Thereafter, as the exercise continues, it normally remains at this level. However, where the pattern of breathing is constrained by the flow–volume curve (Section 28.8.1) the maximal tidal volume may not be maintained. In this case, if the exercise is continued, the tidal volume decreases and the end expiratory lung volume rises. This change has the effect of maximising the lung elastic recoil and hence the calibre of the small airways of the lungs. Concurrently, the breathing frequency increases so the ventilation minute volume continues to rise despite the tidal volume becoming smaller. However, the ventilation per minute of the anatomical deadspace also rises, so there may be no improvement in alveolar ventilation except when the work of breathing is reduced by the patient inhaling a bronchodilator aerosol [28].

28.4.8 Maximal exercise ventilation

Healthy persons utilise most or all of their maximal breathing capacity when they exercise maximally (see Section 12.2 for definitions). Hence, a useful guide to the maximal ventilation during exercise ($\dot{V}_{E,max.ex}$) is the maximal voluntary ventilation (MVV) measured directly or estimated from forced expiratory volume (Section 12.2.2). Usually the ratio $\dot{V}_{E,max.ex}$/MVV is approximately 0.8 [52], but it is near to 1.0 in some athletes, including in middle distance runners and cyclists. At high altitude, due to the reduced air density and viscosity, the MVV and hence the $\dot{V}_{E,max.ex}$ are in excess of the values at sea level (Section 34.2). Converse changes occur under conditions of raised ambient pressure or if the airway is restricted by breathing through a mask or in other ways. In all these circumstances the $\dot{V}_{E,max.ex}$ reflects the available ventilatory capacity during exercise. In some medical conditions, for example exercise-induced asthma or progressive pulmonary congestion from mitral stenosis, the MVV on exercise may be less than at rest. In cardiac and respiratory disorders the relationship of $\dot{V}_{E,max.ex}$ to forced expiratory volume (Fig. 28.13) or to MVV can illuminate the causes of breathlessness and exercise limitation (These aspects are reviewed in Sections 28.7 and 28.8).

28.5 Cardiac output and stroke volume

28.5.1 Cardiac output

Oxygen is delivered from the lungs to individual tissues in proportion to their blood flow. The total flow is the cardiac output; it reflects the metabolic demand from all organs and tissues in the prevailing circumstances. Blood flow to the brain normally has the highest priority. The priority of the muscles is high during exercise but low at other times. Similarly, the flow to the skin has a high priority during exposure to heat. By contrast, the requirement of the gastrointestinal tract for blood flow in relation to meals has a lesser priority.

During exercise the increase in cardiac output results from an augmented return of blood back to the heart. This is as a consequence of veno-constriction from enhanced autonomic activity, expulsion of blood from the spleen and other blood depots, redistribution of body fluid and changes in intravascular pressure consequent on contraction and relaxation of muscles and changes in intrathoracic pressure [54]. The increase in cardiac output bears a nearly linear relationship to oxygen uptake, e.g.

$$\dot{Q}t = 6.1\,\dot{V}O_2(\text{or } 0.137\,\dot{n}O_2) + 3.4, \quad \text{SD } 0.9\,\text{l min}^{-1} \quad (28.1)$$

where $\dot{Q}t$ and $\dot{n}O_2$ are, respectively, the output of the heart and the rate of consumption of oxygen [55]. The relationship is remarkably stable with respect to age, gender, physical fitness and clinical condition (e.g. [54, 56], see also further reading); this has implications for interpretation of exercise cardiac frequency (see below).

The coefficient term in eqn. 28.1 is the increase in cardiac output per unit increase in oxygen uptake; its numerical value in SI units is 0.137 l mmol^{-1} and in traditional units 6.1 l per litre. These quantities can be interpreted as evidence that during normal exercise effectively all the additional cardiac output goes to the active muscles (including to the heart itself). However, when conditions are not conducive to dispersal of body heat (as in a hot or humid environment) some of the additional blood flow is directed to the skin [39].

The maximal cardiac output ($\dot{Q}t$ max) defines the capacity of the cardiovascular system. It varies with body size, declines with age and is increased by physical training. As a result the normal range for $\dot{Q}t$ max is relatively wide, from some 10 l min^{-1} in a small sedentary individual to 35 l min^{-1} in a top athlete.

Practical considerations. Measurement of cardiac output is described in Section 17.3. Knowledge of the outcome is essential for a full description of the physiological response to exercise and for understanding the extent of some cardiovascular disorders. In other circumstances, including assessment of most respiratory patients, sufficient information can be obtained from measurements of cardiac frequency and oxygen uptake during a progressive exercise test. Where appropriate the test may need to be continued up to the symptom limited maximum.

28.5.2 Stroke volume

Cardiac output is the product of stroke volume (SV) and cardiac frequency. Stroke volume is at its maximal value in a supine posture when it is normally in the range 50–100 ml, or 150 ml in athletes. It decreases when the subject is upright. In this posture during progressive exercise starting from rest, the SV increases and approaches its maximal value at an oxygen uptake of approximately 40% of the maximal oxygen uptake (Fig. 28.14). Hence, up to this level of exercise an increase in stroke volume contributes to the increase in cardiac output. With increasing age the stroke volume increases and, as a result, maintains a normal cardiac output during exercise in the presence of a reduction in cardiac frequency [54, 56].

Physique and physical condition help to determine the stroke volume. The association extends to the quantity of muscle in the two ventricles, but more particularly the left; both are increased by physical training. However, the training does not affect the relationship of cardiac output to oxygen uptake; hence, the increase in SV is accompanied by a reduction in exercise cardiac frequency. This aspect is referred to below (Section 28.12.1).

28.6 Exercise cardiac frequency

28.6.1 Numerical values

During exercise of increasing intensity the cardiac output is increased mainly by an increase in cardiac frequency. An increase in stroke volume also contributes during mild exercise (see above), but not when the exercise is performed in a supine posture. Then, due to an increased venous return the SV is already nearly maximal. In other circumstances the increase in frequency reflects change in the balance of stimuli that act on the cardiac pacemaker, including a diminution in parasympathetic (vagal) tone with respect to sympathetic tone and an increase in the plasma concentration of catecholamines. This method of control has the consequence that cardiac frequency responds rapidly to anticipation of exercise, to changes in the thermal environment and to emotional, sensory and physical stimuli. Proper interpretation of the cardiovascular response to exercise is only possible when these factors are controlled. Allowance should also be made for medication that may influence the frequency, including sympathomimetic antagonists and drugs that block calcium channels.

Long-term changes in autonomic control occur with chronic hypoxia and in some endocrine disorders. The pacemaker is also affected by local ischaemia and by ageing. The latter is associated with a reduced frequency at rest and throughout exercise, including maximal exercise. The decline in *maximal cardiac frequency with age* is traditionally described by the following relationship:

$$fc\text{max} = 210 - 0.65\ \text{age (year)}, \quad \text{SD } 19\,\text{min}^{-1} \quad (28.2)$$

where fcmax is maximal cardiac frequency [1]. However, for many populations a lower maximum is more appropriate [18, 59]. The maximal frequency is nearly independent of the physical condition of the subject, but tends to be low in those with an above average quantity of cardiac muscle.

Physical training reduces the cardiac frequency during submaximal exercise (Fig. 28.15). However, as with ageing, the relationship of cardiac output to uptake of oxygen remains nearly constant. This has the important consequence that, at any level of submaximal exercise, a change in frequency associated with training or de-training (or with ageing) reflects a converse change in stroke volume. This can be represented as

$$\dot{Q}t = k = (SV + \Delta SV) \times (fc + \Delta fc), \quad (28.3)$$

hence ΔSV is negatively correlated with Δfc

where the delta values are the changes in stroke volume and frequency. With ageing and with physical training Δfc has a negative sign.

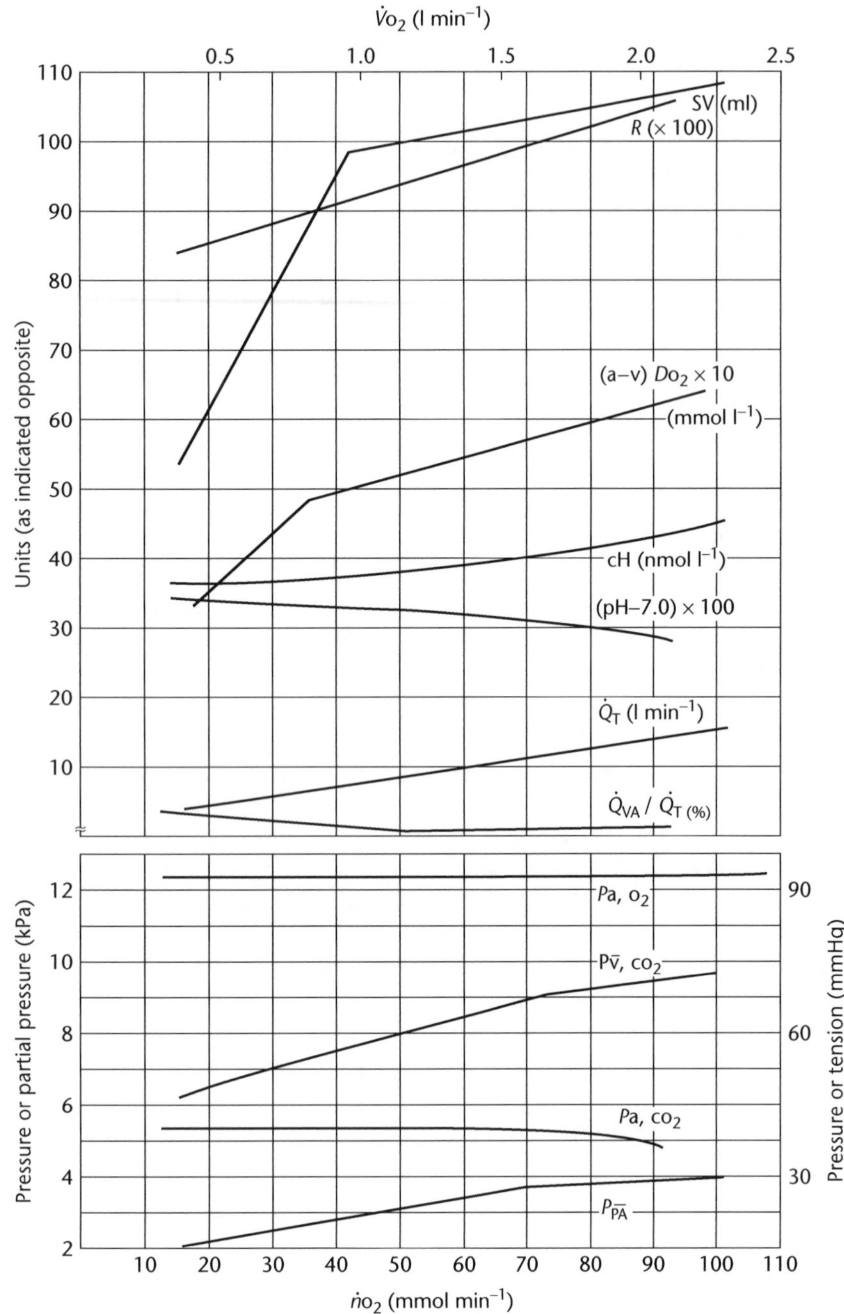

Fig. 28.14 Relationships of indices of cardio-pulmonary function to consumption of oxygen during exercise in an upright posture. The data are for untrained male subjects. The pulmonary arterial pressures are measured from the xiphoid process; lower pressures are recorded when the reference point is the fourth rib at the sternum. Source: Adapted from [57, 58]

Cardiac frequency during progressive exercise from rest is related to the uptake of oxygen in a nearly linear manner (Fig. 28.16). The relationship is the basis for indices of exercise cardiac frequency.

28.6.2 Indices of *f*Csubmax

Oxygen pulse. This traditional index describes cardiac frequency in terms of its contribution to oxygen transport as the oxygen uptake per heart beat in ml STPD. There is no SI equivalent. The index has the form:

$$\text{OP (ml STPD)} = \dot{V}o_2/fc = \text{(stroke volume)} \times \text{(arterio-venous O}_2\text{ difference)} \tag{28.4}$$

Oxygen pulse can be used in the analysis of oxygen transport [16]. However, there is no unique value such as might be used to describe the cardiac frequency response to exercise. This is because the relationship of cardiac frequency to oxygen uptake during progressive exercise is a linear regression, not a

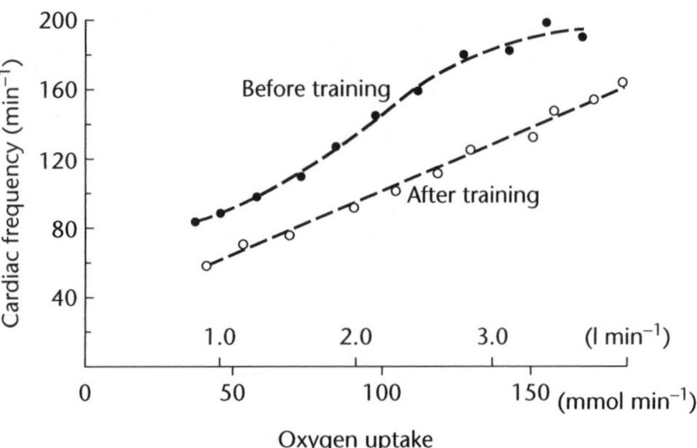

Fig. 28.15 Mean data for exercise cardiac frequency relative to uptake of oxygen of fire brigades men before (●) and after (o) eleven weeks of physical training. The training affected the mean level of cardiac frequency (*f*c) to a greater extent than the slope of the relationship. Training increased the fat free mass (FFM), see Table 4.4 on page 37. On the assumption that the relationship of *f*c to FFM between subjects also applied within subjects, approximately half the reduction in fc_{45} could be accounted for by additional muscle and the remainder by improved contractility. Source: [60]

direct proportionality (i.e.the line does not pass through the origin). As a result the ratio $\dot{V}O_2/fc$ varies depending on the oxygen uptake (Fig. 28.16, also Section 5.3.2). Oxygen pulse does not make a worthwhile contribution to routine exercise testing. A related term, asymptotic oxygen pulse, has been used to describe the slope of the linear relationship of cardiac frequency on uptake of oxygen, but a descriptive term is less ambiguous [62]. Information is needed on the usefulness of the index.

Linear model. This method of presentation describes the linear relationship of exercise cardiac frequency to uptake of oxygen in terms of the slope and intercept of the regression line. Reference values for the slope have been reported [62] and the index can provide an approximate estimate of stroke volume [63]. However, the slope on its own gives an incomplete description as it neglects the intercept of the regression equation, which in some circumstances summarises more of the information present in the relationship. This is apparent in Fig. 28.15 that illustrates the effect on cardiac frequency of physical training. Hence, one parameter on its own is of limited usefulness whilst to report them both can mislead as they are not independent.

Standardised indices. The cardiac frequency response to submaximal exercise can be summarised by the frequency at a specified oxygen consumption representative of moderate exercise, for example an O_2 uptake of 45 mmol min^{-1}(1.0 l min^{-1}). The resulting index is designated in SI units fc_{45} and in traditional units $fc_{1.0}$ [18] (e.g. Fig. 28.16). Other levels of oxygen consumption (e.g. 22, 33 or 67 mmol min^{-1}, equivalent to 0.5. 0.75 and 1.5 l min^{-1}) can also be used. This approach combines in a single index much of the information contained in the slope and the intercept of the relationship of cardiac frequency on uptake of oxygen. Reference values are available (Table 29.15, page 433) and the result can be interpreted in conjunction with indices of lung function. A similar approach is used above to describe submaximal exercise ventilation and tidal volume.

The index fc_{45} ($fc_{1.0}$) is negatively correlated with and provides a measure of stroke volume without the approximations inherent in the slope method described above. This is because the cardiac output at any level of oxygen uptake is relatively constant (Section 28.5.1). Hence, for an oxygen uptake of 45 mmol min^{-1} (1.0 l min^{-1}) eqn. 28.3 becomes

$$\dot{Q}t_{45} = fc_{45} \times SV = k, \quad \text{or } fc_{45} = k/SV \qquad (28.5)$$

The cardiac frequency standardised for O_2 uptake reflects the stroke volume and the determinants of SV; these include age, the

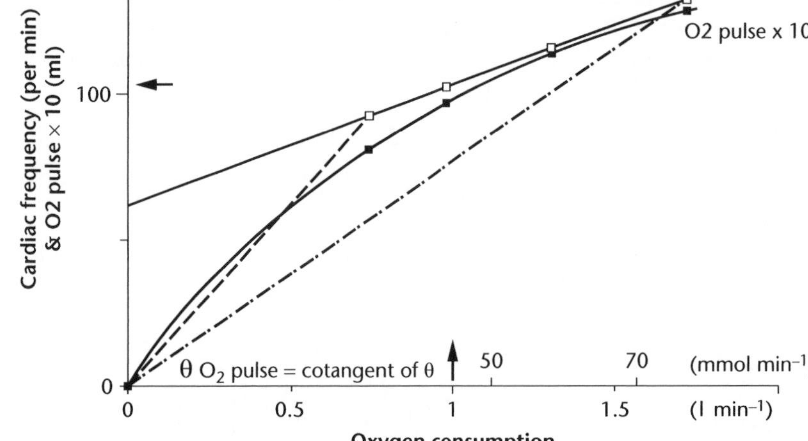

Fig. 28.16 Mean relationships of exercise cardiac frequency (open squares) and oxygen pulse (closed squares) to uptake of oxygen for healthy coal miners [61] (for interpretation see text). The derivation of fc_{45} ($fc_{1.0}$ in traditional units) is indicated by arrows.

quantity of body muscle and the physical condition. The latter attributes can be described respectively by fat-free body mass (FFM, Section 4.7.1) and the rating for habitual activity (i.e. the score for the amount of exercise that the subject takes regularly). These and related indices can be used as reference variables (Table 29.15, page 433).

28.6.3 Clinical applications

A value for f_{C45} that exceeds the reference value may be due to apprehension. If so, the frequency is relatively high at the start of exercise. It then often reverts to a level that is representative of the subject (Fig. 29.8, page 427). Other causes for a raised f_{C45} are hypoxaemia (as with a material transfer defect, Table 29.11, case 8, page 429), impaired cardiac function (Table 28.5), toxaemia from any source, anaemia, dosage with a pharmacologically active drug and loss of physical condition (Fig. 28.15). A patient who is unfit may benefit from an exercise rehabilitation programme (Section 44.4.1). However, in many respiratory patients the f_C is normal for the uptake of oxygen (Table 28.6).

28.7 Breathlessness on exertion

28.7.1 Sensation of dyspnoea

Dyspnoea is an undue awareness that breathing is difficult and requires increased effort. There may be a foreboding that the effort could become unbearable.

Healthy persons vary in their awareness of dyspnoea [65] and this may influence the intensity of the sensation in the event of the lungs becoming abnormal. In addition, the intensity can be enhanced by psychiatric illness or by a psychological difficulty, for example a claim for industrial compensation.

The quality of the sensation can also vary depending on the cause; this is partly because pulmonary abnormalities differ in their effects on the components of each breath (pattern of breathing [66]) and the amount of respiratory effort that breathing entails. Thus, dyspnoea can be used to describe respiratory distress, wheeze, respiratory effort, rapid breathing or sighing [67]. A patient who experiences such symptoms is likely to restrict his or her activities. This can further reduce the exercise tolerance and hence aggravate the symptom.

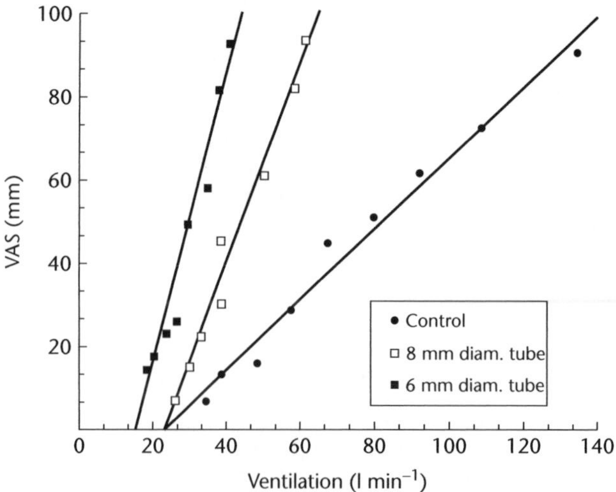

Fig. 28.17 Breathlessness during a progressive exercise test rated using a visual analogue scale (VAS, see Fig. 29.7, page 425). Scoring was each min using an illuminated scale controlled by one finger. The figure shows a normal response (right) and the effect of breathing through one of two resistances. A moderate resistance (e.g. a tube diameter 8 mm, length 25 mm) increased the slope of the relationship whilst a high resistance also reduced the threshold level of ventilation at which breathlessness was first experienced. Source: [68]

Dyspnoea is a feature of most chronic disorders of the lungs and its recognition can contribute to diagnosis. This process is assisted by an observer witnessing the evolution of breathlessness during the course of a standardised exercise test and noting the subject's description at the time (Section 29.3.4).

Minor degrees of dyspnoea are described as breathlessness and the two sensations are regarded as one for purposes of rating. This is done using a questionnaire, visual analogue scale, modified Borg scale or psychological tests (e.g. Fig. 29.7 and Table 29.9, pages 425 and 426, respectively). A typical breathlessness profile for a healthy subject during progressive exercise is given in Fig. 28.17.

28.7.2 Mechanisms of breathlessness

In healthy subjects the intensity of breathlessness at a given level of isocapnoeic ventilation depends on the precise circumstances.

Table 28.5 Mean physiological response to exercise (O_2 uptake 22 mmol min^{-1}, 0.5 l min^{-1}) in 20 female patients before and after valvulotomy for relief of mitral stenosis. Outcome was assessed using clinical criteria.

	Reference	Improvement ($n = 12$)		No improvement ($n = 8$)	
Index	value	Before	After	Before	After
$V_{E\,22}$ (l min^{-1})	13.0	21.1	17.3**	18.5	18.4
Vt_{30} (l)†	1.2	1.05	1.14 *	1.09	1.07
f_{C22}(min^{-1})	104	125	102**	122	133

* $p < 0.02$, ** $p < 0.01$.
† see also Fig. 28.12.
Source: [64].

The symptom is stronger when ventilation is driven by hypercapnia or hypoxia than by exercise. When the stimulus is exercise, cycling can cause more intense breathlessness than walking on a treadmill. By such studies Adams and colleagues were able to dissociate the ventilatory responses from the blood gas tensions; they demonstrated an association between ventilation and breathlessness but not between peripheral carbon dioxide drive and breathlessness [69]. In the case of oxygen the possibility that hypoxia contributed directly to breathlessness could not be ruled out.

Breathlessness is unaffected by local anaesthesia of the airways, and still occurs after heart–lung transplantation, so the symptom is not necessarily dependent on afferent information from the lungs. It can occur following neuromuscular blockade and is not completely dependent of the activity of respiratory muscles [70]. In healthy persons the sensation is greater when ventilation is stimulated physiologically than when the same ventilation is achieved voluntarily [71]. Thus, the evidence suggests that in healthy persons the mechanisms are in the brain, not the lungs or muscles and reflect the degree of reflex activation of the medullary respiratory complex [72]. The symptom is amenable to conditioning, Section 23.7.2 [73, 74].

28.7.3 Clinical aspects

Dyspnoea is an intensely personal experience. In a clinical context it is often the immediate reason for a patient having a reduced exercise capacity, consulting a respiratory physician and attending at a lung function laboratory. Hence, how it is managed is of the greatest importance. Inhalation of oxygen can reduce the ventilation (Section 28.8.1) and bronchoconstriction can be alleviated by bronchodilatation (Chapter 15). However, more than one factor may be involved. For example, in pulmonary sarcoidosis breathlessness can be due to shallow breathing from stimulation of pulmonary receptors. In this event, the dyspnoea and associated tachypnoea can be dramatically reduced by interruption of the vagus nerves [75]. In dogs vagal section eliminated tachypnoea caused by inhalation of histamine [76]. A similar mechanism contributes to breathlessness in conditions that give rise to pulmonary congestion either at rest or on exercise, including coronary ischaemia and mitral stenosis.

28.7.4 Speculations

Susceptibility to breathlessness varies between individuals [65]. In addition, relative insensitivity can be an adaptive response to pulmonary disease that might lead to an affected person being slow to seek medical help. It could also lead to him or her not making an adequate respiratory response to chronic airways obstruction compared with other patients with above average sensitivity. In this event a person's place on the sensitivity spectrum could influence the chances of becoming what is colloquially described as a 'pink puffer' (Type 1 response), or of developing respiratory hypercapnia (designated type 2 or 'blue bloater', Section 38.5). It might also be a factor in sleep apnoea (Section 35.2).

28.8 Limitation of exercise

Exercise becomes maximal when each structure and system in the body is contributing its maximum in the prevailing circumstances. As a result no individual system has sole responsibility for the exercise being terminated. This section reviews some of the primary factors. Assessment of exercise limitation is discussed in Chapter 30.

28.8.1 Ventilatory limitation (including use of oxygen)

Exercise is normally limited by the rate of delivery of oxygen to muscles that are active. There can be a high level of ventilation consequent on lactacidaemia, but for the ventilation to be the primary cause of limitation it should encroach on the ventilatory capacity; this is not normally the case in healthy individuals. Ventilatory limitation occurs in respiratory patients in whom the ventilatory capacity is reduced whilst the ventilatory cost of exercise is increased. A high ventilatory cost alone is the principal limiting factor in persons with normal respiratory control exposed to a hypoxic environment as occurs at high altitude.

Flow–volume loops. The extent of any ventilatory limitation can be assessed by comparing single tidal flow–volume loops obtained during exercise with maximal flow volume curves obtained before or just after exercise [77–79], also Section 12.5. The method entails the assumptions that maximal curves obtained at rest are relevant for exercise and that the loops can be superimposed appropriately. Matching is normally done at total lung capacity and to this end a measurement of inspiratory capacity is made during the exercise. Matching at functional residual capacity is inappropriate as patients with airflow limitation may raise their end expiratory level when they exercise. Matching at residual volume is impracticable. A model showing how the maximal flow–volume curve might constrain the respiratory flows on exercise is given in Fig. 28.18. In this circumstance the pattern of breathing is spontaneously modified with respect to frequency, tidal volume and functional residual capacity in order to maximise the ventilation (Section 28.4.5).

The limitations to this approach include uncertainty as to the comparability of the two sets of loops, neglect of the effects of dynamic compression unless the instantaneous lung volume is measured concurrently by a plethysmographic method (Section 14.6.2) and various practical difficulties. Alternatives are to look for expiratory flow limitation by observing the response of expiratory flow to brief suction applied to the airway (Section 13.6), or using another method as in Section 29.8.2.

Dyspnoeic index. The propensity to breathlessness can be expressed as the ratio of ventilation during exercise to the

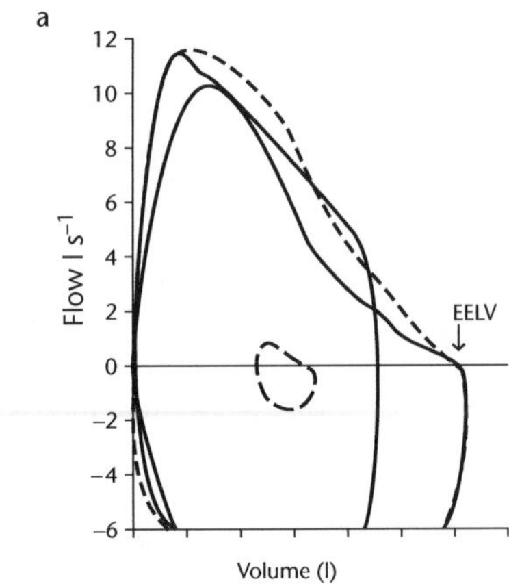

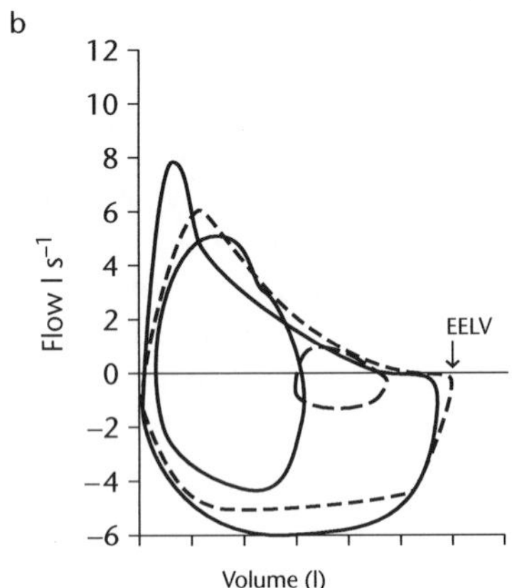

Fig. 28.18 Illustrative flow-volume (f–v) curves from a study showing an increase in end-expiratory lung volume (EELV) on maximal exercise in patients with mild airflow limitation (b) compared with a decrease in control subjects (a) (average changes respectively +5% TLC and –8% TLC). Bold and dashed lines are maximal and composite f–v curves, thin lines are for maximal exercise and small loops are for rest. The exercise curves encroached on the f–v envelopes to a somewhat greater extent in the patient than the control subject. Source: [79, also Further reading].

ventilatory capacity; the ratio was introduced as the dyspnoeic index [52].

$$\text{Dyspnoeic index} = \frac{\text{Exercise ventilation}}{\text{Maximal voluntary ventilation}} \times 100\% \qquad (28.6)$$

The usual denominator is the maximal voluntary ventilation (MVV) measured at rest or estimated from FEV_1 via the relationship of Gandevia and Hugh-Jones [80]:

$$\text{Indirect maximal breathing capacity (l min}^{-1}) = 35\ FEV_1(l) \qquad (28.7)$$

However, this is inappropriate because the relationship of MVV to FEV_1 is not a proportionality and the pattern of maximal breathing can differ between rest and exercise. For patients with chronic airway obstruction these difficulties can be overcome by using as denominator for eqn. 28.6 an estimate of maximal exercise ventilation under conditions of maximal breathlessness obtained from FEV_1 [53]. Then:

$$\text{Dyspnoeic index} = \text{Exercise ventilation} \times 100/(33.1 \times FEV_1^{0.73}) \qquad (28.8)$$

where the denominator is maximal exercise ventilation estimated from FEV_1 (Fig. 28.13).

In most healthy persons the dyspnoeic index at the breaking point of exercise is in the range 70–90% but is often higher in athletes. It rises to, or may exceed 100% if the density of the air is reduced by ascent to altitude or the nitrogen is replaced by helium. A comparable increase can occur during hyperbaria, but maximal exercise in this circumstance should be approached with caution (Section 35.5.1).

In respiratory patients a dyspnoeic index that approaches or exceeds 100% is normally evidence for exercise being limited by ventilatory capacity. The commonest cause is chronic respiratory impairment as given in Table 28.6 (see also Footnote 28.2).

As well as respiratory disease a high dyspnoeic index can result from functional hyperventilation such as might arise from anxiety; in this circumstance RER is increased, cf. Section 28.4.4. A low dyspnoeic index is observed when exercise is limited by a non-ventilatory factor, for example the delivery of oxygen to mitochondria (Table 28.7). However, the MVV that is used in the calculation should be achievable on exercise. This is usually the case in patients with chronic airway narrowing after bronchodilatation. The MVV at rest may not be appropriate if the lung elasticity is low as in emphysema or the exercise alters the mechanical characteristics of the lungs or causes pulmonary congestion. In any of these circumstances the dyspnoeic index is of limited usefulness.

Table 28.6 Physiological features at maximal exercise in COPD. Mean data for 12 men (3 for $f$cmax). Age 57 years, FEV_1 0.94 l, FVC 1.50 l. Predicted $\dot{V}$Emax,ex (from eqn. 28.8) 31.6 l min^{-1}.

Mode of exercise	Cycling		Hand cranking
Inspired gas	Air	O_2	Air
Work rate (W)	50*	68*	40*
$\dot{V}$Emax,ex (l min^{-1})	30.8	29.6	30.5
Dyspnoeic index (%)	97	95	97
Vt,max,ex × 100 ÷ VC (%)	43	45	44
fR,max,ex (min^{-1})	30	28	29
fC,max,ex (min^{-1})	105	111	109

* Maximal work rates differed significantly, $p < 0.05$.

Footnote 28.2. In men with chronic lung disease who are limited on exercise by breathlessness the contributions of ventilatory cost of exercise ($\dot{V}_{E45}$) and FEV_1 to capacity for exercise can be described empirically. The relationship (Table 29.15, page 433) can sometimes be used to confirm a measurement of maximal oxygen uptake in similar patients (Section 30.5.2).

Table 28.7 Physiological features of the breaking point of exercise by mode of limitation.

Limiting feature	Oxygen delivery	Ventilatory capacity
Symptoms	Dyspnoea and fatigue: recovery is slow	Dyspnoea: recovery is rapid
Dyspnoeic index	40–100%	60–130%
Cardiac output	Maximal	Not maximal
Cardiac frequency	150–200 min^{-1}	<150 min^{-1}
Blood lactic acid concentration	6–14 mmol l^{-1}	<6 mmol 1^{-1}
Arterial blood gases		
Pa,O_2	Normal (or reduced)	Normal or reduced
Pa,CO_2	Reduced (cH increased)	Raised, normal or reduced
Diaphragmatic EMG	Usually normal	Evidence of fatigue
Ventilation and oxygen intake during recovery	Decline slowly	Return rapidly to resting level

Effects and use of oxygen. Breathing air enriched with oxygen increases the exercise capacity. This is usually due to the oxygen reducing the chemoreceptor drive to breathing, hence reducing the exercise ventilation and associated breathlessness. The response is apparent with mild hypoxaemia (Sao_2 > 91%) [81]. The correction of any covert hypoxaemia may also reduce breathlessness independent of the change in ventilation (Section 28.7.2), but this appears to be a second order effect. The reduction in ventilation is followed by a rise in arterial tension of carbon dioxide that might be expected to reverse the hypoventilation. In healthy persons it does so at rest but not during exercise (Fig. 23.4, page 292). In respiratory patients the reduction occurs in both circumstances.

The beneficial effect of oxygen on exercise capacity is apparent in normal persons at sea level. It is even more conspicuous at altitude and in some respiratory patients. Amongst patients that benefit, the inhalation of 30–50% oxygen during exercise can postpone the onset of incapacitating breathlessness and permit activities that would otherwise not be possible (Fig. 28.19, also [83]). The response provides a physiological basis for portable oxygen therapy, but not all breathless patients benefit from oxygen, so an assessment should be carried out by comparing the distance a patient can walk breathing air and air enriched with oxygen. The procedure is indicated in the figure.

Patients whose exercise capacity is increased by oxygen are candidates for portable oxygen therapy, but not all in this category find the equipment helpful. A person who does so often has an important task outside the house that can only be performed breathing oxygen. An example is a person with an upstairs office that he or she can only reach by using portable apparatus. Stairs at home can be mounted with help from oxygen delivered via a long flexible tube from a domiciliary supply (Section 35.7.1).

In addition to reducing the ventilation, breathing 100% oxygen rapidly increases the quantity of oxygen dissolved in the blood plasma from 0.3 to 2.0 ml dl^{-1}. When exercise is limited by the quantity of oxygen that can be delivered to tissues the additional oxygen is beneficial because it delays the onset of rapid glycolysis and lactacidaemia. This is equivalent to a small increase in cardiac output. A rise in haemoglobin concentration consequent on a stay at high altitude can exert a comparable effect.

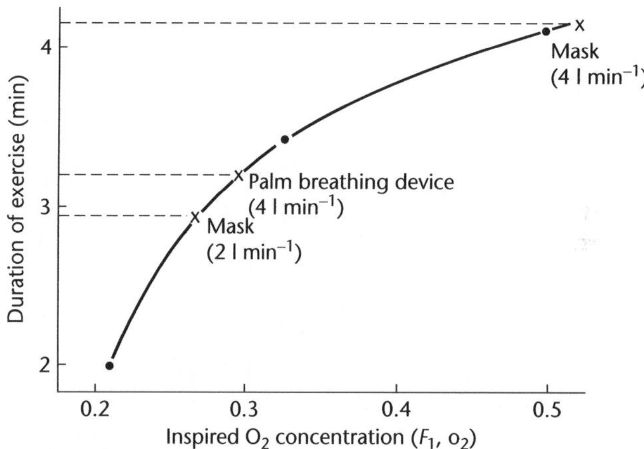

Fig. 28.19 Relationship of the duration of exercise on a treadmill to the dosage of oxygen for 6 patients with chronic lung disease. The speed and slope of the treadmill were adjusted so that each patient was obliged to stop on account of incapacitating breathlessness after 2 min when breathing air. The curve is drawn through the points for mixtures of oxygen and nitrogen. The interrupted lines are the times for a palm breathing device and a mask with reservoir bag and valve to prevent re-breathing; the equivalent concentrations of oxygen can be read off the curve. Source: [82]

28.8.2 Pulmonary gas exchange

This stage in the oxygen transport chain contributes to limitation of exercise in normal subjects at high altitude or breathing a hypoxic gas mixture [84, 85]. It is due to hypoxaemia caused by insufficient gas transfer (Sections 21.3). The principal cause is that gas exchange is taking place on the steep part of the oxygen dissociation curve. A contributory cause is that the time during which the capillary blood is in contact with alveolar gas (i.e. the transit time) is often reduced. By contrast, at sea level the great majority of healthy persons maintain their blood oxygen level during exercise, so pulmonary gas exchange is not a factor limiting exercise. The occasional person who desaturates is usually an athlete with a blunted ventilatory response to exercise [86] or one in whom the ventilation is impeded by a resistance in the airway or by strapping applied to the chest. In these circumstances the hypoxaemia is due to ventilation–perfusion inequality but the reduction in oxygen saturation is normally small. This is because at sea level, unlike at altitude, exchange of gas is taking place on the upper flat part of the haemoglobin dissociation curve.

28.8.3 Cardiac output and muscle blood flow

The three components of the delivery of blood to muscles are the cardiac output, the proportion of the output that can be directed to the muscles and the size of the vascular bed available to receive it. The components each have their own determinants and any one of them can limit exercise in appropriate circumstances. Within limits all of them can be improved by physical training (Section 28.12).

The maximal cardiac output is dependent on the quantity and condition of the muscle of the heart and the adequacy of the coronary circulation. These factors were formerly considered to be the principal determinants of exercise capacity [87], but this view has been modified on account of interdependence between the different components of the oxygen transport chain.

The share of cardiac output available to the muscles depends mainly on whether or not there is a competing demand for blood flow to the skin. The latter can have priority when there is a high external heat load or the air is nearly fully saturated with water vapour [39]. Of the other contenders for blood flow, that for the brain is inviolate whilst the renal requirement can usually be deferred; in most circumstances this is also the case for flow to the gastrointestinal tract, but not when much food is present in the stomach.

The size of the muscle vascular bed depends mainly on the extent to which the muscle is used, so in most circumstances it is appropriate to the requirement.

The distribution of muscle blood flow is towards muscles that are active. This is effected both centrally and via locally produced metabolites that stimulate the local autonomic nervous system [88]. Thus, during exercise, cardiac output increases and vessels to non-essential structures constrict. The changes increase the flow to muscles that are active by up to 20 times compared with the blood flow at rest. The increase is necessary for effective tissue transfer of oxygen (see below).

The muscle blood flow is reduced by any condition that impairs the cardiac output or alters its distribution. Diseases and abnormalities of the heart, ingestion of alcohol and pregnancy are common examples.

28.8.4 Tissue transfer of oxygen

The processes whereby oxygen is unloaded from haemoglobin are the opposite of those that operate in the lungs (Section 21.3). They are assisted by the local temperature, hydrogen ion concentration and tension of carbon dioxide being higher than in the alveoli. The surface area for gas exchange within the muscle fibres is that of the capillary endothelium and sarcolemma and is relatively small. This can be a factor limiting the diffusion of oxygen during maximal exercise. The low membrane diffusing capacity is compensated for by the transfer gradient being relatively large. This is due to two processes. First, the oxygen tension throughout the muscle vascular bed is maximised by free diffusion of oxygen between arterioles, capillaries and venules [89]. Thus, the model of Krogh that postulated a gradient of oxygen tension both along the capillaries and within the muscle from a high point at the start of the muscle capillary has been superseded. Second, the back tension is very low, much less than that in venous blood. This is due to the oxygen being both distributed rapidly by myoglobin and taken up rapidly by cytochrome C present in the mitochondria, where the oxygen is utilised. The mitochondria are numerous and have a large surface area, approximately 200 times that of the muscle capillary membrane, so they take up oxygen rapidly [90].

Myoglobin is an oxygen-carrying protein of molecular weight 17,000. It has a single haem and polypeptide chain and combines with oxygen in a hyperbolic manner (Fig. 28.20).

As well as its small size, the myoglobin molecule has a hydrophilic surface. These properties lead to myoglobin being highly mobile within the sarcoplasm, where its diffusivity is as much as one tenth of that of molecular oxygen. The high diffusivity and the high capacity for oxygen make myoglobin an efficient distributor of oxygen within muscle fibres in normal circumstances [92]. However, the molecule shares with haemoglobin the limitation that its retention of carbon monoxide greatly exceeds

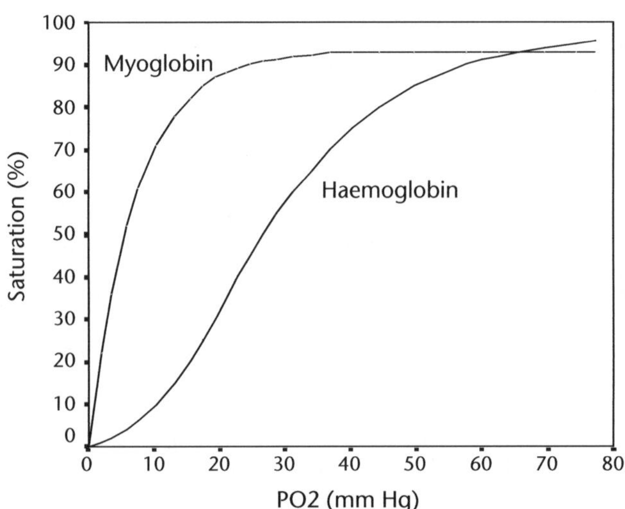

Fig. 28.20 Oxygen dissociation curve for myoglobin. This resembles the first stage in the reaction of oxygen with haemoglobin. It is the absence of subsequent stages that leads to the curve being hyperbolic rather than S shaped (Section 21.2.2). Source: [91]

Table 28.8 Femoral muscle capillary oxygen tension at rest and during cycle ergometry at three inspired oxygen concentrations. The results are means for six non-smoking males (mean age 23.8 years). For symbols and interpretation see text.

Inspired oxygen concentration:		0.21		0.15	0.12
Exercise level:	Rest	Submax	Max	Max	Max
O_2 uptake (mmol min^{-1})	NR	123	199	157	124
(l min^{-1})		2.75	4.46	3.53	2.79
Pa,O_2 (kPa)	11.9	12.4	12.7	7.4	5.0
(mm Hg)	89.0	93.4	95.4	55.5	39.8
$Pc.mu,O_2$ (kPa)	NR	NR	5.1	4.0	3.3
(mm Hg)			38.5	30.3	24.5
$Pv.mu,O_2$ (kPa)	3.8	2.6	2.2	1.9	1.6
(mm Hg)	28.5	19.5	16.8	14.4	12.0
$\dot{V}_E$ l min^{-1}	NR	70	151	136	126
fc min^{-1}	87	149	184	180	176

NR = not recorded. Source: [94]

that of oxygen by a factor of approximately 400. As a result, muscle weakness is a feature of carbon monoxide poisoning.

The oxygen tension in muscle fibres varies with their activity. In one study of dog gracilis muscle the average tension at 25% of maximal oxygen uptake was 2 kPa (13 torr), falling to 0.2 kPa (1.7 torr) at 95% of the maximum [93]. Concurrently, the range of tensions throughout the muscle diminished and at maximal exercise the tension was effectively identical throughout. The observed tensions exceeded those required for oxidative metabolism in the mitrochondria; the latter is less than 0.07 kPa (0.5 torr) and probably of the order of 0.01 kPa (0.1 torr). Thus, even during maximal exercise at sea level the metabolism is not limited by the oxygen tension falling below the critical level for electron transport and oxidative phosphorylation. This has implications for traditional views on anaerobic metabolism in muscle (Section 28.4.6, see also Further reading).

The remarkably high efficiency with which muscle tissue utilises oxygen has the consequence that the transfer gradient for oxygen is effectively the mean oxygen tension of muscle capillary blood. The gradient is defended by both the oxygen delivery, that in trained subjects is high, and by the low oxygen tension at which the muscles operate. Inevitably at low ambient oxygen tensions the demands on the system can exceed the capacity. This has been demonstrated in healthy male subjects performing exercise at different ambient oxygen concentrations when the maximal oxygen uptake was *proportional* to the muscle mean capillary oxygen tension ($Pc.mu,O_2$) calculated using a Bohr integration; the uptake was linearly related to tensions of oxygen in both the blood leaving the exercising muscles ($Pv.mu,O_2$) and the mixed venous blood (Table 28.8).

28.9 Events in muscles

28.9.1 Muscle metabolism

Muscular contraction is effected by the combination of two contractile proteins, actin and myosin. The reaction is triggered by calcium ions migrating from the sarcoplasmic reticulum into the sarcoplasm where they activate myofibular ATPase. The migration is due to nerve stimulation. The reaction consumes energy supplied by breakdown of adenosine triphosphate (ATP) or other phosphate compound having a high energy of hydrolysis. The reaction with ATP can be represented as:

$$\text{ATP} + \text{actin} + \text{myosin} + \text{H}_2\text{O} \overset{\text{Ca}^{++}}{\rightleftharpoons} \text{Actinomysin} + \text{Pi} + \text{ADP} + \text{energy} \quad (28.9)$$

where Pi is inorganic phosphate and ADP is adenosine diphosphate. ADP can be used to generate more ATP but at the cost of reducing the energy that is available in the fibre:

$$2\,\text{ADP} \underset{\text{kinase}}{\overset{\text{adenyl}}{\rightleftharpoons}} \text{ATP} + \text{AMP} \quad (28.10)$$

where AMP is adenosine monophosphate.

The quantity of ATP in skeletal muscle is approximately 7×10^{-3} mol kg^{-1} and is sufficient for only a very brief contraction. The ATP can be replaced instantly by transfer of high-energy phosphate contained in creatine phosphate:

$$\text{CP} + \text{ADP} \underset{\text{kinase}}{\overset{\text{creatine}}{\rightleftharpoons}} \text{ATP} + \text{C} \quad (28.11)$$

where C is creatine and P is phosphate. However, the molar concentration of creatine phosphate in muscle is only about four times that of ATP so replenishment of ATP from this source is inevitably of short term. In the long term the energy for replenishment is effected by oxidation of glycogen, glucose and free fatty acids. However, in the short term ATP can be utilised at a faster rate than it can be renewed by oxidative phosphorylation alone. Thus, during the first half minute of most periods of exercise and during more strenuous or explosive exercise an additional source of energy is needed. This is provided by the rapid breakdown of glucose by a process that does not involve

Table 28.9 Stages in glycolysis.

glucose + ATP	
⇅	
ADP + glucose 6 phosphate ⇌	fructose 6 phosphate + ATP
dihydroxy acetate phosphate	⇅ *
⇅	
glyceraldehyde 3 phosphate ⇌	fructose 1, 6 diphosphate + ADP
⇅ + Pi + NAD	
1.3-diphosphoglycerate + NAD2H	
⇅ + ADP	
ATP + 3 phosphoglycerate	phosphoenol pyruvate
	⇅ + ADP
lactate + NAD ⇌ (NAD2H)	pyruvate + ATP

NAD is nicotinamide adenine dinucleotide, also called coenzyme; in its reduced form this substance is designated NADH or more correctly NAD_2H. The rate limiting step (indicated by *) is controlled by the activation of phosphofructokinase (PFK). This process and also the other abbreviations are described in the text.

oxygen. The process was formerly called anaerobic glycolysis but 'nonaerobic' and 'rapid glycolysis' are more appropriate terms (Section 28.4.6, also see below).

The generation of energy for muscular contraction can be said to have two stages. In the first stage each molecule of glucose is split in two and converted into pyruvate plus reduced coenzyme (NAD_2H), with the formation of four molecules of ATP. Of these, two are replacements for molecules that were expended during the metabolic process. Up to this point the rate-limiting step is the phosphorylation of fructose 6-phosphate by activation of phosphofructokinase (PFK) (Table 28.9).

The second stage entails the disposal of the molecules of pyruvate and reduced coenzyme that were end products from the first stage. In oxidative glycolysis the substances are oxidised with the formation of additional ATP. The process entails transfer of the hydrogen ions from association with NAD to association with oxygen via an electron transport chain within the mitochondrial membrane. The chain involves flavoprotein and a series of cytochromes. It can be represented as

$$NAD_2H + 1/2\,O_2 \underset{\text{flavoprotein}}{\overset{\text{cytochrome}}{\leftrightarrows}} NAD + H_2O + \text{energy} \quad (28.12)$$

The transfer is effected via the Krebs cycle (also known as tricarboxylic or citric acid cycle) through the mediation of oxidative enzymes including succinate dehydrogenase [95]. Other enzymes increase the concentrations of intermediate substances, e.g. alanine aminotransferase [96] that controls the reaction:

glutamate + pyruvate = alanine + 2-oxyglutarate

The enzymes are present in mitochondria, particularly those of slow twitch (type 1) muscle fibres.

In rapid glycolysis the NAD_2H is reoxidised to NAD at the expense of the pyruvate. The latter is reduced to lactate and no ATP is formed. Rapid glycolysis is mediated by lactate dehydrogenase present in the cytoplasm of the muscle fibres, particularly that of fast twitch (type 2) fibres. The different fibre types and subtypes can be identified histologically through stains that are specific for the different enzymes. Features of the different types of fibre and the metabolic processes that they support are summarised in Table 28.10.

28.9.2 Lactate and pyruvate

See also Section 28.4.6.

Most of the lactate produced during the initial rapid glycolysis remains in the muscle. Any lactate that is not metabolised *in situ* passes into the blood where the concentration rises. It is then taken up by the liver or used as substrate by the heart [97]. During mild exercise the lactate concentration and the related concentration of pyruvate are either unchanged from their resting levels or fall slightly if the subject has been fasting [34]. During moderate exercise the concentration often rises transiently due to rapid glycolysis at the start of exercise. For lactate and pyruvate the increases from resting levels are approximately 0.9 and 0.04 mmol l^{-1} (8 mg dl^{-1} and 0.4 mg dl^{-1}), respectively. During strenuous exercise the lactate concentration rises progressively to reach a level of 6–14 mmol l^{-1} (50–130 mg dl^{-1}) at the breaking point of exercise. Most of the increase reflects the insufficient capacity of the mitochondrial enzymes to recycle NAD_2H; the latter is closely related to but not identical with the ability of the oxygen

Table 28.10 Features of two types of effort.

	Explosive effort	Sustained effort
Activity	Turn, lift, throw	Climb, swim, build
Determinants	Muscle strength, skill	High oxidative capacity of muscle
Muscle fibres		
Fibre type	2 (A and B), fast twitch	1 and 2, slow twitch
Enzyme site	Cytoplasm	Mitochondria
Enzyme types	Lactate dehydrogenase Myokinase	MyosinATPase Succinate dehydrogenase
Oxidative capacity	Low	High
Recovery	Slow	Rapid if aerobic throughout
Metabolic pathway		
inital	CP + ADP → C + ATP*	Carbohydrate + NAD → Pyruvate + NAD_2H + ATP*
Final	Lactate dehydrogenase → Lactate + NAD	Krebs cycle + substrate cytochrome chain + O_2 → CO_2 + H_2O + NAD + ATP*
Respiratory component	Small; oxygen debt afterwards	Depends on lung function and muscle blood flow

* (→ ADP + muscle contraction).
CP = phosphocreatine; C = creatine; NAD = nicotinamide-adenine-dinucleotide; ADP = adenosine diphosphate; ATP = adenosine triphosphate.

transport chain to deliver oxygen to the mitochondria. However, some of the increase is due to lactate being in equilibrium with pyruvate, which also becomes more plentiful. The amount can be calculated on the assumption that the ratio of the concentrations of oxidised to reduced coenzyme is the same during exercise as it is at rest. The *excess lactate* is that which cannot be accounted for in this way [98]; its relevance is less than was at one time thought.

28.9.3 McArdle's disease

Patients with this disease are deficient in muscle phosphorylase, hence are unable to oxidise muscle glycogen [99]. The condition is associated with low levels of muscle-NADH, an inability to produce lactate and reduced availability of pyruvate during exercise. The condition is important on account of demonstrating that the presence of lactic acid cannot be the reason for the changes in ventilation during exercise that have been attributed to it (Section 28.4.6). In McArdle's disease the alternative metabolic pathway involves an accumulation of ADP and its breakdown products (e.g. inorganic phosphorus, AMP, inosine 5′-monophosphate, ammonia and adenosine). These substances cause reflex vasodilatation in the active muscles and hence, via the carotid sinus reflex, increase the cardiac output; they may also contribute to fatigue and muscle cramps [100], also [35] and [36] on page 503. The cause of the increased exercise ventilation is probably accumulation of metabolites (Section 28.4.6), but a loss of muscle power leading to increased central drive to respiration may also contribute [101]. The exercise capacity can be improved and the exercise cardiac output restored towards normal by provision of alternative substrates including glucose or fructose by intravenous infusion and free fatty acids by mobilisation from fat depots. This can be achieved by administration of noradrenaline.

28.10 Role of gender

The responses to exercise differ quantitatively between the sexes, with women usually having a higher ventilation and cardiac and respiratory frequency than men, but smaller tidal volume and maximal oxygen uptake. The differences reflect the respective physique, lung sizes, body composition (balance between fat and muscle), activity patterns, haemoglobin concentrations and hormone levels of males and females of all ages. Most of the differences disappear when the relevant variables are allowed for.

Many of the variables that affect the exercise performance also influence the lung function and the two topics are reviewed together in Section 25.7 (see also [102]).

28.11 Effects of age

The physiological response to exercise is usually maintained into middle life and thereafter deteriorates. This process is preceded by progressive deterioration in the structure and function of the lungs. The loss of exercise capacity is contributed to by accumulation of body fat and loss of physical condition from a reduction in the level of habitual activity. Subsequently, there is a more generalised deterioration reflecting changes in most systems of the body. These aspects are reviewed together in Section 25.10 (see also [103]).

28.12 Habitual activity and physical training

28.12.1 Overview of effects

Compared with a sedentary lifestyle maximal training can increase the aerobic capacity by approximately 20%. This is approximately half the variation between individuals due to constitutional differences. Conversely, being confined to bed for 3 weeks can reduce the capacity to only a little above the basal level. Discontinuing a physical training programme has an intermediate effect [104]. The changes affect mainly active skeletal muscles [105] together with the organs and systems that serve them including the heart, the blood [106] and the balance between parasympathetic and sympathetic activity within the autonomic nervous system [107, 108]. Muscles that are inactive or do not participate in a training programme do not benefit from training. This has consequences for rehabilitation (Section 44.4.1). The principal effects of training and an active lifestyle are summarised in Table 28.11; some of them are due to exercise facilitating the release of growth hormone into the blood [109].

Physical training also affects the lungs. Additional growth hormone released by prolonged exercise contributes to their growth in young persons, though not in adults. In addition, at all ages use of the accessory muscles of respiration increases the inspiratory capacity and hence the vital capacity. Consequently the level of habitual activity and type and extent of physical training

Table 28.11 Summary of the changes that result from physical training or an increase in habitual activity. Their combined effect is to increase the ability to perform dynamic exercise. The level of habitual activity is a reference variable for maximal oxygen uptake (Table 29.15, page 433).

Organ/system	Structural changes	Functional changes
Lungs*	Lung size ↑†	Respiratory muscle strength ↑
	Transfer factor ↑†	Vital capacity ↑
		Maximal breathing capacity ↑
Respiratory control	–	Sensitivity to hypoxia ↓ ↓
Exercise ventilation		Submaximal ↓‡
		Maximal ↑
Blood	Total body haemoglobin ↑	Blood volume ↑
		Blood pressure ↓
Heart	Muscle hypertrophies	Contractility ↑
		Stroke volume ↑
		Cardiac frequency ↓
		O_2 uptake at $[La] = 4$ mmol l^{-1} ↑
Muscle capillaries	Number ↑	Blood flow ↑‡
		Mean oxygen tension ↑‡
Muscle fibres	Diameter ↑	Power ↑
	Number ↑	
	Proportion of type 1 ↑¶	
Mitochondria	Number ↑	Oxidative capacity ↑
	Oxidative enzymes ↑	
Gastro-intestinal tract and metabolism	Body fat ↓	
	Basal metabolism ↑	
	Gastro-intestinal motility ↑	
Skeleton	Bone diameter ↑ †	Strength ↑
	Mineral content ↑	
	Cartilage thickness ↑	

* Section 25.5.2
† During period of growth, not subsequently [110]
‡ At constant O_2 uptake
¶ These slow twitch (red) fibres (rich in myosin adenosine triphosphatase) are developed by endurance training.

should be taken into account when interpreting the lung function (Section 25.5.2). For residents at high altitude the effects of activity associated with the terrain and low environmental temperature are supplemented by those of hypoxia (Section 34.2).

The response to training depends on the intensity and duration of the activity. For exercise of high intensity, 30 min per day 3 days a week, for up to 15 weeks, is very effective [108, 111], but for low intensity exercise, for example walking, or where the training is for endurance, longer times are preferable. The beneficial effects of training are apparent at all ages, so old age alone is not a contraindication to taking exercise or engaging in a rehabilitation programme (Section 44.4.1).

28.12.2 Implications for clinical exercise testing

Ventilation. The possession of an above average VC shifts the pattern of breathing towards a relatively large tidal volume and low respiratory frequency. This pattern is associated with a high maximal exercise ventilation, both in absolute terms and relative to the maximal voluntary ventilation (ventilatory capacity). The slower deeper pattern of breathing also reduces the ventilation per minute that is needed to flush the anatomical deadspace; this reduces the ventilation minute volume but at low levels of oxygen uptake (below Owles point, as shown in Figs 28.5 and 28.21)

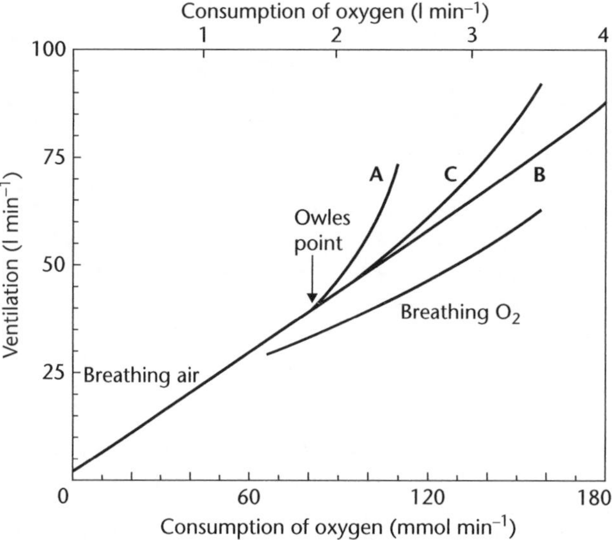

Fig. 28.21 Relationship of ventilation to consumption of oxygen during progressive treadmill exercise up to the maximum which the subjects could achieve. At the time subject *A* was untrained and had a low capacity for exercise, subject *B* was a world class middle distance runner, subject *C* who was assessed by Asmussen and Nielsen [112] was well trained; his response to breathing oxygen was also recorded. During moderate exercise breathing air the ventilatory responses were similar for all three subjects; the responses diverged during strenuous exercise due to the onset of rapid glycolysis at different rates of work which reflected the exercise capacities of the subjects. The ventilation was reduced by breathing oxygen (cf. Figs 23.3 and 23.4, pages 292).

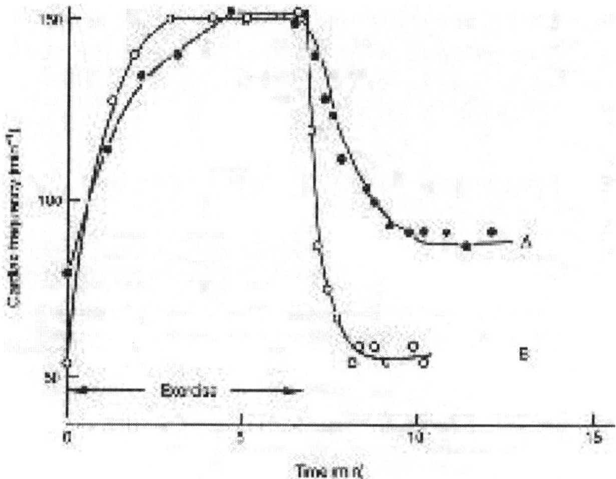

Fig. 28.22 The cardiac frequency during exercise of comparable severity in a world-class athlete (B) and a subject having a low capacity for exercise (A). In the athlete the frequency rises faster at the start of exercise and declines sooner once it is over. Other data are illustrated in Fig. 28.21.

the reduction is small. At higher oxygen uptakes the ventilation is reduced by Owles point being displaced to the right. The displacement is a consequence of improved delivery of oxygen to the muscles and the traditional explanation is that the onset of lactacidaemia is delayed (Fig. 28.10). However, this hypothesis is no longer tenable (Section 28.4.6) and there is a need for more research. The reduced ventilation has the important consequence that during progressive exercise the onset of breathlessness is postponed to a relatively higher rate of work.

Cardiac frequency. Exercise training increases the speed with which the circulation adapts to and recovers from exercise. Hence, the rates of rise and fall in cardiac frequency are increased (Fig. 28.22). Training does not increase and may even reduce the maximal cardiac frequency; the latter provides more time during diastole for perfusion of what is now a more massive heart.

The contractility of the cardiac muscle is also improved by training (see caption to Fig. 28.15) and the two effects together can cause a material increase in stroke volume. There is a corresponding reduction in exercise cardiac frequency and hence no change in cardiac output relative to uptake of oxygen. Training does, however, increase the effectiveness of oxidative metabolism in active muscles by improving their capillary blood supply, increasing the availability of oxidative enzymes and in other ways indicated in Table 28.10.

The reduction in cardiac frequency relative to uptake of oxygen is apparent at rest as well as on exercise, indeed it affects the position to a greater extent than the slope of the relationship ([113], also Fig. 28.15). This observation is a reason for using as an index of the exercise cardiac frequency the value at one level of oxygen uptake (when it can be standardised for body muscle) and not the slope or the position of the relationship (Section 28.6.1). The reduction in frequency is mainly due to diminished sympathetic activity. Increased parasympathetic activity can also contribute, particularly at the start of exercise. The changes lower the blood pressure and have therapeutic applications [106, 107]. The benefits are most apparent in persons with a sedentary lifestyle including the elderly, those with chronic illnesses and persons who are temporarily immobilised by acute illness or injury. The specificity of the effects of activity and physical training to the muscle groups that are used has the important consequence that test exercise in the laboratory should involve the same muscle groups. This usually implies that an exercise test should involve walking as on a treadmill, a 6-min walk or shuttle running and not cycle ergometry (Section 29.4.1).

28.13 References

1. Åstrand P-O, Rodahl K. *Textbook of work physiology.* 3rd ed. London: McGraw-Hill, 1986.
2. Cotes JE. Ventilatory cost of activities. *Br J Ind Med* 1975; **32:** 220–223.
3. Roca J, Whipp BJ, eds. *Clinical exercise testing. Eur Respir Monogr* 1997; **6:** 1–164.
4. Cotes JE, Reed JW, Mortimore IL. Determinants of capacity for physical work. In: Harrison GA, ed. *Energy and effort.* London: Taylor and Francis. *Symposia of Society for Study of Human Biology,* 1982; **22:** 39–64.
5. Cotes JE, Davies CTM, Edholm OG et al. Factors relating to the aerobic capacity of 46 healthy British males and females, ages 18 to 28 years. *Proc R Soc Lond B* 1969; **174:** 91–114.
6. Hugh-Jones P, Lambert AV. A simple standard exercise test and its use for measuring exertion dyspnoea. *BMJ* 1952; **1:** 65–71.
7. Weissman ML, Jones PW, Oren A et al. Cardiac output increase and gas exchange at the start of exercise. *J Appl Physiol* 1982; **52:** 236–244.
8. Krogh A, Lindhard J. The regulation of respiration and circulation during the initial stages of muscular work. *J Physiol (Lond)* 1913; **47:** 112–136.
9. Eldridge FL, Millhorn DE, Kiley JP, Waldrop TG. Stimulation by central command of locomotion, respiration and circulation during exercise. *Respir Physiol* 1985; **59:** 313–337.
10. Adams L, Frankel H, Garlick J et al. The role of spinal cord transmission in the ventilatory response to exercise in man. *J Physiol* 1984; **355:** 85–97.
11. Ozyener F, Rossiter HB, Ward SA, Whipp BJ. Influence of exercise intensity on the on- and off-transient kinetics of pulmonary oxygen uptake in humans. *J Physiol* 2001; **533:** 891–902.
12. Matell G. Time-courses of changes in ventilation and arterial gas tensions in man induced by moderate exercise. *Acta Physiol Scand* 1963; **58**(Suppl 206): 1–53.
13. Durand D, Sadoul P. Etude des paramètres respiratoires au cours des épreuves d'exercises musculaires de durée moyenne à puissance constante chez le sujet sain. Entretiens de *Pathophysiol Respir* 3rd series. Pneumon et Coeur 1959; **9:** 897–940.
14. Grodins FS. Analysis of factors concerned in regulation of breathing in exercise. *Physiol Rev* 1950; **30:** 220–239.
15. Owles WH. Alterations in the lactic acid content of the blood as a result of light exercise and associated changes in the CO_2 combining power of the blood and in the alveolar CO_2 pressure. *J Physiol (Lond)* 1930; **69:** 214–237.
16. Roca J, Whipp BJ. (co-chairmen). Clinical exercise testing with reference to lung diseases: indications, standardization and interpretation strategies. *Eur Respir J* 1997; **10:** 2662–2689.
17. Beaver WL, Wasserman K, Whipp BJ. A new method for detecting anaerobic threshold by gas exchange. *J Appl Physiol* 1986; **60:** 2020–2027.
18. Cotes JE. Response to progressive exercise: a three-index test. *Br J Dis Chest* 1972; **66:** 169–184.
19. Weller JJ, El-Gamal FM, Parker L et al. Indirect estimation of maximal oxygen uptake for study of working populations. *Br J Ind Med* 1988; **45:** 532–537.
20. Gulsvik A, Beckett LA, Bakke P et al. Standardized submaximal exercise testing in never smokers: a normative study. *Clin Physiol* 2001; **21:** 629–636.
21. Allied Dunbar National Fitness Survey. The Sports Council and the Health Education Authority. Northampton, UK. 1992. Data courtesy University of Essex.
22. Kay JDS, Petersen ES, Vejby-Christensen H. Mean and breath-by-breath pattern of breathing in man during steady-state exercise. *J Physiol (Lond)* 1975; **251:** 657–669.
23. Henke KG, Sharratt M, Pegelow D, Dempsey JA. Regulation of end-expiratory lung volume during exercise. *J Appl Physiol* 1988; **64:** 135–146.
24. Jensen JI, Lyager S, Pedersen OF. The relationship between maximal ventilation, breathing pattern and mechanical limitation of ventilation. *J Physiol (Lond)* 1980; **309:** 521–532.
25. Hey EN, Lloyd BB, Cunningham DJC et al. Effects of various respiratory stimuli on the depth and frequency of breathing in man. *Respir Physiol* 1966; **1:** 193–205.
26. Jones NL, Rebuck AS. Tidal volume during exercise in patients with diffuse fibrosing alveolitis. *Bull Eur Physiopathol Respir* 1979; **15:** 321–327.
27. Tomalak W, Cotes JE. Does gender influence tidal volume and respiratory frequency during exercise? *Eur Respir J* 2002; **20**(Suppl 38): 489s.
28. O'Donnell DE, Lam M, Webb KA. Spirometric correlates of improvement in exercise performance after anticholinergic therapy in chronic obstructive pulmonary disease. *Am J Respir Crit Care Med* 1999; **160:** 542–549.
29. Wasserman K, Hansen JE, Sue DY et al. *Principals of exercise testing and interpretation.* 3rd ed. Philadelphia: Lippincot Williams & Wilkins, 1999.
30. Connett RJ, Honig CR, Gayeski TEJ, Brooks GA. Defining hypoxia: a systems review of VO2, glycolysis, energetics, and intracellular PO2. *J Appl Physiol* 1990; **68:** 833–842.
31. Ward S in Whipp BJ, Sargeant AJ eds. *Physiological determinants of exercise tolerance in humans.* Cambridge: Physiological Society. *Studies in Physiology* 1999; **4:** 121–123.
32. Brooks GA. Lactate production under fully aerobic conditions: the lactate shuttle during exercise and recovery. *Fed Proc* 1986; **45:** 2924–2929.
33. Mortimore IL. *The aerobic capacity of healthy people.* PhD Thesis, University of Newcastle upon Tyne, 1982.

34. Reed JW, Parker L. Lactate balance during low levels of exercise. In: Swanson TD, Grodins FS, Hughson RL, eds. *Respiratory control: a modelling perspective.* New York: Plenum,1989: 165–270.
35. Myers J, Ashley E. Dangerous curves. A perspective on exercise lactate, and the anaerobic threshold. *Chest* 1997; **111**: 787–795.
36. Wasserman K, Whipp BJ, Koyal SN et al. Effect of carotid body resection on ventilatory and acid–base control during exercise. *J Appl Physiol* 1975; **39**: 354–358.
37. Paterson D. Potassium and ventilation in exercise. *J Appl Physiol* 1992; **72**: 811–820.
38. McLoughlin F, Popham P, Linton RA et al. Exercise-induced changes in plasma potassium and the ventilatory threshold in man *J Physiol (Lond)* 1994; **479**: 139–147.
39. Williams CG, Bredell GAG, Wyndham CH et al. Circulatory and metabolic reactions to work in heat. *J Appl Physiol* 1962; **17**: 625–638.
40. Belman MJ, Epstein LJ, Doornbos D et al. Non-invasive determinations of the anaerobic threshold. Reliability and validity in patients with COPD. *Chest* 1992; **102**: 1028–1032.
41. Sue DY, Wasserman K, Moricca RB, Casaburi R. Metabolic acidosis during exercise in patients with chronic obstructive lung disease. Use of V-slope method for anaerobic threshold determination. *Chest* 1988; **94**: 931–938.
42. Cotes JE, Fulton HS, King B et al. Relationship of lung function to x-ray reading (ILO) in patients with asbestos-related lung disease. *Thorax* 1988; **43**; 777–783.
43. Reed JW, Ablett M, Cotes JE. Ventilatory responses to exercise and to carbon dioxide in mitral stenosis before and after valvulotomy; causes of tachypnoea. *Clin Sci* 1978; **54**: 9–16.
44. Cotes JE, Gilson JC, McKerrow CB, Oldham PD. A long-term follow-up of workers exposed to beryllium. *Br J Ind Med* 1983; **40**: 13–21.
45. Nordenfelt I, Svensson G. The transfer factor (diffusing capacity) as a predictor of hypoxaemia during exercise in restrictive and chronic obstructive pulmonary disease. *Clin Physiol* 1987; **7**: 423–430.
46. Thin AG, Dodd JD, Gallagher CG et al. Effect of respiratory rate on airway deadspace ventilation during exercise in cystic fibrosis. *Respir Med* 2004; **98**: 1063–1070.
47. Diaz O, Villafranca C, Ghezzo H et al. Breathing pattern and gas exchange at peak exercise in COPD patients with and without tidal flow limitation at rest. *Eur Respir J* 2001; **17**: 1120–1127.
48. Kosmas EN, Milic-Emili J, Polychronaki A et al. Airflow limitation, dynamic hyperinflation and exercise capacity in patients with bronchial asthma. *Eur Respir J* 2004; **24**: 378–384.
49. Cotes JE, Reed JW. Tidal volume during submaximal exercise as an index of lung function: results for men with chronic lung diseases. *Eur Respir J* 2003; **22**: Suppl 45, 88s.
50. Paintal AS. Vagal sensory receptors and their reflex effects. *Physiol Rev* 1973; **53**: 159–227.
51. Kappagoda CT, Ravi K, Teo KK. Effect of pulmonary venous congestion on respiratory rate in dogs. *J Physiol* 1989; **408**: 115–128.
52. Wright GW. Disability evaluation in industrial pulmonary disease. *JAMA* 1949; **141**: 1218–1222.
53. Cotes JE, Posner V, Reed JW. Estimation of maximal exercise ventilation and oxygen uptake in patients with chronic lung disease. *Bull Eur Physiopathol Respir* 1982; **18**(Suppl 4): 221–228.
54. Rowell LB. *Human cardiovascular control.* New York: Oxford University Press, 1993.
55. Reeves JT, Grover RF, Blount SG, Jr, Filley GF. Cardiac output response to standing and treadmill walking. *J Appl Physiol* 1961; **16**: 283–288.
56. Rodeheffer RJ, Gerstenblith G, Becker LC et al. Exercise cardiac output is maintained with advancing age in healthy human subjects: cardiac dilatation and increased stroke volume compensate for a diminished heart rate. *Circulation* 1984; **69**: 203–213.
57. Damato AN, Galante JG, Smith WM. Hemodynamic response to treadmill exercise in normal subjects. *J Appl Physiol* 1966; **21**: 959–966.
58. Higgs BE, Clode M, McHardy GJR et al. Changes in ventilation, gas exchange and circulation during exercise in normal subjects. *Clin Sci* 1967; **32**: 329–337.
59. Fairbarn MS, Blackie SP, Mc Elvaney NG et al. Prediction of heart rate and oxygen uptake during incremental and maximal exercise in healthy adults. *Chest* 1994; **105**: 1365–1369.
60. Brown A, Cotes JE, Mortimore IL, Reed JW. An exercise training programme for firemen. *Ergonomics* 1982; **25**: 793–800.
61. Boni E, Grassi V, Sorbini GA, Tantucci C. In: Serra R. (Coordinator). Research to standardize exercise tests for early detection on respiratory and cardio-respiratory impairment in coal- and steel-workers of ECSC. *Health and Safety at Work* ECSC-EEC-EAEC, Brussels, Luxembourg, 1997: 131–159.
62. Neder JA, Newry LE, Peres C, Whipp BJ. Reference values for dynamic responses to incremental cycle ergometry in males and females aged 20 to 80. *Am J Respir Crit Care Med* 2001; **164**: 1481–1486.
63. Whipp BJ, Higgenbotham MB, Cobb FC. Estimating exercise stroke volume from asymptotic oxygen pulse in humans. *J Appl Physiol* 1996; **81**: 2674–2679.
64. Reed JW. *Mechanisms of tachypnoea.* PhD Thesis, University of Wales 1975.
65. Adams L, Chronos N, Lane R, Guz A. The measurement of breathlessness induced in normal subjects: individual differences. *Clin Sci (Lond)* 1986; **70**: 131–140.
66. Marshall R, Stone RW, Christie RV. The relationship of dyspnoea to respiratory effort in normal subjects, mitral stenosis and emphysema. *Clin Sci* 1954; **13**: 625–631.
67. Elliott MW, Adams L, Cockcroft A et al. The language of breathlessness. Use of verbal descriptors by patients with cardiopulmonary disease. *Am Rev Respir Dis* 1991; **144**: 826–832.
68. Craik MC. *Physiological and clinical aspects of breathlessness assessed using the visual analogue scale.* PhD Thesis, University of Newcastle upon Tyne, 1988.
69. Adams L, Guz A, eds. *Respiratory sensation.* New York: Marcel Dekker, 1996.
70. Banzett RB, Lansing RW, Reid MB et al. 'Air hunger' arising from increased P_{CO_2} in mechanically ventilated quadriplegics. *Respir Physiol* 1989; **76**: 53–67.
71. Lane R, Adams L, Guz A. The effects of hypoxia and hypercapnia on perceived breathlessness during exercise in humans. *J Physiol* 1990; **428**: 579–593.
72. Isaev G, Murphy K, Guz A, Adams L. Areas of the brain concerned with ventilatory load compensation in awake man. *J Physiol (Lond)* 2002; **539**: 935–945.
73. Cooper SJ, Coates JC, Wardrobe-Wong N, Reed JW. Effects of respiratory muscle training on breathlessness during exercise in healthy young adults. *J Physiol (Lond)* 1999; **520**: 57P.
74. Mahler DA, ed. *Dyspnea.* New York: Marcel Dekker, 1998.

75. Guz A, Noble MIM, Eisele JH, Trenchard D. Experimental results of vagal block in cardiopulmonary disease. In: Porter R, ed. *Breathing: Hering-Breuer centenary symposium*. London: Churchill, 1971: 315–329.
76. Schelegle ES, Mansoor JK, Green JF. Interaction of vagal lung afferents with inhalation of histamine aerosol in anesthetized dogs. *Lung* 2000; **178**: 41–52.
77. Potter WA, Olafsson S, Hyatt RE. Ventilatory mechanics and expiratory flow limitation during exercise in patients with obstructive lung disease. *J Clin Invest* 1971; **50**: 910–919.
78. Babb TG, Rodarte JR. Estimation of ventilatory capacity during submaximal exercise. *J Appl Physiol* 1993; **74**: 2016–2022.
79. Babb TG, Viggiano R, Hurley B et al. Effect of mild-to-moderate airflow limitation on exercise capacity. *J Appl Physiol* 1991; **70**: 223–230.
80. Gandevia B, Hughes-Jones P. Terminology for measurements of ventilatory capacity. *Thorax* 1957; **12**: 290–293.
81. Snider GL. Enhancement of exercise performance in COPD patients by hyperoxia: a call for research. *Chest* 2002; **122**: 1830–1836.
82. Cotes JE, Matthews CR, Tasker PM. Continuous versus intermittent administration of oxygen during exercise in patients with chronic lung disease. *Lancet* 1963; **1**: 1075–1077.
83. Garrod R, Paul EA, Wedzicha JA. Supplemental oxygen during pulmonary rehabilitation in COPD patients with exercise hypoxaemia. *Thorax* 2000; **55**: 539–543.
84. Wagner PD. Determinants of maximal oxygen transport and utilisation. *Ann Rev Physiol* 1996; **58**: 21–50.
85. Wagner PD. New ideas on limitation of Vo_2max. *Exerc Sport Sci Rev* 2000; **28**: 10–14.
86. Dempsey JA, Wagner PD. Exercise-induced arterial hypoxemia. *J Appl Physiol* 1999; **87**: 1997–2006.
87. Noakes TD. Physiological models to understand exercise fatigue and the adaptations that predict or enhance exercise performance. *Scand J Med Sci Sports* 2000; **10**: 123–145.
88. O'Sullivan SE, Bell C. The effects of exercise and training on human cardiovascular reflex control. *J Auton Nerv Syst* 2000; **81**: 16–24.
89. Ellsworth ML, Pittman RN. Arterioles supply oxygen to capillaries by diffusion as well as by convection. *Am J Physiol* 1990; **258**: H1240–1243.
90. Hoppeler H, Weibel ER. Structural and functional limits for oxygen supply to muscle. *Acta Physiol Scand* 2000; **168**: 445–456.
91. Roughton FJW Respiratory function of blood. In: Boothby WM, ed.: *Handbook of Respiratory Physiology*. Texas: USAF School of Aviation Medicine, 1954: 51–102.
92. Gayeski TEJ, Connett RJ, Honig CR. Oxygen transport in rest-work transition illustrates new functions for myoglobin. *Am J Physiol* 1985; **248**: H914–H921.
93. Gayeski TE, Honig CR. Intracellular Po_2 in long axis of individual fibers in working dog gracilis muscle. *Am J Physiol* 1988; **254**: H1179–H1186.
94. Roca J, Hogan MC, Storey D et al. Evidence for tissue diffusion limitation of Vo_2 max in normal humans. *J Appl Physiol* 1989; **67**: 291–299.
95. Kornberg H. Krebs and his trinity of cycles. *Nat Rev Mol Cell Biol* 2000; **1**: 225–228.
96. Gibala MJ. Regulation of skeletal muscle amino acid metabolism during exercise. *Int J Sport Nutr Exerc Metab* 2001; **11**: 87–108.
97. Brooks GA. Intra- and extra-cellular lactate shuttles. *Med Sci Sports Exerc* 2000; **32**: 790–799.
98. Huckabee WE. Relationships of pyruvate and lactate during anaerobic metabolism. *J Clin Invest* 1958; **37**: 244–271.
99. Beynon RJ, Bartram C, Flannery A et al. Interrelationships between metabolism of glycogen phosphorylase and pyridoxal phosphate-implications in McArdle's disease. *Adv Food Nutr Res* 1996; **40**: 135–147.
100. Lewis SF, Haller RG. The pathophysiology of McArdle's disease: clues to regulation in exercise and fatigue. *J Appl Physiol* 1986: **61**: 391–401.
101. Hagberg JM, King DS, Rogers M et al. Exercise and recovery ventilatory and VO2 responses of patients with McArdle's disease. *J Appl Physiol* 1990; **68**: 1393–1398.
102. Olfert IM, Balouch J, Kleinsasser A et al. Does gender affect pulmonary gas exchange during exercise? *J Physiol* 2004; **557**: 529–541.
103. Tanaka H, Seals DR. Dynamic exercise performance in Masters athletes: insights into the effects of primary human aging on physiological functional capacity. *J Appl Physiol* 2003; **95**: 2152–2162.
104. Mujika I, Padilla S. Cardiorespiratory and metabolic characteristics of detraining in humans. *Med Sci Sports Exerc* 2001; **33**: 413–421.
105. Hawley JA. Adaptations of skeletal muscle to prolonged, intense endurance training. *Clin Exp Pharmacol Physiol* 2002; **29**: 218–222.
106. Shaskey DJ, Green GA. Sports haematology. *Sports Med* 2000; **29**: 27–38.
107. Goldsmith RL, Bloomfield DM, Rosenwinkel ET. Exercise and autonomic function. *Coron Artery Dis* 2000; **11**: 129–135.
108. Krieger EM, Da Silva GJ, Negrao CE. Effects of exercise training on baroreflex control of the cardiovascular system. *Ann NY Acad Sci* 2001; **940**: 338–347.
109. Cathy JP-R, Wideman L, Weltman JY et al. Gender governs the relationship between exercise intensity and growth hormone release in young adults. *J Appl Physiol* 2002; **92**: 2053–2060.
110. Reuschlein PS, Reddan WG, Burpee J et al. Effect of physical training on the pulmonary diffusing capacity during submaximal work. *J Appl Physiol* 1968; **24**: 152–158.
111. Lemura LM, von Duvillard SP, Mookerjee S. The effects of physical training on functional capacity in adults. Ages 46 to 90: a meta-analysis. *J Sports Med Phys Fitness* 2000; **40**: 1–10.
112. Asmussen E, Nielsen M. Pulmonary ventilation and effect of oxygen breathing in heavy exercise. *Acta Physiol Scand* 1958; **43**: 365–378.
113. Clausen JP. Effect of physical training on cardiovascular adjustments to exercise in man. *Physiol Rev* 1977; **57**: 779–815.

Further reading

Altose MD, Kawakami Y. *Control of breathing in health and disease* (chapters on exercise). New York: Marcel Dekker, 1999.
Brooks GA, Fahey TD. *Exercise physiology: human bioenergetics and its application.* New York: Wiley, 1984.
Dempsey JA, Vidruk EH, Mitchell GS. Pulmonary control systems in exercise: update. *Fed Proc* 1985; **44**: 2260–2270.
Jones NL. *Clinical exercise testing*, 4th ed. Philadelphia: Saunders, 1997.
Gimenez M, Saunier C. *Muscular exercise in chronic lung disease.* Oxford: Pergamon Press, 1980.

*McDonough P, Behnke BJ, Padilla DJ et al. Control of microvascular oxygen pressures in muscles comprised of different fibre types. *J. Physiol* 2005; **563**: 903–913.

Scano G, Stendardi L, Grazzini M. Understanding dyspnoea by its language. Series "Respiratory monitoring: revisiting classical physiological principles with new tools". *Eur Respir J* 2005; **25**: 380–385.

*Vogiatzis I, Georgiadou O, Golemati S et al. Patterns of dynamic hyperinflation during exercise and recovery in patients with severe chronic obstructive pulmonary disease. *Thorax* 2005; **60**: 723–729.

*Recent reference.

CHAPTER 29

Exercise Testing and Interpretation, including Reference Values

This chapter is about exercise testing including interpretation, so is a sequel to Chapter 28 that describes the physiology and clinical physiology of exercise. Exercise capacity and disability are discussed in Chapter 30 and exercise testing in children in Chapter 31.

29.1 Introduction

Most parts of the body contribute to exercise and impairment of almost any part can give rise to symptoms, particularly breathlessness on exertion. An exercise test can identify the underlying features, including any compensatory mechanisms and can help in diagnosis, treatment and other aspects of managing the condition. Thus, exercise testing can be approached at a number of levels and can have any of several objectives. Of these, overall performance is often the least informative. Prior to the assessment there is need to identify what is likely to be useful. A choice can then be made of procedure (ergometric, non-ergometric or field test), protocol and any additional information that may be required to further the objectives of the test [1].

Exercise testing requires that the subject trusts and cooperates with the operator who is both responsible for safety and for obtaining subjective as well as objective information. As a result, working in an exercise laboratory is a demanding occupation, but one that can bring satisfaction to those who are involved.

29.2 Reasons for an exercise test

29.2.1 In apparently fit persons

1 Epidemiology (submaximal test): to assess physical condition of a general population [2] or occupational group [3], or screen for a particular functional defect (see below).
2 Stress cardiography (near maximal test): to look for evidence of coronary insufficiency (page 418) or latent systemic hypertension (systolic BP > 200 mm Hg, diastolic BP > 100 mm Hg or their equivalents in other units). The test procedure has additional applications.
3 Measure maximal oxygen uptake (maximal test): to assess physical condition and performance of athletes [4], monitor

fitness for a particular activity (e.g. mine rescue, deep sea diving), obtain reference values for disability assessments.

29.2.2 In respiratory and other patients

1 Assessment of breathlessness from any cause (symptom limited test): as well as respiratory disease, the cause might be congenital or acquired heart disease, anaemia or a metabolic or endocrine disorder [1, 5].
2 Use as a lung function test:
to complete the diagnosis of a respiratory syndrome (e.g. defective gas transfer [6–8]),
to assess impaired control of breathing [9],
to determine the causes and appropriateness of shallow breathing (Sections 28.4.5 and 28.4.7),
to investigate breathlessness that is disproportionate to the loss of lung function (the latter is a poor guide to exercise capacity) ([10, 11] also Section 30.2),
to apportion the causes of dyspnoea in a patient who has more than one disorder,
to provide additional information on prognosis [12].
3 Investigate features that cannot be demonstrated at rest e.g.:
failure of the transfer factor to increase on exercise [13],
reduction in oxygen saturation during exercise [14],
airways obstruction brought on by exercise (exercise challenge testing) [15, 16], also Section 15.8.3,
ischaemic pain (angina or pain in calf) brought on by exercise (S-LET, Section 29.3.3).
4 Contribute to treatment:
to assess response to bronchodilator therapy where there is apparent benefit but ventilatory capacity is not improved at rest (Section 15.7.2),
preoperative assessment especially in relation to thoracic or cardiac surgery [17], also Sections 43.1–43.5,
to assess need for and monitor portable oxygen therapy (Fig. 28.19 and associated text),
to assess need for and monitor pulmonary rehabilitation [18, 19], also Section 44.4.
5 Make assessments in relation to employment:
to assess the extent of respiratory disability, including any functional component [20], also Chapter 30,
to assess residual exercise ability with view to re-employment [21], also Section 30.6.

29.3 Exercise protocols

29.3.1 Submaximal progressive protocol

The exercise is of progressively increasing intensity, up to a predetermined end point (Table 29.1).

A submaximal protocol is recommended for circumstances where there is a need for high acceptance and completion rates amongst subjects who may be reluctant to perform an exercise test. Hence, the endpoint should be set at the lowest level that is compatible with the aims of the study rather than the maximum that can be attained. The applications include respiratory surveys and making serial observations.

Table 29.1 Some end points for a submaximal progressive exercise test.

Endpoint
Specified rate of work e.g. 60 W on a cycle ergometer.
Fraction of maximal work rate or O_2 uptake *, e.g. 80%
Specified O_2 uptake e.g. $\dot{V}O_2 = 1.0\ l\ min^{-1}$, ($\dot{n}O_2 = 45$ mmol min^{-1})
Specified cardiac frequency e.g. 100 min^{-1}
Fraction of maximal cardiac frequency*, e.g. 85%
Specified respiratory exchange ratio, e.g. 1.0

* The maximum can be measured or estimated.

The immediate objective is to obtain measurements of ventilation, cardiac frequency and other variables with a view to their being standardised in an appropriate manner (e.g. Fig. 29.1).

The mode of exercise can be progressive submaximal, multiple steady state submaximal or symptom limited (maximal) exercise. To avoid fatigue the protocol should normally lead to the desired end point being achieved in approximately 5–10 min. Examples of protocols suitable for respiratory patients exercising on a treadmill and cycle ergometer are given under these headings below. The two forms of ergometry yield significantly different results (Table 29.2).

29.3.2 Submaximal steady state protocol

The procedure is used to create stable conditions for measurement of cardiac output, pulmonary arterial pressure and certain other variables. Exercise is performed at a constant, submaximal rate of work and a steady state is usually considered to have been achieved by the 5th min. The measurements are then made in the 5th and 6th min. The procedure can also be used to assess 'on' and 'off' transients at the beginning and end of exercise and for this purpose the physiological variables are monitored each breath. If the recovery is of interest the monitoring is continued for an appropriate time after exercise. The time for a response variable (e.g.ventilation) to reach its plateau or recovery value during steady state exercise is usually considered to be exponential. In this event the exponent (the time constant τ) is the time to reach 63% of the equilibrium value. Then:

$$\text{Value at time } t = \text{plateau value } (1 - e^{-t/\tau})$$

29.3.3 Symptom-limited exercise test (S-LET)

A progressive protocol is adopted and is continued until symptoms occur that are of sufficient intensity to terminate the exercise. The symptom will normally be incapacitating

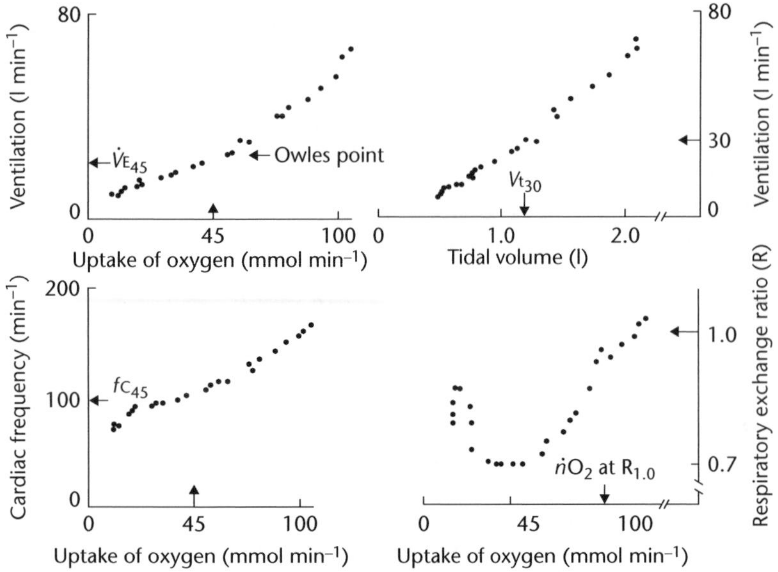

Fig. 29.1 Data obtained during the course of a submaximal progressive exercise test in a healthy subject. The arrows indicate the indices fC$_{45}$, $\dot{V}$E$_{45}$ and Vt$_{30}$, also $\dot{n}$O$_2$ at R = 1.0 and Owles point. These and other indices are described subsequently. An O_2 uptake of 45 mmol min^{-1} is 1.0 l min^{-1} in traditional units.

Table 29.2 Comparison of treadmill and cycle ergometry.

Aspect	Treadmill vs cycle
All subjects	
Max. o_2 uptake and ventilation	Greater*
Extent of desaturation	More marked
Submax Vt	Higher
COPD patients	
Principal symptom	Breathlessness vs fatigue
Submaximal $\dot{V}$E and fC	Similar

* See cycle ergometry, Section 29.4.3.
Source: [3, 22–24].

Table 29.3 Cardiovascular indications for discontinuing an exercise test. Several of the contraindications have more than one cause, so any association with cardiovascular disease should be verified [25].

Appearance	Pallor with sweating Ischaemic pain (angina, pain in leg)
Electrocardiogram	ST depression >0.2 mV Ventricular ectopic beats *If* { coupled 2 or more consecutive >2 single >7 per minute
Blood pressure	Failure to increase with load Excessive increase (>210/150 mm Hg) Decline (Δ BP systolic >10 mm Hg)

breathlessness, but might be fatigue, coughing, bronchospasm or ischaemic pain. Occasionally the exercise will need to be terminated by the operator. In this event the commonest indication is a cardiovascular one (Table 29.3). To avoid fatigue the increments of work should be adjusted so that the patient develops the symptoms in approximately 10 min. The procedure combines measurement of the physiological response to submaximal exercise with observing the patient experience the symptom that limits exercise. From a clinical perspective the record of symptoms can be the most important outcome of the test. S-LET is the first choice for assessment of most patients, particularly where there is a need to find the physiological causes for a patient's breathlessness. For this application a test that entails walking is usually preferable to other forms of ergometry (Section 29.4.1).

29.3.4 Nearly maximal exercise test (ergocardiography, bronchial lability)

This procedure is used in the management of suspected ischaemic heart disease and for assessing fitness for heavy work. It entails progressive exercise that is started from rest. A positive test is one that is terminated because of an electrocardiographic or related abnormality (Table 29.3). Other end points are attainment of a predetermined cardiac frequency, usually 80–85% of the predicted maximal frequency (eqn. 28.2, page 399), or reaching a nearly maximal work rate (usually 80% of the expected $\dot{V}o_2$ max).

The test is commonly undertaken on a treadmill with a standard protocol (e.g. Bruce, Table 29.4). The associated energy expenditures (oxygen uptakes) are indicated in Fig. 29.2. When a cycle ergometer is used the rate of work is usually increased in a linear manner (e.g. 10 or 20 W min^{-1}).

Nearly maximal exercise can form the first part of a two-stage procedure for measurement of aerobic capacity (Section 29.3.5 below). It can also be used to test for exercise-induced airflow limitation (Section 15.8.3).

29.3.5 Maximal exercise test (aerobic capacity)

The procedure entails a submaximal progressive, followed by nearly maximal exercise (stages 1 and 2, respectively). It is used to

Table 29.4 Treadmill protocols for cardiovascular stress testing (ergocardiography); the stages are of 3 min duration except where indicated. Sources: [26, 27], see also [4].

	Bruce [26]		Wolthuis [27]		Balke [26]	
Time (min)	Speed (mph)	Incline (%)	Speed (mph)	Incline (%)	Speed (mph)	Incline (%)
0	1.7*	10	3.3†	0	3.3‡	1‡
3	2.5	12		5		4
6	3.4	14		10		7
9	4.2	16		15		10
12	5.0	18		20		13
15	5.5	20		25		16

* 3.3 mph is 5.3 kph (the conversion factor is 1.61, Table 6.6, page 56).
† One or more stages at lower speeds are recommended for subjects who are not robust.
‡ Incline is increased at 1% per minute.

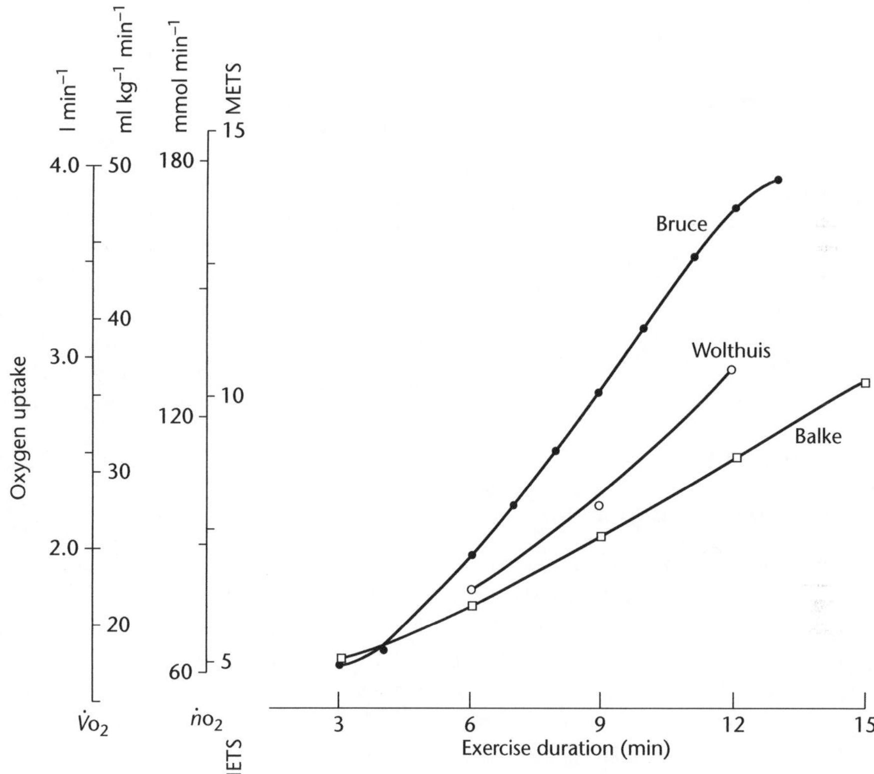

Fig. 29.2 Approximate relationships of oxygen uptake to exercise duration using the protocols listed in Table 29.4. They are for men of mean body mass 80 kg. For these subjects, the resting metabolic rate, referred to as one metabolic equivalent (MET) was 12.5 mmol min^{-1} (0.28 l min^{-1}, equivalent to 3.5 ml kg^{-1} min^{-1}).

measure aerobic capacity, also known as maximal oxygen uptake (Section 28.1, page 386). The index is commonly reported in traditional units (l min^{-1}) for which the appropriate symbol is $\dot{V}O_2$max. This quantity is often used to define the capacity of the cardio-respiratory-muscle system. However, the maximal oxygen uptake varies with the quantity of muscle participating in the exercise and hence the type of ergometry (Table 29.5).

Maximal exercise is appropriate for persons engaging in athletics and other activities requiring a high level of energy expenditure, but is poorly tolerated and sometimes resented by those who are not athletic. Maximal exercise in respiratory patients is used in assessment for portable oxygen therapy (Section 28.8.1), rehabilitation (Chapter 44), rating respiratory disability (Section 30.5.2) and assessing the potential for re-employment (Section 30.6).

The submaximal stage in the measurement of aerobic capacity is used to obtain the relationship of cardiac frequency to uptake of oxygen and/or rate of work. The relationship should be based on several data points and extrapolated to the average maximal frequency for age of *similar* subjects (e.g. eqn. 28.2, page 399). Extrapolation from a single work rate, e.g. [29] is less accurate. The corresponding oxygen uptake and work rate provides an indication of the aerobic capacity. Either quantity can be used as a guide to the initial work level for the second stage of the

Table 29.5 Dependence of aerobic capacity on type of ergometer.

Type of ergometer	$\dot{V}O_2$ max relative to treadmill
Ladder mill	>1.0
Cycling + hand cranking	>1.0
Treadmill	1.0
Cycle ergometer	0.89–0.93*
Hand cranking	0.6 (approx)

* >1.0 in highly trained cyclists.
Source: [28].

test. This should preferably start at an intermediate point on a standard protocol, usually two or three increments of work below the expected maximum. Strong exhortation should be given. The end point is when an increase in rate of work no longer increases the oxygen uptake by >150 ml min^{-1} [30]. In favourable circumstances the end point is reached in 4 or 5 min. However, many subjects find the procedure disagreeable and discontinue exercise without achieving a plateau. In this circumstance the extrapolation procedure should be repeated using the results for stage 2. The aerobic capacity is then either the observed or extrapolated value [2]. When reporting the result the method of derivation should be stated [28]. Additional information is given in Sections 28.1 (Units of measurement), 28.8 (Potential limiting factors) and 30.5 (Interpretation).

29.4 Ergometry

29.4.1 Choice of ergometer

Cycle ergometry is now the preferred choice of both the American Thoracic and European Respiratory Societies [1,5]. However, the defining criteria are administrative and at odds with the physiological evidence; this favours use of a treadmill because this form of exercise usually reproduces the symptoms experienced by a respiratory patient whereas cycle ergometry often does not (Table 29.6, also [24]). Cycle ergometry may be more suitable for cardiac patients. It is appropriate for persons who cycle regularly including many children and those who undertake cycle ergometry as a means of keeping fit.

29.4.2 Treadmill

Treadmill exercise simulates walking and running. These are familiar activities and can extend over a wide range of energy expenditure. The energy cost varies with the velocity and the angle of incline of the belt. When out of doors the energy expenditure also varies with the terrain. For any combination of these variables the energy cost is proportional to the subject's mass including that of any load (Figs 29.3 and 29.4 (right)). The energy cost is reduced by practice through the acquisition of a more economical style of locomotion [34]. Theoretically this could be a problem for serial measurements, but in practice no difficulty appears to have been reported.

A treadmill was formerly driven passively by the subject. Now it is usually a continuous belt that is driven across a flat surface by an electric motor fitted with a continuously variable gear. The minimal surface dimensions should be 2 m × 0.5 m and the belt speed 0–14 kph. The incline (i.e. the sine of the angle to the horizontal expressed as a percentage) should be capable of continuous adjustment from horizontal to at least 15%. The speed and incline indicators should be calibrated. The treadmill should be electrically earthed, and equipped with handrails, safety harness or rear safety chain. It should also have the means for rapid deceleration, capable of being operated either automatically or by the subject or observer. There should be an adjacent platform to provided access and a gantry for supporting the mouthpiece or face mask. Agile subjects can be instructed to step onto the belt when it is moving using the handrails for support. Inexperienced or frail subjects should stand on the belt before it is set in motion, which should be done gradually. The subject should be instructed to walk as naturally as possible in an upright posture with head erect, eyes looking ahead and initially taking relatively long steps. At the start one hand can rest on the rail, but once the predetermined speed has been achieved the arms should be allowed to swing. This encourages the subject to breathe naturally and reduces variability in oxygen uptake because no physical work is then done by the arms. At the end of exercise, either the

Table 29.6 Relative merits of different types of ergometer.

Criterion	Treadmill	Cycle*	Step
Cost	Medium	Medium	Low
Space needed	Considerable	Modest	Modest
Safety requirements	Extra care	Normal care	Extra care
Convenience	Moderate	High	Low
Estimate of external work	Approximate [31]†	Precise	Precise
Symptoms at breaking point	Relevant to patient's experience	Not relevant	Fairly relevant

* Results can be qualitatively different from those for treadmill exercise (Table 29.2).
† Divergent views are expressed as to the clinical usefulness of this information!

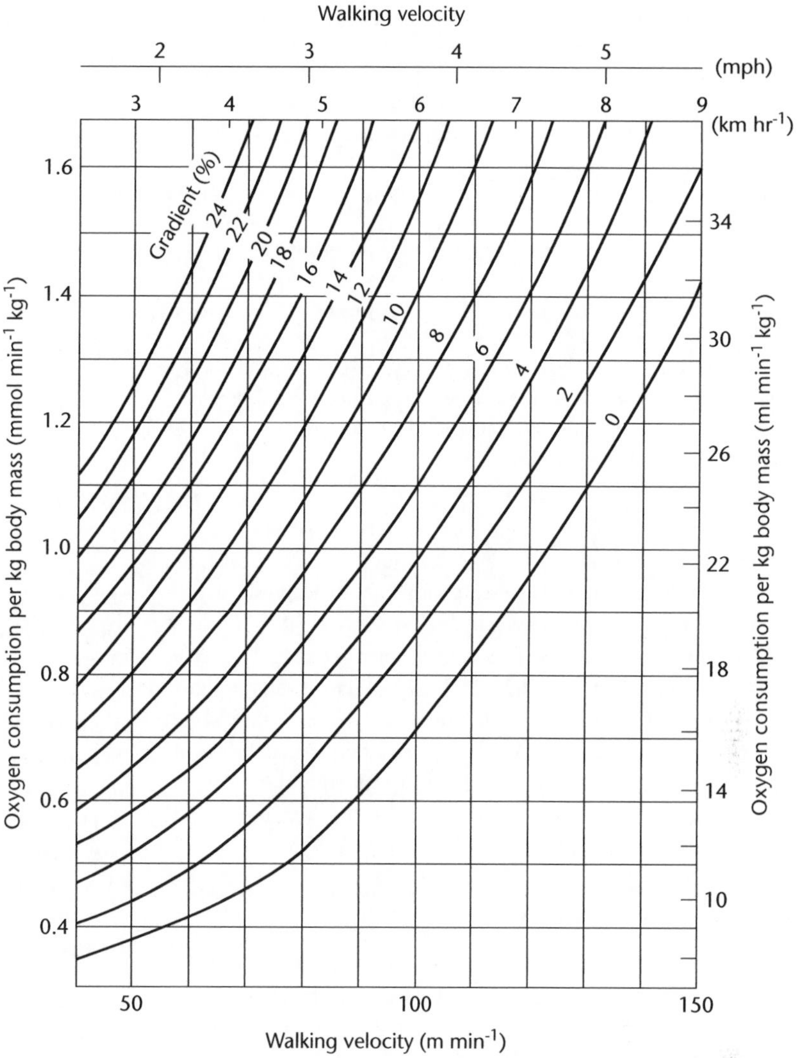

Fig. 29.3 Graphical solution to the relationship of Givoni and Goldman describing the oxygen cost of treadmill walking per kg body mass:

$$\dot{n}o_2 = \frac{44.6}{294}\eta M[2.3 + 0.32(V - 2.5)]^{1.65} + G[0.2 + 0.07(V - 2.5)]$$

RSD 4.86 mmol min^{-1}

where $\dot{n}o_2$ is oxygen uptake in mmol min^{-1}; η is the terrain factor which for treadmill walking is 1.0, M is body mass (kg), G is gradient as percentage (100 × sine of angle of incline), V is velocity (km h^{-1}). To convert to oxygen uptake in traditional units (l min^{-1}) divide by 44.6 and to kcal h^{-1} multiply by 294. Source: [31].

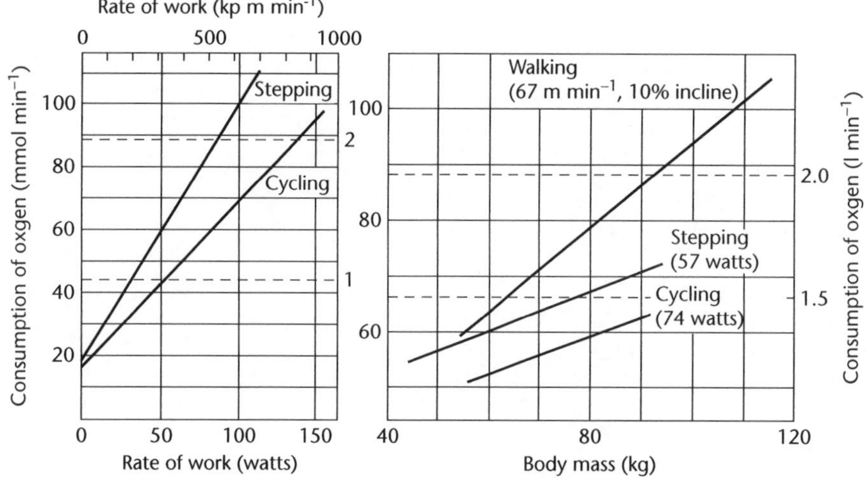

Fig. 29.4 Oxygen cost of exercise for healthy men.
Left. Relationships to rate of work. For cycling, the work is that done in overcoming the restraint applied to the flywheel. For walking and stepping, it is the product of body mass, the vertical movement of the centre of gravity of the body per step and step frequency. The additional cost of stepping reflects that of restraining the body during stepping down (negative work).
Right. Average relationships of the consumption of oxygen to body mass for subjects performing standardised exercise: walking at 67 m min^{-1} (2.5 mph) up an incline of 1 in 10, stepping at 57 W (350 kp m min^{-1}) and cycling at 73.5 W (450 kp m min^{-1}). Sources: [32, 33].

Table 29.7 Progressive protocols for treadmill and cycle ergometry.

	Cycle ergometer			Treadmill			
	Healthy person		Patient	Healthy person		Patient	
Test	Submax	Max	Symptom limited	Submax	Max	Symptom limited	
Starting point	Rest – 20 W	W at RER = 1.0	Rest	3 kph	Incline ≥4°	2.0 kph	Incline 4°
Increment per minute	15 W	20 W	10 W	1 kph 1°*	1°	0.5 kph	1°
End point	Rest = 1.0	$\dot{n}O_2$max	$\dot{n}O_2$max (SL)†	RER = 1.0	$\dot{n}O_2$max	4 kph	$\dot{n}O_2$max (SL)†

W = watts; kph = kilometres per hour; SL = symptom-limited.
* From 4 kph onwards increments of velocity and incline can alternate.
† Exercise may also be terminated at $\dot{n}O_2 = 45$ mmol min^{-1}.
Source: [35], see also Fig. 29.2.

belt is decelerated or the subject quickly gets off by gripping the handrails then placing the feet astride the belt. Exercise protocols for ergocardiography and assessing the physiological response to exercise are given, respectively, in Tables 29.4 and 29.7.

The outcome of the test is usually in terms of oxygen uptake and other physiological indices (Table 29.8). However, for ergocardiography (e.g. Table 29.4) the time into the test or the stage reached can be used instead. For this to be representative of the subject's exercise tolerance the treadmill should have been set precisely and the exercise performed in the recommended manner.

29.4.3 Cycle ergometry

A cycle ergometer is a stationary bicycle with the front wheel removed and the rear wheel restrained in a controlled manner; the restraint is usually electromagnetic, formerly it was mechanical. The cycling rate should be displayed for the subject to see but a metronome should not be used because it can influence the respiratory frequency. The loading should be capable of continuous variation from zero to the equivalent of 1 kW when the subject is cycling at 1 Hz. The work rate will usually be in watts but may be in kilopond metres per minute (see Footnote 29.1). The work rate meter should be calibrated [36, 37].

The restraint on the flywheel is usually controlled by a servomechanism set to maintain either a pre-set steady work rate or one that increases by linear or logarithmic increments. A setting for zero work can also be incorporated. The increases are usually either continuous (triangular or ramp protocol) or incremental each minute. The physiological responses are similar.

Formerly 3-min increments were used on account of combining the features of progressive and nearly steady state exercise (staircase exercise). However, for studying responses to steady state exercise longer increments (e.g. 5 or 6 min) are necessary. The size of the increment will normally be in the range 10 W–30 W min^{-1} and chosen with a view to the subject achieving the chosen end point within 10 min. The end point will usually be a predetermined rate of work or the symptom-limited maximum. The former can constitute either a complete test or be the first stage of a maximal exercise test (Section 30.4.1).

The oxygen cost of cycling is influenced by the work done in moving the legs; this is a function of the mass of the legs and hence of body mass (Fig. 29.5). The work also depends on the subject's familiarity with cycling and with the cycling frequency that is adopted. The overall efficiency is the rate of external work relative to the total energy output as measured by direct calorimetry or estimated from oxygen consumption (indirect calorimetry). The efficiency is approximately 25%.

Cycle ergometry has the merits that the subject is seated throughout the test, the noise level is low and the work rate can be specified. However, the latter can be only an approximate guide to the energy expenditure for the reason given above. Many ergometers can be adapted for use with the arms. Cycling has the disadvantage that for most subjects it is an unfamiliar form of exercise and can cause undue fatigue [24, 40]. Except in trained cyclists the maximal oxygen uptake is less than when a treadmill is used; for most subjects the difference is approximately 10%. Responses to the two forms of exercise also differ in some other respects (Table 29.2).

29.4.4 Stepping exercise

In the traditional step test the subject steps up onto and off a box, using both feet to a count of four, in time with a metronome [41]. The energy expenditure is then linearly related to the work done; this will normally be the product of the height of the step, frequency of stepping and body mass. However, the estimate of work is critically dependent on the subject raising his or her

Footnote 29.1 One kilopond (kp) is the force acting on one kg at the normal acceleration of gravity, hence:

$$1 \text{ kp m min}^{-1} = 9.81/60 = 0.1635 \text{ W}$$

where 9.81 is the gravitational acceleration in cgs units, 60 converts from second to minute and W is rate of work in watts (also see Table 6.6, page 56).

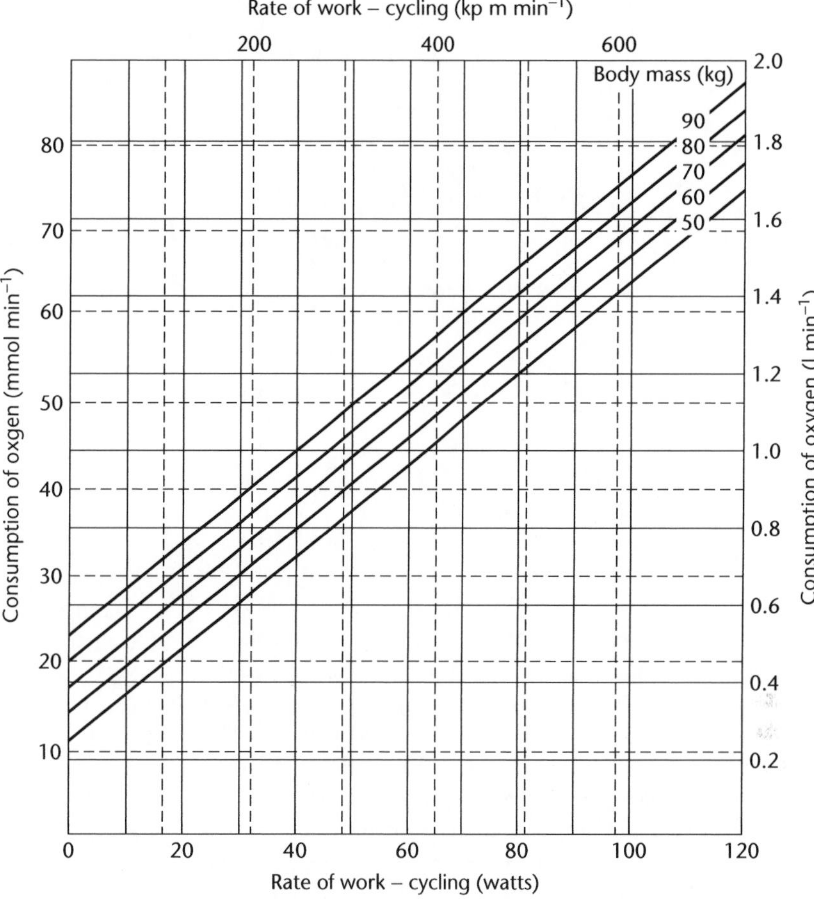

Fig. 29.5 Relationship of oxygen consumption to rate of work and body mass during cycling. A comparable relationship is given in Table 29.15. Source: [38], see also [39].

body mass up and down over the full height of the step and not reducing the rate of work by gripping a handrail. The test is normally performed at a single work level but can be adapted for progressive exercise [42].

The energy expenditure of stepping exercise is greater than that for cycle ergometry at the same rate of external work (Fig. 29.4). The difference is mainly due to the energy expended during stepping down (negative work). Stepping exercise has the disadvantages that the subject may stumble and the movement can dislodge the measuring equipment. The latter disadvantage does not apply to the Harvard pack test of exercise capacity (Section 29.9.4).

Table 29.8 Measurements for routine ergometry in respiratory patients. The procedures are outlined in this section. Measurements for non-ergometric and field tests are in Section 29.9.

Essential	Selected cases
Ventilation and gas exchange	Oxygen saturation
Cardiac frequency	Transfer factor
Electrocardiogram (chest lead)	$\dot{V}$–V curve
Symptoms at termination	End-expiratory lung volume
Fat-free body mass	Systemic blood pressure
FEV_1 and FVC	Cardiac output
	Pulmonary arterial pressure
	Other (e.g. $\dot{V}_A/\dot{Q}$, diaphragmatic emg)

29.5 Measurements

29.5.1 What should be measured?

The measurements should be appropriate to the test, the subject (often a patient) and the local facilities (Table 29.8). Where facilities are limited the investigation of patients who are considered to be at moderately high risk might need to be undertaken elsewhere.

29.5.2 Overview of equipment

The equipment (Fig. 29.6) measures the responses to exercise either over successive periods of half or 1 min or breath by breath.

In most routine laboratories gas is sampled distal to a gas mixing chamber and analysed using instruments that respond relatively slowly, for example an infrared analyser for carbon dioxide and paramagnetic analyser for oxygen (see Section 7.7). Using

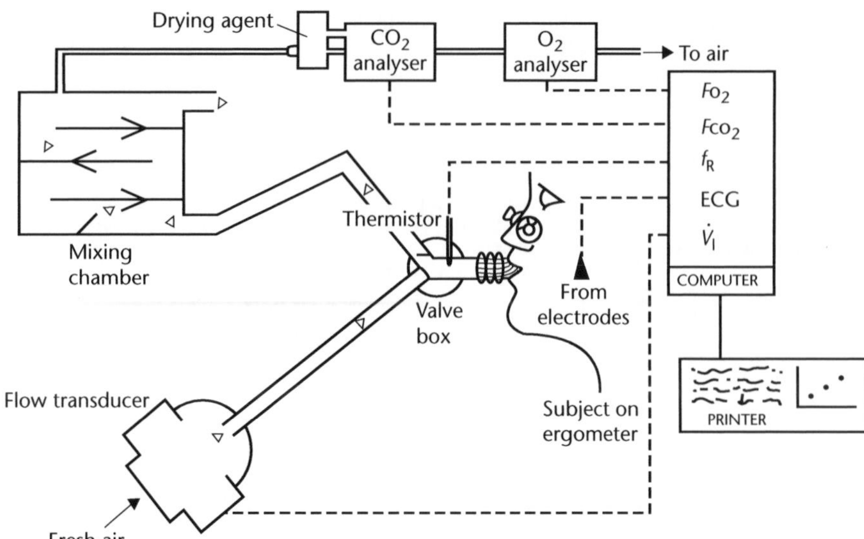

Fig. 29.6 Essential equipment for assessing the physiological response to exercise. For many assessments a pulse oximeter will be used as well.

this approach the results are stable and the equipment is relatively inexpensive. Modern equipment often incorporates gas analysers that respond rapidly, for example a respiratory mass spectrometer. This provides nearly instantaneous analysis of expired gas leaving the lungs, so can be used to provide integrated results for each breath; a gas mixing chamber is not required then. In some equipment the mass spectrometer is also used for other tests.

An electrocardiogram is used to monitor the patient during the exercise (Table 29.3) (*q.v.*). Usually it also provides cardiac frequency. Alternatively, if a pulse oximeter is used to measure arterial oxygen saturation (Section 7.10) the frequency can be obtained concurrently. Other procedures that can be incorporated in the test include flow–volume or simple spirometry [43], arterial blood sampling, cardiac catheterisation and diaphragmatic electromyography (Section 9.5). However, these procedures introduce additional complexity and, depending on circumstances, may not be appropriate for a basic protocol.

29.5.3 Ventilation minute volume

This will normally be measured using a pneumotachograph or rotating vane anemometer and an appropriate integrator (Section 7.3). The sensor will also provide respiratory frequency. It should be located proximal to the inspiratory port of the valve box. The accuracy and resistance to flow, also the methods for calibration, should conform to current recommendations (see Section 7.3). The valve box should have a small deadspace (preferably 10–15 ml, maximum 50 ml). When measurements are over 30 s intervals the expiratory port is connected to a gas-mixing chamber (capacity ~5 l) from which gas is sampled continuously for analysis. The ventilation signals should be in phase with those for gas analysis (see below, 'Breath-by-breath procedures').

In older equipment, expired gas is collected in *Douglas bags* (Fig. 1.3, page 10 and associated text). The method is now used mainly to check other equipment.

Ventilation is reported in litres BTPS per min ($\dot{V}_E$) and per breath (V_t). The circumstances should be stated, for example maximal exercise, symptom-limited exercise or submaximal exercise. If it is the last, the index used should be defined (Section 28.4.3).

29.5.4 Gas analysis

This will usually be by a paramagnetic or zirconium cell analyser for oxygen and an infrared analyser for carbon dioxide. A respiratory mass spectrometer can also be used. With the former methods, water vapour in the expired gas is absorbed prior to the analyses. An allowance must then be made for the changes in partial pressures of the other gases. The corrected gas concentrations are used to calculate O_2 uptake and CO_2 output (see Section 7.8).

Breath-by-breath procedures. The essential features are that the response times for all the instruments are short and the resulting signals are synchronised to allow for differences in response times and in the time taken for the gas to reach the analysers (sampling delays, Section 7.15, page 76). It is helpful if gas analysis is by mass spectrometry as the signals for oxygen and carbon dioxide then have the same characteristics. Gas analysis should be accurate to within 1% [1, 5] and to achieve this the channels for oxygen and carbon dioxide should each be calibrated daily using three test gas mixtures of known composition. The use of two test mixtures is not adequate [44] (see Section 7.7).

The fluctuations in gas flow and composition over the course of each breath should be allowed for by electrical integration of the individual signals. The variability between breaths can be reduced by the calculation of running averages over 5 or 10 breaths. Averaging over time periods, for example 15 s or 30 s, is less satisfactory. The method that is used should be indicated and its accuracy confirmed by comparison with the Douglas bag method [1]; this calibration should be repeated after the equipment has been moved [4] and in other circumstances at regular intervals with a log kept of the results. In addition, at weekly intervals a biological check should be carried out by a member of the laboratory staff [45]. The results should be displayed on a wall chart and any divergent results investigated.

Results for consecutive whole breaths (obtained without averaging) provide information about the 'on' and 'off' transients at the beginning and end of exercise. However, interpretation of transients is still not established [46].

29.5.5 Other measurements

Cardiac frequency. This is best obtained from the electrocardiogram (ECG) that is used to monitor the patient's condition. The electrodes are placed over the upper sternum and cardiac apex (CM5 configuration, [25]), with an earth lead at the base of the sternum and another on the ergometer. The frequency is obtained from the R waves and its accuracy is checked by counting the radial pulse.

Anthropometric measurements. The proportion of body mass which is fat and hence the fat-free mass are obtained by measurements of body mass and subcutaneous fat. The latter is usually measured as skinfold thickness using skin calipers but other methods are also appropriate (Section 4.7.2, page 37). The observer should have received appropriate training and the instrument should have been calibrated. The information is necessary for interpretation of submaximal exercise cardiac frequency and maximal oxygen uptake and on this account should form part of the protocol for ergometry.

Pulse oximetry. Arterial oxygen saturation is usually measured by a pulse oximeter applied to a finger or lobe of the ear. The part should be maximally vasodilated and the sensor should be secure to avoid movement relative to the skin (Section 7.10, page 67).

A change in saturation, for example between rest and exercise, is measured with greater accuracy than an absolute level. Accuracy is best if the oximeter is calibrated using the subject's own arterial blood.

Blood pressure. Manual measurements are expensive in technician time so an automated method should be used where possible.

Flow–volume ($\dot{v}$–V) curve. The method is described in Section 12.5.1 and the procedure for comparing the curve obtained during exercise with that over the same lung volumes at rest in Section 28.8.1.

Transfer factor (Tl). The measurement on exercise is usually made during cycle ergometry. A single breath (breath holding) method (Section 20.4, page 237), with a shortened breath holding time (e.g. 6 s) is recommended [47]. The intra-breath method (Section 20.6) can also be used [48]. Several determinations are made, each at the end of a 5-min period of exercise of constant intensity. The result is interpolated to a standard uptake of oxygen (usually 45 mmol min^{-1}, 1.0 l min^{-1}) or a standard cardiac frequency (usually 100 min^{-1} [13]).

29.5.6 Respiratory symptoms

The procedure for observing and recording the signs and symptoms that a patient experiences is described in Section 29.6. The principal symptom (usually breathlessness) is rated on a visual analogue scale [49] (Fig. 29.7, also Fig. 28.17, page 402) or a Borg scale of perceived exertion or breathlessness (Table 29.9). The scales can be automated for use during, as well as at the end of exercise [52]. Additional scales for assessing respiratory disability are given in Table 8.6 (page 90).

29.6 Conduct of the test

The quality of the test result is influenced by the technical, interpersonal and observational skills of the technician. This is particularly so when the procedure includes assessment of disability and is considered under this heading (Section 30.4.3).

Safety. The laboratory should have a safety protocol that must be adhered to, a resuscitation trolley and an alarm bell for summoning the resuscitation team. The trolley should be checked regularly to ensure that the defibrillator works, the valves of the resuscitator have not stuck and the drugs are not time-expired. Depending on the types of patient that are assessed the resuscitation equipment may be used occasionally, rarely or not at all. Consequently, the safety protocol should specify the training and checking procedures. Conformity with the protocol should be recorded and signed for by a responsible person on a regular basis. More general considerations are discussed in Section 30.3.1.

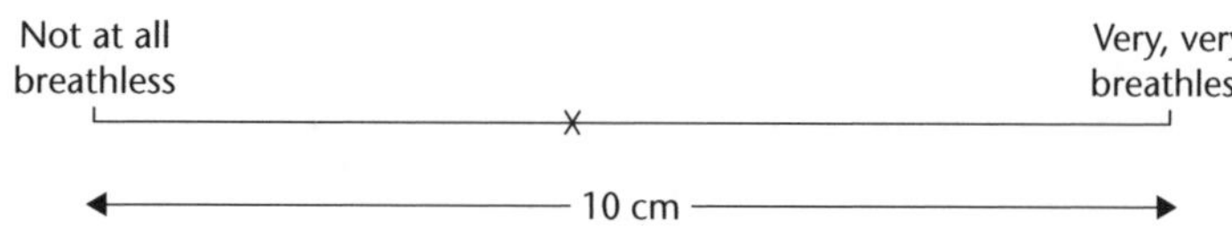

Fig. 29.7 Visual-analogue scale of breathlessness. The subject marks a 10-cm line at the point which reflects the intensity of breathlessness. The distance from the origin can be measured by hand; alternatively the scale can be a chain of lights controlled by a potentiometer. A result is given in Fig. 28.17, (page 402).

Table 29.9 Scores and descriptions used in Borg scales.

Perceived exertion*		Breathlessness†	
Score	Description	Score	Description
7	Very very light	0	Nothing at all
9	Very light	0.5	Very, very slight (just noticeable)
11	Fairly light	1	Very slight
13	Somewhat hard	2	Slight
15	Hard	3	Moderate
17	Very hard	4	Somewhat severe
19	Very very hard (the limit)	5	Severe
20	Beyond endurance	6	
		7	Very severe
		8	
		9	Very, very severe (almost maximal)
		10	Maximal

* Score has a linear scale (0.1 × average cardiac frequency for that level of effort).

† Score has a proportional scale. A similar scale can be used for perceived exertion.

Source: [50, 51].

The technician conducting the test should be competent to monitor the electrocardiogram, be alert to any symptoms that the subject may develop and have access both to the controls of the treadmill if one is used and means for summoning assistance. He or she should have received training in electrocardiography and in cardiorespiratory resuscitation but need not be a physician. However, if the patient has any evidence of ischaemic heart disease a physician should be in close call.

Some cardiovascular indications for terminating the exercise test are given in Table 29.3. Very often the presence of these abnormalities are a result of anxiety not disease, and do not reappear when the exercise in repeated.

Conditions for the test. The ventilatory and cardiovascular responses to exercise are influenced by the condition of the subject, environmental temperature, time of day and time since the last meal. The measurements should normally be made at a neutral temperature (usually 17–23 °C), with the subject relaxed, in a post-absorptive state and not within 2 h of a heavy meal. To eliminate error due to carboxyhaemoglobin, the subject should be instructed not to have smoked or been otherwise exposed to carbon monoxide on the day of the test. The instructions should also detail loose clothing and shoes with soft soles and flat heels. Spectacles will normally be worn but false teeth removed.

A clinical evaluation, anthropometric measurements and assessment of lung function will normally precede the exercise test. The assessment should include measurement of ventilatory capacity and transfer factor. In addition, depending on the clinical history, there may be a need for a 12 lead electrocardiogram. However, cardiovascular disease, unless it is recent, unstable or very advanced, should not preclude an exercise test if the patient is ambulant and there is a clear respiratory indication [1]. Where there is doubt a cardiological opinion should be sought.

Preliminaries. The technician will ensure that the equipment is in good order, with appropriate parts sterile (Section 7.13), toiletries to hand and the instruments calibrated (Chapter 7). He or she should study the request form, have a good idea of the clinical features, check that these have not deteriorated recently or contraindicate exercise and establish the reasons for the test. If an inhaler is used the time of the last dose should be noted and, if appropriate, repeated. Spirometry may need to be repeated and measurements made of body mass and skinfold thickness.

The subject should be instructed on how to perform the exercise, how to communicate symptoms to the laboratory staff and how to discontinue exercise in the event of needing to do so suddenly (see Sections 29.4.2 and 29.4.3). If practicable, the instruction should be given on a preliminary visit during which the subject tries out the equipment.

During the test. The technician's prime responsibility is to keep a close eye on the subject, provide instruction and encouragement as appropriate and, if the subject does not do so, decide when the exercise should be terminated. The decision will be influenced mainly by interaction with the subject and also from the displays of the measuring instruments. In high risk cases the latter should be monitored by a second observer.

At the end of exercise the technician should immediately remove the mouthpiece, quickly seat the subject in a chair (if not already seated), ask the reasons for stopping and observe the extent of breathlessness before and during the reply. Subsequently, the subject should rate the stated symptom using an appropriate scale (Table 29.9). This procedure is necessary because when exercise is limited by symptoms their nature and severity are often the most important outcomes of the test. Accuracy is lost if the information is only obtained after a period of 'winding down'.

29.7 Data processing

A progressive exercise test yields an enormous amount of information. In modern equipment signals are processed online to obtain flows, volumes, gas concentrations and frequencies and then ventilation, tidal volume, respiratory and cardiac frequencies, oxygen uptake and carbon dioxide output and respiratory exchange ratio. Each of these steps involves the use of a mathematical model with coefficient and constant terms (paramenters) of which some are general (as in Section 6.6, page 55) whilst others are specific to the equipment. Before the equipment is brought into use and again after any items have been replaced the models and parameters should be checked carefully as any errors will cause faults in the data that can seldom be corrected retrospectively (Section 7.16, page 79).

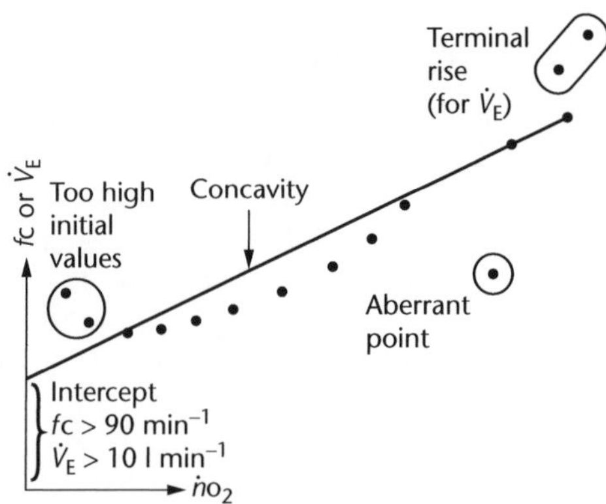

Fig. 29.8 Example of a fault that should be detected by scrutiny of an intermediate result. In most instances the exercise should be repeated, but it may be sufficient to exclude one or two points.

Next, selected indices are related to each other as *x*/*y* plots (e.g. Fig. 29.1, also Fig. 28.5, page 391). The plots should be scrutinised immediately so the quality of the information can be assessed and a decision made as to whether the result is acceptable or if the test should be repeated. Factors to be taken into account include evidence for anxiety such as initial hyperventilation or tachycardia (Fig. 29.8), more than one ventricular ectopic beats and fluctuations in any of the measured variables. The fluctuations are usually due to a leaking mouthpiece or poor electrode contact with the skin.

After the data have been checked the physiological response is reviewed. In one commonly used system of exercise testing the review is based on nine graphs, of which three have two sets of axes, making 12 graphs in all [38]. Some of the graphs are included to permit estimation of the anaerobic threshold (see Table 28.3, page 396). However, the indirect method is not valid for respiratory patients (Section 28.4.6) and some graphs can be omitted on this account. Even so, interpretation of such a large quantity of information is not easy and the results cannot readily be incorporated into a lung function report. In the preceding chapter a case is made for confining the result of a basic exercise test to the symptoms and a limited number of physiological indices (e.g. Table 29.10): these are ones that can be defined without ambiguity and for which reference values are available. Ventilation equivalent and oxygen pulse do not meet these criteria.

29.8 Interpretation of data

29.8.1 Submaximal exercise

Where the patient can achieve an oxygen uptake of at least 33 mmol min^{-1} (0.75 l min^{-1}) the data can be used to explore the reason for an increased exercise ventilation. The exploration is best undertaken one step at a time.

Table 29.10 Data recommended for use in the report on a routine exercise test.

	Submaximal exercise	At symptom limitation
Basic information	Age, fat-free mass, Fat% (or height and weight), FVC	Ditto, also grade of habitual activity, smoking status and FEV_1
Ventilation* Respiratory exchange ratio Cardiac frequency	At specified O_2 uptake (e.g. 45 mmol min^{-1} i.e. 1.0 l min^{-1} In men, possibly less in women)	Maximal attained values for all variables
Tidal volume	At ventilation 30 l min^{-1}	Shape of Hey plot
Saturation by oximetry	Per cent before, during and at end of exercise	Ditto
Symptoms	Score on visual analogue scale	Comment and scores describing condition

* Measurement of flow–volume curve and end-expiratory lung volume should be considered for specialist and research laboratories.

Step 1. Ventilation. Establish if the exercise ventilation is within the normal range (e.g. for $\dot{V}_{E45}$ in men 19–27 l min^{-1} [53]. If it is then, subject to the symptoms and level of ventilatory capacity, there is unlikely to be a respiratory problem.

If the ventilation is abnormal, can it be brought within the normal range by making allowance for the subject's RER and Vt_{30}? If 'yes' any abnormality is unlikely to reside in the lungs. If 'no' this may be because the adjustments for RER and Vt_{30} were inappropriate in the circumstances, alternatively the lungs are responding abnormally. The cause for the increased exercise ventilation should now be explored.

Step 2. RER and SaO_2. Inspection of these variables can point to (but not confirm) the likely mechanism for an increased ventilation. If RER is normal (e.g. $RER_{45} \leq 0.91$) most of the extra ventilation will be to parts of the lungs that are not making a big contribution to gas exchange (high $\dot{V}_A/\dot{Q}$ ratio). This site will usually be alveoli that are poorly perfused (alveolar deadspace). However, if breathing is shallow and rapid (low Vt_{30}) there will be additional ventilation of the airway deadspace as well.

If RER is increased, much of the excess ventilation is of alveoli that are making a material contribution to gas exchange. The commonest cause is lactacidaemia. The increased RER is then likely to reflect either that the work level is high for that subject or he or she is taking relatively little exercise for social reasons (i.e. is unfit) or there is a respiratory, cardiac or other medical condition. In many of these patients the SaO_2 will not have deviated much from the initial level. If the saturation rises the likely causes include uneven lung function and functional overbreathing, possibly superimposed on an organic disorder. If the saturation falls there may be a defect of gas transfer. In this event the transfer factor is likely to be reduced at rest and may fall further when measured during exercise. The common causes include generalised emphysema and alveolitis or diffuse interstitial fibrosis (Sections 40.3 and 40.4, pages 548 and 554). If the patient has airways obstruction, the features represent a Type 1 and not a Type 2 response (patient pink and puffing, not potentially blue and bloated (Sections 38.5, page 535). If the abnormality is mainly in the lung parenchyma it might fit the somewhat inappropriate designation of 'alveolar capillary block syndrome'. However, these syndromes develop progressively and may not be prominent in their early stages.

Step 3. Pattern of breathing. In the present scheme, the pattern is interpreted in terms of Vt_{30} and f_{R30} (for which purpose the ventilation minute volume needs to be at least 30 l min^{-1}). An alternative approach is to consider instead the times of inspiration and expiration and the relationship between them (Section 28.4.5). If Vt_{30} is normal with respect to the reference value (based on forced vital capacity) the pattern of breathing is unremarkable, but if it is abnormal (either high or low) the cause should be identified (Section 28.4.7). In a person with normal lungs a high Vt_{30} often reflects a high level of physical fitness now or in the past. In other circumstances it can be associated with asthma in remission or labile airways obstruction. A Vt_{30} that is reduced relative to vital capacity can be the principal or a subsidiary cause of an increased ventilation leading to breathlessness on exertion. The mechanism is likely to be mechanical, reflex or functional. Dynamic shallow breathing can result from pleural thickening or excess soft tissue on the anterior thorax. Reflex shallow breathing (tachypnoea) arises from receptors in the pulmonary circulation or lung parenchyma (J receptors). Functional shallow breathing is a feature of anxiety and malingering. In all these circumstances the subject is likely to be worried by the symptom, which in the case of respiratory patients is often out of proportion to the deterioration in lung function. Some clinical examples are in Tables 29.11 and 29.12, also Figs 28.11 and 28.12 (pages 397 and 398).

The breathing pattern can be explored further if information is available on the relationship of forced expiratory flow to lung volume during exercise. Shallow breathing accompanying an increase in end-expiratory lung volume and displacement of the flow–volume loop in the direction of total lung capacity (Fig. 28.18, page 404) are evidence for exercise being limited by respiratory factors, see also the following step.

Step 4. Cardiac frequency. The f_C at the chosen uptake of oxygen should be compared with that expected for the subject's muscularity as assessed by fat-free mass or related variable (Fig. 29.11). In a respiratory patient the frequency will usually be relatively normal (Tables 28.6 and 28.7, pages 404 and 405). A high cardiac frequency may indicate that the patient is unfit, experiencing hypoxaemia or toxaemia, or is anxious. Alternatively, it may be a consequence of coexisting cardiac disease.

29.8.2 Exercise limitation

The cause of limitation will be included in the medical report. It is usually either mainly respiratory or mainly circulatory in origin. Other causes are skeleto-muscular difficulties, anaemia, toxaemia and portal cirrhosis. In addition, a possible contribution from apprehension, anxiety or malingering should be borne in mind. Thus, the scrutiny of the data (Table 29.10) should be broadly based and follow that for submaximal exercise reviewed above.

Step 1. Review the symptoms for clues as to the mode of limitation, including: (a) the operator's impression of the condition of the subject at the point of termination, (b) the patient's symptoms and (c) the scores for breathlessness and effort. If the limitation was likely to have been of cardiopulmonary origin, the scrutiny should indicate if the subject experienced incapacitating breathlessness. If so, the physiological response was probably maximal. If the recovery appeared to be slow and the patient was obviously fatigued, the limitation might have been cardiovascular.

Step 2. Look for evidence of cardiovascular limitation. If this was the case the maximal observed cardiac frequency should be similar to its reference value (Eqn 28.2, page 399). Information to this effect might already have been obtained from the electrocardiogram. In addition, there might be evidence for a raised blood concentration of lactic acid, including a progressively increasing respiratory exchange ratio towards or above unity, slow recovery of ventilation after exercise (suggesting an oxygen debt) and a high blood concentration of lactic acid (Section 28.4.6).

Step 3. If the limitation was not cardiovascular, was there evidence for ventilatory limitation, e.g. did the exercise ventilation approximate to the maximum expected for the level of FEV_1 (Fig. 25.13, page 398), (dyspnoeic index near to or in excess of 100%)? Did the flow–volume curve show evidence for exercise limitation (Fig. 28.18, page 404)?

Step 4. Consider what might be learned from the pattern of breathing at near the breaking point of exercise. Here a characteristic pattern is of the terminal part of the Hey plot not being vertical, but inclined to the left (Fig. 29.9). This can indicate progressive shallow breathing associated with air trapping and a rise in end expiratory lung volume at near to the breaking point of exercise. The sequence suggests ventilatory insufficiency.

Many of the changes that have been indicated in this section can be demonstrated more elegantly in other ways but to do so require additional manoeuvres (e.g. [11, 43]) that the patient may not be able to perform (see Footnote 29.2).

Footnote 29.2 A cost benefit analysis into the resource implications, success rates and clinical utility of the alternative procedures might be helpful.

Table 29.11 Examples of exercise test results (post bronchodilator, using treadmill) in men. Reference values for exercise indices are in parentheses.

Diagnosis	COPD		Emphysema		Asthma		Functional over-breathing	
Patient details	Fitter (smoker) with irreversible airflow limitation. TLC and *Tl* both normal		Furnace operator (smoker) with airways obstruction, large TLC, high compliance and low *Tl*		Baker with asthma, apparently controlled by inhaled salbutamol. TLC and *Tl* both normal		Coalminer with pneumoconiosis and undue breathlessness. Normal lung function	
Age (year)	62		57		39		52	
FEV_1 (l)	1.17	(2.69)	1.48	(2.89)	3.75	(3.69)	2.44	(2.99)
Clinical grade (BMRC)*	4 (750 m)		5 (40 m)		2		4	
$\dot{V}_{E45}$ (l min^{-1})†	38	(24)	46	(24)	20	(24)	61	(24)
RER	0.77	(0.79)	0.89	(0.79)	0.76	(0.79)	1.0	(0.79)
V_{t30} (l)‡	0.81	(1.1)	1.75	(1.45)	2.43	(1.4)	0.73	(1.3)
f_{C45} (min^{-1})†	104	(108)	103	(111)	103	(105)	98	(115)
Sa_{O_2}	No desaturation		No desaturation		No desaturation		No desaturation	
Limitation to exercise	Breathlessness ($\dot{V}_{Emax}$ 48 l min^{-1}), dyspnoeic index 113%		Intense breathlessness (Dyspnoeic index 104%)		Tightness of the chest associated with fall in FEV_1 to 3.0 l		Dizziness	
Comment	V_{E45} increased by a large alveolar deadspace. Normal airway deadspace and alveolar ventilations (V_{t30} and RER both normal)		Deep breathing (high V_{t30}) and mild hyperventilation (RER 0.89) maintained a normal saturation (hence 'pink puffer')		Deep breathing (high V_{t30}) contributed to a normal response to submaximal exercise. The patient had exercise-induced airflow limitation		The high $\dot{V}_{E45}$ was due to increased airway deadspace ventilation low V_{t30} (raised f_R) plus hyperventilation (high RER)	

Diagnosis	Obesity		Pleural thickening		Pulmonary fibrosis		Portal cirrhosis	
Patient details	Lagger who was breathless. He had normal lung function but was overweight (BMI 31 kg m^{-2}).		Shipwright (smoker) who was breathless despite normal lung function and quantity of body fat.		Fitter (smoker) with reduced TLC, compliance and *Tl*. No airways obstruction.		Lorry driver with low transfer factor and mild airways obstruction. Normal TLC.	
Age (year)	53		60		70		41	
FEV_1 (l)	4.2	(3.60)	3.21	(3.13)	2.0	(2.81)	2.8	(3.87)
Clinical grade (BMRC)	3		4 (375 m)		4 (375 m)		4	
$\dot{V}_{E45}$ (l min^{-1})	24.7	(24)	50	(24)	38	(24)	60	(24)
RER	0.61	(0.79)	0.83	(0.79)	0.95	(0.79)	1.13	(0.79)
V_{t30} (l)	0.8	(1.52)	1.03	(1.43)	1.02	(1.11)	2.1	(1.4)
f_{C45} (min^{-1})	101	(90)	88	(102)	100	(111)	117	(94)
Sa_{O_2}	No desaturation		No desaturation		96 → 88 → 95		92 → 79	
Limitation to exercise:	Exercise 'somewhat hard'		Stopped because of breathlessness		Exercise limited by fatigue and moderate breathlessness.		Patient extremely breathless.	
Comment:	Normal $\dot{V}_{E45}$ due to alveolar hypoventilation compensating for increased ventilation of airway deadspace. Breathlessness possibly due to hypercapnia and shallow breathing.		Raised ventilation and hence breathlessness due to both shallow breathing and alveolar hyperventilation.		Ventilation increased by large alveolar deadspace (V_A/Q), increased hypoxic drive and ? other factors.		Gross hyperventilation (also tachycardia) secondary to hypoxaemia resulting from transfer defect. Abnormalities were corrected by breathing oxygen.	

* British Medical Research Council. Breathless grades are in Table 38.3. Stated walking distance is in brackets.

† 45 mmol min^{-1} is 1.0 l min^{-1}.

‡ tidal volume at a ventilation of 30 l min^{-1}.

Table 29.12 Examples of exercise test results (post bronchodilator) in women. Reference values for exercise indices are in parentheses.

	Functional hyperventilation		COPD		Pleural thickening		Diffuse interstitial fibrosis	
	Asbestos worker (smoker) with some airways obstruction and reduced transfer factor.		Reversible airways obstruction in former asbestos worker. Lung function was otherwise normal		Previous asbestos worker with COPD and rather small total lung capacity. Normal transfer factor		Previous asbestos worker (smoker) with small lungs and low transfer factor	
Age (year)	44		63		62		65	
FEV_1 (l)	1.75	(2.06)	1.31	(1.97)	1.68	(2.28)	1.17	(1.96)
Clinical Grade (BMRC)*	3		3		4 (275 m)		3	
$\dot{V}E_{22}$ (l min $^{-1}$)†	36	(14)	15.5	(14)	18	(14)	24	(14)
RER	1.28	(<0.9)	0.72	(<0.9)	0.76	(<0.9)	0.82	(<0.9)
Vt_{30} (l)‡	1.4	(1.1)	NA		0.45	(1.15)	0.68	(1.06)
fC_{22} (min $^{-1}$)†	91	(115)	92	(112)	78	(99)	96	(106)
SaO_2	No desaturation		No desaturation		No desaturation		97 → 87 → 95	
Limitation to exercise:	Exercise limited by dizziness.		The patient found exercise 'fairly light'.		Exercise 'somewhat hard'. Rapid shallow breathing.		Exercise limited by breathlessness (dyspnoeic index 112%).	
Comment:	This lady started to hyperventilate half way through the exercise. The result was not helpful in coming to a diagnosis.		Exercise test did not suggest that the minor radiographic abnormalities were of functional significance.		Dynamic shallow breathing was the main cause of disability. It was likely to have been of occupational origin.		Dynamic shallow breathing, hypoxaemia and uneven lung function contributed to increased exercise ventilation.	

* British Medical Research Council. Breathless grades are in Table 38.3 (page 532). Stated walking distance is in brackets.

† 22 mmol min^{-1} is 0.5 l min^{-1}.

‡ tidal volume at a ventilation of 30 l min^{-1}.

Practical outcome. Once the nature of the physiological response to submaximal exercise and the cause of exercise limitation have been established, the therapeutic and other implications should be reviewed and discussed with the patient. Some examples are given in Tables 29.11 and 29.12. The procedure for estimating the extent of exercise limitation (respiratory disability) and the residual exercise capacity with a view to re-employment are considered in Chapter 30.

29.9 Non-ergometric and field tests

29.9.1 Observational tests

A member of the medical team watches the patient move about in the building, accompanies him or her on a walk or when mounting stairs to a higher floor. Covert observation may be appropriate if there is uncertainty as to the extent of a patient's impairment (Section 30.5.3).

29.9.2 Walking tests

6 min (or 12 min) walking test, 6 MWT. This is a simple test of functional capacity for respiratory patients who are limited to exercise by breathlessness or other symptom [54]. It is not recommended for healthy subjects as their walking speed is limited by mechanical considerations [33], so reference values are of limited usefulness. The outcome is the distance walked in the time. The test is mainly employed to monitor the response to therapy, for example bronchodilator therapy, portable oxygen therapy or a programme of rehabilitation. For these applications the outcome is the change in the distance walked between two tests performed before and when under the influence of the relevant procedure. Provided the conditions on the two occasions are comparable, a change of 54 m can be meaningful [55]. The test can also be used to assess the outcome of a controlled trial (e.g. [18]). The protocol should take account of the several factors that influence the distance walked (Table 29.13) and be adhered to. Local conditions may influence what is practicable and the case for a universal protocol (e.g. [56]) has still to be made.

29.9.3 Shuttle tests

A shuttle format can be adapted to almost any circumstance. For example, it can be used to assess exercise capacity [40, 57], be a

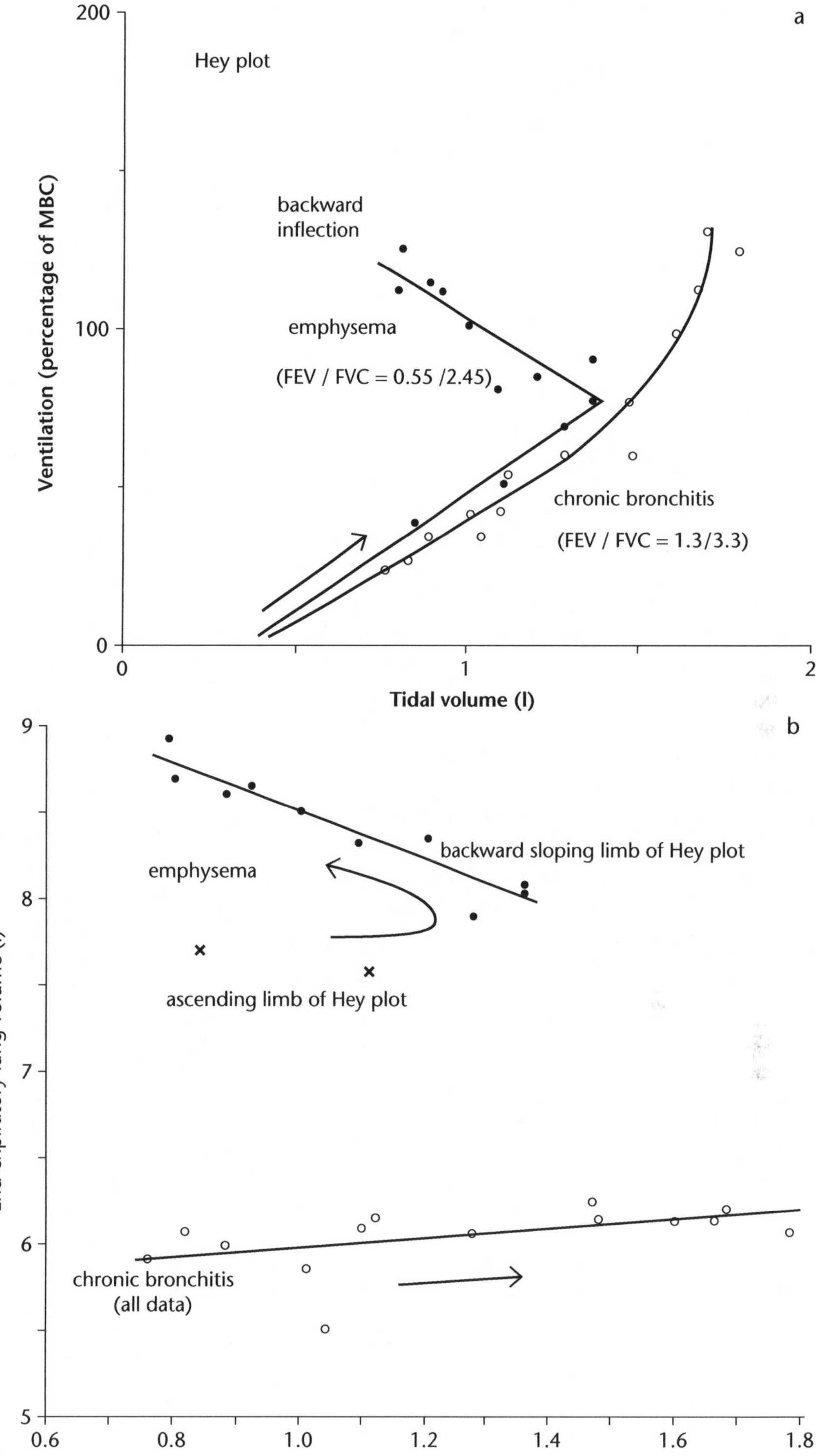

Fig. 29.9 Use of Hey plot to detect a rising end-expiratory lung volume (EELV) during progressive treadmill exercise in a patient with gross emphysema. (a) Hey plot for a patient with emphysema who developed dynamic hyperinflation on exercise compared with a patient with chronic bronchitis who did not. The rise in EELV led to a reduction in tidal volume (*V*t) shown as a backward inflection on the Hey plot. The reduction reflected accurately the increase in EELV shown in (b), a plot of end-expiratory lung volume versus tidal volume. The result is compared with that for a patient with chronic bronchitis who also had hyperinflation but without aggravation on exercise. In this patient the Hey plot was of normal shape (cf. Fig. 29.10). In both men the maximal observed tidal volume was approximately 55% of FVC.
Source: Redrawn with permission from Leaver DG. Airway obstruction in chronic bronchitis and emphysema. MD thesis; University of Cambridge, 1973.

Table 29.13 Conditions for 6-or 12-min walking test (6 or 12 MWT).

Variable	Options	Recommendation
Duration	6 or 12 min	6 min
Surface	Corridor or road	Corridor (100 m long)
Familiarisation	None, 1 or 2 practice walks	One practice
Definitive walks	1 or mean of two	One (1 h after the practice)
Supervisor	At start, beside or at side of and behind patient	At side and slightly behind
Encouragement	None, mild or maximal, with or without standard phrases	Mild encouragement by same supervisor on both occasions

provocation test for bronchial hyper-reactivity, or a means for physical training.

To perform the test the subject walks or runs between and round two traffic cones placed at a predetermined distance apart. In shuttle-walking tests for respiratory patients the distance can be 9 m, in which case each shuttle is 10 m [58]. The speed of walking is dictated by a series of auditory signals (bleeps) played from a pre-recorded compact disk (CD) and delivered via head microphones. The signal is reinforced at the end of each level of exercise to indicate that the speed is about to be increased.

In an incremental test the subject completes three shuttles in the first minute. Thereafter, he or she aims to complete one additional shuttle each minute for 10 or 12 min. In an endurance test the shuttle frequency is usually a predetermined fraction of the maximum achieved during a previous incremental test. The end point is the time when the subject cannot maintain the shuttle frequency or exhibits previously defined features of over loading of the cardiovascular system.

29.9.4 Harvard pack test

This traditional test is used to assess physical fitness for very strenuous work. It is based on the observation that the recovery of cardiac frequency after exercise is faster in well trained than in untrained subjects (Fig. 28.22, page 411). The equipment required is a stopwatch, metronome and box of height 50 cm (20 in) for men and 43 cm (17 in) for women. A pack weighing one third of body weight may be worn on the back in which case handrails are provided. To perform the test, the subject steps on and off the box 30 times per minute. Each step up should end with the subject standing erect. The duration is 5 min unless the subject is obliged to stop sooner; the time is recorded. In the simplest form of the test, the pulse is counted at the wrist for a period of 30 s starting 1 min after the end of exercise. The physical fitness index (PFI) is given by

$$\mathrm{PFI} = \frac{\text{duration of exercise in seconds} \times 100}{5.5 \times \text{number of heart beats}} \quad (29.1)$$

Table 29.14 Reference variables for the physiological response to exercise.

Index		Reference variables*	Comment
Ventilation	below Owles point	O_2 uptake, gender, respiratory exchange ratio and frequency, (smoking)	Contribution of gender is small and the mechanism is unclear
	above Owles point	Habitual activity	
	maximal	Ventilatory capacity	
Tidal volume		Vital capacity, gender, thoraco-abdominal fat	Maximal V_t = approx 60% of FVC
Cardiac frequency	submaximal	O_2 uptake, stroke volume (hence quantity of muscle and habitual activity), age, (smoking)	Greatly influenced by ambient temperature. f_C at a specified O_2 uptake reflects the stroke volume
	maximal	Age	
Cardiac output		O_2 uptake	Relationship relatively constant between subjects
Maximal O_2 uptake		Physique (fat and muscle), habitual activity, age, (smoking)	Type of ergometer influences result. Few reference values relate to below average fitness

* Smoking (yes or no) should be a reference variable in appropriate circumstances (see text). Additional adjustments may be needed if measurements are made under unusual conditions of temperature or barometric pressure.

Table 29.15 Empirical relationships that describe the physiological response to exercise of men and women in an erect posture.

Aspects of function	Gender	Relationship	SD or C of V	Source and other references
(a) Healthy subjects				
Ventilation on O_2 uptake	M,	$\dot{V}_E$ (l min^{-1}) = 0.5 $\dot{n}O_2$† (22 $\dot{V}O_2$) + 2	5.4	Unpublished also [2, 61]
	(for F add 10%)	$\dot{V}_{E45}$ (l min^{-1}) = 19.5 + 0.095 age + 0.87 if SM	2.81	[3]
		$\dot{V}_{E45}$ (l min^{-1}) = 17.1 RER_{45} + 0.19 f_{R30}‡ + 4.48	2.02	[53]*
Tidal volume on vital Capacity	M and F	V_{t30}(l) = 0.16 VC (l) + 0.80	0.22	[62]
		V_t max (l) = 0.64 VC (l) −0.64	0.21	[63] (Fig. 29.10)
Oxygen uptake during cycling	M	$\dot{n}O_2$ (mmol min^{-1}) = 0.53 W (watts) + 0.31 BM − 4.1	4.0	[34, also 39]
Cardiac frequency (submax)	F, ages 20–49	f_C (min^{-1}) = 73.8 + 45.3 V_{O_2}	15%	[65]
	F, ages 50–80	f_C (min^{-1}) = 65.3 + 55.8 V_{O_2}	15%	[65]
	M, ages 20–69	f_C (min^{-1}) = 65.6 + 34.7 V_{O_2}	14%	[65]
	M and F	f_C (min^{-1}) = 34 + (1590 + 58 $\dot{n}O_2$†). FFM^{-1}	12%	[64] (Fig. 29.11)
	M	f_{C45} (min^{-1}) = 71.6 − 5.47 Age + 1812 FFM^{-1} + 0.35% fat	10.8	[3]
	F	f_{C45} (min^{-1}) = 67.5 − 0.39 Age + 3071 FFM^{-1}	17(13%)	[66]
Maximal cardiac frequency (f_C max)	M and F	f_C (min^{-1}) = 210 − 0.65 age [80% of f_C max = 168 −0.52 age]	19	[4]
	F	f_C (min^{-1}) = 209 − 0.86 age	12	[65]
	M	f_C (min^{-1}) = 207 −0.78 age	13	[65]
Cardiac output on oxygen uptake	M	$\dot{Q}t$ (l min^{-1}) = 0.37 $\dot{n}O_2$† (or 6.1 $\dot{V}O_2$) + 3.4	0.9	[67] *also* [68]
Maximal O_2 uptake	M	$\dot{n}O_2$ max (mmol min^{-1}) = 1.11 St + 0.84 BM + 6.7AS −1.03 age + 103	18.5	[68]
	M	$\dot{n}O_2$ max (mmol min^{-1}) = 70 + 1.43 FFM + 6.3 AS −0.95 age (−8.1 if SM)	17.3	[3]
	M	$\dot{n}O_2$ max (mmol min^{-1}) = 70.1 + 0.63 ($\dot{n}O_2$ @ $RER_{1.0}$) + 0.78 FFM −0.29 f_{C45} −0.86 %fat	12.1	[3]
	M	$\dot{n}O_2$ max (mmol min^{-1}) = 44.6 [1.86 St − 0.03 Age + 0.59]	44.6[0.36]	[69]
	F	$\dot{n}O_2$ max (mmol min^{-1}) = 44.6 [0.85 St − 0.02 Age + 0.95]	44.6[0.22]	[69]
Six minute walk (6 MWD)	M	757 St − 5.02 Age − 1.76 BM − 309	93	[70]
	F	211 St − 2.29 BM − 5.78 Age + 667	85	[70]
(b) Men with respiratory impairment				
Maximal exercise ventilation	M	$\dot{V}_E$ max,ex, (l min^{-1}) = 33.1 $(FEV_1)^{0.73}$	18%	[71] (Fig. 28.13)
Maximal O_2 uptake	M	$\dot{n}O_2$ max (mmol min^{-1}) = 66.4 + 13.4 FEV_1(l) − 0.94 $\dot{V}_{E45}$ (l min^{-1}) + 0.45 FFM − 0.31 age (year)	11.6	[10]
Maximal O_2 uptake as per cent of predicted	M	% $\dot{n}O_2$ max = 52.3 + 0.44 %FEV_1 − 0.78 $\dot{V}_{E45}$ + 0.16%$T_{l,co}$ + 52.3	7.3	[10]

* Ventilation is at subject's spontaneously chosen RER_{45} and V_{t30}.

† $\dot{n}O_2$ is uptake of oxygen in SI units (mmol min^{-1}). Coefficient on V_{O_2} (l min^{-1}) is in brackets [conversion factor is $\dot{n}O_2$ = 44.6 V_{O_2}, Table 6.6, page 56].

‡ f_{R30} is 30/V_{t30}.

M, male; F, female; BM, body mass (kg); FFM, fat-free mass (kg); St, stature (m); SM, smoker.

Activity scores: AS 1 inactive to 4 very active. AG 1 inactive to 3 very active. RER = respiratory exchange ratio.

% FEV_1 and % T_l, co are indices expressed as percentages of predicted values.

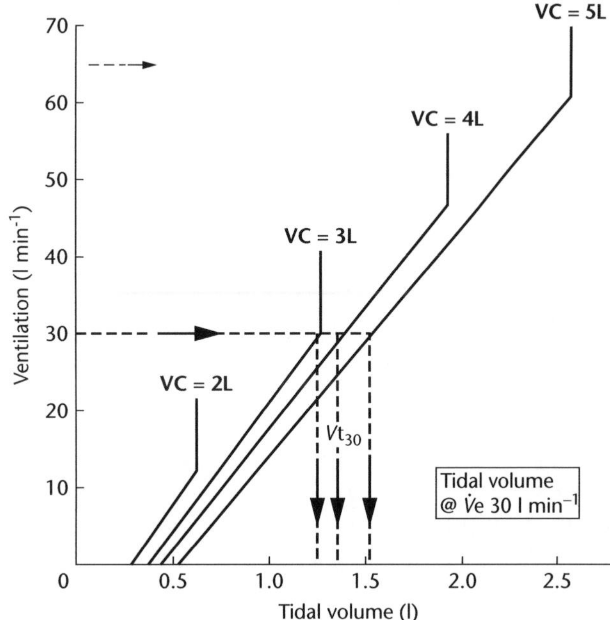

Fig. 29.10 Average relationships of exercise ventilation to tidal volume and vital capacity for men and women of European descent. Sources: [62, 63].

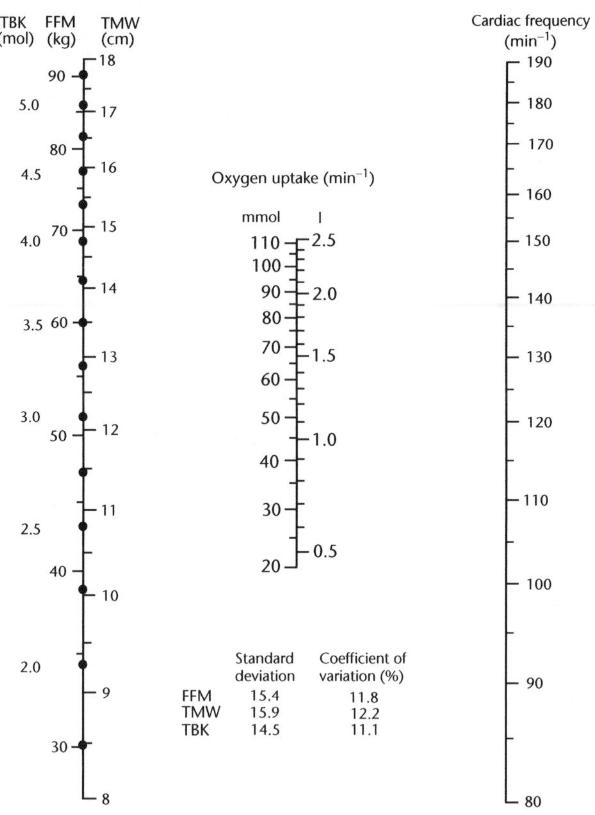

Fig. 29.11 Nomogram for determining the cardiac frequency of young adults of both sexes from oxygen uptake and an index of body muscle (fat-free body mass (FFM, kg), thigh muscle width (TMW cm) or total body potassium (total K) (Section 4.7.1). The data are for cycling (ambient temperature 20°C). Results for walking on a treadmill are similar (Table 29.2). Source: [64], see also Table 29.15.

In subjects of average physical ability the index is in the range 80–50. Higher and lower values are found, respectively, in 'fit' and 'unfit' subjects [59]. Maximal oxygen uptake or a submaximal test, e.g. [60], can provide similar information more objectively (Section 29.3.1).

29.10 Reference values for ergometry in adults

In healthy adults the lung function is mainly determined by anatomical dimensions, gender, ethnic group, environmental exposures and age. The contributions of muscle strength and other manifestations of the level of habitual activity are relatively small. By contrast, for exercise, habitual activity now and in the past can greatly influence the result. This has the effect that, where traditional reference variables are used, the published normal ranges are wide and often of limited usefulness for interpreting the findings in patients. The ranges can be narrowed by the use of additional reference variables, including indices of body composition (fat and muscle) and habitual activity (Table 29.14). Whether or not the subject smokes can be a reference variable in circumstances when the effects of smoking are incidental to the main purpose of the investigation. Allowing for individual variations in the physiological responses (e.g. respiratory exchange ratio or tidal volume) can refine the reference value for $\dot{V}_{E45}$ in defined circumstances ([53] and Table 29.15). Reference values for the physiological response to exercise values are given in Table 29.15, Figs 29.10 and 29.11.

29.11 References

1. ATS-ACCP Statement on cardiopulmonary exercise testing. *Am J Respir Crit Care Med* 2003; **167**:211–277. Erratum, *Am J Respir Crit Care Med* 1451–1452.
2. Gulsvik A, Beckett LA, Bakke Per et al. Standardized submaximal exercise testing in never smokers: a normative study. *Clin Physiol* 2001, **21**: 629–636.
3. Weller JJ, El-Gamal FM, Parker L et al. Indirect estimation of maximal oxygen uptake for study of working populations. *Br J Ind Med* 1988; **45**: 532–537.
4. Åstrand P-O, Rodahl K. *Textbook of work physiology*. 3rd ed. London: McGraw-Hill, 1986.
5. Rocca J, Whipp BJ. (co-chairmen). Clinical exercise testing with reference to lung diseases: indications, standardization and interpretation strategies. *Eur Respir J* 1997; **10**: 2662–2689.
6. Baldwin E de F, Cournand A, Richards DW Jr. Pulmonary insufficiency; 1. Physiological classification, clinical methods of analysis, standard values in normal subjects. *Medicine (Baltimore)* 1948; **27**: 243–278.
7. British Thoracic Society. The diagnosis, assessment and treatment of diffuse parenchymal lung disease in adults. *Thorax* 1999; **54**(Suppl 1): S1–S28.

8. Harris-Eze AO, Sridhar G, Clemens RE et al. Role of hypoxaemia and pulmonary mechanics in exercise limitation in interstitial lung disease *Am J Respir Crit Care Med* 1996; **154**: 994–1001.
9. Bradley GW, Crawford R. Regulation of breathing during exercise in normal subjects and in chronic lung disease. *Clin Sci* 1976; **51**: 575–582.
10. Cotes JE, Zejda J, King B. Lung function impairment as a guide to exercise limitation in work-related lung disorders. *Am Rev Respir Dis* 1988; **137**: 1089–1093.
11. O'Donnell DE, Revill SM, Webb KA. Dynamic hyperinflation and exercise intolerance in chronic obstructive pulmonary disease. *Am J Respir Crit Care Med* 2001; **164**: 770–777.
12. Myers J, Gullestad L, Vagelos R et al. Cardiopulmonary exercise testing and prognosis in severe heart failure: 14 ml/kg/min revisited. *Am Heart J* 2000; **139**: 78–84.
13. Chu SS, Cotes JE. Lung transfer and *K*CO at cardiac frequency 100 beats/min as a guide to impaired function of lung parenchyma. *Thorax* 1984; **39**: 524–528.
14. Nordenfeld I, Svensson G. The transfer factor (diffusing capacity) as a predictor of hypoxaemia during exercise in restrictive and chronic obstructive pulmonary disease. *Clin Physiol* 1987; **7**: 423–430.
15. Silverman M, Konig P, Godfrey S. Use of serial exercise tests to assess the efficacy and duration of action of drugs for asthma. *Thorax* 1973; **28**: 574–578.
16. Schwaiblmair M, Beinert T, Vogelmeier C, Fruhmann G. Cardiopulmonary exercise testing following hay exposure challenge in farmer's lung. *Eur Respir J* 1997; **10**: 2360–2365.
17. Bolliger CT, Jordan P, Soler M et al. Exercise capacity as a predictor of postoperative complications in lung resection candidates. *Am J Respir Crit Care Med* 1995; **151**: 1472–1480.
18. Cockcroft AE, Saunders MJ, Berry G. Randomised controlled trial of rehabilitation in chronic respiratory disability. *Thorax* 1981; **36**: 200–203.
19. Casaburi R, Patessio A, Ioli F et al. Reductions in exercise lactic acidosis and ventilation as a result of exercise training in patients with obstructive lung disease. *Am Rev Respir Dis* 1991; **143**: 9–18.
20. Cotes JE. Rating respiratory disability: a report on behalf of a working group of the European Society for Clinical Respiratory Physiology. *Eur Respir J* 1990; **3**: 1074–1077.
21. Nader JA, Jones PW, Nery LE, Whipp BJ. Determinants of the exercise endurance capacity in patients with chronic obstructive pulmonary disease. The power-duration relationship. *Am J Respir Crit Care Med* 2000; **162**: 497–504.
22. King B, Craik MC, Stevenson IC et al. Validation of progressive exercise in respiratory patients. *Clin Sci* 1987; **73**(Suppl17): 3P.
23. Palange P, Forte S, Onorati P et al. Ventilatory and metabolic adaptations to walking and cycling in patients with COPD. *J Appl Physiol* 2000; **88**: 1715–1720.
24. Man WD, Soliman MG, Gearing J et al. Symptoms and quadriceps fatigability after walking and cycling in chronic obstructive pulmonary disease. *Am J Respir Crit Care Med* 2003; **168**: 562–567.
25. Fletcher GF, Froelicher VE, Hartley LH et al. Exercise standards: a statement from health professionals from the American Heart Association. *Circulation* 1990; **82**: 2286–2322.
26. Pollock ML, Bohannon RL, Cooper KH et al. A comparative analysis of four protocols for maximal treadmill stress testing. *Am Heart J* 1976; **92**: 39–46.
27. Wolthuis RA, Froelicher VF Jr, Fischer J et al. New practical treadmill protocol for clinical use. *Am J Cardiol* 1977; **39**: 697–700.
28. Howley ET, Bassett DR Jr, Welch HG. Criteria for maximal oxygen uptake: review and commentary. *Med Sci Sport Exerc* 1995; **27**: 1292–1301.
29. Astrand I. Aerobic capacity of men and women with special reference to age. *Acta Physiol Scand* 1960; **49**(Suppl 169): 1–92.
30. Taylor HL, Buskirk E, Henschel A. Maximal oxygen uptake as an objective measure of cardiorespiratory performance. *J Appl Physiol* 1955; **8**: 73–80.
31. Givoni B, Goldman RF. Predicting metabolic energy cost. *J Appl Physiol* 1971; **30**: 429–433.
32. Cotes JE, Meade F. The energy expenditure and mechanical energy demand in walking. *Ergonomics* 1960; **3**: 97–119.
33. Cotes JE, Davies CTM, John C. Relationship of oxygen uptake, ventilation and cardiac frequency to body weight during different forms of standardized exercise. *J Physiol (Lond)* 1967; **190**: 29P–30P.
34. Cotes JE, Meade F. Physical training in relation to the energy expenditure of walking and to factors controlling respiration during exercise. *Ergonomics* 1959; **2**: 195–206.
35. Cotes JE, Steel J. *Work-related lung disorders.* Oxford: Blackwell Scientific Publications, 1987.
36. Russell JC, Dale JD. Dynamic torquemeter calibration of cycle ergometers. *J Appl Physiol* 1986; **61**: 1217–1220.
37. Van Praagh E, Bedu M, Roddier P, Coudert J. A simple calibration method for mechanically braked cycle ergometers. *Int J Sports Med* 1992; **13**: 27–30.
38. Cotes JE. Relationships of oxygen consumption, ventilation and cardiac frequency to body weight during standardised exercise in normal subjects. *Ergonomics.* 1969; **12**: 415–427.
39. Wasserman K, Hansen JE, Sue DY et al. *Principles of exercise testing and interpretation.* 3rd ed. Philadelphia: Lippincot, Williams and Wilkins, 1999.
40. Mahoney C. 20-MST and PWC170 validity in non-Caucasian children in the UK. *Br J Sports Med* 1992; **26**: 45–47.
41. Hugh-Jones P, Lambert AV. A simple standard exercise test and its use for measuring exertional dyspnoea. *BMJ* 1952; **1**: 65–71
42. Nagle FJ, Balke B, Naughton JP. Gradational step tests for assessing work capacity. *J Appl Physiol* 1965; **20**: 745–748.
43. Gelb AF, Gutierrez CA, Weisman IM et al. Simplified detection of dynamic hyperinflation. *Chest* 2004; **126**: 1855–1860.
44. Chinn DJ, Naruse Y, Cotes JE. Accuracy of gas analysis in lung function laboratories. *Thorax* 1986; **41**: 133–137.
45. Revill SM, Morgan MD. Biological quality control for exercise testing. *Thorax* 2000; **55**: 63–66.
46. Peunte-Maestu L, Sanz ML, Sanz P et al. Reproducibility of the on-transient cardiopulmonary responses to moderate exercise in patients with chronic obstructive pulmonary disease. *Eur J Appl Physiol* 2001; **85**: 434–441.
47. Kendrick AH, Laszlo G. CO transfer factor on exercise: age and sex differences. *Eur Respir J* 1990; **3**: 323–328.
48. Huang YC, O'Brien SR, MacIntyre NR. Intrabreath diffusing capacity of the lung in healthy individuals at rest and during exercise. *Chest* 2002; **122**: 177–185.
49. Aitken RCB. Measurement of feelings using visual analogue scales. *Proc R Soc Med* 1969; **62**: 989–993.
50. Borg G. Subjective effort and physical activities. *Scand J Rehab Med* 1978; **6**: 108–113.

51. Borg G. A category scale with ratio properties for intermodal and interindividual comparisons. In: Geissler HS, Petzold P, ed. *Psychophysical judgement and the process of perceptions. Proceedings of the 22nd International Congress of Psychology.* Amsterdam: North-Holland, 1980: 25–34.
52. Adams L, Chronos N, Lane R, Guz A. The measurement of breathlessness induced in normal subjects: validity of two scaling techniques. *Clin Sci* 1985; **70**: 7–16.
53. Cotes JE, Reed JW. Inter-subject differences in spontaneously chosen respiratory frequency contribute to normal variation in ventilation during submaximal exercise. *Eur Respir J* 2001; **18**(Suppl): 81s.
54. McGavin CR, Artvinli M, Naoe H, McHardy GJR. Dyspnoea, disability and distance walked: comparison of estimates of exercise performance in respiratory disease. *BMJ* 1978; **11**: 241–243.
55. Solway S, Brooks D, Lacasse Y, Thomas S. A qualitative systematic overview of the measurement properties of functional walk tests used in the cardiorespiratory domain. *Chest* 2001; **119**: 256–270.
56. American Thoracic Society. ATS statement: guidelines for the six-minute walk test. *Am J Respir Crit Care Med* 2002; **166**: 111–117.
57. Bradley J, Howard J, Wallace E, Elborn S. Reliability, repeatability, and sensitivity of the modified shuttle test in adult cystic fibrosis. *Chest* 2000; **117**: 1666–1671.
58. Singh SJ, Morgan MDL, Scott S et al. Development of a shuttle walking test of disability in patients with chronic airways obstruction. *Thorax* 1992; **47**: 1019–1024.
59. Sloan AW. The Harvard step test of dynamic fitness. *Triangle* 1962; **5**: 358–363.
60. Robertshaw SA, Reed JW, Mortimore IL et al. Submaximal alternatives to the Harvard pack index as guides to maximal oxygen uptake (physical fitness). *Ergonomics* 1984; **27**: 177–185.
61. Spiro SG, Juniper E, Bowman P, Edwards RHT. An increasing work rate test for assessing the physiological strain of submaximal exercise. *Clin Sci* 1974; **46**: 191–206.
62. Tomalak W, Cotes JE. Does gender influence tidal volume and respiratory frequency during exercise? *Eur Respir J* 2002; **20**(Suppl 38): 489s.
63. Jones NL, Rebuck AS. Tidal volume during exercise in patients with diffuse fibrosing alveolitis. *Bull Eur Physiopathol Respir* 1979; **15**: 321–327.
64. Cotes JE, Berry G, Burkinshaw L et al. Cardiac frequency during submaximal exercise in young adults; relation to lean body mass, total body potassium and amount of leg muscle. *Q J Exper Physiol* 1973; **58**: 239–250.
65. Fairbarn MS, Blackie SP, Mc Elvaney NG et al. Prediction of heart rate and oxygen uptake during incremental and maximal exercise in healthy adults. *Chest* 1994; **105**: 1365–1369.
66. Cotes JE, Hall AM, Johnson GR et al. Decline with age of cardiac frequency during submaximal exercise in healthy women. *J Physiol* 1973; **238**: 24–25P
67. Reeves JT, Grover RF, Blount SG Jr, Filley GF. Cardiac output response to standing and treadmill walking. *J Appl Physiol* 1961; **16**: 283–288.
68. Jones NL, Makrides L, Hitchcock C et al. Normal standards for an incremental progressive cycle ergometer test. *Am Rev Respir Dis* 1985; **131**: 700–708.
69. Cooper CB, Storer TW. *Exercise testing and interpretation. A practical approach.* Cambridge: Cambridge University Press; 2001.
70. Enright PL, Sherrill DL. Reference equations for the six-minute walk in healthy adults. *Am J Respir Crit Care Med* 1998; **158**: 1384–1387.
71. Cotes JE, Posner V, Reed JW. Estimation of maximal exercise ventilation and oxygen uptake in patients with chronic lung disease. *Bull Eur Physiopathol Respir* 1982; **18**: 221–228.

Further reading

Jones NL. *Clinical exercise testing.* 4th ed. Philadelphia: Saunders, 1997.
Also references 1, 4, 5, 39, 69.

CHAPTER 30

Assessment of Exercise Limitation, Disability and Residual Ability

The assessment of exercise limitation has for too long been more an art than a science. This chapter indicates how the procedure can be improved. Exercise testing is discussed in Chapter 29.

30.1 Terminology

Prior to evaluating any loss of respiratory and exercise capacity there is need for a vocabulary that can describe a person's present function with respect to normal and to indicate any inability to undertake specified tasks. Some terms are listed in Table 30.1.

30.1.1 Respiratory impairment

The World Health Organisation (WHO) has defined impairment as any loss or abnormality of psychological, physiological or anatomical structure or function [1]. As applied to the lungs the term describes the extent to which a person's lung function is subnormal. The abnormality often starts with one aspect of function but inevitably impinges on others. For this reason, impairment was formerly defined in terms of its effects on the levels of arterial blood gases. Now, forced expiratory volume (FEV_1), forced vital capacity (FVC) and transfer factor (Tl or Dl) are commonly used. The level of function is with respect to a set of reference values that should be appropriate to both the subject and the question that is being asked (see Section 26.1.5).

The result for each test is best expressed as a centile or number of standard deviations below the predicted mean value (Z-score or SD unit). The percentage reduction or Z-score can be used to classify the impairment as mild, moderate or severe according to agreed criteria. Traditionally a simpler approach has been used, with both American Thoracic Society (ATS) and the European Respiratory Society (ERS) having broadly similar criteria. The present criteria of the two organisations differ in the definition

Table 30.1 Terminology for a reduction in function relative to normal.

	WHO, 1980 [1]	USA, 1986 [2]	WHO, 1999 [3]
Lung function	Impairment	Impairment	Impairment
Exercise capacity	Disablement	Impairment	Activity limited
Lifestyle	Handicap	Disablement	Participation restricted

Impairment category	Criterion – with respect to reference value (except where stated) ERS	ATS
None (normal)	Within 1.64 RSD	>80% for FVC, FEV_1 and *Tl* (*D*lco) >75% (absolute) for FEV% (FEV_1/FVC)
Slight	Not normal but >60%	
Moderate	In range 59–40% (50% for FVC)	
Severe	<40% (<50% for FVC)	

Table 30.2 Categories of respiratory impairment of the European Respiratory Society (ERS) and American Thoracic Society (ATS). The categories relate to FVC, FEV_1, FEV% and *Tl* (*D*lco). Sources: [4, 2].

of the lower limit of normal and the treatment of FEV_1/FVC (Table 30.2).

The two classifications also differ in that whilst ERS is purely descriptive, the ATS classification purports to quantify the reduction in exercise capacity. The fallacy in this approach is described below.

30.1.2 Respiratory limitation of exercise

Respiratory limitation of exercise is loss of exercise capacity resulting from impaired function of the lungs or associated structures. The limitation is described as respiratory disability in countries where the WHO terminology is used. The term indicates the presence of both exercise limitation and impaired lung function, but does not require that the two features are linked quantitatively. In the United States the terminology assumes that the exercise limitation is closely linked to the respiratory impairment so no separate term is needed to describe it (Table 30.2). This is manifestly untrue [5, 6] and many who use the American terminology recognise the difficulty [7, 8] but the terminology is written into State Laws rather than codes of practice, so cannot easily be revised.

30.1.3 Respiratory handicap (participation restricted)

In countries that accept the WHO terminology, the terms 'respiratory handicap' and 'restricted participation' are used to describe the social disadvantage that results from a respiratory disorder. In the USA the term 'disability' is used instead (Table 30.1). The handicap or restriction is with respect to social intercourse, recreation or employment. The link with exercise limitation need not exclude a role for other factors, for example the ageing process, mental prowess, the requirements of a particular employment or the extent of social support. In some circumstances handicap can occur without exercise limitation. For example, early progressive massive fibrosis in a coal miner would normally lead to him giving up his job even if he had a normal exercise capacity. In this event, he might still undertake heavy work in another occupation.

30.2 Causes of respiratory disablement

Respiratory disablement is usually a consequence of chest illness. This will have had a principal cause that may have been reinforced by aggravating factors and inadequate treatment. Many of the factors are interdependent (Fig. 30.1). On this account their separate contributions can often only be identified with difficulty. They include intrinsic factors [10–12], for which the susceptibility varies widely between individual persons [13].

The contribution of psychological factors to disablement is influenced by a person's mood and mental attitude to ill health [14]. This mental dimension is enhanced if the subject experiences either a sense of injustice or self-reproach (or both) in relation to the cause or management of the disablement, including the process whereby compensation might or might not be awarded. The resultant anxiety can cause a genuine deterioration in the medical condition and influence the physiological result (Fig. 30.2). The findings usually improve once the claim has been settled, even if the amount of the settlement is below the claimant's expectations. Meanwhile the procedure for assessment should be directed to overcoming the psychological stress that is incurred (Sections 30.4.2 and 30.4.3).

Compared with cross-sectional studies the contribution of mental factors is less in longitudinal studies in which the reference values are the initial results for each subject (e.g. Table 30.3).

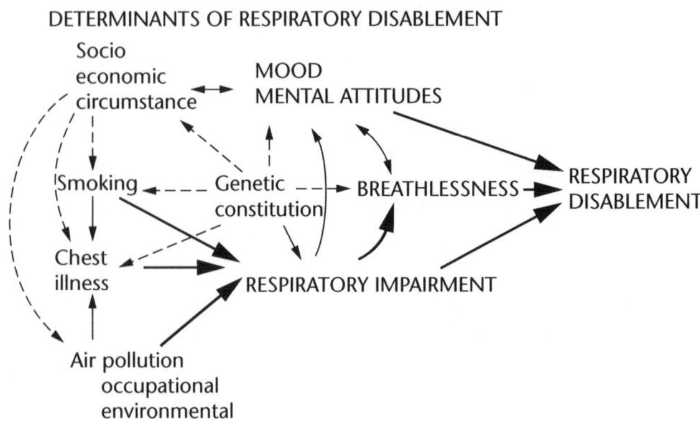

Fig. 30.1 Inter-relations between intrinsic and environmental factors contributing to respiratory disablement. Source: [9].

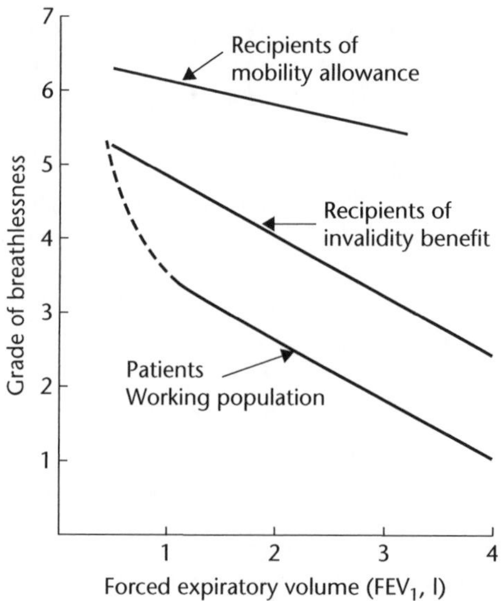

Fig. 30.2 Relationship of grade of breathlessness to FEV_1 in men with chronic bronchitis and/or emphysema assessed in different circumstances, *top* recipients of a mobility allowance, *middle* recipients of invalidity benefit, *bottom* other hospital patients (for whom the relationship was similar to that for men working in a shipyard). In some men breathlessness was enhanced by angina, obesity or another condition. After taking this into account, many of the men in receipt of an allowance were considered to have disproportionate breathlessness. Source: [15].

30.3 Preliminaries to the assessment

30.3.1 Medical considerations

The subject will normally have experienced a reduction in his or her ability to take exercise. In this event there should be evidence for a current or previous medical condition of the lungs or thoracic cage. Alternatively, if the impairment is of minor extent (e.g. <30% disability) the condition is likely to be asymptomatic [16]. The subject will then not be handicapped, but may nonetheless be eligible for compensation [17].

The first stage in any assessment is a clinical interview for recording the symptoms, medical and occupational history, exposure to other respiratory hazards and the present ability to take exercise (Table 30.4, also Fig. 30.3). Much of the information can be obtained using a standard questionnaire (e.g. Fig. 8.2, page 88) with additional questions. Permission to view previous medical results should be obtained. Depending on circumstances a medical examination may be undertaken, including chest radiography and measurement of lung function. If the subject requires or is receiving treatment this may need to be reviewed. Assessment should be delayed until the subject is in optimal health and has recovered from any acute exacerbation.

Table 30.4 Indicators of present ability to take exercise.

Method	Source
BMRC Grade of breathlessness (Fletcher)	Table 38.3, page 532 [cf. 18]
Activity diagram	Fig. 30.3
Previous non-ergometric or field test	Section 29.4

30.3.2 Review of the lung function

The first stage is to establish that the test results conform to accepted criteria e.g. with respect to successive forced expirations (Section 12.6.2) and the shapes of spirograms obtained whilst measuring *Tl* (Section 20.4). The results should be checked for internal consistency. Thus, values for vital capacity obtained in the course of measuring ventilatory capacity, lung volumes, and transfer factor (also lung compliance if it is measured) should bear a sensible relationship to each other.

For rating disability the relevant lung function results are those after maximal bronchodilatation. They should be compared with reference values that are appropriate for the question being asked. Thus, for assessing occupational disability in an occupational group, values for asymptomatic smokers and non-smokers in that industry are often preferred to values for lifetime non-smokers from a rural environment [20]. The latter values are appropriate when the assessment is for life assurance [21]. The reference variables will include age, stature, gender and ethnic group. If the physique is abnormal, as with morbid obesity, the body composition should be taken into account, for example using indices of body fat and muscle (Fat% and fat-free mass) to predict the expected lung function [22], (also Section 26.5, Table 26.18, page 352).

The diagnosis of respiratory impairment will depend on the lung function being below the lower limit of normal; this is usually expressed at the 5% level of probability as (reference value − 1.64 RSD, Table 5.7, page 50). The alternative limit at 80% of the

Table 30.3 Significant factors associated with an increase in breathlessness on exertion over 9 years in 111 coal miners with pneumoconiosis. Source: [16].

Longitudinal analysis	Cross-sectional analysis (follow-up data)
Δ body mass * + Δ residual volume + Δ score for chronic bronchitis* − Δ FVC*	Age + closing volume + *V*-iso $\dot{v}$–sGaw − *K*co*

* These variables together accounted for 82% of the variance in grade of breathlessness at follow-up.

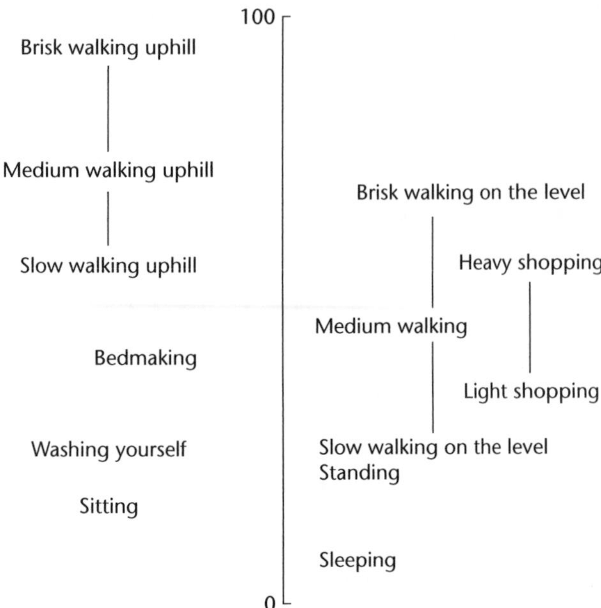

Fig. 30.3 Activity diagram of McGavin and colleagues. The score is indicated by where the subject marks the vertical line. Source: [19].

reference value is not recommended. It is only appropriate when the deviation about the reference equation is a proportional one and this is seldom the case (Section 5.3). Categories of impairment are in Table 30.2 but they are unreliable guides to disability (Section 30.1.2).

30.3.3 When is an exercise test needed?

Respiratory limitation implies that the lung function is impaired, so one or more of the standard lung function tests, forced expiratory volume, vital capacity and transfer factor (diffusing capacity) should have been measured and found to be abnormal. The impairment should be partial because in this circumstance an exercise test can contribute relevant information that cannot be deduced from lung function tests [23]. By contrast, when the lung function after bronchodilatation is markedly impaired a formal exercise test is unlikely to contribute relevant information. An exercise test may also be contraindicated on medical grounds [7]; these overlap with the indications for discontinuing a test (Table 29.3, page 418, also Section 29.6).

30.4 Conduct of the exercise test

30.4.1 Practical considerations

The objectives are to identify the mode of exercise limitation and, if respiratory, to obtain information from which the percentage disability can be calculated. To this end the exercise should involve large muscle groups and be of a type with which the subject is familiar. By this criterion treadmill, stepping and shuttle tests are appropriate. Few subjects with chronic lung disease use a bicycle or undertake cycle ergometry, so this type of exercise is only suitable for a minority, yet is used in most exercise laboratories. The protocol should be for a symptom-limited test (Section 29.3).

The measurements should normally include cardiac frequency, ventilation and gas exchange. The symptoms should be monitored and a close watch kept for possible markers of non-cooperation (Section 30.5.3). The test should be performed under electrocardiographic surveillance (Section 29.3.3).

The condition of the subject at the point when exercise is terminated is an essential outcome of the test. It should be monitored and reported as described previously (Section 29.3.3).

30.4.2 Avoiding non-cooperation

Claimants for compensation are often apprehensive since much can depend on how they perform at the assessment. The anxiety can lead to deliberate or unconscious under-performance of tests of lung function and exercise limitation. This effect can be minimised if the measurements are made as part of a medical consultation, not at a tribunal. At consultation it is possible to discuss with the patient how the findings of his assessment can be used to promote his health or to select suitable employment. This approach builds up confidence and can lead to obtaining the patient's full cooperation.

30.4.3 Special role of the person conducting the test

Preferably the same technician should oversee both the measurements of lung function and the exercise test as this helps to build up trust with the subject. The technician should be informed about the medical condition, including symptoms and any psychological difficulties. Prior to the test he or she should check that the subject is in the usual state of health and has taken the prescribed medication at the appropriate time, including any bronchodilator drug. If the bronchodilator has been omitted the subject should be requested to use the inhaler and any non-compliance noted.

The technician should administer the tests with a subtle blend of sympathy and authority and be alert for evidence of faulty cooperation. Protocols should be adhered to meticulously and in other respects the tests should be performed in the recommended manner. During the exercise test all the data (including the submaximal data) should be recorded and particular attention paid to the condition of the subject at the point when exercise is discontinued (Section 29.3.3).

30.5 Interpreting the exercise test

30.5.1 Type of limitation

For the test to be reliable there should be reasonable consistency in the minute-by-minute results during the exercise (e.g.

Fig. 29.1, page 418). In most circumstances the maximal exercise tidal volume should be appropriate for the FVC (Fig. 29.10, page 434). The maximal exercise ventilation should be appropriate for the level of FEV_1 (Fig. 28.13, page 398) and the respiratory exchange ratio should not be unduly high in relation to the other features (Section 28.4.4). The symptoms, clinical signs, function tests and performance of exercise should be consistent with one another. However, this is not always the case. Material inconsistencies or limitation by coughing can be indications for repeating the test.

Exercise limitation is when the symptom-limited maximal oxygen uptake is below the reference value (Mean – 1.64 RSD). The latter should normally be based on appropriate reference variables, for example fat-free mass (reflecting quantity of muscle, also Table 4.2, page 33), current level of habitual activity (reflecting physical condition), age and cigarette consumption [24]. The cigarette consumption can be replaced by alveolar carbon monoxide concentration and blood haemoglobin concentration. More usual reference variables are age, stature and body mass [25], but they are less discriminatory. When exercise is limited from respiratory causes the features at the point of discontinuing exercise should include those listed in Table 30.5. The principal one is incapacitating breathlessness with or without wheeze. Subjects who do not meet the requirements for respiratory limitation often experience cardiovascular insufficiency as do most healthy persons; the features are in Table 28.7 (page 405). Other subjects will be limited by giddiness, ischaemic pain, or any of a number of other symptoms of which the commonest is tiredness.

Amongst applicants with presumed respiratory disability who have been referred for assessment with a view to compensation, the proportion who actually meet the criteria can be of the order of 20% [5, 26, 27]. Other subjects may have a respiratory component to their disability.

If the limitation is respiratory the appropriateness of the observed maximal oxygen uptake can sometimes be checked using submaximal data obtained during the course of the test (Subject A, Table 30.6). Alternatively, the method can be used to estimate the respiratory component of limitation when there is under achievement (Subject B in whom the respiratory component was estimated as 29%) or another factor is dominant (Subject C). Additional problems arise if there is a possibility of malingering (Section 30.5.3 below).

Table 30.5 Criteria for respiratory limitation of test exercise.

Subject is breathless talking to the observer (saying he or she is breathless is not sufficient)
Ventilation is maximal with respect to FEV_1 and the $\dot{V} - V$ curve.
Exercise cardiac frequency (fC) is below maximum for age*
Blood lactic acid concentration [LA] is submaximal*
After exercise the ventilation ($\dot{V}E_{max}$) usually recovers within 5 min*

* With cardiovascular limitation fC and [LA] are maximal. Recovery is slow (>10 min) due to a need to repay an oxygen debt.

30.5.2 Scoring loss of exercise capacity (disability)

The 'disability' can be scored on a linear scale. It is zero when the maximal recorded oxygen uptake is at the lower limit of normal (i.e. reference value minus 1.64 RSD). The disability is 100% when the exercise capacity is at a defined minimal level [28]. For the European Respiratory Society the level is twice the resting level (2 metabolic equivalents or METS, where 1 MET is an oxygen uptake of 3.5 ml kg^{-1} min^{-1} or its equivalent in SI units). It reflects that the person is no longer able to live semi-independently. For the American Thoracic Society 100% disability is set at 4 METS [2] and the person is no longer considered able to undertake work away from home. The conventions used for defining the limits affect the outcome (e.g. Table 30.6) and should be stated. The percentage disability can be represented on a diagram (Fig. 30.4). The outcome is the overall disability; it should be compatible with the stated exercise capacity (Table 30.4). Where the limitation is respiratory the symptom-limited maximal oxygen uptake will be similar to that estimated from submaximal data (Footnote to Table 30.7). Alternatively, if the estimated value materially exceeds the observed value the former can be used to indicate the approximate limitation from respiratory factors.

In one study, the method of rating was validated by comparing the objective scores for disability based on treadmill exercise with those obtained independently by an experienced clinician who based his score on clinical grade of breathlessness, forced expiratory volume and the appearance of the chest radiograph. A significant correlation was observed ($R^2 = 0.5$, [28]). This result not only indicated a 50% overlap in the information obtained by the two methods but also important differences that arose from the clinician using radiographic as well as functional criteria.

Ideally the accuracy of the estimated disability should be indicated by the provision of confidence intervals, but these appear not to be available. Alternatively, the ratings can be grouped into grades (Table 30.8). Grades based on the measured exercise capacity are inevitably more reliable than those extrapolated from the lung function (Tables 30.2 and 30.7).

30.5.3 Under performance

In most physicians' experience the misrepresentation of symptoms is relatively common, especially in the setting of a tribunal, but there may be mitigating factors (Section 30.2). Submaximal effort, hyperventilation and features of anxiety are also quite common, as is failure to take medication effectively, especially bronchodilators. To avoid the latter, a subject who has been prescribed an inhaler should normally use it in the presence of the technician, prior to the assessment. Subtle manipulation of the performance of physiological tests is rare. Some features that should be watched for are listed in Table 30.9. The principal safeguards are to adhere to protocols, bear in mind that they can be manipulated and look for inconsistencies in the results.

Table 30.6 Illustrative cases giving observed and estimated scores for respiratory disability. Results are for treadmill exercise after full bronchodilatation. Values for $\dot{V}O_2$max in traditional units and disability calculated using ATS criteria are in italics. Reference values are in brackets.

Subject	(A) Storeman (smoker) with calcified plaques and pleural thickening	(B) Labourer (smoker) with COPD, claiming for asbestosis	(C) Coal miner (smoker, asbestos exposure). Multiple pathology
Personal details: age (year)	66	62	58
grade of breathlessness (BMRC)	4–5	4–5	2
activity grade (scale 1–4)	2	2	2
fat free mass (kg)	64	44	53
Lung function: FEV_1 (l)	2.1 (3.0)	0.9 (2.7)	3.1 (2.9)
FVC (l)	3.7 (4.2)	2.9 (3.8)	4.1 (4.0)
TLC (l)	6.4 (7.0)	7.1 (6.0)	5.2 (6.2)
RV (l)	2.6 (2.5)	4.0 (2.1)	1.2 (2.1)
Cstat (mean, l kPa^{-1})	1.8 (2.8)	2.7 (2.7)	3.5 (2.5)
Tl (mmol min^{-1} kPa^{-1})	9.1 (9.1)	7.2 (8.2)	5.9 (8.7)
VA′/VA	0.97 (>0.85)	0.78 (>0.85)	1.07 (>0.85)
Comment	Mild airways obstruction, dynamic restriction to lung expansion (cf. page 397).	Material airways obstruction, not asbestosis	Transfer defect
Response to exercise $\dot{V}_{E45}$ (l min^{-1})*	38 (24)	32 (24)	30 (24)
RER_{45}	0.76 (0.85)	0.88 (0.85)	0.78 (0.85)
SaO_2(%)	95 → 92 → 97	94 → 91 → 96	98 → 93 → 97
Vt_{30} (l)	0.71 (1.3)	0.90 (1.2)	1.1 (1.4)
fc_{45}*	103 (100)	111 (126)	95 (113)
$\dot{n}O_2$ max (mmol min^{-1}) $\dot{V}O_2$ max (l min^{-1})			
observed (with reference value)	63 (104) ... *1.41 (2.33)*	44 (79) ... *0.99 (1.77)*	72 (101) ... *1.61 (2.26)*
reference less 1.64 RSD (same units)	(76) ... *(1.70)*	(51) ... *(1.14)*	(73) ... *(1.63)*
estimated respiration limited max.†	62 ... *1.39*	49 ... *1.10*	85 ... *1.90*
Symptom at termination	struggling to breathe	slight breathlessness	legs tired (quite breathless)
Self reported effort	hard	somewhat hard	hard
Comment	breathing very shallow	not ventilation-limited	not ventilation-limited
Respiratory disability		did not meet criteria	
observed‡	24% ...	7%	did not meet criteria
estimated§	41% (confirms observed result)	29%	none¶

*Ventilation and cardiac frequency at $\dot{V}O_2$ = 1.0 l min^{-1}.
†Calculated as 66.4 + 13.4 FEV_1 (l) – 0.94 $\dot{V}_{E45}$ (l min^{-1}) + 0.45 FFM – 0.31 age (year) (Table 29.15, page 433).
‡100 (76 – 63)/(76 – 22) and 100 (1.7 – 1.41)/(1.7 – 1.0) where 22 and 1.0 are 100% disability [4, 2] (see also Table 30.7).
§Calculation as in *a* but using estimated value for maximal O_2 uptake.
¶ Respiration limited maximal O_2 uptake exceeds (reference – 1.64 RSD).

Rating scale for respiratory disability

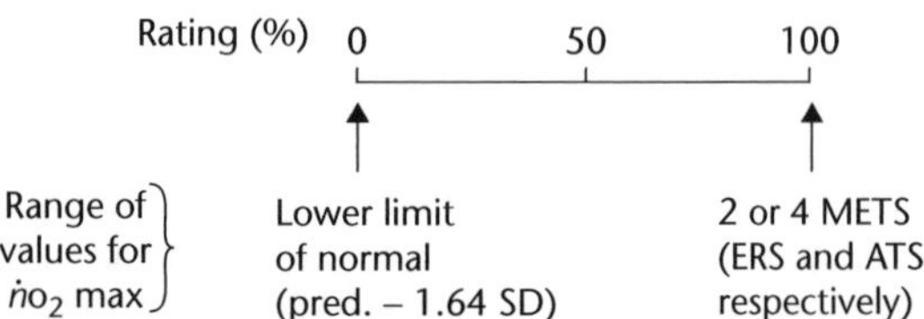

Fig. 30.4 Diagram indicating the derivation of the percentage disability. Source: [29].

30.6 Residual ability

Residual ability is important for daily living but is not the converse of disability. This is partly because exercise capacity decreases with age. Hence, in healthy persons without 'disability', an activity that was easy in youth can become impossible by old age [30] (see e.g. Fig. 25.3, page 329). In addition, the ability to undertake exercise has different determinants depending on its duration and whether the mode of limitation is respiratory, from which recovery is rapid, or cardiovascular, where recovery is slow (Section 28.8), or a mixture of the two.

Table 30.7 Calculation of percentage disability from the observed maximal O_2 uptake, the lower limit of normal (predicted less 1.64 RSD, designated LLN) and the criterion used for 100% disability (see text).*

% disability	100 × (LLN – subject's measured max. O_2 uptake) / (LLN – O_2 uptake at 100% disability)
0% (none)	Maximal O_2 uptake exceeds LLN
100% (total)	Maximal O_2 uptake less than uptake at 100% disability (2 or 4 METS as appropriate)
Reference value for max O_2 uptake based on	age, level of habitual activity, fat free mass (FFM), smoker (yes/no)
If mixed aetiology:	respiration-limited $\dot{V}O_2$max is estimated from: FEV_1, $\dot{V}E$ (submax. ex.), age and FFM (Table 29.15).

* For disability to be respiratory the exercise capacity must be limited by respiratory impairment (Table 30.5). Source: [28].

Table 30.8 Grades of respiratory disability: distribution amongst 157 men who met the criteria for respiratory limitation of exercise [5].

% Disability	Grade	Description	Number of men
0	0	None	44
1–39	1	Slight	59
40–59	2	Moderate	40
60–100	3	Severe	14

For whole body exercise *that is limited by cardiovascular factors* the work level that can be sustained for a period of hours is approximately 40% of maximal oxygen uptake [31]. Hence, this is a useful threshold against which to compare the energy cost of any particular exercise (see Fig. 28.1, page 387). If the exercise entails raising the centre of gravity of the body, as in walking (Section 28.2), the energy cost is proportional to body mass. This has led the American Thoracic Society to categorise sustainable work in terms of oxygen uptake per kg body mass [2]. The threshold for a person required to perform a range of physical tasks is set at an oxygen uptake of 15 ml min^{-1} kg^{-1}, equivalent to an oxygen uptake of 1.05 l min^{-1} for a person weighing 70 kg. For the work to be sustainable this level of $\dot{V}o_2$ should be less than 40% of maximal oxygen uptake, hence $\dot{V}o_2$max should exceed 37.5 ml min^{-1} kg^{-1}(i.e. 15 × 100/40), equivalent to a maximal oxygen uptake of 2.6 l min^{-1} for a man weighing 70 kg. On a superficial view the criterion seems reasonable. However, had it been applied to men in regular employment as welders and other tradesmen in a British shipyard, more than one third would have been excluded as having an insufficient exercise capacity (Fig. 30.5).

The discrepancy was due to $\dot{V}o_2$max per kg body mass not being independent of mass (Section 28.1.1) and to heavy shipyard tasks being performed intermittently. Thus, the method is not satisfactory even when the limitation to exercise is cardiovascular. It is also not applicable to respiratory patients in whom exercise is limited by breathlessness. In both sets of circumstances the ability to undertake a particular task can best be assessed by the subject trying it to see if he or she can cope. However, sometimes this information will have been obtained during the preliminary assessment (Section 30.3.1).

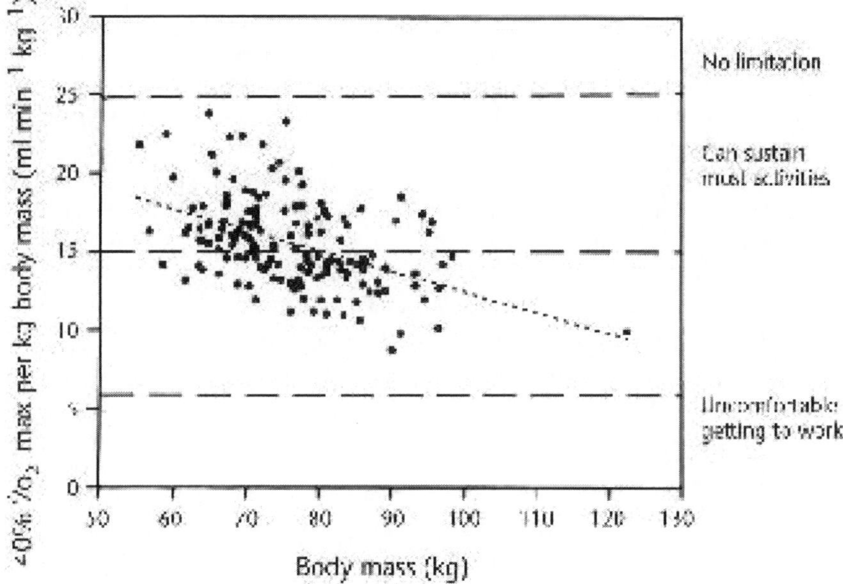

Fig. 30.5 Irrelevance of rigid criteria of suitability for strenuous work. The data points relate 40% $\dot{V}o_2$max to body mass for tradesmen in a shipyard [24]. As in other studies [32], the points are negatively correlated with body mass. The horizontal lines are arbitrary boundaries between different categories of task [2]. The boundaries are unrelated to the ability of the men to perform their work. Source: [33].

Table 30.9 Some types of non-cooperation (deliberate cheating is rare).

Spirometry	Inhaler not used, bronchoconstriction induced, previous inspiration not completed, expiration impeded, leaked or restrained
Transfer factor	Valsalva manoeuvre performed during test
Exercise test	state of agitation induced, ventilation unduly deep or shallow, end-point contrived, symptoms misrepresented
Detection	Observation, repetition, checks for internal inconsistencies in the physiological indices

30.7 Relevance for compensation

In respiratory patients the extent of exercise limitation (disability) is an important factor in awarding compensation. Another consideration is the likely prognosis. This is related to the loss of lung function both at one point in time and longitudinally. Thus, for purposes of compensation the response to exercise and the lung function make inter-related but partly separate contributions to the outcome. The two components of the assessment can also contribute to medical treatment and subsequent clinical management, so a holistic approach has practical utility as well as contributing to the quality of the measurements (Section 30.5.3).

30.8 Summary

The assessment of respiratory limitation of exercise (respiratory disability) poses a challenge to the respiratory team as it combines a need for high professional and technical standards with the vigilance of a good detective. The procedures include clinical appraisal, assessment of lung function especially dynamic spirometry and transfer factor, and, where appropriate, the performance of a symptom-limited maximal exercise test. The exercise should be of a type that the subject performs regularly. For most subjects this entails walking using a treadmill and not cycling using a stationary bicycle. From the results the percentage and grade of disability and the proportion attributable to respiratory insufficiency can be calculated. The information necessary for the assessment can also be used to make allowance for co-existing cardiovascular disease and, in some instances, to overcome the effects of incomplete cooperation by the subject. The assessment of residual ability can make use of the same information, but this topic is best approached empirically.

30.9 References

1. World Health Organisation. *International classification of impairments, disabilities and handicaps.* Geneva: WHO, 1980.
2. American Thoracic Society. Evaluation of impairment/disability secondary to respiratory disorders. *Am Rev Respir Dis* 1986; **133**: 1205–1209.
3. World Health Organisation.*International classification of functioning and disability.* Beta-2 Draft. Geneva: WHO, 1999.
4. De Coster A. Respiratory impairment and disablement. *Bull Eur Respir Pathophysiol Respir* 1983; **19**: 1P–3P.
5. Cotes JE, Zejda J, King B. Lung function impairment as a guide to exercise limitation in work-related lung disorders. *Am Rev Respir Dis* 1988; **137**: 1089–1093.
6. O'Donnell DE, Lam M, Webb KA. Measurement of symptoms, lung hyperinflation, and endurance during exercise in chronic obstructive pulmonary disease. *Am J Respir Crit Care Med* 1998; **158**: 1557–1565.
7. ATS/ACCP statement on cardiopulmonary exercise testing. *Am J Respir Crit Care Med* 2003; **167**: 211–277.
8. Smith DD. Pulmonary impairment/disability evaluation: controversies and criticisms. *Clin Pulm Med* 1995; **2**: 334–343.
9. Cotes JE, Steel J. *Work-related lung disorders.* Oxford: Blackwell Scientific, 1987.
10. Morgan AD, Peck DF, Buchanan DR, McHardy GJR. Effects of attitudes and beliefs on exercise tolerance in chronic bronchitis. *BMJ* 1983; **286**: 171–173.
11. Sprake CM, Cotes JE, Reed JW. Correlates of 6 min walking distance and maximal oxygen uptake in chronic lung disease. *Clin Sci* 1984; **66**: 57P.
12. Hesselink AE, Penninx BW, Schlosser MA et al. The role of coping resources and coping style in quality of life of patients with asthma or COPD. *Qual life Res* 2004; **13**: 509–518.
13. Rosser R, Guz A. Psychological approaches to breathlessness and its treatment. *J Psychosom Res* 1981; **25**: 439–447.
14. King B, Cotes JE. Relation of lung function and exercise capacity to mood and attitudes to health. *Thorax* 1989: **44**: 402–409.
15. Pearce SJ, Posner V, Robinson AJ et al. "Invalidity" due to chronic bronchitis and emphysema: how real is it? *Thorax* 1985; **40**: 828–831.
16. Musk AW, Bevan C, Campbell MJ, Cotes JE. Factors contributing to the clinical grade of breathlessness in coalminers with pneumoconiosis. *Bull Eur Physiopathol Respir* 1979; **15**: 343–353.
17. Wright GW. Disability evaluation in industrial pulmonary disease. *JAMA* 1949; **141**: 1218–1222.
18. Bestall JC, Paul EA, Garrod R et al. Usefulness of the Medical Research Council (MRC) dyspnoea scale as a measure of disability in patients with chronic obstructive pulmonary disease. *Thorax* 1999; **54**: 581–586.
19. McGavin CR, Artvinli M, Naoe H, McHardy GJR. Dyspnoea, disability and distance walked: comparison of estimates of exercise performance in respiratory disease. *BMJ* 1978; **11**: 241–243.
20. Quanjer PhH, editor. Standardized lung function testing. *Bull Eur Physiopathol Respir* 1983; **19**(Suppl) 5: 1–95.
21. American Thoracic Society. Lung function testing; selection of reference values and interpretative strategies. *Am Rev Respir Dis* 1992; **145**: 1202–1218.
22. Cotes JE, Chinn DJ, Reed JW. Body mass, fat percentage, and fat free mass as reference variables for lung function: effects on terms for age and sex. *Thorax* 2001; **56**: 839–844.
23. Gallagher CG. Exercise limitation and clinical exercise testing in chronic obstructive pulmonary disease. *Clin Chest Med* 1994; **15**: 305–326.

24. Weller JJ, El-Gamal FM, Parker L et al. Indirect estimation of maximal oxygen uptake for study of working populations. *Br J Ind Med* 1988; **45**: 532–537.
25. Jones NL, Makrides L, Hitchcock C et al. Normal standards for an incremental progressive cycle ergometer test. *Am Rev Respir Dis* 1985; **131**: 700–708.
26. Oren A, Sue DY, Hansen JE et al. The role of exercise testing in impairment evaluation. *Am Rev Respir Dis* 1987; **135**: 230–235.
27. Agostoni P, Smith DD, Schoene RB et al. Evaluation of breathlessness in asbestos workers. Results of exercise testing. *Am Rev Respir Dis* 1987; **135**: 812–816.
28. Cotes JE, Chinn DJ, Reed JW, Hutchinson JEM. Experience of a standard method for assessing respiratory disability *Eur Respir J* 1994; **7**: 875–880.
29. Cotes JE. Rating respiratory disability: a report on behalf of a working group of the European Society for Clinical Respiratory Physiology. *Eur Respir J* 1990; **3**: 1074–1077.
30. Cotes JE. Assessment of disablement due to impaired respiratory function. *Bull Eur Physiopathol Respir* 1975; **11**: 210P–217P.
31. Christensen EH. Physiological valuation of work in Nykroppa steel works. In: Floyd WF, Welford AT, eds. Ergonomics Research Society, *Symposium on fatigue.* London: HK Lewis, 1953: 93–108.
32. Åstrand P-O, Rodahl K. *Textbook of work physiology.* 3rd ed. London: McGraw-Hill, 1986.
33. Cotes JE, Reed JW. Relationship of maximal oxygen uptake ($\dot{V}O_2$max) to body mass (BM), implications for rating exercise ability. *Eur Respir J* 1999; **14**(Suppl 30): 491s.

Further reading

Williams RGA, Johnston M, Willis LA, Bennett AE. Disability: a model and measurement technique. *Br J Prev Soc Med* 1976; **30**: 71–78.

CHAPTER 31

Exercise in Children

The physiological responses to exercise and the methods of assessment in children closely resemble those in adults (Chapters 28 and 29). This short chapter indicates some of the special features.

31.1 Physiological responses to exercise in children

31.1.1 Effects of size

The smaller size of children compared with adults inevitably influences the responses to exercise. However, many of the underlying physiological responses are numerically similar in the two age groups, for example alveolar ventilation on uptake of oxygen, cardiac output on uptake of oxygen [1–3] and maximal cardiac frequency on age [1]. Apart from young children (age <10 years), the similarity extends to the mechanical efficiency of cycle ergometry [2].

The relatively small lungs leads to children having smaller exercise tidal volumes than adults. This difference is solely due to size as the relationships of exercise tidal volume (Vt_{30}) to forced vital capacity in boys and girls separately are each similar to those for adults of the same gender [4], see also Fig. 31.1. The smaller breaths are compensated for by a higher breathing frequency compared with adults.

The first part of each breath is expended in flushing the anatomical deadspace, so the higher breathing frequency raises the deadspace ventilation per minute and hence the ventilation minute volume. As a result the ventilation for a given oxygen uptake is greater than in adults. The ventilation declines at adolescence, especially in boys amongst whom the adolescent growth spurt markedly increases the vital capacity and exercise tidal volume. This change reduces the frequency of breathing and hence the volume of air per minute used to flush the anatomical deadspace. As a result the ventilation per minute comes down to the adult level (Fig. 31.2).

In girls the changes in exercise ventilation with age are smaller than in boys. This is partly because the adolescent growth spurt and associated increase in vital capacity are usually also less in girls (Section 25.3, page 320). The difference continues into adult life where it contributes to the ventilation during submaximal exercise being somewhat greater in women than in men. An additional factor increasing the average exercise ventilation of small children compared with bigger ones, and women compared with men, is a smaller stroke volume

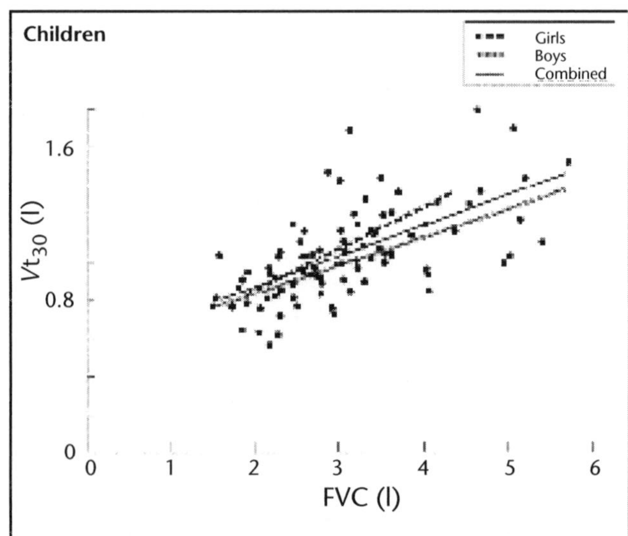

Fig. 31.1 Data relating Vt_{30} to FVC in Caucasian children. The slopes of the relationships differ between the sexes to a small but significant extent. Source: [4].

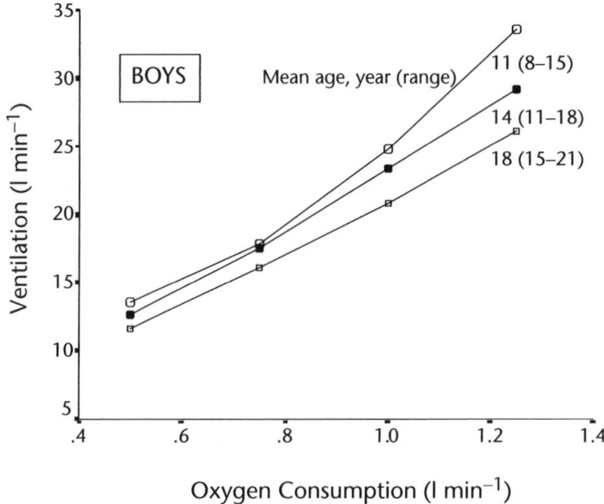

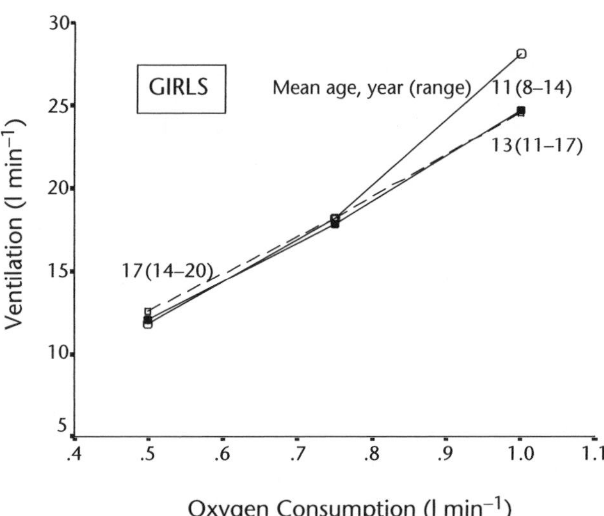

Fig. 31.2 Mean longitudinal values for ventilation during submaximal cycle ergometry relative to uptake of oxygen in 18 boys and 18 girls initially aged 8–15 years. Ventilation decreased at adolescence in the boys but not in the girls who were studied concurrently (cf. Figs 31.3 and 31.4). The curvilinearity in the relationships for girls and young boys but not for older boys at the same levels of oxygen uptake is evidence for Owles point occurring at a relatively lower rate of work in the former subjects, (cf. Fig. 28.5, page 391). Source: [5].

and maximal cardiac output. These features are associated with Owles point occurring at relatively lower levels of oxygen uptake (Section 28.4.6).

Similar considerations apply to cardiac frequency during submaximal exercise [6]. The frequency is higher in children than in adults due to the small size of the heart limiting the stroke volume. The stroke volume (SV) increases as the children get older and, as a result, the frequency for a specified oxygen uptake decreases with increasing age (Figs 31.3 and 31.4). The change is progressive and unlike that for ventilation in boys is not conspicuously related to puberty. The relationships with age are no longer significant after allowance has been made for fat-free mass (FFM) indicating that the decline in fc with age is largely structural in origin (Fig. 31.5, cf. Figs 31.3 and 31.4). The regression relationships on FFM in children are of similar form to that for adults of both sexes (Table 31.1 cf. Table 29.15 and Fig. 29.11, pages 433 and 434), but the magnitudes of the coefficient terms

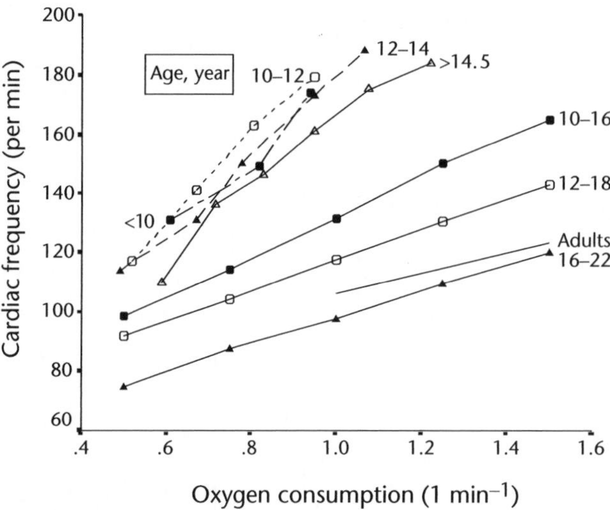

Fig. 31.3 Relationships of exercise cardiac frequency to uptake of oxygen during submaximal exercise in boys. The upper cluster of relationships was obtained during measurement of cardiac output by a rebreathing method [2]. The lower cluster was for 10 Caucasian boys, initially aged 10–16 years who were assessed on three occasions over 6 years. Their cardiac frequency declined progressively [5]. The frequency had reached the level typical of adult men by the end of the period of follow up (cf. Table 29.15, page 433).

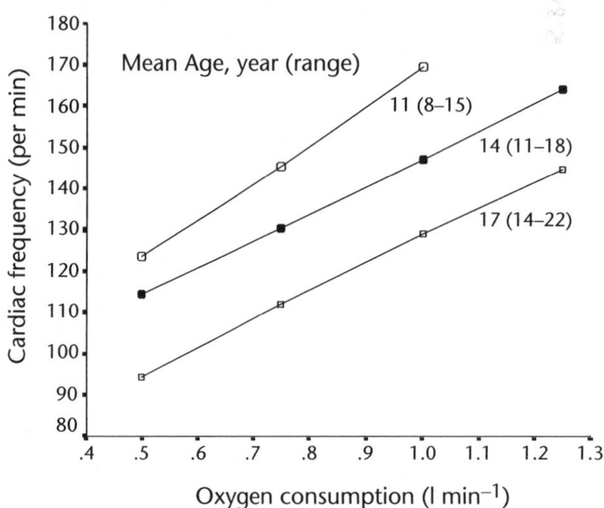

Fig. 31.4 Relationship of exercise cardiac frequency to uptake of oxygen during submaximal exercise in 18 girls who were invited to attend on three occasions over 6 years. The decline with age was significant. Source: [5].

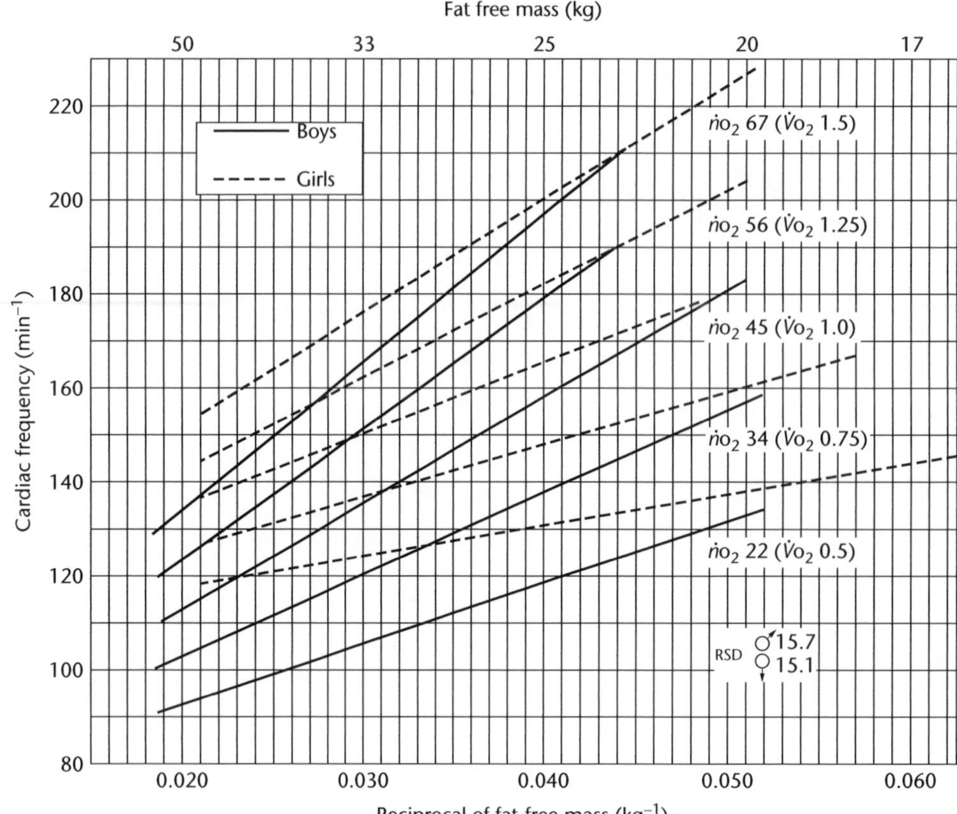

Fig. 31.5 Exercise cardiac frequency in relation to the reciprocal of fat free mass for boys and girls aged 8–16 years at different levels of oxygen uptake ($\dot{n}O_2$ in mmol min^{-1}, $\dot{V}O_2$ in l min^{-1}). cf. Fig. 29.11, page 434). Source: [5].

(parameters) are different. This may reflect imperfect calibration of the anthropometric method for estimating FFM in children.

The maximal cardiac frequency in children is only slightly higher than in young adults [1] so, since the stroke volume is small, the maximal cardiac output is also low. This affects the maximal work rate (exercise capacity), maximal oxygen uptake and the oxygen uptake at Owles point (also the anaerobic threshold, Section 28.4.6), all of which are reduced. The differences from adults diminish progressively during growth. Some trends in the responses are illustrated in the figures. A summary is given in Table 31.2.

31.1.2 Puberty

Onset of puberty increases the exercise capacity, particularly of boys. This is apparent in Fig. 31.6 where the slope of the relationship of $\dot{V}O_2$max on age appears to reach its peak at a later age in boys than in girls, consistent with a later onset of puberty.

31.1.3 Gender

The effects of this variable are difficult to separate from those of body size. Girls on average are smaller, their adolescent growth

Table 31.1 General reference equations for cardiac frequency during submaximal exercise in young people.

	Equation	
Males	$fC = 68.4 + 238/\text{FFM}\ (1 + (8.56/44.6)\dot{n}O_2)$	RSD 15.7, C of V 10.6%
Females	$fC = 103.4 - 193/\ \text{FFM}\ (1 - (9.0/44.6)\dot{n}O_2)$	RSD 15.1, C of V 11.1%

Note: The frequency at a specified oxygen uptake is indicated in Figs 31.3 and 31.4, see also Fig. 29.11, page 434.
FFM = fat-free mass in kg; $\dot{n}O_2$ = is oxygen uptake in mmol min^{-1}. To convert to traditional units (l min^{-1}) the factor 44.6 is omitted.
Source: [5].

Table 31.2 Features of physiological responses to exercise in children.

Feature	Structural component	Functional component
Comparison with adults	Children have a smaller tidal volume and stroke volume	Maximal ventilation and cardiac output ($\dot{Q}t$) are less, exercise capacity and O_2 uptake at Owles point are lower. Submaximal exercise cardiac frequency is higher. Submaximal ventilation (below Owles point) is slightly higher $\dot{Q}t$ relative to O_2 uptake is independent of age
Effect of puberty	Quantity of body muscle increases, especially in boys	Stroke volume and exercise capacity increase
Gender differences (both intrinsic and via association with habitual activity)	On average boys have more muscle than girls; this affects stroke volume and tidal volume (Vt_{30})	Maximal cardiac output and related variables are greater and submaximal cardiac frequency is less in boys Relationship of Vt_{30} to FVC is nearly the same in the two sexes

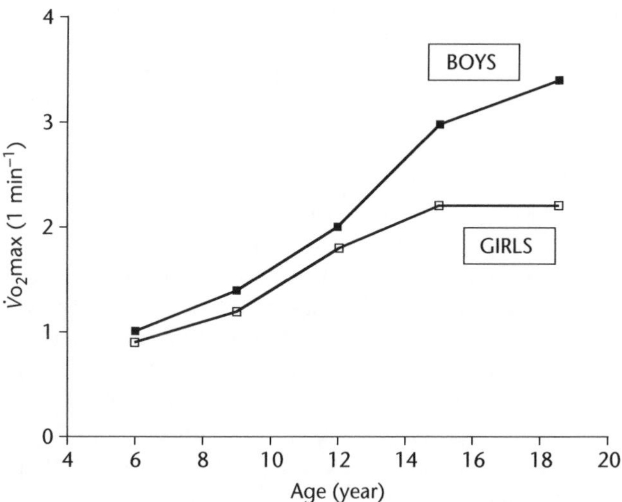

Fig. 31.6 Average maximal oxygen uptake in relation to age for boys and girls. Source: [7].

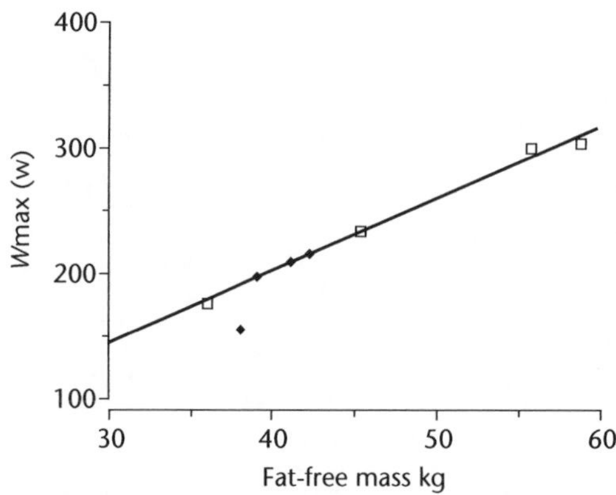

Fig. 31.7 Exercise capacity of boys (open squares) during cycle ergometry, expressed as mean values (W) relative to mean fat-free mass, with data for girls (closed diamonds) superimposed [8].

spurt occurs earlier and it is of shorter duration than in boys. These differences have profound consequences for body size, lung size and responses to exercise (described above). The evidence for gender-specific differences is limited to a few variables and mainly relates to after puberty. They include differences in muscle strength, exposure to respiratory drive from progesterone and the blood concentration of haemoglobin. The relationship of exercise tidal volume (Vt_{30}) to forced vital capacity is only marginally different between the sexes [4], whilst there is no gender difference in the relationship of exercise capacity to fat-free mass (Fig. 31.7) [8, 9]. For both relationships the pattern for adults is the same (Section 25.7.5).

Currently many young people of both sexes are experiencing a conspicuous increase in height compared with their predecessors and the consequences for the lung function and responses to exercise are currently being documented. The phenomenon appears not to be related to gender [10].

31.2 Exercise testing in children

31.2.1 Indications

Most exercise testing in children is in relation to physical recreation and for assessing the cardio-respiratory consequences of cardiac disorders (e.g. [11]). Respiratory exercise testing was formerly used mainly as a provocation test for exercise-induced airways obstruction (e.g. [12]) and management of children with cystic fibrosis (e.g. [13]), including the possibility of lung transplantation. The resulting increased familiarity with exercise testing in children has overflowed into the management of other disorders that may affect the lungs (e.g. [14]). As a result the indications for respiratory exercise testing in children are nearly as wide as those for adults (Section 29.2).

31.2.2 Making the measurements

Introduction. Children usually enjoy physical activity so they tolerate exercise tests well. However, the approach should be child-orientated, preferably in a dedicated laboratory with its own staff. In this event child-size equipment can be used, but equipment for adults (Fig. 29.6, page 424), supplemented with a few additional items is usually satisfactory. If a general exercise laboratory is used some screens and posters for children can help to set the scene.

The exercise can be presented as a game appropriate to the procedure. For example, if shuttle running is to be used to test for exercise-induced airflow limitation [12], the child might be a footballer undergoing physical training. If the respired gas is to be monitored via a mouthpiece the child might be engaged in underwater exploration using a snorkel. The images should be presented in a low-key manner to avoid undue excitement.

Ergometry. Unlike for adults, the choice of ergometer is probably not critical for children (cf. Section 29.4.1, page 420). Where a cycle is used its dimensions should match those of the intended user [15]. The loading on the pedals should be capable of automatic variation to accommodate different rates of pedalling. Where practicable the loading should be increased continuously rather than in discrete increments. Treadmill exercise is appropriate for older children [16], especially boys who often feel challenged by the new experience. Before being connected to any equipment, the child should try out the ergometer. The work level should be increased very gradually.

Connecting to the equipment. Electrodes on the chest are usually tolerated well, but the connection necessary for measuring ventilation may need to be presented imaginatively along the lines indicated above. Where a mask is to be used, more than one shape and a range of sizes should be available and care taken to ensure a close fit along the line of contact with the face. Particular attention should be paid to the fit round the nose.

Once the connections have been made the child should try out the equipment at rest and on exercise, but any measurements at this stage may not be representative on account of excitement, leading to a high cardiac frequency. A frequency that is much above the child's usual level should preferably lead to the test being postponed.

31.3 Reference values for exercise in children

Published reference values for the physiological responses to exercise in children exhibit considerable variation between laboratories. This reflects different protocols and objectives, also alternative views as to how the results should be presented. As a result local reference values based on results for healthy children assessed in the laboratory should be used where possible. The conditions should conform to the criteria described earlier in this chapter. Alternatively, published values should be calibrated to suit local circumstances. Values obtained in a different laboratory are best not applied uncritically. This is particularly the case for exercise cardiac frequency and related variables, since these indices are subject to variation depending on the protocol by which they were obtained (see e.g. Fig. 31.3). Results obtained by an exacting protocol or expressed in terms of an inappropriate model (Section 28.6.2, page 400) are best avoided. For some indices reference values for adults are suitable for children. Where this is not the case the adult values (Table 29.15, page 433) are usually attained at or soon after the end of adolescence.

Examples of the responses to be expected for healthy white children assessed using the present recommended methods are given in Table 31.3. Values for another ethnic group obtained by similar methods are included as well.

Table 31.3 Data on responses to exercise in healthy children obtained by standard methods.

Index	Reference variable	Location
Ventilation (submax)	O_2 uptake	Fig. 31.2 [5] In Caribbean children [17]
Cardiac frequency (submax)	O_2 uptake	Table 31.1 and Figs 31.3 and 31.4 [5]
	FFM	Fig. 31.5 [5] In Caribbean children [17]
Cardiac frequency (max)	Age	Table 29.15 (page 433)
Tidal volume (Vt_{30})	FVC	Fig. 31.1 and Table 29.15
Physiological deadspace	Tidal volume	Eqn. 31.1
Cardiac output	O_2 uptake	Table 29.15
Maximal O_2 uptake	Age	Fig. 31.6
Exercise capacity	FFM and customary activity	Fig. 31.7 (more data needed)

Physiological deadspace. In children and young adults the recommended reference variables are tidal volume and body mass (eqn. 31.1). Then:

$$Vd = 1.54\,BW + 0.049\,Vt + 2(\mathrm{SD}\,22\,\mathrm{ml}) \quad (31.1)$$

where Vd and Vt are physiological deadspace and tidal volume (ml) and BW is body mass (kg) [1]. Stature can also be used.

Other aspects of exercise that are appropriate for children are discussed in Chapters 28 and 29.

31.4 References

1. Godfrey S, Davies CTM, Wozniak E, Barnes CA. Cardio-respiratory response to exercise in normal children. *Clin Sci* 1955, **14:** 419–431.

2. Rosenthal M, Bush A. Haemodynamics in children during rest and exercise: methods and normal values. *Eur Respir J* 1998; **11**: 854–865.
3. Reeves JT, Grover RF, Blount SG, Jr, Filley GF. Cardiac output response to standing and treadmill walking. *J Appl Physiol* 1961; **16**: 283–288.
4. Tomalak W, Cotes JE. Does gender influence tidal volume and respiratory frequency during exercise? *Eur Respir J* 2002; **20**(Suppl 38): 489s.
5. Kagamimori S, Robson JM, Heywood C, Cotes JE. Genetic and environmental determinants of the cardio-respiratory response to submaximal exercise – a six year follow-up study of twins. *Ann Hum Biol* 1984; **11**: 29–38.
6. Vinet A, Nottin S, Lecoq AM, Obert P. Cardiovascular responses to progressive exercise in healthy children and adults. *Int J Sports Med* 2002; **23**: 242–246.
7. Shvarty E, Reibold RC. Aerobic fitness norms for males and females aged 6 to 75 years. *Aviat Space Environ Med* 1990; **61**: 3–11.
8. Cotes JE, Gulsman VAM, de Meer K, Reed JW. Reference values for maximal work capacity in healthy children. Correspondence. *Eur Respir J* 1998; **11**: 791.
9. Rump P, Verstappen F, Gerver WJ, Hornstra G. Body composition and cardiorespiratory fitness indicators in prepubescent boys and girls. *Int J Sports Med* 2002; **23**: 50–54.
10. Cole TJ. The secular trend in human physical growth: a biological view. *Econ Hum Biol* (www.sciencedirect.com) 2003; **1**: 161–168.
11. Zajac A, Tomkiewicz L, Podolec P et al. Cardiorespiratory response to exercise in children after modified fontan operation. *Scand Cardiovasc J* 2002; **36**: 67–68.
12. Burr ML, Butland BK, King S, Vaughan-Williams E. Changes in asthma prevalence: two surveys 15 years apart. *Arch Dis Child* 1989; **64**: 1452—1456; see also comment *Arch Dis Child* 1990; **65**: 646.
13. Cropp GJ, Pullano TP, Cerny FJ, Nathanson IT. Exercise tolerance and cardiorespiratory adjustments at peak work capacity in cystic fibrosis. *Am Rev Respir Dis* 1982; **126**: 211–216.
14. Mlcak RP, Desai MH, Robinson E et al. Increased physiological deadspace/tidal volume ratio during exercise in burned children. *Burns* 1995; **21**: 337–339.
15. Martin JC, Malina RM, Spirduso WW. Effects of crank length on maximal cycling power and optimal pedalling rate in boys aged 8–11 years. *Eur J Appl Physiol* 2002; **86**: 215–217.
16. Silverman M, Anderson SD. Metabolic cost of exercise in children. *J Appl Physiol* 1972; **33**: 696–698.
17. Miller GJ, Saunders MJ, Gilson RJC, Ashcroft MT. Lung function of healthy boys and girls in Jamaica in relation to ethnic composition, test exercise performance, and habitual physical activity. *Thorax* 1977; **32**: 486–496.

Further reading

Godfrey S. *Exercise testing in children.* London: Saunders, 1974.

Figueroa-Colon R, Hunter GR, Mayo MS et al. Reliability of treadmill measures and criteria to determine $\dot{V}O_2$max in prepubertal girls. *Med Sci Sports Exerc.* 2000; **32**: 865–869.

Prioux J, Matecki S, Amsallem F et al. Ventilatory response to maximal exercise in healthy children (Article in French). *Rev Mal Respir.* 2003; **20**: 904–911.

PART 5
Breathing During Sleep

CHAPTER 32

Investigation and Physiology of Breathing During Sleep

Hypoxia during sleep has important medical and social consequences. This chapter gives a practical account of the physiology and clinical pathology. The assessment and treatment of sleep related breathing disorders are in Chapter 33.

32.1 Introduction

The association of somnolence and obesity was recognised in the late 19th century and dramatised by Dickens' description of the sleepy fat boy Joe [1]. The topic was reawakened in 1972 when Lugaresi and colleagues [2] and then Guilleminault [3] reported systematic studies of sleep related breathing disorders. In 1981 Sullivan described the use of nasal continuous positive airway pressure as a realistic treatment for obstructive sleep apnoea (OSA) [4]. This work brought OSA into clinical medicine and led to intensive study of the causative factors. The present text gives a practical account. Full coverage is provided in excellent books by Stradling [5], Martin [6], and Shneerson [7].

32.2 Terminology and definitions

Apnoea
: Cessation of ventilation for at least 10 s.

Apnoea/Hypopnea Index (AHI)
: The number of apnoeas or hypopnoeas occurring per hour of sleep that cause at least a 4% reduction in arterial saturation.

Arousal
: Electroencephalogram (EEG) and electromyogram (EMG) changes suggesting a return to wakefulness that lasts for more than 1.5 s.

Bradypnoea
: Reduced frequency of breathing.

Central apnoea
: Cessation of ventilation for at least 10 s (apnoea) due to failure to make any ventilatory effort. This is due to failure of the central controller.

Hypopnea
: Reduced tidal volume that leads to an arterial desaturation of at least 4%.

Hypoventilation
: Reduced level of ventilation due to smaller tidal volume and/or reduced frequency of respiration that leads to hypercapnia.

Mixed apnoea
: Cessation of ventilation for more than 10 s with no evidence of respiratory effort followed by evidence of effort with no ventilation, all within the same apnoeic episode.

Obstructive apnoea
: Cessation of ventilation for at least 10 s due to occlusion of the airway in the presence of ventilatory effort in terms of thoracic and abdominal movement consistent with appropriate muscle activation.

Polysomnography
: Recording multiple variables during sleep, which include electro-encephalogram (EEG), electro-oculogram (EOG), mouth and nasal flow, thoracic and abdominal movement.

Upper Airway Resistance Syndrome
: Arousal due to increased effort of breathing without cessation of breathing or desaturation.

32.3 Investigative techniques

32.3.1 Sleep staging

Staging sleep requires the recording of an electro-encephalogram (EEG) using three electrodes applied to the head. One electrode is placed on one mastoid process and another on the contralateral hemisphere. The difference in signal between these two is recorded using the signal from the other mastoid as a reference. Detection of rapid eye movement (REM) sleep requires the recording of an electro-oculogram (EOG) using electrodes placed close to each eye. Muscle tone changes with sleep and because its effect on the upper airway is deemed significant it is customary to record a surface electro-myogram (EMG) from muscles under the chin.

32.3.2 Nasal and mouth flow

In most applications it is only necessary usually to measure ventilatory flow qualitatively. For this purpose thermistors or thermocouples taped close to the mouth and to the nose can give readings that indicate if a subject is inhaling or exhaling. The duration of each part of the cycle can then be determined. To obtain an absolute measurement of ventilation it is possible to apply occlusive masks with one of a variety of flow meters attached. These devices need to have a very low resistance to avoid disturbing the subject's breathing whilst asleep; pneumotachographs have been widely used although an ultrasonic flow meter may also be suited for this purpose (Section 7.3.2). However, all these devices will influence the subject's ability to sleep as it is not possible to move the head freely with them attached. Furthermore, the deadspace of the device will change the subject's ventilation and response to various stimuli. Occlusive masks can be applied to a subject whilst they are asleep by remotely inflating a cuff or by direct application of a mask by a sleep technician. These methods have been used to good effect in particular experimental protocols [8].

32.3.3 Abdominal/thoracic movement

Inductance plethysmography using a Respitrace^{TM} (Section 7.3.1) can be used to assess respiratory movements of the trunk. Most importantly this device can separate the thoracic and abdominal components of ventilation but only qualitatively. This recording device can demonstrate the presence of abdominal movement and paradoxical thoracic movement at a time of no

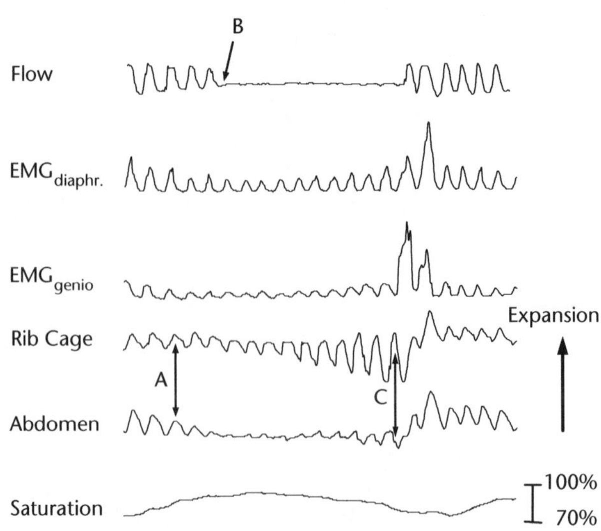

Fig. 32.1 Obstructive apneoa. recordings of mouth flow, EMG of the diaphragm and the genioglossus muscle, movement of the rib cage and the abdomen from a Respitrace^{TM}, and the arterial saturation. At point A during normal breathing the ribcage expansion is in phase with the abdominal expansion. At point B mouth flow ceases whilst rib cage movement continues and gradually increases in amplitude. Flow remains zero since the airway is occluded despite increasing rib cage movement. At point C the rib cage and abdominal movements are now out of phase with sucking in of the abdomen and rib cage expansion. As no air is inhaled the expansion of the rib cage is at the expense of volume loss in the abdomen. Immediately after this there is a burst of EMG activity in the genioglossus followed by restoration of mouth flow and return of rib cage and abdominal movements in phase.

nasal or mouth flow, thus confirming that the upper airway must be occluded (Fig. 32.1).

Numerous other transduction methods have been applied including strain gauges, plethysmographs, and magnetometers (Sections 7.3 to 7.6).

32.3.4 Arterial saturation

Capillary pulse oximetry (Section 7.10.1) is the simplest way to estimate a patient's oxygenation whilst asleep. Early devices applied probes to the pinna of the ear, but now probes attached to a single digit yield satisfactory readings. These can be recorded in a quasi-continuous way so that changes in ventilation can be matched to oxygenation.

32.3.5 Pa,o_2 and Pa,co_2

True arterial oxygenation can only be ascertained from an indwelling arterial catheter with repetitive sampling. This is invasive and for a full overnight study might involve withdrawal of considerable volumes of blood. A transcutaneous method has been devised to estimate arterial Pa,o_2 (Section 7.10.2). An electrode for Pa,co_2 is also available. These devices require the skin to be heated and a principle drawback is that after about 4 h a skin burn may develop that can leave a permanent scar. Moving the electrodes during a study requires a technician in attendance throughout the night and when the electrode is changed the sleep may be disturbed. These electrodes do not give an exact match to arterial $P\text{O}_2$ and $P\text{CO}_2$ but will accurately follow trends so that, during an apnoea any fall in $P\text{O}_2$ and rise in $P\text{CO}_2$ can be tracked to confirm that hypoventilation is occurring.

32.3.6 Snoring

Excessive snoring is a cardinal symptom and sign for various sleep related breathing disorders. Snoring can be a normal phenomenon in many subjects and does not necessarily indicate a pathological process. If snoring is due to pathological airway closure it is necessary to demonstrate (i) that it coincides with evidence of upper airway changes that are consistent with partial obstruction and (ii) that at the time of any apnoea the snoring ceases. A simple microphone can be attached to the neck by tape and the signal recorded for this purpose.

With polysomnography it is possible to record the temporal relationship between snoring, airflow and the changes in abdominal and thoracic movements. Some systems have used video recording of the patient together with sound monitoring to demonstrate the relationship between snoring, cessation of snoring, thoracic and abdominal movement and the increase in limb movement with the subsequent arousal.

32.3.7 Heart rate

Heart rate and blood pressure are not constant during REM sleep but vary. If there is cyclical desaturation due to airway occlusion then the variability of the heart rate and blood pressure may increase and will follow the periodic cycle of the airway occlusion that is causing the additional variability. It can be helpful to record the ECG by three electrodes together with the other inputs. Then, spectral analysis of the heart rate variability can track changes due to airway obstruction while asleep.

32.3.8 Movement

Piezoelectric devices can be used to record limb movements. An alternative is to record a patient sleeping using a video camera which can give information on snoring through sound recording, limb movement and thoracic and abdominal movement. Limb movements occur during REM sleep and during arousal. Video recordings do not readily lend themselves to automated numerical analysis.

32.3.9 Sleepiness

The clinical importance of sleep related breathing disorders is defined by symptoms. Many patients snore without having any other symptoms to suggest disturbance of their sleep so it is necessary to estimate 'sleepiness' and the effects of sleep deprivation. The Epworth sleepiness score is widely used as a reliable and reproducible index [9]. The subject estimates on a scale from 0 to 3 how likely she/he is to doze under eight defined circumstances (Table 32.1). A score above 12 suggests a high likelihood of there being OSA, narcolepsy, or idiopathic insomnia. Two of these circumstances relate to aspects of driving or being in a car which may reduce the value of the score in those subjects with no access to a car, or those whose replies might implicate them in their job. However, subjects are instructed to imagine how they would be affected under the given circumstances even if they have not experienced them directly.

Table 32.1 Epworth Score to assess daytime sleepiness.

Question: "How likely are you to doze off or fall asleep in the following situations, in contrast to feeling just tired?"

Use the scale below to score your response to each of the following eight situations with the most appropriate number from your experience in the last month.

0 = would *never* doze
1 = *slight* chance of dozing
2 = *moderate* chance of dozing
3 = *high* chance of dozing

A	Sitting and reading
B	Watching TV
C	Sitting, inactive in a public place, e.g. a theatre or a meeting
D	As a passenger in a car for an hour without a break
E	Lying down to rest in the afternoon when circumstances permit
F	Sitting and talking to someone
G	Sitting quietly after lunch without alcohol
H	In a car, while stopped for a few minutes in the traffic

The Epworth Score is the sum of the individual scores

Source: [9]

The Epworth score and other scoring systems that have been tried are subjective measures being reliant on the patient's assessment. An alternative, more objective method is to measure how long it takes for a subject to fall asleep when placed in optimal surroundings. The multiple sleep latency test (MSLT) is one such test where the time to fall asleep is measured at several times across the day [10]. The sleep state is defined by EEG and so the test is not simple to carry out. Furthermore, there is considerable overlap between the time taken for normal subjects to fall asleep and those with sleep deprivation, so the MSLT cannot easily discriminate between individuals but can indicate within-subject changes.

The converse is to determine the subject's resistance to falling asleep. Tests have been devised using boring tasks and estimating when a subject's attention lapses. Another test measures how long a subject can stay awake; this is called the maintenance of wakefulness test (MWT) [11] and records the EEG to define when sleep occurs. More recently the Oxford sleep resistance test (OSLER) was devised which is similar to the MWT but identifies lapses in repeated button pressing in response to visual stimuli as the measure of when sleepiness supervenes [12]. Thus, the OSLER avoids the technical complexity of the MWT. Whilst these objective measures are closer to what patients complain about, none of them have been shown to be superior to the subjective assessment by the Epworth score in the study of sleep related breathing disorders [13].

32.4 Respiratory physiology in sleep

32.4.1 Sleep levels

A full description of the various stages of sleep as defined by the electro-encephalogram (EEG) is beyond the scope of this text.

In the awake state the EEG is characterized by high frequency (>30 Hz) and low voltage activity. As the person progresses into sleep two types of slow waves become more prominent, delta waves and spindle waves. Delta waves are 0.5–4 Hz oscillations that are particularly prominent during deep sleep (stages 3 and 4). Spindle waves are 1–3 s duration epochs of 'waxing' and 'waning' 6–15 Hz oscillations. Figure 32.2 shows the various type of EEG wave. Sleep stages are outlined in Table 32.2 and can be divided broadly into light sleep (stages 1 and 2 on EEG staging),

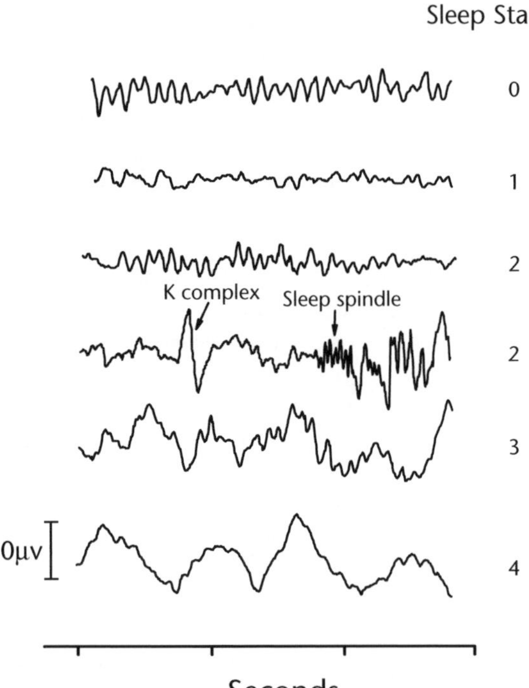

Fig. 32.2 Types of EEG wave seen during wakefulness and sleep.
Stage 0 wakefulness with continuous alpha activity (8–12 Hz)
Stage 1 sleep low amplitude record with some theta activity (3.5–7.5 Hz)
Stage 2 sleep with beta activity (12–14 Hz) with an example of a K complex and sleep spindles
Stage 3 sleep with some slow wave delta activity (0.5–2 Hz) and theta activity
Stage 4 deep sleep with predominantly slow wave delta activity.

Table 32.2 Sleep stages.

	EEG	Features
Wakefulness	high frequency (8–12 Hz) random activity	
REM sleep	EOG	Autonomic activity Limb movement
Stage 1	theta waves (3–7 Hz)	
Stage 2	spindles, K complexes	Absent movement
Stages 3 and 4	slow delta waves (0.5–2 Hz)	Absent movement

deep sleep which is slow wave sleep (stages 3 and 4) and rapid eye movement (REM) sleep which coincides with dreaming, the purpose of which is still debated. Adequate duration of deep slow wave sleep appears necessary for a subject to wake refreshed from sleep.

With the onset of deep sleep breathing becomes more regular and minute ventilation falls by about 10% with Pa,co_2 rising by up to 1 kPa (7.5 mm Hg). Heart rate and blood pressure also tend to fall. Arousal from deep sleep tends to be more difficult than from the other stages and may leave the subject feeling perplexed for a few moments. As one moves from light sleep to deep sleep there is a loss of resting tone in muscles that have tonic activity [14] and EMG activity falls.

During REM sleep there is further reduction in muscle tone associated with a lack of body and limb movement. A centre in the pons oversees this reduction in muscle tone [15]. Conversely, autonomic activity increases leading to marked fluctuations in breathing, heart rate, and blood pressure.

Wakefulness is an actively maintained state whereby the cortex is tonically excited from the reticular activating system (RAS) and this leads to a low amplitude EEG with high frequency random activity at between 8 and 12 Hz, called alpha activity. In slow wave sleep large, low frequency (0.5–2 Hz) delta waves are apparent.

Fundamental to the study of sleep disordered breathing is the definition of an arousal from sleep. When an event occurs that stresses the system an arousal response occurs with RAS activity raising the sleep level transiently. This is often associated with movement of the limbs and change in posture; this can be measured as a surrogate for arousal. The duration of the arousal may be very brief (Fig. 32.3) and methods of sleep state analysis that break the data into 30 s epochs and quote the dominant sleep stage for this duration may not report on significant but brief arousals. Arousal patterns on EEG and EMG suggesting a change to wakefulness that lasts for more than 1.5 s have been shown to relate to poor daytime performance [16]. Differences occurring in the various sleep stages are outlined in Table 32.3.

In humans the cough reflex is inhibited during sleep [17] and the effect of intrapulmonary receptors remain uncertain. However, higher centres continue to influence the respiratory centres in humans during sleep. In the transition between wakefulness and sleep both the frequency of breathing and tidal volume can vary [18]. During stable non-REM sleep ventilation usually becomes stable and very rhythmic. During REM sleep the

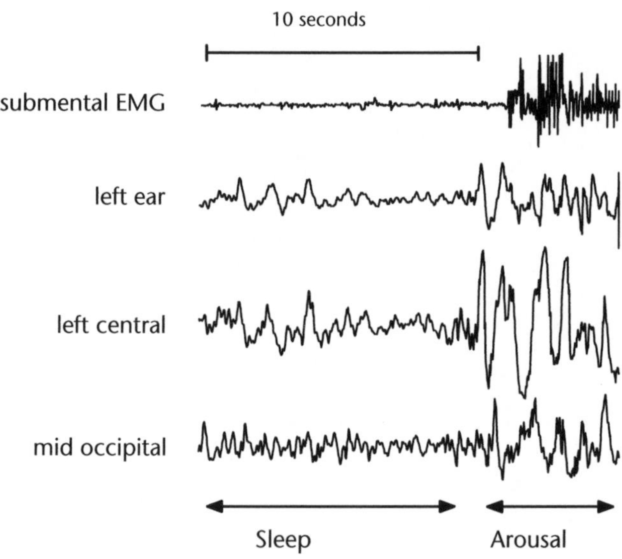

Fig. 32.3 Arousal response. recordings from the submental EMG and three EEG electrodes (left ear, left central and mid occipital). The record shows 10 s of sleep pattern followed by the first few seconds of an arousal response.

Table 32.3 Some features of different sleep states compared with being awake.

	Non-REM stage 2	Non-REM stages 3–4	REM
EEG voltage	–	↑	–
EEG frequency	–	↓	–
Arousal	↓↓	↓↓↓	↓
Muscle tone	↓	↓↓	nil
Tidal volume	↓	↓	↓↓
Rib cage contribution	↑	↑	↓↓
Respiratory frequency	–	–	↑
Hypercapnia/hypoxaemia	↑	↑	↑↑
Respiratory responsiveness	↓↓	↓↓	↓↓↓↓

ventilatory pattern becomes very irregular with small tidal breaths during the period of actual rapid eye movement [19]. Thus, in normal subjects periods of hypopnoea and apnoea are occurring as a natural phenomenon.

32.4.2 The CO_2 and O_2 responses

There are several reasons for the initial changes in ventilation occurring during deep sleep. Tidal volume falls with deeper non-REM sleep but the respiratory frequency remains unchanged or is slightly increased [20]. There is reduced sensitivity to $P\text{CO}_2$ at the respiratory centre [8] both in terms of slope and intercept of the relationship as shown in an idealised plot in Fig. 32.4. This is likely to be due to the reduction in the cortical influences of wakefulness on the respiratory centre rather than a more complex change. There is a similar reduction in O_2 sensitivity when asleep

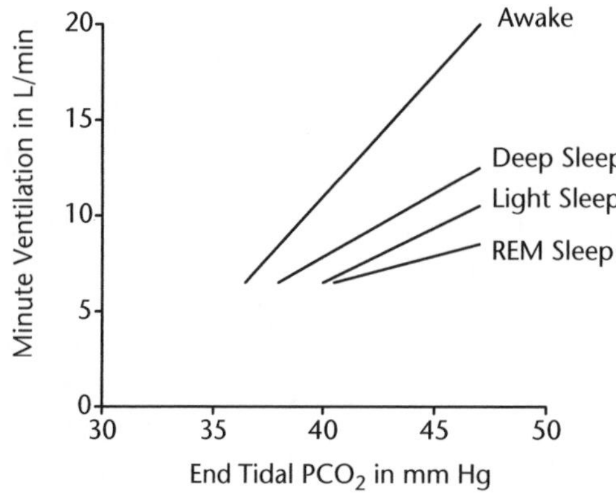

Fig. 32.4 Responses to hypercapnia during different sleep stages.

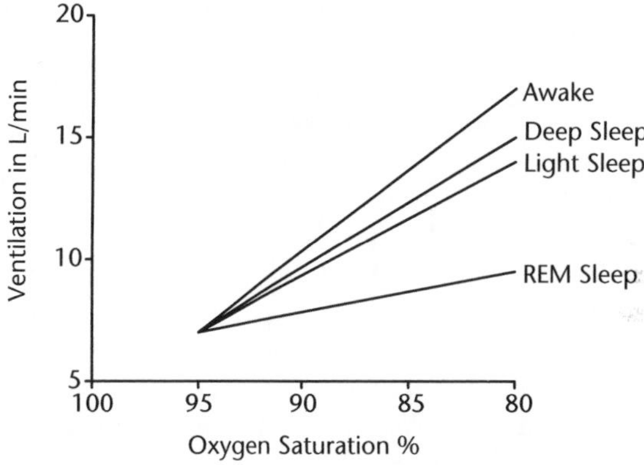

Fig. 32.5 Responses to hypoxia during different sleep stages.

[21] but this is only seen in terms of change in slope (Fig. 32.5). The slight rise in $P\text{CO}_2$ during sleep could be due to an increased production of CO_2, but evidence indicates that metabolic rate and CO_2 production are reduced during sleep [22]. When REM sleep commences the set point for the CO_2 threshold for control does not seem to change, as shown by experiments on subjects being artificially ventilated [23].

32.4.3 Upper airway

Breathing through the nares with the mouth closed is associated with a higher airway resistance than when breathing with the mouth open. If the anterior nares become blocked a subject may revert to mouth breathing, but this is not so comfortable because of drying of the upper airway when the humidification from the nares is lost.

With diaphragmatic descent negative pressures occur in the upper airway and hypopharynx. Atmospheric pressure on the neck and cheeks leads to a tendency for the upper airway to collapse. Cartilage in the trachea resists this force but in the hypopharynx it requires activity in the pharyngeal dilator muscles to prevent the pharyngeal tent from collapsing. Several muscle groups are involved. There are those that regulate the position of the hyoid bone (geniohyoid, sternohyoid), those that influence the position of the tongue (genioglossus) and those that influence the position of the soft palate (tensor palatini and levator palatini). The muscles are driven from the central respiratory pattern generating neurones located in the ventral medulla (Section 23.2) which primes genioglossus before the onset of diaphragm contraction and so prepares the upper airway prior to the onset of inspiration [24]. This inspiratory phasic activation of genioglossus [25] is quite different from the more tonic activation of muscles such as tensor palatini [26].

These muscles can be further activated by a rapid reflex response to a fall in intrapharyngeal airway pressure [27]. This reflex is locally derived as it can be largely abolished by topical local anaesthesia [28]. In the awake state the patency of the upper airway is thus adequately defended. With the onset of sleep there is at first a small drop in the inspiratory phasic activation of genioglossus which quickly recovers [29] and, as non-REM sleep supervenes this negative pressure reflex is substantially impaired [30]. The generalised reduction in muscle tone occurring in slow wave sleep dramatically affects those upper airway muscles which are under tonic activation, such as levator palatini. During stage 4 sleep the activation of these muscles may be only 25% of that during wakefulness [26], which increases the pharyngeal resistance of the upper airway. This can lead to collapse of the pharyngeal tent in normal subjects [31] with a resulting increased resistance that leads to a drop in minute ventilation that is not properly corrected. This contributes to the hypoventilation and rise in $P\text{CO}_2$ that occurs in normal sleep.

When awake the level and mode of ventilation rapidly adapts to increasing loads and resistance. When asleep this protective mechanism is diminished. If additional resistive loading is added to subjects whilst in non-REM sleep there is a rapid reduction in minute ventilation which is proportional to the load [32]. The reduction may be more than 50%, it may take several minutes to improve and full recovery is not assured.

32.4.4 Thorax

The normal recruitment of respiratory muscles is altered when asleep. The reduction in muscle tone leads to a reduction in the amount of abdominal movement occurring with diaphragm contraction. This is thought to be due to increased compliance of the thorax consequent upon the reduction in tone in the intercostal muscles. Reduced muscle tone can also be anticipated to lead to a small fall in FRC. This will have little consequence in normal subjects, but in those with abnormal configurations of the chest wall the changes in lung volume may become significant with consequences for arterial oxygenation.

32.5 Respiratory pathophysiology in sleep

Abnormalities in breathing whilst asleep fall into three major categories: those relating to airway closure, those relating to failure of central control, and mixed disorders with features of both.

A

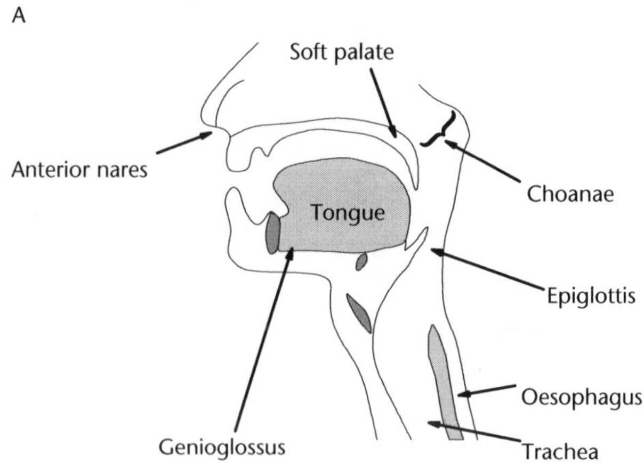

B

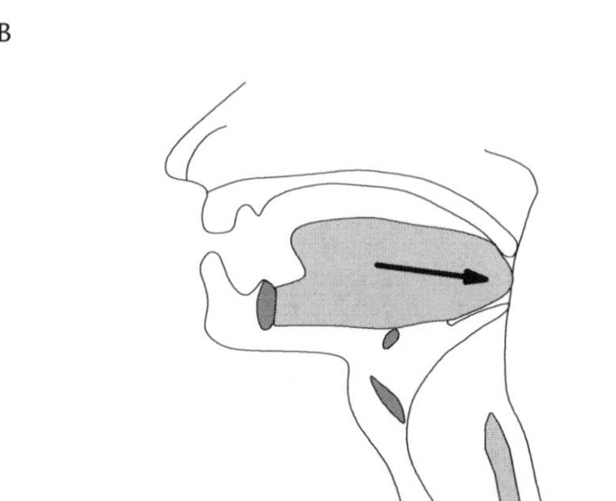

Fig. 32.6 A. Schematic diagram of the mouth and upper airway. B. Schematic diagram of the mouth and upper airway during airway collapse.

32.5.1 Upper airway control

The factors that influence the ability to maintain a patent upper airway are the anatomy and the tonic discharge to the pharyngeal dilator muscles.

Anatomy. The section of the upper airway between the choanae and epiglottis is susceptible to collapse (Figs 32.6a and b). Above and below there is cartilage or bone to defend the airway. The factors that make this area vulnerable are the position of the tongue and the compliance of the pharyngeal muscles. Subjects with a short jaw are particularly at risk of the airway closing as the usual activity within the genioglossus is insufficient to keep the tongue forward. In children enlarged tonsillar tissue will also reduce the airway lumen and make airway closure more likely [33].

Obesity is associated with obstructive sleep apnoea and deposits of fat around the pharyngeal area contribute to reducing the available volume in this critical part of the airway. Several different techniques, including acoustic reflection, CT scanning, and MRI scanning have shown that the pharyngeal volume is smaller in patients with obstructive sleep apnoea (OSA) [34, 35]. Not only is the volume of the upper airway smaller in subjects with OSA but the shape of the airway tends to be longer than it is wide [36] which makes it much more likely to collapse [37]. The lateral pharyngeal wall volume and the tongue volume are independently related to the risk for developing OSA [38].

Muscle activity. Subjects with OSA have a smaller upper airway than those without and this leads to them requiring a greater level of activation of the above muscles in wakefulness to overcome this limitation. This increased drive to the muscles includes both the reflex activity due to negative pressure in the airway [39] and the tonic non-phasic activity [40]. When asleep the usual reduction in muscle activity is even greater in patients with OSA [41] and this makes their airways very susceptible to collapse.

The normal neuronal control of these muscles is not completely understood. Accordingly, the factors that predispose some subjects to having a low activity are unknown. It is also unclear to what extent subjects develop collapse of the pharyngeal airway because of poor coordination between the recruitment of inspiratory muscles and the upper airway muscles. If the activation of inspiratory muscles is out of phase with that for the upper airway muscles then the pharyngeal airway would be rendered more susceptible to collapse just when the greatest negative airway pressure is being produced.

32.5.2 Central control

The medullary respiratory centres bring about rhythmical activation of the respiratory muscles to effect ventilation. There are various inputs to help control this system (see Chapter 23). These include (i) arterial chemoreceptors (ii) intrapulmonary stretch receptors (iii) metabolic influences, (iv) behavioural influences from higher centres. The behavioural influences act by different pathways from the autonomic and chemical control of the medullary centre and so different patterns of abnormality may emerge.

Central sleep apnoea syndrome (CSAS) may be broadly divided into that associated with hypercapnia and that with hypocapnia.

With CSAS associated with hypercapnia the problem is due to a reduced CO_2 responsiveness, or if the ventilatory pump fails due to muscle or chest wall abnormalities. Under these circumstances the subject tends to hypoventilate whilst awake and this becomes more profound when asleep. The loss of autonomic control of breathing is often most profound as soon as sleep starts when there is non-REM sleep. At this time the normal stable rhythmic ventilation is purely driven by autonomic control. Such a patient may have little difficulty whilst awake but develop profound hypoventilation once asleep. Vascular damage, infection, plaques of multiple sclerosis, tumour, or trauma at critical areas in the brain stem can lead to this development. Very rare degenerating conditions of the autonomic system (such as multi-system atrophy or

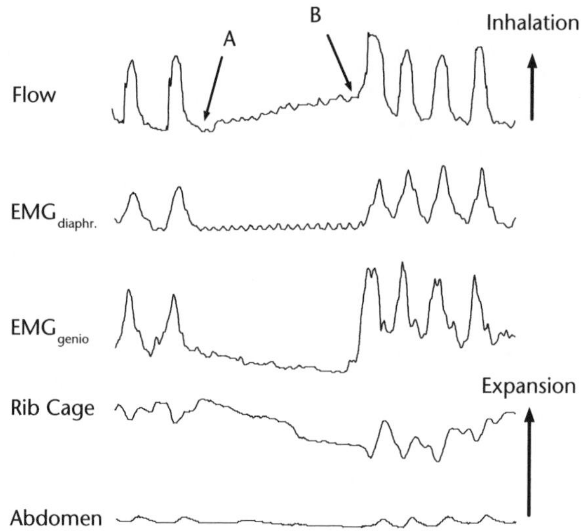

Fig. 32.7 Central apnoea. recordings of mouth flow, EMG from the diaphragm and genioglossus, and the rib cage and abdominal movement. At point A in expiration mouth flow ceases, together with a cessation in EMG activity and the cyclical rib cage and abdominal movement. The rib cage gradually deflates further and at point B inhalation occurs with resumption of EMG activity.

Shy–Drager syndrome) can also affect autonomic control. Fig. 32.7 shows a recording of a central apnoea.

CSAS associated with hypocapnia is seen in heart failure [42] and when residing at high altitude [43] (Section 34.2, page 474). The breathing pattern whilst asleep tends to be periodic with tidal volume being small, then increasing to a maximum before declining again to a period of total apnoea. The cycle then repeats itself and is called Cheyne–Stokes breathing. This situation may arise because of a delay in signal processing of the feedback loop for the control mechanism such that an increase in tidal volume is driven by the hypercapnia that arises from the apnoea; this then causes hypocapnia and a further apnoea occurs as there is a lag in the system. Another potential and more plausible cause is that the gain of the response to CO_2 is inappropriately high and an overshoot in response then occurs. Recent evidence indicates this loop gain is present in some patients with OSA and contributes to the problem by making the respiratory control system unstable [44]. The response of the respiratory controller to CO_2 is enhanced by circulating hormones such as adrenaline and noradrenaline [45] and is diminished by dopamine [46], benzodiazepines and opiate drugs.

The periodic breathing characteristically seen in subjects who move to high altitudes relates to increased gain on the hypercapnic response because the subject is hypoxic. On arrival at altitude the hypoxia leads to hyperventilation and hypocapnia. Whilst falling asleep the CO_2 threshold rises and the prevailing arterial $P\text{co}_2$ is so low that apnoea occurs. The ensuing hypoxia leads to an arousal response, and as the arterial CO_2 rises during the apnoea the increased gain in response to this rise leads to an exaggerated response and periodic breathing can follow. When

Cheyne–Stokes breathing is seen in left heart failure the resting arterial $P\text{CO}_2$ tends to be low. This is in part due to increased controller gain with respect to CO_2 [47], and possibly also due to increased ventilation consequent from activation of C fibre (J) receptors by pulmonary venous congestion stretching the tissues. The low arterial $P\text{CO}_2$ may fall below the apnoeic threshold and concomitant hypoxia may steepen the CO_2 response as above. Slow circulation time has been suggested as a cause of a lag in the feedback loop but evidence for this has not been found [48].

There are a number of reflexes in the upper airway that produce inhibition of the central respiratory drive when a subject is asleep. Both laryngeal [49] and pharyngeal [50] stimulation when asleep can inhibit ventilation. This may account for more complex abnormalities of combined obstructive and central apnoeas in some subjects [51].

32.6 References

1. Minutes from the Clinical Society of London. *Br Med J* 1889; **1**: 358.
2. Coccagna G, Mantovani M, Brignan F et al. Continuous recording of the pulmonary and systemic pressure during sleep in syndromes of hypersomnia and periodic breathing. *Bull Eur Physiopathol Respir* 1972; **8**: 1159–1172.
3. Guilleminault C, Tilkian A, Dement WC. The sleep apnoea syndromes. *Ann Rev Med* 1976; **27**: 465–484.
4. Sullivan CE, Issa FG, Berthon-Jones M, Eves L. Reversal of obstructive sleep apnoea by continuous positive airway pressure applied through the nares. *Lancet* 1981; **1**: 862–865.
5. Stradling JR. *Handbook of sleep-related breathing disorders.*. Oxford: Oxford University Press, 1993.
6. Martin RJ. Ed. *Cardiorespiratory disorders during sleep.*. 2nd ed. Futura Publishing: New York, 1990.
7. Shneerson JM. *Handbook of sleep medicine.* Oxford: Backwell Science, 2000.
8. Douglas NJ, White DP, Weil JV et al. Hypercapnic ventilatory response in sleeping adults. *Am Rev Respir Dis* 1982; **126**: 758–762.
9. Johns MW. A new method for measuring daytime sleepiness: the Epworth sleepiness scale. *Sleep* 1991; **14**: 540–545.
10. Carskadon MA, Dement WC, Mitler MM et al. Guidelines for the multiple sleep latency test (MSLT): a standard measure of sleepiness. *Sleep* 1986; **9**: 519–524.
11. Poceta JS, Timms RM, Jeong DU et al. Maintenance of wakefulness test in obstructive sleep apnoea syndrome. *Chest* 1992; **101**: 893–897.
12. Bennett LS, Stradling JR, Davies RJO. A behavioural test to assess daytime sleepiness in obstructive sleep apnoea. *J Sleep Res* 1997; **6**: 142–145.
13. Engelman HM, Douglas NJ. Sleepiness, cognitive function, and quality of life in obstructive sleep apnoea/hypopnoea syndrome. *Thorax* 2004; **59**: 618–622.
14. Jacobson A, Kales A, Lehmann D et al. Muscle tonus in human subjects during sleep and dreaming. *Exp Neurol* 1964; **10**: 418–424.
15. Jouvet M, Delforme F. Locus coeruleus et sommeil paradoxal. *C R Soc Biol* (Paris) 1965; **159**: 895–899.
16. Cheshire K, Engleman H, Deary I et al. Factors impairing daytime performance in patients with the sleep apnoea/hypopnoea syndrome. *Arch Int Med* 1992; **152**: 538–541.
17. Power JT, Stewart IC, Connaughton JJ et al. Nocturnal cough in patients with chronic bronchitis and emphysema. *Am Rev Respir Dis* 1984; **130**: 999–1001.
18. Block AJ, Boysen PG, Wynne JW et al. Sleep apnea, hypopnea, and oxygen desaturation in normal subjects. *N Engl J Med* 1979; **300**: 513–517.
19. Kline LR, Hendricks JC, Davies RO et al. Control of activity of the diaphragm in rapid eye-movement sleep. *J Appl Physiol* 1986; **61**: 1293–1300.
20. Douglas NJ, White DP, Pickett CK et al. Respiration during sleep in normal man. *Thorax* 1982; **37**: 840–844.
21. Douglas NJ, White DP, Weil JV et al. Hypoxic ventilatory response decreases during sleep in normal men. *Am Rev Respir Dis* 1982; **125**: 286–289.
22. Robin ED, Whaley RD, Crump CH et al. Alveolar gas tensions, pulmonary ventilation and blood pH during physiologic sleep in normal subjects. *J Clin Invest* 1958; **37**: 981–989.
23. Ingrassia TS, Nelson SB, Harris CD, Hubmayr RD. Influence of sleep state on CO_2 responsiveness. A study of the unloaded respiratory pump in humans. *Am Rev Respir Dis* 1991; **144**: 1125–1129.
24. Van Lunteren E. Muscles of the pharynx: structural and contractile properties. *Ear Nose Throat J* 1993; **72**: 27–29, 33.
25. Tangel DJ, Mezzanotte WS, Sandberg EJ, White DP. The influence of sleep on the activity of tonic postural versus inspiratory phasic muscles in normal men. *J Appl Physiol* 1992; **73**: 1053–1066.
26. Tangel DT, Mezzanotte WS, White DP. The influence of sleep on tensor palatini EMG and upper airway resistance in normal subjects. *J Appl Physiol* 1991; **70**: 2574–2581.
27. Horner RL, Innes JA, Murphy K, Guz A. Evidence for reflex upper airway dilator muscle activation by sudden negative airway pressure in man. *J Physiol* 1991; **436**: 15–29.
28. Horner RL, Innes JA, Holden HB, Guz A. Afferent pathway(s) for pharyngeal dilator reflex to negative pressure in man: a study using upper airway anaesthesia. *J Physiol* 1991; **436**: 31–44.
29. Worsnop C, Kay A, Pierce R et al. Activity of the respiratory pump and upper airway muscles during sleep onset. *J Appl Physiol* 1998; **85**: 908–920.
30. Wheatley J, Mezzanotte W, Tangel D et al. Influence of sleep on genioglossus muscle activation by negative pressure in normal man. *Am Rev Respir Dis* 1993; **148**: 597–605.
31. Wiegand L, Zwillich CW, White DP. Collapsibility of the human upper airway during normal sleep. *J Appl Physiol* 1989; **66**: 1800–1808.
32. Wiegand L, Zwillich CW, White DP. Sleep and the ventilatory response to resistive loading in normal man. *J Appl Physiol* 1988; **64**: 1186–1195.
33. Arens R, McDonough JM, Corbin AM et al. Upper airway size analysis by magnetic resonance imaging of children with obstructive sleep apnea syndrome. *Am J Respir Crit Care Med* 2003; **167**: 65–70.
34. Mortimore IL, Marshall I, Wraith PK et al. Neck and total body fat deposition in nonobese and obese patients with sleep apnoea compared with that in control subjects. *Am J Respir Crit Care Med* 1998; **157**: 280–283.
35. Schwab RJ, Gupta KB, Gefter WB et al. Upper airway and soft tissue anatomy in normal subjects and patients with sleep-disordered

breathing. Significance of the lateral pharyngeal walls. *Am J Respir Crit Care Med* 1995; **152**: 1673–1689.

36. Leiter C. Upper airway shape: is it important in the pathogenesis of obstructive sleep apnea? *Am J Respir Crit Care Med* 1996; **153**: 894–898.
37. Malhotra A, Huang Y, Fogel RB et al. The male predisposition to pharyngeal collapse: importance of airway length. *Am J Respir Crit Care Med* 2002; **166**: 1388–1395.
38. Schwab RJ, Pasirstein M, Pierson R et al. Identification of upper airway anatomic risk factors for obstructive sleep apnea with volumetric magnetic resonance imaging. *Am J Respir Crit Care Med* 2003; **168**: 522–530.
39. Mezzanotte WS, Tangel DJ, White DP. Waking genioglossal EMG in sleep apnea patients versus normal controls (a neuromuscular compensatory mechanism). *J Clin Invest* 1992; **89**: 1571–1579.
40. Fogel R, Malhoyta A, Pillar G et al. Genioglossal activation in patients with obstructive sleep apnea versus control subjects. Mechanism of muscle control. *Am J Respir Crit Care Med* 2001;**164**: 2025–2030.
41. Mezzanotte WS, Tangel DJ, White DP. Influence of sleep onset on upper airway muscle activity in apnea patients versus controls. *Am J Respir Crit Care Med* 1996; **153**: 1880–1887.
42. Köhnlein T, Welte T, Tan LB, Elliott MW. Central sleep apnoea syndrome in patients with chronic heart disease: a critical review of the current literature. *Thorax* 2002; **57**: 547–554.
43. West JB, Peters RMJ, Asknes G et al. Nocturnal periodic breathing at altitudes of 6,300 and 8,050 m. *J Appl Physiol* 1986; **61**: 280–287.
44. Younes M, Ostrowski M, Thompson W et al. Chemical control stability in patients with obstructive sleep apnea. *Am J Respir Crit Care Med* 2001; **163**: 1181–1190.
45. Weil JV, Byrne-Quinn E, Sodal IE et al. Augmentation of chemosensitivity during mild exercise in normal man. *J Appl Physiol* 1972; **33**: 813–819.
46. Van de Borne P, Oren R, Somers VK. Dopamine depresses minute ventilation in patients with heart failure. *Circulation* 1998; **98**: 126–131.
47. Javaheri S. A mechanism of central sleep apnea in patients with heart failure *N Eng J Med* 1999; **341**: 949–954.
48. Sin DD, Fitzgerald F, Parker JD et al. Risk factors for central and obstructive sleep apnea in 450 men and women with congestive heart failure. *Am J Respir Crit Care Med* 1999; **160**: 1101–1106.
49. Mathew OP, Sant'Amrogio FB. Laryngeal reflexes. In: Mathew OP, Sant' Ambrogio G, eds. *Respiratory function of the upper airway. Lung biology in health and disease.* New York: Marcel Dekker, 1988: 259–302.
50. Mathew OP, Farber JP. Effect of upper airway negative pressure on respiratory timing. *Respir Physiol* 1983; **54**: 259–268.
51. Issa FG, Sullivan CE. Reversal of central sleep apnea using nasal CPAP. *Chest* 1986; **90**: 165–171.

CHAPTER 33

Assessment and Treatment of Sleep Related Breathing Disorders

The assessment and treatment of sleep related breathing disorders is one of the recent success stories of respiratory medicine. This chapter provides an overview. The underlying physiology and methods are in Chapter 32.

33.1 Introduction

Clinically important sleep-related breathing disorders are common with an estimated prevalence of about 2% in middle-aged women, 4% in middle-aged men [1] and 3% in pre-school children [2]. The estimates of prevalence vary according to the definitions used and populations studied. Furthermore, moderate to severe sleep apnoea syndrome is largely undiagnosed in the general population [3, 4]. Accordingly, the impact on public health is large and the cost-benefit aspects of the management of Obstructive Sleep Apnoea (OSA) have been vigorously debated [5, 6].

33.2 Sleep studies

In a clinical setting there are a number of options for performing sleep studies. The British Thoracic Society and several international bodies have issued guidelines on the investigation and treatment of these conditions in adults [7–11] and in children [12, 13]. There is a balance to be made between adopting a perfect but technically and logistically demanding approach and being pragmatic. The former requires sleep studies with polysomnography, usually under laboratory conditions, and the latter uses limited data acquisition whilst the patient sleeps at home.

Recent work investigated use of a compromise algorithm using a two-step approach for screening commercial drivers [14]. An apnoea prediction questionnaire based on symptoms, age, gender and body mass index was used to stratify subjects into high, intermediate and low risk categories with respect to the sleep apnoea syndrome. Those with high scores were predicted to have OSA that was later confirmed by polysomnography. Those with intermediate scores had oximetry and any with a raised oximetry desaturation index (based on the number of desaturations $\geq$3% divided by test duration in hours) had polysomnography. The use of a screening questionnaire in all subjects, with oximetry provided in a subset, had a sensitivity and specificity of 91% for identifying drivers with severe apnoea defined as an AHI of $\geq$30 events per hour. The algorithm had a false-positive rate of 8.9%, a false-negative rate of 0.5% and a negative predictive value of 99%, so it could be useful for identifying those with a high likelihood of having severe OSA without the need for full polysomnography.

33.2.1 Polysomnography

Polysomnography involves the simultaneous recording of many diverse signals in order to obtain a full picture of all aspects of sleep and ventilation (Table 33.1). These studies are usually undertaken by specific packages that can automatically analyse, interpret and store the information obtained. The physical size of all the recording equipment dictates that they are kept in a

Table 33.1 Details of the signals recorded during a polysomnographic study for sleep apnoea.

Signal*	Transducer	Information
EEG, EOG, EMG	Surface electrodes	Sleep staging and arousal detection
Oral and nasal flow	Thermistor, thermocouple	Qualitative ventilation
Thoraco-abdominal movement	Respitrace™ inductance plethysmograph	Respiratory effort
Snoring	Microphone	Timing of upper airway obstruction
Arterial saturation	Pulse oximeter	Detection of desaturation
Posture	Video camera	Detection of arousal
Movement	Piezo electric actigraph	Sleep staging and arousal detection
ECG	Surface electrodes	Detection of responses to arousal and hypoxia

* EEG, electroencephalogram; EOG, electro-oculogram; EMG, electromyogram; ECG, electrocardiogram.

specially designed sleep laboratory and cannot be readily used for home studies. A sleep technician is required to set up all the equipment and connect it to the subject. The technician may also oversee the study throughout the night in case any faults arise or electrodes become detached. Necessarily these are expensive tests to organise and do not lend themselves for screening large numbers of subjects. However, they are essential for investigating complex abnormalities of breathing during sleep and for deciding how these should be managed.

33.2.2 Limited sleep studies

Pragmatists believe that with limited resources for the treatment of OSA most attention should be focussed on investigating those with the severest problems. Except for upper airway resistance syndrome the hallmark of the other three types of sleep related disordered breathing is nocturnal hypoxaemia. Thus, a screening test to determine if there is significant nocturnal hypoxaemia using pulse oximetry alone, or perhaps with simultaneous microphone recording for snoring, is all that may be required.

A study comparing this approach with polysomnography found the simple oximetry test had 100% specificity if there were at least 15 dips of 4% saturation per hour in bed [15]. However, the sensitivity in detecting true sleep apnoea syndrome was only 31%, so the predictive value of a negative test was only 63%. It was recommended that polysomnography was required for all negative oximetry screening tests where the index of suspicion from symptoms was high.

A study in the patient's home used a portable polysomnographic system to record nasal airflow, chest wall impedance, oximetry, heart rate, snoring, and posture [16]. A criterion of 10 apnoeic or hypopnoeic spells per hour had a specificity of about 85% and a sensitivity of about 60% for identifying patients with sleep apnoea/hypopnoea syndrome. This was considered cost effective for diagnosing sleep disordered breathing problems despite the extra cost in technician time that was required for the 56% of subjects who were unable to set up the equipment in their own home.

33.3 Sleep apnoea clinical syndromes

These have been classified into (i) obstructive, where airflow ceases due to airway occlusion, (ii) central, where respiratory drive ceases, (iii) mixed, where there are components of both, and (iv) a syndrome of disturbed sleep where increased respiratory resistance leads to arousal without cessation of ventilation.

33.3.1 Obstructive

The characteristic finding is of cessation of airflow with continued respiratory effort as evinced by thoraco-abdominal excursion leading to desaturation and an arousal response (see Figs 32.1 and 32.3, pages 456 and 459). Usually this is accompanied by snoring and is repeated in cycles. Frequent arousals lead to poor quality sleep and the subject then suffers with daytime somnolence. An apnoea/hypopnoea index (AHI) of more than 15/h was considered clinically significant and likely to be associated with debilitating symptoms [17]. More recently an AHI of greater than 5/h apnoeas has been accepted as abnormal [18]. Associated causative factors include obesity, abnormalities of the jaw such as micrognathia and retrognathia, macroglossia, and swellings in the pharyngeal space such as enlarged tonsils.

33.3.2 Central

In this instance there is cessation of ventilation due to reduced or absent evidence of respiratory effort as evinced by absent thoraco-abdominal movement and reduced EMG activity in respiratory muscles (see Fig. 32.7, page 461). The ensuing hypoxia causes an arousal response, which leads to the onset of ventilation again. Associated causative factors include neurological conditions affecting autonomic function and their regulation in

Table 33.2 Conditions that can affect the autonomic and central control of breathing.

Autonomic function	Brain stem	Drugs
Dysautonomia	Medullary infarction	Barbiturates
Diabetes mellitus	High cervical cord transection	Opiates
Multi-system atrophy	Poliomyelitis	
Shy–Drager syndrome	Motor neurone disease	
	Raised intracranial pressure	

the brainstem, and agents acting as cerebral depressants which include alcohol and many sedative drugs (Table 33.2).

33.3.3 Mixed

In some subjects there are features of both obstructive and central apnoeas. Some of this may relate to the inhibitory reflexes in the larynx and pharynx being activated by obstructive collapse of the pharyngeal tent. Treatment of the obstructive component can in some cases abolish the central apnoeas as well [19].

33.3.4 Upper airway resistance syndrome

This syndrome has been proposed to account for subjects with clinical symptoms of excessive daytime sleepiness with no evidence of airway obstruction or loss of central drive but an increased effort required to breathe [20]. The proposed mechanism is that in some subjects an increased airway resistance alone is sufficient to lead to an arousal response and so disturb sleep architecture. Characteristically, there are increasingly negative oesophageal pressure swings, indicating an increased respiratory effort against a resistance, which suddenly reverses at the time of arousal. However, not all these events have been found to be associated with arousal. Analysis of EEG spectra have shown an increase in delta activity in relation to the oesophageal pressure reversals [21] suggesting a central neural mechanism, short of full arousal, that is able to overcome the raised airway resistance and so protect sleep.

33.4 Treatment of sleep apnoea

There has been considerable debate about the cost-benefit relation for the treatment of sleep related breathing disorders [22]. The clinical view is that if patients have an AHI of greater than 15/h, are symptomatic and derive relief from treatment then this is clinically worthwhile [17]. Many of the treatments are in themselves unpleasant with adherence rates of about 40% [23], so they are only likely to be tolerated by those who obtain definite benefit.

All provocative factors should be addressed, particularly the management of obesity [24]. This is necessary since, arising from one study, a 10% weight gain over 4 years predicted an approximately 32% increase in AHI and a 10% weight loss predicted a 26% decrease in AHI [25]. The consumption of alcohol at night should be reduced [26, 27], and that of respiratory depressant drugs phased out progressively [28].

33.4.1 Obstructive

Continuous positive airways pressure (CPAP). The first description of CPAP was by Sullivan [29] who found it to be immediately effective in relieving symptoms of daytime sleepiness due to obstructive sleep apnoea. Since then randomised placebo [30] or sham [31] controlled studies have confirmed this benefit. These studies have shown considerable learning and placebo effects emphasising the need for properly designed studies to demonstrate any benefit from CPAP.

The original method was to insert a tube into the nose and seal it in place so a positive pressure could be applied to support the pharynx and prevent it from closing. Current methods use a mask to apply over the nose with the seal made to the face around the nose. Leakage from the mouth can be minimised by use of a chin strap.

Patients with obstructive sleep apnoea should have a sleep study performed on CPAP therapy to demonstrate that the obstructive episodes are prevented. Failure to prevent the obstruction may be due to insufficient inflation pressure. Not all patients can tolerate high inflation pressures and some CPAP machines slowly ramp up the inflation pressure so the final pressure is only reached when the subject is asleep.

Mandibular advancement devices. A small number of patients have correctable anatomical reasons for developing OSA. There are many studies indicating the importance of cross sectional area available in the pharynx to allow free breathing during the night. Whilst obesity and an enlarged neck circumference are the most common predisposing factors [32, 33] the other anatomical aspects to consider are shortening and posterior positioning of the mandible, a low and posteriorly positioned hyoid bone, and abnormalities of the soft palate [34]. Repetitive snoring vibrates the soft palate and can lead to it becoming swollen and reddened. Hence, the swelling may result from the OSA and then exacerbate it. If the jaw is underdeveloped with retrognathia, the chin is behind the frontal plane of the forehead and this makes OSA more likely.

A number of devices have been used to help bring forward the jaw and tongue. Simple mechanical devices are sometimes helpful in milder cases of OSA [35, 36]. A mandibular advancement device has been found to be effective and more acceptable to patients with mild OSA than nasal CPAP [37]. However, in another study the 3-year adherence with such a device was only 50%, whilst 40% of subjects experienced problematic symptoms [38]. Acromegaly is associated with OSA in which macroglossia may play a part. These patients tend to have prognathism, with the lower jaw overlapping the upper jaw, rather than retrognathism. Patients with acromegaly and OSA have increased vertical (dolichofacial) growth of the mandible relative to the anterior growth [39]. This indicates how complex the relationship is between the anatomy of the jaw and the tendency to develop OSA.

Surgery. Tracheostomy was the initial treatment for OSA [40]. Whilst being highly effective it has so many psychological and medical disadvantages that it is no longer recommended. If the cause is chronic gross tonsillar enlargement then corrective surgical treatment can be effective [41, 42].

Following the same logic of mandibular advancement devices (see above) a surgical extension of the jaw can be undertaken [43], but this is a complex procedure and on its own may not alleviate the symptoms.

Surgical removal of tissue around the tonsillar pillars, the uvula and soft palate was first tried in the 1950s to help cure problematic snoring. This procedure might increase the pharyngeal volume and alter the compliance of the structures operated on. Modifications of this operative technique, now referred to as uvulopalatopharyngoplasty (UPPP), have been tried enthusiastically in the USA for the management of OSA. The consensus now is that the response rate is only around 50% [44] and it is difficult to predict in advance which patient is likely to benefit. The procedure has a number of drawbacks including marked post-operative pain, nasal regurgitation, and voice alteration, so the indications for UPPP are limited.

Drug Treatment. Protriptyline reduces the duration of REM sleep and increases the duration of the deeper stages of non-REM sleep [45]. This response was also seen with fluoxetine [46] which, like protriptyline, can help reduce apnoeas but with a paradoxical tendency to increase the number of arousals. Another effect of this class of drug is to increase peak inspiratory genioglossus activity but without influencing the AHI [47]. Respiratory stimulants can be used, but they may lead to insomnia which defeats the purpose of the treatment, though aminophylline can alleviate Cheyne–Stokes ventilation found in heart failure [48]. Medroxyprogesterone (MPA) may be effective for daytime hypoventilation with hypercapnia and, in the context of sleep apnoea exacerbated by alcohol, it improves oxygenation without changing the number or length of events [49]. A review of drug treatments for sleep disordered breathing concluded that MPA was indicated for hypercapnic failure in obesity, thyroxine was helpful in those with myxoedema, acetazolamide was helpful for central apnoea and theophylline for Cheynes–Stokes respiration [50]. However, a subsequent Cochrane systematic review of evidence concluded there was little to justify drug therapy in obstructive sleep apnoea [51].

33.4.2 Central

Central apnoea may arise from a number of diseases affecting the central nervous system and these can require non-invasive ventilation to overcome the problem. Acetazolamide renders the patient acidaemic as a means for driving respiration and can help overcome central apnoea [52]. A simpler treatment for patients with eucapnic central apnoea (patients with cardiac disease and/or stroke) is to administer oxygen which has been associated with a reduction in AHI from a mean of 34/h to 5/h [53]. Central apnoea is common in patients with heart failure and the symptom can be improved by increasing the cardiac output. In one study this was achieved by over-drive pacing to raise overnight heart rate from a mean of 57/min to 72/min [54]. An alternative, beneficial treatment for these patients is to administer continuous positive airway pressure (CPAP) [55]; this can reduce the mitral regurgitation fraction, increase the left ventricular ejection fraction and reduce the circulation atrial natriuretic peptide, ANP [56].

33.5 Respiratory conditions affected by sleep

33.5.1 Asthma

The diurnal variation in bronchial tone in asthma is well recognised and covered elsewhere (Section 40.2.1).

33.5.2 COPD

An early study identified COPD patients who suffered precipitous drops in oxygen saturation during REM sleep [57]. However, subsequent studies indicated that daytime hypoxaemia can predict the level of nocturnal hypoxaemia [58, 59]. Thus, sleep studies may not contribute additional information as to which patients should receive long-term supplemental oxygen therapy.

COPD may co-exist with the obstructive sleep apnoea syndrome, so a history of snoring and excessive daytime somnolence are indications for performing a sleep study.

33.5.3 Neuromuscular and skeletal disorders

Conditions where the prevailing chest wall and lung compliance are very low (i.e. a rigid system) can result in the neuromuscular drive to ventilation being insufficient to produce adequate ventilation; this will lead to hypoventilatory failure. The first indication will appear at night when a sleep study may detect hypoxia and hypoventilation that is not evident in the day. Ultimately, such subjects develop daytime hypoventilation as well. The conditions where this may occur are given in Table 33.3. An annual sleep study is recommended to monitor these patients so that, if hypoventilation is detected, night time artificial ventilatory support can be provided [60]. By resting the respiratory muscles in this way the muscles may perform better during the day [61].

Table 33.3 Disorders where hypoventilatory failure at night can be the first clinical problem. This can be detected by a sleep study. The disorders are separated into whether they primarily affect chest wall compliance, lung compliance or muscle power.

Chest wall compliance	Lung compliance	Neuro-muscular disorders
Kyphoscoliosis	Pulmonary fibrosis	Myasthenia gravis
Thoracoplasty		Polymyositis
Fibrothorax		Guillain–Barre syndrome
		Muscular dystrophies
		Poliomyelitis
		Myopathies
		Acid maltase deficiency
		Spino-cerebellar degeneration
		Motor neurone disease

33.6 References

1. Young T, Palta M, Dempsey J et al. The occurrence of sleep-disordered breathing among middle-aged adults. *New Eng J Med* 1993; **328**: 1230–1235.
2. Gislason T, Benediktsdottir B. Snoring, apneic episodes, and nocturnal hypoxemia among children 6 months to 6 years old. An epidemiologic study of lower limit of prevalence. *Chest* 1995; **107**: 963–966.
3. Ohayon MM, Guilleminault C, Priest RG et al. Snoring and breathing pauses during sleep: telephone interview survey of a United Kingdom population sample. *BMJ* 1997; **314**: 860–863.
4. Young T, Evans L, Finn L, Palta M. Estimation of the clinically diagnosed proportion of sleep apnea syndrome in middle-aged men and women. *Sleep* 1997; **20**: 705–706.
5. Gibson GJ. Public health aspects of obstructive sleep apnoea. *Thorax* 1998; **53**: 408–409.
6. Rodenstein DO. Sleep apnoea syndrome: the health economics point of view. *Monaldi Arch Chest Dis* 2000; **55**: 404–410.
7. The American Thoracic Society. Indications and standards for cardiopulmonary sleep studies. *Am Rev Respir Dis* 1989; **139**: 559–568.
8. Douglas NJ, Calverley PMA, Catterall JR et al. Facilities for the diagnosis and treatment of abnormal breathing during sleep including nocturnal ventilation. *BTS News* 1990; **5**: 7–10.
9. Executive summary on the systematic review and practice parameters for portable monitoring in the investigation of suspected sleep apnea in adults. ATS Statement. *Am J Respir Crit Care Med* 2004; **169**: 1160–1163.
10. Scottish Intercollegiate Guidelines Network. *Management of obstructive sleep apnoea/hypopnoea syndrome in adults.* Guideline 73, 2003. Edinburgh: Royal College of Physicians. http://www.sign.ac.uk
11. American Thoracic Society. Indications and standards for use of nasal continuous positive airway pressure (CPAP) in sleep apnea syndromes. *Am J Respir Crit Care Med* 1994; **150**: 1738–1745.
12. American Thoracic Society. Standards and indications for cardiopulmonary sleep studies in children. *Am J Respir Crit Care Med* 1996; 153: 866–878.
13. American Thoracic Society. Cardiopulmonary sleep studies in children. Establishment of normative data and polysomnographic predictors of morbidity. *Am J Respir Crit Care Med* 1999; **160**: 1381–1387.
14. Gurubhagavatula I, Maislin G, Nkwuo JE, Pack AI. Occupational screening for obstructive sleep apnea in commercial drivers. *Am J Respir Crit Care Med* 2004; **170**: 371–376.
15. Ryan PJ, Hilton MF, Boldy DAR et al. Validation of British Thoracic Society guidelines for the diagnosis of the sleep apnoea/hypopnoea syndrome: can polysomnography be avoided? *Thorax* 1995; **50**: 972–975.
16. Parra O, Garci-Esclasans N, Montserrat JM et al. Should patients with sleep apnoea/hypopnoea syndrome be diagnosed and managed on the basis of home sleep studies? *Eur Respir J* 1997; **10**: 1720–1724.
17. Douglas NJ. Systematic review of the efficacy of nasal CPAP. *Thorax* 1998; **53**: 414–415.
18. Stradling JR, Davies RJO. Sleep 1: Obstructive sleep apnoea/hypopnoea syndrome: definitions, epidemiology, and natural history. *Thorax* 2004; **59**: 73–78.
19. Issa FG, Sullivan CE. Reversal of central sleep apnea using nasal CPAP. *Chest* 1986; **90**: 165–171.
20. Guilleminault C, Stoohs R, Clerk M et al. A cause of excessive daytime sleepiness: the upper airway resistance syndrome. *Chest* 1993; **104**: 781–787.
21. Black JE, Guilleminault C, Colrain IM, Carrillo O. Upper airway resistance syndrome. Central electroencephalographic power and changes in breathing effort. *Am J Respir Crit Care Med* 2000; **162**: 406–411.
22. Wright J, Johns R, Watt I et al. Health effects of obstructive sleep apnoea and effectiveness of continuous positive airways pressure: a systematic review of the research evidence. *BMJ* 1997; **314**: 851–860.
23. Loube DI. Technologic advances in the treatment of obstructive sleep apnea syndrome. *Chest* 1999; **116**: 1426–1433.
24. Suratt PM, McTier RF, Findley LJ et al. Changes in breathing and the pharynx after weight loss in obstructive sleep apnea. *Chest* 1987; **92**: 631–637.
25. Peppard PE, Young T, Palta M et al. Longitudinal study of moderate weight change and sleep-disordered breathing. *JAMA* 2000; **284**: 3015–3021.
26. Taasan VC, Block AJ, Boysen PG, et al. Alcohol increases sleep apnea and oxygen desaturation in asymptomatic men. *Am J Med* 1981; **71**: 240–245.
27. Remmers JE. Obstructive sleep apnea: a common disorder exacerbated by alcohol. *Am Rev Respir Dis* 1984; **130**: 153–155.
28. Dolly FR, Block AJ. Effect of flurazepam on sleep-disordered breathing and nocturnal oxygen desaturation in asymptomatic subjects. *Am J Med* 1982; **73**: 239–243.
29. Sullivan CE, Issa FG, Berthon-Jones M, Eves L. Reversal of obstructive sleep apnoea by continuous positive airway pressure applied through the nares. *Lancet* 1981; **1**: 862–865.

30. Engleman HM, Martin SE, Kingshott RN et al. Randomised, placebo-controlled trial of daytime function after continuous positive airway pressure (CPAP) therapy for the sleep apnoea/hypopnoea syndrome. *Thorax* 1998; **53**: 341–345.
31. Montserrat JM, Ferrer M, Hernandez L et al. Effectiveness of CPAP treatment in daytime function in sleep apnea syndrome: a randomized controlled study with an optimized placebo. *Am J Respir Crit Care Med* 2001; **164**: 608–613.
32. Davies RJ, Stradling JR. The relationship between neck circumference, radiographic pharyngeal anatomy, and the obstructive sleep apnoea syndrome. *Eur Respir J* 1990; **3**: 509–514.
33. Brander PE, Mortimore IL, Douglas NJ. Effect of obesity and erect/supine posture on lateral cephalometry: relationship to sleep-disordered breathing. *Eur Respir J* 1999; **13**: 398–402.
34. Lowe AA, Gionhaku N, Takeuchi K, Fleetham JA. Three dimensional CT reconstructions of tongue and airway in adult subjects with obstructive sleep apnea. *Am J Orthod* 1986; **90**: 364–374.
35. Lowe A, Fleetham J, Ryan F, Mathews B. Effects of a mandibular repositioning appliance used in the treatment of obstructive sleep apnea on tongue muscle activity. *Prog Clin Biol Res* 1990; **345**: 395–404.
36. Ng AT, Gostopoulos H, Quan J, Cistulli PA. Effect of oral appliance therapy on upper airway collapsibility in obstructive sleep apnea. *Am J Respir Crit Care Med* 2003; **168**: 238–241.
37. Bennett LS, Davies RJ, Stradling JR. Oral appliances for the management of snoring and obstructive sleep apnoea. *Thorax* 1998; **53**(Suppl 2): S58–S64.
38. Clark GT, Sohn JW, Hong CN. Treating obstructive sleep apnoea and snoring: assessment of an anterior mandibular positioning device. *J Am Dent Assoc* 2000; **131**: 765–771.
39. Hochban W, Ehlenz K, Conradt R, Brandenburg U. Obstructive sleep apnoea in acromegaly: the role of craniofacial changes. *Eur Respir J* 1999; **14**: 196–202.
40. Guilleminault C, Simmons FB, Motta J et al. Obstructive sleep apnea syndrome and tracheostomy. *Arch Int Med* 1981; **141**: 985–988.
41. Guilleminault C, Eldridge FL, Simmons FB et al. Sleep apnea in eight children. *Pediatrics* 1976; **58**: 23–239.
42. Potsic WP, Pasquariello PS, Baranak CC et al. Relief of upper airway obstruction by adenotonsillectomy. *Otolaryngol Head Neck Surg* 1986; **94**: 476–480.
43. Riley RW, Powell NB, Guilleminault C et al. Maxillary, mandibular, and hyoid advancement: an alternative to tracheostomy in obstructive sleep apnea syndrome. *Otolaryngol Head Neck Surg* 1986; **94**: 1591–1594.
44. Conway W, Fujita S, Zorick F et al. Uvulopalatopharyngoplasty. One year follow up. *Chest* 1985; **88**: 385–387.
45. Sharpley AL, Cowen PJ. Effect of pharmacologic treatments on the sleep of depressed patients. *Biol Psychiatry* 1995; **37**: 85–98.
46. Hanzel DA, Proia NG, Hudgel DW. Response of obstructive sleep apnea to fluoxetine and protriptyline. *Chest.* 1991; **100**: 416–421.
47. Berry RB, Yamaura EM, Gill K, Reist C. Acute effects of paroxetine on genioglossus activity in obstructive sleep apnea. *Sleep* 1999; **15**: 1087–1092.
48. Javaheri S, Parker TJ, Wexler L et al. Effect of theophylline on sleep-disordered breathing in heart failure. *New Eng J Med* 1996; **335**: 562–567.
49. Collop NA. Medroxyprogesterone acetate and ethanol-induces exacerbation of obstructive sleep apnea. *Chest* 1994; **106**: 792–799.
50. Hudgel DW, Thanakitcharu S. Pharmacological treatment of sleep-disordered breathing. *Am J Respir Crit Care Med* 1998; **158**: 691–699.
51. Smith I, Lasserson T, Wright J. Drug treatments for obstructive sleep apnoea. *Cochrane Database Syst Rev* 2002; **2**: CD003002.
52. DeBacker WA, Verbraecken J, Willemen M et al. Central apnea index decreases after prolonged treatment with acetazolamide. *Am J Respir Crit Care Med* 1995; **151**: 87–91.
53. Franklin KA, Eriksson P, Sahlin C, Lundgren R. Reversal of central sleep apnea with oxygen. *Chest* 1997; **111**: 163–169.
54. Garrigne S, Bordier P, Jais P et al. Benefit of atrial pacing in sleep apnea syndrome. *New Eng J Med* 2002; **346**: 404–412.
55. Sin DD, Logan AG, Fitzgerald FS, et al. Effects of continuous airway pressure on cardiovascular outcomes in heart failure patients with and without Cheynes-Stokes respiration. *Circulation* 2000; **102**: 61–66.
56. Tkacova R, Liu PP, Naughton MT, Bradley TD. Effect of continuous positive airways pressure on mitral regurgitation fraction and atrial natriuretic peptide in patients with heart failure. *J Am Coll Cardiol* 1997; **30**: 739–745.
57. Douglas NJ, Calverley PMA, Leggett RJE et al. Transient hypoxaemia during sleep in chronic bronchitis and emphysema. *Lancet* 1979; **1**: 1–4.
58. Connaughton JJ, Catterall RA, Elton RA et al. Do sleep studies contribute to the management of patients with severe chronic obstructive pulmonary disease? *Am Rev Respir Dis* 1988; **138**: 341–344.
59. Little SA, Elkholy MM, Chalmers GW et al. Predictors of nocturnal oxygen saturation in patients with COPD. *Resp Med* 1999; **93**: 202–207.
60. Carroll N, Branthwaite MA. Control of nocturnal hypoventilation by nasal intermittent positive pressure ventilation. *Thorax* 1988; **43**: 349–353.
61. Kerby GR, Mayer LS, Pingleton SK. Nocturnal positive pressure ventilation via a nasal mask. *Am Rev Respir Dis* 1987; **135**: 738–740.

Further reading

American Thoracic Society/American Sleep Disorders Association. Statement on health outcomes research in sleep apnea. *Am J Respir Crit Care Med* 1998; **157**: 335–341.

Martin RJ. Ed. *Cardiorespiratory disorders during sleep.* 2nd ed. New York: Futura Publishing, 1990.

Shneerson JM. *Handbook of sleep medicine.*. Oxford: Blackwell Science, 2000.

Stradling JR. *Handbook of sleep-related breathing disorders.* Oxford: Oxford University Press, 1993.

PART 6

Potentially Adverse Environments

CHAPTER 34

Hypobaria: High Altitude and Aviation Physiology and Medicine

Hypobaria has represented a long-standing challenge to physiologists, physicians, mountaineers and balloonists, also more recently to aviators and travellers in space. This chapter links some basic and applied aspects.

34.1 Introduction

The first studies into the effects of low barometric pressures in man were made from hot air balloons (Section 1.4.4). The measurements established that during ascent the barometric pressure diminishes relative to that at sea level. The gaseous composition of the air is unchanged. The low pressure (*hypobaria*) reduces the partial pressure of oxygen; this constitutes *hypoxia* of hypobaric origin, hence hypobaric hypoxia. The effects on people vary depending on whether the exposure is abrupt, as can occur in aviation or a decompression chamber, is experienced gradually through making an ascent or is permanent in the case of a resident at altitude from birth.

The immediate consequences of exposure to a reduced atmospheric pressure (hypobaria) arise from the lower density and viscosity of the air; some of the changes are later ameliorated by the process of acclimatisation. In addition, the ambient temperature is usually less than at sea level; this raises the metabolic rate and there may be difficulties arising from exposure to cold. Where the exposure is on land the terrain is often rugged, so the level of physical activity and hence the physical fitness are increased. These features increase the requirement for dietary calories and for water to replace that lost by evaporation from the lungs.

Children growing up at altitude and adults who were reared there have additional features that are due to chronic hypoxaemia affecting most aspects of lung function. The effects are summarised in Table 34.1 where they are contrasted with those of hyperbaria. Some of the effects are direct ones; others are indirect due to the inclement environment influencing fertility and survival after conception. Ascent to very high altitudes also carries a short-term risk of mountain sickness that may be subclinical,

Table 34.1 Some effects of alteration in barometric pressure.

	Reduced pressure	Increased pressure
Lungs*		
Total lung capacity	↑†	↑
Ventilatory capacity	↑	↓‡
Transfer factor	↑†	↓§
Respiratory control		
Sensitivity for CO_2	↑	↓
Sensitivity to hypoxia	↓†	–
Exercise ventilation	↑	↓
Cardiac function	↓ (↑†)	–
Blood		
volume	↓	–
[haemoglobin]	↑	–
[2, 3-diphosphoglycerate]	↑	–
arterial O_2 tension	↓‡	(↑)
Muscle oxidative capacity	↑	-
Function of nervous system	↓	↓

* Sections 34.2 and 35.3.1
† effect long term
‡ principal effect (for details see text)
§ after deep saturation dives to >300 m.

acute or chronic. The risk is enhanced after a spell at lower altitude.

When the exposure to low pressure occurs rapidly the gas present in the lungs, middle ear and nasal sinuses may expand faster than it can escape via the trachea and other orifices. The pressure within the cavity then rises relative to the surroundings and can cause *barotrauma.* Failure to equalise pressures can extend to gases dissolved in body fluids, particularly nitrogen. Bubbles of nitrogen form in any of several tissues of the body and can cause *decompression sickness.*

The physiological responses to hypobaria and their implications for life at high altitude and for aviation have excited generations of physiologists [1–3]; classical studies are reviewed in Chapter 1. Present views on the respiratory effects of hypobaria and the implications for persons who are exposed are summarised in this chapter. More detailed reviews into the respective features of high altitude and aviation are available elsewhere e.g. [4, 5]. Imposed changes in gravitational force (G) also affect the lungs; some of the consequences for respiration and gas exchange are considered in Sections 17.1.3 and 18.1.

O_2 and CO_2 partial pressures at altitude. In atmospheric air the partial pressure of oxygen is determined by the barometric pressure. In the lungs the partial pressure of oxygen is also influenced by the presence of carbon dioxide and water vapour. The water vapour pressure is a function of body temperature and is effectively constant at about 6.3 kPa (47 torr). The partial pressure of carbon dioxide is not constant but decreases during hypoxaemia as a result of the increased chemoreceptor drive raising the level of ventilation. A further reduction in $P\text{CO}_2$ occurs as a result of acclimatisation. The average composition of alveolar gas in relation to barometric pressure and altitude in unacclimatised subjects is shown in Fig. 34.1.

34.2 Physiological effects of hypobaria

Maximal ventilation and wind resistance. Hypobaria lowers the density and kinematic viscosity of the respired gas. Both changes reduce the Reynolds number for air flowing through tubes, including those in the lungs and hence the extent to which the flow of air is turbulent (Section 14.3.4). Similar changes occur in instruments for measuring flow [7, 8]. In the lungs the airway resistance is reduced and the maximal voluntary ventilation (MVV) is increased (Fig. 34.2). The increase enables a person to ventilate the lungs with a greater volume of ambient air at altitude than is possible at sea level. During exercise under hypobaric conditions the situation is better than that since the maximal exercise ventilation ($\dot{V}$ Emax,ex) more nearly approaches the MVV than is usually the case at sea level, i.e. the ratio $\dot{V}$ Emax,ex/MVV rises during hypobaria [10]. The change is due to the hypobaria increasing the hypoxic drive to breathing. The increased ventilation leads to work hypertrophy of the respiratory muscles and affects mountaineers on expeditions to high altitude. The effect persists for a period of weeks after the subject has returned to sea level (Pugh LGCE, personal communication).

The changes in ventilation augment the maximal volume of air that can be inhaled per minute, but the energy cost of ventilation rises with minute volume and can exceed the quantity of extra oxygen that is delivered [11]. Exercise is then 'ventilation limited' and the capacity for aerobic exercise is reduced [12]. Performance at some athletic and cycling sprint events may nonetheless be increased at altitudes of up to about 3000 m (10,000 ft), since the reduced gas density lowers the resistance offered by air to forward movement of the body [13, 14].

Respiratory control and acclimatisation. Hypobaria lowers the partial pressure of oxygen in inspired air and results in hypoxaemia. This stimulates ventilation at rest and all levels of exercise. The hyperventilation initiates some of the changes that constitute acclimatisation; it also has consequences for maximal exercise ventilation that are described above.

The immediate effect of hypoxaemia is to augment the peripheral drive to respiration from the carotid bodies. Subsequently, this effect is enhanced by acclimatisation which increases the responsiveness of the glomus cells [15]. The change may be a consequence of inhibition of a local effect of dopamine, but, if so, the mechanism is unclear [16]. It is independent of the cerebral effect of hypoxia, which, normally, is to depress ventilation [17]. Hypoxaemia also lowers cerebral vasomotor tone and increases the local blood flow. As a result the oxygen tension in some parts of the brain is increased. The changes can modify central chemoreceptor drive and the responsiveness of the respiratory motor centres.

The respiratory response to hypoxaemia persists undiminished for many years but eventually becomes 'blunted' in some subjects. The change represents a displacement of the response, which still occurs at lower oxygen tensions [18]. It is associated with a somewhat increased ventilation during normoxia and a paradoxical response to breathing oxygen which then increases ventilation instead of depressing it. Studies in cats chronically exposed to hypoxia suggest that the changes are initiated by stimuli from supra-pontine centres in the brain [19]. The carotid chemoreceptors may also be involved since chronic hypoxia leads to hypertrophy of glomus tissue and to accumulation of dopamine; this might be expected to reduce chemoreceptor activity. However, 'blunting' appears not to be due to dopamine, since the response of the chemoreceptors to stimulation with doxapram is not reduced by lifetime residence at high altitude [20]. Thus, the physiological mechanism remains in doubt. The blunting can be accompanied by a reduced ventilatory response to carbon dioxide (see 'Blunting of the hypoxic response' below).

The onset of hyperventilation, driven by hypoxia, increases excretion of carbon dioxide from the lungs and blood and hence raises plasma pH; this partly inhibits the chemoreceptor drive to respiration (Section 23.5.2). Subsequently, the respiratory alkalosis is corrected by action of the kidneys. The reabsorption of sodium from the renal tubules is reduced, whilst the reabsorption

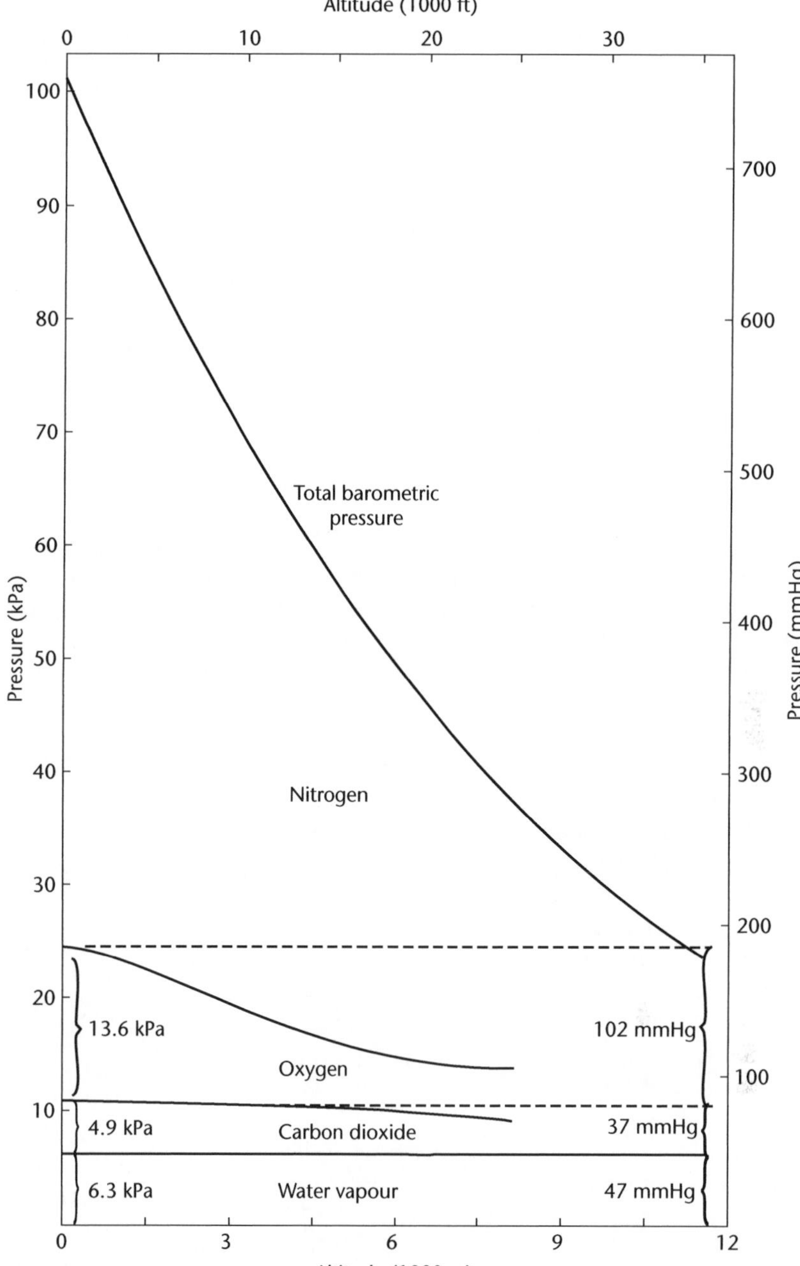

Fig. 34.1 Diagram showing the composition of alveolar gas in unacclimatised subjects under conditions of reduced barometric pressure. The upper line indicates the barometric pressure; this falls exponentially with altitude, the pressure halving every 5.5 km (18,000 ft). The distances between the other lines represent the approximate partial pressures of the alveolar gases. Conditions at sea level are represented by the horizontal lines; the line for oxygen intercepts the curve for barometric pressure at about 10,300 m (34,000 ft). The alveolar oxygen tension of a subject who is breathing oxygen at this altitude is equal to that which obtains while breathing air at sea level. Source: [6].

of $[Cl^-]$ is increased (Sections 22.3.3 and 22.3.4); the urine becomes more alkaline in consequence. The plasma $[H^+]$ then rises gradually and attains the normal sea level value in about a month. At this stage the hypoxic drive to breathing (which is enhanced by the low ambient oxygen partial pressure) is no longer restrained by incipient hypocapnia. Instead, it contributes to a progressive rise in ventilation which is the principal feature of acclimatisation. The additional ventilation raises the alveolar oxygen tension compared with the unacclimatised state. The correction of the respiratory alkalosis also restores the ventilatory response to carbon dioxide (Fig. 23.7, page 295).

Factors that contribute to the processes of acclimatisation operate at the levels of the peripheral and central chemoreceptors, the respiratory reticular formation and higher centres in the brain. The individual effects can be stimulatory or inhibitory and the outcome depends on how they summate.

The effect of hypocapnia is mainly to stimulate central chemoreceptors, but this action is modulated by the acid–base changes in cerebrospinal fluid (CSF) being out of phase with those in blood [21]. The differences are due to the choroid plexuses actively modifying the composition of CSF and preventing ingress of lactic acid. In addition, the local cerebral blood

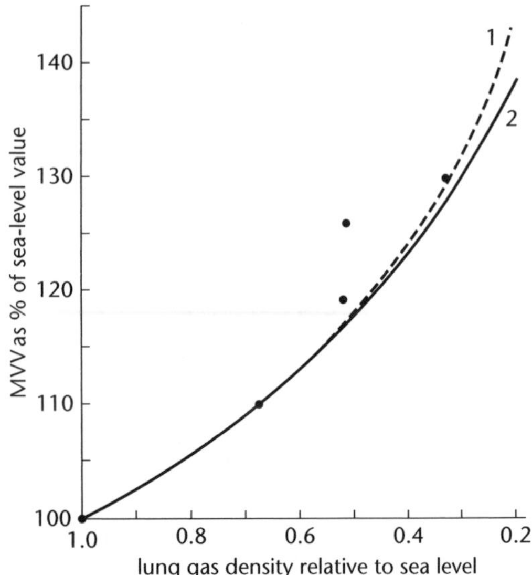

Fig. 34.2 Maximal voluntary ventilation under conditions of reduced barometric pressure; mean values for16 healthy young men. Curves 1 and 2 are the theoretical relationships based on gas density, with and without allowance for gas viscosity. The curve that allows for viscosity describes the data better [9].

flow can be reduced by the hypocapnia increasing cerebral vasomotor tone. Some of these actions are opposed by an increase in non-aerobic glycolysis leading to lactacidaemia (Section 28.9).

The process of acclimatisation varies in its completeness between individuals depending on previous exposures, the age when these took place and the genetic constitution. The consequences are apparent within high altitude communities where relatively few persons have a high susceptibility to hypoxic pulmonary vasoconstriction compared with populations at sea level (Section 17.2.2). In addition, responses to hypoxia are affected by environmental factors (see below, also Section 34.5).

Alveolar gas exchange. The mechanisms whereby during normoxia the blood leaves the alveolar capillaries almost fully saturated with oxygen are described in Section 21.3.2. The most important aspect is that gas exchange is completed on the flat top part of the oxyhaemoglobin dissociation curve (Fig. 21.1, page 260). By contrast, during hypoxia, the middle steeper part of the curve is used. This disadvantage is mitigated by a pronounced shift to the left of the oxygen dissociation curve through the combined effects of respiratory alkalosis, lactacidaemia, increased production of 2,3-diphosphoglycerate and, in some circumstances, a reduction in lung temperature (Fig. 34.3).

However, the displacement only goes a small way to compensate for the very material reduction in inspired oxygen tension that occurs at high altitude. Transfer of gas is further disadvantaged by an increase in cardiac output that is a consequence of hypoxia. The increased flow shortens the time spent by individual red cells in the alveolar capillaries during which exchange of gases can take place. These features result in blood leaving the alveolar capillaries without achieving gaseous equilibrium with the alveolar gas (Fig. 34.4). At an altitude of 3000 m the alveolar to end capillary gradient is small at rest, but increases during exercise when it can exceed 1.3 kPa (10 mm Hg). Larger values occur at higher altitudes. Hence, the oxygenation of arterial blood is diffusion limited, especially at very high altitudes [24, 25]. Uneven distribution of ventilation with respect to perfusion may also occur, but its contribution to hypoxaemia is small except when there is alveolar interstitial oedema [26].

At altitude, in healthy persons the changes combine to maximise the transfer of oxygen from atmospheric air to arterial blood and also in the tissues from capillary blood to mitochondria in skeletal muscle fibres [24, 25]. However, the levels of oxygenation that are achieved are not the same in everybody because of inherited differences in components of the oxygen transport chain. High altitude populations appear to be well endowed in this respect whilst persons at the other end of the distribution are at increased risk of acute mountain sickness (Section 34.5). In addition, in circumstances when gas exchange is already subject to another constraint, for example uneven lung function or defective gas transfer, the normal adjustments to altitude are often insufficient and material hypoxaemia can develop.

Circulatory system. Acute exposure to hypoxia stimulates aortic chemoreceptors to cause an almost immediate increase in cardiac frequency; the tachycardia can be experienced as palpitations. These are often severe in persons who take exercise soon after a rapid ascent to high altitude by train or car and can cause acute distress. Concurrently, there are increases in vasomotor tone [27] and in cardiac output relative to uptake of oxygen. The changes have the effect of increasing the delivery of oxygen to tissues. Less oxygen is then extracted per unit volume of circulating blood, so the tissue and mixed venous oxygen tensions are not as low as would otherwise be the case.

If the exposed person discontinues or slows down their ascent the circulatory changes are normally reversed as part of the process of acclimatisation. The relationship of cardiac output to oxygen uptake then reverts to that at sea level [28]. However, the relative contributions to the output of cardiac frequency and stroke volume remain abnormal, with the frequency increased and the stroke volume reduced. The mechanism is unclear.

In some circumstances, including at very high altitude, the stroke volume may be further reduced as a consequence of fluid depletion. Hypoxic depression of the myocardium appears not to be a contributory factor.

Haemopoietic system. A long-term effect of hypoxaemia is to increase the production by the renal cortices of the hormone erythropoietin [29]. This stimulates the bone marrow to increase the production of erythrocytes. The response is heralded within a few hours by a rise in turnover of iron and, subsequently, by an increase in blood reticulocytes. There is also a reduction in plasma volume. As a result of these changes the red cell count and

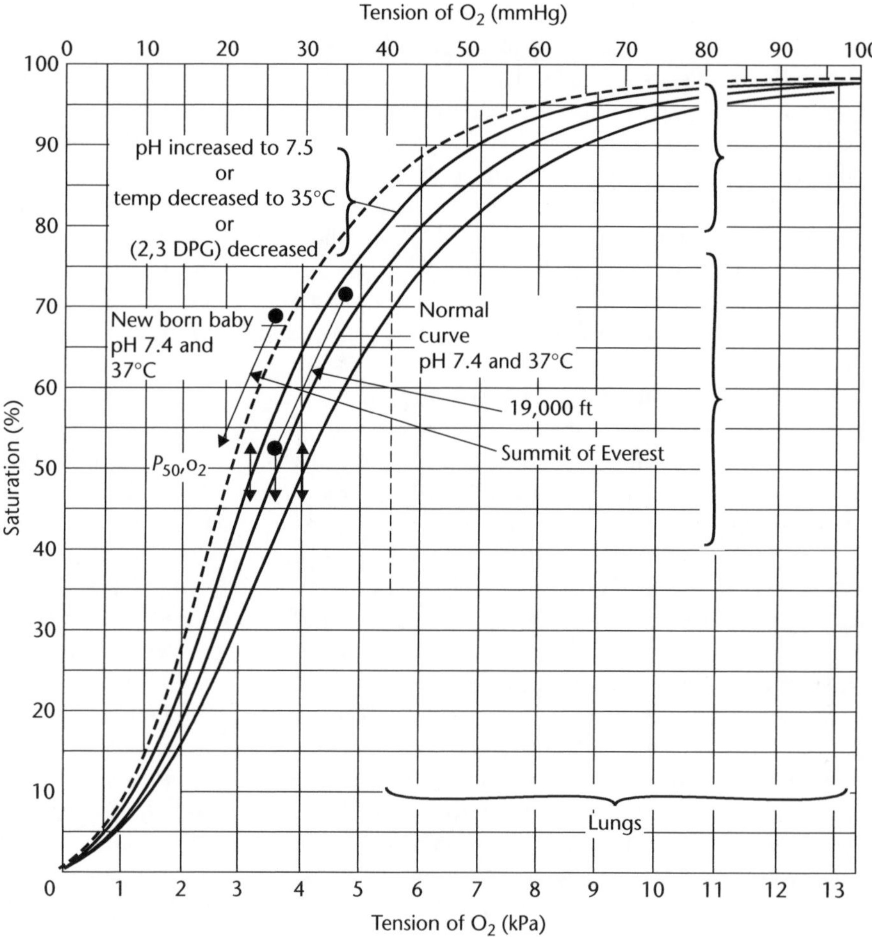

Fig. 34.3 Dissociation curve for oxyhaemoglobin at sea level (Fig. 21.1, page 260), with data for subjects acclimatised to high altitude superimposed. The displacements facilitate gas exchange (see text); they are in the direction of those associated with foetal haemoglobin). Sources: [22, 23]

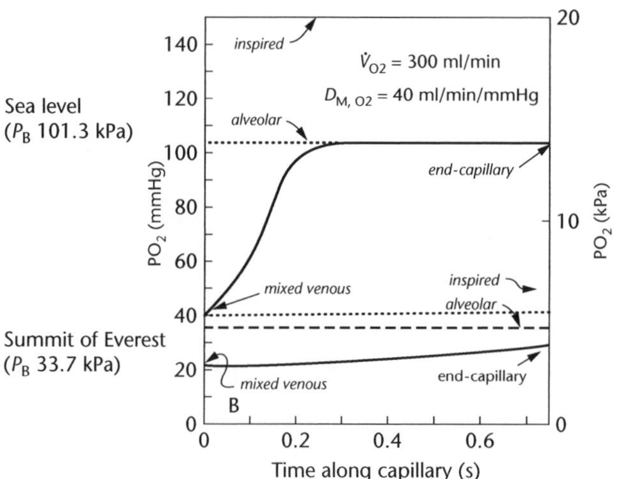

Fig. 34.4 Time course for uptake of oxygen by blood during transit through an alveolar capillary. The upper curve is for conditions at sea level (Fig. 21.2, page 263). The lower curve extends the diagram to conditions at high altitude. Here the oxygen tensions are all lower, gas exchange takes place on the steep part of the oxygen dissociation curve (Fig. 34.3) and blood leaves the capillary still containing oxygen at a lower tension than in alveolar gas. See text. Source: Redrawn from [23].

blood oxygen capacity rise progressively over a period of some 5 weeks [30]; the final improvement can exceed 30% [29].

The polycythaemia is beneficial in that it increases the capacity of blood to deliver oxygen to tissues. This effect persists for a few weeks after return to sea level, so can be a help to athletes who train at altitude for an event at a lower altitude. However, as well as benefits there are also disadvantages to using altitude for training. For example, the maximal intensity of exercise is less at altitude, so the muscle strength is not developed to the extent that it would be when training at sea level. In addition, the polycythaemia is accompanied by a rise in blood viscosity and increased rouleaux formation amongst the red blood cells. The changes can predispose to vascular thromboses, impair gas exchange in both lungs and tissues and be a cause of heart failure. These complications affect particularly those persons in whom the erythropoietic response is at the upper end of the normal distribution. Such people are at increased risk of chronic mountain sickness (Monge's syndrome, Section 34.5).

Exercise at altitude. At altitude the capacity for exercise is reduced, despite effective compensatory mechanisms [24]. The principal one is hyperventilation that in turn initiates the processes of acclimatisation. Other changes include additional myoglobin, increases in the density of capillaries supplying active muscles, proliferation of mitochondria and rises in the concentrations of enzymes that contribute to oxidative metabolism (Section 28.9.1). Hypocapnia activates the enzyme phosphofructokinase, whilst hypoxaemia facilitates rapid glycolysis, a process that is mitigated by acclimatisation [31]. The changes supplement those in gas exchange described above [32]. Together they increase the capacity for exercise by a factor of about four compared with the unacclimatised state. The benefit appears to persist for a few weeks following return to sea level but the evidence is conflicting [33].

Depending on the altitude, the level of training and the intensity of the exercise, unacclimatised persons can develop unpleasant and even life threatening symptoms. These are due to the hypoxaemia driving the ventilation and cardiac frequency to cause intense breathlessness and tachycardia. During very strenuous exercise, the tachycardia can convert to bradycardia on account of a rise in parasympathetic tone [34]. The hyperventilation leads to respiratory alkalosis, which in turn reduces cerebral blood flow to cause giddiness and even loss of consciousness. In acclimatised subjects the ventilation can be sustained and the associated breathlessness becomes the principal factor that limits exercise (see 'Maximal ventilation and wind resistance' above). However, the breathlessness is due to hyperventilation, which in turn is due to increased respiratory drive from hypoxaemia secondary to an inadequate transfer factor. As a result, in acclimatised subjects at high altitude exercise is 'diffusion limited'. At altitudes above the level of acclimatisation, for example at near the summit of Mount Everest the adaptation is incomplete and even mild exercise is incapacitating [23]. At this point the condition of the climber has features in common with the patient with disabling chronic respiratory impairment in whom exercise is also limited by breathlessness (Table 34.2).

Sleep. At altitude the hypoxaemia and resulting hypocapnia modify the changes that occur during normal sleep at sea level (Section 32.4). On the first night following the ascent there is an increase in very light sleep (stage 1), a reduction in slow wave sleep (stages 3 and 4) and an increased number of arousals. The associated periodic breathing, comprising alternating hyperpnoea and apnoea was first described by John Hunter in 1781 [4]. The initial stimulus is hypoxia; this results in more profound hypoxaemia and hence greater peripheral chemoreceptor drive during sleep than when the subject is awake. The increased drive causes hyperventilation that rouses the subject; it also flushes CO_2 out of the lungs and the resulting hypocapnia temporarily eliminates the drive to breathe. During the apnoea the arterial tension of oxygen falls and that of carbon dioxide rises; the changes initiate the next period of hyperventilation. Any severe nocturnal hypoxaemia contributes to high altitude deterioration (Section 34.5).

Blunting of the hypoxic response. . The normal adaptation to high altitude is centred round the process of acclimatisation. This process and the related changes (see 'Respiratory control and acclimatisation' above) go some way to restoring the capacity for exercise and, in the case of acute exposure, permit survival in

Table 34.2 Exercise limitation in a climber under conditions simulating those on the summit of Mt Everest compared with that of a male patient with chronic lung disease who had the same maximal oxygen uptake at sea level.

Subject	Climber (CP)		Patient (male) with COPD	
Age (year)	31		62	
Conditions	6300 m, breathing 14% O_2 in N_2, bicycle		Sea level, air, treadmill	
$\dot{V}O_2$ max (l STPD min^{-1})	1.06	(3.4)	1.06	(2.0)
MVV (l BTPS min^{-1})	190†	(150)	37*	(94)
$\dot{V}E$max,ex (l BTPS min^{-1})	166	(24)	42	(24)
as % of estimated MVV	87%		114%	
RER and HbO_2(Saturation, %)	1.12	45%	0.77	97%
Cardiac frequency (min^{-1}) at $\dot{V}O_2 = 1.06$ l STPD min^{-1}	135	(95)	109	(108)

Reference values are in brackets; those for cardiac frequency include an allowance for physical fitness.

* estimated from FEV_1.

† assuming normal value at sea level.

Note. Both men were limited on exercise by breathlessness caused by a high exercise ventilation relative to MVV. In CP this was due to hypoxic hyperventilation with high RER (Section 28.4.4) and low saturation. In the patient it was due to airways obstruction with normal RER and saturation, but raised ventilation due to $\dot{V}A/\dot{Q}$ inequality. Cardiac frequency was normal for $\dot{V}O_2$ in the patient but increased in CP on account of hypoxia; both values were submaximal. Sources: [23 and unpublished].

conditions that might otherwise be lethal. The driving force is the ventilatory response to hypoxia. This normally persists for many years but can eventually decline; the extent of acclimatisation then diminishes. This was first observed in Andean high altitude natives amongst whom blunting of the ventilatory response to hypoxia usually occurs in early adolescence. In adults who move to high altitude the feature is common after about 20 years. It is reversed by return to sea level. However, the condition is not reversible in all circumstances. For example, in persons with severe hypoxaemia due to cyanotic congenital heart disease the blunting usually persists after the cardiac defect has been corrected. Blunting is also not invariable, e.g. Tibetans are less susceptible than mountain people in the Andes [35]. This suggests that the pattern of adaptation can differ between ethnic groups, reflecting their genetic constitution [36]. A genetic factor has also been invoked to explain an atypical ventilatory response to carbon dioxide in some other high altitude residents (Section 27.1.6).

Blunting of the hypoxic response is accompanied by relative hypercapnia and other features of chronic mountain sickness, including gross polycythaemia (Section 34.5). The syndrome resembles other conditions of chronic hypoventilation including sleep apnoea/hypopnoea syndrome (Chapter 32). However, the associations do not extend to the Himalayan bar-headed goose and the South American llama. These animals, when raised at high altitude, exhibit blunting yet are very tolerant of their situation [37].

34.3 Effects of residence at altitude on lung function

Permanent residents at high altitudes in excess of 3000 m (10,000 ft) usually have larger lungs than dwellers of comparable stature at lower altitudes (cf. Table 25.2, page 319). The change appears to be a consequence of hypoxaemia during childhood influencing the growth of the lung since a similar change occurs in experimental animals. However, most animal studies have entailed exposure to relatively low pressures (simulated altitudes of the order of 5500 m (18,000 ft)) so are not strictly comparable. The increase in size of the lungs, when it occurs, does so during adolescence [38] and some evidence suggests that it may reflect interaction between hypoxaemia and another factor which could be genetic but is possibly a high level of habitual activity. The interaction could explain the relatively large lungs of the Quecha Indians of Peru and the mountain people of the Himalayas including the Bods of Ladakh in Kashmir, the high altitude natives of Nepal and the inhabitants of the Lumana region of Bhutan. The increase in lung size affects the mechanical function of the lungs [39, 40].

Some residents at the intermediate altitude of approximately 1800 m (6000 ft) also have relatively large lungs. This is the case for the highlanders of New Guinea [41] and people who live in the foothills of the Himalayas. However, similar changes have not been seen in Denver, Colorado or in the high Veldt of the Transvaal in South Africa, so the mechanism is uncertain. It could reflect the relatively higher level of habitual activity during childhood of the former subjects or be a consequence of warfare in previous generations leading to the selective elimination of subjects with small ventilatory capacities. Further comparative studies are needed to illuminate these aspects. The mountain dwellers also have an increased potential for gas exchange. This is reflected in an increased transfer factor for carbon monoxide (Table 27.3, page 368). The change is partly due to the hypoxaemia both increasing the reaction rate (θ) of carbon monoxide with oxyhaemoglobin and causing polycythaemia with its attendant rise in blood haemoglobin concentration (cf. Section 20.7). Structural changes associated with having large lungs and an above average capacity for exercise can also contribute. In view of these associations, time spent at high altitude should be taken into account when choosing reference values for lung function in an individual or group of subjects (Section 26.1.5).

34.4 Coping with altitude

General aspects. Any increase in altitude above sea level entails a reduction in ambient oxygen tension. In most circumstances this does not affect people's ability to live normal lives, but performance of skilled tasks is impaired in proportion to the altitude [42]. In addition, the tolerances to carbon monoxide from inhaled tobacco smoke, and to ingested alcohol are reduced.

Bronchitis is relatively common, partly because the air is dry and ciliary function is impaired [43]. Episodes of bronchitis sufficient to cause minor degrees of airways obstruction then result in disproportionate hypoxaemia, particularly in persons with a blunted chemoreceptor response to hypoxia (see above). Hence, patients with chronic obstructive pulmonary disease (COPD) are more likely to develop pulmonary hypertension and right heart failure than at sea level [44]. Persons with responsive pulmonary vessels are particularly at risk (Section 17.2.2). Vascular thromboses are also common on account of polycythaemia. These features have practical implications for transport of patients by air (page 482). Other aspects are considered below.

Low altitudes, up to 1500 m (5000 ft). Able-bodied people who drive or fly to places that are at low altitude usually only experience difficulty if they take very strenuous exercise within a few days of arrival; examples include athletes, ball game players, ballet dancers and rescue workers. Adaptation occurs rapidly. Persons with degenerative vascular disease or medical conditions that predispose to hypoxaemia may have other difficulties. These are described in the next paragraph.

Moderate altitudes in the range 1500–3000 m (5000–10,000 ft). The effects of lack of oxygen are most prominent during exercise and at night. During exercise there may be hyperventilation, giddiness and tachycardia. Alternatively, during very strenuous exercise, the tachycardia can convert to bradycardia on account of a rise in parasympathetic tone. These symptoms can be prevented and the capacity for exercise restored by administration of oxygen at a flow of $2\ l\ min^{-1}$ to $4\ l\ min^{-1}$; a mask fitted with an oxygen reservoir bag or other device that avoids rebreathing and prevents waste of oxygen during expiration should be used.

Insomnia with dreaming and periodic breathing are very common on ascent to altitudes in excess of 1800 m (6000 ft) (see 'Sleep' above). The abnormalities improve with acclimatisation. The disturbed sleep impairs performance during the following day. There can then be lassitude, morning headache and accentuated hypoxaemia, apparently due to subclinical lung pathology [45]. The nocturnal symptoms and subsequent impairment are alleviated by the subject breathing oxygen in low dosage during the night. For this purpose a flow setting of $0.5–1.0\ l\ min^{-1}$ in conjunction with nasal prongs is usually adequate. The symptoms can also be improved by slightly increasing the arterial carbon dioxide tension, for example by breathing through a mask that has a finite deadspace. Periodic breathing can be avoided by prior treatment with acetazolamide (dose in adults 500 mg/day, [46]); this prevents the development of a respiratory alkalosis by promoting the renal excretion of sodium.

During a business trip at altitude a person's performance is enhanced if time is allowed for acclimatisation before work begins. Abstention from smoking and alcohol, eating modestly and adopting a relaxed lifestyle also help. The quality of work can be improved by raising the inspired oxygen partial pressure in the work place. This can be done by pressurisation or with an oxygen concentrator [47, 48].

High altitudes, above 3000 m (10,000 ft). The features of lower altitudes are more pronounced, including anorexia [49], impaired mental function and mountain sickness (see below). In addition, exposure to high altitude can cause long-term mental impairment in susceptible individuals, even in the absence of acute episodes; the extent of the risk is unclear [50, 51].

Climbing Mt Everest without oxygen. To a physiologist such a venture appears fool hardy, especially as up to the time of writing some 160 climbers have died on the mountain. Some sensible precautions are suggested at the end of the next section. Yet in excess of a thousand people have now made the ascent without additional oxygen, and some measures that have made this possible are given in Table 34.3.

Table 34.3 Factors in Messner and Habeler's ascent of Mt Everest without oxygen (1978).

Born and grew up in the Alps
Exceptionally fit, fast climbers
Fully acclimatised
Light, double-layered clothing
Light packs (only 9 kg)
Barometric pressure higher than expected

Source: [52]

34.5 High altitude illness

Introduction. Incautious ascent to high altitude can result in severe illness or death. This became apparent to the early balloonists, some of whom died from hypoxia or exposure to cold. The risk has been rediscovered by generations of travellers to high places. The most frequently occurring condition is acute mountain sickness (AMS). This presents with headache or other symptom within a few hours of the ascent. In the early stages it can be relieved by descent to lower altitude. If untreated the condition can progress to high altitude cerebral oedema (HACE). Independent of these disorders an exposed person can develop high altitude pulmonary oedema (HAPE). This condition typically presents with breathlessness on the 2nd or 3rd day after arrival at altitude. In its early stages it can be relieved by descent to lower altitude or treated by administration of oxygen. In other circumstances the hypoxaemia progresses. This in turn can bring on or exacerbate the other conditions and can cause death. However, where the warning signs are acted on quickly the affected person is likely to make a complete, rapid recovery.

Acute mountain sickness (AMS). Mountain sickness is due to inappropriately rapid ascent to altitudes in excess of 3000 m and formerly occurred mainly in the Andes where this type of ascent was possible. Since the advent of air travel it has become prevalent in other mountainous regions including Kenya and the Himalayas where, depending on circumstances, 10% to 60% of visitors can be affected. Predisposing factors include a relatively young age (not infancy or old age) and exertion soon after the ascent. The level of habitual activity (physical fitness) appears not to be relevant, whilst the role of a reduced ventilatory response to hypoxia is unclear. High altitude residents returning from a visit to low altitudes are at increased risk. The condition usually occurs within 6–12 h after arrival at altitude.

AMS appears to be due to an increase in size of the brain brought about through summation of a number of small changes [53, 54]. These include cerebral vasodilatation caused by hypoxaemia, increases in capillary blood pressure and permeability and changes in permeability of the blood–brain barrier. The extent to which the increase in brain size can be accommodated by displacement of cerebrospinal fluid may also be important. At this stage cerebral oedema is not a conspicuous feature. The initial symptom can be euphoria; but usually the first to be noticed are headache that does not respond to aspirin, nausea, lethargy, dizziness on standing up and disturbed sleep with dreams.

High altitude cerebral oedema (HACE). In the absence of treatment AMS may progress to cerebral oedema. At this stage the subject can experience ataxia and hallucinations, consciousness becomes impaired and the condition is at risk of progressing to coma and death. The physical signs can include papilloedema, retinal haemorrhages and focal cerebral lesions that can affect the cranial nerves.

High altitude pulmonary oedema (HAPE). Onset of undue breathlessness and loss of exercise capacity on the 2nd or 3rd day after an ascent to or above 2500 m is likely to be due to onset of pulmonary oedema. The oedema is initially interstitial when it can be accompanied by a dry (unproductive) cough. The closing volume can be increased [55]. Later, there can be frank pulmonary oedema, with blood stained sputum, mild fever and crackles on auscultation of the chest. The associated hypoxaemia can initiate or aggravate acute mountain sickness or HACE when it can be associated with distressing symptoms, including nausea, anorexia, vomiting and pronounced misery. Fortunately, the condition usually responds well to treatment so seldom progresses to advanced disease.

The pulmonary oedema is associated with a rise in pulmonary capillary pressure (>19 mm Hg) but the mechanism is unclear. It is not due to failure of the left heart [56] or changes in fluid osmotic pressure. The most conspicuous antecedent is vasoconstriction affecting small muscular pulmonary arteries, but by itself this is not a sufficient cause. How it could become such is if the vasoconstriction was uneven, leaving only a small part of the vascular bed to carry the entire cardiac output [53]. This could raise the local intravascular pressure, causing increased permeability from stress failure of the endothelium [57]. A similar mechanism has been proposed to explain the oedema that can occur during maximal exercise at sea level. Precipitating factors include injudicious ascent to altitude, high intensity exercise and exposure to cold. The susceptibility is increased by recent lower respiratory infection and by the possession of an enhanced vasopressor response to hypoxia [58]; the latter is an inherited characteristic and reflects the responsiveness of the renin–aldosterone system to hypoxia [59, 60].

Prevention and treatment. The possibility of mountain sickness should be borne in mind on all journeys to altitudes in excess of about 1500 m. However, it is unlikely below about 3000 m. For ascents to greater altitudes time should be allowed for acclimatisation. This can usually be achieved by not ascending more than 300 m per day, having a pause after every third day and including unallocated days in the itinerary. On general grounds, abstaining from smoking, alcohol and sedative drugs is likely to be beneficial. For prophylaxix against AMS and HACE use can be made of antioxidants [54, 61], acetazolamine (diamox) in the dosage 250 mg bd or tds and dexamethasone (dosage 4 mg bd). These remedies can be combined. For prophylaxis against HAPE slow release nifedipine (dosage 20 mg tds) [62] or an inhaled β agonist such as salmeterol can be useful. These substances can be said to buy time for acclimatisation, but this is best achieved in the manner described.

The mild form of AMS is usually self-limiting, so an appropriate treatment is rest and/or medication. Consideration can be given to temporary descent to a lower altitude. More significant symptoms, including those of impending pulmonary or cerebral oedema are indications for immediate descent towards sea level on a stretcher. Meanwhile, oxygen and appropriate remedies from those given above should be administered and, if equipment is available, the inspired oxygen tension raised by pressurisation using a pressure bag or portable chamber [63]. Morphine or diuretic drugs are not normally recommended. Recovery from mountain sickness is usually rapid and complete but in a few cases may be delayed [64].

The probability of developing an altitude-related illness depends on the objective and timetable of the expedition, the resources available for porterage, the level and incidence of symptoms that are acceptable and the susceptibility of the subjects. As a result, no one level of precautions will fit all expeditions. This is especially true of provision of oxygen, where the choice is between none, oxygen for emergencies and oxygen during exercise and at night. The dividing lines for these levels of commitment might be at 6000 m (20,000 ft) and 7600 m (25,000 ft) but the choice must depend on the circumstances.

34.6 Physiology and medicine of flight

Introduction. Physiological adaptations to hypoxaemia secondary to hypobaria are considered earlier in this chapter. How they can be reconciled with the requirements of aviation and the additional problems associated with barotrauma, atelectasis and decompression sickness are examined here.

The cabin. Aircraft normally fly at altitudes well in excess of 1500 m (5000 ft) so passengers and aircrew require protection from hypoxia. This is normally achieved by raising the pressure in the cabin above that of the surrounding air. Ideally, the pressure should be that at sea level, but the pressure difference from atmospheric pressure would then be large, requiring a strong and hence expensive or heavy airframe for its containment. Instead, a compromise is reached in which the cabin altitude is kept at an intermediate altitude, usually 1850–2150 m (6000–7000 ft). In practice, the cabin altitude is usually allowed to drift upwards as the plane gains altitude. The normal upper limit specified in American Federal Aeronautical Regulations is 2434 m (8000 ft), with a ceiling for breathing air of 3000 m. In practice, higher cabin altitudes (up to 4000 m) have been observed in the past and, whilst this should trigger the release of over-head oxygen masks, a release cannot be relied on. Thus, there may be a risk of significant hypoxia. In addition, an altitude of 2434 m is too high for some patients, so there is need for supplementary oxygen.

Loss of cabin pressure leads to the occupants being exposed to ambient pressure with its attendant hypoxia. The risk is present in all aircraft but especially military ones. To meet it, the pilot and co-pilot usually wear oxygen masks and drop-down masks are supplied for aircrew and passengers. A supply of 100% oxygen is sufficient at altitudes of up to approximately 10,300 m (34,000 ft). At this altitude the barometric pressure minus the partial pressures of carbon dioxide and water vapour is, on average, 14 kPa (105 mm Hg), the same as the alveolar oxygen tension when breathing air at sea level (Fig. 34.1). At higher altitudes hypoxaemia can only be prevented by delivering 100% oxygen to the lungs under positive pressure. This is achieved in military aircraft by using pressurised masks and suits. In civil aircraft the pilot is under instruction to minimise the period of hypoxia by emergency descent.

Assessment of aircrew. Health standards and recommended practices for aircrew are laid down by the International Civil Aviation Organisation, an agency of the United Nations. They are interpreted on a regional basis by, for example the Joint Aviation Authorities of Europe and implemented by national organisations, whose current recommendations should be ascertained. A very high standard of health is required for pilots and air traffic control officers, with slightly lower standards for other aircrew. In the UK supervision is by the Civil Aviation Authority [65]. The requirements include freedom from all respiratory disorders and normal chest X-ray and electrocardiogram. There is an implication that the lung function and response to exercise should also be normal, but what this entails is not specified.

The chances of having an uneventful journey are high and more closely related to the experience of the pilot than to his or her health credentials, so there is a case for an element of discretion in the application of the regulations, particularly as they affect senior personnel [66].

34.6.1 Fitness to fly as a passenger

Persons who are healthy, including the elderly, and most patients are normally fit to fly and the vast majority does so without ill effects. Where there may be difficulties these are now subject to recommendations for best practice [67–69]. The most important topic is venous stasis that, if not prevented can lead to thrombosis in a deep vein in the leg and subsequently to pulmonary embolism [70].

Respiratory disorders. Most patients, including those with asthma and COPD, usually travel well. However, asthmatics should take with them any bronchodilator sprays; these should not be left in luggage destined for the hold of the aircraft [69]. Patients with COPD can experience severe hypoxia so there may be a case for supplementary oxygen. This can be assessed by exposure to hypoxia under controlled conditions in a respiratory laboratory. The alternative of making the assessment in terms of forced expiratory volume or resting arterial oxygen tension at sea-level breathing air [71] appears not to be satisfactory [72]. If oxygen is indicated but not supplied the patient is unlikely to come to immediate harm [73, 74], but the possibility of severe hypoxaemia causing subtle cerebral deterioration cannot be excluded (cf. [50, 51]). Respiratory contra-indications to flying include the existence of a recent pneumothorax (within 6 weeks of correction), recent thoracic surgery and production of copious sputum. Anecdotal evidence suggests that a small fibrosed pneumothorax can be tolerated in some circumstances, but a large cyst probably cannot [69].

Other conditions. Pregnancy is not a contraindication to flying from one lowland area to another [75]. However, a flight to a mountainous district might not be advisable. Patients with symptomatic ischaemic vascular disease, including coronary ischaemia, congenital heart disease, anaemia and related conditions usually travel without incident. Amongst these groups patients at high risk should be identifiable by clinical assessment, possibly supplemented by a hypoxic provocation test. However, no cost benefit analysis of this procedure appears to have been carried out. Unstable heart disease, coronary thrombosis in the recent past (within 1–3 weeks), severe anaemia (Hb $<7.5\ \text{g dl}^{-1}$) and sickle cell disease or thalassaemia can be contraindications to flight (see also Section 34.7). In these and other cases where there may be doubt the airline medical department should be consulted.

Hypoxia inhalation test. The upper limit for cabin altitude when breathing air is 2434 m (8000 ft, see 'The cabin' above); this provides an ambient oxygen tension equivalent to breathing 15% oxygen in nitrogen at sea level. Thus, this gas mixture, or the equivalent pressure in a hypobaric chamber (564 mm Hg), can be used to assess the level of hypoxaemia that a patient is likely to experience during flight. The gas mixture can be prepared in Douglas bags using rotameters, or by the patient breathing air through a 35% Venturi mask supplied with 100% nitrogen [76]. Alternatively, 14% oxygen (523 mm Hg) can simulate conditions at 3000 m. Theoretically, the hypobaric test and that based on an equivalent gas mixture might be expected to yield slightly different results; in practice the results are similar [77].

During the test the blood oxygen level should not be allowed to fall below a predetermined value; if this is reached the test is positive and normoxic conditions should be restored. The critical level has been variously set at 6.7 kPa (50 mm Hg), 7.3 kPa (55 mm Hg) and an oxygen saturation of 90% [75, 78]. Of these standards the last only requires pulse oximetry, not blood sampling. When hypoxia is induced in an exposure chamber or body plethysmograph a positive test should then be repeated with the patient receiving supplementary oxygen from, for example oxygen by nasal prongs at $2\ \text{l min}^{-1}$ or $3\ \text{l min}^{-1}$. Alternatively, if the critical oxygen level is not achieved the test is negative. It should be terminated once the oxygen level has stabilised. The circumstances when the test is necessary as distinct from being appropriate have still to be worked out.

Practical considerations. Once suitability for flying has been established the conditions under which the airline can supply oxygen should be ascertained. Some airlines are more flexible than others and an off peak time may be best. Consideration should also be given to the patient's mobility. Those who can walk 50 m can usually manage with little or no assistance; others may need a wheel chair or require a stretcher [79, 80].

34.7 Barotrauma

Compression of air in the middle ear and nasal sinuses. Compression of gas present in the middle ear or nasal sinuses can cause difficulty for the subject if the rate at which the gas volume is reduced exceeds that at which air enters from the pharynx. This is particularly likely to occur in subjects with an upper respiratory infection, sinusitis or nasal catarrh. The condition usually occurs in an aeroplane during the descent, but also in a compression chamber during the application of pressure or a decompression chamber during recompression. Involvement of the middle ear is relatively common and presents with pain, deafness and a sensation of heaviness on the affected side.

Management. Acute barotrauma is best avoided by prophylactic decongestion as described below, adopting a slow rate of pressure change (less than 0.15 bar min^{-1}) and by the subject opening the eustachian tubes by swallowing, singing or yawning at regular intervals during the time when the pressure is rising (i.e. air in internal cavities is reducing in volume). If symptoms develop, the subject should inhale methedrine or a similar decongestant drug, then take a deep breath, shut the mouth, close the nose with one thumb and forefinger and attempt to exhale. The manoeuvre will usually force air into the middle ear or the sinus that is affected. If it is unsuccessful a solution of 0.5% ephedrine in saline should be applied over the ostium of the appropriate sinus by suitably positioning the head. If this treatment fails resort may be made to politzeration or myringotomy.

Delayed barotrauma. This is a condition of slow onset due to absorbtion of gas from the middle ear or sinuses following breathing 100% oxygen. Precipitating circumstances include an upper respiratory infection and a change in barometric pressure in association with aviation or hyperbaric oxygen therapy.

Expansion of air in an enclosed space. Gas present in a body cavity expands whenever the pressure around the person is reduced. The decompression can cause difficulty if the cavity is a closed one or the pressure drop occurs rapidly; persons who are at risk include those with a pneumothorax, either spontaneous or following thoracic surgery, and lung cysts (Section 35.4). Air can also be present as a consequence of an endoscopic examination. In the eye air can be introduced by retinal surgery. It will expand and cause blindness if the patient travels by air before the gas has been reabsorbed [81].

Very rapid decompression can lead to rupture of the lungs. In a pressurised aeroplane this can occur if cabin pressure drops precipitously as a result of failure of a window, door or airframe. There is a potential risk during work in a decompression chamber or whilst escaping from a submerged submarine (Section 35.4).

Over-expansion of gas anywhere in the body can be treated by immediate recompression. Alternatively, for a tension pneumothorax or similar emergency the pressure can be relieved by cannulation.

Over-inflation or rupture of the lung is a possible complication of oxygen therapy or anaesthesia where the gas is delivered from a cylinder. This hazard can be avoided by having a pressure release valve that operates at a maximal pressure of 6 kPa (45 mm Hg).

Atelectasis during breathing oxygen. Alveoli continue to take up oxygen after the airway that serves them has been occluded. On this account a manoeuvre which, when breathing air would cause the temporary closure of a segmental airway can, when breathing oxygen, lead to the absorption of sufficient gas to prolong the occlusion and give rise to atelectasis. This can affect the lower lung lobes of military flying personnel if they are exposed to positive acceleration whilst breathing 100% oxygen. Atelectasis can also occur in relation to anaesthesia (Section 42.3.4) and during the inhalation of 100% oxygen by patients whose breathing is shallow. The condition is prevented by routinely using oxygen in a maximal concentration of 0.7. When closure occurs the patency of the airway can usually be restored by a single deep inspiration.

Absorbtion of gas from air pockets. The constituent gases in an enclosed pocket of air anywhere in the body are in equilibrium with the adjacent tissues; here the sum of the tensions of the oxygen, carbon dioxide, nitrogen and water vapour is less than atmospheric, so the gas in the pocket is absorbed. A closed pocket of oxygen is absorbed more rapidly than one containing air. This is because the gas tension gradient between the pocket and its surroundings is larger for oxygen than for nitrogen (Fig. 34.1). For this reason oxygen should be used instead of air to delineate organs prior to radiography. It should also be used if a small bubble of gas is to be injected into an artery to promote vasodilatation.

34.8 Decompression sickness

Decompression sickness is due to nitrogen that was formerly in solution appearing in the form of bubbles as a result of the air pressure round the subject being reduced suddenly [82]. The situation resembles that in a bottle of sparkling water when the cap is removed. The condition can occur after rapid ascent (decompression) from sea level to high altitude or a high simulated altitude in a decompression chamber. The risk is related to the pressure gradient for nitrogen between the tissues and the lungs. The pressure in the lungs normally varies with altitude, where the minimal effective change is a halving of the pressure (e.g. from sea level to 5500 m, equivalent to 18,000 ft). The tissue nitrogen tension is normally that at sea level, but can be reduced by the subject breathing oxygen to flush nitrogen from the body (e.g. for 4 h). It is increased if the subject has recently breathed air under pressure as a result of SCUBA diving. The risk of decompression sickness can then be reduced by the diver delaying his or her flight; a pre-flight surface interval of 17 h seems to be optimal [83]. The quantity of dissolved nitrogen is relatively high in obese subjects; this is because the solubility of nitrogen in fat exceeds that in lean tissue (see below). The quantity of body fat usually increases with age, so this is another risk factor.

The chance of a bubble forming at a particular site is determined by the local quantity of nitrogen and the presence of one or more trigger factors. These include the impact of cosmic rays, anatomical anomalies and turbulence in blood vessels. Local turbulence can be caused by exercise and for this reason bubbles form mainly in the limbs. The presenting symptom is pain so the condition is sometimes known as 'the bends' but this term is usually reserved for the analogous condition in divers (Section 35.5.1). The pain is relieved by recompression to sea level.

Bubbles that form in the blood lodge in the lungs where they can cause cough, breathlessness, chest pain and shock ('chokes'). The latter condition can result in death unless alleviated by recompression; this should be to as high a pressure as is practicable, for example 3 atmospheres absolute pressure (ATA).

Clearance of nitrogen from tissues. The speed with which nitrogen moves between individual tissues and the lungs influences susceptibility to decompression sickness, compressed air illness and related conditions. The flow of nitrogen is affected by the blood supply of the tissue and the content of fat, in which nitrogen is 5 times more soluble than in serum. Older subjects usually have a reduced tissue blood flow but more fat compared with younger ones so their clearance times are prolonged. In young men breathing oxygen, the nitrogen is cleared very rapidly from the blood and those organs such as the kidney and the thyroid gland that have a large blood flow in relation to their size (half-times of 1–2 min). For the abdominal viscera, but not the lumina of the intestines, for the grey matter of the brain and spinal cord and for organs that are well perfused with blood the half-time is approximately 5 min. The nitrogen in the muscles and the connective tissues of the body is cleared more slowly with a half-time of 25–30 min, whilst the nitrogen in the depot fat is cleared very slowly with a half-time of 1–4 h. On this account, in order to reduce the risk of decompression sickness to a material extent the period of breathing 90% oxygen in nitrogen should extend to approximately 4 h. Hundred per cent oxygen should not be used as it can promote atelectasis (see above).

Breathing 90% oxygen can be used to promote the reabsorbtion of nitrogen from a pneumothorax, pneumoperitoneum or a region of surgical emphysema, but the process is slow, taking a minimum of 12 h. Flatulence due to paralytic ileus can also be relieved.

34.9 References

1. Barcroft J, Binger CA, Bock AV et al. Observations upon the effect of high altitude on the physiological processes of the human body carried out in the Peruvian Andes chiefly at Cerro de Pasco. *Philos Trans R Soc Lond (Biol)* 1923; **211**: 351–480.
2. West JB, editor. *High altitude physiology. Benchmark papers in human physiology 15.* Stroundsbery, PA: Hutchinson Ross, 1981.
3. Fenn WO, Rahn H, Otis AB. A theoretical study of the composition of alveolar air at altitude. *Am J Physiol* 1946; **146**: 637–653.
4. Ward MP, Milledge JS, West JB, eds. *High altitude medicine and physiology.* 3rd ed. London: Arnold, 2000.
5. West JB. High altitude. In: Crystal RG, Barnes PJ, West JB, Weibel ER, eds. *The lung; scientific foundations,* vol 2, 2nd ed. New York: Lippincott-Raven, 1997: 2653–2666.
6. Committee for Medical Research. *Handbook of respiratory data in aviation.* Washington DC, 1944.
7. Pollard AJ, Mason NP, Barry PW et al. Effect of altitude on spirometric parameters and the performance of peak flow meters. *Thorax* 1996; **51**: 175–178.
8. Jensen RL, Crapo RO, Berlin SL. Effect of altitude on hand-held peak flow meters. *Chest* 1996; **109**: 475–479.
9. Cotes JE. Ventilatory capacity at altitude and its relation to mask design. *Proc Roy Soc B* 1954; **143**: 32–39.
10. Lahiri S, Milledge JS, Sørensen SC. Ventilation in man during exercise at high altitude. *J Appl Physiol* 1972; **32**: 766–769.
11. Cibella F, Cuttitta G, Romano S et al. Respiratory energetics during exercise at high altitude. *J Appl Physiol* 1999; **86**: 1785–1792.
12. Pugh LGCE, Gill MB, Lahiri S et al. Muscular exercise at great altitudes. *J Appl Physiol* 1964; **19**: 431–440.
13. Williams DA. Athletic performance at high altitude. *Nature (Lond)* 1966; **211**: 753.
14. Pugh LGCE. Athletes at altitude. *J Physiol (Lond)* 1967; **192**: 619–646.
15. Vizek M, Pickett C, Weil JV. Increased carotid body hypoxic sensitivity during acclimatization to hypobaric hypoxia. *J Appl Physiol* 1987; **63**: 2403–2410.
16. Pedersen ME, Dorrington KL, Robbins PA. Effects of dopamine and dopmeridone on ventilatory sensitivity to hypoxia after 8 h of isocapnic hypoxia. *J Appl Physiol* 1999; **86**: 222–229.
17. Sato M, Severinghaus JW, Powell FL et al. Augmented hypoxic ventilatory response in men at altitude. *J Appl Physiol* 1992; **73**: 101–107.
18. Weil JV, Byrne-Quinn E, Sodal IE et al. Acquired attenuation of chemoreceptor function in chronically hypoxic man at high altitude. *J Clin Invest* 1971; **50**: 186–195.
19. Ou LC, St John WM, Tenney SM. The contribution of central mechanisms rostral to the pons in high altitude ventilatory acclimatisation. *Respir Physiol* 1983; **54**: 343–351.
20. Forster HV, Dempsey JA, Birnbaum ML et al. Effect of chronic exposure to hypoxia on ventilatory response to CO_2 and hypoxia. *J Appl Physiol* 1971; **31**: 586–592.
21. Saunders KB, Band DM, Ebden P et al. Acid–base status and gas exchange in the anaesthetized dog breathing pure oxygen. *Respiration* 1972; **29**: 305–316.
22. West JB, Lahiri S, Gill MB et al. Arterial oxygen saturation during exercise at high altitude. *J Appl Physiol* 1962; **17**: 617–621.
23. West JB, Hackett PH, Maret KH et al. Pulmonary gas exchange on the summit of Mount Everest. *J Appl Physiol* 1983; **55**: 678–687.
24. Peacock AJ, Jones PL. Gas exchange at extreme altitude: results from the British 40th anniversary Everest expedition. *Eur Respir J* 1997; **10**: 1439–1444.
25. Wagner PD, Sutton JR, Reeves JT et al. Operation Everest II. Pulmonary gas exchange during a simulated ascent of Mt. Everest. *J Appl Physiol* 1987; **63**: 2348–2359.
26. Reeves JT, Groves BM, Sutton JR et al. Operation Everest II: preservation of cardiac function at extreme altitude. *J Appl Physiol* 1987; **63**: 531–539.
27. Bredle DL, Chapler CK, Cain SM. Metabolic and circulatory responses of normoxic skeletal muscle to whole-body hypoxia. *J Appl Physiol* 1988; **65**: 2063–2068.

28. Bebout DE, Storey D, Roca J et al. Effects of altitude acclimatization on pulmonary gas exchange during exercise. *J Appl Physiol* 1989; **67**: 2286–2295.
29. Milledge JS, Cotes PM. Serum erythropoietin in humans at high altitude and its relation to plasma renin. *J Appl Physiol* 1985; **59**: 360–364.
30. Weil JV, Jamieson G, Brown DW, Grover RF. The red cell mass-arterial oxygen relationship in normal man. *J Clin Invest* 1968; **47**: 1627–1639.
31. Brooks GA. Are arterial, muscle and working limb lactate exchange data obtained on men at altitude consistent with the hypothesis of an intracellular lactate shuttle? *Adv Exp Med Biol* 1999; **474**: 185–204.
32. Wagner PD. New ideas on limitation of V_{O_2} max. *Exerc Sport Sci Rev* 2000; **28**: 10–14.
33. Green HJ, Roy B, Grant S et al. Increases in submaximal cycling efficiency mediated by altitude acclimatization. *J Appl Physiol* 2000; **89**: 1189–1197.
34. Hartley LH, Vogel JA, Cruz JC. Reduction of maximal exercise heart rate at altitude and its reversal with atropine. *J Appl Physiol* 1974; **36**: 362–365.
35. Moore LG. Comparative human ventilatory adaptation to high altitude. *Respir Physiol* 2000; **121**: 257–276.
36. Beall CM. Tebetan and Andean patterns of adaptation to high-altitude hypoxia. *Hum Biol* 2000; **72**: 201–228.
37. Brooks JG III, Tenney SM. Ventilatory response of llama to hypoxia at sea level and high altitude. *Respir Physiol* 1968; **5**: 269–278.
38. Beall CM, Baker PT, Baker TS, Haas JD. The effects of high altitude on adolescent growth in Southern Peruvian Amerindians. *Hum Biol* 1977; **49**: 109–124.
39. Cruz JC. Mechanics of breathing in high altitude and sea level subjects. *Respir Physiol* 1973; **17**: 146–161.
40. Brody JS, Lahiri S, Simpser M et al. Lung elasticity and airway dynamics in Peruvian natives to high altitude. *J Appl Physiol* 1977; **42**: 245–251.
41. Cotes JE, Anderson HR, Patrick JM. Lung function and the response to exercise in New Guineans: role of genetic and environmental factors. *Phil Trans R Soc B.* 1974; **268**: 349–361.
42. Tichauer ER. Operation of machine tools at high altitude. *Ergonomics* 1963; **6**: 51–73.
43. Barry PW, Mason NP. O'Callaghan C. Nasal mucociliary transport is impaired at altitude. *Eur Respir J* 1997; **10**: 35–37.
44. Schoene RB. Lung disease at high altitude. *Adv Exp Med Biol* 1999; **474**: 47–56.
45. McElroy MK, Gerard A, Powell FL et al. Nocturnal O_2 enrichment of room air at high altitude increases daytime O_2 saturation without changing control of ventilation. *High Alt Med Biol* 2000; **1**: 197–206.
46. Hackett P. Pharmacological prevention of acute mountain sickness. *BMJ* 2001; **322**: 48–49.
47. West JB. Commuting to high altitude. Recent studies of oxygen enrichment. *Adv Exp Med Biol* 1999; **474**: 57–64.
48. West JB. Safe upper limits for oxygen enrichment of room air at high altitude. *High Alt Med Biol* 2001; **2**: 47–51.
49. Bailey DM, Davies B, Milledge JS et al. Elevated plasma cholecystokinin in high altitude: metabolic implications for the anorexia of acute mountain sickness. *High Alt Med Biol* 2000; **1**: 9–23.
50. Hornbein TF, Townes BD, Schoene RB et al. The cost to the central nervous system of climbing to extremely high altitude. *N Engl J Med* 1989; **321**: 1714–1719.
51. Regard M, Oelz O, Brugger P, Landis T. Persistent cognitive impairment in climbers after repeated exposure to extreme altitude. *Neurology* 1989; **39**: 210–213.
52. Ward MP. *Everest: a thousand years of exploration.* Glasgow: Ernest Press, 2003.
53. Hackett PH. High altitude cerebral oedema and acute mountain sickness. A pathophysiology update. *Adv Exp Med Biol* 1999; **474**: 23–45.
54. Basnyat B, Murdoch DR. High altitude illness (Seminar). *Lancet* 2003; **361**: 1967–1974.
55. Cremona G, Asnaghi R, Baderna P et al. Pulmonary extravascular fluid accumulation in recreational climbers; a prospective study. *Lancet* 2002; **359**: 303–309.
56. Boussuges A, Molenat F, Burnet H et al. Operation Everest 111 (Comex '97): modifications of cardiac function secondary to altitude-induced hypoxia. *Am J Respir Crit Care Med* 2000; **161**: 264–270.
57. West JB, Colice GJ, Lee Y-J et al. Pathogenesis of high-altitude pulmonary oedema: direct evidence of stress failure of pulmonary capillaries. *Eur Respir J* 1995; **8**: 523–529.
58. Archer SL, Weir EK, Reeve HL, Michelakis E. Molecular identification of O_2 sensors and O_2-sensitive potassium channels in the pulmonary circulation. *Adv Exp Med Biol* 2000; **475**: 219–240.
59. Milledge JS, Beeley JM, McArthur S, Morice AH. Atrial natriuretic peptide, altitude and acute mountain sickness. *Clin Sci* 1989; **77**: 509–514.
60. Woods DR, Pollard AJ, Collier DJ et al. Insertion/deletion polymorphism of the angiotensin1-converting enzyme gene and arterial oxygen saturation at high altitude. *Am J Respir Crit Care Med* 2002; **166**: 362–366.
61. Bailey DM, Davies B. Acute mountain sickness; prophylactic benefits of antioxidant vitamin supplementation at high altitude. *High Alt Med Biol* 2001; **2**: 21–29.
62. Antezana AM, Antezana G, Aparicio O et al. Pulmonary hypertension in high-altitude chronic hypoxia: response to nifedipine. *Eur Respir J* 1998; **12**: 1181–1185.
63. Saito S, Aso C, Kinai M et al. Experimental use of a transportable hyperbaric chamber durable for 15 psi at 3700 meters above sea level. *Wilderness Environ Med* 2000; **11**: 21–24.
64. Steinacker JM, Tobias P, Menold E et al. Lung diffusing capacity and exercise in subjects with previous high altitude pulmonary oedema. *Eur Respir J* 1998; **11**: 643–650.
65. Mitchell SJ. Health assessment in aviation medicine: an overview. *Occup Med* 2003; **53**: 3–4.
66. Mitchell SJ, Schenk CP. The value of screening tests in applicants for professional pilot medical certification. *Occup Med* 2003; **53**:15–18.
67. Dowdall N. Customer health: a new role for occupational physicians. *Occup Med* 2003; **53**: 19–23.
68. Aerospace Medical Association medical guidelines taskforce. Medical guidelines for air travel. 2nd ed. *Aviat Space Environ Med* 2003; **74**(Suppl): A1–19.
69. British Thoracic Society. Managing passengers with respiratory disease planning air travel: British Thoracic Society recommendations. *Thorax* 2002; **57**: 289–304.
70. Shepherd L, Edwards SL. The effects of flying: processes, consequences and prevention. *Br J Nursing.* 2004; **13**: 19–29.
71. Dillard TA, Rosenberg AP, Berg BW. Hypoxemia during altitude exposure. A meta-analysis of chronic obstructive pulmonary disease. *Chest* 1993; **103**: 422–425.

72. Christensen CC, Ryg M, Refvem OK, Skjonsberg OH. Development of severe hypoxemia in chronic obstructive pulmonary disease patients at 2,438 m altitude. *Eur Respir J* 2000; **15**: 635–639.
73. Douglas NJ, Calverley PM, Leggett RJE et al. Transient hypoxaemia during sleep in chronic bronchitis and emphysema. *Lancet* 1979; **1**: 1–4.
74. Naeije R. Preflight medical screening of patients. *Eur Respir J* 2000; **16**: 197–199.
75. Newlands JC, Barclay JR. Air transport of passengers of advanced gestational age. *Aviat Space Environ Med* 2000; **72**: 770.
76. Robson AG, Hartburg TK, Innes JA. Laboratory assessment of fitness to fly in patients with lung disease: a practical approach. *Eur Respir J* 2000; **16**: 214–219.
77. Dillard TA, Moores LK, Bilello KL, Phillips YY. The pre-flight evaluation. A comparison of the hypoxic inhalation test with hypobaric exposure. *Chest* 1995; **107**: 352–357.
78. Cramer D, Ward S, Geddes D. Assessment of oxygen supplementation during air travel. *Thorax* 1996; **51**: 202–203.
79. Smeets F. Travel for technology-dependent patients with respiratory disease. *Thorax* 1994; **49**: 77–81.
80. Kramer MR, Jakobson DJ, Springer C, Donchin Y. The safety of air transportation of patients with advanced lung disease. Experience with 21 patients requiring lung transplantation or pulmonary thromboendarterectomy. *Chest* 1995; **108**: 1292–1296.
81. Polk JD, Rugaber GK, Arenstein R, Fallon WF. Central retinal artery occlusion by proxy: a cause of sudden blindness in an airline passenger. *Aviat Space Environ Med* 2002; **73**: 385–387.
82. Ernsting J, Nicholson AN, Rainford DJ. *Aviation medicine.* 3rd ed. Oxford: Butterworth-Herineman, 1999.
83. Vann RD, Gerth WA, Denoble PJ et al. Experimental trials to assess the risks of decompression sickness in flying after diving. *Undersea Hyperb Med* 2004; **31**: 431–444.

Further reading

Bencowitz HZ, Wagner PD, West JB. Effect of change in P_{50} on exercise tolerance at high altitude: a theoretical study. *J Appl Physiol* 1982; **53**: 1487–1495.

Cowell SA, Stocks JM, Evans DG et al. The exercise and environmental physiology of extravehicular activity *Aviat Space Environ Med* 2002; **73**: 54–67.

Hebbel RP, Eaton JW, Kronenberg RS et al. Human llamas. Adaptation to altitude in subjects with high hemoglobin oxygen affinity. *J Clin Invest* 1978; **62**: 593–600.

Pollard AJ, Murdoch DR. *The high altitude medicine handbook.* 2nd ed. Oxford: Radcliffe Medical Press, 1998.

West JB, Elliott AR, Guy HJ, Prisk GK. Pulmonary function in space. *JAMA* 1997; **277**: 1957–1961; also *JAMA* 1998; **279**: 275–276.

Widdicombe JG. Nasal airflow resistance at simulated altitude. Editorial. *Eur Respir J* 2002; **19**: 4–5

CHAPTER 35

Immersion in Water, Hyperbaria and Hyperoxia Including O_2 Therapy

This chapter describes the physiological features and difficulties arising from man's exploration of the sea. The associated hyperoxia links the topic with oxygen therapy which is also treated here.

35.1 Introduction

Immersion. Life on earth evolved in an aquatic environment, so man has inherited features that contribute to his survival in water. These include the diving reflexes, thermal insulation and measures that actively protect against cold. However, their efficacy is limited in the face of the difficulties that the environment presents, especially mechanical instability, adverse effects of water pressure on the body and exposure to cold.

Immersion as in bathing and swimming can be an activity in its own right. Alternatively, it can be a prelude to submersion and breath-hold diving or SCUBA diving, breathing a compressed gas mixture. The latter entails exposure to hyperbaric conditions and carries a risk of decompression sickness (Fig. 35.1). Immersion, decompression, hyperbaria and hyperoxia are considered in the present chapter. Adaptations to heat and cold are discussed in Chapter 36.

Hyperbaria. The evolution of man has not included a hyperbaric phase and tolerance of high pressures has not been necessary for survival. As a result man is poorly equipped to cope with raised barometric pressures. These are experienced mainly during diving, work in caissons and in association with hyperbaric oxygen therapy.

The main stimuli to study of hyperbaric physiology and medicine have been in relation to prospecting and drilling for oil and gas, undersea warfare, underwater archaeology and recreational diving. The techniques for hyperbaric oxygen therapy have largely arisen from this work. Representative pressures are: in caissons and for hyperbaric oxygen therapy 2-3 atmospheres absolute (2-3 ATA), and for diving any pressure from these levels up to 35 ATA or higher. Exposure to the lower pressures is likely to continue, but the effects of very high pressures on the human body will soon be only of academic interest because of increasing use of robots and submersible craft.

Hyperoxia. Projections stimulated by the Gaia hypothesis (Section 1.1) have suggested that living organisms may have been exposed to a hyperoxic phase during evolution. If so, this would explain why human beings are equipped with powerful defences against hyperoxia. These cannot cope with the overwhelming hyperoxia that can accompany hyperbaria but may do so during oxygen therapy. In both sets of circumstances the need to protect against irreversible damage is a major constraint on what can be tolerated.

The defences against hyperoxia are damaged by tobacco smoke and other air pollutants (Sections 37.3 and 37.4).

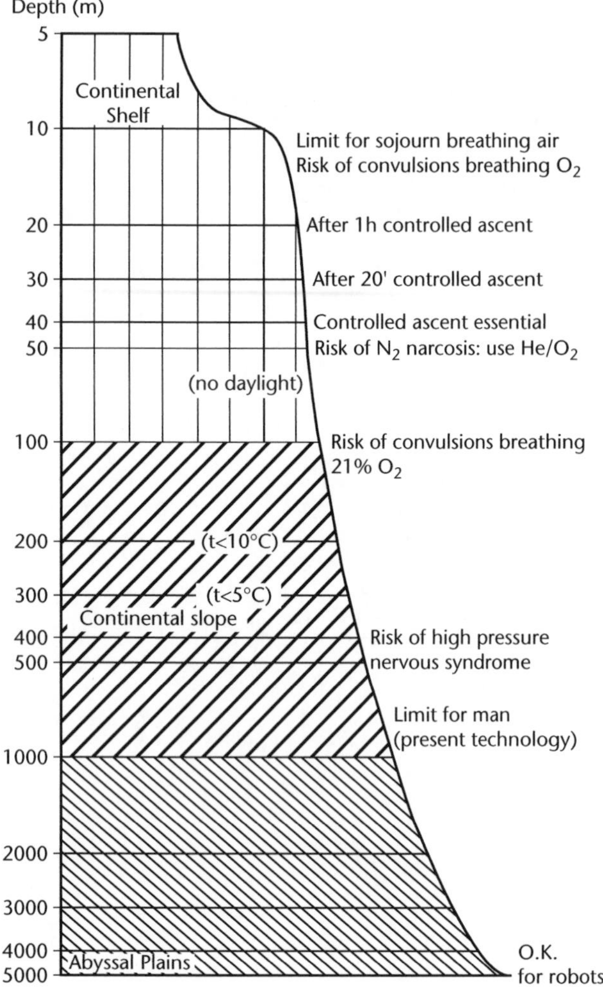

Fig. 35.1 Limitations to human exploration of the sea. Temperatures are for the tropics. Absolute pressure (ATA) is given by (Depth (m)/10.3 + 1). Source: [1].

35.2 Surviving at air–water interface (including drowning)

Buoyancy. The density of the human body is the weighted average of the densities of the constituent organs and tissues, including bones (density in the range 2–3 kg l^{-1}), fat (density 0.7 as in Section 4.7) and air in the lungs where the density approaches zero. The weighted average is nearly one, so the human body has neural buoyancy and usually floats on water. The body rides higher in the water in fat people than in lean ones and in sea water than in fresh water (see also [1, 2]). The possession of relatively large lungs is also an advantage. When the high buoyancy is due to fat this improves the insulation against hypothermia [3].

The normal swimming position is horizontal, but in the absence of volitional control the body adopts a vertical attitude since density of the legs and pelvis exceeds that of the upper regions. This provides limited protection against inhaling water.

Instability. Movement across water entails displacing that which is below the buoyancy line; this requires material expenditure of energy from muscles that non-swimmers may not use normally, so movement is relatively slow. Even a strong swimmer can lose control when in a current or rough water.

Cold immersion. Stimuli arising from immersion in cold water initiate powerful reflex responses (Section 3.3.11, also 'Diving bradycardia' below); these can initiate chain reactions that have the most devastating consequences (Table 35.1). Subsequent cooling of the body can also be incapacitating. These complications of immersion are more frequent in men than in women, the very young and the elderly; they are ameliorated in proportion to the amount of clothing the subject is wearing at the time. The risks associated with immersion are increased by cutaneous vasodilatation as occurs following ingestion of alcohol.

Inhalation of water. Water can be inhaled during the initial reflex gasp that can follow immersion. Alternatively, where immersion causes apnoea, any inhalation may be delayed and only take place after several minutes when the subject is losing consciousness. If water is inhaled the quantity is usually small and insufficient to be a principal cause of death.

The effects of a significant quantity of water entering the acini depend on its osmotic pressure. Influx of fresh water leads to haemolysis of erythrocytes and inactivation of surfactant, both of which exert secondary effects. Influx of sea water attracts lung water into the alveoli and has other consequences. These are indicated in Table 35.1.

Treatment of near drowning. First aid measures include immediate clearance of debris from the mouth, adoption of a 'jack-knife' posture to drain water from the lungs and appropriate assistance to ventilation. Where practicable this is best given under positive pressure via an airway or tracheal tube. The stomach is emptied via a gastric catheter. Subsequent treatment may include exchange transfusion, defibrillation of the heart, measures to alleviate cerebral and/or pulmonary oedema and prophylactic use of antibiotics [4–6].

35.3 Effects of diving on lung function

35.3.1 Immersion and dives with breath holding

Ventilation and respiratory work. Immersion squeezes the chest and anterior abdominal wall. It also displaces blood from lower regions of the body into the lungs. These changes reduce the expiratory reserve volume and inspiratory capacity. As a result the total lung capacity and vital capacity are reduced. This effect is enhanced if the subject has a myopathy or diaphragmatic weakness. Also, because the lungs are less expanded, the airway

Table 35.1 Physiological complications of cold immersion and inhaling water.

Cutaneous reflexes from immersion	Gasp reflex	Immediate inhalation of water
	Vasoconstriction	Pulmonary congestion and oedema, Blood pressure rises
	Diving reflex	Bradycardia; may lead to unconsciousness
	Release of noradrenaline	Risk of ventricular fibrillation, especially in cardiac patients
	Bronchoconstriction	Cold-induced asthma
Airway reflexes	Laryngeal spasm	Subsequent inhalation of water
	Bronchoconstriction	May persist after rescue
Direct effects of inhaling water	Water in airways,...	Airway obstruction,
	......if fresh	delayed atelectasis, $\dot{V}_A/\dot{Q}$ imbalance
	......if sea	pulmonary oedema
	Sea water in blood	Mg^{++} and Ca^{++} ions can cause fibrillation
	Fresh water in blood	Haemolysis releases K^+ions; these can cause fibrillation
	Hypothermia	Additional vasoconstriction, Impaired function of limb muscles etc.

resistance and work of breathing are relatively high. The changes are associated with reductions in forced expiratory volume and forced expiratory flows; these responses are accentuated in persons with mild asthma [7]. Immersion also impedes the movement of the chest wall, so the tidal volume during exercise is reduced (Section 28.4.5). This contributes to respiratory sensation and reduces the capacity for exercise [8].

The adverse mechanical effects of immersion are ameliorated by eliminating the pressure gradient across the chest wall. During immersion to the neck, this is achieved by having the subject breathe air at a positive pressure of 1.0 kPa (10 cm H_2O) with respect to lung centroid pressure [9]. During submersion additional benefit is experienced by exercising in a prone rather than an upright posture [8].

Diving bradycardia. Immersion of the face in cold water (10°C) has been observed to reduce cardiac frequency and raise mean arterial pressure, despite the cardiac output often being reduced. The response is an accentuated form of that observed during breath holding without the face being immersed. It has the effect of conserving oxygen stored in the lungs for the benefit of the brain and other vital organs. The conservation is at the expense of the muscles where the metabolism becomes non-aerobic (Section 28.4.6) so the blood lactic acid concentration rises [10].

The bradycardia has been considered as part of an all-embracing diving reflex such as has been attributed to diving birds and mammals. However, responses to diving vary between species [11], so a holistic approach is not appropriate [12].

Perfusion and gas exchange in lungs. Immersion displaces blood from the lower half of the body into the lungs where it fills the greater part of the vascular bed. As a result the distribution of blood flow becomes relatively uniform and the normal vertical gradient down the lungs disappears (Section 17.1.3) [13]. Concurrently, closing volume is increased, especially in the elderly [14]. This change is associated with less uniform distribution of ventilation with respect to perfusion in older subjects ($\dot{V}_A/\dot{Q}$ inequality) and a somewhat increased shunting of blood across non-ventilated parts of the lungs. However, the changes are to some extent compensated for by an increase in ventilation and, as a result, arterial oxygen tension is relatively normal [15]. Transfer factor (Tlco) is not changed by immersion, except when this is accompanied by imposition of an inspiratory resistance to breathing. The transfer factor is then reduced temporarily [16]. The change may be evidence for interstitial pulmonary oedema. Overt alveolar oedema occurs in a small proportion of subjects [17]. For divers who are unencumbered the risk factors for oedema include immersion in cold water and an increase in blood flow from any cause. However, there may also be a genetic predisposition [18].

Ventilatory sensitivity to CO_2. Immersing the face in cold water causes a modest reduction in ventilatory sensitivity to carbon dioxide [19]. This response is not apparent when the exposure is to hot water. It appears to be a component of the diving reflex. The ventilatory sensitivity is further reduced in persons who dive regularly and, as a result, their ability to hold the breath is prolonged [20].

Breath holding dives to great depths. For centuries, the Ama women of Japan have been harvesting the sea to depths of about 20 m [21] and dives to over 100 m have been performed by exceptional individuals. At these depths the lungs are compressed down to their residual volume despite the influx of up to 1 l of blood displaced from other parts of the body [22]. Other physical hazards include loss of buoyancy due to compression, lung rupture (barotrauma) during the ascent and shallow water blackout. In this condition loss of consciousness is a consequence of severe hypoxaemia in the latter part of the ascent. Unconsciousness is preceded by a strong urge to breathe. The syndrome is caused by the summation of several processes; they include high utilisation of oxygen at depth, reduced alveolar oxygen tension due to the ascent (decompression effect) and consequent reversed diffusion of oxygen from pulmonary capillary blood into the lungs. An additional factor can be inappropriate delay in starting the ascent due to loss of the urge to breathe. This can occur as a result of excessive hyperventilation prior to the dive causing severe hypocapnia. In this circumstance the blood concentration of CO_2 may not return to a level sufficient to produce an urge to breathe before the onset of unconsciousness. In the face of these difficulties, the principal features that make deep dives possible are an appropriate inheritance, much practice and trial by ordeal, leading to selection of depth-tolerant individuals [18].

Post-immersion. After an immersion that is apparently without ill effects the subject may nonetheless experience on-going hypothermia, airway narrowing, a reduced transfer factor and other features of damage to the lung parenchyma [23, 16, 17].

35.3.2 Deep dives

Features of divers. Divers are usually physically very fit, so at the start of their diving careers they usually have above average lung function (ventilatory capacity, lung volumes and transfer factor); they also have a relatively high capacity for exercise. These features are enhanced by work as a diver (Section 28.12). The work develops the muscles of the shoulder girdle which also act as accessory muscles of respiration, so the vital capacity is enlarged [24]. However, the long-term effect on FEV_1 of exposures related to diving is relatively small, so the FEV% is below average [25]. Thus, in this circumstance, unlike in COPD (Section 40.3), the low ratio is evidence for muscular development, not airways obstruction. However, the forced expiratory flow at small lung volume ($FEF_{75\%FVC}$) is also low [26–28]. Part of the explanation may be that many commercial divers are exposed to fumes from welding during their work, but other factors also contribute, including hyperoxia [29], see also Section 35.7.2.

Ventilatory effects of breathing air under pressure. Compression of the respired air raises its density and viscosity. This increases the resistive and inertial components of the work of breathing [30–32]. As a result, for persons briefly exposed to high pressures whilst breathing air the peak expiratory flow, forced expiratory volume, maximal breathing capacity and maximal exercise ventilation are all reduced (Table 35.2). Some of these features of hyperbaria are illustrated elsewhere in the book (see Table 35.3).

Additional features are observed in divers who are exposed to raised pressures for long enough to experience training of the respiratory muscles. This can occur during a saturation dive in which the diver lives for a period of weeks in a hyperbaric environment in which gas density is increased [24, 34]. During such a dive the forced vital capacity can increase as a consequence of training of the respiratory muscles. After return to sea level conditions (1 ATA) the initial level is restored. The half time for recovery is of the order of 4 weeks (Fig. 35.2).

Table 35.2 Effects of breathing air at 3 atmospheres absolute pressure (3 ATA) upon lung function and exercise capacity. Mean results for eight subjects (including one female).

	1 ATA	3 ATA	P*
Forced expiratory volume (FEV_1,l)	4.40	3.79	<0.01
Maximal voluntary ventilation (l min^{-1})	187.5	92.2	<0.01
Maximal exercise ventilation (l min^{-1})	96.4	76.8†	<0.01
Exercise capacity (W)	245	269†	<0.05
Maximal cardiac frequency (min^{-1})	190	191	NS

Source: [33].
* paired *t*-test. NS not significant.
† change from 1 ATA is due to hyperoxia.

Table 35.3 Examples of pressurisation affecting indices of ventilatory capacity.

Aspect	Topic	Location	page
Physical properties of air	Density and viscosity	Table 14.2	154
Dynamic lung function	Maximal breathing capacity	Fig. 14.2	153
	Flow–volume curve	Fig. 14.3	154
Static lung function	Forced vital capacity	Fig. 35.2	490

Physiological effects of hyperoxia. Some physiological systems normally operate under conditions of mild hypoxia. As a result they are affected by a rise in ambient pressure during breathing air as this circumstance raises the oxygen tension of respired gas (Table 35.4).

Hyperoxia associated with hyperbaria lowers the transfer factor by reducing immediately the reaction rate of carbon monoxide with oxyhamoglobin (θ, section 20.7.4). Prolonged hyperoxia reduces erythropoiesis; this is likely to be due to

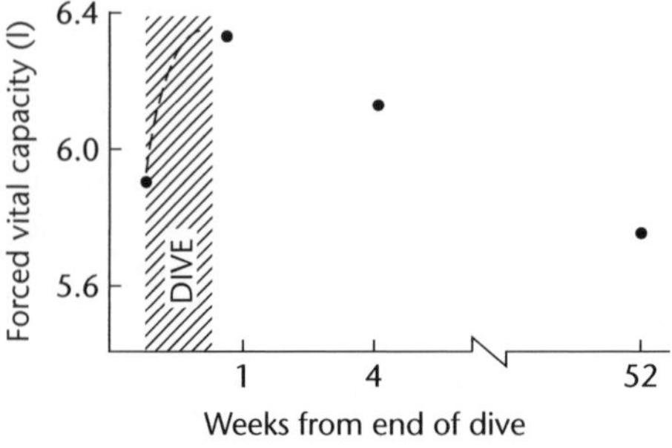

Fig. 35.2 Forced vital capacity in relation to a single saturation dive to 300 m, mean data for 7 men. The half time for recovery was approximately 4 weeks. Source: [34].

Table 35.4 Some physiological consequences of hyperoxia. The pathological consequences are considered subsequently.

Aspect	Effect	Location
Carotid body	Loss of respiratory drive from hypoxia, CO_2, nor-adrenaline, progesterone	Section 23.5 (including Fig. 23.7, page 295)
Oxygen content of blood	Transfer factor (*T*lco) reduced,	Section 20.7.4
	Saturation increases,	Section 21.2.2
	More oxygen in solution,	
	Capacity for exercise increased	This section, also Section 28.8.1
Erythropoietin	Production ceases,	This section
	[Hb] declines slowly	
Cerebral circulation	Loss of hypoxic vasodilatation	Section 23.5.3

suppression of production of erythropoietin [29]. The consequent mild anaemia disappears spontaneously over the weeks after return to sea level conditions.

Exercise during hyperbaria. Most of the features listed in Tables 35.2 to 35.4 impinge on the ability to perform exercise under hyperbaric conditions. The compression of the respired gas reduces the maximal exercise ventilation. Where the gas is air, the compression also raises the oxygen tension and this hyperoxia eliminates chemoceptor drive to breathing. As a result, the ventilation during submaximal exercise is reduced. The ventilation during maximal exercise is also reduced, partly on account of elimination of hypoxic drive, but also because the work of breathing is increased. The changes reduce the excretion of carbon dioxide, so the arterial tension of carbon dioxide is higher than in normal circumstances. At the same time the increased oxygen tension raises the oxygen saturation and the quantity of oxygen carried in solution in arterial blood.

The sequence of events that has been described reduces the volume of blood needed to deliver a given quantity of oxygen to muscle and other tissues. As a result the cardiac frequency and output during submaximal exercise are lower than at atmospheric pressure. However, the maximal frequency and output are not constrained, so the maximal oxygen delivery is greater than in normal circumstances. Hence, during hyperbaria breathing air the maximal oxygen uptake is increased despite a reduction in maximal exercise ventilation. In persons who are habitually exposed to hyperbaria or who do much swimming the exercise capacity is further increased by the training effect of these activities on respiratory and skeletal muscle and the muscle of the heart.

During prolonged exposure to hyperbaric conditions, for example in a man working from a diving support vessel, this sequence of events can be modified by the hyperoxia reducing the production of the red cell promoting hormone erythropoietin. The haemoglobin concentration then falls progressively, but the decline is limited to the duration of the dive which is seldom more than 3 weeks, so the effect on exercise capacity is small. If the work is not physically demanding the associated inactivity is likely to be more detrimental.

35.3.3 Pathological and adaptive changes in the lungs

Acute changes. The principal hazards to the lungs in diving are drowning, (described above), barotrauma from expansion of gas in an enclosed space, decompression sickness that can lead to bubbles lodging in pulmonary capillaries and oxygen toxicity from a rise in oxygen tension. The latter can occur either during a dive or if oxygen is administered during decompression to hasten the elimination of nitrogen. The commonest change is a small reduction in forced vital capacity. In addition, the transfer factor and capacity for exercise can be reduced, usually by an average of 10%–15% [34–36]. The time for restoration of pre-dive values depends on the magnitude of the initial changes and can be 4–6 weeks. There is no apparent evidence for acute changes in forced expiratory flow at small lung volumes.

Long-term changes. Based on results of annual medical examinations, changes in the forced vital capacity of working divers reflect the average depths to which they have been exposed. It increases in men who go progressively deeper and *vice versa* [26]. Conversely, forced expiratory volume can be decreased for a year after a deep dive. In a follow up of men entering initial training courses the transfer factor and flow rate at small lung volume ($FEF_{75\%FVC}$) of 77 professional divers were observed to decline at a faster rate over 6 years of active work compared with policemen of comparable age and physique [27]. The differences were related to the diving exposure, but not to smoking habit or age. These observations suggest that the lung function of professional divers is subject to small long-term changes of occupational origin. The changes in vital capacity may reflect the workload on the muscles of respiration, but for the other changes a toxicological explanation seems probable.

35.4 Barotrauma in divers and submariners

Changes in environmental pressure (either positive or negative) are normally transmitted to gas present in body cavities. This occurs as a result of gas flowing along the normal channel of communication, for example an airway, the Eustachian tube or ostium to a paranasal sinus. Difficulty arises if the channel of communication is restricted or obstructed. Obstruction affecting the middle ear and sinuses, and air in body cavities consequent on recent surgery are considered in Section 34.7.

A lung cyst is another potential cause of difficulty. For the cyst not to be reabsorbed it will have only a limited communication with an airway; this may allow ingress of some air during compression, but not sufficient egress to prevent over-expansion during decompression. In relation to diving the volume changes can be large. For example, during decompression (ascent) from a depth of 30 m (100 ft) to sea level the volume of a closed cyst increases by a factor of four. Where the decompression is rapid the cyst is likely to rupture; air will then escape into the pleura or mediastinum, or into a blood vessel from whence it can become an arterial air embolus (see below). Persons possessing stiff lungs, possibly as a consequence of previous illness, appear to be at particular risk [37, 38]. By contrast, asthmatics can usually dive without incident, though diving is not advised if a subject has experienced asthma symptoms within the previous 48 h or becomes wheezy during exercise or if exposed to cold [39]. Divers and submariners are at high risk of trauma during an emergency ascent from under the sea, for example when escaping from a submarine, or during a training exercise. The effects can be mitigated by slowing the ascent and by conscious expiration whilst it is taking place. However, in susceptible individuals an ascent in shallow water can also be traumatic [38].

35.5 Decompression sickness

35.5.1 Features

Introduction. In divers and caisson workers (tunnellers) decompression sickness can arise from the inert gas constituent of the respired gas; this becomes dissolved in some tissues during exposure to high pressure and is released as bubbles during decompression back to sea level conditions [40, 41]. The commonest gas is nitrogen from breathing compressed air, but in deep saturation dives a helium–oxygen mixture is breathed and the bubbles then contain helium. The organs most likely to be affected are those that are well perfused during pressurisation [42, 43] and are subject to factors such as minor trauma that predispose to the dissolved gas coming out of solution (Section 34.8). Apart from causing local damage, a bubble can enter the blood stream and cause difficulties in the lungs or embolise another part of the body.

The factors that contribute to dissolved gas coming out of solution to form bubbles are as for acute hypobaria (see Section 34.8). However, in hypobaria the source of the bubbles is nitrogen present in solution at sea level and then released as bubbles as a direct consequence of decompression. Much of the nitrogen is dissolved in body fat and the majority of the effects are local ones.

Acute decompression sickness

(i) Occurrence. A reduction in environmental pressure in excess of approximately 50% over a short period of time usually leads to the formation of bubbles; these occur particularly in muscles and in blood vessels, from whence they are carried into the lungs. The bubbles can be visualised by Doppler scans; they are usually asymptomatic.

Symptoms can occur during decompression or during the succeeding 72 h. They usually take the form of localised muscle pains (the bends) which can be intense and incapacitating but not life threatening. Alternatively, bubbles in the lungs can obstruct the pulmonary circulation and cause symptoms including coughing, hence the designation 'the chokes'. The condition may progress to circulatory failure. In addition, the bubbles can give rise to emboli in the systemic circulation. These can lodge anywhere in the body and can either be silent or cause symptoms, depending on the site. Emboli to the brain, retina or spinal cord can be particularly obtrusive. The systemic emboli can be secondary to local pulmonary vasodilatation or the presence of a patent foramen ovale with flow of blood into the left atrium; the latter is a consequence of the bubbles raising the pulmonary vascular pressures [44, 45].

(ii) Treatment. The immediate treatment for acute decompression sickness is to shrink the bubbles by recompression. This should be followed by steps to speed up the elimination of inert gas using one of the methods described below.

In the case of caisson workers and persons operating from diving bells, recompression can be undertaken without delay since the appropriate facilities are at hand. For others, including most divers the treatment will entail travel to a centre where there is a diving compression chamber or high-pressure oxygen chamber. Such centres should be located and contacted in advance of any diving taking place. An applied pressure of 3 ATA is usually appropriate.

(iii) Long-term sequelae of decompression sickness. The sequelae of diving can take any of several forms depending on precipitating factors. The most conspicuous form is in caisson workers who are at a risk of developing aseptic necrosis of the head of the femur. Other joints can also be affected. The condition is due to recurrent emboli consequent on repeated exposure to pressure, plus local trauma. In other workers, repeated small emboli to the central nervous system or spinal cord can cause long-term damage.

35.5.2 Prophylaxis (including saturation dives)

Dives breathing air. Acute decompression sickness is avoided by not exposing susceptible individuals and by limiting the applied pressure to 2 ATA (10-m diving depth). Where higher pressures are used the circumstances should be such that relatively few bubbles form during decompression. For dives performed breathing air under pressure the rate of decompression should match that at which surplus nitrogen is eliminated from the body. To achieve this, the 'ascent' is undertaken in stages according to a predetermined schedule. The first of these was constructed by Haldane [46]. Subsequent commercial schedules have readjusted the balance between risk and economic return to suit local requirements. This process has reached a pinnacle of refinement for very deep dives.

Saturation dives breathing mixtures of three gases. Problems associated with breathing compressed air can be avoided by replacing some of the nitrogen with helium or hydrogen. Both gases have the advantages of having a low density and being relatively insoluble in body tissues; helium is also inert, so is safer to use. The use of a triple gas mixture reduces both the work of breathing and the risks of decompression sickness and nitrogen narcosis compared with using air. Helium has the disadvantages that its presence reduces the clarity of speech, which can become unintelligible. The gas also transmits heat readily, so its use in high concentration can give rise to hypothermia. For these reasons some nitrogen is included in the gas mixture and electrically heated suits may be used. Isolated inner ear decompression sickness is a rare complication [47].

35.5.3 Diving strategies

Diving strategies are determined by the need to avoid the formation of gas bubbles during the return to ambient conditions. Some procedures if not conducted with great care can lead to oxygen toxicity (Section 35.7.2).

There is only a small risk of decompression sickness following dives to a depth of 10 m (2 atmospheres absolute, i.e. 2 ATA), so shallow underwater dives to this depth can usually be of any duration. Dives down to a depth of 50 m (6 ATA), can also be undertaken during breathing air, but the duration must be shorter and the ascent undertaken in stages in order that the quantity of tissue nitrogen is kept within manageable limits. For deeper dives, down to 200 m (20 ATA), this objective is achieved by replacing the ambient air with a gas mixture containing another inert gas, for example helium. The diver is compressed over several days in order to wash out nitrogen and saturate the tissues with the new gas. This is done on shore or in a diving support vessel, from which the divers are transferred under pressure to a diving bell or capsule for operational work. The subsequent return to ambient pressure is undertaken over a period of up to 18 days to allow time for degassing. This process is hastened by breathing oxygen-enriched air in as high a concentration as is considered safe and by reducing the pressure as fast as is practicable. Both procedures have the aim of maximising the proportion of time that divers spend at depth. However, an error of judgement can expose the lungs to damage from hyperoxia [34, 35].

35.6 Screening for fitness to dive

A diver is at risk from a number of potential hazards and may expose others to risk should things go wrong. Hence physical fitness, freedom from pulmonary pathology, training and a diving companion are necessary prerequisite to diving. Health checks should be undertaken annually. Guidelines for recreational diving have been prepared by many interested national societies (e.g. [48]). Commercial and military diving is supervised by official bodies including, in the UK, the Commission for Health and Safety at Work (HSE).

The minimal requirement is for a health questionnaire. Where this is not completely normal, or for greater security, the questionnaire should be supplemented by clinical consultation, measurement of ventilatory capacity (FEV_1 and FVC) and for commercial diving chest radiography. In most circumstances all these investigations should yield normal results [39]. Additional tests, for example measurement of static lung compliance [37], CT scans [49] and a maximal exercise test are normally only recommended in special circumstances.

35.7 Hyperoxia

35.7.1 Summary of O_2 therapy

All tissues of the body depend for their function on an adequate supply of oxygen and elaborate mechanisms exist for this to be achieved. A deficiency that cannot be corrected in an appropriate manner by other means requires relief by administration of oxygen. Some methods are listed in Table 35.5.

Depending on the application, the oxygen is provided at a low, medium or high partial pressure. A modest enrichment of the inspired air is appropriate for patients with respiratory distress syndrome, including premature infants [50, 51] and for respiratory patients. In the latter instance an inspired oxygen concentration in the range 25%–40% is used to correct hypoxaemia due to uneven lung function ($\dot{V}_A/\dot{Q}$ inequality, Section 18.4.4). This dosage is appropriate for acute incidents, ambulatory oxygen (Table 35.6) and long-term domiciliary oxygen therapy (LTOT); the latter is administered for 16–22 h daily to prolong life in patients who are at risk of cor pulmonale [52] (see also Section 36.3). For LTOT the source of oxygen is usually an oxygen concentrator or liquid oxygen supply. The condition of the patient should meet internationally accepted criteria of suitability for treatment (Table 35.6), as the regimen is both costly and demanding and if embarked on without a good prospect of benefit can add to the patient's difficulties.

An enrichment in excess of 30% does not normally confer an additional benefit. This is because gas exchange is now taking place on the flat top part of the oxyhaemoglobin dissociation curve where the oxygen saturation is relatively constant (Section 21.2.2). Additional oxygen may actually cause harm by putting the patient at risk of carbon dioxide narcosis (*q.v.*). However,

Table 35.5 Methods for providing and administering oxygen.

Equipment	Features	Application
Plant producing liquid oxygen	Provides 100% O_2 in transportable form	Most hospitals O_2 trolley for personal use
Compressed O_2 (cylinders)	Convenient but cylinders heavy to move	Most clinics. Back up for concentrator
Oxygen concentrator	Produces 30–90% O_2 on site. Is relatively cheap	Any. Ideal for remote sites, ambulances, domiciliary use
Nasal prongs	Low dosage (2–4 l min^{-1})*	Respiratory and other patients
Needle into trachea	Effective but invasive. Risk of infection	
Venturi mask	Controlled dosage (25–40% O_2)*	Respiratory patients
Mask with bag (no valve)	Allows rebreathing of exhaled CO_2	High altitude
Oxygen visor		
Mask; bag fitted with one-way valve. Other 'demand' systems can have similar features	Is efficient provided mask fits the face without leaks	Can deliver 60% O_2 for general medical use. Use with portable oxygen apparatus (Fig. 28.19, page 405).
Oxygen tent	Is versatile but needs close supervision. Risk of fire	Neonates, infants, patients who are restless
Compression chamber or capsule	Subject breathes oxygen under hyperbaric conditions	Treatment of air embolism, gangrene and other conditions

* Flow during expiration is wasted

Table 35.6 Oxygen for patients with COPD that is clinically stable over 3 weeks.

Method	Indication	Comment
LTOT	$Pa,O_2 < 7.3$ kPa (55 mm Hg) on two occasions 3 weeks apart whilst clinically stable *Or* Pa,O_2 in range 7.3–8 kPa (55–60 mm Hg) + another feature such as: Congestive heart failure Pulmonary hypertension Polycythaemia Nocturnal hypoxaemia ($SaO_2 < 90\%$ for more than 30% of night)	Raising Pao_2 to >8 kPa (60 mm Hg) at night and for >8 h during day prolongs life. Its quality needs to be safeguarded
Ambulatory O_2	Mobility increased and breathlessness decreased by reduction in exercise ventilation (Section 28.8.1) Fall in SaO_2 on exercise is reversed	Patient must be determined to be active outside the house

Source: [53].

this possibility is a reason for vigilance, not for administering too little oxygen, see also Footnote 35.1

A relatively high enrichment to achieve a concentration of approximately 60% O_2 is used for patients with pulmonary oedema or where an increase in the quantity of oxygen in solution in blood would be beneficial. In either of these circumstances a higher enrichment might be desirable on physiological grounds, but carries a risk of oxygen toxicity. Oxygen under pressure (hyperbaric oxygen therapy) can be used for treating a limited number of disorders where the benefits are likely to outweigh the considerable risks that are incurred.

Footnote 35.1. The general advice that chronic respiratory patients are best treated with oxygen in low dosage may not apply to ambulatory oxygen used to increase mobility. In this circumstance an enrichment of 50% can be more effective (e.g. Fig. 28.19, page 405).

35.7.2 Pathological effects of a raised oxygen tension

Carbon dioxide narcosis. Respiration is normally driven by the inherent activity of respiratory and related centres in the brain with supplementary inputs from central and peripheral receptors; these are activated by chemical and other stimuli (see Chapter 23). The most important stimuli are from the carotid bodies which respond particularly to hypoxaemia. Respiratory drive from this source is eliminated by a modest increase above normal in arterial oxygen tension. The loss of hypoxic drive is of little consequence except when other respiratory drives are reduced. One example is the oxygen paradox, described below. More important causes include depression of respiratory drive by morphine or other drug and hypercapnia associated with an increase in work of breathing. In either of these circumstances uncontrolled administration of oxygen can seriously depress respiratory drive, with potentially fatal consequences. The following is a hypothetical example:

> A patient is admitted to hospital with an acute chest illness. He is anxious and talkative and on examination, in addition to having physical signs related to the chest, is cyanosed and is breathless on slight exertion. The heart rate and the frequency of respiration are increased. Arterial P_{O_2} is 5.3 kPa (40 mm Hg), P_{CO_2} is 8 kPa (60 mm Hg) and the blood pH is within normal limits (7.45 to 7.35 pH units). The patient is prescribed antibiotics and oxygen via a non-rebreathing mask (e.g. Hudson). The oxygen improves his colour and relieves his anxiety and breathlessness; he relaxes and is left to sleep undisturbed. It is noted that his colour is a healthy pink, his pulse is full and his hands are warm to touch. Later, the nursing staff find that he is difficult to rouse; the arterial P_{CO_2} is 13 kPa (100 mm Hg) and the blood pH has fallen to 7.20. The life of the patient is now in jeopardy from carbon dioxide narcosis caused by inappropriate oxygen therapy.
>
> *Comment.* The prescription was correct to the extent that oxygen was to be given continuously; intermittent oxygen could have led to cerebral damage from hypoxia. However, supervision was inadequate. A trial of low dosage oxygen (in the range 24%–28%) should have been carried out. In the event of hypercapnia persisting this treatment ought to have been supplemented by measures to increase ventilation.

Oxygen toxicity. A molecule of oxygen is activated by progressively binding four electrons to form a series of reactive substances (reactive oxygen species). These are superoxide anion ($.O_2^-$), peroxide anion which converts to hydrogen peroxide (H_2O_2) and hydroxyl radical (.OH). The addition of another electron leads to the formation of water. The superoxide anion can react with inorganic substances including iron in the ferric state, copper and nitric oxide [54]. It can also disrupt proteins, enzymes and nucleic and fatty acids. These processes are initiated by a rise in the tension of oxygen in inspired gas; they have been investigated in experimental animals and the consequences have been observed in man [55].

The seriously disruptive effects of the reactive species of oxygen have led to the formation of antioxidant defences. Those in tissue cells include the enzymes superoxide dismutase, catalase and glutathione peroxidase and the vitamins C and E (ascorbic acid and α-tocopherol). In the plasma, the enzyme CuZn superoxide dismutase (SOD) has a similar role, whilst the protein albumin can act as a scavenger. However, not all the actions of the reactive species are undesirable. For example, they may contribute to some beneficial effects of hyperbaric oxygen therapy [56].

Exposure to oxygen in excess of about 50 kPa (375 mm Hg) causes congestion and proliferation of pulmonary capillaries; the changes are secondary to destruction of alveolar endothelium and usually progress to pulmonary oedema and to death within 3 to 7 days [57]. Similar histological changes have been observed at postmortem in patients who received prolonged oxygen therapy; the oxygen has usually been given by assisted ventilation [50]. This 'pulmonary respiratory syndrome' is a serious complication of respiratory distress in the newborn [51]. In premature infants the oxygen can also cause spasm of the incompletely developed retinal vessels. This condition is reversible in the early stages, but if the cause is not removed can progress to retrolental fibroplasia. Oxygen toxicity also occurs in divers who are exposed to inappropriately high tensions of oxygen at depth or when oxygen is inhaled during decompression to hasten the elimination of nitrogen (Section 35.5.3).

The early features of oxygen toxicity include cough, retrosternal pain, tracheal inflammation, a reduced velocity of mucus flow and a small diminution in vital capacity. If the condition is not reversed at this stage it can progress to florid respiratory distress syndrome (Section 41.12) and can threaten life. The toxic effects of oxygen are aggravated by a rise in the metabolic rate as a result of exercise, hyperthermia, coexisting viral infection or high blood levels of catecholamines, cortisone and thyroxine. The effects are minimised by adrenergic blockade, anaesthesia and anti-oxidant drugs. Hypercapnia is an additional risk factor, whilst the risk of oxygen toxicity is reduced if the exposure to hyperoxia is intermittent.

The present evidence suggests that subjects at sea level can breathe oxygen in a fractional concentration of 0.7 (70% O_2 in N_2) for up to 24 h and at an F_{I,O_2} of 0.5 (50% O_2) for a period of months without developing symptoms, though anaemia can occur from suppression of the production of erythropoietin. Higher exposures can be unsafe on account of oxygen toxicity. This risk has been modelled in terms of a unit pulmonary toxic dose (UPTD) and the relationship used to construct oxygen tolerance curves for different circumstances [58]. Additional risks from breathing 100% O_2 are atelectasis (Sections 18.4.4, 18.4.5 and 34.7) and that the circumstances constitute a fire hazard.

Oxygen toxicity is seldom a problem for respiratory patients in whom the main requirement is for a low dosage of oxygen to correct hypoxaemia secondary to $\dot{V}_A/\dot{Q}$ inequality (see above). Patients receiving oxygen for treatment of circulatory failure are theoretically at risk of oxygen toxicity since the optimal dosage is at the lower end of the range at which the condition might occur. However, the underlying condition is often self-limiting and, provided the treatment is supervised, the risk to the patient is small.

Oxygen poisoning. Exposure to oxygen at a pressure of 2 bar or above can cause oxygen poisoning in which the subject convulses and loses consciousness. This change is preceded by pallor and an ill-defined sense of unease. The risk of poisoning is related to the pressure that is applied and the duration of exposure. The predisposing and the ameliorating factors are similar to those for oxygen toxicity. The condition is avoidable.

35.7.3 Hyperbaric O_2 therapy

Indications. The use of a hyperbaric chamber permits the recompression of subjects who have developed acute decompression sickness as a result of diving, work in a caisson or in relation to aviation (Section 34.8). The compression is followed by decompression at a slower rate. The process of eliminating nitrogen can be speeded up by combining pressurisation with administration of oxygen. However, in relation to aviation active pressurisation is only likely to be required for the occasional severe case. Re-compression to sea level conditions is normally a sufficient treatment. A hyperbaric chamber can also be used for treating patients with oxygen under pressure.

Hyperbaric oxygen therapy is of confirmed value for cerebral gas embolisation [59], gas gangrene, carbon monoxide poisoning [60] also page 513, delayed radiation injuries [61] and some types of tissue ischaemia. However, for promoting healing of a wound topical oxygen may also be effective [62]. Attempts to demonstrate a worthwhile therapeutic role in multiple sclerosis have yielded mainly negative results [63].

Methods. The treatment can be delivered in a compression chamber such as is normally part of an underwater diving facility. This accommodates both patient and attendants and is suitable for bulk treatments or relatively complex or emergency procedures. But the facility occupies space, is expensive to run and exposes staff to a risk of chronic decompression sickness (Section 35.5.1). In a hospital setting, for example a radiotherapy or paediatric department, a single person capsule is often preferable. The capsule is small, transparent (usually made from 'perspex' which is polymethyl methacrylate) and relatively inexpensive, but access to the patient is restricted. Artificial ventilation and cardiac arrest procedures cannot be carried out during the period of hyperbaria.

The pressure chamber contains air and personnel enter or leave via a pressure lock. The patient is supplied with oxygen via a mask. To avoid leaks this should envelop the face and the oxygen should be supplied under slight positive pressure with respect to the pressure in the chamber. A similar arrangement is also suitable for use with a pressure capsule. Alternatively, the capsule can be filled with 100% oxygen, but there is then a heightened risk of fire. The temperature and humidity in the capsule are controlled by air-conditioning and the exhaled carbon dioxide is removed by re-circulation of the gas in the capsule through a canister containing soda lime. The physical isolation of the patient is partly overcome by the good visual and oral communication with the operator, and by the continuous monitoring of both the patient's respiration and heart rate and the pressure and composition of the gas in the capsule. At a pressure of 2 bar the duration of each treatment can be up to 2 h with a repeat after 1 h. For radiotherapy a pressure of 3 bar and duration of up to 40 min can be employed.

Complications. A routine treatment is normally without incident, but complications can occur from human error, a failure of equipment, a change in the procedure to accommodate unrelated ill health or pathology associated with the medical condition (Table 35.7).

Overall view. An operational hyperbaric chamber should be accessible to centres where diving is carried out. Such a chamber should also be used therapeutically. However, due to the associated drama and high cost there is a tendency for those concerned to emphasise the therapeutic successes and under play the failures. There is an urgent need for more cost/benefit analyses *vis-à-vis* other treatments [64]. For inland centres a decision on whether or not to establish a facility might await the outcome of research now in progress [65].

Table 35.7 Possible complications of hyperbaric oxygen therapy.

Circumstances	Conditions
During pressurisation	Atelectasis, barotrauma affecting nasal sinuses and eustacean tube (for which prophylactic myringotomy can be helpful)
At pressure	Oxygen toxicity, convulsions
Decompression	Pulmonary barotrauma leading to surgical emphysema or pneumothorax Vascular embolism (chokes)
Collateral damage	To target organ (e.g. brain) To adjacent structures (e.g. a facial bone)
Incidental complication	Deep vein thrombosis, injury etc.
Staff in compression chamber	Injury, barotrauma, complication of repeated pressurisation (e.g. necrosis of head of femur)

35.8 References

1. Cotes JE, Steel J. *Work-related lung disorders.* Oxford: Blackwell Scientific, 1987.
2. McLean SP. Hinrichs RN. Influence of arm position and lung volume on the center of buoyancy of competitive swimmers. *Res Q Exerc Sport* 2000; **71**: 182–189.
3. Edholm OG, Weiner JS, eds. *Principles and practice of human physiology.* London: Academic Press, 1981: 111–190.
4. Fenner PJ. Drowning. In: Warrell D, Cox TM, Firth JD, Benz EJ., eds. *Oxford textbook of medicine.* 4th ed. Oxford, UK: Oxford University Press, 2005.
5. Moon RE, Long RJ. Drowning and near-drowning. *Emerg Med (Fremantle)* 2002; **14**: 377–386, also 354–355.
6. Bierens JJ, Knape JT, Gelissen HP. Drowning. *Curr Opin Crit Care* 2002; **8**: 578–586.
7. Leddy JJ, Roberts A, Moalem J et al. Effects of water immersion on pulmonary function in asthmatics. *Undersea Hyperb Med* 2001; **28**: 75–82.
8. Derion T, Roddan WG, Lanphier EH. Static lung load and posture effects on pulmonary mechanics and comfort in underwater exercise. *Undersea Biomed Res* 1992; **19**: 85–96.
9. Taylor NA, Morrison JB. Static respiratory muscle work during immersion with positive and negative respiratory loading. *J Appl Physiol* 1999; **87**: 1397–1403.
10. Andersson JP, Liner MH, Fredsted A, Schagatay EK. Cardiovascular and respiratory responses to apneas with and without face immersion in exercising humans. *J Appl Physiol* 2004; **96**: 1005–1010.
11. Butler PJ, Jones DR. Physiology of diving of birds and mammals. *Physiol Rev* 1997; **77**: 837–899.
12. Manley L. Apnoeic heart rate responses in humans. A review. *Sports Med* 1990; **9**: 286–310.
13. Lopez-Majano V, Data PG, Martignoni R et al. Pulmonary blood flow distribution in erect man in air and during breathhold diving. *Aviat Space Environ Med* 1990; **61**: 1107–1115.
14. Derion T, Guy HJ. Effects of age on closing volume during head-out water immersion. *Respir Physiol* 1994; **95**: 273–280.
15. Derion T, Guy HJ, Tsukimoto K et al. Ventilation-perfusion relationships in the lung during head-out water immersion. *J Appl Physiol* 1992; **72**: 64–72.
16. Thorsen E, Skogstad M, Reed JW. Subacute effects of inspiratory resistive loading and head-out water immersion on pulmonary function. *Undersea Hyperb Med* 1999; **26**: 137–141.
17. Lund KL, Mahon RT, Tanen DA, Bakhda S. Swimming-induced pulmonary oedema. *Ann Emerg Med* 2003; **41**: 251–256.
18. Ferretti G, Costa M. Diversity in and adaptation to breath-hold diving in humans. *Comp Biochem Physiol A Mol Integr Physiol* 2003; **136**: 205–213.
19. Mukhtar MR, Patrick JM. Ventilatory drive during face immersion in man. *J Physiol* 1986; **370**: 13–24.
20. Delapille P, Verin E, Tourny-Chollet C, Pasquis P. Ventilatory responses to hypercapnia in divers and non-divers: effects of posture and immersion. *Eur J Appl Physiol* 2001; **86**: 97–103.
21. Hong SK, Rahn H The diving women of Korea and Japan. *Sci Am* 1967; **216**: 34–43.
22. Stolp BW, Lundgren CEG, Piantadosi CA. Diving and immersion. In: Crystal RG, West JB, Weibel ER, Barnes PJ, eds. *The lung: scientific foundations.* 2nd ed. Philadelphia: Lippincott-Raven, 1997; 2699–2712.
23. Tetzlaff K, Friege L, Koch A et al. Effects of ambient cold and depth on lung function in humans after a single scuba dive. *Eur J Appl Physiol* 2001; **85**: 125–129.
24. Fisher AB, DuBois AB, Hyde RW et al. Effect of 2 months' undersea exposure to N2-O2 at 2.2 Ata on lung function. *J Appl Physiol* 1970; **28**: 70–74.
25. Bouhuys A, Beck GI. Large lungs in divers? *J Appl Physiol* 1979; **47**: 1136–1137.
26. Davey IS, Cotes JE, Reed JW. Relationship of ventilatory capacity to hyperbaric exposure in divers. *J Appl Physiol* 1984; **56**: 1655–1658.
27. Skogstad M, Thorsen E, Haldorsen T, Kjuus H. Lung function over six years among professional divers. *Occup Environ Med* 2002; **59**: 629–633.
28. Tetzlaff K, Friege L, Reuter M et al. Expiratory flow limitation in compressed air divers and oxygen divers *Eur Respir J* 1998; **12**: 895–899.
29. Thorsen E, Segadal K, Kambestad BK. Mechanisms for reduced pulmonary function after a saturation dive. *Eur Respir J* 1994; **4**: 4–10.
30. Vail EG. Hyperbaric respiratory mechanics. *Aerospace Med* 1971; **42**: 536–546.
31. Hesser CM, Linnarsson D, Fagraeus L. Pulmonary mechanics and work of breathing at maximal ventilation and raised air pressure. *J Appl Physiol* 1981; **50**: 747–753.
32. Van Liew HD. Mechanical and physical factors in lung function during work in dense environments. *Undersea Biomed Res* 1983; **10**: 255–264.
33. Craik MC. *Physiological and clinical aspects of breathlessness assessed using the visual analogue scale.* PhD Thesis, University of Newcastle upon Tyne, 1988.
34. Cotes JE, Davey IS, Reed JW, Rooks M. Respiratory effects of a single saturation dive to 300m. *Br J Ind Med* 1987; **44**: 76–82.
35. Thorsen E, Hjelle J, Segadal K, Gulsvik A. Exercise tolerance and pulmonary gas exchange after deep saturation dives. *J Appl Physiol* 1990; **68**: 1809–1814.
36. Dujic Z, Eterovic D, Denoble P et al. Effect of a single air dive on pulmonary diffusing capacity in professional divers. *J Appl Physiol* 1993; **74**: 55–61.
37. Colebatch HJH, Smith MM, Ng CKY. Increased elastic recoil as a determinant of pulmonary barotrauma in divers. *Respir Physiol* 1976; **26**: 55–64.
38. Tetzlaff K, Reuter M, Leplow B et al. Risk factors for pulmonary barotrauma in divers. *Chest* 1997; **112**: 654–659.
39. BTS fitness to dive group. British Thoracic Society guidelines on respiratory aspects of fitness for diving. *Thorax* 2003; **58**: 3–13.
40. Barratt DM, Harch PG, Van Meter K. Decompression illness in divers: a review of the literature. *Neurolog* 2002; **8**: 186–202.
41. Andersen HL. Decompression sickness during construction of the Grerat Belt Tunnel, Denmark. *Undersea Hyperb Med* 2002; **29**: 172–188.
42. Ketty SS. The theory and application of the exchange of inert gas at the lungs and tissues *Pharm Rev* 1951; **3**: 1–41.
43. Srinivasan RS, Gerth WA, Powell MR. Mathematical models of diffusion-limited gas bubble dynamics in tissue. *J Appl Physiol* 1999; **86**: 732–741.
44. Wilmshurst PT, Pearson MJ, Walsh KP et al. Relationship between right-to-left shunts and cutaneous decompression illness. *Clin Sci* 2001; **100**: 539–542.

45. Foster PP, Boriek AM, Butler BD et al. Patent foramen ovale and paradoxical systemic embolism: a bibliographic review. *Aviat Space Environ Med* 2003; **74**: B1–B64.
46. Hamilton FT, Bacon RH, Haldane JS, Lees E. *Report of a committee appointed by the Lords Commissioners of the Admiralty to report upon the conditions of deep water* divin (C.N. 1549). London: HMSO, 1907.
47. Doolette DJ, Mitchell SJ. Biophysical basis for inner ear decompression sickness. *J Appl Physiol* 2003; **94**: 2145–2150.
48. Jenkins C, Anderson SD, Wong R et al. Compressed air diving and respiratory disease. A discussion document of the Thoracic Society of Australia and New Zealand. *Med J Aust* 1993; **158**: 275–279.
49. Millar IL. Should computer tomography of the chest be recommended in the medical certification of professional divers. *Br J Sports Med* 2004; **38**: 2–3.
50. Raghavendran K, Kulaylat MN, Thompson B, Ambrus JL. Respiratory distress syndrome: principles and current therapy. *J Med* 2002; **33**: 147–165.
51. Weinberger B, Laskin DL, Heck DE, Laskin JD. Oxygen toxicity in premature infants. *Toxicol Appl Pharmacol* 2002; **181**: 60–67.
52. Sin DD, McAlister FA, Man SF, Anthonisen NR. Contemporary management of chronic obstructive lung disease: scientific review. *JAMA* 2003; **290**: 2301–2312.
53. Royal College of Physicians. *Domiciliary oxygen therapy services.* London: Royal College of Physicians, 1999: 1–49.
54. Halliwell B, Gutteridge JMC. Oxygen toxicity, oxygen radicals, transition metals and disease. *Biochem J* 1984; **219**: 1–14.
55. Crapo JD, Barry BE, Foscue HA, Shelburne J. Structural and biochemical changes in rat lungs occurring during exposure to lethal and adaptive doses of oxygen. *Am Rev Respir Dis* 1980; **122**: 123–143.
56. Hink J, Jansen E. Are superoxide and/or hydrogen peroxide responsible for some of the beneficial effects of hyperbaric oxygen therapy? *Med Hypothesis* 2001; **57**: 764–769.
57. Folz RJ, Piantadosi CA, Crapo JD. Oxygen toxicity. In: Crystal RG, Barnes PJ, West JB, Weibel ER, eds. *The lung; scientific foundations,* Vol 2. 2nd ed. New York: Lippincott-Raven, 1997: 2713–2722.
58. Clark JM, Lambertsen CJ. Pulmonary oxygen toxicity: a review. *Pharmacol Rev* 1971; **23**: 37–133.
59. Benson J, Adkinson C, Collier R. Hyperbaric oxygen therapy for iatrogenic cerebral arterial gas embolism. *Undersea Hyperb Med* 2003; **30**: 117–126.
60. Gorman D, Drewry A, Huang YI, Sames C. The clinical toxicology of carbon monoxide. *Toxicology* 2003; **187**: 25–38.
61. Feldmeier JJ, Hampson NB. A systematic review of the literature reporting the application of hyperbaric oxygen. *Undersea Hyperb Med* 2002; **29**: 1–3.
62. Gordillo GM, Sen CK. Revisiting the essential role of oxygen in wound healing. *Am J Surg* 2003; **186**: 259–263.
63. Bennett M, Heard R. Hyperbaric oxygen therapy for multiple sclerosis. *Cochrane Database Syst Rev* 2004; **1**: CD003057.
64. Guo S, Counte MA, Romeis JC. Hyperbaric oxygen technology: an overview of its application, efficacy and cost-effectiveness. *Int J Technol Assess Health Care* 2003; **19**: 339–346.
65. Saunders PJ. Hyperbaric oxygen therapy in the management of carbon monoxide poisoning, osteoradionecrosis, burns, skin grafts and crush injury. *Int J Technol Assess Health Care* 2003; **19**: 521–525.

Further reading

Brubakk A, Neuman T, eds. *Bennett and Elliott's physiology and medicine of diving.* 5th ed., London: WB Saunders, 2001.

CHAPTER 36

Cold, Heat and the Lungs

In evolutionary times mankind developed strategies to protect against thermal hazards. The hazards are still present and may increase as a result of environmental changes.

36.1 Outline of thermal physiology

Body temperature

The maintenance of a relatively constant core body temperature enables mammals including man to operate in a wider range of environments compared with other species. The temperature is normally in degrees Celsius; the conversion to Fahrenheit is given in Table 6.6 (page 56). The core temperature is usually recorded in the oesophagus or at the tympanic membrane. Urinary temperature is similar. These temperatures are near to that of the thermal control centres in the hypothalamus, whilst the oral and rectal temperatures are, respectively, lower and higher by approximately 0.3–0.6°C. Within the core the local temperatures vary reflecting both the metabolic activity of different organs and the relative thermal balance of the several parts of the body. During normal living the core temperature is maintained at a steady level within broad limits of approximately 35°C to 41°C. This range is optimal for most enzymatic processes, whilst outside it the function deteriorates so that eventually the cells die. The upper limit for survival is about 42°C, but the lower limit is much less at approximately 25°C [1] when the onset of ventricular fibrillation is the likely terminal event. During exercise the thermal controls are relaxed and the core temperature rises progressively. The limit is determined by hyperthermia depressing the central neural drive to skeletal muscles [2]. The temperature rise associated with exercise is less during pregnancy [3].

Conditioning the inspired air

See Section 3.2.

Autonomous temperature regulation

Temperature is sensed in the hypothalamus and the skin, especially that of the face and the epithelium of the proximal respiratory tract. The thermal information interacts with that from the carotid chemoreceptors at a number of levels. The information is the basis for autonomic regulation of body temperature by variation in the loss of heat from the skin through control of the calibre of arterio-venous anastomotic pathways; these determine the distribution of blood flow as between the skin, and deeper structures.

Heat. In a hot environment heat is dispersed from the skin. Some heat is also lost from the lungs, but except in a cold environment the quantity is small. The situation is different in hairy mammals, amongst whom thermal panting is the principal physiological mechanism for heat loss. In man the principal mechanism for heat loss is active secretion and evaporation of sweat. The stimulus is a rise in core body temperature and the response appears to be mediated by an increase in the secretion of growth hormone by the anterior pituitary gland [4].

In a hot environment the blood flow to the skin and the volume of blood in superficial vessels are increased. The increased flow is achieved by both a rise in cardiac output and diversion of flow from other organs and tissues [1]. The increased cardiac output is associated with an increase in cardiac frequency but, due to the additional blood in the skin the stroke volume is below normal. This affects performance during maximal exercise when the cardiac output is sub-optimal so less blood flow is available for the working muscles. Reduced muscle blood flow is usually the main factor limiting exercise in the heat [5]. In addition the hyperthermia can act directly by impairing the function of the cerebral cortex [2].

Repeated or continuous exposure to heat increases the capacity of the subject to disperse heat by evaporation of sweat. The process of acclimatisation entails a reduction in basal metabolism, an increase in blood volume, hypertrophy of sweat glands and a reduction in the salt content of the sweat. The stimulus is a rise in core temperature independent of skin temperature. The process is remarkably effective since, even in a cold environment, exposure to heat for as short a time as 4 h per day can materially improve heat tolerance [1,6].

Cold. In cold conditions conservation of heat by cutaneous vasoconstriction is supplemented by increased internal production. The principal short-term mechanism is shivering, which is mediated centrally [7]. In infancy additional heat can be produced from subcutaneous brown fat, but this ability is lost during childhood. In the longer term, additional heat is generated by enhanced sensitivity to the calorigenic action of noradrenaline and by increased activity of the thyroid gland leading to a rise in basal metabolism. Hairy mammals can also improve their thermal insulation by pilo-erection, a process that is represented in man by 'goose-flesh'. Acclimatisation to cold only occurs to a limited extent [1] mainly through an increase in metabolic heat production. Additional food intake by increasing the quantity of subcutaneous fat might also be expected to help.

Cold air is dry and when inhaled takes much heat and moisture from the airways. This water vapour is then lost in the exhaled air. Over a period of time the quantity of water lost in this way can become substantial.

Volitional temperature regulation

The autonomic control mechanisms adjust the body to a wide range of thermal environments. They are normally supplemented by voluntary actions taken in response to a person feeling too hot or too cold. The measures can be directed to the environment, the internal heat production and the processes of heat exchange. The effectiveness of the measures can be described quantitatively by thermal balance equations [1]. The principal measures that can be taken are summarised in Table 36.1.

Table 36.1 Volitional temperature regulation.

Aspect	Aspect	Action
Environment	Temperature	Heating or cooling the air
	Radiant heat load	Moving into sun or shade
	Convection	Altering local air flow
	Conduction	Immersion in hot or cold water
	Evaporation	Drying or humidifying the air
Internal heat production	Metabolic	Level of food intake, Stimulant or bland drinks
	Activity	Rest or exercise
	Passive	Hot or cold drinks
Local thermal balance	Thermal insulation	More or less clothing
	Convection	Garments open or tight weave, loose or close fit
	Radiation	Light or dark clothing
	Evaporation	Normal or increased fluid intake, clothing dry or damp

Individual variation

There is considerable individual variation in tolerance of inclement thermal environments. A long, lean physique is an advantage in the heat whilst its converse improves tolerance to cold. The differences are reflected in the traditional physiques of the inhabitants of hot and cold regions of the world. They are also apparent as between men and women and in participants in sports where a particular physique can confer a thermal advantage (e.g. subcutaneous fat in swimmers, Section 35.2). Such differences can be supplemented by traditions and local knowledge, for example amongst the bush people of Southwest Africa and Australian Aboriginals in their traditional environments. Independent of these factors the physiological capacity to tolerate heat is to some extent genetically determined [8].

Age

Tolerance of a sub-optimal thermal environment is reduced in the very young and the elderly. In infants and especially those who are born prematurely the compensatory mechanisms are imperfect and this may contribute to sudden infant death syndrome [9, 10]. In the elderly thermal intolerance is mainly a consequence of somatic and behavioural changes associated with ageing [11]. In addition, there is an age-related deterioration in the control of skin sympathetic nerve activity in response to changes in ambient temperature; the impairment appears not to extend to muscle sympathetic activity, but body fluid distribution during exercise in the heat can be affected [12, 13].

Interaction between thermal regulation and hypoxia

Depending on the circumstances the responses to thermal stimuli and to hypoxia can mutually reinforce or neutralise each other. This is evidence that the two sets of control mechanisms to some extent overlap. Exposure to hypoxia reduces the cutaneous perception of cold [14]. This might lead to a person at altitude or a hypoxic elderly patient not taking appropriate action in response to cold. Hypoxia also diverts blood flow into the splanchnic vascular bed at the expense of blood flow to the skin [15]. This reinforces the immediate cutaneous vasomotor response to cold, but can seriously impair the body's defences against hyperthermia. Other interactions are considered below.

36.2 Normal respiratory responses to cold

36.2.1 Acute effects

Cooling the skin. Sudden cooling of the skin, as by immersion of the trunk in cold water, can cause an immediate inspiration followed by transient hyperventilation [16, 17]. The initial gasp can then lead to inhalation of water and subsequently to apnoea (Section 35.2). A less strong cutaneous stimulus can cause transient hyperventilation that results in hypocapnia sufficient to reduce blood flow to the brain. There is then a risk of the subject becoming disorientated or developing syncope.

Controlled cooling of the skin can be used to suppress a rise in body temperature such as occurs with fever or during exercise. In the latter circumstance, preventing the normal rise in core temperature reduces the ventilation and is accompanied by hypercapnia [18]. This has been taken as evidence for a thermal component to regulation of exercise ventilation. An alternative explanation is given below.

Cooling the face. Cooling that is largely confined to the face may elicit a diving response (Section 35.3.1). This can include pulmonary vasoconstriction that is accentuated by hypoxia; the two effects are additive [19, 20]. Conversely, pulmonary vasoconstriction due to hypoxia can be aggravated by the subject being exposed to cold. In this way the cold can increase the risk of mountain sickness (Section 34.5).

Cooling upper and lower airways. Breathing cold air through the nose stimulates local thermal receptors [21]. Their activation reduces the ventilatory response to hypercapnia including the slope and intercept of the regression of ventilation on arterial tension of carbon dioxide (S and C of eqn. 23.3, page 294). The changes contribute to hypoxaemia that in turn may be a factor in cold-induced pulmonary hypertension (see above). Depending on the species, the principal effect on ventilation can be to reduce either tidal volume, as has been reported in man [21] or respiratory frequency, as in calves [19]. Concurrently the nasal resistance rises.

In healthy persons who are not atopic or exposed to polluted air, the airways resistance and forced expiratory volume are unaffected by breathing cold air through the nose, taking exercise that entails mouth breathing during exercising at subzero temperature or undergoing a cold water challenge test. However, approximately 50% of atopic individuals who are otherwise asymptomatic experience some bronchoconstriction during cold stimulation of the lower airways; in this circumstance their exercise capacity is reduced [22, 23]. Some non-atopic subjects may bronchoconstrict if the air is extremely cold (e.g. –50°C). Any bronchoconstriction increases the work of breathing and this reduces the capacity for exercise. Where cooling is accompanied by peripheral hypothermia this also impairs the ability to perform exercise by reducing the mobility of joints, impairing sensation and reducing the oxidative capacity of enzyme systems in the muscles.

Lowering the core temperature. Lowering the core temperature normally causes shivering. This raises the consumption of oxygen and the ventilation needed to sustain it. With further cooling shivering ceases and the level of ventilation falls. This is part of a generalised deterioration in all bodily functions. The respiratory consequences include hypoxaemia, hypercapnia, respiratory acidosis and bronchodilatation. Respiratory responsiveness to hypoxia and other stimuli is reduced [20]. At this stage the changes can only be reversed by external intervention. At temperatures below 27°C death by ventricular fibrillation is the likely outcome.

Transfer factor. Under quiet resting conditions the transfer factor is increased by exposure to cold insufficient to cause shivering, but not by a cold pressor test when the transfer factor can be reduced. The former response reflects a redistribution of blood volume between the lungs, skin and other organs (Fig. 36.1), whilst the latter could be due to pulmonary vasospasm [24–26]. Both influences might operate for persons taking a sauna when any changes in transfer factor are small [27].

36.2.2 Longer term effects

Prolonged inhalation of cold air in arctic regions or from work in a cold store can have an adverse effect on the lungs. In extreme conditions it can cause frostbite. With lesser cooling the beat frequency of cilia is reduced. This impairs the removal of debris and contributes to an increased prevalence of respiratory symptoms. Concurrently, the resistance of central airways rises and the ventilatory capacity is somewhat reduced. The bronchial reactivity to carbachol has been observed to increase, but not that to breathing cold air [28]. Residents in cold places can experience additional damage to the lungs from smoking and from air pollution consequent on the ventilation of dwelling places being reduced in order to conserve heat.

36.3 Cold in respiratory patients

Some respiratory patients experience bronchoconstriction and breathlessness when exposed to cold air, whilst in others the breathlessness is ameliorated and they feel more comfortable. Others again are unaware of any changes. How an individual patient will respond is likely to reflect the extent and type of respiratory impairment (Type 1 or Type 2, Section 38.5), the mode of exposure to cold (cutaneous or lower respiratory tract), the initial thermal environment (warm, temperate or cold) and the blood oxygen tension.

Bronchoconstriction. Some asthmatic and chronic obstructive pulmonary disease (COPD) patients report that they develop symptoms of chest tightness, wheeze and/or increased breathlessness on exertion if exposed to cold air, for example when leaving a building in cold weather or at night. The changes reduce the ability to take exercise and are ameliorated by measures to promote bronchodilatation (Section 15.7.2). The symptoms are an integrated response to cooling the skin (usually the face and hands) and breathing cold air through the mouth. The relative contributions of these two stimuli appear to vary with circumstances [29–31]. Cold air entering the nose raises the resistance of the nasal passages but probably not that of the lung airways [32]. The cutaneous component of the bronchoconstrictor response is independent of those due to other provocations including metacholine and exercise.

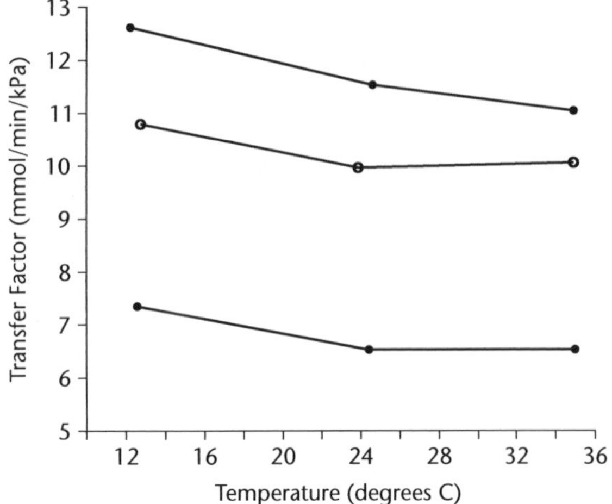

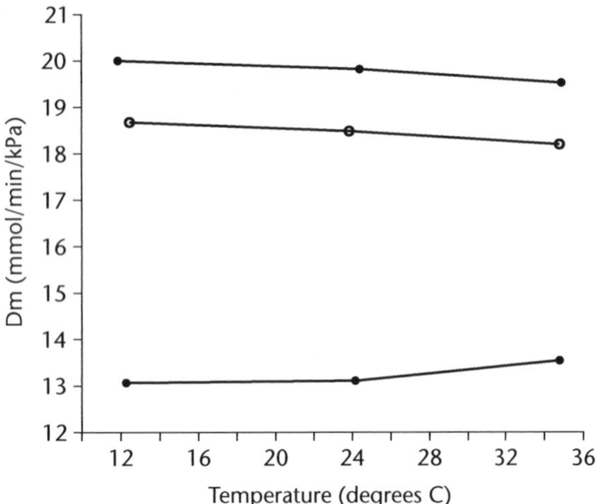

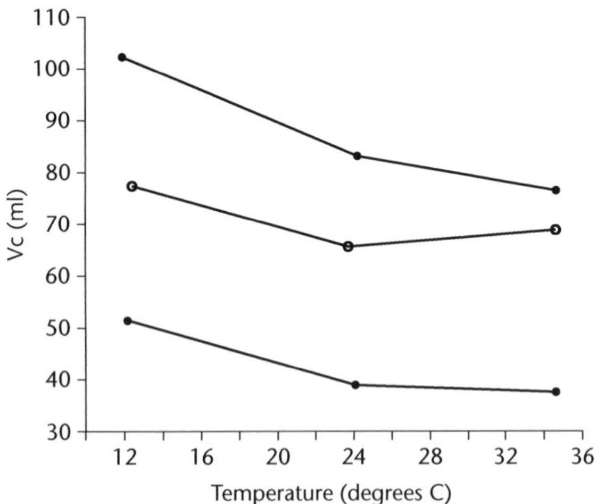

Fig. 36.1 Effect of environmental temperature on *T*l,co, *D*m,co and *V*c. Each point is the mean of two estimates measured in an environmental chamber. Subjects: top lines – white male, age 21, 1.70 m, 65 kg; middle lines – white male, age 37, 1.65 m, 59 kg; bottom lines – Asian female, age 23, 1.52 m, 48 kg. Source: Smith S, Chinn DJ, Aftab NA, Cotes JE (unpublished).

A patient who experiences bronchoconstriction in response to cold is likely to respond by using his or her aerosol inhaler, withdrawing from the cold environment and taking steps to reduce or avoid any future exposure to cold. In the short term some relief is likely to be experienced by adjusting the clothing to cover the face.

Hypoventilation and related features. In healthy persons and some animals an exposure to cold can reduce the hypercapnoeic component of respiratory drive. Part of the evidence is summarised above. It can be relevant for patients who become acutely breathless at night, some of whom will move to an open window or use a fan to relieve their symptoms. A similar reduction in symptoms and an increase in capacity for exercise has been reported in patients with advanced COPD (mean FEV_1 0.99 l) during breathing cold air through the mouth [33]. This effect is secured by the cold stimulus reducing the level of exercise ventilation and hence the dyspnoeic index (Section 28.7). In appropriate circumstances the response is beneficial. However, the benefit is secured at the cost of the hypoventilation causing hypoxaemia; this can interact with cold to aggravate pre-existing pulmonary hypertension due to the disease [34]. The risk to the patient can be increased by the cold also reducing awareness of cold and hence the stimulus to volitional remedial action [14]. As a result the core temperature may fall and the patient is then at imminent risk of death from hypothermia. This hazard is likely to be reduced by long-term oxygen therapy for relief of pulmonary hypertension (LTOT) since the oxygen eliminates the part of the response to cold that is attributable to hypoxia.

36.4 Respiration in a hot environment

In healthy young adults living in a temperate climate the standard indices of lung function at rest, including forced expiratory volume and vital capacity, peak expiratory flow and transfer factor are not much affected by acute exposure to a hot environment (32°C). The calibre of small lung airways is increased, possibly as a consequence of reduced bronchomotor tone [24]. On exercise there can be shallow breathing, alveolar hyperventilation and the related changes reported under autonomous temperature regulation above. Undue fatigue can occur from accumulation of reactive oxygen species in muscles that are active [35, 36].

The shallow breathing and associated increase in respiratory drive reflect the role of thermal panting as a mechanism for disposing of heat via the lungs. The responses are initiated by a rise in temperature in the hypothalamus, but involve the carotid chemoreceptors and dopamine as a chemical mediator [37]. The hyperventilation causes a respiratory alkalosis that displaces to the right the relationship of ventilation to arterial tension of carbon dioxide (Fig. 23.7, page 295).

36.5 References

1. Edholm OG, Weiner JS. Thermal physiology. In: Edholm OG, Weiner JS, eds. *Principles and practice of human physiology.* London: Academic Press 1981; 111–190.

2. Nielsen B, Nybo L. Cerebral changes during exercise in the heat. *Sports Med* 2003; **33**: 1–11.
3. Lindqvist PG, Marsal K, Merlo J, Pirhonen JP. Thermal response to submaximal exercise before, during and after pregnancy: a longitudinal study. *J Matern Fetal Neonatal Med* 2003; **13**: 152–156.
4. Jorgensen JO, Krag M, Kanaley J et al. Exercise, hormones and body temperature. Regulation and action of GH during exercise. *J Endocrinol Invest* 2003; **26**: 838–842.
5. Gonzalez-Alonso J, Calbet JA. Reductions in systemic and skeletal muscle blood flow and oxygen delivery limit maximal aerobic capacity in humans. *Circulation* 2003; **107**: 824–830.
6. Hori S. Adaptation to heat. *Jpn J Physiol* 1995; **45**: 921–946.
7. Doufas AG, Wadhwa A, Lin CM et al. Neither arm nor face warming reduces the shivering threshold in unanesthetized humans. *Stroke* 2003; **34**: 1736–1740.
8. Heled Y, Moran DS, Mendel L et al. Human ACE I/D polymorphism is associated with individual differences in exercise heat tolerance. *J Appl Physiol* 2004; **97**: 72–76.
9. Dollberg S, Demarini S, Donovan EF, Hoath SB. Maturation of thermal capabilities in preterm infants. *Am J Perinatol* 2000; **17**: 47–51.
10. Mitchell EA, Williams SM. Does circadian variation in risk factors for sudden infant death syndrome (SIDS) suggest there are two (or more) SIDS subtypes? *Acta Pediatr* 2003; **92**: 991–993.
11. Kenney WL, Munce TA. Invited review: ageing and human temperature regulation. *J Appl Physiol* 2003; **95**: 2598–2603.
12. Grassi G, Seravalle G, Turri C et al. Impairment of thermoregulatory control of skin sympathetic nerve traffic in the elderly. *Circulation* 2003; **108**; 729–735.
13. Morgan AL, Sinning WE, Weldy DL. Age effects on body fluid distribution during exercise in the heat. *Aviat Space Environ Med* 2002; **73**: 750–757.
14. Golja P, Kacin A, Tipton MJ et al. Hypoxia increases the cutaneous threshold for the sensation of cold. *Eur J Appl Physiol* 2004; **92**: 62–68.
15. Minson CT. Hypoxic regulation of blood flow in humans. Skin blood flow and temperature regulation. *Adv Exp Med Biol* 2003; **543**: 249–262.
16. Keating WR, Nadel J. Immediate respiratory response to sudden cooling of the skin. *J Appl Physiol* 1965; **20**: 65–69.
17. Cooper KE, Martin S, Riben P. Respiratory and other responses in subjects immersed in cold water. *J Appl Physiol* 1976; **40**: 903–910.
18. Cotes JE. The role of body temperature in controlling ventilation during exercise in one normal subject breathing oxygen. *J Physiol (Lond)* 1955; **129**: 554–563.
19. Busch MA, Tucker A, Robertshaw D. Interaction between cold and altitude exposure on pulmonary circulation of cattle. *J Appl Physiol* 1985; **58**: 948–953.
20. Giesbrecht GG. The respiratory system in a cold environment. *Aviat Space Environ Med* 1995; **66**: 890–902.
21. Burgess KR, Whitelaw WA. Effects of nasal receptors on pattern of breathing. *J Appl Physiol* 1988; **64**: 371–376.
22. Millqvist E, Johansson A, Bende M, Bake B. Effect of nasal air temperature on FEV_1 and specific airways conductance. *Clin Physiol* 2000; **20**: 212–217.
23. Helenius IJ, Takkanen HO, Haahtela T. Exercise-induced bronchospasm at low temperature in elite runners. *Thorax* 1996; **51**: 628–629.
24. Aftab N, Chinn DJ, Cotes JE, Smith SL. Effect of ambient temperature on airway function in man. *J Physiol (Lond)* 1987; **391**:65P.
25. Mishra N, Marya RK, Mahajan KK. Effect of cold challenge on alveolar capillary blood volume in normal individuals. *Indian J Physiol Pharmacol* 1990; **34**: 255–258.
26. Gastaud M, Dolisi C, Bermon S et al. Short-term effect of cold provocation on single-breath carbon monoxide diffusing capacity in subjects with and without Raynaud's phenomenon. *Clin Exp Rheumatol* 1995; **13**: 617–621.
27. Kiss D, Popp W, Wagner C et al. Effects of the sauna on diffusing capacity, pulmonary function and cardiac output in healthy subjects. *Respiration* 1994; **61**: 86–88.
28. Jammes Y, Delvolgo-Gori MJ, Badier M et al. One-year occupational exposure to a cold environment alters lung function. *Arch Environ Health* 2002; **57**: 360–365.
29. Koskela HO, Koskela AK, Tukiaineu HO. Bronchoconstriction due to cold weather in COPD. The roles of direct airway effects and cutaneous reflex mechanisms. *Chest* 1996; **110**: 632–636.
30. Skowronski ME, Ciufo R, Nelson JA, McFadden ER Jr. Effects of skin cooling on airway reactivity in asthma. *Clin Sci (Lond)* 1998; **94**: 525–529.
31. Kaminski RP, Forster HV, Bisgard GE et al. Effect of altered ambient temperature on breathing in ponies. *J Appl Physiol* 1985; **58**: 1585–1591.
32. McLane ML, Nelson JA, Lenner KA et al. Integrated response of the upper and lower respiratory tract of asthmatic subjects to frigid air. *J Appl Physiol* 2000; **88**: 1043–1050.
33. Spence DPS, Graham DR, Ahmed J et al. Does cold air affect exercise capacity and dyspnoea in stable chronic obstructive pulmonary disease? *Chest* 1993; **103**: 693–696.
34. Bedu M, Giraldo H, Janicot H et al. Interaction between cold and hypoxia on pulmonary circulation in COPD. *Am J Respir Crit Care Med* 1996; **153**: 1242–1247.
35. Reid MB, Haack KE, Franchek KM et al. Reactive oxygen in skeletal muscle. 1. Intracellular oxidant kinetics and fatigue in vitro. *J Appl Physiol* 1992; **73**: 1797–1804.
36. Moopanar TR, Allen DG. Reactive oxygen species reduce myofibrillar Ca^+-sensitivity in fatiguing mouse skeletal muscle at 37°C. *J Physiol* 2005; **564**: 189–199.
37. Bonora M, Gautier H. Role of dopamine and arterial chemoreceptors in thermal tachypnea in conscious cats. *J Appl Physiol* 1990; **69**: 1429–1434.

CHAPTER 37

Airborne Respiratory Hazards: Features, Protective Mechanisms and Consequences

Human activities and natural phenomena combine to pollute the air we breathe. This chapter describes the defences of the lungs and some consequences of their not being able to respond adequately in all circumstances.

37.1 Introduction

Epidemiological perspective. The volcanic eruption that destroyed the ancient civilisation of Crete is possibly the first where the acute and subacute effects of severe air pollution were recorded at the time (Book of Exodus, Chapters 12 and 13). The causal association was established retrospectively. However, even in those days the dust in mines and quarries was perceived to be harmful. The ill effects were described in increasing detail from the 16th century onwards [1–3], attempts were made to reduce the level of urban air pollution [4] and questions were asked about possible harm from tobacco smoke [5]. The lethal effect of air pollution became apparent in a fog that enveloped London in early December 1952. This coincided with the annual Smithfield cattle show where some cattle died (see Footnote 37.1). Subsequently, it became apparent that thousands of people died as well. Most deaths were respiratory, but mortality from cardiovascular disease was also increased [6].

A subsequent epidemiological survey showed that much respiratory ill health was associated with the presence of small airborne particles (diameter $< 10\mu m$) [7]. The most active fraction

Footnote 37.1. The proportion of deaths was higher for the cattle that won prizes than amongst the others. This was probably due to the prize-winning cattle being kept exceptionally clean, so their stalls contained less ammonia from urine than in the other stalls. The ammonia provided protection by neutralising the acid mist from sulphur dioxide in the air.

Table 37.1 Potential lung contaminants and defences against them.

Class of substance	Constituents	Quasi-physical defence, internal and (external)	Biological defence mechanisms*
Gas Vapour	CO, NO_2, O_3, SO_2 etc Volatile substances	Apnoea, shallow breathing, exhalation	Neutralisation by cellular action (chemical, biochemical or immunological)
Aerosol (mist)	Micro-organisms (e.g. in droplets from a cough or sneeze), chemicals (*as from an inhaler*)	Exhalation (Irradiation of air)	Protective reflexes
Particulate	Spores, debris, desiccated droplets, respirable dusts and fibres, ultrafine particles	Impaction or sedimentation followed by clearance (Dust suppression, precipitation or filtration)	Muco-ciliary escalator Ingestion by macrophages with subsequent disposal

* In some circumstances the responses are themselves harmful.

was possibly ultrafine particles (diameter $< 0.1\mu m$ (100 nm)) that formed during combustion [8]. The effect of the particles can be enhanced by the presence of toxic gases and other inhaled pollutants, including those in exhaust from motor vehicles and in tobacco smoke. Many of these pollutants also act independently [9].

Circumscribed pollution. Some pollutants, for example ultrafine particles and gases that enter the atmosphere pollute the entire planet. Others pollute more locally so might be said to target particular communities. The target can be a whole city, such as Los Angeles or Canterbury, New Zealand where stationary cold air, trapped by inversion of the normal thermal gradient can sometimes act as a blanket. Alternatively, the target population can be people working in a particular industry or occupation that generates a harmful dust or vapour. Particular buildings can be a source if they are contaminated by solvents and other chemicals.

Prevention is usually effective where there is circumscribed pollution that is closely identified with a particular source. This is the case for many occupational airborne pollutants. The associated disorders have largely been eliminated, or the development of new cases prevented by application of research in occupational epidemiology, dust physics and the quantitative relationships of exposure to indices of ill health. These fields of endeavour have, and are being helped by information about respiratory defence mechanisms, epidemiological techniques (Chapter 8) and the effects of inhaled materials on lungs.

Biological perspective. An impressive number of diseases are caused by breathing air that contains potentially harmful particles. These penetrate or evade the lungs' defences and cause damage at the site of deposition or elsewhere. Much of the damage is due to the pollutant or pollutants interacting with each other and with inflammatory cells to release reactive oxygen species in the lungs [10, 11], also Section 35.7.2.

The damage is minimised by biological defence mechanisms that purify the respired gas, dispose of material that comes in contact with airway epithelium and inactivate that which enters the lung parenchyma. The location of the primary defences varies between mammalian species. In rodents they are mainly in the nose, but in man they are shared between the upper and lower parts of the respiratory tract. The classes of substances and the types of defences against each of them are listed in Table 37.1.

37.2 Responses to physical properties of inhaled substances

37.2.1 Reflex responses

Protective reflexes. Sneezing expels substances that alight on receptors in the nose and coughing performs a similar function for material in the larger airways (Sections 3.3.11 and 13.6). The responses are effective against single or clusters of droplets or particles. In the case of a major exposure the reflexes can alert a subject to take appropriate action. In addition, the larynx can close in response to strong local stimulation such as might be provided by a small insect or large particle. The closure is usually followed by forced expiration and coughing. Irritant gases can stimulate pulmonary J receptors (Section 23.3.4) and cause apnoea followed by evasive action. Alternatively, the depth of breathing can be reduced [12]. None of these mechanisms protect against extended exposures.

Bronchoconstriction. Particles that settle or impact on the walls of airways can stimulate receptors to cause reflex bronchoconstriction [13] and hence characteristic changes in lung function (e.g. Fig. 15.1, page 168). The constriction is dose dependent [14] (Fig. 37.12, page 520) and leads to more impaction of particles by increasing their forward velocity. It also promotes sedimentation by reducing the distance through which particles can fall. As a result, cleansing of the inspired air by sedimentation is enhanced

Table 37.2 Clearance of particles and fibres from respired gas

Aerodynamic diameter (μm)	Principal mechanism	Main site*	Clearance (%)
>20	Sedimentation	General atmosphere	100
20–7	Impaction	Nose, oropharynx, carina	100
7–5	Impaction, interception (fibres)	Nose, carina, bronchial bifurcations	80
5–0.5	Sedimentation	Bronchioles, alveoli	50†
0.5–0.05	Diffusion	Alveoli	25
0.05–0.01	Diffusion	Alveoli, bronchioles, bronchi	40

* Particles and most fibres deposited in conducting airways are cleared via muco-ciliary escalator.
† For mouth breathing. With nose breathing the clearance is greater and the alveolar deposition is reduced to approximately 25% (see also Fig. 37.3).
Source: [15].

and particles are deposited more proximally than would otherwise be the case. That this may protect the respiratory epithelium deeper in the lungs can be surmised from the observation that, for a given exposure to antigen, smokers are less likely to develop extrinsic allergic alveolitis than non-smokers (Section 37.7.5). However, other explanations are possible.

37.2.2 Cleansing mechanisms

Droplets either have the characteristics of particles or they are unstable and shrink through evaporation of water. They then become droplet nuclei that remain suspended in air until conditions are right for them to expand through coalescence and taking up water vapour. Such droplets usually drift downwards under the influence of gravity so are removed from the air by sedimentation. The process is often slow as it begins from a position of floating in air and the density of the droplet does not much exceed unity. Solid particles have a higher density and exist in a wide range of shapes and sizes. Their behaviour in airways can be described in terms of their momentum and aerodynamic diameter. The latter is the diameter of a sphere of unit density having the same terminal settling velocity in air as the particle or fibre under consideration. In the case of a spherical particle the aerodynamic diameter is the product of the particle diameter and square root of the density ($D \times \rho^{0.5}$) (see Table 37.3). Fibres behave like particles of similar diameter.

The biologically important range of aerodynamic diameters is 20–0.01μm. Where the aerodynamic diameter exceeds 20μm the particles quickly fall out of the air by sedimentation, so they are only inhaled in exceptional circumstances. Below 0.01μm the particles remain suspended almost indefinitely so are expired (Table 37.2). Relatively large particles (diameters 20–8 μm) deposit in the nose or oropharynx (Fig. 37.1).

Particles of intermediate size enter the respiratory tract; here most are removed from the air stream by the processes of impaction, sedimentation or diffusion. Those that alight on bronchial mucus are transported by cilia to the oro-pharynx (the muco-ciliary escalator). The material is subsequently swallowed or expectorated. Some respirable particles (aerodynamic diameter < 3μm) settle in respiratory bronchioles. These are ingested by phagocytic cells. Some macrophages migrate proximally towards the mouth and join the muco-ciliary escalator, whilst others enter the substance of the lungs. Particles that penetrate the airways can move by diffusion into the alveoli and may then enter the alveolar capillaries or interstitium. The airway cleansing mechanisms in healthy persons are summarised in Table 37.1 and their effectiveness is indicated in Figs 37.2 and 37.3. However, the data do not apply to subjects with impaired ciliary function such as smokers and others with damaged airways (Sections 3.3.3, 37.3 and 41.3.2).

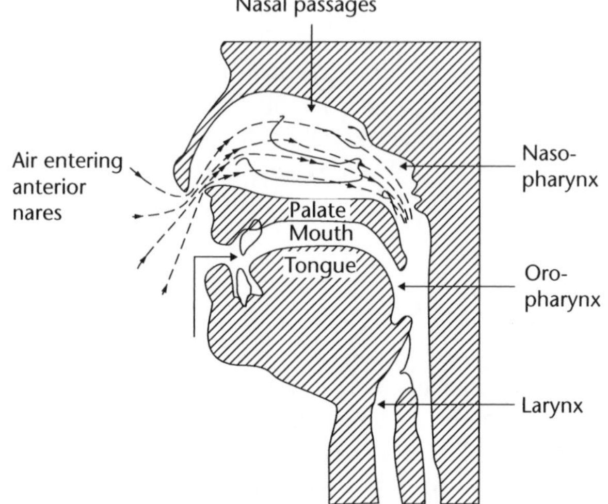

Fig. 37.1 Cross-section of the naso-pharynx. The small cross-sectional area of the anterior nares results in a high linear velocity being imparted to the incoming air. Any associated particles are given a high forward momentum that leads to their impacting on the anterior ends of the turbinate bones. Source: [16].

Impaction. occurs when a particle that enters the lungs fails to follow the line of airflow but carries on under its own momentum

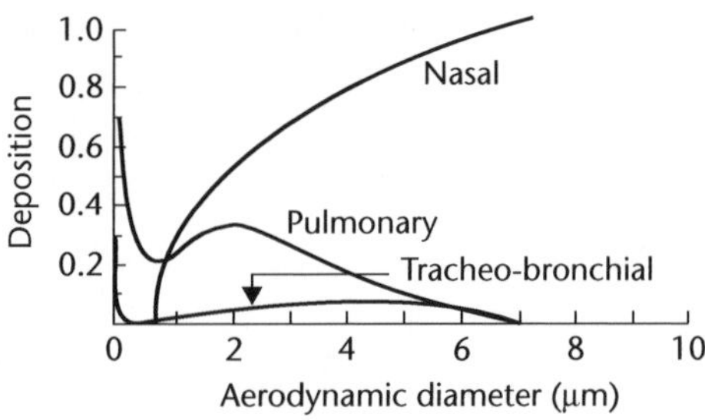

Fig. 37.2 Fractional deposition of particles in the respiratory tract for a subject breathing at a respiratory frequency of 15 min^{-1}, tidal volume 1.45 l. The model is that of the Task Force on Lung Dynamics of the Health Physics Society. Source: [17], see also [18].

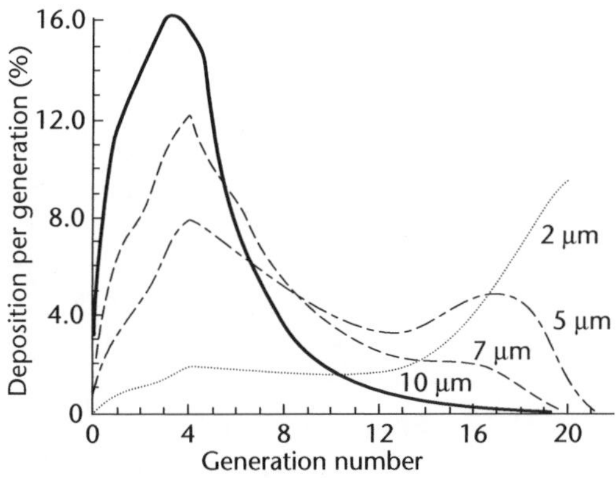

Fig. 37.3 Deposition of inhaled particles by airway generation. Source: [19].

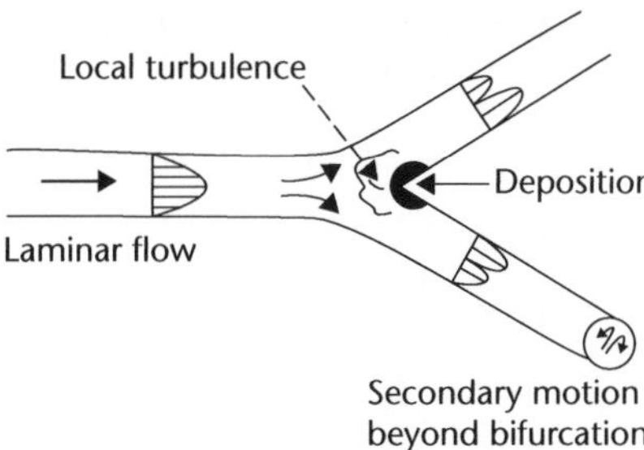

Fig. 37.4 Model airway showing flow profiles and deposition of suspended material at a bifurcation. Source: adapted from [20].

to impact with the respiratory epithelium. In the nose impaction is with the turbinates. In the airways it is with the carinae at the bifurcation of the trachea and the origins of large bronchi (Fig. 37.4).

The process of impaction removes from the inspired gas almost all particles of aerodynamic diameter greater than 7 μm. Nose breathing is rather more effective than mouth breathing, but the difference is small. The probability of impaction varies directly with the velocity of airflow, hence is increased by

Table 37.3 Symbols and abbreviations used in equations.

Symbol	Definition	c.g.s units	SI units
D	Particle diameter	cm	μm
d	Airway diameter	cm	μm
V	Mean air velocity	cm s^{-1}	m s^{-1}
ρ	Density of particle	g cm^{-3}	kg m^{-3}
ρa	Density of air	g cm^{-3}	kg m^{-3}
η	Viscosity of air	g cm^{-1} s^{-1} (poise)	N s m^{-2}
g	Gravitational acceleration	981	–

exercise. It varies inversely with airway diameter, so is enhanced by bronchoconstriction. The relationship between these variables is described by the Stokes number:

$$\text{Stokes number}(N) = \rho D^2 V/9\eta d \quad (37.1)$$

It also varies with the Reynolds number and hence the kinematic viscosity of air ($\eta/\rho a$, Section 14.3.4) [19, 21]. The symbols used in the relationships are given in Table 37.3.

Sedimentation. Particles sediment under the influence of gravity and other factors that contribute to the settling velocity. Then, according to the Stokes law,

$$\text{Settling velocity} = (\rho - \rho a) D^2 g/18\eta \quad (37.2)$$

Sedimentation occurs mainly in the naso-pharynx and smaller bronchi and bronchioles. It affects mainly particles in the size range 5–2 μm of which approximately 30% are deposited and for the most part expectorated (see above). The remainder are exhaled. The balance between sedimentation and exhalation is influenced by airway diameter (see 'Bronchoconstriction' above) and by the time that the material is in the lungs. This in turn is a function of the pattern of breathing, including any breathholding.

Fibres. The settling velocity of a fibre resembles that of a sphere of the same diameter and is nearly independent of fibre length. However, long or curved fibres (e.g. crysotile asbestos) are less likely to negotiate bends in the airways than short, straight ones (e.g. amosite asbestos), so they may deposit on airway walls by interception [22].

Diffusion. Ultrafine particles (aerodynamic diameter less than 0.5 μm) are jostled by other particles (i.e. they exhibit Brownian motion) so are more likely to come into contact with and adhere to the walls of small airways and alveoli as a result of diffusion. The process is time dependent. The trapped particles enter the lung parenchyma and alveolar capillaries. They can be present in vast numbers and can then be an important cause of ill health (Section 37.5).

Table 37.4 Methods of respiratory protection.

Method	Sub-category	Detail
Substitution	Use alternative process or safer materials	
Segregation	Sealed cabinet	Operator uses sleeved gloves or remote sensors
Dust suppression or removal	Exhaust ventilation	
	Water spray or infusion	
	Tools operated at slow speed	
Breathing apparatus	Closed circuit	Absorber for CO_2
		Supply of oxygen
		Circulating fan (optional)
	Open circuit	Supply of clean compressed air (portable air pump or compressed air line)
Respirator	Can need power assistance if filters have high resistance	Physical, electrostatic and/or chemical filters

37.2.3 Hygiene standards and external respiratory protection

Hygiene standards. The body's defences against breathing polluted air can be supplemented by external protection. This has the objective of reducing the concentration of respirable material to a predetermined level (the hygiene standard) that can be tolerated for an appropriate period. The hygiene standard is usually expressed as a recommended exposure limit, but other terminologies are also used, for example 'threshold limit value' (TLV), 8-h time weighted average concentration (for regular work) and short-term exposure limit (e.g. up to 15 min). The approved level is for gases in parts per million and for concentration of respirable particles and fibres (aerodynamic diameter $< 7\mu$m) in mg m^{-3} or fibre count per m^3. Hygiene standards are subject to regular review [23].

Methods of external respiratory protection. Where possible the protection should be directed to the source of pollution and not to the person who is exposed (Table 37.4). However, this may not be practicable in an emergency situation or if the exposure only occurs occasionally, as when cleaning inside a furnace.

Personal protection is provided by use of a respirator or breathing apparatus. The former employs physical or chemical means to purify the respired gas, whilst the latter delivers a supply of clean air to the nose and/or mouth. The method should be appropriate to the circumstances. Any personal equipment should provide a leak-free contact with the subject. This normally entails having face masks in a range of shapes and sizes that can accommodate different facial dimensions, particularly those of the bridge of the nose and around the mouth or chin. The face piece should be fitted individually and preferably tested for leaks. This can often be done by getting the subject to inhale gently whilst the air inlet is obstructed. A more rigorous test is to expose the subject to a test substance, for example an agent that causes lacrimation or one whose presence in the respired gas can be monitored externally. For someone with a beard an air hood may be preferable. A principal requirement is that the equipment should be tolerable and preferably comfortable to wear and not impose too great a resistance to breathing in circumstances when the equipment is to be used. Ideally the resistance should not reduce the ventilatory capacity during heavy exercise (Table 7.2, page 60), but in practice the wearer may have to settle for that which can be tolerated for the required time [24]. In appropriate circumstances a respirator can materially reduce the quantity of dust entering the lungs [25].

37.2.4 Clinical relevance of the dimensions of particles (see also individual substances below)

Material that enters the airways and is not removed by protective mechanisms deposits on the respiratory tract where it can have a local action, an effect elsewhere in the lung or a systemic action. These processes have great clinical importance, including for delivering therapeutic agents (e.g. see Further reading).

Bronchodilatation. The target organ for bronchodilatation is the network of conducting airways containing smooth muscle in their walls. The muscle is relaxed mainly by pharmacologically active particles of diameter 3–6 μm that settle on the airway walls. Maximal sedimentation is achieved by using particles within this size range (monodispersed), taking a relatively deep breath at a not too fast rate and breath holding after the aerosol has been inhaled [26, 27]. However, in clinical practice the aerosol delivery is usually sub-optimal. In addition, the inhaled cloud usually contains particles of a wide range of sizes. Some particles settle out before they enter the lungs and some deposit either in the pharynx or in peripheral parts of the respiratory tract; the latter then enter the blood stream and can cause side effects. Ensuring that a higher proportion of each inhalation reaches its target improves cost-effectiveness and reduces side effects.

Transmission of infection. The common cold, influenza and many bacterial infections are transmitted by droplets that are inhaled. The process entails generation of an aerosol by sneezing or coughing. The droplets so formed can infect an adjacent person by impacting in the anterior nares or settling in the nasopharynx. Other droplets are desiccated to form 'droplet nuclei' that can remain suspended in air for long periods. The process of desiccation kills some viruses but puts other organisms into a form where they can settle in respiratory bronchioles, become ingested into phagocytic cells and enter the substance of the lungs. Pulmonary tuberculosis is usually transmitted in this way.

Droplets can be intercepted at source by use of an oro-nasal mask. The concentration of infected nuclei can be reduced by dilution with fresh air, exposure to sunlight or irradiation with ultraviolet light. Irradiation can be undertaken in the ducts of air conditioning equipment.

Hay fever/asthma. The hypersensitivity reaction is initiated by airborne antigenic material releasing mediator substances in the nasal epithelium or lower respiratory tract. The nose can be affected by particles of a wide range of sizes. Material that enters the lower respiratory tract will have been inhaled as small particles (aerodynamic diameter 1–5 μm). Within this range the larger particles deposit on the walls of conducting airways. The most active particles, such as fragments of house dust mite, cause exudation of enzymes and other pharmacologically active substances that act directly on the bronchial smooth muscle. The smaller particles settle mainly in respiratory bronchioles and some of these are activated after ingestion by phagocytic cells. The risk factors include individual susceptibility, the dose of inhaled antigen (itself influenced by any residual bronchoconstriction) and the effectiveness of the muco-ciliary escalator. Clearance via the escalator is often impaired as part of the allergic reaction.

Occupational dusts and fibres. Industrial processes generate many types of airborne particles and fibres. Those that damage the lungs do so if they accumulate at a vulnerable site. The location is determined by the physical characteristics of the inhaled material (Table 37.5). Some of the consequences are presented in subsequent paragraphs.

37.3 Tobacco smoke (also marijuana)

Overview. Tobacco smoke contains substances that can damage the lungs and cardiovascular system. The changes are most marked in smokers, but also affect non-smokers who are exposed to environmental tobacco smoke (i.e. passive smoking) in places of work, restaurants, public forums and at home. Children of parents who smoke are at greatest risk if they are asthmatic [28]. In utero exposure to tobacco products can damage the lungs both directly and by reducing the body weight at birth [28, 29]. It may have long term consequences (see Further reading).

The practice of smoking usually starts at about the time of puberty, but may begin earlier, for example during the daily bus journey to school. Young people who develop conspicuous airway narrowing then often discontinue, but may persevere on account of pressure from others. They are then at high risk of lung disease in later life, as are those who give up and then resume the habit [30]. The cultural factor is strong in some communities, for example parts of India where there is a high prevalence of childhood emphysema. The use of a mild, low tar, non-irritant tobacco is another risk factor since it is better tolerated, but in many respects is no less harmful than more irritant types of leaf [31, 32].

Table 37.5 Examples of inter-dependence between physical characteristics of airborne material, lung anatomy and lung diseases.

Site	Process	Agent	Disease
Carinae in large airways	Impaction (high momentum)	Asbestos fibres Particles containing tar (e.g. from tobacco)	Carcinoma
Respiratory bronchioles	Sedimentation, ingestion by phagocytes	Mineral particles (diam. 2–5 μm)	Pneumoconiosis
	Smoking causing narrowing of small airways	Clearance of spores and other material is increased	Incidence of EAA is reduced*
Pleura	Entry via lung tissue	Asbestos fibres (chemical effect) Crocidolite or other fine lance-like material (physical effect)	Pleural plaques Mesothelioma
Alveoli	Inhalation into lung parenchyma†	Toxic gases Ultrafine particles†	Alveolitis (acute or chronic) (Atherosclerosis)

* EAA is extrinsic allergic alveolitis (Section 37.7.5).

† Can pass into alveolar capillaries and from there reach other parts of the body.

Classification of smoking status. In most circumstances smoking status can be described as never smoked, current smoker, ex-smoker (quit more than 3 months ago) and passive smoker (Section 8.2.6). The smoking category can be subdivided into light or heavy (>14 cigarettes per day) or by the amount smoked. This can be expressed as grams per day. Additional refinements can include the daily intake of tar, nicotine or carbon monoxide, whether or not the subject inhales, and other features of the pattern of smoking. In most circumstances the variance in lung function attributable to these aspects is small in comparison to that due to whether or not the subject smokes [33]. Duration of smoking can be expressed in years and total cigarette consumption in pack years, where one pack year is a tobacco consumption of 20 cigarettes per day for one year. The term can mislead as it is highly correlated with age (Section 5.6.2). Very recent exposure to tobacco smoke can be assessed from measurement of alveolar carbon monoxide concentration (Section 20.7.1). Smoking over the previous week is reflected in the quantity of cotinine in body fluid, whilst an estimate of cumulative exposure over the preceding months can be obtained from the nicotine content of hair [34].

Pathological effects of tobacco smoke. Tobacco smoke affects the lungs both directly by its physical presence and through the actions of its constituent substances. The aerosol stimulates receptors in lung airways to cause bronchoconstriction. Amongst the constituents of tobacco smoke, carbon monoxide impairs the respiratory function of the blood by combining with haemoglobin, reduces the capacity for exercise, and damages the myocardium (Section 37.4.1). It also affects the measurement of transfer factor by methods based on carbon monoxide (Section 20.7.1). Ultrafine particles cause alveolitis and predispose to intravascular thromboses (Section 37.5). Tar, superoxides, ozone and oxides of sulphur and nitrogen exert an irritant effect upon the bronchial epithelium, affect adversely the cilia, damage the Clara cells that produce CC10 (Clara cell 10 kDa protein) [35] and release proteolytic enzymes from alveolar macrophages. These changes acting in combination enlarge the airspaces by digesting the substance of the lung. The resulting emphysema is particularly conspicuous in persons with an inherited deficiency of α_1-antitrypsin (PiZZ), e.g. [36]. The changes reduce the elastic recoil of the lungs, lead to narrowing of small lung airways and reduce both FEV_1 and the capacity of the lung to transfer gas [37, 38].

In addition to constituents that affect lung function, tobacco tar contains benzo(a)pyrene that can cause cancer. This occurs mainly at bifurcations (carinae) in the larger airways, where concurrent impaction of asbestos fibres can exert a synergistic effect e.g. [39]. The incidence of cancer at many other sites in the body is also higher in smokers than non-smokers.

Magnitude of the effect. The effect of smoking varies with the type of tobacco and the manner of its preparation and use. The response is dose dependent both in cross-sectional studies and longitudinally [40, 41] (Figs 37.5 and 37.6).

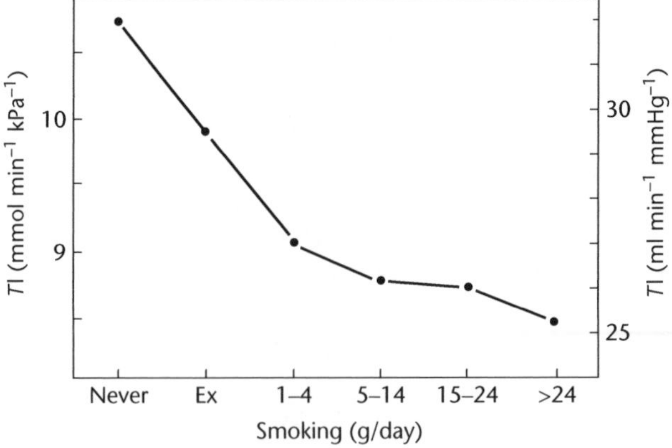

Fig. 37.5 Relationship of transfer factor to smoking category in male dockyard workers. Source: [42].

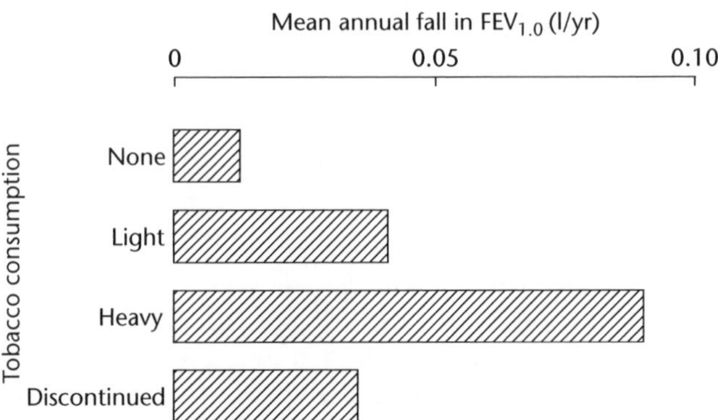

Fig. 37.6 Mean annual decline in forced expiratory volume in men followed for 5 years analysed by smoking category. In this study the dividing line between light and heavy smoking was 14 cigarettes per day. Source: [43].

In a general population the association with dose is particularly strong for lung cancer. Amongst persons who smoke but do not inhale, the practice of smoking a pipe or cigars is less damaging to the lungs than smoking cigarettes.

Acute effects. The inhalation of tobacco smoke causes an immediate rise in the airway resistance that persists for at least an hour. The change is a reflex response to the deposition of particles upon the epithelium of the larynx, trachea and larger bronchi, and is not specific to tobacco smoke. The intensity of the response varies, being greater in subjects with increased bronchial reactivity to histamine and other agents compared with non-responders (Section 15.8.1). It is also greater amongst smokers who regularly bring up sputum. The acute rise in resistance occurs in the larger airways. It reduces the forced expiratory volume (FEV_1) and the maximal expiratory flow at large lung volumes (e.g. $FEF_{50\%\,FVC}$). The flow at small lung volumes ($FEF_{75\%\,FVC}$) is not affected by an acute exposure. The transfer factor is reduced transiently [44]; see also Section 20.7.1.

The immediacy of the responses to tobacco smoke is a reason for routine measurements of lung function not being carried out until at least an hour has elapsed after the completion of smoking a cigarette. In heavy smokers, when it is proposed to measure the transfer factor or, in any smokers to measure the subdivisions of transfer factor, either the back tension of carbon monoxide in the blood should be measured or the subject should not have smoked on the day of the assessment. Abstinence is also desirable prior to the performance of an exercise test.

Subacute effects. Damage to the lungs by tobacco smoke causes changes in lung function at a time when the subject is still asymptomatic. The changes precede the development of chronic bronchitis, emphysema or other complication. This needs to be recognised because asymptomatic smokers are often considered wrongly to have normal function. The impairment is to all aspects of lung function and is described in numerous publications.

The earliest feature is usually narrowing of small airways. This can be detected as an increase in the single breath nitrogen index or in closing volume (Section 16.2.6). Concurrently, the specific compliance and forced expiratory flow ($FEF_{75\%\,FVC}$) are reduced. However the latter change, in particular, has wide confidence limits. The changes were at one time thought likely to presage a reduction in FEV_1 and poor prognosis but this has turned out not to be the case, so a close chronological link between narrowing of small and large airways has not been established [45, 46]. Instead, the next features can be some reduction in arterial oxygen tension and increase in ventilation during submaximal exercise ($\dot{V}E_{45}$), evidence for uneven lung function ($\dot{V}A/\dot{Q}$ inequality). The premature closure of airways increases the residual volume. Thus, by the time the FEV_1 is abnormal there is already substantial impairment of lung function. In some patients the elastic recoil pressure of the lung is then reduced (i.e. lung compliance is increased) and this change may progress as clinically apparent emphysema ensues. Concurrently, there is an increase in the permeability of the alveolar capillary membrane as measured using 99^m Tc-DTPA [47], the transfer factor is reduced (average reduction 1.0 mmol min^{-1} kPa^{-1} i.e. 3 ml $min^{-1}torr^{-1}$) (e.g. Table 37.6), and on exercise the pulmonary arterial pressure is somewhat increased. The effects of smoking on widely used lung function indices are summarised in Table 37.6.

Relation to stage in life

(i) Adolescence and early adulthood. Smoking during adolescence reveals those who develop symptoms. Such persons (other than the ones who are susceptible to peer pressure) are more likely to stop smoking than asymptomatic smokers (hence healthy smoker effect). In young men, continuing to smoke leads to premature cessation in growth of the lungs (Fig. 37.7). It also brings forward the age at which the lung function starts to decline [40, 41], also Table 37.7. As a result young adult smokers have inferior lung function compared with non-smokers.

Table 37.6 Average effect on lung function of smoking 20 cigarettes per day (sm) compared with being a non-smoker of the same age (non-sm). For each index being a smoker significantly impaired the lung function ($p < 0.05$).

		Men		Women	
		non-sm	sm	non-sm	sm
Number of subjects		136	91	97	84
FEV_1	l	3.80	3.42	2.65	2.45
VC	l	5.11	4.80	3.07	2.91
FEV_1/VC	%	77	74	87	84
RV/TLC	%	36	38	–	–
MVV	1 min^{-1}	153	141	–	–
$FEF_{25-75\%}$	1 s^{-1}	3.86	3.12	3.43	3.01
*R*aw	kPa l^{-1} s	0.20	0.23	0.21	0.24
	cm H_2O l^{-1}s	2.0	2.3	2.1	2.4
*T*l,co	mmol $min^{-1}kPa^{-1}$	11.7	10.0*	8.8	7.8
	ml $min^{-1}torr^{-1}$	34.9	29.9	26.2	23.2
*P*a, O_2	kPa	–	–	12.0	11.6
	mm Hg	–	–	90.2	86.9

* See also Fig. 37.5.
Source: [48, 49].

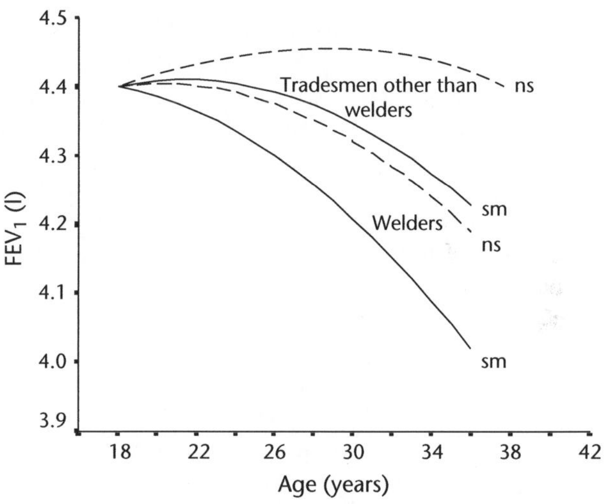

Fig. 37.7 Evolution of FEV_1 in young shipyard workers followed over 8 years. The data are derived from a model of the change in FEV_1 with age, assuming FEV_1 is at its mean level (4.4 l) at 18 years of age. The figure shows the short-term changes attributable to smoking (sm, compared with continuing as a non-smoker ns) and to work as a welder (the latter in smokers and non-smokers separately). Both effects are reversible following discontinuing exposure. Source: [50]

(ii) Middle and later life. Being a smoker enhances the deterioration of all aspects of lung function with age (Section 25.9). The changes are cumulative and over a period of years can lead to material respiratory impairment, disability and premature death from respiratory and other causes in persons who continue to

smoke [51, 52]. The respiratory disabilities are now known as chronic obstructive pulmonary disease (COPD) and the syndrome can include emphysema. The clinical and physiological features are in Section 40.3 and aspects of the response to bronchodilator drugs in Section 15.4.

Giving up smoking. Discontinuing smoking at any stage in life usually results in a small improvement in lung function. The improvement can be concealed if the subject increases his or her body mass to a material extent (Section 25.5.1). In population studies the forced expiratory volume adjusted for age of smokers tends to revert to that of non-smokers as a result of stopping smoking [53, 54]. Improvements have also been reported for transfer factor and lung distensibility [55, 56]. Smoking cessation reduces the risk of developing lung cancer, with this improvement continuing for some 15 years. After this time the risk is reduced to that of non-smokers [57]. The risk of developing ischaemic heart disease is also reduced.

The advantages to smokers of abandoning the habit make a compelling case for their doing so. However, it is not easy. This is partly due to changes in the brain that result in a smoker becoming addicted to nicotine. The changes are linked to pleasurable sensations arising from relaxation of nervous tension. The drug also abates hunger and increases cardiac frequency and blood pressure.

Giving up smoking can be assisted by the subject receiving nicotine from another source (e.g. nicotine patches applied to the skin) in a progressively decreasing dose. Additional actions that can be helpful include a re-iterated declaration to abandon smoking, abrupt cessation, the jettisoning of all tobacco products, lighters and ashtrays, and a dramatic change in lifestyle, for example avoiding the company of smokers. However, success does not come easily and any recipe that is conveyed with enthusiasm can often be a help.

Marijuana (cannabis). Particles present in marijuana smoke cause reflex narrowing of large airways and histopathological changes of acute and chronic bronchitis. There may also be other disadvantages [58]. However, early studies did not show evidence for narrowing of small lung airways or damage to the lung parenchyma [59] and up to the time of writing this finding appears not to have been disputed.

37.4 Gaseous hazards

37.4.1 Carbon monoxide

Introduction. Carbon monoxide is an inconspicuous gas that is responsible for more than half of all cases of fatal accidental poisoning [60]. It is present in fumes from incomplete combustion of carbon, including tobacco smoke, welding fumes, fires in buildings (Section 41.13), some motor exhaust and effluent from domestic grates, braziers, furnaces and many industrial processes.

Poisoning is associated with 'carbon monoxide anaemia' in which the gas progressively displaces oxygen from combination with haemoglobin. The reactions were characterised in the first part of the last century by Haldane, Roughton and colleagues [61, 62] and their work provided the basis for partitioning the transfer factor (Tl,CO) into its component variables (Section 20.7).

Endogenous carbon monoxide (CO) is produced by degradation of haem (heme) that is derived mainly from damaged erythrocytes. The degradation products include carbon monoxide and biliverdin that becomes bilirubin. Both the bile pigments and CO in low concentrations are anti-oxidants and protect the vascular endothelium from oxidative stress [63, 64]. Carbon monoxide has a similar role in the central nervous system where it contributes to neuro-transmission [65]. These actions could have therapeutic implications [66]. They are nonetheless compatible with carbon monoxide in higher concentration having a toxic action [67], whilst intermediate doses might contribute to the damage caused by environmental pollutants [68].

Physiology. Carbon monoxide competes with oxygen for binding sites on the haemoglobin molecule [61, 62]. The relative affinities of the two gases are in the ratio of between 210 and 300 to 1, so when a low concentration of carbon monoxide is breathed for a long time the saturation of haemoglobin with carbon monoxide rises significantly. For example, when breathing air containing carbon monoxide in the fractional concentration of 0.001 the percentage saturations of haemoglobin with oxygen and with carbon monoxide are both 50%. The presence of carbon monoxide displaces the lower part of the haemoglobin dissociation curve to the left and the upper part to the right (Fig. 37.8).

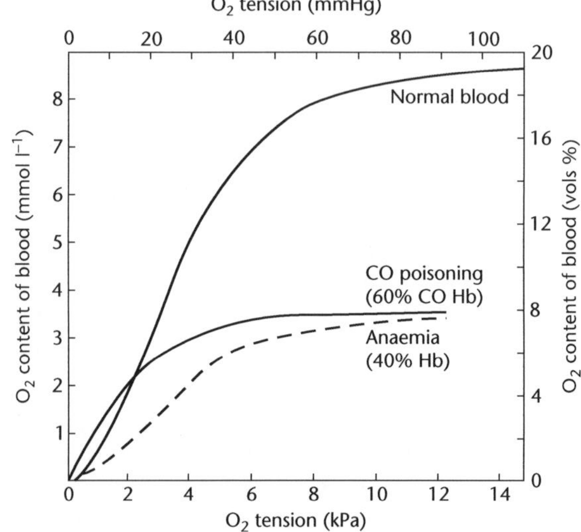

Fig. 37.8 Typical oxygen dissociation curves for blood in which only 40% of the normal quantity of haemoglobin is available for transport of oxygen. When the depletion is due to anaemia the oxygen tension of capillary blood is relatively high, but when due to carbon monoxide it is lower than normal. Source: [69].

Table 37.7 Mean age at start of lung function decline in 488 young shipyard workers analysed by smoking categories.

	Smokers* years	Non-smokers years	
FEV_1	18.5	25.1	$p < 0.05$
FVC	25.8	35.6	$p < 0.05$
PEF	35.0	45.2	$p < 0.05$

* At any time during period of follow up (7.2 year).
Source: [Chinn DJ, Cotes JE. Unpublished.]

As well as combining with haemoglobin, carbon monoxide combines preferentially with myoglobin where the affinity compared with that of oxygen is approximately 22:1. Thus, carbon monoxide reduces the quantity of haemoglobin that is accessible to oxygen, reduces the oxygen tension in tissue capillaries and interferes with the storage and transport of oxygen within muscles. The changes reduce the delivery of oxygen to mitochondria and hence the capacity for exercise. The constraint on aerobic metabolism leads to some energy being obtained by non-aerobic metabolism with associated production of lactic acid (Section 28.9.1). Carbon monoxide appears not to have an acute effect on intracellular respiratory enzymes [70].

Levels of CO in blood. Endogenous production of carbon monoxide from breakdown of haem is approximately 18 nmol h^{-1} (0.4 ml h^{-1}). This is associated with a concentration of carboxyhaemoglobin in blood of approximately 0.7%. Smokers absorb carbon monoxide from cigarette smoke in which it is present in a fractional concentration of up to 0.06; this raises the blood level of carboxyhaemoglobin to an average of 5%. The level is usually less than this in passive smokers, and more (e.g. 14%) in heavy smokers. In city dwellers an additional amount is present as a result of environmental pollution, mainly from petrol engines. This raises the [COHb] in a non-smoker to a figure of between 1% with slight pollution and 30% in exceptional circumstances, for example prolonged exposure at a busy city inter-section or road tunnel. High concentrations of carbon monoxide may also be experienced from exposure to some industrial fumes and flue gases.

Features attributable to COHb

(i) Low level exposure. Features of transient mild exposure can include irritability, lassitude and depression. Further exposure can cause headache and dyspepsia. Pre-existing degenerative vascular disease can be made worse and there may be dementia, especially in persons receiving electro-convulsant therapy. These effects are often undiagnosed, yet they are a notable cause of chronic ill health and can shorten life [71, 72]. Identification of the condition depends on it being included amongst the differential diagnoses and on facilities for measuring the alveolar or blood carbon monoxide concentration being available (Section 20.7.1).

(ii) Acute poisoning. During an acute episode, a rise in the saturation of haemoglobin with carbon monoxide to approximately 15% reduces the visual acuity, the attention level and the manual dexterity. These features affect the ability to drive a motor vehicle [65]. At levels of COHb in the range 20–40% there is likely to be headache, giddiness and weakness. If the exposure continues the victim may become disorientated and in a state of collapse due to cerebral oedema. There may then be tachycardia and rapid breathing, a fall in blood pressure and sudden loss of consciousness. The skin and mucous membranes can have a cherry red appearance due to the presence of carboxyhaemoglobin, but usually the colour is obscured by pallor from the collapse of the circulation. The patient is then cold and sweating and at risk of myocardial infarction [71].

Management of carbon monoxide poisoning. The immediate requirements are to stop further exposure to carbon monoxide and undertake resuscitation. Treatment may also be required for respiratory depression, cardiac arrest or cerebral oedema. Oxygen is administered in as high a concentration as is practicable in order to hasten the elimination of carbon monoxide from the body (Table 37.8). If at all possible the patient should be transferred to a hyperbaric chamber as there is suggestive evidence that such therapy, even as long as 6 h after the collapse, can prevent delayed damage to the brain [71].

Exposure limits. The upper limit for safety is often set at 15% carboxyhaemoglobin (1.4 mmol l^{-1}). However, a [COHb] of 10%, for which the corresponding alveolar concentration is about 50 parts per million (2 μmol l^{-1}), impairs the function of the nervous system, and even lower concentrations can have a long-term effect (cf. Section 34.3). For gas that is breathed continuously the concentration of 50 ppm should not be exceeded. On this basis the safe times for shorter exposures are indicated in Fig. 37.9.

37.4.2 Hypoxia in a confined space

Hypoxia or anoxia can occur in a confined space as a result of the oxygen being removed by metabolism, combustion or other oxidative chemical reaction. In unfavourable circumstances

Table 37.8 Mean half-times for elimination of carbon monoxide from dogs to whom oxygen was administered in different ways. Source: [73].

Inspired gas	Half-time (min)
21% O_2	210*
100% O_2	29.8
5% CO_2 in O_2	20.6
7% CO_2 in O_2	16.3
O_2 at 2 atmospheres	8.6

* Estimated.

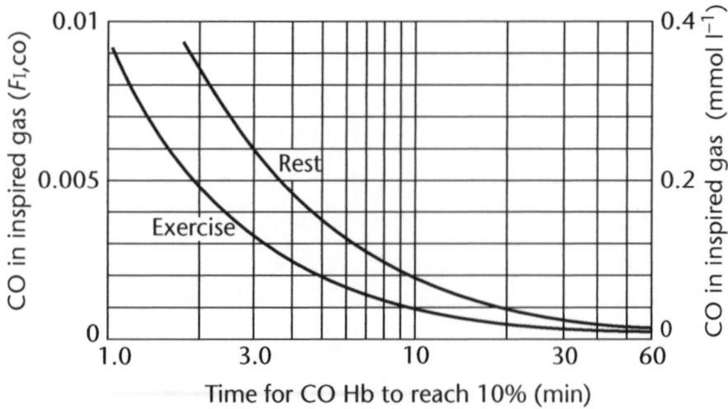

Fig. 37.9 Maximal concentrations of carbon monoxide in air which may be inhaled for different periods of time by healthy subjects without the saturation of Hb with carbon monoxide rising above 10%. The curves for rest and exercise have been constructed for ventilation minute volumes of 10 l min^{-1} and 30 l min^{-1}, respectively.

entry into such an environment can lead to loss of consciousness within 15 s and death within 2 min. In a coal mine or sewer the cause is said to be 'black damp'. The condition can also occur in a tank, ship's hold or silo containing grain. In these instances the local environment contains nitrogen and additional carbon dioxide but little oxygen. Hypoxia without hypercapnia can be experienced in an empty chamber, such as the flotation tank of a ship, from which the oxygen is abstracted by rusting of the iron.

A person entering a space where there is little oxygen needs to be supplied with respirable gas. To achieve this the local gaseous environment can be replaced or improved, or the subject provided with a compressed airline or closed-circuit breathing apparatus (Section 37.2.3).

37.4.3 Ozone

Ozone is tri-atomic oxygen (O_3). It is formed from atmospheric oxygen both naturally by exposure to ultraviolet light from the sun and by an electrical discharge. Ozone formed in the upper atmosphere absorbs additional ultraviolet rays preventing them from reaching the surface of the earth. Thus, ozone provides protection from the skin tumour malignant melanoma. Below the ozone layer the gas is produced during spells of bright sunlight; it can then react with constituents of air pollution, but where the air is clean the concentration rises. This tends to happen in summer rather than in winter and in rural areas, or at sea, compared with towns. The ozone causes damage to the lungs in proportion to the amount that is inhaled. Children in country districts, distance runners, cyclists and agricultural workers are all at increased risk [9]. Their exposure is usually seasonal and causes seasonal changes in forced expiratory volume and other indices of lung function [74]. Some protection can be provided by a dietary supplement of antioxidants [75]; this suggests that the ill effects are due, at least in part, to reactive oxygen species (Section 37.1).

Ozone is produced by an electrical discharge through air in lightning, electrical appliances and electric arc welding. As a result the welding of stainless steel in a confined space can cause pulmonary oedema (Table 37.13, page 521). Poisoning can also occur in conjunction with the use of ozone as a disinfectant or anoxidising agent in the production of plastics, cortisone and related substances.

Breathing ozone causes almost immediate reductions in forced expiratory volume and forced vital capacity but the changes last for only a few hours [76]. They appear to be due to stimulation of receptors in the upper airways [77]. Concurrently, in some subjects there is a more slowly developing inflammatory response with mucosal oedema, an outpouring of neutrophils into the respiratory bronchioles and release of inflammatory mediators, including histamine and reactive oxygen species [78]. This stage in the response can be associated with wheeze and the physiological features of narrowing of small lung airways (e.g. Section 16.2.2). It occurs in up to 20% of subjects, many of whom are asthmatic [79] and is accompanied by increased bronchial reactivity as demonstrated by a bronchoconstrictor response to metacholine. The response is due to sensitisation of bronchopulmonary C-fibre nerve endings by ozone [80].

The changes in small airway function from ozone appear to be cumulative [10, 81] and this raises the possibility that, over time they might contribute to development of chronic lung disease. Another possible contributory factor is ultrafine particles of which the effects can be accentuated by exposure to ozone [82]. Ozone and tobacco smoke interact in their effects on small airways, but not their immediate effects on FEV_1 [10, 83, 84].

37.4.4 Nitrogen oxides

Oxygen reacts with nitrogen in stages to form a series of gases with different properties (Table 37.9). Of these, nitrogen dioxide can seriously affect the lungs both in gaseous form and after hydration to nitrous acid.

Nitrogen dioxide is produced during degradation of substances containing nitrogen compounds, including explosives, synthetic fabrics, ammonium salts and dyes. It is also formed when air is heated to a high temperature. Nitrogen dioxide is a constituent of tobacco smoke, forest fires and urban air pollution, particularly fumes from vehicle exhaust. On this account the exposure can be high in proximity to busy roads. Domiciliary

Table 37.9 Nitrogen oxides.

N_2O	Nitrous oxide (N_2 suboxide)	Inert, anaesthetic gas
NO	Nitric oxide	Pharmacologically active
N_2O_3	Di-nitrogen trioxide	Present in mixtures ($N_2O_3 \rightleftharpoons NO + NO_2$)
NO_2	Nitrogen dioxide	Brown irritant gas (> 21°C)
N_2O_4	Di-nitrogen tetra-oxide	Is unstable ($N_2O_4 \rightleftharpoons 2NO_2$)
N_2O_5	Nitrogen pentaoxide	Decomposes at > −10°C to form O_2, NO and NO_2

pollution can occur in homes were the cooking is by gas [85] or there are gas heating appliances without ducted flues.

High concentrations. Exposure to a high concentration of nitrogen dioxide (>100 ppm) can occur as a result of an industrial accident or unprotected entry into a silo (silofillers disease). The initial consequence is severe bronchospasm that can be fatal. After a few hours or days pulmonary oedema can occur, whilst after a few weeks there is a risk of pulmonary infection. The recovery can be complicated by development of pulmonary fibrosis [86]. Intermediate concentrations of NO_2 (>5 ppm) can give rise to respiratory and other symptoms. Emphysema can be induced in some animal species, but it is uncertain to what extent this risk extends to man.

Low concentrations. Challenge studies using 2 ppm have demonstrated the occurrence of both a transient reduction in ventilatory capacity (FEV_1 and FVC) and inflammatory changes in small lung airways. The latter causes narrowing that can be detected by spirometry, measurement of closing volume (Section 16.2.2) or measurement of recovery of small inhaled particles [87]. In asthmatics the response to allergen challenge can be increased [88].

The chronic effects of NO_2 are mainly due to inflammatory changes affecting neutrophils, Clara cells [89] and other cellular constituents of the walls of small airways. The changes have the effect of interfering with the respiratory defences against viral and bacterial infections [90]. The mechanism is currently unclear, but it is synergistic with those of ozone and sulphur dioxide and differs in not being mainly dependent on oxidative pathways [91].

37.4.5 Sulphur dioxide

SO_2 is formed during combustion of sulphur present in coal or petroleum products, smelting of sulphide ore, including iron pirites, and calcining of natural sulphates. Its main use is in production of sulphuric acid that, in turn, is the starting point for innumerable industrial processes. The gas dissolves in water to form sulphurous acid which is corrosive of body tissues including that of the upper and lower respiratory tract, teeth and clothing.

In the absence of measures to provide clean air, SO_2 is an important component of urban and occupational air pollution and a cause of bronchitis and acute and chronic airways obstruction [92]. It is particularly harmful when adsorbed onto respirable particles of soot, as occurs in smog (sooty fog) [6, 93]. Exposure to SO_2 can precipitate symptoms of asthma in sensitive subjects [94] and can act as a co-carcinogen in the production of lung cancer. Sulphurous acid absorbed via the lungs or intestinal tract can have significant systemic effects both as an acid and through its oxidative properties [95].

Due to control measures, SO_2 is only a minor problem in developed countries [96] and, where measures have been introduced lung function has improved in consequence [97].

37.5 Integrated effects of environmental air pollution

The main primary source of respirable air pollution is combustion of what was at some stage vegetable material, e.g. coal, petroleum product, tobacco, building material or forest flora. On account of this common origin the consequences are broadly similar in different situations [98]. Heterogeneity is introduced by the local climate and geography, proximity to particular

Table 37.10 Some variables that influence the extent and respiratory consequences of air pollution.

Variable	Circumstance	Mechanism or agent
Combustion: Carbonaceous.	See list in text	Particles, gases, vapours (Table 37.1).
Chemical substances, local industry	In containers, manufactured items (e.g. tyres), finishes etc. contaminants	Industrial and agricultural chemicals, toxic minerals, (e.g. arsenic, beryllium, cadmium), sulphur dioxide etc
Latitude	Intensity of sunlight Need for supplementary heat	Ozone, oxides of nitrogen Extent of combustion.
Geography	Wind speed and direction Susceptibility to mist/fog Scope for temperature inversion	Extent to which pollutants are dispersed or concentrated.
Stage of industrialisation	Standards of environmental hygiene. Type and amount of fuel used for transport.	Extent of use of clean fuel and that from renewable sources.
Features of population	Age distribution Smoking habits Uptake of health services Level of habitual activity	Proportion of population who are old, have asthma or chronic airways obstruction. Amount of air inhaled

types of pollution and features of the persons who are exposed (Table 37.10).

The consequences of breathing polluted air include impaired growth in children [99], suboptimal lung function at any stage of life, increased respiratory morbidity and hospital admissions [99] and increased mortality compared with persons in more favourable circumstances [7]. The recorded extent of the changes depends on which indices are used and the local circumstances (Table 37.10). The exposure is usually to more than one pollutant and these can interact within the local environment to generate additional pollutants. Following entry into the body the effects of two or more pollutants can be additive (as in Fig. 37.7) or they can interact by mutually reinforcing each other's action (e.g. smoking and asbestos fibres both causing lung cancer, Section 37.3). In addition, one pollutant can affect the mechanism whereby another pollutant is rendered harmless [100]. Examples of interactive effects include those between ozone and ultrafine particles (Section 37.4.3), between particle deposition and obstructive lung disease [101] and between the dietary intake of ascorbic acid, being a non-smoker and breathing relatively clean air. As a result, observational studies are often of limited usefulness for attributing causation [102]. Intervention studies can be much more informative (Chapter 8).

37.6 Indoor respiratory hazards

The principal air pollutants within buildings are products of combustion from open fires, boilers, cooking stoves and other appliances, smoke from tobacco and neighbourhood pollution, for example from proximity to a busy road [103, 104]. The features of exposures to these pollutants have been described above.

Buildings and their occupants are a potent source of allergic materials. When circumstances are appropriate these can give rise to hypersensitivity disorders, of which the commonest are asthma and extrinsic allergic alveolitis (hypersensitivity pneumonitis). Micro-organisms and unidentified constituents of air within 'sick' buildings can also cause problems.

37.6.1 Asthma of domestic origin

The airborne dust of buildings contains a host of potentially antigenic materials; they include residues from house dust mite that are highly antigenic and dust and danders from domestic pets. Repeated small exposures to such material give rise to sensitisation in susceptible individuals, particularly those who are atopic (Section 15.3). Other domestic allergens include foodstuffs, paints, solvents, medicines and domestic chemicals.

The immediate consequence of becoming sensitised depends on the age at which the sensitisation is acquired. In infancy there may be eczema, in childhood wheezy bronchitis, recurrent conjunctivitis, rhinitis and/or hay fever. If asthma is to develop it usually does so in the second or third decade of life. The condition presents with paroxysmal episodes of breathlessness and wheeze, associated with airways obstruction that is mainly apparent in the large airways. The features of asthma are given subsequently (Section 40.2; also see Section 37.7.6).

37.6.2 Extrinsic allergic alveolitis (arising within a building)

The dust in some buildings contains airborne particles or droplets that can initiate a delayed allergic reaction. The majority of such antigens are imported and are of occupational origin. One group that is specific to individual buildings arises from contaminated air conditioners or humidifiers, hence *humidifier fever, or water droplet antigen disease* [105, 106]. In another, the antigenic material comes from a budgerigar or other bird kept as a pet [106, 107]. This class of conditions is described below (Section 37.7.5). Spores from moulds in a building are a further source of antigen, but any consequences are usually minor if the building is maintained adequately [108].

37.6.3 Micro-organisms

The act of coughing or sneezing generates an aerosol that contains bacteria or viruses. These desiccate to form droplet nuclei that can remain airborne and contaminate the air of the building. Inhalation of the nuclei can result in transmission of a bacterial infection, for example tuberculosis (Section 37.2.4). The nuclei or the droplets from which they form can also transmit viral infections such as influenza. The odds of this happening are increased in the presence of air pollution from nitrogen dioxide (Section 37.4.4). Contamination of lung function equipment is another, but relatively uncommon, source of cross-infection (Section 7.13). Fortunately, infection of a hot water or air conditioning system by legionella pneumophilia is rare [109].

37.6.4 Sick building syndrome

Some buildings are associated with symptoms amongst the people who work there. The symptoms are usually of a general nature, not respiratory. They are elicited by questionnaire, when the scores are reproducible and associated with unfavourable ratings for sickness absence and/or productivity. In a few instances a specific causal substance can be identified, but this is uncommon.

A sick building is usually air conditioned, not ventilated naturally and has a low rate of ventilation with outside air ($<10\,l\,s^{-1}$ per person). The level of internal cleanliness is often low. The treatment appears to be to abandon air conditioning in favour of giving the occupants of the building control of their local environment including the ambient temperature, level of illumination and ventilation with fresh air. The air quality can be further improved by having a high standard of cleanliness and an agreed 'no smoking' policy [110, 111].

37.7 Lung disorders of occupational origin

37.7.1 Introduction

Acute effects. The acute effect of an inhaled dust is dependent on its size distribution (Table 37.2), its nature and the dose. Inert particles impacting on the large airways may produce bronchoconstriction, cough, mucous secretion and a change in the pattern of breathing (Section 37.2.1). Irritant particles impacting on larger airways can cause bronchoconstriction directly (e.g. SO_2 in smog) or by release of mediators such as histamine (e.g. cotton dust). Constriction of larger airways can follow after prior sensitisation to antigenic particles as in an attack of asthma. Inert particles lodging on the gas-exchanging epithelium appear to have no detectable acute effect. Irritant particles can cause alveolitis directly, whilst substances that evoke a delayed allergic reaction can cause extrinsic allergic alveolitis (also known as hyper-sensitivity pneumonitis).

Chronic effects. The chronic effect of inhaled dust on the conducting airways can be to produce cough and sputum (bronchitis), airways obstruction or bronchiectasis. The chronic effect on the parenchyma of the lung is usually of minor proportions. However, inert dusts that are radio-opaque (e.g. oxides of iron and tin) may give rise to characteristic appearances of simple pneumoconiosis on the chest radiograph. More reactive dusts that reach the lung parenchyma may cause pulmonary fibrosis (e.g. asbestosis), with characteristic changes in lung volume, gas transfer and elastic recoil, or granuloma formation (as occurs with quartz, berylium or organic dusts), or pulmonary emphysema (e.g. as part of coal workers pneumoconiosis or from the inhalation of proteolytic materials). These effects are often aggravated by smoking [112], individual susceptibility (e.g. rheumatoid diathesis and progressive massive fibrosis [113], genetic susceptibility to beryllium [114]) or super-imposed extrinsic factors (e.g. tuberculosis in silicosis [15]).

Mechanisms. In most mineral pneumoconioses the damage to the lungs is either a direct toxic effect of the dust or a secondary action. The latter can be via release of oxidants from phagocytic cells that overwhelm the antioxidant defences, activation of macrophages to attract polymorphonuclear leukocytes with resulting inflammation, and secretion of growth factors that lead to scarring [114–117]. The processes can be monitored directly, or indirectly from measurements of bio-available iron in coal [118], blood levels of selenium [119] and other variables.

Epidemiology. The incidence and extent of most dust induced diseases are related to the cumulative exposure to respirable dust. The exceptions include silicosis where peak exposure is important [120], mesothelioma (see below) and beryllium (see 'Chronic effects' above). The prevalence can be reduced by hygiene measures (Section 37.2.3). In countries where these have been applied meticulously the prevalence of the relevant occupational lung diseases has fallen dramatically. However, the prevalence can creep up again if vigilance is relaxed [121]. The prevalence of diseases due to sensitising agents (occupational asthma and extrinsic allergic alveolitis) appears to be increasing and currently this is also the case for mesothelioma.

37.7.2 Asbestos-related lung diseases

Asbestos from the Greek ασβεστος 'unquenchable' is a fibrous silicate that is tough and fire resistant. The fibres, obtained by crushing the ore, have excellent insulating properties, but many of them are respirable (fibre diameter $< 5\mu m$, Section 37.2.2) and can cause lung diseases, including mesothelioma, pleural thickening, asbestosis and lung cancer. For most applications asbestos has now been replaced by less controversial alternatives.

Mesothelioma. This malignant tumour of the pleura is usually a long delayed sequel to inhaling fibres of crocidolite, the blue asbestos. In the UK the use of crocidolite has been banned since 1972, but new cases still occur due to the tumour having a long incubation period [57]. The condition presents with local and general symptoms. On assessment of lung function, the lung expansion and the quantity of air in the lungs are reduced.

Pleural plaques/thickening. These conditions can be a consequence of inhaling fibres of asbestos (usually chrysotile, the white asbestos). Plaques can be fibrous or calcified, when the radiographic appearance can range from a tiny spot to an extensive opacity. In the absence of pleural or pulmonary fibrosis the lung function is usually normal. Pleural thickening with or without plaques often causes a restrictive ventilatory defect, particularly if the lesion involves one or both costophrenic angles [122], see Section 28.4.7 and cases in Tables 37A, 29.11 and 30.6, pages 429 and 442, respectively). On exercise breathing is shallow and this contributes to an increased ventilation with associated breathlessness. The transfer factor can be reduced reflecting the change in total lung capacity, but *Tl*/*V*A is then increased above normal [123], also Section 20.9.

Fibrosis within the lung (asbestosis). Diffuse fibrosis that is clinically significant is usually visible as linear opacities on the chest radiograph. Lesser changes can be apparent on high-resolution computer-assisted tomography (HRCT scan) [124]. The changes are accompanied or occasionally preceded by restriction to lung expansion and reductions in transfer factor and *Tl*/*V*A (Table 37A). The features of chronic airways obstruction may coexist. In addition, asbestosis predisposes to the development of bronchial carcinoma, particularly in smokers [125]. The tumour will occupy space in the thorax and further reduce the total lung capacity.

37.7.3 Beryllium disease

Inhalation of beryllium dust or fumes can give rise to granulomatous lesions in the lungs. The onset is capricious [114] and depends on the dose, the level of susceptibility and the presence of trigger factors including pregnancy or withdrawing from exposure. The features can be those of pulmonary oedema, acute pneumonitis, subacute malaise or chronic breathlessness on exertion either during the course of exposure to beryllium or subsequently. The chest radiograph then shows diffuse small opacities. The impairment of lung function is typical of proliferative disease of the lung parenchyma, including a defect of gas transfer and a ventilatory defect of the restrictive type (Section 38.3.2). Tachypnoea is sometimes a prominent feature and, except when the condition has progressed to interstitial fibrosis, the symptoms and the changes in lung function can be improved by the administration of corticosteroid drugs [126]. An example has been given previously (Fig. 28.11, page 397).

37.7.4 Byssinosis

Byssinosis, named after the Latin word byssin that describes the fine silky filaments of some molluscs, affects cotton mill operatives and others exposed to dust from cotton, flax and soft hemp (cannabis sativa). The operatives develop cough and tightness in the chest on returning to work on a Monday after a weekend away from the dust, or on another day after returning from a holiday. Following repeated exposures symptoms are also experienced later in the week. There is an associated reduction in ventilatory capacity and rise in airway resistance (Fig. 37.10).

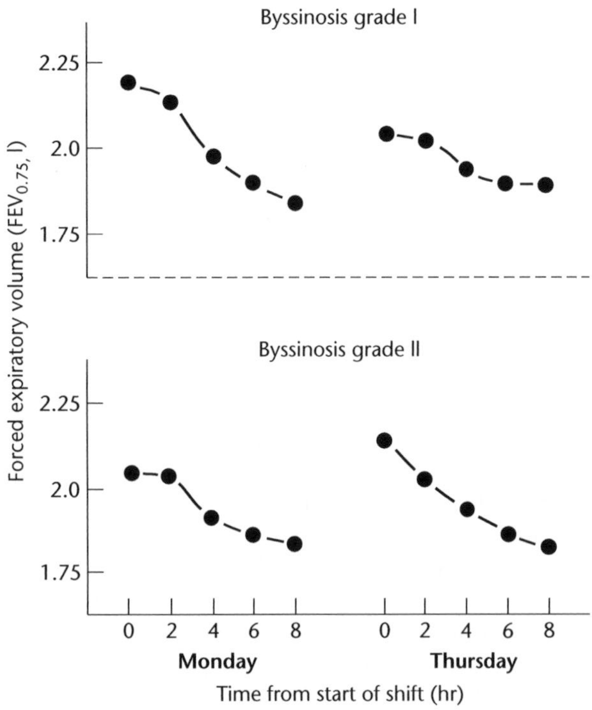

Fig. 37.10 Mean levels of $FEV_{0.75}$ over a working shift for cardroom workers with byssinosis grades I and II. In grade I the decline was most marked on Mondays but in grade II it occurred on other days as well. Source: [127].

The airways obstruction is due to release of histamine from mast cells in the lungs in response to constituents of the dust [128, 129]. The reformation of the histamine is believed to be speeded up by repeated exposures and the rate determines on which days in the week the symptoms occur.

There are no changes in the structure of the lungs and no long-term changes in lung function except where chronic bronchitis and/or emphysema co-exist. A typical case is described as Occupational case B (Table 37B). Byssinosis does not occur with jute, manila hemp, sisal or man-made fibres though the exposure to any of these dusts in high concentration can cause bronchitis.

37.7.5 Extrinsic allergic alveolitis (EAA) including Farmer's lung

Extrinsic allergic alveolitis (also known as hypersensitivity pneumonitis) describes a group of disorders in which an antigen–antibody reaction leads to the formation of multiple granulomata in the lung parenchyma [130]. In farmer's lung the antigen is present on the spores of mouldy hay. In bird handler's lung the antigen is in dust from the feathers or droppings of pigeons, budgerigars or some other birds. Other antigens are listed in Table 37.11.

Repeated exposures to antigen leads to the development of precipitating antibodies in the blood plasma. The titre can be assessed quantitatively using a radioimmunoassay or other specific test. Subsequent exposure to the antigen can then cause a pulmonary reaction 3–6 h later. People who are atopic (and so are predisposed to asthma) can develop an immediate asthma attack as well.

An acute episode of extrinsic allergic alveolitis typically presents as a flu-like illness, reflecting the alveolitis, and breathlessness with shallow breathing. Most aspects of lung function are impaired. The changes are usually maximal some 10 h after exposure and persist into the next day. On the first occasion the affected person usually recovers completely. Repeated mild exposure to antigenic material can cause chronic EAA. Persons at increased risk include working farmers (Occupational case C, Table 37C) and a person (usually an elderly lady living alone) who keeps an infected budgerigar or other bird as a companion [131]. Chronic EAA presents with progressive breathlessness on exertion and the features of diffuse interstitial fibrosis (Section 40.4). There are matching changes in the chest radiograph which are characteristically in the upper zones of the lung fields. Smoking may have a protective effect [132] (see also Section 37.2.1).

37.7.6 Occupational asthma

Immediate onset asthma. A person's occupation may result in exposure to any of hundreds of sensitising agents, including chemical substances and plant or animal residues (Table 37.12). In most instance the sensitisation is mediated via IgE, the affected person is atopic (Section 15.3) and the airway narrowing develops

Table 37.11 Some causes of extrinsic allergic alveolitis.

Source	Condition	Possible cause
(a) Moulds, other micro organisms and spores		
Hay	Farmer's lung	*Micropolyspora faeni*
Grain	Thresher's lung	*Sitophilus granaris*
Straw, thatch	Chaffcutter's lung	*Thermoactinomyces vulgaris**
Dry rot		*Merulius lacrymans**
Bagasse	Bagassosis	*Thermactinomyces vulgaris*
Mushroom compost		*Agaricus hortensis**
Cork	Suberosis	*Penicillium frequentans*
Malt dust		*Aspergillus clavatus*
Maple bark		*Cryptostroma corticale*
Redwood dust	Sequoiosis	*Aureobasidium pullulans*
Cheese washings		*Pencillium sp.*
Paprika		*Mucor liemalis*
Air filters	Air conditionitis	*Thermoactinomyces candidus*
Humidifier sludge	Humidifier fever	*Acanthamoeba*
(b) Animal residues		
Droppings, feathers and serum of pigeons, budgerigars and other birds.		
Bovine and porcine serum and pituitary snuff.		
(c) Chemical substances		
Pyrethrum, some resins*		
Diisocyanates etc		

* These agents can also cause occupational asthma.
Source: [15].

immediately on exposure to the antigen. If the concentration of antigen is small, the effect can be cumulative throughout a shift and can continue into subsequent working days. For such a person to continue in employment the lung function should return to normal during rest days (see e.g. Fig. 15.7, page 177).

Immediate onset asthma of occupational origin is usually recognised early in the illness because the asthma reaction is closely associated with the work place. The sensitisation can often be demonstrated by making a skin prick test (Section 15.3). Serial measurements of peak expiratory flow at the work place

Table 37.12 Examples of substances that can cause occupational asthma.

Category	Immediate response	Dual response
Mammalian and bird residues	Danders: cat, dog, cow etc	Budgerigar, other bird
Arthropods and molluscs	Insects: cockroaches, weevil. Crustacea: prawns, crabs. Mites: cheese, flour, grain	
Tree bark, dust and sap	African maple, zebra wood.	Boxwood, Californian red wood, red cedar, colophony (pine resin)
Vegetable products	Grain pollen and protein, printers' ink	
Micro organisms	–	see Table 37.11
Enzymes	–	Papain, *B. subtilis*
Drugs	Penicillin, tetracycline	Spiramycin, aspirin
Dyes	Reactive dyes	Diazonium salts
Metal salts	Salts of nickel, chromium	Salts of platinum
Other*	–	Isocyanates, epoxy compounds, furfuryl alcohol, formaldehyde

* These substances are used in many industrial processes. They are also non-specific irritants.
Source: [15].

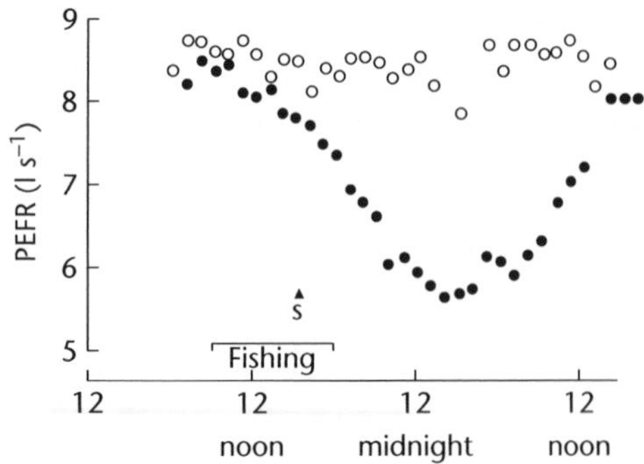

Fig. 37.11 Circadian values for peak expiratory flow in a fisherman who developed delayed onset (IgG mediated) asthma as a result of sensitisation to maggots of the bluebottle fly (*Callifora*) used as bait. Except in the middle of the night, each point is the mean of five daily recordings. S indicates onset of symptoms. Source: [133].

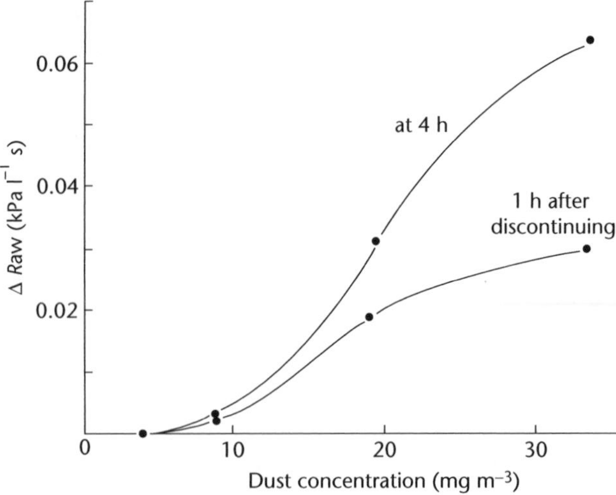

Fig. 37.12 Acute response of airway resistance to breathing coal dust. Source: [14].

can also be used to confirm the diagnosis or provide evidence on the effectiveness of hygiene measures. Challenge testing can be used to demonstrate the intermediate mechanism (see Fig. 15.8, page 178).

Delayed or dual onset asthma. Persons who are not atopic do not become sensitised via the IgE pathway. They may nonetheless develop immediate onset asthma where this is associated with short-term sensitising IgG. More often IgG or another immunoglobulin (IgD or IgM) contributes to delayed onset asthma as part of the syndrome of extrinsic allergic alveolitis (Table 37.11, also Section 37.7.5). In this circumstance airways obstruction usually develops after an interval of 4–12 h (Fig. 37.11).

Occupational asthma of delayed onset is often difficult to identify. The subject may have had respiratory symptoms, including nocturnal wheeze, extending over several years and any acute episodes may not be closely linked with the working environment. In this circumstance use should be made of all available information, including results of a RAS test or challenge test (Section 15.8). A negative result can usually be relied on but a positive result does not exclude that other factors may have contributed to the illness.

37.7.7 Pneumoconiosis of coal workers and other occupational groups

Simple pneumoconiosis. Respirable particles of mineral dust (diameter $> 5\mu m$) accumulate in the lungs where they form foci adjacent to respiratory bronchioles. Foci that overlap cause a fine mottled appearance on the chest radiograph (simple pneumoconiosis). Most cases of simple pneumoconiosis are due to coal, but the condition also occurs with other mineral dusts, including kaolin, Fuller's earth, carbon black, barium, tin oxide, antimony, iron oxide and diatomaceous earth. Where the dust is of coal the affected bronchioles can dilate and this process results in focal emphysema that is visible on a large lung section [134].

Most cases of simple pneumoconiosis, including those due to tin oxide (stannosis) and iron oxide (siderosis) are asymptomatic and the lung function is within normal limits. In coal workers' pneumoconiosis there can be a small reduction in forced expiratory volume (FEV_1) with a lesser change in forced vital capacity (FVC). The change in FEV_1 starts off as an acute response that is initially fully reversible (Fig. 37.12). The subsequent decline is related to duration of exposure to dust and is in addition to any changes due to smoking and/or to chronic bronchitis [135].

Focal emphysema in coalminers is associated with the small p type of radiological opacities (diameter less than 1.5 mm). The transfer factor is likely to be reduced, the residual volume somewhat increased and the arterial oxygen tension below the normal range. Pulmonary arterial pressure can be increased. In some men the changes give rise to breathlessness and can shorten life [136, 137].

Progressive massive fibrosis (PMF). Where much dust is present in the lungs the dust foci coalesce to form space occupying lesions. The lesions can enlarge by a process of avascular necrosis, whilst the intervening tissue then becomes stretched and emphysematous (compensatory emphysema). In some cases the changes distort the airways, thrombose some pulmonary arteries and contribute to the occurrence of chronic bronchitis, pulmonary hypertension and congestive cardiac failure. The massive lesions can liquefy and rupture into bronchi from whence the contained black material is expectorated as melanoptysis. The presenting symptom is usually breathlessness on exertion. Disability is due to the combined effects of the reduced ventilatory capacity and increased ventilatory cost of exercise [138]. The features of PMF are exemplified in occupational case D (Table 37D).

37.7.8 Silicosis

Silicon in the form of silicon dioxide is a principal constituent of the earth's crust. As a result of crushing or abrasion it forms a

Table 37.13 Some additional circumstances that can damage the lungs.

Process or agent	Effect on the lung
Refining aluminium	Pot room asthma [141, 142].
Handling chlorine*	Chronic airflow obstruction.
Deep sea diving.	Section 35.3.3
Enzyme detergents*	Emphysema (if heavy exposure), asthma.
Fire fighting*	Any, depending on what is burnt.
Foundry work*	Asthma, chronic airflow obstruction, silicosis.
Producing tungsten carbide	Hard metal disease (Occupational case E, Table 37E, also [143]).
Lipid aerosol, oil mist.	Lipid pneumonia [144, 145].
Nitrogen dioxide*	Section 37.4.4
Organophosphates	e.g. parathion poisoning.
Ozone*	Section 37.4.3
Paraquat	Respiratory distress syndrome (Section 41.12)
Sulphur dioxide*	Section 37.4.5
Welding steel (especially in shipbuilding) *	Respiratory symptoms, airflow obstruction, ozone poisoning (stainless steel)

* Effects summate or interact with those of smoking.
Source: [15].

toxic, respirable dust that gives rise to nodular lesions in the lungs. These differ from those of simple pneumoconiosis of coal workers in being relatively avascular and containing more macrophages and fibrous tissue. The lesions occur along lymphatics and in the lung tissue. Heavy exposure, as from unprotected sandblasting, causes acute silicosis which is a diffuse interstitial pneumonitis [139]. Silicosis also occurs in subacute, progressive and chronic forms and the lesions can coalesce to give rise to massive fibrosis.

In simple silicosis the lung function resembles that in simple pneumoconiosis of coal workers [140]. However, the airways obstruction and reduction in transfer factor are usually more marked and can progress following cessation of exposure. In acute silicosis the pattern of function is that of a disease of the lung parenchyma (Section 40.4).

37.7.9 Other occupational lung diseases

Some conditions not described individually above are listed in Table 37.13.

37.8 References

1. Georg Bauer (Agricola) *De Re Metallica* Bohemia, 1556.
2. Ramazzini*De Morbis Artificum Diatriba* Padua, 1700.
3. Thackrah CT. *The effects of the principal arts, trades and professions on health and longevity*, 2nd ed. London, 1832.
4. Evelyn J. Diary entry for 14th September 1661. In: Francis P, ed.*John Evelyn's Diary*, ed.. London: Folio Society, 1963.
5. King James 1. A Counterblaste to Tobacco. London, 1603
6. Ministry of Health. *Mortality and morbidity during the London fog of December 1952.* London: HMSO, 1954.
7. Dockery DW, Pope CA, Xu XP et al. An association between air pollution and mortality in 6 United States cities. *N Eng J Med* 1993; **329**: 1753–1759.
8. Seaton A, MacNee W, Donaldson K, Godden D. Particulate air pollution and acute health effects. *Lancet* 1995; **345**(8943): 176–178.
9. Carlisle AJ, Sharp NC. Exercise and outdoor ambient air pollution. *Br J Sports Med* 2001; **35**: 214–222.
10. Churg A Interactions of exogenous or evoked agents and particles: the role of reactive oxygen species. *Free Radic Biol Med* 2003; **34**: 1230–1235.
11. Yuan Z, Schellekens H, Warner L et al. Reactive nitrogen species block cell cycle re-entry through sustained production of hydrogen peroxide. *Am J Respir Cell Mol Biol* 2003; **28**: 705–712.
12. Cole TJ, Cotes JE, Johnson GR et al. Ventilation, cardiac frequency and pattern of breathing during exercise in men exposed to O-chlorobenzylidine malononitrile (CS) and ammonia gas in low concentrations. *Q J Exp Physiol* 1977; **62**: 341–351.
13. DuBois AB, Dautrebande L. Acute effects of breathing inert dust particles and of carbachol on the mechanical characteristics of the lungs in man; changes in response after inhaling sympathomimetic aerosols. *J Clin Invest* 1958; **37**: 1746–1755.
14. McDermott M. Acute respiratory effects of the inhalation of coal-dust particles. *J Physiol* 1962; **162**: 53P.
15. Cotes JE, Steel J. *Work-related lung disorders.* Oxford, UK: Blackwell Scientific, 1987.
16. Swift DL, Proctor DF. Access of air to the respiratory tract. *In:* Brain JD, Proctor DF, Reid LM Eds. *Respiratory defence mechanisms: Part 1. Lung biology in health and disease.* New York: Marcel Dekker 1977; **5**: 63–93.
17. Task group on lung dynamics. Committee II of International commission on radiological protection. Deposition and retention models for internal dosimetry of the human respiratory tract. *Health Phys* 1966; **12**: 173–208.
18. Boecker BB. Reference values for basic human anatomical and physiological characteristics for use in radiation protection. *Radiat Prot Dosimetrey.* 2003; **105**: 571–574.
19. Gerrity TR, Lee PS, Hass FJ et al. Calculated deposition of inhaled particles in the airway generations of normal subjects. *J Appl Physiol* 1979; **47**: 867-873.
20. Schroter RC, Sudlow MF. Flow patterns in models of the human bronchial airways. *Respir Physiol* 1969; **7**: 341–355.
21. Brain JD, Proctor DF, Reid LM, eds. *Respiratory defence mechanisms: Part 1. Lung biology in health and disease*, vol 5.New York: Marcel Dekker, 1977: 1–488.
22. Timbrell V. Deposition and retention of fibres in the human lung. *Ann Occup Hyg* 1982; **26**: 347–369.
23. Health and Safety Executive. EH40/2002. Substances hazardous to health. Supplement 2003. Occupational exposure limits. London: HMSO.
24. Brown RC. Protection against dust by respirators. *Int J Occup Saf Ergon* 1995; **1**: 14–28.
25. Howie RM, Walton WH *in* Ballantyne B, Schwabe PH. Eds. *Respiratory protection: principles and applications.* London: Chapman Hall. 1981.
26. Usmani OS, Biddiscombe MF, Nightingale JA et al. Effects of bronchodilator particle size in asthmatic patients using monodisperse aerosols. *J Appl Physiol* 2003; **95**: 2106–2112.

27. Bennett WD, Scheuch G, Zenan KL et al. Regional deposition and retention of particles in shallow, inhaled boluses: effect of lung volume.*J Appl Physiol* 1999; **86**: 168–173.
28. Li U-F, Gilliland FD, Berhane K et al. Effects of *in utero* and environmental tobacco smoke exposure on lung function in boys and girls with and without asthma. *Am J Respir Crit Care Med* 2000; **162**: 2097–2104.
29. Barker DJP. *Mothers, babies and health in later life.* Edinburgh: Churchill Livingstone, 1998.
30. Sherrill DI, Enright P, Cline M et al. Rates of decline in lung function among subjects who restart cigarette smoking. *Chest* 1996; **109**: 1001–1005
31. Anderson HR, Anderson JA, Cotes JE. Lung function values in healthy children and adults from highland and coastal areas of Papua New Guinea. *Papua New Guinea Med J* 1974; **17**: 165–167
32. Harris JE, Thun MJ, Mondul AM, Calle EE. Cigarette tar yields in relation to mortality from lung cancer in the cancer prevention study II prospective cohort,1982-8. *BMJ* 2004; **328**: 72–76.
33. Krzyzanowski M, Sherrill DL, Paoletti P, Lebowitz MD. Relationship of respiratory symptoms and pulmonary function to tar, nicotine, and carbon monoxide yield of cigarettes. *Am Rev Respir Dis* 1991; **143**: 306–311.
34. Jaakkola MS, Jaakkola JJK. Assessment of exposure to environmental tobacco smoke. *Eur Respir J* 1997; **10**: 2384–2397.
35. Shijubo N, Itoh Y, Yamaguchi T et al. Serum and BAL Clara cell 10 kDa protein (CC10) levels and CC10 – positive bronchiolar cells are decreased in smokers. *Eur Respir J* 1997; **10**: 1108–1114.
36. Piitulainen E, Eriksson S. Decline in FEV_1 related to smoking in individuals with severe α_1-antitrypsin deficiency (PiZZ). *Eur Respir J.* 1999; **13**: 247–251.
37. Hogg JC, Wright JL, Wiggs BR et al. Lung structure and function in cigarette smokers. *Thorax* 1994; **49**: 473–478.
38. Tylen U, Boijsen M, Ekberg-Jansson A et al. Emphysematous lesions and lung function in healthy smokers 60 years of age. *Respir Med* 2000; **94**: 38–43.
39. Lee PN. Relation between exposure to asbestos and smoking jointly and the risk of lung cancer. *Occup Environ Med* 2001; **58**: 145–153.
40. Jaakkola MS, Jaakkola JJK, Ernst P, Becklake MR. Ventilatory lung function in young cigarette smokers: a study of susceptibility. *Eur Respir J* 1991; **4**: 643-650.
41. Sherrill DL, Lebowitz DM, Knudson RJ, Burrows B. Smoking and symptom effects on the curves of lung function growth and decline. *Am Rev Respir Dis* 1991; **144**: 17–22.
42. Harries PG. *The effects and control of diseases associated with exposure to asbestos in Devonport dockyard.* MD Thesis, University of London, 1970; 226.
43. Higgins ITT, Oldham PD. Ventilatory capacity in miners. A five-year follow up study. *Br J Ind Dis* 1962; **19**: 65–76.
44. Rajikin MH, Etta KM. Transfer factor in smokers and non-smokers after smoking two cigarettes. *Med J Malaysia* 1989; **44**: 23–29.
45. Becklake MR, Permutt S. Evaluation of tests of lung function for screening for early detection of chronic obstructive lung disease. In: Macklem PT, Permutt S, eds. *The lung in the transition between health and disease.* New York: Marcel Dekker, 1979: 345–387.
46. Stanescu DC, Rodenstein DO, Hoeven C, Robert A. "Sensitive tests" are poor predictors of the decline in forced expiratory volume in one second in middle-aged smokers. *Am Rev Respir Dis* 1987; **135**: 585–590.
47. Jones JG, Minty BD, Lawler P, Hulands et al. Increased alveolar epithelial permeability in cigarette smokers. *Lancet* 1980; **1**: 66–68.
48. Krumholz RA, Hedrick EC. Pulmonary function differences in normal smoking and nonsmoking, middle-aged, white-collar workers. *Am Rev Resp Dis* 1973; **107**: 225–230.
49. Woolf CR, Suero JT. The respiratory effects of regular cigarette smoking in women. *Am Rev Respir Dis* 1971; **103**: 26–37.
50. Chinn DJ, Cotes JE, El-Gamal FM et al. Respiratory health of young shipyard welders and other tradesmen studied cross-sectionally and longitudinally. *Occup Env Med* 1995; **55**: 33–42.
51. Fletcher C, Peto R, Tinker C, Speizer FE. *The natural history of chronic bronchitis and emphysema.* Oxford, UK: Oxford University Press, 1976.
52. Calverley PM, Walker P. Chronic obstructive pulmonary disease. *Lancet* 2003; **362**: 1053–1061.
53. Camilli AE, Burrows B, Knudson RJ et al. Longitudinal changes in forced expiratory volume in one second in adults: effect of cigarette smoking and respiratory symptoms. *Am Rev Respir Dis* 1987; **135**: 794–799.
54. Scanlon PD, Connett JE, Waller LA et al. Smoking cessation and lung function in mild-to-moderate chronic obstructive pulmonary disease. The lung health study. *Am J Respir Crit Care Med* 2000; **161**: 381–390.
55. Knudson RJ, Kaltenborn WT, Burrows B. The effects of cigarette smoking and smoking cessation on the carbon monoxide diffusing capacity of the lung in asymptomatic subjects. *Am Rev Respir Dis* 1989; **140**: 645–651.
56. Colebatch HJH, Greaves IA, Ng CKY. Exponential analysis of elastic recoil and ageing in healthy males and females. *J Appl Physiol* 1979; **47**: 683–691.
57. Peto R, Darby S, Deo H. et al. Smoking, smoking cessation and lung cancer since 1950: combination of national statistics with two case-control studies. *BMJ* 2000; **321**: 323–329.
58. Taylor RD, Hall W. Respiratory health effects of cannabis: position statement of the Thoracic Society of Australia and New Zealand. *Intern Med J* 2003; **33**: 310–313.
59. Tashkin DP, Coulson AH, Clark VA et al. Respiratory symptoms and lung function in habitual heavy smokers of marijuana alone, smokers of marijuana and tobacco, smokers of tobacco alone, and nonsmokers. *Am Rev Respir Dis* 1987; **135**: 209–216
60. Omaye ST. Metabolic modulation of carbon monoxide toxicity. *Toxicology* 2002; **180**: 139–150.
61. Roughton FJW. Respiratory functions of blood. In: Boothby WM, ed.*Respiratory physiology in aviation.* Randolph Fields, TX. USAF School of Aviation Medicine. 1954.
62. Roughton FJW. Transport of oxygen and carbon dioxide. *Handbook of physiology,Vol 1: Respiration* (Section 3). Bethesda, MD: American Physiological Society, 1964: 767–825.
63. Durante W. Carbon monoxide and bile pigments: surprising mediators of vascular function. *Vasc Med* 2002; **7**: 195–202.
64. Paredi P, Kharitonov SA, Barnes PJ. Analysis of expired air for oxidation products. *Amer J Respir Crit Care Med* 2002; **166**: S31–37.
65. Raub JA, Benignus VA. Carbon monoxide and the nervous system *Neurosci Biobehav Rev* 2002; **26**: 925–940.
66. Abraham NG. Therapeutic applications of human heme oxygenase gene transfer and gene theapy. *Curr Pharm Des* 2003; **9**: 2513–2524.

67. Wagener FA, Volk HD, Willis D et al. Different faces of the heme-heme oxygenase system in inflammation. *Pharmacol Rev* 2003; **55**: 551–571.
68. McGrath JJ. Biological plausibility for carbon monoxide as a copollutant in PM epidemiologic studies. *Inhal Toxicol* 2000; **12**(Suppl 4): 91–107.
69. Roughton FJW, Darling RC. Effect of carbon monoxide on oxyhemoglobin dissociation curve. *Am J Physiol* 1944; **141**:17–31.
70. Haab P. The effect of carbon monoxide on respiration. *Experimentia* 1990; **46**: 1202–1206.
71. Gorman D, Drewry A, Huang YL, Sames C. The clinical toxicology of carbon monoxide. *Toxicology* 2003; **187**: 25–38.
72. Townsend CL, Maynard RL. Effects on health of prolonged exposure to low concentrations of carbon monoxide *Occup Environ Med* 2002; **59**: 708–711.
73. Douglas TA, Lawson DD, Ledingham I McA et al. Carbon monoxide poisoning: a comparison between the efficiencies of oxygen at one atmosphere pressure, of oxygen at two atmosphere pressure, and of 5% and 7% carbon dioxide in oxygen. *Lancet* 1962;**1**: 68–69.
74. Kopp MV, Bohnet W, Frischer T et al. Effects of ambient ozone on lung function in children over a two-summer period. *Eur Respir J* 2000; **16**: 893–900.
75. Grievink L, Jansen SMA, van't Veer P, Brunekreef B. Acute effects of ozone on pulmonary function of cyclists receiving antioxidant supplements. *Occup Environ Med* 1998; **55**: 13–17.
76. Schelegle ES, Siefkin AD, McDonald RJ. Time course of ozone-induced neutrophilia in normal humans. *Amer Rev Repir Dis* 1991; **143**: 1353-1358.
77. Hazucha MJ, Bates DV, Bromberg PA. Mechanism of action of ozone on the human lung. *J Appl Physiol* 1989; **67**: 1535–1541.
78. Mudway IS, Kelly FJ. Ozone and the lung: a sensitive issue. *Mol Aspects Med* 2000; **21**: 1–48.
79. Bosson J, Stenfors N, Bucht A et al. Ozone-induced bronchial epithelial cytokine expression differs between healthy and asthmatic subjects. *Clin Exp Allergy* 2003; **33**: 777–782.
80. Lee LY, Widdicombe JG. Modulation of airway sensitivity to inhaled irritants: role of inflammatory mediators. *Environ Health Perspect* 2001; **4**: 585–589.
81. Frank R, Liu MC, Spannhake EW et al. Repetitive ozone exposure of young adults. Evidence for persistent small airway dysfunction. *Am J Respir Crit Care Med* 2001; **164**: 1253–1260.
82. Oberdorster G. Pulmonary effects of inhaled ultrafine particles. *Int Arch Occup Environ Health* 2001; **74**: 1–8.
83. Frampton MW, Morrow PE, Torres A et al. Ozone responsiveness in smokers and nonsmokers. *Am J Respir Crit Care Med* 1997; **155**: 116–121.
84. Voter KZ, Whitan JC, Torres A et al. Ozone exposure and the production of reactive oxygen species by bronchoalveolar cells in humans. *Inhal Toxicol* 2001; **13**: 465–483.
85. Moran SE, Strachan DP, Johnston ID, Anderson HR. Effects of exposure to gas cooking in childhood and adulthood on respiratory symptoms, allergic sensitization and lung function in young British adults. *Clin Exp Allergy*. 1999; **29**: 1033–1041.
86. Bauer U, Berg D, Kohn MA et al. Acute effects of nitrogen dioxide after accidental release. *Public Health Rep* 1998; **113**: 62–70.
87. Devlin RB, Horstman DP, Gerrity TR et al. Inflammatory response in humans exposed to 2.0 ppm nitrogen dioxide. *Inhal Toxicol* 1999; **11**: 89–109.
88. Barck C, Sandstrom T, Lundahl J et al. Ambient level of NO_2 augments the inflammatory response to inhaled allergen in asthmatics. *Respir Med* 2002; **96**: 907–917.
89. Barth PJ, Mullet B. Effects of nitrogen dioxide exposure on Clara cell proliferation and morphology. *Pathol Res Pract* 1999; **195**: 487–493.
90. Becker S. Soukup JM. Effect of nitrogen dioxide on respiratory viral infection in airway epithelial cells. *Environ Res* 1999; **81**: 159–166.
91. Blomberg A, Krishna MT, Helleday R et al. Persistent airway inflammation but accommodated antioxidant and lung function responses after repeated daily exposures to nitrogen dioxide. *Am J Respir Crit Care Med* 1999; **159**: 536–543.
92. Piirila PL, Nordman H, Korhonen OS, Winblad I. A thirteen-year follow-up of respiratory effects of acute exposure to sulfur dioxide. *Scand J Work Environ Health* 1996; **22**: 191-196.
93. Jakab GJ, Clarke RW, Hemenway DR et al. Inhalation of acid coated carbon black particles impairs alveolar macrophage phagocytosis. *Toxicol Lett* 1996; **88**: 243–248.
94. Gong H Jr, Lachenbruch PA, Harber P, Linn WS. Comparative short-term health responses to sulfur dioxide exposure and other common stresses in a panel of asthmatics. *Toxicol Ind Health* 1995; **11**: 467–487.
95. Meng Z. Oxidative damage of sulfur dioxide on various organs of mice: sulfur dioxide is a systemic oxidative damage agent. *Inhal Toxicol* 2003; **15**: 181–195.
96. Tunnicliffe WS, Harrison RM, Kelly FJ et al. The effect of sulphurous air pollutant exposures on symptoms, lung function, exhaled nitric oxide and nasal epithelial lining fluid antioxidant concentrations in normal and asthmatic adults. *Occup Environ Med* 2003; **60**: e15
97. Frye C, Hoelscher B, Cyrys J et al. Association of lung function with declining ambient air pollution. *Environ Health Perspect* 2003; **111**: 383–387.
98. Wong CM, Atkinson RW, Anderson HR et al. A tale of two cities: effects of air pollution on hospital admissions in Hong Kong and London compared. *Environ Health Perspect* 2002; **110**: 67–77.
99. Horak F Jr, Studnicka M, Gartner C et al. Particulate matter and lung function growth in children: a 3-yr follow-up study in Austrian schoolchildren. *Eur Respir J* 2002; **19**: 838–845.
100. Oehme FW, Cooppock RW, Mostrom MS, Khan AA. A review of the toxicology of air pollutants: toxicology of chemical mixtures. *Vet Hum Toxicol* 1996; **38**: 371–377.
101. Brown JS, Zeman KL, Bennett WD. Ultrafine particle deposition and clearance in the healthy and obstructed lung. *Am J Respir Crit Care Med*. 2002; **166**: 1240–1247.
102. Schwela D Air pollution and health in urban areas. *Rev Environ Health* 2000: **15**: 13–42.
103. Bruce N, Perez-Padilla R, Albalak R. Indoor air pollution in developing countries; a major environmental and public health challenge. *Bull World Health Organ* 2000; **78**: 1078–1092.
104. Shima M, Adachi M. Indoor nitrogen dioxide in homes along trunk roads with heavy traffic. *Occup Environ Med* 1998; **55**: 428–433.
105. Edwards JH, Cockcroft A. Inhalation challenge in humidifier fever. *Clin Allergy* 1981; **11**: 227–235.
106. Bourke SJ, Dalphin JC, Boyd G et al. Hypersensitivity pneumonitis: current concepts. *Eur Respir J* 2001; Suppl **32**: 81s–92s.
107. Ohtani Y, Saiki S, Sumi Y et al. Clinical features of recurrent and insidious chronic bird fancier's lung. *Ann Allergy Asthma Immunol* 2003; **90**: 604-610, also *Ibid* 579–580.

108. Hardin BD, Kelman BJ, Saxon A. Adverse human health effects associated with moulds in the indoor environment. *J Occup Environ Med* 2003; **45**: 470–478.
109. Gould D. Legionaires' disease. *Nurs Stand* 2003; **17**: 41–44.
110. Skyberg K, Skulberg KR, Eduard W et al.Symptoms prevalence among office employees and associations to building characteristics. *Indoor Air* 2003; **13**: 246–252.
111. Burge PS. Sick building syndrome. *Occup Environ Med* 2004; **61**: 185–190.
112. Elmes PC. Relative importance of cigarette smoking in occupational lung disease. *Br J Ind Med* 1981; **38**: 1–13.
113. Ondrasik M. Caplan's syndrome *Baillieres Clin Rheumatol* 1989; **3**: 205–210.
114. Kelleher P, Pacheco K, Newman LS. Inorganic dust pneumonias: the metal-related parenchymal disorders. *Envirn Health Perspect* 2000; **108**: 685–696.
115. Schins RP, Borm PJ. Mechanisms and mediators in coal dust induced toxicity: a review. *Ann Occup Hyg* 1999; **43**: 7–33.
116. Castranova V, Vallyathan V. Silicosis and coal workers' pneumoconiosis. *Environ Health Persp* 2000; **108**: 675–684.
117. Kamp DW, Panduri V, Weitzman SA, Chandel N. Asbestos-induced alveolar epithelial cell apoptosos: role of mitochondrial dysfunction caused by iron-derived free radicals. *Mol Cell Biochem* 2002; **234-235**: 152–160.
118. Khang Q, Dai J, Ali A et al. Roles of bioavailable iron and calcium in coal dust-induced oxidative stress: possible implications in coal workers' lung disease. *Free Radic Res* 2002; **36**: 285–294.
119. Nadif R, Oryszczyn MP, Fradier-Dusch M et al. Cross sectional and longitudinal study on selenium, glutathione peroxidase, smoking and occupational exposure in coal miners. *Occup Environ Med* 2001; **58**: 239–245.
120. Buchanan D, Miller BG, Soutar CA. Quantitative relations between exposure to respirable quartz and risk of silicosis. *Occup Environ Med* 2003; **60**: 159-164.
121. Markowitz G, Rosner D. The reawakening of national concern about silicosis. *Public Health Rep* 1998; **113**: 302–311.
122. Cotes JE, King B. Relationship of lung function to radiographic reading (IOL) in patients with asbestos related lung disease. *Thorax* 1988; **43**: 777–783.
123. Wright PH, Hanson A, Kreel L, Capel LH. Respiratory function changes after asbestos pleurisy. *Thorax* 1980; **35**: 31–36.
124. Rudd RM. New developments in asbestos-related pleural disease. *Thorax* 1996; **51**: 210–216.
125. McDonald JC. Asbestos and lung cancer: has the case been proven? *Chest* 1980; **78**: 374s–376s.
126. Cotes JE, Gilson JC, McKerrow CB, Oldham PD. A long-term follow-up of workers exposed to beryllium. *Br J Ind Med* 1983; **40**: 13–21.
127. McKerrow CB, McDermott M, Gilson JC, Schilling RSF. Respiratory function during the day in cotton workers: a study in byssinosis. *Br J Ind Med* 1958; **15**:75–83
128. McL Niven R, Pickering CA. Byssinosis: a review. *Thorax* 1996; **51**: 632–637.
129. Rylander R. Diseases associated with exposure to plant dusts: focus on cotton dust. *Tuber Lung Dis* 1992; **73**: 21-26.
130. Wild LG, Lopez M. Hypersensitivity pneumonitis: a comprehensive review. *J Investig Allergol Clin Immunol* 2001; **11**: 3–15.
131. Ohtani Y, Saiki S, Sumi Y et al. Clinical features of recurrent and insidious chronic bird fancier's lung. *Ann Allergy Immunol* 2003; **90**: 604–610.
132. Murin S, Bilello KS, Matthay R. Other smoking-affected pulmonary diseases. *Clin Chest Med* 2000; **21**: 121–137.
133. Stockley RA, Hill SL, Drew R. Asthma associated with a circulating IgG antibody to *Calliphora* maggots. *Clin Allergy* 1982; **12**: 151–155.
134. Cockcroft A, Seal RME, Wagner JC et al. Post-mortem study of emphysema in coal workers and non-coal workers. *Lancet* 1982; **ii**: 600–603.
135. Rogan JM, Attfield MD, Jacobsen M et al. Role of dust in the working environment in development of chronic bronchitis in British coalminers. *Br J Ind Med* 1984; **41**: 217–226.
136. Cockcroft AE, Wagner JC, Seal RME et al. Irregular opacities in coal-workers' pneumoconiosis-correlation with pulmonary function and pathology. *Ann Occup Hyg* 1982; **26**: 767–787.
137. Bauer TT, Schultze-Werninghaus G. KollmeierJ et al. Functional variables associated with the clinical grade of dyspnoea in coal miners with pneumoconiosis and mild bronchial obstruction. *Occup Environ Med* 2001; **58**: 794–799.
138. Gilson JC, Hugh-Jones P, Oldham PD, Meade F. Lung function in coal workers' pneumoconiosis. Medical Research Council (Lond). *Spec Rep Ser* 1955; **290**: 1–266.
139. Xipell JM, Ham KN, Price CG, Thomas PD. Acute silicoproteinosis. *Thorax* 1977; **32**: 104–111.
140. Glover JR, Bevan C, Cotes JE et al. Effects of exposure to slate dust in North Wales. *Br J Indr Med* 1980; **37**: 152–162.
141. Field GB. Pulmonary function in aluminium smelters. *Thorax* 1984; **39**: 743–751.
142. Fritschi L, Sim MR, Forbes A et al. Respiratory symptoms and lung function changes with exposure to five substances in aluminium smelters. *Int Arch Occup Environ Health* 2003; **76**: 103–110.
143. Tan KL, Lee HS, Poh WT et al. Hard metal disease-the first case in Singapore. *Ann Acad Med Singapore* 2000; **29**: 521–527.
144. Health effects of mineral oil mist and metalworking fluids. *Symposium. Appl Occup Environ Hyg* 2003; **18**: 815–975.
145. Miller GJ, Ashcroft MT, Beadnell HMSG et al. Tle lipoid pneumonia of black fat tobacco smokers of Guyana. *Quart J Med* 1971; **40**: 457–470.

Further reading

Becklake MR, Ghezzo H, Ernst P. Childhood predictors of smoking in adolescence: a follow-up study of Montreal school children. *CMAJ* 2005; **174**: 377–379.

Laube BL. The expanding role of aerosols in systemic drug delivery, gene delivery and vaccination. *Respir Care* 2005; **50**: 1161–1176.

Appendix: Illustrative cases of occupational lung disorders

Table 37.A. Occupational cases A: lung function in three men exposed to asbestos (reference values are in brackets).

Index	Diffuse pleural disease		Asbestosis
	Extensive calcified plaques	Fibrosis	
Age (a)	60	42	50
Height (m)	1.87	1.80	1.69
Weight (kg)	85	93	59
FEV_1 (l)	3.3 (3.5)	1.9 (3.8)	1.2 (3.1)
FVC (l)	4.1 (4.8)	2.9 (4.8)	2.1 (4.1)
FEV_1%	81 (69)	64 (76)	57 (73)
TLC (l)	5.9 (7.7)	4.0 (7.1)	4.3 (6.1)
RV (l)	2.0 (2.6)	1.4 (2.1)	1.8 (2.0)
Cstat (l kPa^{-1})	1.7 (3.1)	1.1 (2.8)	1.0 (2.4)
(l cm H_2O^{-1})	0.17 (0.31)	0.11 (0.28)	0.10 (0.24)
Pmax (kPa)*	5.0 (2.5)	3.5 (2.5)	5.1 (2.5)
(cm H_2O)	50 (25)	35 (25)	51 (25)
Tl (mmol min^{-1} kPa^{-1})	8.6 (10.5)	7.6 (10.9)	3.4 (9.1)
(ml min^{-1} mm Hg^{-1})	25.8 (31.5)	22.8 (32.7)	10.2 (27.3)
Kco (Tl/VA)	1.6 (1.4)	1.9 (1.7)	0.9 (1.5)
$\dot{V}_{E45}$ (l min^{-1})	33 (24)	34 (24)	42† (24)
Vt_{30} (l)‡	1.0 (1.5)	1.0 (1.5)	0.8 (1.4)
Sa_{O_2} (rest/ex.%)	96/96	NA	91/84
Pattern	Mild restrictive	Restrictive, mild obstructive	Mixed

* Maximal recoil pressure, upper limit of normal is 3.7 kPa (37 cm H_2O).
† Extrapolated.
‡ Reference values for Vt_{30} are based on predicted FVC.

These patients all had a reduced total lung capacity associated with a low compliance and high recoil pressure. The low TLC contributed to reductions in exercise tidal volume (Vt_{30}) and in transfer factor; in asbestos pleural disease the latter effect was partly compensated for by an increase in Kco. In all the patients the exercise ventilation was increased, mainly on account of shallow breathing and an enlarged physiological deadspace. Exercise desaturation contributed to respiratory drive in the patient with asbestosis. For further cases see Tables 29.11 and 29.12, pages 429 and 430.

Table 37.B. Occupational case B: respiratory impairment in late stage byssinosis.

Mr. B, aged 66 years, worked for 51 years in the cotton industry, mainly on jobs connected with carding. During this time he developed symptoms of chest tightness, especially on Monday afternoons. He also noticed breathlessness on exertion which was most marked after work and during episodes of bronchitis secondary to head colds. Subsequent to his retirement, which was on account of redundancy, his symptoms improved. At that time he smoked half an ounce of pipe tobacco per day and had moderate breathlessness on exertion (clinical grade 3, see page 532). On clinical examination the area of cardiac dullness was diminished and fine crackle were present at both lung bases posteriorly. The chest X-ray showed a large lung, a flat diaphragm and loss of vascular markings. The ECG showed evidence of right ventricular preponderance. On assessment of lung function the forced expiratory volume was reduced and represented a small proportion of the forced vital capacity. The total lung capacity and the residual volume were increased; the proportion of the vital capacity which could be expelled by forced expiratory effort was diminished on account of air-trapping which was present on the spirogram. The transfer factor (diffusing capacity) for the lungs and the tension of oxygen and carbon dioxide in the arterial blood were all within normal limits. The response of ventilation to exercise was increased both when breathing air and when breathing oxygen. The airway resistance was increased but the static lung compliance was within normal limits.

These findings were evidence for chronic obstructive pulmonary disease with airways obstruction, though the normal value for the lung volume index of uneven ventilation was an inconsistent feature. This was not an artefact due to under-estimation of the residual volume by the closed-circuit method since measurements of lung volume by plethysmography yielded a similar result. The high level of ventilation during exercise reflected an enlarged physiological deadspace.

	Mr B	Reference value
Age (a)	66	–
Height (m)	1.72	–
Weight (kg)	77	–
FEV_1 (l)	1.33	2.77
FVC (l)	2.75	3.89
FEV_1%	48	67
TLC (l)	8.23	6.4
IVC (l)	4.32	3.9
FRC (l)	4.68	3.7
RV (l)	3.91	2.3
RV%	48	39
Air-trapping	Yes	–
T_L† (single breath)	9.3 (28)	8.4 (25)
V_{Aeff}/V_A	0.90	>0.85
P_{a,O_2}†	11.2 (84)	12 (89)
P_{a,CO_2}†	5.9 (44)	<6 (46)
$\dot{V}_E$, ex air (l min^{-1})	43.1	24
$\dot{V}_E$, ex O_2 (l min^{-1})	43.1	22
C_{stat}, inspn†	1.9 (0.19)	2.5 (0.26)
R_{aw} (Interrupter method on inspiration)†	0.48 (4.8)	0.09 (0.9)

† The data are given in SI units with traditional units in brackets, e.g. for P_{a,O_2} kPa (torr), T_l mmol min^{-1} kPa^{-1} (ml min^{-1} $torr^{-1}$), for C_{stat} l kPa^{-1} (l cm H_2O^{-1}) and for R_{aw} kPa l^{-1}s (cm H_2O l^{-1}s). The conversion factors are given in Table 6.6 (page 56).

Table 37.C. Occupational case C: farmer's lung.

History. The patient and her husband, who was a quarry man, looked after three cows on a smallholding in mid-Wales. One summer, for the first time, they used a bailer for their hay. The hay was subsequently found to be mouldy. The following spring the patient (age 51 years, height 1.57 m) experienced an acute febrile illness with breathlessness and expectoration of some greenish, blood-flecked sputum.
Examination. Mid- to late inspiratory crackles were heard at the lung bases. The chest X-ray showed some diffuse mottling of both lung fields, and the ECG showed evidence of left ventricular hypertropy. The blood pressure was 160/105 mm Hg.
Lung function (see below). The compliance, total lung capacity and subdivisions were slightly reduced but the ventilatory capacity, FEV_1 and airflow resistance were normal. The transfer factor (Tl) and its membrane component (Dm) were reduced and the exercise ventilation was increased to a greater extent breathing air than oxygen.
Diagnosis. The diagnosis of disease of the lung parenchyma due to farmer's lung was supported by the findings of precipitating antibodies against *M. faeni.*
Subsequent course. The condition cleared up during the summer and the advice to change over to making silage was rejected. However, after an illness the following winter the patient agreed to use a fine dust respirator which was carefully chosen to fit her face. This prevented further episodes.

	Subacute	3 months later	Reference value
Forced expiratory volume (FEV_1 l)	2.30	2.45	2.25
Forced vital capacity (FVC l)	2.73	3.05	3.2
FEV_1/FVC (%)	84	80	75
Total lung capacity (TLC l)	4.46	4.94	4.9
Residual volume (RV l)	1.49	1.65	1.7
Transfer factor (Tl)*	4.5 (13)	6.7 (20)	7.7 (23)
Diffusing capacity of alv. Membrane (Dm)*	6.7 (20)	14.4 (43)	15 (45)
Vol. of blood in alv. caps. (Vc ml)	43	43	56
Lung compliance (Cstat, l kPa^{-1} and l cm H_2O^{-1})	1.2 (0.12)	1.4 (0.14)	2.0 (0.20)
Airway resistance (kPa l^{-1}s and cm H_2O l^{-1}s)	0.11 (1.1)	0.11 (1.1)	0.12 (1.2)
Exercise ventilation ($\dot{V}e_{45}$, l min^{-1}):			
Air	39	24	25
O_2	30	24	24

* mmol min^{-1} kPa^{-1} (ml min^{-1} mm Hg^{-1})

Table 37.D. Occupational cases D and E: PMF and hard metal disease.

Complicated pneumoconiosis (PMF). Mr. D., an ex-coalminer aged 63 years, had worked underground for 31 years as a collier and then an overman. He gave a history of shortness of breath on exertion since age 45 years. At that time an X-ray showed numerous dust foci throughout the lung with superimposed areas of coalescence, typical of progressive massive fibrosis (category 3/B, 2/2 on the International classification). He was transferred to a less dusty occupation. However, his capacity for exercise continued to deteriorate and he developed chronic bronchitis. At the time of assessment Mr D was recovering from an acute chest illness. For this he was treated with digoxin and diuretics as well as bronchodilator and antibiotic drugs. On examination of the chest there were few abnormal physical signs, but the breath sound conduction and the tactile vocal fremitus were reduced. There was no cardiac failure. The ECG showed prominent *P* waves but was otherwise normal. On assessment of lung function (see below) the forced expiratory volume was reduced and represented a small proportion of the forced vital capacity; both volumes were labile and increased after the inhalation of a bronchodilator aerosol. The total lung capacity was on the low side of normal but the residual volume was increased. The forced vital capacity was equal to the two stage vital capacity and there was no evidence of air-trapping on the spirogram. The transfer factor (diffusing capacity) for the lung was reduced with diminution in the membrane component. The lung volume index of uneven ventilation showed evidence of abnormality. The tension of oxygen in the arterial blood was reduced at rest, but the tension of carbon dioxide was normal. However, during exercise when the patient was breathing oxygen the tension of carbon dioxide increased and at this time the ventilation was markedly reduced. The lung was less compliant that normal and the airway resistance was increased.

The findings were evidence for impairment of all aspects of lung function and were consistent with a space-occupying lesion (*i.e.* progressive massive fibrosis) plus airway obstruction. However, with a different industrial history, they could have been due to the combination of the latter condition with interstitial pulmonary fibrosis, though a lower value for the transfer factor would then have been expected. The relatively large bronchodilator response suggested that the patient was not receiving adequate therapy at the time of assessment. The improvement in the capacity for exercise during breathing oxygen suggested that the patient might be considered for portable oxygen therapy.

Hard metal disease. Mr. E, aged 64 years, had worked in the tungsten carbide industry where he was exposed to cobalt dust. For 11 years his job had been cleaning the insides of furnaces. He presented with breathlessness on exertion and recurrent bouts of bronchitis. At assessment he was breathless on moderate exertion (clinical grade 3, see page 532) but was otherwise in good health. On examination of the chest a few fine crackles were heard at both lung bases with some wheezes. The chest radiograph showed diffuse nodulation. The ECG was normal. On assessment of lung function (see below) the forced expiratory volume and the forced vital capacity were somewhat reduced but the lung volumes were otherwise within normal limits. The $FEV_1\%$ was normal and there was no air-trapping on the spirogram. The transfer factor (diffusing capacity) for the lung was reduced, due mainly to a diminution in the membrane component. The tensions of oxygen and carbon dioxide in the arterial blood were both low at rest. On exercise the Pa,o_2 fell further when breathing air and ventilation was abnormally high. The airway resistance and the compliance were relatively normal.

These findings were evidence for disease affecting the lung parenchyma. In view of the history they were probably occupational in origin (see also [143]).

Subject/condition	Mr D/PMF	Reference value	Mr E/hard metal disease	Reference value
Age (a)	63	–	64	–
Height (m)	1.63	–	1.76	–
Weight (kg)	54	–	79	–
FEV_1 (l)	1.23	2.5	2.03	3.0
Change with bronchodilator (%)	+17	<10	+7	<10
FVC (l)	2.71	3.5	2.90	4.1
$FEV_1\%$	45	68	70	68
TLC (l)	5.01	5.6	5.98	6.8
IVC (l)	2.40	3.5	3.37	4.1
FRC (l)	3.59	3.7	3.73	3.8
RV (l)	2.61	2.0	2.61	2.4
RV%	52	38	44	38
Air-trapping	No	–	No	–
Tl* (single breath)	6.7 (20)	7.5 (22)	4.4 (13)	9.0 (27)
Dm* (single-breath)	9.7 (29)	14 (42)	8.0 (24)	16 (47)
Vc (ml)	58	70	43	86
V_{Aeff}/V_A	0.64	>0.85	–	>0.85
Pa,o_2*	8.3 (62)	12 (89)	9.6 (72)†	12 (89)
Pa,co_2*	5.6 (42)	<6(46)	4.3(32)	<6(46)
$\dot{V}_E$, ex air (l min^{-1})	32	24	56	24
$\dot{V}_E$, ex o_2 (l min^{-1})	23	22	35	22
$Cstat$, inspn*	1.1 (0.11)	2.2 (0.23)	1.8 (0.18)	2.7 (0.27)
Raw (plethysmograph)*	0.25 (2.5)	0.1 (1.0)	0.14 (1.4)‡	0.1 (1.0)

* For units see footnote to Table 37.B.

† On exercise 8.3 (62).

‡ Interrupter method on inspiration.

PART 7
Lung Function in Clinical Practice

CHAPTER 38

Patterns of Abnormal Function in Lung Disease

38.1 Introduction

Numerous medical conditions affect the lungs either directly or by involving the pulmonary circulation. The responses usually conform to one of a limited number of syndromes of disordered lung function (Table 38.1). The syndromes can usually be identified by measurement of the ventilatory capacity, lung volumes and transfer factor, but in some instances the mechanical function of the lungs or the physiological response to exercise must also be assessed.

The presence of a particular syndrome constitutes a functional diagnosis. This will reflect, and in some instances indicate precisely, the underlying changes in structure. Lung function tests can provide information on causation only if there is a unique feature, such as a bronchoconstrictor response to a specific allergen. The tests can be used to measure disability, monitor the course of the condition and its response to treatment, assess residual exercise capacity and indicate prognosis. In these ways the lung function laboratory makes an important contribution to respiratory medicine. The contribution is most effective when there is full exchange of information between the clinician and the laboratory on why assessments have been requested and, subsequently, on their contribution to the clinical outcome. This information should include any morbid anatomical findings which may influence lung function.

Table 38.1 Syndromes of disordered lung function.

Disorder		Subtype
Ventilatory defect	(a) Obstructive	(i) Reversible
		(ii) Fixed
		(iii) Small airways syndrome
	(b) Non-obstructive	(i) Restrictive
		(ii) Hypodynamic
Defect of gas transfer		
Sleep disordered breathing		
Bronchial hyperresponsiveness		(i) Non-specific
		(ii) Specific

Referral to the lung function laboratory will usually be for a suspected condition of the airways or parenchyma of the lungs (Table 38.2). Less often the main point of interest will be the chest wall, respiratory control system or pulmonary circulation. Patients with acute respiratory infections should rarely be referred since the results will not be a fair reflection of the true underlying function. Lung function tests readily detect changes due to diseases of the airways which may be localised, e.g. goitre, tumour or polyp, or be more generalised, e.g. asthma. Generalised conditions of the airways can present with cough and expectoration of phlegm, with wheeze which may be episodic, or with breathlessness on exertion. The common causes are chronic bronchitis, asthma and emphysema (Chapter 40, see page 545). However, these conditions may co-exist and all can be associated with airflow limitation so the distinction between them is not always clear cut. This has led to use of the term chronic obstructive pulmonary disease (COPD). Some argue that using the term

Table 38.2 Disorders of the lungs that often lead to patients being referred to the lung function laboratory.

Condition	Common presentation	Features
Chronic bronchitis	Chronic cough and sputum	Mucous gland hyperplasia, bronchial wall inflammation
Asthma	Episodic airflow limitation, wheeze, nocturnal cough	Bronchial wall inflammation, eosinophilic bronchiolitis
Emphysema	Breathlessness on exertion and later at rest	Alveolar destruction, enlarged airspaces
COPD	Progressive airflow limitation	
Diseases of lung parenchyma	Breathlessness with shallow breathing (initially on exertion)	
Restrictive disorders	Shallow breathing, breathlessness	
Disorders of pulmonary circulation	Breathlessness, chest pain, syncope, right heart failure	
Pneumoconiosis	Cough, breathlessness	

obstruction is semantically incorrect since obstruction is often not present but there is airflow limitation due to narrowing of bronchi. However, the ATS and ERS have embraced the use of COPD and the term is widely accepted.

38.2 Symptoms and function

Respiratory function is impaired when it is demonstrably inferior to that of reference subjects at one point in time or when observed longitudinally (Chapter 26, e.g. page 358). Because the lungs have considerable functional reserve, some impairment can be present without any symptoms and it may then be difficult to detect (Section 30.3.1). The likelihood of recognition is increased if the subject is habitually more breathless on exertion than others of the same age and sex. For a subject who is accustomed to walking out of doors the clinical grade of breathlessness can be assessed using the four-point scale of Fletcher, or an extended version of it (Table 38.3).

For a subject who is not accustomed to taking much exercise the degree of respiratory insufficiency can be assessed in terms of his or her daily activity. For example a subject might be breathless (experience dyspnoea) when mounting stairs, walking whilst carrying a basket of shopping, walking from one room to the next at home, towelling down after a bath or shower, dressing or undressing, during meals or in conversation at rest. The ability to perform some of these activities is encapsulated in the oxygen cost diagram of McGavin and colleagues (Fig. 30.3, page 440). To make a more precise assessment the capacity for exercise should be determined in the manner described in Chapter 29.

A subject with respiratory impairment is in a state of respiratory failure if the tensions of oxygen and carbon dioxide in the arterial blood lie outside the range of normal variation. In the case of carbon dioxide, a tension at sea level that is consistently more than 6.3 kPa (47 mm Hg) is regarded as abnormal. However, the definition does not apply to subjects breathing oxygen during strenuous exercise when the tension of carbon dioxide is normally increased (Section 28.8.1). While breathing air the lower limits of oxygen tension are the same at rest and on exercise. At age 20 a tension of oxygen of slightly less than 11 kPa (83 mm Hg) and at age 60 of less than 10 kPa (76 torr) indicates mild respiratory failure. The corresponding oxygen saturations are 95% and 93%, respectively. The tension of oxygen that indicates a serious derangement of lung function varies with circumstances; at sea level a reduction on account of lung disease to less than 8 kPa (60 mm Hg) is always a cause for concern (see also Section 29.8).

Table 38.3 Clinical grades of breathlessness of Fletcher [1] with example of their application for Welsh coal miners aged 50–75 years.

Description	Clinical grade	ability score	FEV_1
Is living: needs help with feeding	–	8	0.3
With help can dress and sit out of bed	–	7	0.5
Can converse, walk 10 m, bath with help	–	6	0.7
Can walk 100 m, sing, climb 8 stairs	–	5	1.1
Can walk 400 m	4	4	1.6
Can walk unlimited distance at slow pace	3	3	2.1
Can walk at normal pace on level ground without becoming breathless	2	2	2.6
Can hurry on level ground and walk uphill without undue breathlessness	1	1	3.1

Note: The grades are assessed using the MRC Questionnaire on Respiratory Symptoms where comparison is made with a healthy man of the same age (Fig. 8.2, page 88). Alternative scoring systems are also used (Table 44. 1, page 612). The corresponding FEV_1 has wide confidence limits and is greatly influenced by the pathological diagnosis (cf. Tables 29.11 and 12, pages 429 and 430).
Source: Cotes, unpublished.

38.3 Ventilatory defect

Performance of exercise requires increased minute ventilation. A wide range of conditions can limit a person's ability to obtain sufficient air for exercise or to undertake the activities of daily living without experiencing dyspnoea (Section 28.7). These conditions affect the mechanics of ventilation and are usually detected by recording the maximal forced expiratory manoeuvre. The typical changes in this manoeuvre are classified into an obstructive or non-obstructive pattern, and of which the latter can be subdivided into restrictive and hypodynamic types. Some of the causes of airway obstruction are in Table 14.3 (page 155).

38.3.1 Obstructive defect

An obstructive type of ventilatory defect is usually diagnosed from a reduced $FEV_1\%$ (FEV_1/FVC) or from a reduced peak expiratory flow associated with a prolonged forced expiratory time. The condition is associated with reduced airway calibre, hence lower expiratory flow and also with premature closure of airways during expiration; the closure has implications for other aspects of lung function (Section 12.5.1). Because the expiration is forced the airway closure is accentuated by dynamic compression, and this reduces the forced vital capacity relative to the inspiratory vital capacity (IVC). As a result the $FEV_1\%$ is reduced to a lesser extent than the Tiffeneau index (FEV_1/IVC), which is widely used for diagnosis of airflow limitation in some western European countries.

Reversible versus fixed. The obstructive type of ventilatory defect can be described as reversible or fixed (irreversible). The criteria for reversibility of FEV_1 following administration of a bronchodilator drug are that the change must exceed the random variation (0.16–0.19 l, Section 15.7.2, also [2].), and be clinically meaningful for the patient. On the latter count the ERS recommends that a change should exceed 12% of the predicted value [3], whilst the ATS accept an increase of at least 12% of baseline as significant [4]. However, airflow limitation that does not initially respond to a bronchodilator aerosol may do so following corticosteroid therapy. In addition, some patients may have no significant response at one point in time but at some later stage demonstrate significant reversibility. Thus, the distinction between reversibility and irreversibility is often not clear cut. Reversibility originally served to distinguish asthma from other types of airflow limitation; it is now used mainly for assessing the likely benefit of bronchodilator therapy.

The site of airflow limitation may be within the lung parenchyma (intrapulmonary) or external to it (extrapulmonary) and may be within the thorax (intrathoracic) or outside the thorax (extrathoracic). The forces acting on the airways to cause obstruction in these different locations can be deduced from the shapes of maximal flow–volume loops obtained in the lung function laboratory. Fig. 38.1 shows a curve for a patient with advanced emphysema. Curves for patients with other types of obstruction are included in Section 41.2.

Small airways obstruction. Care must be taken in defining conditions affecting small airways solely from lung function tests. The initial paper suggesting the index $FEF_{25-75\%}$ was a sensitive

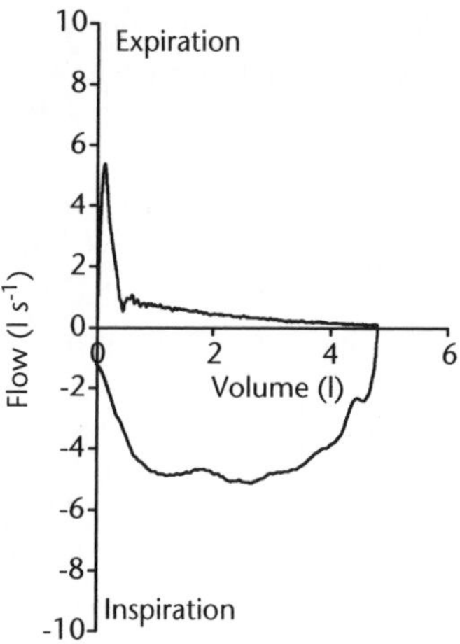

Fig. 38.1 Flow–volume loop of a patient with emphysema who expired for 17 s to deliver an FVC of 4.8 l. After expiration of approximately 0.5 l the expiratory flow declined abruptly due to pressure dependent collapse of airways. The subsequent low flow was due to low elastic recoil and grossly narrowed airways, giving an almost straight tail to the loop.

test of small airways disease, used a threshold of 80% of the predicted value for defining abnormality [5]. However, at the 10% level of probability [3] the normal ranges are wide, 66%–134% for a man aged 25, of average height, and 45% to 154% for a man aged 70. In view of the wide range the index is of limited usefulness. More informative indices are the alveolar nitrogen slope, closing volume and the frequency dependence of compliance all of which have been shown to be associated with disease of small airways as assessed by histological analysis [6].

Stanescu [7] has described a small airways obstruction syndrome where there is a decrease in VC and FEV_1, with a normal FEV_1/VC ratio and a normal TLC, together with an increase in RV and RV/TLC ratio. The condition is attributed to premature closing of airways leading to air trapping. VC and not FVC should be used for its identification since FVC can be reduced by dynamic expiratory airflow obstruction [8]. The presence of focal air trapping in this condition was demonstrated by HRCT scans [9], but the finding did not correlate with the results of any other lung function tests.

38.3.2 Restrictive defect

A restrictive ventilatory defect of pulmonary origin is usually due to a decrease in the distensibility of the lung (i.e. the lung compliance is reduced and elastic recoil increased). The reduction can be due to an increase in the quantity of interstitial tissue in the lung, for example interstitial pneumonitis, fibrosis, infiltration or oedema. Alternatively, the reduced lung compliance can be due to fibrosis of the visceral pleura and sub-pleural tissue. Any of these changes can increase the retractive force exerted on the walls of lung airways; the retraction reduces the airways resistance and increases the $FEV_1\%$. In this circumstance the peak expiratory flow can be well preserved or even supramaximal early in the disease process but, once lung volume becomes severely reduced the PEF also declines because it is then measured at a relatively small lung volume.

A restrictive defect of intrapulmonary origin can be mimicked by a space-occupying lesion of the lung or pleura, such as pneumothorax or pleural effusion which reduces the lung volumes and FEV_1. These conditions can also reduce the ventilation and perfusion of the affected part of the lungs.

When the restrictive defect arises in the chest wall, the compliance of the lungs is normal, but the compliance of the chest wall is reduced. This change can be a consequence of severe obesity, or a disease process affecting the ribs or the vertebral column, for example in ankylosing spondylitis or kyphoscoliosis (Section 41.7). The shallow breathing increases the respiratory frequency and hence the volume of air per minute used to ventilate the physiological deadspace. The ventilation minute volume is increased in consequence, especially that during exercise (Section 28.4.7).

38.3.3 Hypodynamic defect

A hypodynamic type of ventilatory defect occurs when the vital capacity is diminished by a reduction in the maximal force that can be exerted by the respiratory muscles. The force generated by the weak muscles is insufficient to move the chest wall and expand the lungs fully against their elastic recoil, so TLC is reduced. During expiration the weakness affects the ability to compress the chest wall much below its usual relaxation point, so RV is increased. Thus, VC is small due to limitation at both ends of the manoeuvre. The principal diagnostic feature is a low maximal inspiratory pressure (Section 9.9). As a result, all lung function indices that are dependent on lung volume or respiratory effort are impaired to some extent.

38.4 Gas exchange defect

Defective gas transfer is characterised by a reduced transfer factor; this leads to the blood leaving the alveolar capillaries without its full complement of oxygen. In the absence of complicating factors the ventilatory response to exercise is increased and there may also be exercise hypoxaemia (see e.g. Table 29.11, page 429 also Section 40.4.4). Reduced gas transfer may be due to abnormalities of the lung parenchyma including interstitial pneumonitis, interstitial fibrosis and emphysema, or due to pulmonary vascular disease such as pulmonary emboli. With interstitial fibrosis there is also likely to be a restrictive type of ventilatory defect, whilst with emphysema there is often intrapulmonary airflow limitation (Sections 40.3 and 40.4).

Hyperventilation on exercise may be the first indication of the condition, and the presence of progressive hypoxaemia on exercise shows that the diffusing capacity of the lungs for oxygen is reduced. This finding initially led to the theory that the syndrome was due to insufficient diffusion of oxygen across the thickened alveolar membranes, hence the term 'alveolar capillary block'. Because oxygen has a very high diffusivity this aspect of gas exchange is unlikely to be seriously impaired except with pulmonary oedema and so the term alveolar capillary block syndrome may not be appropriate. The reduction of transfer factor with associated hypoxaemia on exercise can be due to splinting or enlargement of the respiratory bronchioles increasing the path length for diffusion in the airspaces (e.g. Fig. 3.5, page 26, cf. Fig. 19.2 page 229), or to blockage or destruction of alveolar capillaries causing an increase in the flow of blood and consequent reduction in transit time through the remaining capillaries. The time for which the red cells are in contact with the alveolar gas can then be too short for gas exchange to continue to equilibrium (Fig. 21.2, page 263). Thus, exercise hypoxaemia can be attributed to imperfect matching between the alveolar surface available for the exchange of gas and lung volume (Tl/V_A inequality), blood flow ($Tl/\dot{Q}_C$ inequality) and lung capillary blood volume (Tl/V_C inequality). Hypoxaemia from these causes occurs principally on exercise (Section 21.4.5). In addition, the structural changes were believed to cause maldistribution of ventilation with respect to perfusion ($\dot{V}_A/\dot{Q}$ inequality) leading to hypoxaemia at rest (Section 21.5.2). Recent work has largely confirmed this dual explanation for the hypoxaemia, but the relative contributions of the distributive and diffusive components are still in doubt e.g. [10].

The features of defective gas transfer can be obscured by any coexisting mechanical derangement of the lungs. Where this is minimal, as in some pulmonary infiltrations, the hypoxaemia and possibly other factors increase the drive to respiration causing marked hyperventilation at rest as well as on exercise. The hyperventilation partly corrects the hypoxaemia; it also leads to hypocapnia and to a compensatory readjustment to the acid–base balance of the body (Section 22.3.3). In other patients there is a material restrictive, obstructive or hypodynamic type of ventilatory defect; these reduce the ventilatory response to exercise and accentuate the ventilation–perfusion inequality. The degree of exercise desaturation is then increased. Thus, the effects of defective gas transfer upon exercise ventilation and the arterial oxygen tension can be represented by a continuum with the ventilatory and blood gas components being to some extent negatively correlated.

38.4.1 Reduction in size or number of lung units

Some conditions affecting the lungs reduce the size or number of effective lung units without major change in the way other units are able to effect gas exchange. Under these circumstances the alveolar volume is reduced. Examples include causes of lung collapse or consolidation (e.g. occluded bronchus, pneumonia) and causes of extrapulmonary restriction, for example myopathy, pleural disease or chest wall disease. Intrapulmonary changes in compliance due to fibrosis can lead to reduction in V_A with little change in gas exchange in effective units. This can be seen in some cases of non-active pulmonary fibrosis. With this abnormality the Tl is low due to reduced lung size (i.e. V_A is low), but the

Tl/*V*A is often normal or spuriously high. The change can be allowed for empirically (Section 20.9.1).

38.4.2 Defective lung units

Lung conditions that alter the $\dot{V}_A/\dot{Q}$ balance of ventilated alveoli compromise the gas exchange characteristics. In conditions causing an alveolitis the alveoli may remain ventilated but gas exchange is poor. Under these circumstances the alveolar volume (V_A) may be little affected but *Tl* is reduced substantially and *Tl*/*V*A is low . This may occur early in extrinsic allergic alveolitis or in drug induced lung disease.

38.5 Respiratory failure

The mechanisms for ventilatory control are described in Chapter 23 (see page 285). When the lungs fail in their role of gas exchange two patterns are recognised. In type 1 failure arterial P_{O_2} is low but arterial P_{CO_2} is within the normal range when breathing air. In type 2 failure the P_{O_2} is low and P_{CO_2} is high due to hypoventilation. The differences in the ventilation and perfusion of the lungs that underlie these conditions are shown in Fig. 40.6 (page 551). The approximate levels of arterial blood gases are given in Table 38.4.

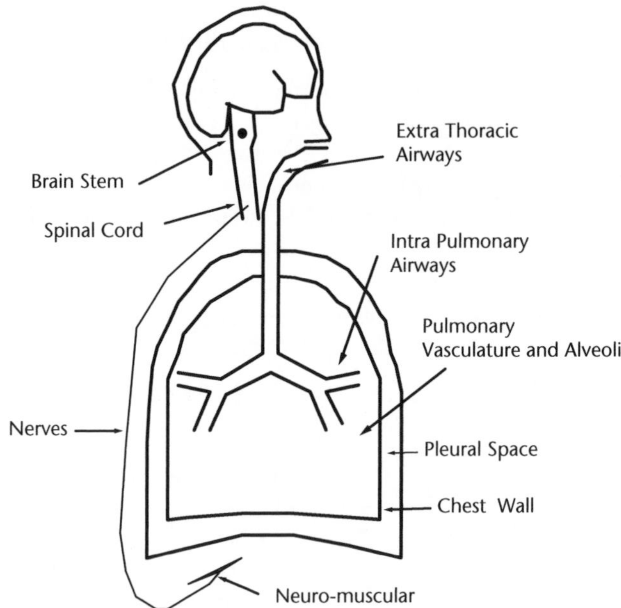

Fig. 38.2 Cartoon of the pulmonary system for considering conditions that affect its function.

38.5.1 Type 1 respiratory failure

This type of respiratory failure is commonly due to $\dot{V}_A/\dot{Q}$ imbalance, not failure of ventilatory control and the drive for ventilation is strong. In addition to lung disorders the condition can be due to shunting of blood from the right side of the heart to the left. In this circumstance the hypoxaemia does not improve with oxygen therapy. When the hypoxaemia is due to an intracardiac shunt the function of the lungs may be normal. However, pulmonary hypertension may develop progressively and if so the intracardiac shunt can reverse from being a left to right shunt, such as an atrial septal defect, to a right to left shunt. In this circumstance the ability of the lungs to oxygenate the blood may also be impaired.

38.5.2 Type 2 respiratory failure

There are many causes for type 2 respiratory failure (Fig. 38.2), in which there is hypoxaemia and hypoventilation relative to the metabolic needs of the subject. The condition can develop acutely, in which case there is an acidosis with normal blood bicarbonate levels (hence *acute type 2 failure*). By 24 to 36 h the renal compensatory mechanisms have had time to retain sodium bicarbonate to offset the acidaemia, hence *compensated or persistent type 2 respiratory failure* in which the acidosis is ameliorated by a rise in blood sodium bicarbonate. Many patients with COPD are in this state. They tolerate a raised P_{CO_2} and, because of the renal compensation, have a normal pH and chronically high bicarbonate level. Their respiratory drive may then be governed solely by their reduced P_{O_2} and so they are at risk of profound apnoea if their chronic hypoxia is relieved with the administration of supplemental oxygen (Section 35.7.2). Patients in stable chronic type 2 respiratory failure remain at risk of further respiratory infections or episodes of increased airflow limitation and in these circumstances they may then experience acute or chronic type 2 failure with a return of the acidaemia consequent from an acute rise in P_{CO_2} (Table 38.4).

Table 38.4 Examples of arterial gas samples in respiratory failure taken whilst breathing air.

	PH	P_{a,O_2}		P_{a,CO_2}		HCO_3^- mmol/l
Normal ranges breathing air:	7.35–7.45	kPa 9.5–13.0	mm Hg 71–97.5	kPa 4.2–5.5	mm Hg 31.5–41	23–27
Type 1 respiratory failure	7.41	5.5	41	4.8	36	24
Acute type 2 respiratory failure	7.11	5.6	42	10.4	78	25
Compensated type 2 respiratory failure	7.39	6.7	50	9.8	73.5	33
Acute on chronic type 2 respiratory failure	7.20	6.4	48	11.3	85	36

38.6 Bronchial hyperresponsiveness

In this syndrome a subject is at risk of developing bronchoconstriction in response to non-specific or specific stimuli. The former include inhaling a bronchoconstrictor aerosol of histamine or methacholine, taking strenuous exercise and breathing cold air. The latter include dust from disintegrated house dust mites, grass pollen and any of a host of airborne allergens, including occupational allergens (Sections 15.8, 37.7.6 and 40.2).

38.7 Examples of abnormal lung function

Table 38.5a–f contain examples of typical patterns of lung function abnormality.

Table 38.5 Examples of lung function in common lung conditions, (a) asthma, (b) COPD, (c) emphysema, (d) lung fibrosis. (e) obesity (f) myopathy.

(a)

Asthma			Observed lung function	Reference value	Standardised residual	After bronchodilator		
						FEV_1	Diff.	% Pred.
Gender	M	FEV_1	2.70	4.03	−2.6	3.88	1.18	29*
Age	48	FVC	4.70	5.00	−0.5	5.05	0.35	7
Height (m)	1.84	FEV%	57	78.6	−3.0			
Weight (kg)	73	PEF	6.10	9.40	−2.7			
BMI	22	FRC	4.20	3.65	0.9			
		RV	3.50	2.24	3.1			
		TLC	8.30	7.62	1.0			
		RV%	42	32.7	1.7			
		*T*lco (SI)	13.5	11.2	1.6			
		(Trad)	40.2	33.4				
		*K*co (SI)	1.89	1.58	1.2			
		(Trad)	5.63	4.71				

* As reported. 36% when expressed in the form $\Delta x/\bar{x}$ (Section 15.7.2).

Comment. Marked airflow limitation with significant reversibility are evidence for asthma. The above average TLC and *T*l in association with a linear physique suggest a previous high level of habitual activity. Further examples are in Tables 40.1 and 29.11, pages 549 and 429.

(b)

COPD			Observed lung function	Reference value	Standardised residual	After bronchodilator		
						FEV_1	Diff.	% Pred.
Gender	M	FEV_1	1.48	2.84	−2.7	1.55	0.07	2*
Age	58	FVC	2.33	3.53	−2.0	2.36	0.03	1
Height (m)	1.63	FEV_1%	64	76.8	−1.9			
Weight (kg)	80	PEF	5.50	7.68	−1.8			
BMI	30	FRC	5.80	3.25	4.3			
		RV	4.00	2.18	4.4			
		TLC	7.50	5.94	2.2			
		RV%	53	36.6	3.1			
		*T*lco (SI)	9.30	8.25	0.7			
		(Trad)	27.7	24.6				
		*K*co (SI)	1.43	1.45	−0.1			
		(Trad)	4.26	4.32				

* As reported. 4.6% when expressed in the form $\Delta x/\bar{x}$ (Section 15.7.2).

Comment. A heavy smoker (65 pack year exposure) with COPD who has airflow limitation and no significant reversibility. The VC (TLC-RV) exceeds the FVC indicating dynamic gas trapping during the forced expiratory manoeuvre. In COPD the trapping is typically secondary to inflammatory changes in small lung airways. The normal gas transfer argues against significant emphysema. Further examples are given in Tables 40.2, 29.11, and 29.12 (pages 553, 429 and 430).

Table 38.5 *(Continued)*

(c)

Emphysema		Observed lung function		Reference value	Standardised residual
Gender	M	FEV_1	0.56	3.25	−5.3
Age	54	FVC	1.65	4.04	−3.9
Height (m)	1.7	FEV%	34	77.5	−6.1
Weight (kg)	63	PEF	2.50	8.28	−4.8
BMI	22	FRC	7.10	3.37	6.2
		RV	5.22	2.19	7.4
		TLC	9.08	6.50	3.7
		RV%	57	35.0	4.1
		*T*lco (SI)	2.48	9.29	−4.8
		(Trad)	7.39	27.7	
		*K*co (SI)	0.44	1.50	−3.9
		(Trad)	1.31	4.47	

Comment. A heavy cigarette smoker (82 pack years) with severe obstructive defect, large volume lungs and low gas transfer, consistent with severe emphysema. VC (i.e. TLC-RV) is greatly in excess of FVC indicating dynamic gas trapping during the forced expiratory manoeuvre; in emphysema (unlike in typical COPD) this is due to the lung elasticity being greatly reduced (as in Table 40.2, page 553).
A further example that includes the findings on exercise is given in Table 29.11 (page 429).

(d)

Pulmonary fibrosis		Observed lung function		Reference value	Standardised residual
Gender	F	FEV_1	1.96	2.66	−1.8
Age	52	FVC	2.52	3.11	−1.4
Height (m)	1.66	FEV%	74	79.1	−0.7
Weight (kg)	68	PEF	7.50	6.47	1.1
BMI	25	FRC	2.18	2.77	−1.2
		RV	1.08	1.84	−2.2
		TLC	3.64	5.17	−2.5
		RV%	30	36.6	−1.2
		*T*lco (SI)	3.49	8.29 (6.75)*	−4.1
		(Trad)	10.4	24.7 (20.1)	
		*K*co (SI)	1.05	1.71	−3.3
		(Trad)	3.13	5.10	

* Value expected for observed *V*A′ (*T*l′/*K*co) is in brackets (see Section 20.9.1).
Comment. A patient with SLE (systemic lupus erythromatosus; Section 41.19.2) on prednisolone and azathioprine with moderate restrictive defect and impaired gas transfer consistent with pulmonary fibrosis seen on chest radiograph. Note the high PEF due to the fibrotic lung stretching airways open on full inspiration (a result of increased elastic recoil as shown in Table 40.4, page 556). With disease progression the lung volume decreases further so PEF will ultimately drop. The small RV is probably due to cellular infiltration into the lung parenchyma. The small *T*l is due to both reduced lung expansion (restriction) and damage to the lung parenchyma. A similar pattern is observed in pulmonary fibrosis from other causes (e.g. sarcoidosis). Further examples including the findings on exercise are given in Tables 29.11 and 29.12 (pages 429 and 430).

Table 38.5 *(Continued)*

(e)

Gross obesity		Observed lung function		Reference value	Standardised residual
Gender	F	FEV_1	2.70	3.19	−1.3
Age	29	FVC	2.92	3.66	−1.7
Height (m)	1.65	FEV%	90	83.5	1.0
Weight (kg)	129	PEF	6.70	7.10	−0.4
BMI	47	FRC	2.60	2.73	−0.3
		RV	1.50	1.45	0.1
		TLC	4.50	5.10	−1.0
		RV%	33	28.8	0.8
		*T*lco (SI)	8.90	9.34	−0.4
		(Trad)	26.5	27.8	
		*K*co (SI)	2.02	1.87	0.8
		(Trad)	6.02	5.57	

Comment. Results are essentially normal except for a mild restrictive defect consistent with an effect from the patient's obesity; expect minor reductions in FEV_1, FVC and TLC, with slight rise in RV and gas transfer. The lung function can be interpreted with greater confidence when separate allowances are made of body fat and muscle (Section 4.7.2 and Table 26.18, page 352). A further example that includes exercise is given in Table 29.11 (page 429).

(f)

Myopathy		Observed lung function		Reference value	Standardised residual
Gender	F	FEV_1	0.86	1.97	−2.9
Age	59	FVC	0.88	2.35	−3.4
Height (m)	1.53	FEV%	98	77.8	3.1
Weight (kg)	74	PEF	3.00	5.54	−2.8
BMI	32	FRC	2.40	2.49	−0.2
		RV	1.90	1.71	0.5
		TLC	2.80	4.31	−2.5
		RV%	68	39.0	4.9
		*T*lco (SI)	7.20	6.88 (5.57)*	0.3
		(Trad)	21.4	20.5 (16.6)	
		K co (SI)	3.10	1.66	7.2
		(Trad)	9.24	4.94	

* Value expected for observed *V*A′ (*T*l′/*K*co) is in brackets (see Section 20.9.1).

Comment. A restrictive defect with normal transfer factor but very high *K*co. The PEF and mouth pressures are low, suggesting a myopathy (mouth pressures are not included in the Table). On review, *T*l is abnormally high for the lung volume (see reference value adjusted for *V*A′ in brackets). The explanation is probably that FVC was below that needed for a technically satisfactory measurement (Section 20.4.1).

38.8 References

1. Fletcher CM. The clinical diagnosis of pulmonary emphysema – an experimental study. *Proc R Soc Med* 1952; **45**: 577–584.
2. Tweeddale PM, Alexander F, McHardy GJR. Short term variability in FEV_1 and bronchodilator responsiveness in patients with obstructive ventilatory defects. *Thorax* 1987; **42**: 487–490.
3. Quanjer PhH, Tammeling GJ, Cotes JE et al. Standardized lung function testing. Lung volumes and forced ventilatory flows. *Eur Respir J* 1993; **6**(Suppl 16): 5–40.
4. American Thoracic Society. Standardization of spirometry. 1994 update. *Am J Respir Crit Care Med* 1995; **152**: 1107–1136.
5. Leuallen EC, Fowler WS. Maximal midexpiratory flow. *Am Rev Tuberc* 1955; **72**: 783–800.
6. Cosio M, Ghezzo H, Hogg JC et al. The relations between structural changes in small airways and pulmonary-function tests. *N Engl J Med* 1977; **298**: 1277–1281.
7. Stanescu D. Small airways obstruction syndrome. *Chest* 1999; **116**: 231–233.
8. Pellegrino R, Violante B, Selleri R et al. Changes in residual volume during induced bronchoconstriction in healthy and asthmatic subjects. *Am Rev Respir Dis* 1994; **150**: 363–368.
9. Vikgren J, Bake B, Ekberg-Jansson A et al. Value of air trapping in detection of small airways disease in smokers. *Acta Radiol* 2003; **44**: 517–524.
10. Agusti R, Roca J, Rodriguez-Roisin R et al. Different patterns of gas exchange response to exercise in asbestosis and idiopathic pulmonary fibrosis. *Eur Respir J* 1988; **1**: 510–516.

CHAPTER 39

Strategies for Assessment

39.1 Introduction

There are many different ways of investigating a clinical respiratory problem and often these will be specific to particular patients taking into account their wishes and expectations. The tests available to help diagnose and monitor pulmonary disorders will be outlined here and will include some tests in clinical practice that do not necessarily assess function but may describe an anatomical change which can be extremely helpful in establishing a diagnosis.

The clinical utility of tests depends on their repeatability. The day-to-day repeatability within a laboratory is much better than the repeatability between laboratories. The day-to-day repeatability is critically important when monitoring patients for the activity of their disease or response to treatment. The between laboratory repeatability is important with regard to multi-centre studies. In one study when this was assessed using three test subjects the between laboratory variation was best for vital capacity (VC) at 13% of the maximal value recorded, and worst for *T*lco and residual volume (RV), at 46% and 51% of maximal value, respectively [1]. The differences were due more to procedural factors, protocols and reference values than to errors in instrument calibration, and were reduced substantially following a review [2]. Thus consultations between laboratories should be on going.

Very few pulmonary disorders can be diagnosed from lung function tests alone. Usually the diagnosis will require a comprehensive approach that includes the patient's history, clinical findings, chest radiography and possibly other procedures. The decision on which lung function tests to apply should take account of all this information, so where the choice is made by laboratory staff they should have access to it.

39.2 Techniques available

Various respiratory function techniques will be discussed in the context of their value in assessing lung function in a clinical setting. Research techniques are included where they have added to our understanding of how to evaluate patients. The repeatability of the various tests is an important determinant of their clinical utility.

39.2.1 Spirometry and flow–volume loops

These tests are extremely informative in many pulmonary disorders and form the mainstay of investigation. Spirometry is the first and sometimes only test of lung function undertaken and no patient assessment is complete without an FEV_1 and VC. Furthermore, measurement of VC is a component of many tests and serves as a useful quality control check between instruments when judging patient effort.

Many laboratories would not necessarily include flow–volume loops ($\dot{v}$–V curves, Section 12.5.1) as part of their routine assessment, perhaps only using these in certain circumstances. FV loops can improve the quality control aspects of patient testing by, for example helping to distinguish a poorly co-ordinated manoeuvre from a hypodynamic manoeuvre or a restricted manoeuvre. Upper airway obstruction is one of the few conditions that can be diagnosed solely from lung function testing and flow volume loops are the most important test in this context (Section 41.2). Peak expiratory flow (PEF) monitoring is key to the diagnosis of asthma in some patients and in the majority of cases of occupational asthma. The use of data logging meters may be necessary in the latter setting because of the tendency of some subjects to present inaccurate records [3, 4].

Airflow limitation is the commonest problem in clinical respiratory medicine and the spirogram and flow–volume loop are crucial for the assessment and management of these patients. The tests may be performed to exclude airflow limitation and its reversibility prior to use of a diagnostic algorithm to identify further investigative tests. The tests are reviewed in Chapter 12 and assessment of bronchodilatation in Section 15.7.2.

39.2.2 Airways resistance

The resistance to flow in airways is increased when there is material narrowing of lung airways. Thus, measurement of airways resistance (*R*aw) was formerly considered promising, especially as the test was performed during quiet tidal breathing and removed the necessity for an effort-dependent forced expiratory manoeuvre. However, the measurement has not found a place in routine testing of patients as the overall resistance was found to contain a variable (and sometimes large) component from the larynx and glottic aperture (Section 14.3.4).

Airway resistance is intimately related to the lung volume at which the measurement is made. Accordingly, *R*aw should be standardised for lung volume. The simplest method, though not the most accurate, is to express the resistance as specific airways conductance (s*G*aw) which is the reciprocal of *R*aw per litre of thoracic lung volume (TGV, see Fig. 14.1, page 152). Measurement of instantaneous TGV is made by whole body plethysmography (Section 14.6) and this influences the practical logistics of using *R*aw in routine patient testing. Forced oscillometry and interruption techniques are also used for obtaining *R*aw but the methods cannot yield the TGV so *R*aw cannot be standardised for lung volume. Initially, it was anticipated that the measurement of Raw at different frequencies during forced oscillometry would help distinguish the component of resistance from central and peripheral airways [5]. However, artefacts due to dissipation of the oscillatory signal in the upper airways, cheeks and mouth confound the interpretation of the result unless a hood technique is used to apply the forced oscillation simultaneously to the outside of the head and neck [6]. The full clinical applicability of this test is yet to be defined.

The measurement of *R*aw using the interruptor method (*R*int) may have applications when testing very young children who cannot perform spirometry reliably.

In conclusion, *R*aw and s*G*aw are not used routinely for patient management but are most often utilised in specialised clinical testing or in a research setting.

39.2.3 Airways responsiveness

Most subjects with symptomatic asthma show bronchial hyperresponsiveness (BHR). Accordingly, a test of BHR should help in the differential diagnosis of patients with airflow limitation. However, about 10% of the population have increased BHR and only half of these may have asthma. Thus, the clinical utility of the test is diminished by its lack of specificity. Tests of BHR are often used in epidemiological studies to elucidate features relating to clinical asthma and to study its natural history. However, the role of specific challenge testing is more secure in testing subjects with suspected occupational asthma to establish a causal relationship. The procedure may be supplemented by skin allergen testing (Sections 15.3 and 15.8).

39.2.4 Static lung volumes

These tests are helpful and show different patterns of disturbance in patients with airflow limitation compared to those with restrictive disease. Large volume lungs (that is, large TLC) and high RV are found in COPD and emphysema. The helium dilution method for determining TLC may underestimate the volume in patients with marked airflow limitation. In asthma the TLC may be large and RV is often increased. In patients with severe airflow limitation the usual finding of a low FEV_1 with respect to VC is less marked than expected as the VC and forced vital capacities (FVC) are reduced due to airway closure. Under these circumstances the RV is much increased and its measurement helps distinguish airways disease from a restrictive defect that is also associated with a reduced VC.

In restrictive disease the TLC and RV tend to be reduced. Thus, static lung volumes have a critical role in determining the pattern of defect (Chapter 10).

39.2.5 Compliance

Static lung compliance is calculated from the relationship of recoil pressure to lung volumes using an indirect procedure in which the pressure is that recorded from a balloon in the oesophagus (Section 11.8). The subject relaxes all respiratory muscles whilst the lung volume is held constant by occluding the mouth tube with a shutter. Under these circumstances the mouth pressure is assumed to be equal to alveolar pressure and so the recoil pressure from the lungs can be obtained independent of that of the chest wall. The shape of the upper half of the plot of elastic recoil pressure curve of the lungs against lung volume can be fitted to a single exponential given by eqn 11.2 (page 122):

$$V = \mathrm{A} - \mathrm{B}e^{-kPst}$$

where V is lung volume, Pst is the recoil pressure of the lungs, the exponent k is a shape factor to describe the exponential curve and A and B are constants. The value k relates to the volume change per unit recoil pressure change and is a measure of lung compliance. It is increased in emphysema and reduced in interstitial lung disease (Sections 40.3 and 40.4). However, the assumption that mouth pressure is equal to alveolar pressure is not secure in the presence of airflow limitation. In addition, HRCT can now be used to visualise any anatomical abnormality.

Measurement of static compliance is technically demanding, can be unpleasant for the patient and is not widely used. This is also the case for dynamic compliance when the same procedure is applied during tidal breathing (see also Section 11.10).

39.2.6 Pulse oximetry

The use of pulse oximetry has increased dramatically since the early 1990s. It is frequently used for real time estimation of arterial saturation during anaesthesia, in endoscopy procedures, and post operatively. Pulse oximetry assesses the oxygenation of a patient but any tendency to type 2 respiratory failure with CO_2 retention cannot be assessed and must always be considered. During emergencies a normal oxygen saturation whilst breathing air can exclude significant respiratory failure. However, if respiratory failure is suspected then reliance on oximetry alone is not recommended and arterial gases must be obtained.

Pulse oximetry can be used during exercise test regimens (Section 29.5.1). For patients with normal spirometry who complain of dyspnoea on exercise, rapid arterial desaturation by oximetry during a step test or simply walking up and down a corridor can alert the clinician to an underlying gas exchange problem.

39.2.7 Arterial gases

Investigation of arterial gases is essential in all patients admitted with respiratory distress or where respiratory failure is considered. Direct arterial puncture is the best method for a reliable estimate with immediate measurement in a blood gas analyser. Arterialised capillary blood from an ear lobe is sometimes used but the results are more prone to errors (Sections 7.9 onwards).

Arterial gas samples are required for assessment for long-term oxygen therapy (LTOT) and assessment of fitness to travel in commercial aircraft.

LTOT assessment. With the patient in a stable clinical state arterial gas samples taken at least 3 weeks apart must show a $P\text{O}_2$ of 7.3 kPa (55 mm Hg) or less whilst breathing air and when repeated on continuous oxygen therapy the $P\text{O}_2$ must increase by at least 1 kPa (7.5 mm Hg) without a deleterious effect on $P\text{CO}_2$ (Section 35.7.1). If these criteria are met then LTOT may improve life expectancy by reducing the risk of the patient developing severe pulmonary hypertension. If the patient is a current smoker no benefit is obtained and the presence of 100% oxygen around the patient can make ordinary clothing extremely flammable. Other clinical criteria are also involved in the decision to prescribe LTOT (Section 35.7.1 also [7]).

Flight assessment. Increasingly patients who have respiratory disability are wishing to use flying as a means of transport. Commercial aircraft are pressurised to an altitude of about 8000 ft so for normal subjects the arterial $P\text{O}_2$ may expect to fall to between 7 and 8.5 kPa (52–64 mm Hg) [8]. For respiratory patients there is no absolute safe level but the $P\text{O}_2$ should not remain below around 7 kPa (52 mm Hg) which is on the point of the oxygen–Hb dissociation curve where further reductions in $P\text{O}_2$ lead to a disproportionate fall in the amount of oxygen carried (Section 21.2.2). The assessment of fitness to fly is described in Section 34.6.

39.2.8 Gas transfer factor

The single breath CO gas transfer factor is one of the most widely used tests to assess gas exchange in the lung. It can be influenced by many factors both technical and biological and these must be considered when interpreting a low result (Section 20.9). The measurement is not as reproducible as spirometry [9] but is entirely adequate if attention is paid to calibration and other details of the measurement (Section 20.4). Also fewer subjects are able to give acceptable measurements of gas transfer than for spirometry, being as low as 68% in one population study [10]. However, the test is attractive in epidemiological studies and can also yield an estimate of TLC. In clinical applications the test is used routinely for following patients with interstitial lung diseases and for estimating the functional deficit in emphysema.

39.2.9 Mouth pressures

Simple devices are available for the measurement of maximal inspiratory and expiratory pressures (Section 9.9). The range of normal values is wide and so, on their own these estimates are not reliable in making a diagnosis. However, taken together with other lung function data, such as a flow–volume loop, measurement of respiratory pressures can help confirm a diagnosis of myopathy.

39.2.10 $\dot{V}/\dot{Q}$ isotope scans

Simultaneous ventilation and perfusion scans using isotopes and γ camera scintigraphy yields a graphic representation of ventilation and perfusion abnormalities in the lungs. Modern scanners can undertake numerical analysis to yield estimates of regional $\dot{V}/\dot{Q}$. This technique has been used principally in the diagnosis of pulmonary embolism where perfusion defects in the absence of ventilation defects (mismatch) indicate the likelihood of embolism (Sections 7.12 and 18.6).

A further use of isotope scans has been to predict post lung resection ventilatory function on the basis of pre-operative estimates of perfusion to the lung that is not to be resected (Section 43.2).

39.2.11 Multiple inert gas elimination technique

The Multiple inert gas elimination technique (MIGET) for describing $\dot{V}/\dot{Q}$ relationships in the lungs has been of inestimable help in investigating many lung diseases. However, only a few institutions have the necessary equipment or are able to perform the tests reliably (Section 18.2), so its use is principally for research.

39.2.12 Exercise tests

The lungs have tremendous reserve of function that are encroached on during exercise so a patient usually first experiences dyspnoea when he or she is active. Dyspnoea present at rest is invariably made worse by exercise. Thus, exercise testing offers a means for early identification of lung disease and estimating the true extent of impairment, including disorders of gas exchange and disturbances to the pattern of breathing. Exercise tests that include expired gas analysis can help distinguish respiratory from cardiovascular causes of dyspnoea.

One limitation to exercise testing, particularly when performed by a non-cyclist on a cycle ergometer, is that the symptoms may not be those experienced during daily living. A test that entails walking e.g. Treadmill exercise, 6-min walk or shuttle test should be used where possible (Section 29.4.1). Exercise testing contributes greatly to the assessment of patients with chronic lung disorders, including COPD and occupational disorders, and for assessing patients for lung resection. It also helps in rehabilitation reviews. The procedures and interpretation are in Chapter 29. Other aspects are in Chapters 30 and 31.

39.2.13 Sleep studies

Sleep studies are indicated for patients where significant sleep disordered breathing is likely to be present. The tests are described in Chapters 32 and 33.

Normal subjects who are symptom free, when they perform sleep studies may have abnormalities that appear not to have clinical significance. Thus, symptoms of daytime somnolence, fatigue and unrefreshing sleep should be present before considering these tests in the clinical setting. Patients with severe kyphoscoliosis, thoracoplasty, or progressive myopathy who are at risk of nocturnal hypoventilatory failure may also need regular sleep studies.

If patients are found to have significant obstructive sleep apnoea they may be treated successfully with continuous positive airways pressure (CPAP). Repeat studies may need to be performed to titrate the level of CPAP required to overcome an individual's airway closure (Section 42.5.1 also [11]).

39.2.14 Radiology

Most respiratory patients are investigated by postero-anterior chest radiography for the information it provides on anatomical features and the distributions of disease processes. The features of the X-ray can contribute to the interpretation of lung function tests, particularly the appearance of the lung fields, pleura and diaphragm, also whether or not there is pleural effusion, lung collapse or other abnormality. The report may comment on the size of the lungs and, by adding a lateral film, the TLC can readily be assessed (Section 10.3.4, also [12]).

The advent of high-resolution computerised tomography (HRCT) of the lungs has added increased anatomical detail of how different diseases affect the lungs. Conditions such as lymphangioleiomyomatosis and lymphangitis carcinomatosis for example have characteristic and diagnostic features. Estimates of the degree and distribution of emphysematous change on HRCT can be an important correlate to aid the interpretation of lung function tests [13]. Furthermore, imaging at different levels of inspiration can help describe regional ventilation.

Spiral CT demonstration of pulmonary emboli resident in pulmonary arteries has also changed the investigation of this condition [14], which in the past has relied solely on isotope lung scans or full pulmonary angiography.

39.3 Strategies for diseases

In general, the strategy for assessment should be patient-centred. However, templates of tests and monitoring regimens for certain common clinical syndromes exist though care must be taken with choice of predicted values and interpretative strategies (Sections 26.1 and 26.8, also [15, 16, 17]). Common conditions and the tests used for their assessment are summarised in Table 39.1.

A retrospective study of lung function tests on over 1500 subjects attending a routine lung function laboratory found that the usual diagnostic categories of chronic airflow limitation, asthma and interstitial lung disease could be separated from each other, and from heart disease and miscellaneous disorders by using just spirometry, static lung volumes and gas transfer factor (FEV_1 and FVC, TLC and *T*lco) [18]. Inclusion of more indices did not improve the specificity of the classifications. This indicates the clinical utility of a limited number of routine tests. However, for patients who experience breathlessness or somnolence facilities for excercise and sleep studies should be readily available.

39.3.1 Airflow limitation

The diagnosis of asthma is usually made on the basis of clinical symptoms plus serial measurements of PEF. The pathological diagnosis from bronchial histology is not usually undertaken and lung function testing makes an essential contribution.

PEF monitoring may show characteristic within day variations (Section 40.2), but for the pattern to be unambiguous the patient should not be aware of what is being looked for (i.e. naïve). Unfortunately, where compensation may be an issue some patients deliberately alter their readings. Consequently, blinded, coded or data logging meters may be needed to ensure that a reliable diagnosis can be made (Section 39.2.1).

Spirometry and/or PEF measurements are also essential in order to discover if airflow limitation is reversible (Section 15.7.2).

Table 39.1 Tests and procedures that are most helpful for the diagnosis and management of common conditions affecting the lungs.

Condition	Function tests	Additional test or procedure
Asthma	FEV_1 and FVC, reversibility, PEF monitoring	Bronchial hyper-responsiveness, skin tests, IgE
COPD	FEV_1 and FVC, reversibility, TLC*, *T*lco	HRCT, exercise test
Emphysema	FEV_1 and FVC, TLC*, *T*lco, exercise test	HRCT, static lung compliance
Bronchiectasis	FEV_1 and FVC, reversibility	HRCT, *T*lco
Interstitial	FEV_1 and FVC, TLC*, *T*lco, exercise test	HRCT, static lung compliance, lung biopsy
Sarcoidosis	FEV_1 and FVC, reversibility, TLC*, *T*lco	Lung biopsy
Myopathy	FEV_1 and FVC, mouth pressures, supine VC	EMG, muscle biopsy
Pulmonary embolism	arterial gases	$\dot{V}/\dot{Q}$, CT pulmonary angiogram
Goitre/UAO (upper airway obstruction)	FV loops	HRCT, *s*Gaw
Pneumonia	arterial gases	Chest X-ray, blood and sputum culture
Acute lung injury	arterial gases	CT

* including subdivisions.

By contrast, testing for bronchial hyperresponsiveness is seldom helpful in making a secure diagnosis for asthma, except in the setting of occupational asthma where specific bronchial challenge testing may be needed (Section 15.8.5). In paediatric practice brief exercise challenges are used to diagnose exercise induced asthma (EIA, Section 15.8.3).

Unsupervised home PEF monitoring can help some patients to make adjustments to their treatment during exacerbations. They include those with persistent asthma that requires oral steroids [19] and patients at risk of frequent exacerbations who can have a poor perception of deteriorating symptoms [20]. Not all patients require this level of intervention and for many it is sufficient

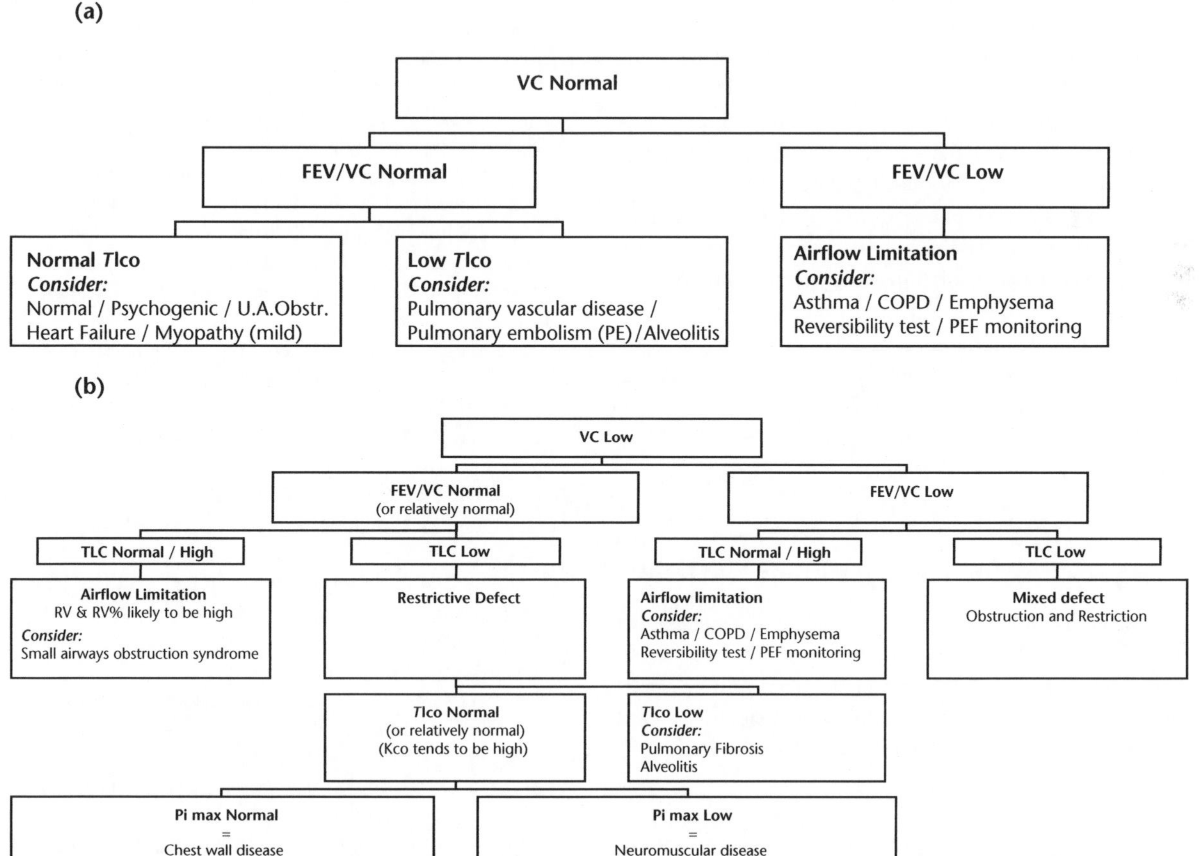

Fig. 39.1 Flow diagram for determining the cause of dyspnoea on the basis of lung function tests.
(a) Subject presents with dyspnoea but has a normal VC. (b) Subject presents with dyspnoea and has a low VC. Source: [23].

to record spirometry and PEF during clinic visits; alternatively they may be helped by systematic monitoring of symptoms [21]. PEF monitoring during hospital treatment of exacerbations is essential to help determine when the patient is fit for discharge and when a reduction in corticosteroid dose can be undertaken.

In COPD and emphysema FEV_1, FVC and VC monitoring is generally more helpful than following PEF.

39.3.2 Interstitial lung disease

For these conditions dynamic forced manoeuvres, static lung volumes and gas transfer are the minimum requirement for testing function. Estimation of arterial blood gases or oximetry and an exercise test may also be required. Some conditions causing interstitial lung disease can progress rapidly over weeks and tests may need to be repeated every two weeks or so during treatment. In many subjects with either cryptogenic fibrosing alveolitis or sarcoidosis the disease may progress in a more indolent fashion and then monitoring every 8 weeks or so for adjustment to treatment may be appropriate.

39.3.3 Neuro-muscular disease

Significant respiratory muscle weakness leads to a reduction in vital capacity in the supine position. Dynamic forced expiratory testing, static lung volumes and gas transfer are all likely to be required initially together with measurement of expiratory and inspiratory mouth pressures. In some circumstances the dynamic forced expiratory tests are all that can be undertaken, for instance in Guillain Barré syndrome. Monitoring of VC or FVC may be all that is required to assess response to treatment, or progression and requirement for ventilation. For example if VC is less than 15 $ml\ kg^{-1}$ then artificial ventilation is likely to be required [22]. Although PEF is also affected, the measurement of VC is more reliable and repeatable in this context.

Measurement of mouth pressures can be easily undertaken but the reference ranges for normal subjects are very wide. This limits their use as a diagnostic test but they can be helpful for monitoring disease progress or response to treatment.

39.4 Algorithm for the dyspnoeic patient

If, having taken a full history and undertaken a clinical examination, there is some doubt about why a patient is breathless, then an algorithm may help decide if there is a pulmonary cause (Fig. 39.1). This approach is not infallible as cardiac disease can produce changes in lung function tests (see Chapter 41).

39.5 References

1. Mushtaq M, Hayton R, Watts T et al. An audit of pulmonary function laboratories in the West Midlands. *Respir Med* 1995; **89**: 263–270.
2. Dowson LJ, Mushtaq M, Watts T et al. A re-audit of pulmonary function laboratories in the West Midlands. *Respir Med* 1998; **92**: 1155–1162.
3. Verschelden P, Cartier A, L'Archeveque J et al. Compliance with and accuracy of daily self-assessment of peak expiratory flows (PEF) in asthmatic subjects over a three month period. *Eur Respir J* 1996; **9**: 880–855.
4. Malo JL, Trudeau C, Ghezzo H et al. Do subjects investigated for occupational asthma through serial peak expiratory flow measurements falsify their results? *J Allergy Clin Immunol* 1995; **96**: 601–607.
5. Pimmel RL, Tsai MJ, Winter DC, Bromberg PA. Estimating central and peripheral respiratory resistance. *J Appl Physiol* 1978; **45**: 375–380.
6. Peslin R, Duvivier C, Didelon J, Gallina C. Respiratory impedance measured with head generator to minimize upper airway shunt. *J Appl Physiol* 1985; **59**: 492–501.
7. British Thoracic Society. Guidelines on the management of COPD. *Thorax* 1997; 52(Suppl 5): S1–S28.
8. British Thoracic Society Standards of Care Committee. Managing passengers with respiratory disease planning air travel: British Thoracic Society recommendations. *Thorax* 2002; **57**: 289–304.
9. Clausen J, Crapo R, Gardner R. Interlaboratory comparisons of pulmonary function testing. *Am Rev Respir Dis* 1984; **129**: A37.
10. Well I, Eide GE, Bakke P, Gulsvik A. Applicability of the single-breath carbon monoxide diffusing capacity in a Norwegian community study. *Am J Respir Crit Care Med* 1998; **158**: 1745–1750.
11. Scottish Intercollegiate Guidelines Network. Management of obstructive sleep apnoea/hypopnea syndrome in adults. A national clinical guideline. 2003. http://www.sign.ac.uk
12. Rodenstein DO, Sopwith T, Denison DM, Stanescu DC. Reevaluation of the radiographic method for measurement of total lung capacity. *Bull Eur Physiopathol Respir* 1985; 21: 521–525.
13. Gevenois PA, De Vuyst P, de Maertelaer V et al. Comparison of computed density and microscopic morphometry in pulmonary emphysema. *Am J Respir Crit Care Med* 1996; **154**: 187–192.
14. Kim KI, Muller NL, Mayo JR. Clinically suspected pulmonary embolism: utility of spiral CT. *Radiology* 1999; **210**: 693–697.
15. The European Respiratory Society. Standardized lung function testing. *Eur Resp J* 1993; **6**(Suppl 16): 5–40.
16. The American Thoracic Society. Lung function testing: selection of reference values and interpretive strategies. *Am Rev Respir Dis* 1991; **144**: 1202–1218.
17. Pellegrino R, Viegi G, Enright P et al. Interpretative strategies for lung function tests. *Eur Respir J* 2005; **26**: 948–968.
18. Laszlo G, Lance GN, Lewis GT, Hughes AO. The contribution of respiratory function tests to clinical diagnosis. *Eur Respir J* 1993; **6**: 983–990.
19. Grampian Asthma Study of Integrated Care (GRASSIC). Effectiveness of routine self monitoring of peak flow in patients with asthma. *BMJ* 1994; **308**: 564–567.
20. Veen JC, Smits HH, Ravensberg AJ et al. Impaired perception of dyspnea in patients with severe asthma. Relation to sputum eosinophils. *Am J Respir Crit Care Med* 1998; **158**: 1134–1141.
21. D'Souza W, Crane J, Burgess C et al. Community-based asthma care: trial of a 'credit card' asthma self-management plan. *Eur Respir J* 1994; **7**: 1260–1265.
22. Ropper AH, Kehne SM. Guillain-Barre syndrome: management of respiratory failure. *Neurology* 1985; **35**: 1662–1665.
23. Laszlo G. *Pulmonary Function: A Guide for Clinicians.* New York: Cambridge University Press, 1994.

CHAPTER 40

Lung Function in Asthma, COPD, Emphysema and Diffuse Lung Fibrosis

The conditions described in this chapter are common causes of impaired lung function and a reduced exercise capacity. They are here subjected to detailed scrutiny. Community and occupational aspects of the conditions are in chapter 37.

40.1 Introduction

Much has been written on the common respiratory diseases that afflict Western societies. In the present account the main emphasis has been on evidence from the most recent literature to give the reader a contemporary entry into the subject. A clinical text should also be consulted. The space devoted to a particular condition does not reflect its prevalence or its clinical or respiratory importance.

40.2 Asthma

40.2.1 Spirometry and peak expiratory flow

Asthma is defined as a condition with airflow limitation that varies over short periods of time, either spontaneously or in response to treatment, and is associated with inflammation in the airways [1]. Thus, there is usually evidence of airflow limitation with a reduced PEF, FEV_1 and a low FEV_1/VC. Variability of the airflow limitation is characteristic and a patient with asthma may have normal function when well, but markedly reduced function during the course of an attack. This is usually, but not invariably precipitated by exposure to an airborne antigen to which the patient is sensitive (hence *extrinsic asthma*). Some aspects of susceptibility are in Section 15.3 and some of the antigens are in Sections 37.6.1 and 37.7.6.

The variability in airflow limitation can be demonstrated by the characteristic diurnal variation in peak expiratory flow (PEF) [2, 3] with morning dipping (Fig. 40.1 also Figs 15.6 and 15.7, pages 176 and 177). The within day variation in PEF may increase in a subject as their asthma deteriorates (Fig. 40.2) and subsequently reduce as it responds to treatment (Fig. 40.3). The natural variability in PEF in the population has been defined and, when expressed as a per cent of the mean, a variability of more than 20% suggests the presence of asthma [4]. The characteristic drop in PEF whilst asleep is now thought to reflect increased cross latching of smooth muscle that occurs during sleep when the tidal volumes are lower and deep sighs and larger

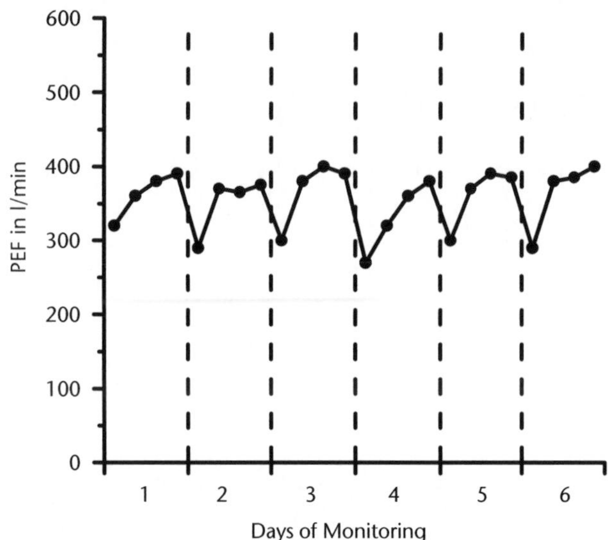

Fig. 40.1 Within-day variability of peak expiratory flow in a patient with asthma showing a greater than 25% drop each morning.

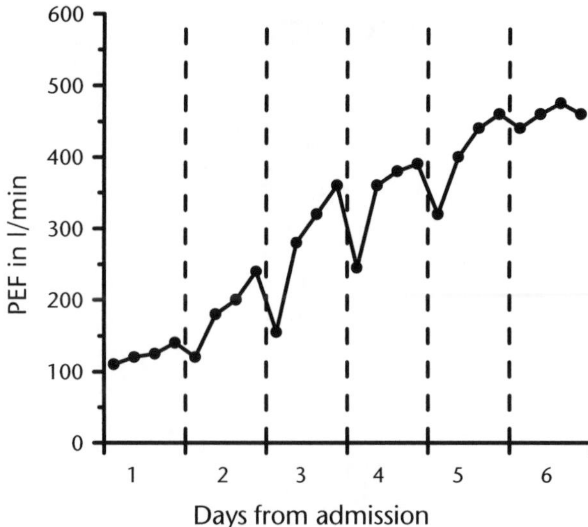

Fig. 40.3 Within-day variability in peak expiratory flow during recovery following an admission with severe asthma.

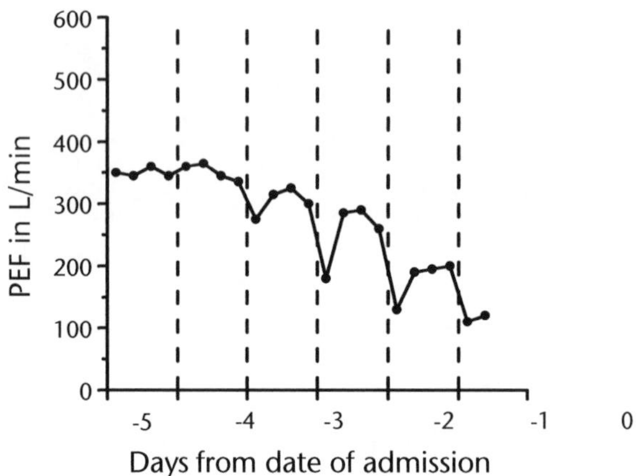

Fig. 40.2 Peak expiratory flow in the 5 days prior to admission where the patient did not adjust treatment during the beginning of an asthma attack that was due to an upper respiratory tract viral infection.

breaths are much less common [5] (Section 25.6). When smooth muscle contracts it becomes stiff due to the binding of myosin to actin, and due to temporary bridging with the cytoskeletal matrix. These latter bridges do not turn over very quickly. The rhythmical pattern of tidal breathing and deep sighs that form part of normal breathing whilst awake disrupt these bridges.

Patients with asthma are best monitored during exacerbations by PEF, as performing the full maximal expiratory manoeuvre to derive FVC often leads to severe coughing and increasing airflow limitation. In stable asthma the PEF and FEV_1 with FVC should be recorded. One disadvantage of using PEF or the maximal forced expiratory manoeuvre to monitor function is that the inspiration to TLC has an effect on the bronchial tone. In normal subjects the muscle tone in the bronchi is reduced by a full inspiration but in asthma there may be a paradoxical rise [6]. Hence, the measurement technique may influence the findings [7]. Measurement of specific conductance can demonstrate the constrictor effect of a deep inhalation in asthmatics and the bronchodilating effect in normal subjects (Section 14.3.4).

40.2.2 Airways resistance and bronchial hyperresponsiveness

Airways resistance (Section 14.3.4) is increased in asthma and can be measured without the need for a volitional effort or a deep inspiration as required for measurement of PEF or FEV_1. Measurement of airways resistance is not a routine test and can be technically demanding. The assessment is subject to error on account of airflow limitation and, in general, its use is limited in the clinical setting because it has a much larger variation on repeated testing than does either the FEV_1 or PEF. The method requires body plethysmography or a forced oscillation technique. The latter method can be relatively easier to use in a clinical setting and may help in the assessment of small children who find forced expiratory manoeuvres difficult to perform [8]. The technique can be useful in a research setting for detecting short term within subject changes because it is more sensitive to changes than PEF or FEV_1.

The lung volume at which small airways collapse occurs at a much higher volume in patients who have frequent exacerbations compared with those with more stable asthma [9]. Hence, the closing volume and closing capacity (Section 16.2.5) are larger even though TLC and RV may be comparable between the groups. This suggests continued inflammation of the airways changes the characteristics of small airway performance which may become permanent with airway remodelling [10].

The variable degree of airflow limitation characteristic of asthma is reflected in an increased responsiveness of the airways to various inhaled agents and, in some cases to exercise. An exercise-induced component is common in childhood asthma and appears to reflect a loss of water from the airway-lining layer. The resulting change in osmolality leads to movement of water from cells and triggers release of mediators that cause bronchoconstriction [11]. Change in osmolality may also explain the effect of fog and nebulised distilled water or hyperosmolar solutions in causing bronchoconstriction in asthma [12, 13]. Challenge studies using histamine or methacholine to determine the degree of airway responsiveness have been widely employed in clinical and epidemiological studies [14]. The response is a unimodal continuum with asthmatics being more responsive at lower provoking doses. However, an arbitrary cut off point is used for diagnosis which can restrict its use in individual subjects. Bronchial challenge testing using specific agents can be undertaken for the diagnosis of occupational asthma and this is often done using a specially ventilated room where the ambient air can be mixed with the putative agent. The procedure is not without hazard.

Procedures for assessing susceptibility to the several forms of bronchial hyperresponsiveness are described in Sections 15.8.1 to 15.8.5.

40.2.3 Reversibility

A distinguishing feature of asthma is the short-term nature of changes in airflow limitation either due to the disease process or response to treatment. Thus, a test of reversibility of the airflow limitation using bronchodilator drugs can be helpful. For a change after bronchodilator to be significant the improvement in FEV_1 should be more than about 160 ml for this to exceed the natural short-term variation in performing the test [15], also Section 15.7.2. In addition, the improvement should be more than a specified proportion of the subject's predicted FEV_1 for it to be clinically meaningful in distinguishing asthma from a poorly reversible disease process such as chronic obstructive pulmonary disease (COPD) or bronchiectasis (Sections 15.5 and 38.3.1, also [16]).

40.2.4 Lung volumes

Early studies on lung volumes using plethysmography suggested that during the onset of an attack of asthma the TLC increased acutely and substantially. This finding has been shown to be largely incorrect, as one of the principles of the measurement was violated, namely that the recorded mouth pressure reflected alveolar pressure [17]. However, studies using helium dilution have shown that TLC and RV can be increased in patients admitted during an asthma attack and will reduce with successful treatment [18]. In asthmatic patients the inspiratory muscles continue to be under tonic contraction throughout the breathing cycle and this contributes to the hyperinflation [19,20]. Acute bronchial challenge with methacholine sufficient to cause a significant drop in FEV_1 does not induce any change in TLC [21]. Early work suggested a change in static pressure–volume curves in asthma but a recent study failed to find a significant change in elastic recoil compared to normal controls [22]. Intrabronchial studies have shown that in young asthmatics the central airways are less compliant than in normal subjects ([23] also Section 11.9) suggesting that chronic inflammation causes a stiffer elastic property in the airways. The inflammation leads to increased evolution of nitric oxide from the lung parenchyma and should be allowed for when $Tl_{,NO}$ is measured (Section 20.10).

40.2.5 $\dot{V}A/\dot{Q}$ changes and gas transfer

The shape of the flow–volume curve in asthma is concave upwards with a curved appearance suggestive of unequal lung emptying, with different units having different time constants due to the patchy and varied reduction in airway calibre throughout the lungs. Ventilation scans confirm the patchy nature of the disease [24] and nitrogen washout studies confirm that areas of the lungs are emptying with different time constants [25]. This aspect has been best illustrated by the MIGET technique (Section 18.2) in that $\dot{V}A/\dot{Q}$ distribution is abnormal which contributes to the hypoxia that develops during attacks [26]. In acute severe asthma there is a bimodal distribution of $\dot{V}A/\dot{Q}$ with areas of lung still perfused that are poorly ventilated and areas well ventilated but not adequately perfused (Fig. 40.4). In milder asthma the $\dot{V}A/\dot{Q}$ is the usual unimodal form but with a broadened perfusion distribution [28]. These $\dot{V}A/\dot{Q}$ changes cause the hypoxia that is not directly related to changes in FEV_1 [29]. The use of β_2 agonists and 100% oxygen can reduce the reflex hypoxic pulmonary vasoconstriction that is helping to correct local $\dot{V}A/\dot{Q}$, so these therapies may exacerbate the $\dot{V}A/\dot{Q}$ mismatch [26]. Thus, as an attack of asthma develops there is a relative increase in ventilation to those areas of the lungs that do not have marked bronchoconstriction. This has little effect on improving oxygenation, because of the shape of the oxygen–haemoglobin dissociation curve (Fig. 21.1, page 260), but it will lead to reduction in Pa,CO_2 because of the relationship between carriage of CO_2 in the blood and alveolar ventilation (Fig. 21.3, page 267). However, as an attack worsens with more widespread and severe airflow limitation developing, then hypoventilation occurs with a rising Pa,CO_2 (Fig. 40.5). Thus, when monitoring a patient with asthma using arterial blood gases a change from a low Pa,CO_2 to one within the normal range may either be due to improvement or deterioration of the asthma. Other indicators are therefore required to interpret these findings, such as PEF measurement or the patient's ability to talk freely. A Pa,CO_2 above the normal range in asthma is a danger sign and indicates type 2 respiratory failure. A continued rise in Pa,CO_2 above the normal range despite adequate therapy is an indication for considering artificial ventilation.

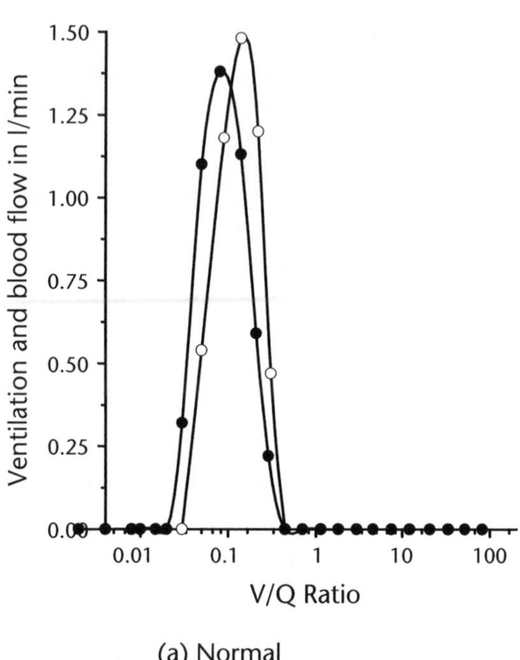

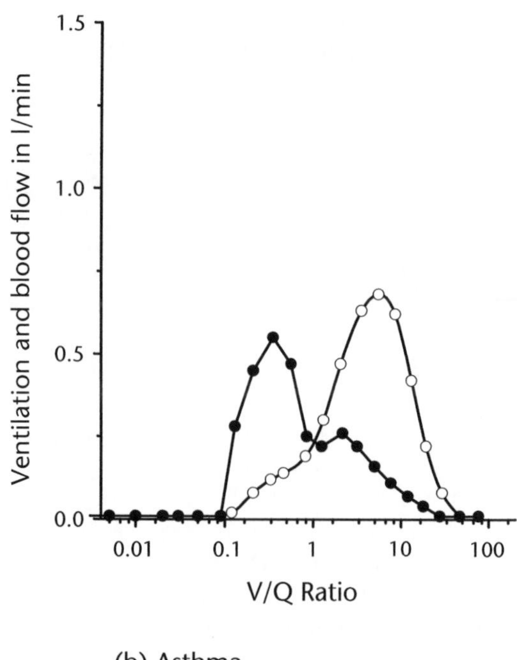

Fig. 40.4 Ventilation (open circles) and perfusion (closed circles) distribution found in (a) normal subject and (b) a patient with asthma during an acute attack. Source: Adapted from [27].

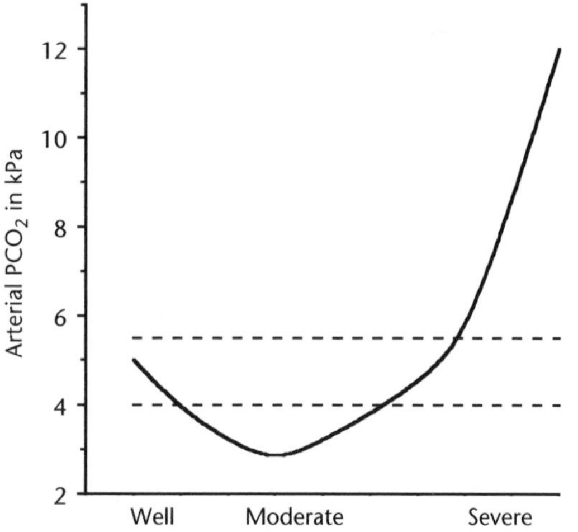

Fig. 40.5 Schematic relationship between the arterial $P\text{CO}_2$ and the severity of an asthma attack. The dashed lines show the normal range for the $P\text{a,CO}_2$. Source: Adapted from [30]

Total lung gas transfer factor (Tl,co) and Tlco/VA can be higher than predicted by, on average, 17% in those with mild asthma [31] due to better perfusion of the apices than in normal subjects. In more severe cases the transfer factor is reduced as a consequence of the $\dot{V}\text{A}/\dot{Q}$ imbalance. In the general population a high transfer factor is found in obese subjects, those with a high body surface area or a large total lung capacity and those with asthma [32]. Transfer factor can increase in response to bronchodilator therapy [33] as this may improve $\dot{V}\text{A}/\dot{Q}$ matching (cf. Table 20.5, page 244).

40.2.6 Control of breathing

Whilst asthma patients in remission tend to have higher levels of ventilation and lower $P\text{a,CO}_2$ values than normal subjects there is no abnormality in their ventilatory response to CO_2 [34]. However, when bronchoconstriction supervenes the response includes an increase in lung volume (hyperinflation) that might stimulate, but also modify the reflex function of pulmonary stretch receptors. This could explain why asthma patients with a history of very severe attacks have a reduced ability to sense the changes in their airways resistance and ventilatory control [35].

40.2.7 Illustrative cases

The pattern of lung function during a severe attack of asthma, and following treatment is illustrated in Table 40.1. Lung function in a patient presenting for the first time is given in Table 38.5, Case a (page 536) and the response to exercise in a baker with stable asthma is given in Table 29.11 (page 429).

40.3 Chronic obstructive pulmonary disease and emphysema

Chronic obstructive pulmonary disease (COPD) is defined as poorly reversible airflow limitation that is slowly progressive, irreversible and does not change markedly over several months [36, 37]. The condition is usually due to breathing fumes from cigarette smoke and/or severe atmospheric pollution for a period of months or years (Sections 37.3 and 37.5).

Table 40.1 Lung function in a patient with asthma.
Asthma. Mr. A, a non-smoker aged 57 years, had left the police force after 25 years service on account of late onset of asthma. There was a past history of nasal polyps and a strong family history of asthma. The patient was admitted to a hospital on the tenth day of his third significant exacerbation at which time he was severely ill with marked hypercapnia and respiratory acidosis. The sputum contained eosinophils and hyperinflation was evident on the chest radiograph. Lung function measurements were made on the third day of admission at which time there was a gross obstructive type of ventilatory defect with very material air trapping. The physiological deadspace and the alveolar–arterial tension difference for oxygen were increased and there was a small intrapulmonary shunt. This was evidence that some acini were perfused but not ventilated. However, the transfer factor was normal. Following treatment the measurements were repeated 8 days later at which time most indices had reverted to normal.
The findings were considered to be typical of status asthmaticus.

Subject:	Mr A	
	Asthma	
Condition:	Relapse	Remission
Age (year)		57
Stature (m)		1.85
Body mass (kg)		83
FEV_1 (l)	0.6	2.7
FVC (l)	2.6	5.3
FEV_1%	23	51
TLC (l)	8.97	6.72
FRC (l)	5.63	3.83
RV (l)	4.31	1.58
RV/TLC%	48	23.5
Tl (single breath)*	11.4 (34)	11.4 (34)
Vd/*Vt* (%)	52	32
A-aDo_2*	6.7 (50)	1.2 (9)
$\dot{Q}s/\dot{Q}t$ (%)	5.7	3.4
Pa,o_2*	8.0 (60)	13.1 (98)
Pa,co_2*	4.9 (37)	4.7 (35.5)
$\dot{V}_E$, rest air (l min^{-1})	17.5	12.7
f_R (min^{-1})	19.7	14.3

* The data are given in SI units with traditional units in brackets, e.g. for Pa,o_2 kPa (torr), *Tl* mmol min^{-1} kPa^{-1} (ml min^{-1} $torr^{-1}$), for *C*stat and *C*dyn l kPa^{-1} (l cm H_2O^{-1}) and for *R*aw kPa l^{-1}s (cm H_2O l^{-1}s). The conversion factors are given in Table 6.6 (page 56).

Pathology. The fumes affect the epithelium of respiratory bronchioles where they give rise to increased secretion of mucus, inflammation and thickening of the subepithelial tissue, damage to cilia, increased bronchomotor tone and destruction of alveoli present in the walls of these small airways. The destruction is effected by proteolytic enzymes (elastases) that are liberated by polymorphonuclear leucocytes attracted to the locality by secretions from alveolar macrophages. The affected tissue disappears and is replaced by air spaces that are located in the centres of acini, hence *centriacinar emphysema* (also known as *centrilobular emphysema*). Centrilobular emphysema usually occurs in the upper lobes and apical segments of the lower lobes. It is traditionally more common in tall than in short subjects and in men than in women. These circumstances share the common feature of a relatively big vertical gradient of pleural pressure down the lungs (Sections 11.2 and 16.1.8). The susceptibility to emphysema is increased by local scarring, as in silicosis (Section 37.7.8), or by disruption of the lung from accumulation of coal dust (*focal emphysema*, Section 37.7.7). Centrilobular emphysema can often be improved if the volume of the lungs is reduced by surgery (lung volume reduction surgery, Section 43.2.2).

In centrilobular emphysema the provoking agents enter the lungs via the airways. The agents can also enter via the pulmonary venous blood. This is the case when emphysema is caused by elastases in the blood that have escaped destruction as a result of deficiency or inactivation of the protective enzyme α_1 antitrypsin (Section 41.4.1). The blood borne elastases destroy alveoli throughout the acini, hence the name *panacinar emphysema.* The distribution of the lesions is mainly to the bases of the lungs matching the distribution of blood flow. The small airways are normally intact but their calibre is diminished because the presence of emphysema reduces the elastic recoil of the lungs, and hence the traction exerted on the airway walls (Section 11.2).

Clinical features. The symptoms of COPD are chronic cough and phlegm, increased susceptibility to acute chest illnesses (chronic bronchitis) and increased breathlessness on exertion. These features can be identified and quantified using the BMRC questionnaire on respiratory symptoms (Fig. 8.2, page 88). The presence of material emphysema is not invariable and because it is a pathologically defined condition the diagnosis formerly needed confirmation from lung biopsy, or at postmortem. The advent of high resolution CT scanning has allowed a high level of certainty in the diagnosis on the basis of changes in attenuation on the scans. Objective measures of emphysema using the relative area occupied by pixels below a threshold level of attenuation have been proposed [38]. The measures are strongly and negatively correlated with gas transfer per unit alveolar volume ($r = -0.86$), weakly correlated with FEV_1 but uncorrelated with lung elastic recoil [39] which is reduced in emphysematous lungs [40].

Where emphysema is present the lung function changes in COPD can reflect some loss of alveolar surface area as well as airflow limitation and $\dot{V}A/\dot{Q}$ imbalance. The latter is partly compensated for by pulmonary vasoconstriction (Section 17.2.2). This raises the pulmonary arterial pressure, increases the work of the right ventricle and can progress to right heart failure (cor pulmonale). The condition can be reversed temporarily by long-term oxygen therapy (LTOT, Section 35.7.1).

40.3.1 Spirometry and peak expiratory flow

The presence of airflow limitation is fundamental to the diagnosis of COPD with patients showing a reduced PEF and FEV_1, with a low FEV_1/VC ratio. The absolute level of FEV_1 relates to prognosis [41] with a 5-year survival of only about 30% when the absolute FEV_1 is below 0.75 l. In advanced disease the VC and FVC may be reduced as well as the FEV_1 due to premature airway closure during the dynamic manoeuvre. Under these circumstances the RV is greatly increased, thus distinguishing the finding of a low FEV_1 and FVC due to airflow limitation and not due to a restrictive disease process. Since FVC is poorly reproducible in these subjects it has recently been suggested that FEV_6 may be used as a surrogate for FVC [42]. The ratio FEV_1/FEV_6 had a sensitivity and specificity of over 95% for the diagnosis of airflow limitation in COPD. Flow–volume loops tend to show a pressure dependent collapse of airways on expiration with a relatively normal inspiratory limb (Fig. 38.1, page 533). COPD and emphysema often co-exist in the lungs of these patients, which is reflected in the results of lung function studies.

The global initiative for obstructive lung disease (GOLD) has defined severity of COPD using arbitrary thresholds of FEV_1 expressed as per cent predicted [43]. Use of per cent predicted does not remove the age, height and sex bias from lung function tests [44, 45] so the method may falsely label some older [46] and shorter subjects into inappropriate categories of severity. The GOLD classification has been criticised for not being evidence based [47] and previous studies with validated survival have been based on absolute values of FEV_1 [41, 48].

The possible causes for airflow limitation in COPD and emphysema include airway oedema from infection, reduced alveolar driving pressure due to loss of elastic recoil and increased collapsibility of the airways. The reduced elastic recoil not only reduces the alveolar driving pressure but also reduces the support to the airways. Study of resected lungs from patients with COPD found that it was the reduced elastic recoil and reduced upstream conductance that related best to airflow limitation [49].

Considerable interest has been shown in the accelerated annual decline in FEV_1 in subjects with COPD [50]. However, it is only possible to derive reliable estimates of decline from large numbers of subjects using sophisticated statistical techniques. The short- and medium-term variability of FEV_1 in these patients is large so it is not possible to estimate reliably the rate of decline for an individual subject unless about 10 years of data are obtained. Observations obtained more frequently than every 3 months to a year are not helpful [51] due to the high degree of autocorrelation of the measurements. Analysis of the nitrogen slope (Section 16.2.6) is now rarely undertaken in clinical practice but an increased phase 3 slope has been found to predict more rapid decline in FEV_1 in smokers over a 13-year period [52].

40.3.2 Reversibility

COPD is defined as a condition of poorly reversible airflow limitation. Hence, short-term reversibility is, by definition, below that which might define asthma. However, many patients with COPD derive subjective benefit from the use of bronchodilators without showing significant reversibility on spirometry. This has led to a search for other objective measures that better match the subjective benefit. The 6-min walk test, bronchial hyperresponsiveness and tests of alveolar mixing have all failed to reflect convincing benefit from bronchodilators. In patients with COPD an increase in FEV_1 of 4% or more of the predicted value following bronchodilator is associated with perceived benefit [53]. This improvement is less than the 9% of predicted value that is the threshold for defining asthma [16]. However, when FEV_1 reversibility is tested repeatedly in a group of patients fulfilling ERS criteria for COPD the responses fit a normal distribution with no clear cut-off point [54]. The absolute increase in FEV_1 did not relate to the initial FEV_1, and when arbitrary threshold values to define responder status were applied many subjects changed responder status on repeated testing. Hence, as the definition of COPD relies on poor reversibility this remains a vexed issue.

40.3.3 Lung volumes

Static volume changes in COPD and emphysema include an increased RV, FRC and TLC at rest. Measuring the TLC by helium dilution may not show as large an increase as that measured by plethysmography as some areas of lung may not be in continuity with the airways. Any elevation of TLC implies some loss of elastic recoil due to concomitant emphysema. Elevation of FRC may occur at rest for the same reason but in patients without such a change this may occur during exercise and is termed dynamic hyperinflation (Section 40.3.6). Loss of elastic recoil, airway oedema and increased intrinsic airway compliance all lead to an increased tendency for airways to collapse during expiration. This raises the closing volume, thus worsening gas exchange, and increases RV. Inspiratory capacity is reduced (Section 40.3.6).

40.3.4 $\dot{V}A/\dot{Q}$ changes and gas transfer

In COPD the gas transfer factor will be reduced where there is coexistent emphysema. A low *T*l,co with severe airflow limitation [41] and/or hypoxaemia is associated with a much poorer prognosis [55]. However, where lung function is uneven the interpretation of *T*l,co can be uncertain if, as is usually the case the measurement is made using the single breath estimate of lung volume. A meaningful estimate is more likely to be obtained if the patient is fully bronchodilated first (Table 20.5, page 244). The cause of the hypoxaemia in COPD has been shown by MIGET to be due to $\dot{V}A/\dot{Q}$ imbalance [56] with no evidence for true shunt or diffusion limitation being involved. Two patterns of abnormality were found (Fig. 40.6), one with areas of very low $\dot{V}A/\dot{Q}$ (compatible with chronic bronchitis) and another with areas of high $\dot{V}A/\dot{Q}$ (compatible with emphysema). This latter finding was subsequently confirmed from resected lung specimens [57].

On exercise (see below) the degree of $\dot{V}A/\dot{Q}$ imbalance does not change in patients with severe disease but, in those with milder disease the $\dot{V}A/\dot{Q}$ maldistribution improves with resulting improvement to gas exchange [58].

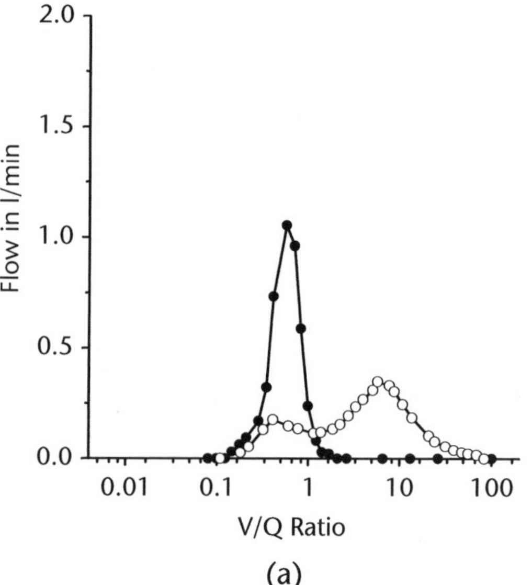

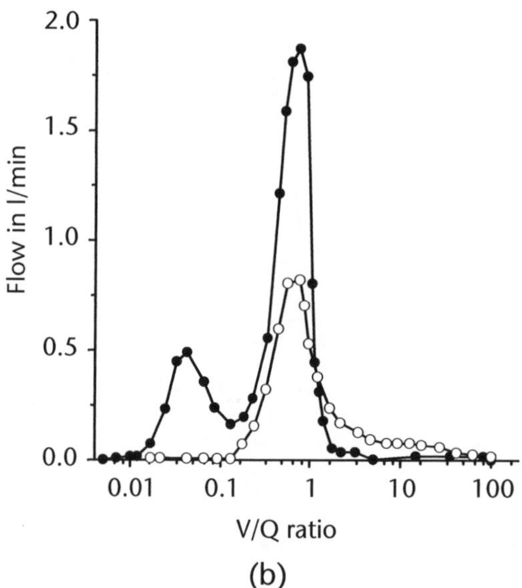

Fig. 40.6 Ventilation (open circles) and perfusion (closed circles) distribution found in two patients with COPD. In (a) the findings are compatible with emphysema showing significant areas with very high $\dot{V}_A/\dot{Q}$. In (b) there are areas with very low $\dot{V}_A/\dot{Q}$ which will predispose to hypoxia.

40.3.5 Muscle function

Low body mass index (BMI $< 23\,kg\,m^{-2}$) is an independent predictor of mortality in advanced COPD [48], and underweight patients report a poorer quality of life and are less physically active [59]. However, these patients are also more dyspnoeic and this accounts for the difference. In another study increased dyspnoea in underweight patients with COPD was related to a reduced gas transfer and lower ventilatory capacity [60]. This has led to interest in the possibility that muscle function influences outcome and symptoms in COPD. Changes in peripheral muscles are likely to be due to atrophy from inactivity due to the patient taking less habitual activity because of their pulmonary insufficiency [61]. When patients with moderate COPD undertook a symptom-limited maximal exercise test there was no evidence of diaphragm contractile fatigue [62].

An earlier study has shown that in patients with severe COPD (average FEV_1 of 0.8 l) (i) maximal mouth pressures at rest are reduced, (ii) the accessory muscles and not the diaphragm increase their contribution on exercise, (iii) exercise capacity was negatively correlated to the patient's ability to make their inspiratory pleural pressure more negative, (iv) exercise capacity was positively correlated to maximum oxygen pulse (that is $\dot{V}O_2$/heart rate) [63]. The third observation relates to an increased FRC with no increase in TLC on exercise, and the fourth observation suggests that the increasingly negative pleural pressure on exercise reduces stroke volume, as the cardiac output response is normal in COPD with a lower stroke volume but higher heart rate response [64]. When COPD patients with and without type 2 respiratory failure were exercised it was found that both groups had similar exercise capacity and muscle recruitment indicating that it was the inability to increase ventilation and not respiratory muscle function that explained the hypercapnia in these patients [65].

40.3.6 Exercise

If exercise is limited in COPD by an inability to increase alveolar ventilation sufficiently why is ventilation limited? In normal subjects tidal volume increases during progressive exercise with both a drop in FRC and a rise in end inspiratory volume [66]. In older subjects the tidal flow at volumes below FRC may become maximal for this lung volume [67]. In COPD, where maximal flows at any given lung volume are lower, the FRC during exercise becomes dynamically reset at a level higher than that at rest in order to help maintain expiratory flow and so allow the minute ventilation to increase in line with demand. This dynamic hyperinflation reduces the inspiratory capacity (IC). During tidal breathing at rest the FRC of COPD patients can be higher than the relaxation volume (elastic equilibration volume) which in normal subjects and those with restrictive disease are the same [68]. Thus, in COPD both FRC (end expiratory volume) and end inspiratory volume (EIV) rise on exercise until EIV reaches TLC and no further increase is possible. The work of breathing under these circumstances is much increased compared to normal subjects. This dynamic hyperinflation during exercise in COPD has recently been shown to impinge on the tidal volume response to exercise [69] and to correlate with exercise dyspnoea [70], see also Sections 28.4.7, 28.7, 28.8 and 29.8.2 (step 4).

An interesting new technique of suddenly applying a negative pressure at the mouth during tidal breathing (NEP) has been used to demonstrate whether subjects are truly flow limited at rest or on exercise during tidal breathing [71]. In normal subjects the added negative pressure can increase the flow since flow is usually set by the subject's driving pressure (now increased) and not by any limitation from the airways. In patients with intrapulmonary airflow limitation the added driving pressure from the NEP cannot increase the flow since in these circumstances flow is limited by impaired airway function. Figure 40.7 shows the

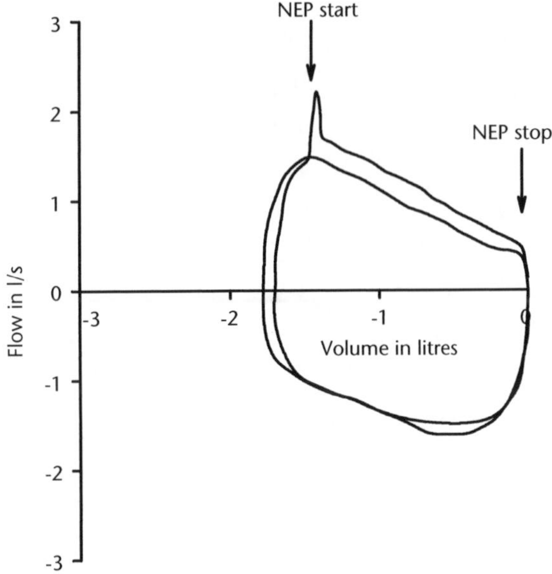

Fig. 40.7 Two full tidal flow–volume loops are shown for a patient with COPD at rest with volume expressed relative to FRC. An initial full tidal loop is shown with NEP started at the arrow on the next tidal breath and stopped as FRC was approached. Expiratory flow was increased by NEP indicating flow was not limited by airway characteristics. Source: Adapted from [72].

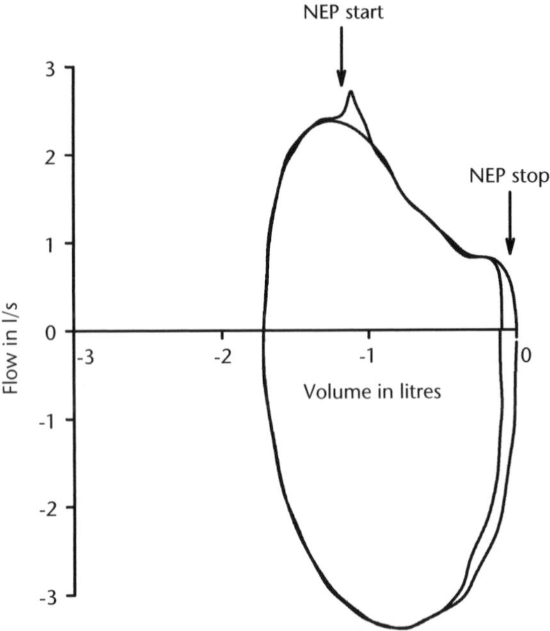

Fig. 40.8 Two full tidal flow–volume curves are shown for the same patient as in Fig. 40.7, now during exercise. An initial full tidal loop is shown with NEP started at the arrow on the next tidal breath and stopped as FRC was approached. Expiratory flow was now unchanged by NEP indicating flow was limited during exercise by airway characteristics. Source: Adapted from [72].

application of NEP to a patient with COPD at rest. The transient rise in flow at the onset of NEP is due to slight collapse of the cheeks and upper airway followed, in this case, by an increase in expiratory flow indicating no airflow limitation. In Fig. 40.8 the same subject is tested during exercise when there is no increase in flow indicating intrapulmonary airflow limitation.

However, this technique can lead to major collapse of the upper airway in some subjects that falsely suggests intrapulmonary airflow limitation. A technique has been proposed using manual abdominal compression (MAC) to enhance the driving pressure at the beginning of a spontaneous tidal expiration, and so avoid any difficulty from upper airway collapse [73]. MCA increased expiratory flow in all normal subjects but half of the patients with COPD had flow limitation demonstrated during tidal breathing by this technique. NEP and MAC have the advantage of avoiding any interference from the previous volume history in assessing airflow limitation [6] and are of interest in detecting the effect of therapeutic interventions in COPD.

Exercise limitation is universally found as COPD progresses. This has led to the development of training programmes that may improve exercise tolerance and quality of life (Section 44.4).

40.3.7 Control of breathing

The natural history of advanced COPD leads to chronic type 2 respiratory failure with hypercapnia in many patients. The measurement of ventilatory drive to changes in O_2 and CO_2 in the presence of airflow limitation is affected by the degree of airflow limitation present. Measurement of the $P_{0.1}$ is used to assess neural drive (Section 23.9.6). When comparing severe COPD patients, who were either normocapnic or hypercapnic, with normal subjects the resting $P_{0.1}$ was higher in patients than controls, but the increase in $P_{0.1}$ per unit increase in $P\text{CO}_2$ was similar for each of the three groups [74]. However, the ventilatory response to a unit increase in $P\text{CO}_2$ was lower in the hypercapnic group and only a lower FEV_1 and higher diaphragmatic load were predictive of hypercapnia. A separate, earlier and smaller study found that $P_{0.1}$ as a per cent of MIP was not different between the three groups of subjects [75]. However, the change in $P_{0.1}$ per unit increase in $P\text{CO}_2$ was lower in the hypercapnic group (but the same as the other groups when standardised for MIP) suggesting the involvement of impaired inspiratory muscle function.

Concern about treating COPD patients with oxygen and causing worsening hypercapnia has centred on the possibility of the oxygen therapy switching off the hypoxic drive (Section 35.7.2, page 494). A study of stable COPD patients with hyperoxia found the degree of ensuing hypercapnia was related to the FEV_1 and not to any measure of CO_2 or O_2 drive, nor to resting $P\text{CO}_2$ or $P\text{O}_2$ [76]. The major reason for hyperoxic hypercapnia in these patients was impaired gas exchange and changes in deadspace ventilation.

40.3.8 Illustrative cases

The pattern of lung function in COPD is shown for three illustrative cases in Table 40.2. Lung function in new cases presenting with COPD and with emphysema are given in Table 38.5 b and c page 536, and examples of the response to exercise are shown in Figs 28.13, 28.18, 28.19 and 29.9, also Table 29.11.

Table 40.2 Lung function in patients with COPD.

Mild. Mr. B, aged 51 years, was a machine fitter, who, 18 months before the consultation, developed a head cold which went to his chest. Before this he coughed occasionally but was otherwise in good health; subsequently he had a persistent cough with morning sputum and episodes of wheeze and tightness of the chest. He smoked 20 cigarettes per day. The remaining medical history was unexceptional, as was the physical examination, the chest X-ray and the electrocardiogram. On assessment of lung function the FEV_1 was reduced and represented a smaller proportion than normal of the forced vital capacity (FEV_1% reduced). The FVC was less than the IVC; this was evidence for dynamic compression during forced expiration. The FEV_1 was increased following the inhalation of a bronchodilator aerosol. The dynamic lung compliance was less than the static measurement. The other indices of lung function were within normal limits. The findings were typical of moderate airway obstruction in a patient with bronchitis. In this instance the sputum and wheeze disappeared and the FEV_1 increased to 2.41 after a course of antibiotic drugs; the patient was advised to give up smoking.

Advanced. Mr. C entered the coal mines at the age of 13 years. He was a light smoker. At the age of 23 he had the first of many episodes of bronchitis and at 34 he moved from the mines into light employment. He gave up work at the age of 49. Two years later during an acute chest illness Mr. B was observed to have a severe productive cough, an audible wheeze and coarse rhonchi and crackles over both lung bases. His chest radiograph did not show specific changes; bronchograms were negative for bronchiectasis. The cardiac outline, the ECG and the haemoglobin concentration were within normal limits. Assessment of lung function showed evidence of gross obstruction to the lung airways but with a normal transfer factor. Five years later, at the age of 56, Mr. B developed congestive cardiac failure during an acute chest illness. The ECG then showed the features of pulmonary heart disease and the mean pressure in the pulmonary artery at rest was 39 mm Hg. The haemoglobin concentration was increased. These conditions responded to treatment which included long-term oxygen therapy. Oxygen from a portable apparatus and later from an oxygen line improved the capacity for exercise.

For the last 4 years of his life Mr. C had marked hypoxaemia and hypercapnia $Pa,O_2 < 5.3$ kPa ($<$ 40 mm Hg), $Pa,CO_2 > 8.0$ kPa ($>$ 60 mm Hg) and frequent acute exacerbations of his respiratory and cardiac failure; in several of these he required assisted ventilation for the treatment of carbon dioxide narcosis. He died suddenly at the age of 65 following an injury sustained at home.

At postmortem the bronchi exhibited evidence of chronic inflammation and the pulmonary arteries showed atheroma and thickening of their walls; an old thrombus partly occluded the left main pulmonary artery. The lung contained emphysematous bullae at the apices and along the fissures, but the parenchyma was relatively intact.

Emphysema. Mr. D, aged 48 years, was a Civil Servant, who presented with breathlessness on exertion (Grade 3) and recurrent episodes of cough and sputum of 7 years duration. He gave a history of being chesty as a child, but his symptoms cleared up completely during adolescence. As a young man he passed the medical examination for the RAF as Grade 1 and he lost only a very few days from work prior to the onset of breathlessness. It was after this that he developed bronchitis. He smoked 14 cigarettes per day, reducing to 6 per day during periods of chest illness. On examination he was breathless, cyanosed and underweight; his chest was held in an inspiratory position and the percussion note was hyper-resonant. The breath sounds were faint, expiration was prolonged and soft expiratory wheeze was present at both bases posteriorly. The chest X-ray showed increased transradiancy and the vascular markings in the periphery of the lung fields were reduced. The ECG showed deep *S* waves in *V*6 but was otherwise normal.

On assessment of lung function the FEV_1 was greatly reduced, but increased in response to a bronchodilator aerosol; the FVC was within normal limits. The total lung capacity was enlarged in association with a very high static lung compliance and low recoil pressure. The residual volume was increased proportionally more than the TLC so the RV% was increased as well. The airway resistance was high especially during expiration reflecting the low static recoil pressure. The transfer factor (diffusing capacity) for the lung was much reduced despite the enlarged total lung capacity. The reduction was associated with a very low Tl/V_A. The arterial carbon dioxide tension was low on account of hyperventilation and the oxygen tension was low at rest, falling further during exercise.

The patient was diagnosed as having emphysema together with chronic airflow limitation, which was partly reversible. He was treated with bronchodilator and antibiotic drugs and was able to increase his capacity for exercise by use of portable oxygen equipment.

Over the next 3 years there was little alteration in the indices of lung function, apart from the transfer factor which fell to a low level. This change was associated with an increase in breathlessness and a reduction in the capacity for exercise; the patient was then confined to bed. He died from respiratory failure 12 years after the onset of his symptoms. At postmortem the lung was large with peripheral bullae and did not deflate when the chest was opened. The large lung sections showed gross panacinar emphysema with extensive loss of lung tissue, including the vascular bed. The features were those of deficiency of $\alpha 1$ antitrypsin with additional reversible airflow limitation.

Subject:	Mr. B	Mr. C	Mr. D
Condition:	Mild airway disease	Advanced airway disease	Emphysema
Age (a)	51	57* → 65	48 → 51*
Stature (m)	1.70	1.64	1.83
Body mass (kg)	77	50	53
FEV_1 (l)	1.8	0.7	0.8
Response to bronchodilator (%)	+17	+10	+45
FVC (and IVC) (l)	3.4 (3.95)	1.55	4.7
FEV%	53	45	17
TLC (l)	6.30	6.18	9.81
RV (l)	2.35	3.86	5.09

(*Continued*)

Table 40.2 *(Continued)*

Subject:	Mr. B	Mr. C	Mr. D
Condition:	Mild airway disease	Advanced airway disease	Emphysema
RV%	37	62	52
Cstat†	3.1 (0.31)	1.4 (0.14)	6.0 (0.6)
Cdyn†	1.6 (0.16)	–	3.4 (0.34)
*R*aw (inspiration) †	0.082 (0.82)	–	0.54 (5.4)
*R*aw (expiration) †	–	–	0.78 (7.8)
*T*l,co†	7.9 (24)	7.7(23) → 4.7(14)	5.8(23) → 3.0(9)
Pa,O_2†	12.8 (96)	8.0(60) → 4.9(37)	8.0(60)‡
Pa,CO_2†	5.1 (38)	5.3 (40) → 10.7 (80)	4.5 (34)
$\dot{V}_E$, ex air (l min^{-1})§	36.5 (2.5/10)	23 (1.0/0)	33 (2.0/0)
$\dot{V}_E$, O_2 (l min^{-1})	31.l	16	21
Dyspnoeic index (air)	–	107	125
Hb concentration (g dl^{-1})	–	14.7 → 18.7	– → 17.3

* 1 year after onset of cardiac failure. Arrow indicates passage of time.
† For units see footnote to Table 40.1.
‡ On exercise the Pa,O_2 fell to 5.7 kPa (43).
§ Walking, speed (mph) and incline (%) in brackets.

40.4 Diffuse lung fibrosis (diffuse interstitial lung disease)

This group of conditions embraces idiopathic pulmonary fibrosis (IPF), also known as cryptogenic fibrosing alveolitis, and various forms of interstitial fibrosis or pneumonitis (Table 40.3). The conditions differ in the extent to which cellular and fibrotic changes predominate. In all of them there is a reduced transfer factor and increased ventilation at rest and on exercise. The presenting symptom is breathlessness on exertion and this is usually associated with shallow breathing.

40.4.1 Spirometry and peak expiratory flow

The development of fibrosis in the alveolar interstitium increases the static recoil of the lung and so reduces lung compliance [77, 78]. Early in the disease process, before there is marked restriction of the lung volumes, the maximal expiratory flows are increased due to increased traction on the airways leading to higher achievable flows early within the dynamic forced expiratory manoeuvre [79]. As the disease progresses the TLC and VC decrease and maximal flows early in the expiratory manoeuvre are reduced; this is because the diminished lung volume is associated with relatively small airways. However, when compared to normal lungs the airways at any given lung volume tend to have a larger diameter because they are subject to a greater elastic recoil. This can lead to traction bronchiectasis evident on CT scanning [80]. Subjects with IPF tend to have supramaximal PEF and mid-expiratory flows early on in the disease process; these then decline as TLC becomes markedly reduced. The extra traction on airways ensures they do not collapse so easily during a forced expiratory manoeuvre, so contributing to a reduction in RV.

Table 40.3 Interstitial lung diseases which give rise to characteristic findings on assessment of lung function

(a) *Systemic diseases which can involve the lung:*
Sarcoidosis, beryllium disease
Disorders of connective tissue, including:
progressive systemic sclerosis, rheumatoid arthritis , lupus erythematosus, polyarteritis nodosa
Coeliac disease
Schistosomiasis (bilharzia)
Xanthomatoses, including eosinophilic granuloma
Disseminated tuberculosis, carcinomatosis, neurofibromatosis and other conditions
Chronic interstitial oedema (from left ventricular failure, hexamethonium, uraemia etc.)

(b) *Diseases which primarily involve the lung:*
Interstitial pneumonitis, including Hamman Rich Syndrome (diffuse fibrosing alveolitis)
Extrinsic allergic alveolitis
Nitrous fume exposure (e.g. silo-filler's disease)
Virus pneumonia
Drug sensitivity (e.g. to nitrofurantoin, bleomycin, busulphan)
Chronic interstitial fibrosis, including: cases of interstitial pneumonitis, asbestosis, talcosis, hard metal disease, acute silicosis, radiation fibrosis
Bronchiolar or alveolar cell carcinoma, lymphomatous infiltrate
Alveolar proteinosis and micro-lithiasis; pulmonary muscular hyperplasia leiomyomatosis and other conditions.

Prediction of survival in IPF from results of lung function tests is best made using VC and TLC, whilst resting gas exchange and PO_2 are uninformative [81]. FEV_1 as a proportion of FVC is often increased, so this index needs to be interpreted with circumspection.

40.4.2 Lung volumes

Reduction in TLC and FRC, followed later by RV, is usual as the disease progresses [82–84]. Lone IPF has been found to deteriorate more than if the interstitial fibrosis is associated with collagen vascular diseases (see Section 41.19)) [85].

The increased static elastic recoil, which is the hallmark of this condition, can be measured (Section 11.8.2) and the static pressure volume curve fitted to an exponential with an exponent k describing the distensibilty of the available lung units (Section 11.8.3). When compared to normal subjects those with IPF have a reduced value for k such that the maximal recoil pressure at full inspiration is about twice that expected in normal subjects [86]. The technique is now seldom used in routine clinical practice but can have application in research studies.

40.4.3 $\dot{V}A/\dot{Q}$ changes and gas transfer

IPF predominantly affects the lower lobes so it is possible for patients to have orthodeoxia [87] which arises because, in the upright posture lung perfusion is distributed under gravity more to the affected lower lobes, but on lying supine the perfusion is redistributed to the less affected upper zones, and so oxygenation may improve. In IPF there is only a small change in $\dot{V}A/\dot{Q}$ ratios (using MIGET) but a degree of shunt is often present. About 19% of the A-aD_{O_2} seen with the subject at rest is due to a true diffusion limitation with the remainder due to $\dot{V}A/\dot{Q}$ imbalance [88].

In a study of patients under treatment for IPF measurement of gas transfer, P_{O_2}, A-aD_{O_2} and spirometry found a drop of 10% or more in FVC after 1 year was the only significant predictor of survival [89]; others have confirmed that VC and TLC best predict survival in IPF [81].

40.4.4 Exercise

On exercise A-aD_{O_2} increases in patients with IPF with 40% of this difference due to impaired diffusion with little change in $\dot{V}A/\dot{Q}$ mismatching [88]. However, in one study when IPF was compared to asbestosis the A-aD_{O_2}, P_{O_2} and Vd/Vt were comparable at rest, but gas transfer was lower in IPF [90]. On exercise the $Pa,_{O_2}$ fell in patients with IPF but not asbestosis, suggesting that the form of interstitial fibrosis in IPF might affect the pulmonary vasculature more than other types of fibrosis (cf. Section 37.7.2). It appears that structural changes in the pulmonary vasculature and not hypoxic vasoconstriction (reversible by the administration of oxygen) are the main cause for the pulmonary hypertension [88]. This feature can be associated with a lower $Pa,_{O_2}$ on exercise and worse $\dot{V}A/\dot{Q}$ mismatching. Comparisons between patients with IPF and sarcoidosis have also found greater reduction in gas transfer and differences in exercise limitation with IPF [91].

The increased ventilation reflects an increased hypoxic drive to breathing and shallow breathing leading to an increased minute volume being expended in ventilating the physiological deadspace (Section 28.4.7). In some related conditions the shallow breathing is in excess of that expected for the reduction in FVC (e.g. Fig. 28.11, page 397). Where the ventilation is increased at rest, the patient experiences a respiratory alkalosis that further enhances the ventilation during exercise.

40.4.5 Control of breathing

Patients with IPF tend to breath with shallow frequent breaths; this will optimise the energy cost of breathing when the lung elastic recoil is increased, and so help reduce dyspnoea [92]. No specific abnormality of ventilatory control is associated with IPF but it has been found that IPF patients who have a significant desaturation at night tend to have a low sensitivity to hypercapnia and a lower resting arterial saturation while awake [93]. Where the condition is primarily a pneumonitis the shallow breathing is enhanced by activation of pulmonary J receptors (Section 23.3.4).

40.4.6 CT correlated with function

HRCT scanning has increasingly been used in the diagnosis and follow up of patients with IPF [94]. The overall extent of IPF on HRCT was negatively correlated with FVC and gas transfer, and P_{O_2} at peak exercise [95]. The extent of ground glass pattern, suggesting active alveolitis, was negatively correlated with FVC and P_{O_2} at peak exercise but not correlated with gas transfer. A possible explanation for this finding comes from another study on 68 patients with IPF, of whom 14 were found to have unexpected HRCT evidence of concomitant emphysema [96]. These subjects had relative preservation of lung volumes and worse gas transfer compared to the other subjects. A further study found HRCT evidence of emphysema in patients with IPF and relatively preserved lung volumes [97], and highlighted the difficulty of interpreting gas transfer measurements in IPF if the degree of any associated emphysema is not known. A normal HRCT can be found in patients with functional impairment and biopsy proven IPF [98]. Thus, lung function tests are more sensitive than HRCT in detecting mild changes due to IPF.

40.4.7 Illustrative cases

The patterns of lung function in patients with pulmonary fibrosis are shown in Table 38.5d (page 536), the appendix to Chapter 37 (pages 525 to 528) and Table 40.4. Further cases are given in Tables 29.11 and 29.12 (pages 429 and 430).

Table 40.4 Lung function in two patients with diffuse fibrosing alveolitis.

Uncomplicated disease. Mr. E, aged 42 years, presented with breathlessness on exertion of 3 months' duration which was rapidly getting worse. He had a dry, unproductive cough. He gave a history of apparently trivial exposure to a number of noxious chemicals and of a recent nervous breakdown. On examination he was overweight. There were a few coarse crackles at the right base. The blood pressure was 150/110 mm Hg. The chest X-ray showed mottled opacities throughout both lung fields and elevation of the right diaphragm. The ECG showed left axis deviation. The Mantoux reaction was positive at 1/1000; the serum proteins were normal. The physical signs were consistent with fibrosing alveolitis affecting particularly the right lung. However, in view of the history of psychosomatic illness, the patient was referred for assessment of lung function with a view to obtaining confirmatory evidence for the diagnosis.

On assessment of lung function the forced expiratory volume and forced vital capacity were both reduced, as were all the components of the total lung capacity. The ratios FEV_1/FVC and RV/TLC were within normal limits. The transfer factor (diffusing capacity) for the lung was diminished due to a reduction in the membrane component. The lung volume index of uneven ventilation was within normal limits. The tensions of oxygen and carbon dioxide in the arterial blood when breathing air at rest were on the low side of normal. The ventilation on exercise was increased both when breathing air and when breathing oxygen. The lung compliance was greatly reduced and the airway resistance was low. The findings were considered typical of interstitial pulmonary fibrosis and this diagnosis was confirmed at lung biopsy. The low compliance was also noted by the anaesthetist who experienced difficulty in maintaining the ventilation of the lung by manual compression of the anaesthetic bag. The patient subsequently received steroid therapy which improved his symptoms, but the transfer factor and total lung capacity continued to deteriorate.

Complicated by airways obstruction. Mr. F, aged 51 years, was charge-hand in a flour mill where he had worked for 16 years. Before that he worked as a cleaner in the railways and served in the army, but did not go outside the continent of Europe. He presented with breathlessness of recent origin and a history of recurrent winter bronchitis; he was otherwise in good health and had no sputum at the time of investigation. He smoked 10–20 cigarettes per day. On examination he was overweight; coarse crackles and wheeze were heard on auscultation of the chest. The Mantoux reaction was strongly positive and the sputum contained aspergillus; no tubercle bacilli were detected. The plasma proteins were normal. The precipitin reaction for aspergillia and the Casoni test were both negative. The chest X-ray showed an enlarged heart, prominent pulmonary arteries, diffuse mottling in both lung bases and what appeared to be a small pleuropericardial cyst in the left cardio-phrenic angle. The ECG was within normal limits. The patient was referred for assessment of lung function, as a case of obstructive lung disease with some atypical features.

The findings on assessment of lung function included reductions in the forced expiratory volume and FEV_1%; the total lung capacity was somewhat reduced but the residual volume as a percentage of total lung capacity was normal. Some air trapping was evident on the spirogram. The transfer factor (diffusing capacity) for the lung was reduced as were both its components. The tension of oxygen in the arterial blood was reduced and that of carbon dioxide was on the low side of normal. The ventilation during exercise was increased when breathing air and markedly reduced when breathing oxygen. The dynamic compliance was less than the static compliance and the airway resistance was increased.

The changes in the ventilatory capacity, airway resistance and dynamic lung compliance were evidence for airways obstruction, but the combination of a low transfer factor with a small total lung capacity and a normal residual volume was not typical of this condition. These latter observations were interpreted as evidence for associated fibrosing alveolitis and this diagnosis was confirmed at lung biopsy. The patient was treated with corticosteroid drugs and his symptoms improved.

Subject:	Mr. E	Reference values	Mr. F	Reference values
Diffuse fibrosing alveolitis:	Uncomplicated		Mixed	
Age (a)	42		51	
Height (m)	1.72		1.69	
Weight (kg)	92		75	
FEV_1 (l)	1.78	3.5	1.20	3.1
change with bronchodilator (%)	0	<10	0	<10
FVC (l)	2.18	4.4	2.50	4.1
FEV_1%	82	76	48	73
TLC (l)	2.80	6.4	5.08	6.2
IVC (l)	1.94	4.4	3.25	4.1
FRC (l)	1.68	2.6	2.72	4.0
RV (l)	0.86	1.9	1.83	2.0
RV%	31	31	36	34
Air trapping	No	No	Yes	No
Tl (single breath)†	4.7 (14)	10 (30)	5.5 (17)	9.0 (27)
VA'/VA	0.95	>0.85	0.85	>0.85
Pa,O_2†	11 (82)	12.5 (94)	9.3 (70)	12 (92)
Pa,CO_2†	4.7 (35)	4.8–6.3 (36–47)	4.8 (36)	4.8–6.3 (36–47)
$\dot{V}E$, ex, air (l min^{-1})	44.8	37	44.7	37
$\dot{V}E$, ex, O_2 (l min^{-1})	34.6	35	30.9	35
Cstat (inspiration)†	0.5 (0.05)	2.4 (0.24)	2.6 (0.26)	2.4 (0.24)

Table 40.4 (*Continued*)

Subject:	Mr. E	Reference values	Mr. F	Reference values
Diffuse fibrosing alveolitis:	Uncomplicated*		Mixed	
Cdyn[†]	0.4 (0.04)	2.4 (0.24)	1.6 (0.16)	2.4 (0.24)
*R*aw (plethysmograph)[†]	0.076 (0.76)	0.1 (1.0)	0.30 (3.0)	0.11 (1.1)

[†] For units see footnote to Table 40.1.

40.5 References

1. The British Thoracic Society. Guidelines for the management of asthma: a summary. *BMJ* 1993; **306**: 776–782.
2. Turner-Warwick M. On observing patterns of airflow obstruction in chronic asthma. *Br J Dis Chest* 1977; **71**: 73–85.
3. Hetzel MR, Clark TJH. Comparison of normal and asthmatic circadian rhythms in peak expiratory flow rate. *Thorax* 1980; **35**: 732–738.
4. Higgins B. Peak expiratory flow variability in the general population. *Eur Respir J* 1997; **24**(Suppl): 45S–48S.
5. Fredberg JJ, Inouye DS, Mijailovich SM, Butler JP. Perturbed equilibrium of myosin binding in airway smooth muscle and its implications in bronchospasm. *Am J Respir Crit Care Med* 1999; **159**: 959–967.
6. Pellegrino R, Sterk PJ, Sont JK, Brusasco V. Assessing the effect of deep inhalation on airway calibre: a novel approach to lung function in bronchial asthma and COPD. *Eur Respir J* 1998; **12**: 1219–1227.
7. Burns GP, Gibson GJ. The apparent response of airway function to deep inspiration depends on the method of assessment. *Respir Med* 2001; **95**: 251–257.
8. Delacourt C, Lorino H, Fuhrman C et al. Comparison of the forced oscillation technique and the interrupter technique for assessing airway obstruction and its reversibility in children. *Am J Respir Crit Care Med* 2001; **164**: 965–972.
9. in 't Veen JC, Beekman AJ, Bel EH, Sterk PJ. Recurrent exacerbations in severe asthma are associated with enhanced airway closure during stable episodes. *Am J Respir Crit Care Med* 2000; **161**: 1902–1906.
10. Beckett PA, Howarth PH. Pharmacotherapy and airway remodelling in asthma? *Thorax* 2003; **58**: 163–174.
11. Anderson SD, Daviskas E. The mechanism of exercise-induced asthma. *J Allergy Clin Immunol* 2000; **106**: 453–459.
12. Brannan JD, Koskela H, Anderson SD, Chew N. Responsiveness to mannitol in asthmatic subjects with exercise- and hyperventilation-induced asthma. *Am J Respir Crit Care Med* 1998; **158**: 1120–1126.
13. Wojnarowski C, Storm Van's Gravesande K, Riedler J et al. Comparison of bronchial challenge with ultrasonic nebulized distilled water and hypertonic saline in children with mild-to-moderate asthma. *Eur Respir J* 1996; **9**: 1896–1901.
14. Chinn S, Sunyer J. Bronchial hyperresponsiveness. *Eur Respir Mon* 2000; **15**: 199–215.
15. Tweeddale PM, Alexander F, McHardy GJ. Short term variability in FEV1 and bronchodilator responsiveness in patients with obstructive ventilatory defects. *Thorax.* 1987; **42**: 487–490.
16. Dales RE, Spitzer WO, Tousignant P et al. Clinical interpretation of airway response to a bronchodilator. Epidemiologic considerations. *Am Rev Respir Dis* 1988; **138**: 317–320.
17. Shore S, Milic-Emili J, Martin JG. Reassessment of body plethysmographic technique for the measurement of thoracic gas volume in asthmatics. *Am Rev Respir Dis* 1982; **126**: 515–520.
18. Woolcock AJ, Read J. Lung volumes in exacerbations of asthma. *Am J Med* 1966; **41**: 259–273.
19. Martin J, Howell E, Shore S et al. The role of respiratory muscles in the hyperinflation of bronchial asthma. *Am Rev Respir Dis* 1980; **121**: 441–447.
20. Muller N, Bryan AC, Zamel N. Tonic inspiratory muscle activity as a cause of hyperinflation in asthma. *J Appl Physiol* 1981; **50**: 279–282.
21. Kirby JG, Juniper EF, Hargreave FE, Zamel N. Total lung capacity does not change during methacholine stimulated airway narrowing. *J Appl Physiol* 1986; **61**: 2144–2147.
22. Bogaard JM, Overbeek SE, Verbraak AF et al. Pressure-volume analysis of the lung with an exponential and linear-exponential model in asthma and COPD. Dutch CNSLD Study Group. *Eur Respir J* 1995; **8**: 1525–1531.
23. Brackel HJL, Pedersen OF, Mulder PGH et al. Central airways behave more stiffly during forced expiration in patients with asthma. *Am J Respir Crit Care Med* 2000; **162**: 896–904.
24. Vernon P, Burton GH, Seed WA. Lung scan abnormalities in asthma and their correlation with lung function. *Eur J Nucl Med* 1986 ;**12**: 16–20.
25. Cooper DM, Mellins RB, Mansell AL. Ventilation distribution and density dependence of expiratory flow in asthmatic children. *J Appl Physiol.* 1983; **54**: 1125–1130.
26. Ballester E, Reyes A, Roca J et al. Ventilation-perfusion mismatching in acute severe asthma: effects of salbutamol and 100% oxygen. *Thorax* 1989; **44**: 258–267.
27. Rodriguez-Roisin R. Acute severe asthma: pathophysiology and pathobiology of gas exchange abnormalities. *Eur Respir J* 1997; **10**: 1359–1371.
28. Rodriguez-Roisin R, Roca J. Contributions of multiple inert gas elimination technique to pulmonary medicine. 3. Bronchial asthma. *Thorax* 1994; **49**: 1027–1033.
29. Roca J, Ramis LI, Rodriguez-Roisin R et al. Serial relationships between ventilation-perfusion inequality and spirometry in acute severe asthma requiring hospitalization. *Am Rev Respir Dis* 1988; **137**: 1055–1061.
30. McFadden ER, Lyons HA. Arterial blood gas tension in asthma. *New Eng J Med* 1968; **278**: 1027–1032.
31. Collard P, Njinou B, Nejadnik B et al. Single breath diffusing capacity for carbon monoxide in stable asthma. *Chest* 1994; **105**: 1426–1429.
32. Saydain G, Beck KC, Decker PA et al. Clinical significance of elevated diffusing capacity. *Chest* 2004; **125**: 446–452.

33. Akesson U, Dahlstrom JA, Wollmer P. Changes in transfer factor of the lung in response to bronchodilatation. *Clin Physiol* 2000; **20**: 14–18.
34. Hormbrey J, Jacobi MS, Patil CP, Saunders KB. CO_2 response and pattern of breathing in patients with symptomatic hyperventilation, compared to asthmatic and normal subjects. *Eur Respir J.* 1988; **1**: 846–851.
35. Kikuchi Y, Okabe S, Tamura G et al. Chemosensitivity and perception of dyspnea in patients with a history of near-fatal asthma. *New Eng J Med* 1994; **330**: 1329–1334.
36. Siafakas NM, Vermeire P, Pride NB et al. Optimal assessment and management of chronic obstructive pulmonary disease (COPD). *Eur Respir J* 1995; **8**: 1398–1420.
37. American Thoracic Society. Standards for the diagnosis and care of patients with chronic obstructive pulmonary disease (COPD) and asthma. *Am Rev Respir Dis* 1987; **136**: 225–244.
38. Müller NL, Staples CA, Miller RR, Abboud RT. "Density mask": an objective method to quantitate emphysema using computed tomography. *Chest* 1988; **94**: 782–787.
39. Baldi S, Miniati M, Bellina CR et al. Relationship between extent of pulmonary emphysema by high-resolution computed tomography and lung elastic recoil in patients with chronic obstructive pulmonary disease. *Am J Respir Crit Care Med* 2001; **164**: 585–589.
40. Boushy SF, Abounrad MH, North LB, Helgason AH. Lung recoil pressure, airways resistance, and forced expiratory flows related to morphological emphysema. *Am Rev Respir Dis* 1971; **104**: 551–561.
41. Burrows B, Earle RH. Course and prognosis of chronic obstructive lung disease. *New Eng J Med* 1969; **280**: 397–404.
42. Swanney MP, Jensen RL, Crichton DA et al. FEV_6 is an agreeable surrogate for FVC in the spirometric diagnosis of airway obstruction and restriction. *Am J Respir Crit Care Med* 2000; **162**: 917–919.
43. National Institutes of Health, National Heart, Lung and Blood Institute. Global strategy for the diagnosis, management, and prevention of chronic obstructive pulmonary disease. NHLBI/WHO Workshop Report. Update 2004. www.goldcopd.com
44. Sobol BJ, Weinheimer A. Assessment of ventilatory abnormality in the asymptomatic subject: an exercise in futility. *Thorax* 1966: **21**: 445–449.
45. Miller MR, Pincock AC. Predicted values: how should we use them? *Thorax* 1988; **43**: 265–267.
46. Hardie JA, Buist AS, Vollmer WM et al. Risk of over-diagnosis of COPD in asymptomatic elderly never smokers. *Eur Respir J* 2002; **20**: 1117–1122.
47. Kerstjens HAM. The GOLD classification has not advanced understanding of COPD. *Am J Resp Crit Care Med* 2004; **170**: 212–213.
48. Gorecka D, Gorzelak K, Sliwinski P et al. Effect of long term oxygen therapy on survival in patients with chronic obstructive pulmonary disease with moderate hypoxaemia. *Thorax* 1997; **52**: 667–668.
49. Tiddens HAWM, Bogaard JM, de Jongste JC et al. Physiological and morphological determinants of maximal expiratory flow in chronic obstructive lung disease. *Eur Respir J* 1996; **9**: 1785–1794.
50. Fletcher C, Peto R. The natural history of chronic airflow limitation. *BMJ* 1977; **i**: 1645–1648.
51. Dirksen A, Holstein-Rathlou N-H, Madsen F et al. Long-range correlations of serial FEV_1 measurements in emphysematous patients and normal subjects. *J Appl Physiol* 1998; **85**: 259–265.
52. Stanescu D, Sanna A, Veriter C, Robert A. Identification of smokers susceptible to development of chronic airflow limitation: a 13-year follow-up. *Chest* 1998; **114**: 416–425.
53. Redelmeier DA, Goldstein RS, Min ST, Hyland RT. Spirometry and dyspnoea in patients with COPD. When small differences mean little. *Chest* 1996; **109**: 1163–1168.
54. Calverley PM, Burge PS, Spencer S et al. Bronchodilator reversibility testing in chronic obstructive pulmonary disease. *Thorax* 2003; **58**: 659–664.
55. Dubois P, Machiels J, Smeets F et al. CO transfer capacity as a determining factor of survival for severe hypoxaemic COPD patients under long-term oxygen therapy. *Eur Respir J* 1990; **3**: 1042–1047.
56. Wagner PD, Dantzker DR, Dueck R et al. Ventilation-perfusion inequality in chronic obstructive pulmonary disease. *J Clin Invest* 1977; **59**: 203–216.
57. Barberà JA, Ramirez J, Roca J et al. Lung structure and gas exchange in mild chronic obstructive pulmonary disease. *Am Rev Respir Dis* 1990; **141**: 895–901.
58. Barberà JA, Roca J, Ramirez J et al. Gas exchange during exercise in mild chronic obstructive pulmonary disease. Correlation with lung structure. *Am Rev Respir Dis* 1991; **144**: 520–525.
59. Shoup R, Dalsky G, Warner S et al. Body composition and health-related quality of life in patients with obstructive airways disease. *Eur Respir J* 1997; **10**: 1576–1580.
60. Sahebjami H, Sathianpitayakul E. Influence of body weight on the severity of dyspnea in chronic obstructive pulmonary disease. *Am J Respir Crit Care Med* 2000; **161**: 886–890.
61. Bernard S, LeBlanc P, Whittom F et al. Peripheral muscle weakness in patients with chronic obstructive pulmonary disease. *Am J Respir Crit Care Med* 1998; **158**: 629–634.
62. Mador MJ, Kufel TJ, Pineda LA, Sharma GK. Diaphragmatic fatigue and high-intenstiy exercise in patients with chronic obstructive pulmonary disease. *Am J Respir Crit Care Med* 2000; **161**: 118–123.
63. Montes de Oca M and Celli BR. Respiratory muscle and cardiopulmonary function during exercise in very severe COPD. *Am J Respir Crit Care Med* 1996; **154**: 1284–1289.
64. Light RW, Mintz HM, Linden GS, Brown SE. Hemodynamics of patients with severe chronic obstructive pulmonary disease during progressive upright exercise. *Am Rev Respir Dis* 1984; **130**: 391–395.
65. Montes de Oca M and Celli BR. Respiratory muscle recruitment and exercise performance in eucapnic and hypercapnic severe chronic obstructive pulmonary disease. *Am J Respir Crit Care Med* 2000; **161**: 880–885.
66. Babb TG, Rodarte JR. Lung volumes during low-intensity steady-state cycling. *J Appl Physiol* 1991; **70**: 934–937.
67. Johnson BD, Reddan WG, Pegelow DF et al. Flow limitation and regulation of functional residual capacity during exercise in physically active ageing population. *Am Rev Respir Dis* 1991; **142**: 960–967.
68. Morris MJ, Madgwick RG, Lane DJ. Difference between functional residual capacity and elastic equilibrium volume in patients with chronic obstructive pulmonary disease. *Thorax* 1996; **51**: 415–419.
69. O'Donnell DE, Revill SM, Webb KA. Dynamic hyperinflation and exercise intolerance in chronic obstructive pulmonary disease. *Am J Respir Crit Care Med* 2001; **164**: 770–777.
70. Marin JM, Carrizo SJ, Gascon M et al. Inspiratory capacity, dynamic hyperinflation, breathlessness, and exercise performance during the 6-minute-walk test in chronic obstructive disease. *Am J Respir Crit Care Med* 2001; **163**: 1395–1399.
71. Koulouris NG, Valta P, Lavoie A et al. A simple method to detect expiratory flow limitation during spontaneous breathing. *Eur Respir J* 1995; **8**: 306–313.

72. Koulouris NG, Dimopoulou I, Valta P et al. Detection of expiratory flow limitation during exercise in COPD. *J Appl Physiol* 1997; **82**: 723–731.

73. Ninane V, Leduc D, Kafi SA et al. Detection of expiratory flow limitation by manual compression of the abdominal wall. *Am J Respir Crit Care Med* 2001; **163**: 1326–1330.

74. Montes de Oca M, Celli BR. Mouth occlusion pressure, CO_2 response and hypercapnia in severe chronic obstructive pulmonary disease. *Eur Respir J* 1998; **12**: 666–671.

75. Scano G, Spinelli A, Duranti R et al. Carbon dioxide responsiveness in COPD patients with and without chronic hypercapnia. *Eur Respir J* 1995; **8**: 78–85.

76. Sassoon CS, Hassell KT, Mahutte CK. Hyperoxic-induced hypercapnia in stable chronic obstructive pulmonary disease. *Am Rev Respir Dis* 1987; **135**: 907–911.

77. Gibson GJ, Pride NB. Pulmonary mechanics in fibrosing alveolitis. *Am Rev Respir Dis* 1977; **116**: 637–647.

78. Murphy DM, Hall DR, Petersen MR, Lapp NL. The effect of diffuse pulmonary fibrosis on lung mechanics. *Bull Physiopathol Respir* 1981; **17**: 27–41.

79. Tan CSH, Tashkin DP. Supernormal maximal mid-expiratory flow rates in diffuse interstitial lung disease. *Respiration* 1981; **42**: 200–208.

80. Desai SR, Wells AU, Rubens MB et al. Traction bronchiectasis in cryptogenic fibrosing alveolitis: associated computed tomographic features and physiological significance.*Eur Radiol* 2003; **13**: 1801–1808.

81. Erbes R, Schaberg T, Loddenkemper R. Lung function tests in patients with idiopathic pulmonary fibrosis. Are they helpful for predicting outcome? *Chest* 1997; **111**: 51–57.

82. Jezek V, Fucik J, Michaljanic A, Jezkova L. The prognostic significance of functional tests in cryptogenic fibrosing alveolitis. *Bull Eur Physiopathol Respir* 1980; **16**: 711–720.

83. Schwartz MI, Whitcomb ME, French JB. Significance of an isolated reduction in residual volume. *Am Rev Respir Dis* 1971; **103**: 430–432.

84. Yernault JC, de Jonghe M, de Coster A, Englert M. Pulmonary mechanics in diffuse fibrosing alveolitis. *Bull Physiopathol Respir* 1975; **11**: 213–244.

85. Agusti C, Xaubet A, Roca J et al. Interstitial pulmonary fibrosis with and without associated collagen vascular disease: results of a two year follow up. *Thorax* 1992; **47**: 1035–1040.

86. Thompson MJ, Colebatch HJ. Decreased pulmonary distensibility in fibrosing alveolitis and its relation to decreased lung volume. *Thorax*. 1989; **44**: 725–731.

87. Tenholder MF, Russell MD, Knight E, Rajagopal KR. Orthodeoxia: a new finding in interstitial fibrosis. *Am Rev Respir Dis* 1987; **136**: 170–173.

88. Agusti AG, Roca J, Gea J et al. Mechanisms of gas-exchange impairment in idiopathic pulmonary fibrosis. *Am Rev Respir Dis* 1991; **143**: 219–225.

89. Hanson D, Winterbauer RH, Kirtland SH, Wu R. Changes in pulmonary function test results after 1 year of therapy as predictors of survival in patients with idiopathic pulmonary fibrosis. *Chest* 1995; **108**: 305–310.

90. Agusti AG, Roca J, Rodriguez-Roisin R et al. Different patterns of gas exchange response to exercise in asbestosis and idiopathic pulmonary fibrosis. *Eur Respir J* 1988; **1**: 510–516.

91. Spiro SG, Dowdeswell IR, Clark TJ. An analysis of submaximal exercise responses in patients with sarcoidosis and fibrosing alveolitis. *Br J Dis Chest* 1981; **75**: 169–180.

92. Brack T, Jubran A, Tobin MJ. Dyspnea and decreased variability of breathing in patients with restrictive lung disease. *Am J Respir Crit Care Med* 2002; **165**: 1260–1264.

93. Tatsumi K, Kimura H, Kunitomo F et al. Arterial oxygen desaturation during sleep in interstitial pulmonary disease. Correlation with chemical control of breathing during wakefulness. *Chest* 1989; **95**: 962–967.

94. Terriff BA, Kwan SY, Chan-Yeung MM, Muller NL. Fibrosing alveolitis: chest radiography and CT as predictors of clinical and functional impairment at follow-up in 26 patients. *Radiology* 1992; **184**: 445–449.

95. Xaubet A, Agusti C, Luburich P et al. Pulmonary function tests and CT scans in the management of idiopathic pulmonary fibrosis. *Am J Respir Crit Care Med* 1998; **158**: 431–436.

96. Wells AU, King AD, Rubens MB et al. Lone cryptogenic fibrosing alveolitis: a functional-morphological correlation based on extent of disease on thin-section computed tomography. *Am J Respir Crit Care Med* 1997; **155**: 1367–1375.

97. Doherty MJ, Pearson MG, O'Grady EA et al. Cryptogenic fibrosing alveolitis with preserved lung volumes. *Thorax* 1997; **52**: 998–1002.

98. Orens JB, Kazerooni EA, Martinez FJ et al. The sensitivity of high-resolution CT in detecting idiopathic pulmonary fibrosis proved by open lung biopsy. A prospective study. *Chest* 1995; **108**: 109–115.

CHAPTER 41

How Individual Diseases Affect Lung Function (Compendium)

41.1 Introduction

Common respiratory disorders (asthma, COPD, emphysema and fibrosis) are discussed in Chapter 40. In this compendium other clinical conditions that affect the lungs are reviewed briefly. The conditions are classified using a systems approach, but the space allocation does not reflect the prevalence of the topics or their clinical or respiratory importance. Attention is focused on the recent literature to give the reader a contemporary entry into the subjects. For other information a clinical text should be consulted.

41.2 Extrapulmonary airways

The airways are the essential conduit for the movement of gas by bulk flow from the environment to the alveoli for gas exchange. Problems can arise at any point causing airflow limitation. The airways can be classified as to being extrathoracic or intrathoracic, where the latter are exposed to intrapleural pressure changes during breathing. The intrathoracic airways can be extrapulmonary or intrapulmonary. The latter are invested within the lung where they are influenced by lung elastic recoil.

The extrapulmonary airways include the mouth, pharynx, larynx, trachea and initial parts of the major bronchi. If there is severe obstruction to the extrapulmonary airways above the main carina then type 2 respiratory failure can ensue with hypoxia and hypercapnia; peak expiratory flow (PEF) is usually more affected than forced expiratory volume in 1 s (FEV_1) (Section 38.5.2). Diseases affecting the extrapulmonary airways are considered in their anatomical sequence.

Oedema in the oropharynx. Oedema can have many causes, including infection, trauma, burns, insect stings, C1 esterase inhibitor deficiency and allergy. The oedema can cause airway occlusion and the subject can present with type 2 respiratory failure. Thus, monitoring of minute ventilation, and arterial gases is needed. Intermittent airway obstruction in the oropharynx can lead to sleep apnoea syndrome (Section 33.3). Tumours of the larynx can also cause obstruction with stridor and characteristic flow–volume loop abnormalities [1].

The upper trachea. The first part of the trachea, like the larynx and oropharynx, is extrathoracic and so on inspiration tends to collapse because the intraluminal pressure is negative with respect to atmospheric pressure. Narrowing of the trachea is commonly due to goitre [2] and can be asymptomatic. Stridor is usually only found in extreme obstruction. With lesser obstruction the energy cost to breathing is increased due to increased resistance. PEF is reduced relative to FEV_1 [3] such that their ratio (FEV_1 in ml divided by PEF in $l\ min^{-1}$) is greater than 10. The extramural pressure of a goitre can cause thinning of the cartilaginous structure in the trachea, so if the goitre is removed it can leave an unsupported floppy segment of trachea. This effect may also be seen in relapsing polychondritis. Thus, on inspiration the extrathoracic tracheal wall can collapse giving inspiratory airflow limitation and stridor.

The lower trachea. This structure is intrathoracic so is subject to pleural pressure. As a result the airway expands on inspiration and tends to collapse on expiration, the exact opposite of the extrathoracic portion. The site of any obstruction (upper or lower trachea or both) can be indicated by the flow–volume loop (Fig. 41.1). One cause of lower obstruction is a goitre behind the sternum (retrosternal goitre).

Tumours of the trachea are a rare mural cause of airway obstruction (either intra- or extrathoracic). Another rare cause in old people is tracheobronchopathia osteochondrodysplastica; this is associated with cartilageneous projections into the lumen of the large cartilaginous bronchi. Flow–volume loops can show evidence of upper airway obstruction in this condition [4].

Pathological enlargement of the trachea in tracheobronchomegaly is associated with bronchiectasis. Thus, the

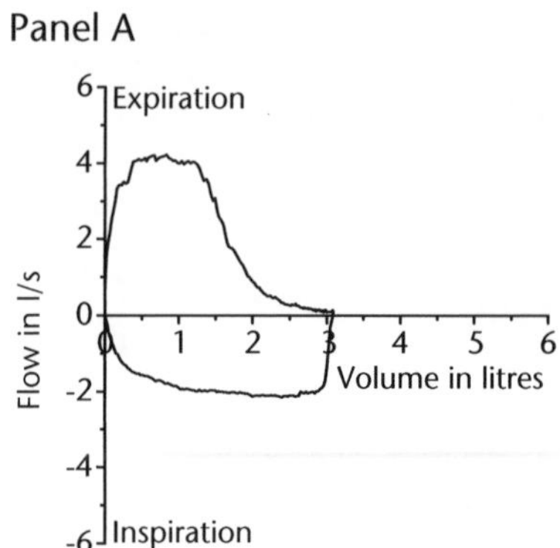

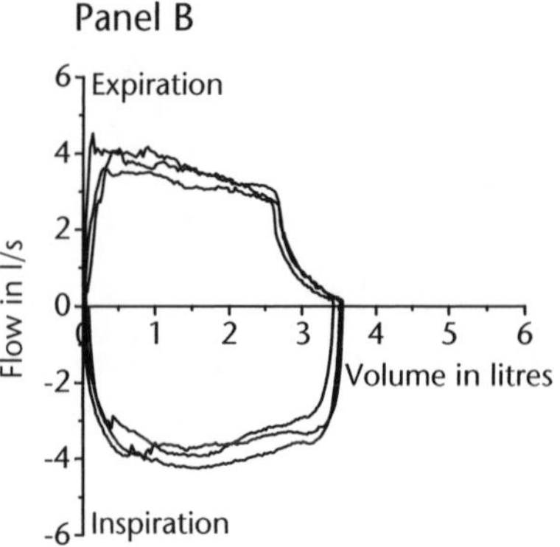

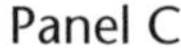

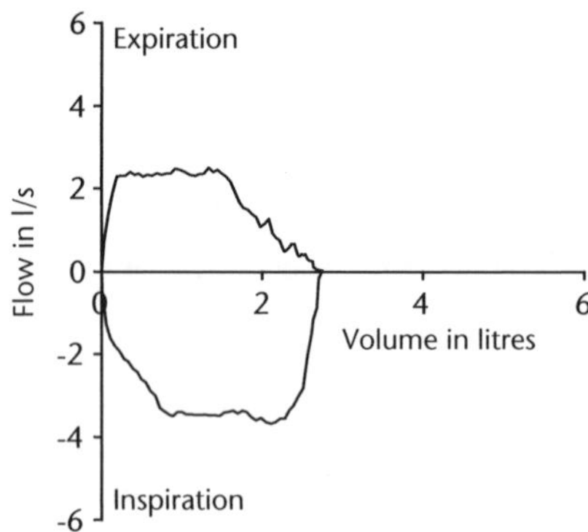

Fig. 41.1 Panel A shows flow–volume loop of subject with an extrathoracic upper airway obstruction due to goitre. The inspiratory limb is flow limited at around 2 l s^{-1} which is much less than the expiratory limitation at around 4 l s^{-1}. This suggests the limiting segment is collapsing on inspiration and so is variable extrathoracic. Panel B shows repeatable limitation with both expiratory and inspiratory limbs limited at around 4 l s^{-1} suggesting fixed upper airway obstruction. Panel C shows flow limited to about 2 l s^{-1} in the expiratory limb but is better at around 4 l s^{-1} on the inspiratory limb suggesting variable upper airway obstruction with flow limitation in the intrapulmonary position. Source: [5] on page 141.

intrapulmonary airflow limitation from the bronchiectasis masks any tendency for a higher PEF due to the larger upper airway. A larger trachea in acromegaly may lead to a larger PEF.

41.3 Intrapulmonary airways

Overview. Intrapulmonary airways are subjected to both pressure swings within the thorax and elastic forces within the lung that maintain their patency in expiration. Generalised airway narrowing is commonly due to structural changes as with COPD, increased tone in the muscle of the airway as in asthma and loss of lung elasticity in emphysema (Sections 40.2 and 40.3). Other conditions (either general or local) cause airflow limitation. Isolated or non-homogeneous conditions tend to cause type 1 respiratory failure but when generalised and severe can lead to type 2 respiratory failure.

41.3.1 Bronchiectasis

Characteristically in this condition the small and medium sized airways are dilated, inflamed and have excessive mucus. The changes can be visualised by HRCT. They are associated with airflow limitation; the reduction in FEV_1 is related to the extent of the structural abnormality rather than the quantity of mucus. [5]. The bronchiectatic segments can exhibit features of emphysema; this is probably due to proteolytic enzymes released by the inflammatory process. In one study, subjects with emphysema had significantly more severe airflow limitation and lower transfer factor than patients without CT evidence of emphysema [6]. In another study the presence of airflow limitation at rest, identified using the negative expiratory pressure technique, was associated with more severe dyspnoea and exercise limitation [7].

A number of studies have suggested that there is increased bronchial hyperresponsiveness (BHR) to histamine and methacholine, but no excess atopy or asthma [8]. In this study, unlike in others [9, 10], the responsiveness was not related to baseline FEV_1.

41.3.2 Cystic fibrosis

Cystic fibrosis (CF) is an autosomal recessively inherited defect of epithelial secretory cells throughout the body. The principal organs affected are the lungs, gastrointestinal tract and skin sweat glands. In the lungs there is an increase in the viscosity of bronchial secretions; this impairs the function of cilia and leads to recurrent bronchial infection. The condition affects about 1 in 3000 live births in Europe and North America. The commonest gene mutation (>70% cases) is on delta F508 of the CF gene protein product, called CF transmembrane regulator.

CF usually causes childhood bronchiectasis with concomitant airflow obstruction. The FEV_1 and FEV_1% are reduced and residual volume (RV) increased. The airflow limitation is usually poorly reversible. However, management of the condition has improved and some 35% of patients now survive into adulthood. As a result, reference equations for lung function that is continuous through adolescence to adulthood should be used (Section 26.7.2). The condition is progressive, consequently FEV_1 declines more rapidly than does the forced vital capacity (FVC) [11]. The decline has been found to be moderated by male gender, pancreatic sufficiency and some non-delta F508 gene mutations [12]. In growing children the disease process leads to the lung function increasing at a slow rate relative to the increase in stature; the shortfall can be demonstrated on charts showing percentiles (Section 26.3.5). In adults FEV_1 can decline whilst body mass and peak oxygen uptake on exercise are unchanged [13]. A low FEV_1 is associated with a high radiological score for disease severity [14, 15].

The forced oscillation technique has been used in children with CF to test for increased total respiratory resistance (Rrs) and the results compared with those found in asthmatics [16]. There was concordance between a low FEV_1 and high Rrs at 10 Hz in asthma, but in CF a low FEV_1 was usually associated with normal Rrs suggesting the technique at 10 Hz did not reflect changes due to the effects of more peripheral airways obstruction in CF. Between 24% [17] and 58% [18] of patients with CF have been found to have BHR; this reflects the severity of the CF and not the presence of co-existing asthma.

Assessing young children using tests that rely on voluntary effort can be unreliable and so there has been recent interest in using multi-breath inert gas washout as a measure of ventilation inhomogeneity [19, 20] (see Section 16.2.7). These studies found that, compared with FEV_1, the method was more sensitive in detecting abnormality and functional progression with time.

Gas transfer becomes impaired in CF and this relates to measures of disease severity [21] including airflow limitation [22]. Subjects with a low FEV_1 and low gas transfer are those likely to desaturate on exercise [23]. Tests of positional changes in gas transfer in CF showed little change compared to normal subjects when breathing air, but did so when breathing 100% oxygen [24]. This indicated that local hypoxic vasoconstriction responded to breathing oxygen and was not due to fixed vascular damage.

The disease progresses at a variable rate with some subjects surviving to middle age and beyond. By that time they are usually in severe respiratory failure and potential candidates for lung transplantation (Section 43.3.1).

41.3.3 Bronchiolitis obliterans and organising pneumonias

These conditions are characterised by variable degrees of scarring, narrowing and obliteration of small (<1 mm) airways, also organising exudate within bronchioles, alveolar ducts and alveoli. The spectrum of disease includes obliterative bronchiolitis with or without an organising pneumonia (BOOP or OB), and chronic (cryptogenic) organising pneumonia (COP) where obliteration of airways is not obvious. OB is the usual finding in lung transplant rejection [25] but is also seen in bone marrow transplantation, rheumatoid arthritis and after inhalation of fumes or toxic gases. The condition can follow viral and other infections [26]. Airflow limitation is present, with both FEV_1 and $FEF_{25-75\%}$ being reduced. HRCT shows mosaic areas of air trapping on expiratory scans, but not on inspiratory scans consistent with small airway obstruction. This pattern has been observed with OB (including that associated wth transplant rejection), bronchiectasis and asthma [27].

The reported proportion of patients with COP or BOOP who exhibit a restrictive defect with low gas transfer and hypoxaemia (type 1 failure) varies widely between studies. In some almost all are affected [28, 29] whereas in others the proportion is less (e.g. 9 patients out of 15 [30]), or only the severe cases [31]. The diversity reflects the extent of alveolar involvement versus bronchial obliteration.

Summary: VC↓ FVC↓ Tlco↓ Pa,O_2 ↓
RV↑ if obliterative bronchiolitis is dominant.

41.4 The alveoli

Conditions that affect the alveolar membrane influence the gas-exchanging properties of the lungs. They may also alter the volume of lung tissue or the distribution of fluid within the lung parenchyma and this can affect the dynamic and static lung volumes. Often both aspects are affected (e.g. in pneumonia the process of consolidation reduces the air-containing volume and the surface for gas exchange; see Sections 41.9.1 and 41.9.2). With emphysema the enlargement of airspaces is a consequence of destruction of alveolar walls (see 'Chronic obstructive pulmonary disease and emphysema', Section 40.3). Alveolitis due to allergic or inhalational injury may reduce the compliance of the alveoli and affect $\dot{V}A/\dot{Q}$ relationships in the lung parenchyma. The primary change in lung function can then be hypoxaemia due to reduced gas transfer with little change in static or dynamic volumes. If fibrosis supervenes the overall elastic recoil of the lungs is increased leading to increased patency of airways and reductions in all compartments of total lung capacity (TLC) (see 'Diffuse lung fibrosis', Section 40. 4).

41.4.1 α_1-antitrypsin deficiency

α_1-antitrypsin is an enzyme that enters the circulation from the liver and has the role of protecting the lung tissue from proteolytic enzymes. Deficiency of the enzyme is associated with emphysema (see introduction to Section 40.3). The deficiency is autosomal recessively inherited. Coding for α_1-antitrypsin is on chromosome c14q with the deficient gene (Z allele) present in 3% of the population of northern Europe. The terminology for the condition uses PiZ phenotype to refer to ZZ or ZNull genotypes, PiM for MM or MNull, and so on. PiZ phenotype is associated with the most severe enzyme deficiency and with lung disease. PiM and PiS phenotypes do not seem to be associated with lung disease nor do PiMZ, PiSZ or PiMS.

A person deficient in α_1-antitrypsin (α_1AT) cannot fully protect their lungs from proteolytic enzymes. These come from two sources: first, pancreatic trypsin from the gut that enters the lung in the mixed venous blood and is distributed mainly to the lung bases, second, elastases and proteases from leucocytes that are attracted to the lungs by noxious stimuli, especially tobacco smoke. The first route gives rise to emphysema that is panlobular and basal, the second to COPD and to emphysema that is centriacinar and mainly affects the cranial half of the lungs (see 'Pathology' at the start of Section 40.3). The initial descriptions were of basal, panlobular emphysema, material airflow limitation and large lungs with air trapping (TLC and RV increased) [32]. The transfer factor might be normal [33].

The recent use of HRCT has shown that the distribution of the emphysema associated with deficiency of α_1AT is often predominantly in the upper lobes [34]. In such patients a reduction in transfer factor can be the main physiological feature [35]. The suggested explanation for the difference is that basal disease may allow better $\dot{V}_A/\dot{Q}$ matching, with the option of diversion of blood to the apices where the vessels provide additional surface for gas exchange. This option may not be available when the disease is mainly apical since the basal vessels are likely to be already full as a result of the operation of gravity.

41.4.2 Interstitial lung disease

See Section 40.4

41.5 Pulmonary vascular disease

Since the purpose of the lungs is to effect exchange of O_2 and CO_2 between air and blood it is evident that diseases affecting the pulmonary arterial and venous circulation, including pulmonary embolism, can profoundly affect lung function. There is an arterial supply to the bronchi from the aorta. This can be the source of bronchial arterial bleeding and even massive haemoptysis. Inflammation of the pulmonary circulation occurs in a variety of diseases (e.g. Wegener's granulomatosis, Section 41.16). Connective tissue diseases can also affect the pulmonary vasculature (Section 41.19, see also Further reading).

41.5.1 Pulmonary Embolism

Venous thromboemboli to the lungs are usually an acute and sudden phenomenon, but can be chronic and insidious. Acute occlusion of the pulmonary arteries with emboli of thrombus from the deep veins leads to wasted ventilation to the areas affected. On its own this is of little consequence. However, the redistribution of the remaining perfusion to vessels that are still patent causes local over-perfusion and $\dot{V}_A/\dot{Q}$ inequality; this leads on to hypoxia and hypocapnia [36]. Estimates of alveolar deadspace as a percentage of tidal volume have been found to correlate well with the extent of the perfusion deficit also expressed as a percentage. In one study the two quantities were on average 43% and 38%, respectively (R^2 0.59) [37].

Pleuritic pain from pulmonary embolism (PE) plus stimulation of slowly adapting stretch receptors can result in rapid shallow breathing, yet such is the drive to respiration that the level of alveolar ventilation can be increased. CO_2 is then more than adequately washed out from lung areas that retain perfusion and can cause respiratory alkalosis (Section 22.3.3). If the embolisation is massive the pulmonary circulation can be effectively blocked leading to systemic hypotension and a poor peripheral circulation. The mixed venous oxygen tension is then very low and this also contributes to the arterial hypoxaemia. The low cardiac output contributes to the $\dot{V}_A/\dot{Q}$ inequality [38] and to the alveolar–arterial oxygen tension difference (A-aD_{O_2}) which is increased in proportion to the severity of the condition [39]. However, an increased A-aD_{O_2} is also found in other conditions, whilst up to 10% of patients with PE have a normal A-aD_{O_2} [40], so the measurement contributes little to diagnosis.

Multiple very small emboli can recur over a prolonged period of time. Each embolus often has little immediate effect but cumulatively they produce pulmonary hypertension. A study of patients with thromboembolic hypertension found a normal vital capacity (VC), hypoxia in the most severely affected patients and changes in gas transfer, but these features did not correlate with the severity of the pulmonary hypertension [41] or with the prognosis [42].

Summary
Acute: $P_{a,O_2}\downarrow$ $P_{a,CO_2}\downarrow$ $T_{lco}\downarrow$ $K_{co}\downarrow$ normal spirometry if not inhibited by pain.
Chronic: $P_{a,O_2}\downarrow$ $T_{lco}\downarrow$ $K_{co}\downarrow$ pulmonary hypertension

41.5.2 Fat embolism

Fracture of long bones or the pelvis can lead to embolisation of fat from marrow into the pulmonary arteries via the venous circulation. The condition is characterised by tiny haemorrhages into the skin (petechiae), fat droplets in the urine and hypoxaemia. An increased number of macrophages in fluid from a broncho-alveolar lavage can be diagnostic (e.g. sensitivity 85% and specificity 82% in one study [43]. A prospective study of single fractures found fat embolisation in 11% of patients [44], rising to 35% with multiple fractures [45]. The emboli can show up as a diffuse subsegmental mottled appearance on isotope lung perfusion scans [46]. The associated hypoxaemia and hyperventilation can result in an A-aD_{O_2} in excess of 100 mm Hg (13 kPa).

41.5.3 Primary pulmonary hypertension

This is a very rare condition of unknown aetiology that most commonly affects women up to middle age [47]. Pulmonary vascular resistance is high and patients become hypoxic, particularly on exercise. This has been shown to be due to poor perfusion of adequately ventilated lung [48]. Prostacyclin infusion can improve survival, and recently inhaled prostacyclin has been shown to improve exercise tolerance but not resting hypoxaemia [49]. The 6-min-walk test has been found to be a good non-invasive predictor of survival with a distance of less than 332 m being linked to a much lower survival [50]. A study of conventional lung function tests in this condition found that in half of the 79 patients there was a reduction in lung volumes and in three quarters there was reduction in gas transfer [51]. As expected the changes in gas transfer best correlated with dyspnoea and objective measurement of exercise performance. In a larger study that focussed on the ventilatory effects of PPH in 171 patients there was no change in TLC, but a raised RV and RV/TLC and reduced VC suggesting narrowing of small lung airways (Section 38.3.1); its severity mirrored that of the hypertension [52].

41.5.4 Pulmonary veno-occlusive disease

In this rare condition some pulmonary veins and venules are obstructed by fibrosis of their intima but without plexiform lesions. The patients develop pulmonary hypertension, pleural effusions and interstitial changes in the lung parenchyma; these are seen as septal lines on the chest radiograph. The pulmonary wedge pressure is normal [53], as are the results of spirometry and of ventilation scans. The static lung volumes are often reduced [54]. There is a progressively developing transfer defect with hypoxaemia and a reduced transfer factor [55]. Lung perfusion scanning is usually normal [56] but there may be evidence for pulmonary embolism [57].

41.5.5 Arterio-venous malformations

The condition may be congenital in origin or develop during the course of hepatic disease (Section 41.20). Patients with pulmonary arterio-venous malformations (AVM) show hypoxaemia due to an increased shunt fraction [58]. The hypoxaemia is not corrected by breathing 100% oxygen. The patients tend to hyperventilate (e.g. portal cirrhosis, Table 29.11, page 429) and have an abnormally high physiological deadspace. The transfer factor is usually reduced. In the study reported here embolisation of the pulmonary circulation improved oxygenation by reducing the shunt fraction but the transfer factor and deadspace were unchanged.

Some patients with pulmonary AVM due to hereditary haemorrhagic telangiectasia develop pulmonary hypertension that is indistinguishable from the primary form [59, 60]; the condition has a hereditary component [61].

41.5.6 Foreign body vasculitis (intravenous drug abusers)

Intravenous drug abusers may attempt to dissolve drugs formulated for oral use that contain talc or cellulose. This particulate matter leads to embolisation in the lungs and the development of foreign body granulomas [62, 63]. A study of 23 narcotic addicts, most of whom had no respiratory symptoms, found a low gas transfer in 42%. All of them had abnormal lung perfusion scans and nearly half were hypoxic at rest [64]. The remaining 58% had normal lung function and chest radiographs. A larger prospective study of IV drug abusers found low gas transfer (<75% of predicted value) in 42% of subjects. In most this was the only abnormality of function, with no evidence of increased deadspace or shunting [65].

41.6 The pleura

Pleural diseases limit the extent to which the lungs can expand. This can be due to pain from pleurisy, the presence of fluid in the pleural space, reduced coupling of chest wall to the lungs by pneumothorax, or compliance of the chest wall being reduced secondary to pleural thickening or mesothelioma. The shallow breathing increases the volume of air used per minute to ventilate the physiological deadspace, so the ventilation minute volume is increased. The shallow breathing is partly structural but may be partly dynamic, particularly with pleural adhesions (but not discrete pleural plaques). The tachypnoea increases the ventilation minute volume and can cause profound breathlessness on exertion (example given in Table 29.11, page 429). Pleural disease due to asbestos is discussed in Section 37.7.2.

With diseases of the pleura the FVC and TLC are reduced (as they are in other restrictive diseases), and the function of the inspiratory muscles is impaired [66]. If the condition is mainly unilateral the perfusion of the affected lung may be reduced; this response mitigates the hypoxaemia (Section 17.2.2). However, if the lung is materially underventilated the condition can progress to type 2 respiratory failure (Section 38.5.2). A study of the effect of pleural fluid removal has shown that with per litre of fluid removed TLC increased by 0.58 l, FVC increased by 0.33 l and gas transfer increased by 20% [67].

A pneumothorax is due to a tear or penetration injury of the lung and usually presents with pain and/or dyspnoea. However, if the tear acts as a one-way valve (ball valve) the pressure within the pneumothorax can be raised by coughing. In this circumstance the mediastinum can be displaced and the cardiac output reduced leading to shock and death unless the tension is relieved.

Summary

Mild:	TLC↓ RV↓ FEV_1 ↓ FVC↓ Tl/V_A ↑ $\dot{V}_{E,ex}$↑
Severe:	TLC↓ RV↓ FEV_1 ↓ Pa,O_2 ↓ Pa,CO_2 ↑ $\dot{V}_{E,ex}$↑
Monitor:	FVC or VC, arterial gases.

41.7 The chest wall

The integrity of the chest wall is essential for the respiratory pump to be effective. The action is mainly due to the descent of the diaphragm reducing the pressure in the thorax with respect to atmospheric pressure so air is forced into the lungs causing them to expand (Section 9.7). The three components of the pump are the muscles, the physical properties of the thorax and the airways.

41.7.1 Flail segment, sucking pneumothorax

A penetrating wound of the chest wall can cause a sucking pneumothorax whilst blunt trauma can cause a segment of chest wall to be sucked inwards on inspiration (flail chest). Both these problems can lead to hypoventilation and, if the wound is not closed, to type 2 respiratory failure. The conditions are medical emergencies, so lung function tests (such as evidence for reduced maximal pressures) are rarely undertaken. Arterial gas monitoring is essential since the presence of respiratory failure indicates a need for artificial ventilation. Surgical stabilisation is then undertaken using reconstruction plates. The outcome is usually satisfactory. However, in one study a ventilatory defect was still apparent 6 months after the operation [68].

41.7.2 Pectus excavatum and pectus carinatum

A depressed sternum (pectus excavatum) is due to imperfect development of the chest wall. It is largely a cosmetic problem but pulmonary and cardiac function can be impaired. Often there is a mild restrictive ventilatory defect that is not much improved (or is made worse) following surgical correction [69], However, the operation is likely to improve the capacity for exercise [70]. Approximately half the patients have normal spirometry. Many of the others have an increased residual volume (RV and RV/TLC) that tends to return to normal as the child grows up [71].

Pectus carinatum, in which the sternum is unduly prominent, usually develops following prolonged respiratory problems in childhood. The changes in lung function include a raised TLC and are due to the underlying lung condition.

41.7.3 Kyphoscoliosis

Spinal deformity such as scoliosis can have a serious effect on the configuration of the lungs within the chest and reduces the effectiveness of the respiratory muscles [72]. The static lung volumes are then reduced and often there is airflow limitation [73]. Ventilation is more severely effected on the side with the greatest spinal convexity but there is less effect on perfusion. The resulting $\dot{V}_A/\dot{Q}$ imbalance leads to hypoxia and increased A-aD_{O_2} [74]. Surgical correction of scoliosis has been shown to lead to a further reduction in FVC [75, 76]. In the long term the mechanical disadvantage of the kyphoscoliosis leads eventually to respiratory failure. The optimal treatment is likely to include nocturnal nasal intermittent positive pressure ventilation and long-term oxygen therapy (LTOT), [77]. See also Section 41.7.6.

41.7.4 Sternotomy/thoracotomy

Surgical exploration of the chest for any reason leads to a scar on the chest wall that alters chest wall compliance (Section 43.4.1). The lung function is seldom affected. However, failure of a median sternotomy to heal can lead to painful rocking of the sternum and a reduced ventilatory capacity.

41.7.5 Thoracoplasty

Thoracoplasty was a surgical procedure that immobilised the lung of a patient with pulmonary tuberculosis by removing upper thoracic ribs. Other procedures that had the same objective were artificial pneumoperitoneum, artificial pneumothorax, phrenic nerve crush and inserting space-occupying material (plombage). The logic was to prevent ventilation of cavitating tuberculous lesions and so stop the spread of the disease to other parts of the lungs and to other people. The treatment was usually effective and as a result there are still patients alive who had unilateral or bilateral thoracoplasty. The procedure brought about the collapse of regions of the lungs and also altered how the respiratory muscles operated. It reduced the lung volumes and could progress to airflow limitation [78, 79], see Section 41.9.4.

41.7.6 Ankylosing spondylitis

Patients with ankylosing spondylitis usually have a mild restrictive ventilatory defect with otherwise normal airway function [80]. In this they differ from patients with kyphoscoliosis in whom the restriction to lung expansion is usually greater and the respiratory elastance and resistance are increased [81].

Ankylosing spondylitis can be complicated by upper zone fibrosis that enhances the restrictive defect. In one study of 30 patients the averages for lung function indices with respect to predicted value were VC and FEV_1 approximately 80%, transfer factor 88% and K_{CO} 114% [82]. In another study P_{Emax} and P_{Imax} were, respectively, 56% and 76% of predicted values; the changes were correlated with but proportionally greater than those in the lung volumes. This suggested that there might be some intercostal muscle atrophy [83]. P_{Imax} has been found to be the principal predictor of exercise capacity [84]. Optoelectronic plethysmography has been used to show that activity of the muscles is co-ordinated to optimise the expansion of the thoraco-abdominal compartment [85].

41.7.7 Obesity

Obesity alters the chest wall compliance and reduces the effectiveness of respiratory muscle action. In one study the changes increased the energy cost of breathing by approximately 14% [86]. Additional fat in the abdomen raises the diaphragm and this reduces the functional residual capacity (FRC) and expiratory reserve volume (ERV) (Section 25.5.1, also Table 26.18, page 352). The lung bases are therefore poorly ventilated which contributes to hypoxaemia [87]. Other conventional tests of lung function are usually relatively normal. On exercise there can be dynamic shallow breathing that increases the ventilatory cost of exercise (Section 28.4.7, also illustrative case in Table 29.11, page 429). Obesity in children is increasingly becoming a problem and a reduced FRC and transfer factor have been found [88] (also Table 25.4, page 320), together with an increased persistence of symptomatic wheeze beyond puberty [89]. In adults self reported asthma is more common in the obese, but obese patients were less likely to have objective evidence of airflow limitation [90].

Obese patients often under ventilate their lungs, but the hypoventilation of morbid obesity is not well correlated with mass *per se*, suggesting that other factors are involved as well. Obesity is associated with sleep apnoea or hypopnoea syndrome (Section 33.3).

Summary

Mild:	TLC↓ RV↔ FEV_1 ↓
Severe:	TLC↓ RV↓↑ FEV_1 ↓ Pa,O_2 ↓ Pa,CO_2 ↑
	PEmax↓ PImax↓ $\dot{V}$E,ex↑ Vt_{30} ↓
Monitor:	FVC, VC, FEV_1, annual sleep study.

41.8 Neuro-muscular disease

Failure of the respiratory muscles (particularly failure of the diaphragm) will lead to hypoventilation and type 2 respiratory failure. The problem can arise anywhere in the nerve pathway from the higher centres of the brain to the respiratory muscles (Fig. 23.1, page 286) or in the muscles themselves.

A spinal cord transection at the level of C3 or above interrupts all the pathways, so is not compatible with spontaneous ventilation. Such a lesion is fatal unless artificial ventilation is applied. Lesions below C4 and C5 preserve the roots of the phrenic nerve and hence the function of the diaphragm. A transection at this level allows spontaneous ventilation that is usually sufficient to support gas exchange at rest, but not during exercise (Section 9.5).

41.8.1 Brain stem failure

The regular nerve impulses travelling in the phrenic nerve arise from the brain stem. This signal can be affected by direct damage to the brain stem by trauma, haemorrhage, compression or tumour. Drugs that depress brain function overall, such as barbiturates, lead to reduced output from the respiratory centre and hypoventilation ensues. Opiate drugs have a more specific effect in depressing the respiratory centre leading to bradypnoea and hypopnea. Administration of oxygen can exert a synergistic effect. There are rare brain diseases that seem to affect this aspect of brain function. Multi-system atrophy can reduce the respiratory output of the brain stem particularly during sleep or when the subject is distracted. Ventilatory abnormalities during sleep are also common in other complex neurological disorders affecting the brain stem (e.g. Steel–Richardson–Oslzewski syndrome [91]).

Hypoventilation is the main result, so the tidal volume and frequency of breathing are reduced. There is then hypoventilatory failure with Pa,O_2 reduced and Pa,CO_2 increased.

41.8.2 Disease of the α motor neurone

Epidemics of poliomyelitis were common prior to the widespread use of oral vaccination. They left many patients with chronic type 2 respiratory failure on account of paralysis of the diaphragm [92]. This was secondary to destruction of phrenic α motor neurones in the cervical cord at levels 3 to 5. Motor neurone disease (MND), also known as amyotrophic lateral sclerosis, can affect the same motor neurones and cause terminal respiratory failure. A preceding weakness of the diaphragm can be assessed in several ways (Section 9.9); one is to measure the change in VC on adopting a supine posture [93]. Measurement of arterial gases (or saturation) and sleep studies can help predict if and when ventilatory support might be appropriate [94, 95]. Such tests can also be used to assess prognosis. Measuring sniff nasal inspiratory pressure to assess diaphragm weakness found that a value less than 40 cm of water had a 97% sensitivity in predicting 6-month mortality but only a 79% specificity. FVC less than half of the predicted value had a 58% sensitivity and 96% specificity [96], (Section 9.9). Time taken to achieve PEF and peak cough flow have also been proposed as effective measures for monitoring patients with MND [97, 98].

41.8.3 Phrenic neuropathy, Guillain–Barré syndrome

The phrenic nerve may be affected by neuropathies of which the post-infective ascending polyneuropathy of Guillain–Barré is the most common. This neuropathy ascends from the legs upwards. It therefore affects the intercostal muscles before the phrenic nerve roots and hence the diaphragm, at which point artificial ventilation is required. The need for intervention can be assessed by frequent measurement of arterial gases, but this is seldom a reliable method because progression of the illness can be rapid. Continuous recording of saturation or clinical observation and frequent measurement of VC can also be used. In one study the intervention point was when VC had fallen below the region of 12 to 15 ml kg^{-1} (around 1 l for a 70 kg patient) [99]. In a retrospective analysis of 196 patients with Guillain–Barré syndrome who had their FVC monitored, a value of <60% of predicted had an odds ratio of 2.9 for predicting the need for ventilation [100]. However, an inability to raise the head off the pillow had an odds ratio of 5.0, so clinical assessment should be used as well.

In needle EMG studies of the diaphragm the amplitude of the compound action potentials related to the need for ventilation. An abnormal phrenic nerve conduction time was also found in some but no all of those requiring ventilation [101]. Thus, this sophisticated procedure appears not to have superceded spirometry.

41.8.4 Myasthenia, myopathy, muscular dystrophies, myositis

In myasthenia there is a failure of the neuromuscular junction to deliver sufficient transmitter for normal muscle action. The condition can be confined to the ocular muscles and in this circumstance the lung function is not impaired. By contrast, when the condition is generalised there can be weakness of the respiratory muscles and this reduces the ventilatory capacity (FVC, FEV_1, *P*Imax and *P*Emax all reduced). The *P*Imax showed improvement after neostigmine [102]. However, in another study there was no relationship between the grade of myasthenia or the consequent dyspnoea and any measure of muscle strength [103]. In severe myasthenia hypoventilation and type 2 respiratory failure can ensue.

In myopathies and dystrophies the muscle fibres are defective in producing sufficient force and in myositis this is due to acute inflammation of the muscle fibres. The result is peripheral muscle weakness that can affect the respiratory muscles and so lead to type 2 respiratory failure. Measurement of mouth pressure during phrenic nerve stimulation found 78% of 23 consecutive patients with either dermatomyositis, polymyositis or inclusion body myositis had diaphragm weakness (<10 cm water pressure), with the weakness tending to be more severe in those with dermatomyositis [104]. It has been estimated that in patients with myopathy or polymyositis if *P*Imax and/or *P*Emax are less than 30% of predicted value and VC is less than 55% of predicted value then type 2 failure is likely [105]. Because interstitial lung disease is quite common in these disorders, a restrictive ventilatory defect may be present that is not due to myopathy *per se* [106].

Mitochondrial myopathies can be due to disorders of mitochondrial metabolism leading to reduced ATP generation. This reduces the ability to take exercise. In one study patients with mitochondrial disease were found to have relatively normal static and dynamic volumes and gas transfer. However, *P*Imax and *P*Emax were significantly reduced, as was Pdi_{max}. Patients had a higher heart rate response to exercise and a higher ventilatory response for a given oxygen consumption when compared to controls, although the maximal ventilation achieved was lower and maximum heart rates were equivalent [107]. The cause was not identified but suggested possibilities included altered sensitivity of chemoreceptors in the muscle [108] or changes to mechanoreceptors.

In these disorders monitoring the VC or FVC can indicate when artificial ventilation may be necessary (Section 41.8.3). However, where the dystrophy is likely to be progressive, sleep studies may also be necessary since the hypoventilation is likely to become critical at night. On this account, patients with Duchenne dystrophy have been offered nasal intermittent ventilatory support with benefit to arterial gases [109]. Lung function in terms of VC continued to deteriorate and required treatment with tracheostomy and full artificial ventilation.

41.8.5 Parkinsonism

Parkinson's disease is associated with lesions in the caudate nucleus and putamen where there are fewer nerve cells and a subnormal quantity of dopamine. The presenting features are tremor and poverty of movement that affects all muscle groups. The fingers move as if rolling a pill, there is a tottering gait and speech is liable to lapse in the middle of a sentence. This is due to failure of the control mechanisms independent of impaired lung function [110]. The breathing tends to be shallow and rapid, such that the overall minute volume is increased when compared to control subjects [111]. This could be due to a reduced compliance of the rib cage relative to the abdomen. The changes predispose to pneumonia.

In one study, amongst 58 patients with Parkinson's disease there were important reductions in FVC, FEV_1, Pa,o_2 and increased values for RV and total airways resistance [112]. Some patients had a restrictive pattern that was related to difficulties with turning in bed, walking and falling, whereas others had an obstructive defect that was related to difficulty with hand movements. Polysomnography conducted in 15 patients with Parkinson's disease showed significant sleep disordered breathing when compared to matched controls with nine showing obstructive and one central sleep apnoea syndrome [113]. A few patients treated with bromocriptine or its cogeners can develop pleural disease with effusions, pleural thickening or even parenchymal disease [114]. This possibility should be remembered when interpreting lung function tests from such patients.

41.8.6 Stroke

Loss of motor function after a hemiparesis leads to immobility and risk of pneumonia. Interest has been shown in whether the function of the lungs is affected by a hemiparesis. Studies have shown a restrictive picture with normal lung compliance and resistance [115]. Inspiratory capacity was found to decrease over 6 months and it was suggested this might be due to changes in the thoracic cage resulting from immobility [115, 116]. A recent study looked at diaphragm movement by ultrasound [117] and found that VC was low (average 79% predicted value) and RV high (average 123% predicted value) after stroke with no change in TLC or FRC. Diaphragm movement was normal during spontaneous breathing but was reduced during volitional inspiration. Optoelectronic plethysmography [118] has shown that ventilation on the paretic side was not reduced for tidal breathing but was reduced compared to the other side for voluntary manoeuvres. However, the response to hypercapnia was greater on the paretic side indicating that the various pathways for ventilatory control are not all affected to the same extent.

Summary: VC↓ RV↑ TLC and FRC normal.

41.8.7 Multiple sclerosis

In this condition demyelination of nerve fibres results in neurological symptoms which can relapse and remit, but in most cases the neurological damage is progressive and after a number of years causes disability. In advanced multiple sclerosis respiratory impairment occurs as a result of weakness of the muscles of respiration. Pneumonia is a frequent complication as is aspiration due to bulbar weakness. Reversible neuro-muscular failure can occur earlier in the disease. One study found that the greater the functional disability, the greater the impairment of lung function with reduction in VC to an average of about 80% and *T*lco to about 83% of predicted values. *P*Emax was reduced to an average of 30% and *P*Imax to about 50% of predicted values. Desaturation at night occurred in 70% of the patients tested [119].

41.9 Pulmonary infections

41.9.1 Bronchitis and upper respiratory tract infections

Acute viral upper respiratory tract infections (URTI) have been associated with changes in lung function in some but not all studies. FEV_1, FVC and PEF were unchanged in two studies [120, 121] but there were increases in frequency dependence of both compliance and resistance suggesting changes in peripheral airways. A longitudinal study in children did find convincing evidence for impaired spirometric function during URTI [122]. A prospective study of 15 subjects who developed the condition found no change in spirometry or BHR [123] whereas a cross sectional study reported increased BHR with no increase in resting airways resistance [124]. Another study found a drop in spirometric indices that improved over 5 weeks after the infection [125]. It is usually recommended to avoid lung function tests within 4 weeks of an URTI.

41.9.2 Pneumonia

Consolidation of a lobe or lobule reduces the alveolar volume commensurately. There is reflex reduction in blood supply to the affected lobe but this is often incomplete so hypoxia due to low $\dot{V}_A/\dot{Q}$ is common. Conventional lung function tests are not usually undertaken in such patients and arterial gas estimation and circulatory status drive clinical decision making on management. Type 1 respiratory failure can supervene leading to the need for artificial ventilatory support. Markers of severity and poorer prognosis include pre-existing lung disease (such as COPD, cystic fibrosis, and bronchiectasis, all of which are associated with airflow limitation) and moderate or severe hypoxaemia (P_{a,O_2} <8 kPa or 60 mm Hg) [126, 127].

41.9.3 Pneumocystis jiroveci pneumonia

This rare form of pneumonia is usually seen in patients with marked cellular immune deficiency, e.g. patients on immunosuppressive therapy or with acquired immune deficiency syndrome (AIDS). Most such patients are now on prophylactic chemotherapy to help prevent pneumocystis jiroveci pneumonia (PCP).

The possibility that a change in lung function might precede other evidence of clinical deterioration has attracted interest. In a follow-up study of 1300 patients who were at risk, some 6% when still asymptomatic had a decline in gas transfer of ≥20% of their predicted value but in none was PCP found to be the cause [128]. A different study on over 450 subjects [129] found that gas transfer fell in both those who developed PCP (from 68% to 44% of predicted) and in those who did not develop the condition (from 71% to 57% of predicted value). The fall was significantly greater in those with PCP and predated the diagnosis of PCP by up to 2 months. However, a fall in gas transfer of at least 5% from the start value only had a sensitivity of 75% and specificity of 28% in predicting the onset of PCP.

A group of 19 patients with a primary episode of PCP were studied to determine the recovery of lung function with treatment [130]. Both FVC and FEV_1 were reduced to a median of 61% of the predicted value, but FEV_1 recovered within a week and FVC within a month of starting treatment. Gas transfer was reduced to 43% of predicted value initially and recovered only to 64% of predicted by 9 months.

41.9.4 Tuberculosis

One of the earliest applications of lung function tests was in relation to pulmonary tuberculosis [131] where a low VC was found to indicate a poor prognosis. However, studies of patients with active disease were soon curtailed on account of the risk of cross-infection. The lesions heal by fibrosis so at this stage in the disease there are reductions in TLC, FRC and RV with FVC and FEV_1 reduced to a similar extent. A study of over 25,000 South African miners found an FEV_1 below 80% of predicted value in 18% following a single episode of pulmonary tuberculosis (TB) and in up to 35% of those who had suffered three episodes [132]. A prospective study of patients treated for TB found relatively little functional impairment; this was related to the number of segments affected and the volume of cavities [133]. Progressive disease can be complicated by chronic respiratory failure. The presence of nocturnal desaturation is then a bad prognositc feature. By contrast age, FVC, FEV_1 and P_{a,CO_2} are unhelpful in this respect [134]. Patients whose pulmonary TB was treated with thoracoplasty (see 41.7.5) have reduced lung volumes; they may develop significant airflow limitation [78] and nocturnal hypoventilation [135]. Annual sleep studies can be a help in indicating when effective therapy should be started [136].

Extensive pleural disease following pleural effusion due to TB can lead to marked restriction to movement of an otherwise effective lung. Under these circumstances TLC, FRC, RV, FVC and *T*lco are reduced, but *K*co is normal or increased (cf. Section 20.9.1).

41.9.5 Pulmonary mycoses

Fungal infections of the lungs (fungimycoses) can be caused by any of a number of organisms of which the commonest are coccidioidomycosis, blastomycosis and histoplasmosis. A study of children infected with blastomycosis found that most, but not all, had normal lung function several years after successful treatment [137]. During the acute illness a restrictive ventilatory defect is found, with low lung compliance and evidence for narrowing of small airways [138]; the changes are reversed by treatment. In another series restrictive and obstructive patterns were seen [139] as well as a gas transfer defect. The obstructive defect was first to recover. The presence of airways obstruction apparently complicating paracoccidioidomycosis can reflect an underlying COPD rather than the infection [140]. With very severe infections respiratory failure and acute lung injury can occur [141, 142].

41.10 Occupational lung diseases

See Section 37.7

41.11 Lung tumours

Primary tumours of the lungs are commonly related to fume from smoking cigarettes but may be caused by other inhaled dusts or vapours, for examples asbestos fibres, radon gas or other ionising agent, arsenic, polycyclic hydrocarbons, chromium and probably silica. The lungs are also the site for metastases from other organs and tissues, including the breast, the contra-lateral lung, the gastro-intestinal tract and sarcomas from any sites.

Primary tumours occupy space within the lung and this may influence its function. More troublesome is if a bronchus is occluded as this is followed by collapse and consolidation distal to the blockage. FEV_1 and FVC are then reduced and FEV_1 is reduced further where there is coexisting COPD, as is the case in most smokers (Sections 37.3 and 40.3).

The blood supply to the lung tissue affected by a central tumour is usually reduced. This can be revealed by $\dot{V}_A/\dot{Q}$ scanning. The information can help to determine the extent of any resection that may be contemplated (Section 43.3.1)

Multiple small metastases can cause few problems initially, but as they grow and increase in number the lung becomes less compliant, gas exchange is affected and dyspnoea ensues. Spread of tumour to the pleura can cause a pleural effusion (see above). A more severe effect on lung function is seen with spread of tumour tissue into the lymphatics draining the lungs (hence lymphangitis carcinomatosa). The lungs develop a restrictive defect with a very low static compliance, reduced static and dynamic lung volumes and a very low transfer factor with attendant hypoxaemia.

41.12 Acute lung injury

The term adult respiratory distress syndrome (ARDS) was first used in 1967 to define a condition where serious gas exchange abnormalities coexisted with a low lung compliance not due to pulmonary congestion from left heart failure [143]. Heart failure was to be excluded on the basis of a normal or low pulmonary capillary wedge pressure. The syndrome is now thought to reflect one end of a spectrum of conditions where the function of the lungs has been compromised. The broader term acute lung injury (ALI) is also used. A consensus definition of ARDS includes the following items [144]: acute onset of respiratory failure, the ratio of Pa,O_2 in mm Hg to FI,O_2 of less than 200 (regardless of PEEP), diffuse bilateral pulmonary infiltrates on the chest radiograph and pulmonary capillary wedge pressure less than 18 cm H_2O. The above ratio $Pa,O_2/FI,O_2$ in SI units is <27 kPa. A cardinal feature of ALI is that the permeability of the alveolar–capillary barrier and hence the total lung water are increased [145]. It has been suggested that the diagnosis is made based on an acute lung injury score, the presence of a clinical disorder that can cause ALI, the absence of left heart failure and the presence of non-pulmonary organ failure.

Acute lung injury is also called non-cardiogenic pulmonary oedema. It can be caused by many insults to the lungs; e.g. oxygen toxicity, paraquat poisoning, pancreatitis, post-cardiac bypass shock lung, trauma (particularly crush injuries), irradiation and inhalation injuries.

A clinical ALI score can be derived for each patient [146] and the elements considered in the score indicate how lung function is affected. There is alveolar consolidation that is measured on CXR, and problems with gas exchange that are quantified by the ratio of PO_2 (in kPa) divided by FI,O_2, with >40 being deemed normal and <13 very severe. With the patient ventilated it is relatively easy to measure respiratory compliance, with >80 ml cm H_2O^{-1} being normal and <20 ml cm H_2O^{-1} being severe. The level of positive end expiratory pressure required to maximise oxygen delivery is given a score, with <5 cm H_2O being normal and >15 cm H_2O being very severe. Pressure–volume curves can be constructed for assessing lung compliance and to help in optimising alveolar recruitment by adjusting ventilator settings. It is suggested that these curves should be measured allowing for a variable level of PEEP rather than at constant PEEP as the latter method leads to predictions for unnecessarily high ventilatory pressures to achieve satisfactory recruitment [147], (also Section 42.5).

In the acute phase the patient is generally too ill to undergo routine lung function testing and artificial ventilation is commonly required. The increased alveolar–capillary permeability can be assessed in a number of ways. The accumulation in the lungs of intravenously administered radiolabelled proteins such as indium labelled transferrin [148] can be assessed by scintillation counting over the lungs. However, a correction is needed for the volume of blood in the lungs. This is achieved by also counting for separately labelled red cells. The technique has the limitations that it may not detect the earliest changes in ALI and cannot distinguish protein leak from alveolar haemorrhage.

An alternative is to use the clearance of inhaled technetium labelled diethylenetriamine penta-acetate (DTPA). The material is administered as an aerosol of particle diameter less than 1 μm and the decay of the deposited isotope is obtained after making an allowance for the natural decay [149]. A normal clearance (approximately 1% per minute) is thought to exclude significant alveolar damage. The technique is very sensitive e.g. it can be abnormal after application of PEEP [150] or after smoking a cigarette [151], (also Section 7.12).

Positron emission tomography has been used to assess the distributions of lung water content (LWC) and of pulmonary blood flow in patients with ALI. The study demonstrated that there was inadequate diversion of pulmonary perfusion away from oedematous areas. This suggested that diminished hypoxic vasoconstriction in these areas contributes to the hypoxaemia and unfavourable $Pa,O_2/F_I,O_2$ratio [152].

Recovery from ALI was originally reported as being complete [153, 154] but long-term follow-up studies indicate that functional impairment can persist [155, 156]. Almost all survivors tend to have abnormal lung function at 4 weeks from discharge and in two thirds the transfer factor is still abnormal at 1 year. However, the lung volumes tend to return to normal [157]. A study of 52 survivors of severe ALI [158] showed good improvement by 3 months, with a little more recovery by 6 months and a relatively static period after that, such that TLC reached over 80% of predicted value, with FVC and gas transfer only reaching 70–75% of predicted values. The rate of recovery was slower for those subjects with the highest acute lung injury scores as indicated by an abnormal $Pa,O_2/F_I,O_2$ ratio, the level of required PEEP and the lung compliance.

41.13 Inhalation effects

Noxious substances when they are inhaled can increase alveolar capillary permeability and cause pulmonary oedema and ALI, see Section 37.4. Similarly, cigarette smoke can increase the permeability [151] and attract neutrophils into the lungs where they cause local destruction leading to COPD (Sections 37.3 and 40.3).

The noxious substances include chlorine gas and NO_2. Some gases also increase bronchial responsiveness and lead to wheeze which some workers have called reactive airways dysfunction syndrome [159]. Other gases, for example smoke from fires, as well as causing pulmonary and mucosal oedema [160] can give rise to airflow limitation, either obstructive or restrictive [161–163], also Further reading. Normal spirometry probably excludes significant smoke inhalation injury. The effects from carbon monoxide inhalation are discussed in Section 37.4.1

41.13.1 Ozone

The effects of breathing this gas are described in Section 37.4.3. Additional references are given below [164–167].

41.13.2 Aspiration

Inhalation of kerosene, paraffin or mineral oils can cause an alveolitis with associated lipoid laden macrophages. Single case reports indicate that a restrictive ventilatory defect can develop associated with severe exertional dyspnoea [168, 169]. See also 'Gastro-oesophageal reflux', Section 41.22.1.

41.13.3 Marijuana

In one longitudinal study the regular inhalation of marijuana without tobacco was found not to cause a decline in FEV_1 [170] but the effects of the tobacco and marijuana can be additive [171]. Chronic smoking of marijuana alone has been found to have no effect on transfer factor, closing volume and slope of phase III of the single breath nitrogen washout curve. These findings suggest that there is no harmful effect on small airway function; however, airway resistance was increased indicating an effect on large airways [172]. Acute exposure to marijuana induces a mild bronchodilatation [173] but has no effect on pulmonary alveolar permeability [174], also Section 37.3.

41.13.4 Cocaine, heroin

Smokers of 'freebase' cocaine have been found to have a reduced transfer factor [175–177] for which the cause is not known. Increased pulmonary alveolar permeability has been found after inhaling crack cocaine [178]. A recent study of over 200 users of inhaled crack cocaine found no independent effect of the cocaine on gas transfer whereas there was a definite tobacco effect where the two were taken together [179]. Heroin smoking leads to histamine release and will exacerbate asthma [180].

41.14 Hyperventilation syndrome

Hyperventilation has been defined as breathing that is in excess of the metabolic requirement; hence, RER is increased (Section 28.4.4). The end expiratory lung volume is often elevated and the breathing is usually more thoracic than diaphragmatic in character. The excessive elimination of CO_2 results in a respiratory alkalosis (Section 22.3.3). Hyperventilation syndrome can arise in otherwise normal subjects or be a feature of anxiety, malingering and personal adequacy; some features are in Section 30.5.3, also [181]. A provocation test can be used, but many workers think both the test and the term to be unhelpful [182–184].

41.15 Immunological lung disease

41.15.1 Sarcoidosis

Sarcoidosis is a systemic immunological disorder of unknown aetiology that causes accumulations of CD4+ T_{H1} lymphocytes throughout the lungs and elsewhere in the body. The lesions progress to form granulomas. In Europe and the United States the condition affects one person per 2500 to 10,000. In the early stages it may have little observable effect on lung function, but when there are extensive lung infiltrations the VC and gas transfer are reduced.

The radiological changes of pulmonary sarcoidosis include hilar adenopathy on its own (stage I) or evidence of parenchymal change with or without hilar adenopathy. (stages II and III, respectively) Transbronchial biopsy undertaken in stage I disease has a high probability of revealing granulomas in relation to alveoli and small airways. Spirometry can be normal [185], but in approximately 50% of subjects there are increases in the nitrogen alveolar slope, the RV and the closing capacity, whilst the dynamic compliance can be reduced [186]. However, in stage I disease a reduced transfer factor may be the only abnormality [187]. The change is progressive and accompanied by a reduction in VC [187, 188], but in stage 1 the static compliance and mouth pressures can be normal [186].

Many of the physiological features are suggestive of narrowing of small airways; this is accompanied by air trapping that is apparent on HRCT scans of the lungs in the majority of subjects, even some who have relatively normal lung function. Many of the changes are intercorrelated [189, 190]. Airflow limitation was found in more than half of a series of over 100 patients with various stages of sarcoidosis [191]. All those patients were deemed to have evidence of small airways disease.

Endobronchial sarcoidosis can be present [192] or develop even in patients with stage I disease [193]; the lesions are accompanied by an obstructive type of ventilatory defect that is not reversed by short-acting bronchodilators. In patients who experience dyspnoea there is often desaturation on exercise, the extent of which is inversely related to the patient's transfer factor [194]. However, the chest radiograph staging and VC were poor predictors of exercise capacity.

Sarcoidosis is a multi-system disease and involves the respiratory muscles. The consequences have been investigated in patients with dyspnoea and more advanced disease amongst whom FVC, TLC, RV and gas transfer were all reduced. *P*Imax and *P*Emax were greatly reduced as well [195] and, compared with conventional lung function tests, the levels were more closely associated with dyspnoea.

The natural progression of sarcoidosis and the effect of treatment can be monitored using the VC and transfer factor. The changes in lung function occur relatively slowly so assessment is only necessary every 2–3 months.

41.15.2 Extrinsic allergic alveolitis

This group of conditions is referred to as hypersensitivity pneumonitis as well as extrinsic allergic alveolitis (EAA). They are reactions to a variety of allergens such as bird protein and various fungi. The conditions are reviewed in Section 37.7.5, see also [196–201].

41.15.3 Allergic bronchopulmonary aspergillosis

Allergic bronchopulmonary aspergillosis (ABPA) arises in asthmatic subjects and in up to 2% of patients with cystic fibrosis [202]. ABPA causes a central bronchiectasis due to an immunological response to *Aspergillus fumigatus* species. Subjects with ABPA and asthma will have the typical airflow limitation associated with asthma but the degree of acute reversibility may be less than expected. However, in up to 10% of patients with ABPA and cystic fibrosis there is no evidence of significant airflow limitation [202].

41.16 Rare pulmonary diseases

41.16.1 Swyer–James syndrome or Macleod's syndrome

The defining feature is radiological hyperlucency in one lung. It is thought to follow a viral infection of the lower respiratory tract in infancy that causes a constrictive bronchiolitis with associated airflow limitation and oligaemia in one lung [203, 204]. CT scanning has shown that the condition may not be strictly unilateral [205] and bronchiectasis is often also present [206]. Differential lung function studies using radioisotope techniques and broncho-spirometry showed in one case that the affected lung had less ventilation, reduced air flow and reduced perfusion [207].

41.16.2 Microlithiasis

In this rare condition small bony nodules with a layered onion skin-like structure (micronodular ossifications) are present in the lungs. The disorder appears to be familial especially amongst Turkish people [208]. Patients can have a restrictive defect [209] that deteriorates slowly. One case showed reduced FEV_1 and FVC with a low TLC by helium dilution (about 50% of predicted value) but normal TLC by plethysmography [210]. This suggested substantial areas of lung not communicating with airways. *K*CO was about half that predicted and the patient had type 1 respiratory failure. The hypoxaemia was due to $\dot{V}_A/\dot{Q}$ inequality in the presence of pulmonary hypertension. Both features were improved by the use of nasal CPAP.

41.16.3 Pulmonary alveolar proteinosis

In this rare condition amorphous material (comprising mainly fat and protein) fills the alveolar spaces; it is more common in males than females and presents in middle life with dyspnoea and cough [211]. FEV_1 and FVC are reduced to a similar degree [212], consistent with functional loss of alveoli. Gas transfer is often reduced to a greater extent than expected from the degree of the restrictive defect [213] and hypoxia occurs due to $\dot{V}_A/\dot{Q}$ imbalance. Isotope studies on a patient undergoing lung lavage treatment have shown improved $\dot{V}_A/\dot{Q}$ ratios in response to therapy [214].

41.16.4 Histiocytosis X

In this pulmonary disorder the alveolar septa and bronchial walls are infiltrated by histiocytes and eosinophils. The lesions progress to diffuse pulmonary fibrosis and cystic honeycombing in the lungs. Similar lesions can develop in other organs, e.g. eosinophilic granulomas affect bones. Letterer–Siwe disease is a diffuse multi-system disease in children, and Hand–Schuller–Christian disease affects neuroendocrine function and also bones.

In histiocytosis X the spirometry findings are variable, with evidence for airways obstruction indicating a poor prognosis e.g. $FEV_1/FVC < 0.66$ and $RV/TLC > 0.33$ [215]. A low transfer factor is usual and associated with poor exercise performance [216], as is the presence of pulmonary hypertension. The hypertension can develop independent of the extent of impairment of lung fuction [217].

41.16.5 Tuberous sclerosis

This is a rare inherited disorder (autosomal dominant) in which there is mental deficiency, epilepsy and adenoma sebaceum. A few, mainly female patients (<1%), develop diffuse pulmonary fibrosis [218] and there can be lymphangioleiomyomatosis [219]. The pulmonary function defect is one of irreversible airflow limitation with a high RV/TLC and reduced gas transfer factor [220, 221]. A slow inexorable decline in lung function is usual.

41.16.6 Lymphangioleiomyomatosis

This is a rare condition in women of childbearing age in which abnormal smooth muscle tissue is present around bronchi, blood vessels and lymphatics in the lungs. Common presentations include dyspnoea, haemoptysis, pneumothorax and chylous effusions. CT shows multiple small discrete cystic lesions [222]. The patients can have large lungs (TLC 114% predicted value, RV 200% predicted value) and low transfer factor (57% predicted value) [223]. Static lung compliance can be increased, likewise the airway resistance. The latter is due to airway narrowing, not loss of elastic recoil.

There is a progressive decline in FEV_1 (mean 106 ml $year^{-1}$) that reflects the transfer factor at the time of diagnosis [224] and there is progressive hypoxaemia, particularly on exercise. This needs to be assessed directly as hypoxaemia appears not to be related to the levels of transfer factor and FEV_1 at rest [225]. Treatment can be monitored with dynamic and static lung volumes and transfer factor.

41.16.7 Wegener's granulomatosis

This condition is one of a group of vasculitides characterised by the triad of granulomatous inflammation, vasculitis of the upper and lower airways and glomerulonephritis. In one study the most common abnormality was airflow obstruction affecting the trachea or lobar bronchi [226]. The lung volumes were small on account of diffuse and focal infiltrates and cavitating lesions. The nose and glottis can also be affected, the latter being detected by flow–volume loop tests for upper airway obstruction (Section 14.3.6), [227]. Treatment (by immunosuppression) can improve the airflow limitation and lung volumes but a low transfer factor is less responsive.

41.16.8 Bronchocentric granulomatosis

This condition involves a granulomatous necrotising process in peripheral airways that is thought to be due to an immunological reaction to aspergillus species. No special lung function changes have been reported, but half of the affected patients are asthmatic and in many subjects this condition is a complication arising on a background of bronchopulmonary aspergillosis.

41.16.9 Lymphomatoid granulomatosis

This is a rare form of pulmonary vasculitis characterised by necrotising angiocentric and angiodestructive lymphoid infiltrates of uncertain aetiology. A restrictive defect has been reported in a single case with infiltrative disease [228]. A report on a series of patients found frequent revisions of diagnosis and suggest this condition may be a transient histological picture on the way to becoming a lymphoma [229].

41.16.10 Castleman's disease

This is a lymphoproliferative disorder that may be a response to infection with human herpes virus type 8. It can be multicentric, with sheets of tissue embracing mediastinal structures. No special lung function abnormalities have yet been conclusively attributed to this condition.

41.16.11 Behçets disease

This is a rare chronic multi-system vasculitis that can affect many organs including the skin and eyes, also the central nervous system. There can be oral or genital ulceration. Intrathoracic involvement includes thromboses of the superior vena cava, pulmonary arteries and pulmonary veins, and can progress to pulmonary infarction [230]. $\dot{V}_A/\dot{Q}$ abnormalities occur with extensive disease [231]. There are few case reports. One study found airflow limitation and raised RV with associated hypoxaemia [232]. Another of 29 cases failed to find any relation between lung function tests and the presence of pulmonary lesions on HRCT [233].

41.16.12 Idiopathic pulmonary haemosiderosis

This condition is a rare cause for iron deficiency anaemia, which is from recurrent episodes of diffuse alveolar haemorrhage, often with haemoptysis. Presentation is usually in childhood. The underlying defect is in the alveolar capillary basement membrane and is different from that in Goodpasture's syndrome. There is increasing evidence for an association with coeliac disease [234, 235]. Airflow limitation with low gas transfer is found [234]. Serial studies show airflow limitation and ultimately a restrictive defect [236, 237]. During the haemorrhages hypoxia is usual and gas transfer can be high if there is free blood in the airways.

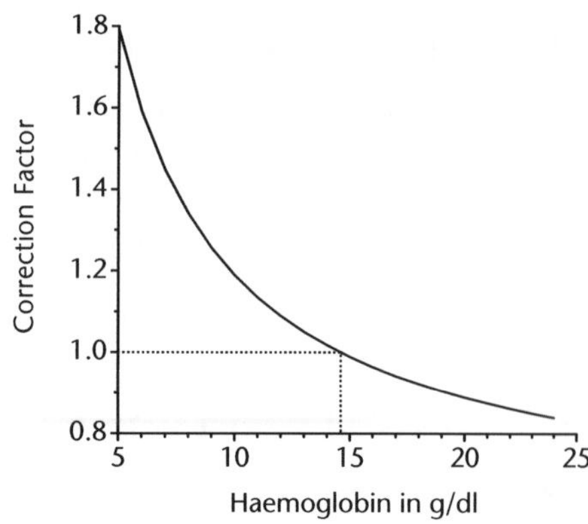

Fig. 41.2 Plot of correction factor for gas transfer factor against haemoglobin (Hb) concentration. The value for Hb of 14.6 g dl^{-1} is marked with a dotted line.

Pulmonary fibrosis can supervene, also pulmonary hypertension that is secondary to the chronic hypoxia [238].

41.17 Haematological diseases

41.17.1 Anaemia and polycythaemia

These conditions affect the quantity of oxygen that can be carried by blood and hence the blood flow and mixed venous oxygen tension that are appropriate for delivering a given quantity of oxygen to the tissues. Lung function is only affected indirectly. However, the haemoglobin concentration is a component of the reaction rate of carbon monoxide with blood and influences the transfer factor for carbon monoxide on this account [239]. The underlying relationships and a method for standardising *Tl*,co for [Hb] is discussed in Section 20.7.2, see also Fig. 41.2.

41.17.2 Methaemoglobinaemia

For haemoglobin (Hb) to carry oxygen it must be in the reduced ferrous (Fe^{2+}) state (Section 21.2.1). If the Hb is oxidised to methaemoglobin the haem iron is in the ferric (Fe^{3+}) state and is incapable of binding oxygen. This can occur due to hereditary abnormalities of Hb, with several types of methaemoglobin (MetHb) now described, or to cytochrome b_5 reductase deficiency. More commonly the condition is acquired due to the action of toxins or drugs such as nitrites, nitrates, aniline dyes and sulphonamides.

The effect of methaemoglobin is greater than just a reduction in the quantity of Hb available to transport oxygen, since the conformation of methaemoglobin causes a left shift of the O_2–Hb dissociation curve. As a result, whilst (in the absence of other disease) the Pa,o_2 will be normal, a reduced quantity of O_2 is unloaded from HbO_2 for a given fall in tissue Po_2, e.g. if approximately 35% of the total Hb is in the form of MetHb the patient will show symptons of headache, weakness and breathlessness. A level above 80% is life threatening. There is the additional consequence that a relatively small quantity of MetHb results in cyanosis e.g. 1.5 g dl^{-1} of MetHb gives rise to the same level of cyanosis as 5 g dl^{-1} of deoxygenated Hb. The altered light absorption affects pulse oximeters that give a reading approaching 85% irrespective of the true underlying arterial saturation [240] see also Section 7.10.1.

41.17.3 Carboxyhaemoglobinaemia

Carbon monoxide is a poisonous gas that combines with haemoglobin. It is present in tobacco smoke, coal gas and many fumes from combustion. The environmental, epidemiological and occupational implications, the long-term consequences for health and the symptoms and treatment of poisoning are discussed in Section 37.4.1.

Carbon monoxide is harmful in at least four ways: (i) CO reacts with Hb and myoglobin to limit O_2 uptake and this has a particularly bad effect on the myocardium, (ii) a raised HbCO level shifts the Hb–O_2 dissociation curve for the remaining Hb to the left so that for a given tissue Po_2 less O_2 is released to tissues (Fig. 37.8, page 512), (iii) CO inhibits the mitochondrial electron transfer chain, particularly inhibiting cytochrome b and aa_3, (iv) CO binds to and inhibits intracellular enzyme systems containing Fe, for example cytochrome P_{450} and NADPH.

Arterial gas sampling on a patient with marked CO poisoning can reveal normal arterial partial pressures for O_2 whilst the true arterial saturation is extremely low. Furthermore, pulse oximeters using just two wavelengths of light will not correctly reflect the low saturation and will give a misleading overestimate (Section 7.10.1).

41.17.4 Sulphaemoglobinaemia

In this condition haemoglobin takes up sulphide groups that are present in the blood as a consequence of drug ingestion (e.g. sulphonamides or phenacetin). The resulting sulphaemoglobinaemia causes intense cyanosis, such that just 0.5 g dl^{-1} in this form gives equivalent cyanosis to 1.5 g $dl^{-1}$of methaemoglobin or 5g $dl^{-1}$of deoxygenated Hb. The clinical effect of sulphaemoglobin is less than might be expected because there is a shift of the Hb–O_2 dissociation curve to the right so more O_2 is unloaded for a given fall in tissue Po_2 [241]. As for methaemoglobin the partial pressure of O_2 in arterial gases can be normal whilst the underlying arterial saturation is very low and double wavelength pulse oximeters do not give accurate readings.

41.17.5 Sickle cell disease

Sickle cell disease is due to an abnormal haemoglobin (HbS). The condition is inherited as a recessive gene so the carrier state exists. It presents as acute episodes due to the red cells becoming deformed (sickle shaped) and in this form blocking capillaries throughout the body including the lungs. Factors that predispose to sickling include infections and hyperventilation and/or hypoxia (e.g. during flight). The resulting acute chest syndrome (ACS) is a major and potentially fatal pulmonary complication of sickle cell disease. Vaso-occlusive disease is also found elsewhere in the body. Infections can cause ACS to develop but undiagnosed fat embolism is a compounding factor [242], It can be diagnosed from fat droplets in macrophages obtained by bronchoalveolar lavage. Regional hypoxia within the lungs is a predisposing factor that can be ameliorated by incentive spirometry [243, 244]. Upper abdominal surgery has been shown to predispose to acute chest syndrome with onset between 24 and 96 h post-operatively [245]. The lower lobes on the same side as the surgery was the commonest site with pleural effusion present in half the cases.

The level of hypoxia is often greater than expected from the degree of shadowing on the chest radiograph and the level of alveolar–arterial oxygen gradient correlates with severity [246]. This is due to micovascular occlusion that can be seen on thin section CT scans in acute chest syndrome [247]. Increased airways resistance and lower expiratory flow rates have been found and these relate to the number of episodes of ACS [248, 249]. Contrary to one's intuition the transfer factor was higher in subjects who experienced several episodes of ACS [248].

Sickle cell chronic lung disease (SCLD) is a prime cause of mortality in the long term, and involves both perfusion and diffusion defects with a restrictive pattern and generalised fibrosis [250]. The number of episodes of ACS was found to be a significant risk factor for developing SCLD. This restrictive picture has been found to start developing in children with sickle cell disease [251].

41.17.6 Thalassaemia major

Thalassaemia major is an inherited haemoglobinopathy in which the abnormality is in the globin moiety. The condition is associated with splenomegaly and microcytic hypochromic anaemia that requires frequent transfusions. The patients commonly have a restrictive ventilatory defect [252–256]. A reduced transfer factor is usual [252, 255, 257] but not invariable [253]. The cause for these changes is uncertain. Some have found no relation between the degree of iron overload from repeated blood transfusion and the abnormality in lung function [255, 257, 258], whereas others have found worse function with more severe iron overload [252, 254]. A confounding issue is that intravenous deferoxamine, used as a chelator for iron, has been reported to cause a pulmonary syndrome [259].

A comprehensive study of 17 patients found restrictive defects with reduced compliance, increased airway conductance and an increase in Kco [260]. Autopsy evidence from other thalassaemic subjects had shown no evidence of fibrosis. A possible explanation for these findings was of dysynapsis in lung growth, with smaller air spaces relative to both the vascular bed and the major airways.

41.17.7 Transfusion reaction

Acute haemolytic transfusion reaction due to incompatible blood can cause circulatory collapse, tachypnoea, haemoglobinaemia and haemoglobinuria. The condition can lead on to acute lung injury (ALI), particularly where HL-A specific leukocyte antibodies in the donor blood bind to the recipient leukocytes [261]. Dyspnoea and pulmonary infiltrates occur.

41.17.8 Bone marrow transplantation

There are several reasons why lung function may deteriorate after bone marrow transplantation (BMT). These broadly separate into those consequent from the preparation for BMT, post-transplant infectious complications, and non-infectious lung complications associated with graft-versus-host disease (GVHD) that may be acute or chronic.

Recipient preparation. Depending on the BMT recipient's underlying disease and the donor's genetic match it may be necessary to eradicate the recipient's underlying disease and immunosuppress them to enhance the chance of a successful transplant. Regimens may include receiving whole body irradiation, high dose cyclophosphamide and/or busulphan and other cytotoxic drugs. Nearly all these agents can cause pulmonary damage that is seen as an idiopathic pneumonia 2–10 weeks post-transplant. Longitudinal studies of BMT survivors have shown a mild restrictive defect that develops within 3–6 months and recovers beyond 1 year [262, 263]. A multivariate analysis indicated that preparatory radiation dose was one of the factors involved [262]. FVC, FEV_1, TLC and gas transfer were all reduced but expiratory flows and $FEV_1\%$ were not affected.

Graft-versus-host disease. Donor cells can cause an immunological reaction with host tissues that is termed graft-versus-host disease (GVHD); it is characterised by skin rash, raised bilirubin, also diarrhoea, and is either acute (within the first 3 months, hence aGVHD) or chronic after this time (hence cGVHD). The occurrence of GVHD gives rise to the transient restrictive and gas transfer defects mentioned above [262, 263]. It is also a factor delaying or reducing the recovery of lung function [262].

A persistent pulmonary syndrome characterised by late onset cough, dyspnoea and pulmonary infiltrates has been found in nearly 20% of bone marrow transplanted patients [264–266]. There is associated airflow limitation of an obstructive type, for which chronic GVHD is the major risk factor [264]. Open biopsy on a few of these patients showed bronchiolitis obliterans and patchy interstitial pneumonitis [266]. An earlier larger series of patients found low $FEV_1\%$ at 1 year that related to cGVHD and to use of methotrexate but not to the dose of conditioning irradiation or aGVHD [267].

Onset of airflow limitation in the first 4 months after BMT was a predictor of a subsequent progressive decline in lung function that might end in death [268]. cGVHD and use of busulphan therapy were associated factors [269]. By contrast, a reduction in transfer factor was common, benign and not related to mortality.

41.17.9 Leukaemia

Patients with leukaemia and exceptionally high white cell counts can have normal oxygen saturations by pulse oxymetry but hypoxaemia when a specimen of arterial blood is analysed [270]. This artifact is due to the high metabolic activity of the white cells [271]. The effect can be reduced by minimising the delay before analysis and by storing the blood sample in ice. Metabolic activity can be halted by adding cyanide to the sample.

Intravascular leukostasis has been described with extremely high white cell counts that caused severe hypoxic respiratory failure. The failure was reversed by reducing the white cell count [272]. The cause for the impaired gas exchange could be capillary obstruction; alternatively it might be endothelial damage by enzymes from the stationary leukocytes.

Long-term survivors of childhood acute lymphoblastic leukaemia have been found to have a restrictive ventilatory defect [273, 274] and reduced transfer factor. The *K*co was normal which, in the presence of a reduced lung volume, was further evidence for a persisting transfer defect (Section 20.9.1). The factors implicated included craniospinal irradiation, cyclophosphamide therapy and pulmonary complications during treatment [273]. However, it might have been that the growth of the lungs was impaired [274].

41.17.10 Myeloma

The principle effects of multiple myeloma on lung function are secondary pulmonary infections and the deposition of amyloid (Section 41.23.2).

41.18 Cardiac disease

In longitudinal surveys FEV_1 is an independent predictor of all cause mortality [275] including deaths from ischaemic heart disease. The effects of cardiac dysfunction on lung function are explored here, but not the converse effect of lung diseases causing heart failure.

41.18.1 Left heart failure

Left heart failure from any cause and also mitral stenosis are associated with a raised pressure in pulmonary veins and a high pulmonary capillary wedge pressure; the high pressures distend pulmonary capillaries, increase the volume of interstitial fluid in the lungs, stimulates C-fibre receptors to cause shallow breathing (Section 23.3.4) and can result in pulmonary oedema.

The model of mitral valve disease has been extensively investigated; it shows a raised RV due to transudation of fluid leading to closure of small airways and reduced TLC, FVC, FEV_1, FEV_1/FVC and transfer factor [276]. The reduced VC is secondary to pulmonary congestion and physical enlargement of the heart. The congestion reduces the lung compliance, particularly at the lung bases, so the regional distribution of ventilation to the bases is low [277–279]. By contrast, in aortic valve disease the pulmonary circulation is spared any effect until the left ventricle fails, so few changes are seen until this occurs. Patients with left heart failure often wheeze. Successful treatment of the heart failure reverses these changes [280]. Thus, ipratropium bromide had a significant bronchodilator effect before treatment of the heart failure but not afterwards, suggesting the failure results in a reversible increase in cholinergic bronchial tone. Orthopnoea (breathlessness when lying down) is a common symptom in heart failure and the associated rise in respiratory resistance has been found to be also related to posture [281].

Studies of patients with chronic heart failure who proceed to have heart transplantation have helped determine which effects on lung function can be corrected. VC, TLC and gas transfer were all reduced in a group of patients pre-transplant and 1 year post-transplant the VC and TLC had improved from 76% to 94% predicted value and 79% to 98% of predicted value, respectively, whereas transfer factor remained low at 64–67% of predicted value [282]. Others have confirmed these results, even finding a fall in gas transfer [283]. This may be related to the patients having a high vascular resistance from which recovery can be slow since 2 years post-valve surgery the gas transfer has been found to increase [284].

In severe heart failure muscle strength (as assessed by *P*Emax and *P*Imax) is reduced and this may influence the response to exercise [285, 286]. In normal subjects on exercise end expiratory lung volume (EELV) increases with higher ventilation, but in heart failure EELV remained close to RV leading to greater airflow limitation [287]. It appears that the reduced respiratory muscle strength significantly contributes to dyspnoea in cardiac failure [288]. Another factor is shallow rapid breathing that can be reversed when pulmonary congestion is relieved (Fig. 28.12, page 398).

Patients with left heart failure and pulmonary congestion frequently have disturbed breathing at night and cyclical Cheynes–Stokes breathing is common (Section 32.5, also page 378).

41.18.2 Congenital heart disease

Congenital heart disease may lead to pulmonary hypertension, chronic hypoxia and polycythaemia. In children with ventricular septal defect and pulmonary hypertension a positive correlation between mean pulmonary artery pressure and static lung elastic recoil pressure has been found [289]. In children with left-to-right cardiac shunting this lower lung compliance has been confirmed [290] together with smaller tidal volumes and higher airways resistance, and these changes correlated with echocardiographic measurement of the ratio of pulmonary artery size to aortic size, which is a surrogate for pulmonary artery pressure.

41.19 Joint and connective tissue diseases

The main connective tissue diseases are each associated with a slightly different pattern of lung involvement.

41.19.1 Rheumatoid disease

Rheumatoid disease may affect the airways, interstitium, pulmonary vasculature, pleura and respiratory muscles. Pleural effusions are not uncommon and lead to a restrictive disorder with high gas transfer per unit of accessible volume. Lung nodules can arise that may be prominent on chest radiography and have been shown to be associated with a reduced pulmonary capillary volume with no change in transfer factor [291].

Recent studies have clarified the frequency of the various pulmonary complications. About 20% of 150 consecutive patients with rheumatoid arthritis had HRCT evidence of fibrosing alveolitis [292]. Amongst these patients the majority (82%) had an isolated transfer defect and 14% had a restrictive ventilatory defect. In another study approximately 8% had evidence of small airways disease as evinced by reduced $FEF_{25-75\%}$ and increased phase III slope from the single breath nitrogen washout [293]. However, HRCT evidence of small airways disease was found in two thirds of those patients who had normal lung function. Airflow limitation (low FEV_1% attributable to rheumatoid arthritis, not smoking) was found in 16% of subjects [294]. A possible reason for a restrictive defect was a reduction in chest wall compliance [295].

Respiratory muscle weakness (reduced P_I,max and P_E,max) in association with reduced values for FVC and PEF have been observed in children and adults [296, 297]. In the adults the changes were related to corticosteroid usage. Other drug therapy such as gold and penicillamine can lead to a restrictive defect and reduced transfer factor; the response to gold was reversible on drug cessation [298].

A syndrome of obliterative bronchiolitis with increased TLC, RV and RV%, severe airflow limitation, a low transfer factor and hypoxaemia was described in 1977 [299]. More cases have since been confirmed [300]. HRCT showed a mosaic pattern on expiration indicating small airways disease leading to air trapping [301].

41.19.2 Systemic lupus erythematosus

In this auto-immune connective tissue disorder a surprising manifestation is the 'shrinking lungs syndrome'. This is associated with marked elevation of the diaphragm for which the cause is unclear (it might be either diaphragm weakness or chest wall restriction) [302]. In one case there was diaphragm paralysis associated with bilateral damage to the phrenic nerves [303] but other cases had diaphragmatic weakness for voluntary contractions but not for artificial stimulation [304]. An effect of systemic lupus erythematosus (SLE) on muscle performance has been found to account for exercise limitation and a reduced ventilatory response to CO_2 [305, 306].

Systemic lupus erythematosus can affect nearly all parts of the respiratory system [307], for example HRCT scanning often shows diffuse interstitial disease with honeycombing. The transfer factor is usually reduced [308] and the chest radiograph may show a 'ground glass' appearance. The transfer defect affects particularly the membrane component (Dm); it can be accompanied by nail fold capillary changes [309] and Raynaud's phenomenon [310]. Radiographic evidence for pleural disease can be accompanied by a restrictive ventilatory defect (see Illustrative case, Table 38.4d, page 537). Patients with SLE often develop primary pulmonary hypertension at a relatively early stage in the disease [311].

41.19.3 Sjogren's syndrome

Patients with this auto-immune disease often have narrowing of small airways, with reduced values for $FEF_{50\%}$ and $FEF_{75\%}$ and CT evidence of segmental bronchial thickening; the FEV_1 can be relatively normal [312]. HRCT scans have produced features suggestive of air trapping and bronchial wall thickening (in 50% and 32% of cases, respectively) [313]. Bronchial hyperresponsiveness has been reported in over 50% of patients [314, 315]. The residual volume can be increased [316]. Over a 4-year period PEF increased slightly whilst the transfer factor fell slightly [317]. In another longitudinal study that included HRCT and bronchiolar–alveolar lavage a subpleural line CT pattern was present in 28% of subjects. BAL neutrophil predominance was associated with an accelerated reduction in transfer factor [318].

41.19.4 Scleroderma

Scleroderma patients exhibit a thickened stiff skin. The condition can be associated with pulmonary vascular changes and interstitial involvement leading to fibrosing alveolitis. Amongst 34 patients, 12 reported dyspnoea and in 17 (50%) the chest radiograph was abnormal [319]. In 6 patients there was an isolated reduction in transfer factor, whilst in 14 patients (41%) a restrictive ventilatory pattern was found. The same proportion has been found in other studies [320, 321]. In 40 patients followed over 3 years a fall in gas transfer was related to increasing areas of honeycombing on HRCT [322]. Where there is severe oesophageal motor disturbance the gas transfer can be greatly reduced [323].

Exercise testing has identified patients who had a raised deadspace to tidal volume ratio, but normal transfer factor [324] and others with pulmonary hypertension [325]. Increased pulmonary capillary permeability has been demonstrated using a DTPA clearance test. The procedure is an alternative means for identifying the extent to which the lungs are affected in these patients [326].

41.19.5 Marfan's syndrome

Marfan's syndrome is an inherited disorder that can feature kyphoscoliosis and/or pectus excavatum (Sections 41.7.2 and 41.7.3). Amongst 79 children with the condition the only changes in lung function were those attributable to the chest wall abnormalities [327]. However, bronchial hyperresponsiveness has been reported [328], also two cases of pneumothorax and changes in lung function characteristic of emphysema [329].

41.19.6 Ehlers–Danlos syndrome and cutis laxa

Hereditary abnormalities of collagen and elastin formation can affect the lungs. In Ehlers–Danlos syndrome there can be tracheomegaly and chest wall deformities without specific changes in lung function [330]. In one case with tracheobronchomegaly there was irreversible airflow limitation [331]. Case reports indicate that cutis laxa is associated with early onset emphysema [332, 333].

41.20 Liver disease

The best recognised effects of liver disease on the lungs are secondary to ascites and dilated blood vessels. The exact cause of the latter is uncertain but failure of the liver to metabolise low levels of circulating hormones that can influence vascular structures has been mooted. The pulmonary hepatic vascular disorders discussed below have recently been reviewed in detail [334].

41.20.1 Ascites

In liver disease and in malignant diseases of the abdomen, fluid (ascites) can accumulate in the peritoneal space. A large volume will distend the abdomen and splint the diaphragm so that it works at a disadvantage. Several studies have looked at the effect on lung function of removing a large volume (up to 5 l) by paracentesis. Nearly all studies show increases in TLC, VC, FEV_1 and ERV with no change in the FEV_1/VC ratio [335–337]. An increase in *T*l,co after paracentesis has been found with improved Pa,O_2 [335, 338] but other studies have failed to show this effect [336, 337]. Paradoxical reduction in *T*l,co has been found when subjects with ascites were tested supine [339], whilst the increase in *T*l,co measured erect after paracentesis was accompanied by a reduction in *K*co [335] suggesting that ventilation to well perfused lung bases had been improved.

Because of a potential connection through the diaphragm, a pleural effusion may occur secondary to the ascites and independently affect lung function.

41.20.2 Hepatopulmonary syndrome

The hepatopulmonary syndrome (HPS) occurs in about 20% of patients with chronic liver disease or portal hypertension. Diagnosis can be based on a triad of liver cirrhosis, arterial hypoxaemia due to an increase A-a,DO_2 and intrapulmonary vascular dilatation [340, 341] The dilatation is in pre-capillary pulmonary vessels and its effect on gas exchange is that of an AV shunt. Alternative criteria for HPS are (i) presence of chronic liver disease, (ii) absence of other cardiac or pulmonary disease, (iii) A-a,DO_2, $\geq$ 2 kPa (15 mm Hg) when breathing air and (iv) *either* the appearance of radiolabelled microspheres in the extrapulmonary vasculature after IV injection *or* evidence for intrapulmonary vascular abnormalities on a positive contrast enhanced echocardiogram [342]. Pulmonary vasodilatation in these patients has been found to relate to circulating levels of progesterone [343]. Dyspnoea can be severe (e.g. Case 8, page 429).

A common finding is *orthodeoxia*, where arterial saturation falls on moving from the supine to erect position. If abnormal connections between the pulmonary venous and arterial system are evenly distributed within the lungs then on adopting the erect posture more perfusion will go to the bases and this can increase the shunt fraction compared with the supine position. In a study of 20 patients with mild to moderate HPS, 25% had orthodeoxia with worsening of $\dot{V}A/\dot{Q}$ [344]. Orthodeoxia can also occur with a patent foramen ovale and in pulmonary fibrosis where, in the supine position, more perfusion is directed away from the predominantly affected bases.

The multiple inert gas elimination technique (MIGET) has shown that in HPS the desaturation is related to an increased dispersion of $\dot{V}A/\dot{Q}$ [344] with up to 15% of total perfusion going to areas of low $\dot{V}A/\dot{Q}$ ($\dot{V}A/\dot{Q} < 0.01$), and an increased right-to-left shunt where up to 28% of perfusion went to areas of $\dot{V}A/\dot{Q} < 0.005$ [345]. These effects on the pulmonary vasculature are not permanent since they reverse within 2–6 months after liver transplantation [346].

41.20.3 Portopulmonary hypertension

A study of over 1000 patients referred for liver transplant found that approximately 9% had pulmonary hypertension, including some 2% with moderate or severe hypertension [347]. The condition presents with haemodynamic failure, but unlike with HPS there is no hypoxaemia and the condition appears not to be reversible after transplantation. In addition, severe portopulmonary hypertension (PPHT) has a higher post-transplant mortality [347]. Diagnosis of PPHT in liver patients is made by Doppler echocardiography with a sensitivity of 97% and a specificity of 77% [348]. The occurrence of the condition is not related to the severity of liver failure [340].

41.20.4 Primary biliary cirrhosis

Primary biliary cirrhosis is a complex autoimmune disease that can be associated with, and has similar pulmonary manifestations to, Sjogren's syndrome [349]; see Section 41.19.3. A study of 61 patients without respiratory symptoms found an isolated reduction in transfer factor in 24 of them (39%). This feature was related to other abnormalities some of which occur in scleroderma (Section 41.19.4) and collectively go by the acronym CREST syndrome [350].

41.21 Renal disease

41.21.1 Pulmonary haemorrhagic syndromes

A number of conditions can lead to alveolar haemorrhage. They include Goodpasture's syndrome, Henoch–Schonlein purpura and acute glomerulonephritis. When these conditions are active transfer factor is chronically reduced [351, 352] and this reverses on complete resolution of the underlying abormality. In addition, if there is fresh blood in the airways the transfer factor (Tl,co) is increased due to uptake of CO by the blood in the airways [353]. Kco can be 50% or more above baseline in subjects followed serially during acute haemorrhage.

41.21.2 Dialysis and chronic renal failure

Chronic renal failure can be complicated by anaemia, acid–base disturbance and a tendency of fluid overload leading to left heart failure all of which can influence lung function. The fluid might contribute to bronchial hyperresponsiveness but the evidence is conflicting [354–356].

Lung function was assessed in 80 patients on differing forms of renal support (no support, haemodialysis, peritoneal dialysis or post transplantation) [354]. Spirometry was relatively normal but transfer factor was diminished in all groups and especially in those on chronic ambulatory peritoneal dialysis [357]. After renal transplant residual volume was reduced whilst transfer factor remained low. The changes did not relate to duration of renal failure, but chronic subclinical pulmonary oedema might have led to a degree of interstitial fibrosis, e.g. in a study of patients who had been dialysed for 5 years or more transfer factor was reduced compared with patients pre dialysis or within 1 year of starting dialysis [358]; no differences were found in other lung function indices (TLC, RV, FEV_1).

The effect of instilling 2 l of dialysate into the peritoneum of ambulant patients (CAPD) has been shown to reduce RV but not affect FEV_1, gas transfer or distribution of ventilation [359], so this therapy can be applied to patients with poor lung function. In patients having chronic CAPD the diaphragm develops an increased force as its length is increased following instillation of dialysate. The change was not seen in normal subjects [360], suggesting that chronic enforced diaphragm lengthening induced an adaptive response to help cope with the changed circumstances.

Hypoxia can occur during haemodialysis [361]. The response is related to the type of membrane and the composition of the dialysate, with bicarbonate resulting in less hypoxaemia than acetate [362].

41.22 Gastrointestinal disease

41.22.1 Gastro-oesophageal reflux

A relationship between gastro-oesophageal reflux (GOR) and asthma has been suggested and evidence from oesophageal pH monitoring has suggested that GOR can trigger bronchoconstriction via a vagally mediated reflex [363]. Some studies suggest that the reflex can be blocked by atropine [364, 365]. In another study GOR was found in a third of asthma patients amongst whom the occurrence of bronchial hyperresponsiveness was related to the frequency with which reflux was occurring [366]. FVC, VC and FEV_1 can be reduced in such patients, suggesting that silent aspiration may have been responsible [367]. Aspiration of meconium at birth can be followed by airflow limitation and bronchial hyperresponsiveness during childhood [368, 369] but the evidence is ambiguous [370]. The capacity for exercise of such children has been reported as normal [368].

41.22.2 Coeliac disease and inflammatory bowel disease

A study comparing lung function in patients with coeliac disease (CD) and patients with inflammatory bowel disease (IBD) found airflow limitation in IBD but not in CD [371]. However, pulmonary permeability measured by DTPA clearance was increased only in CD. No evidence for interstitial lung disease was found in an earlier study of 18 patients with CD [372], but the patients did have airflow limitation (reduced FEV_1 and $FEF_{50\%}$).

Amongst patients with IBD some workers have found that between one third and one half had impaired lung function, with raised FRC and RV or reduced transfer factor [373, 374]. The changes seemed to relate to disease activity and could revert to normal. A larger study found no difference in spirometry but gas transfer was significantly lower in patients with active disease [375]. A reduced gas transfer was found in about half of a group of 32 patients with ulcerative colitis despite lack of HRCT change, and the reduction was found to relate to the histopathological staging of the colitis [376]. The impairment of lung function has been found to be greater in those with active disease [377]. A possible cause for these changes is that granulocytes are activated in IBD and isotope studies have shown an increased granulocyte pool in the lungs, which correlated with activation. Patients with increased granulocyte migration in the lungs had increased DTPA clearance suggesting alveolar permeability changes [378].

41.22.3 Pancreatitis

Pancreatitis is a cause of acute lung injury (ALI) leading to lung function changes with hypoxia and low transfer factor [379, 380], see Section 41.12. Pleural effusion can also occur and of all patients dying with acute pancreatitis 94% have pulmonary complications [381].

41.23 Metabolic disease

41.23.1 Diabetes mellitus

It was formerly thought that diabetes did not affect the lungs. However, in the mid 1980s the FVC, FEV_1, TLC, FRC and RV were observed to be reduced in diabetics with limited joint mobility [382]. There was no evidence of airflow limitation. The finding was attributed to a reduction in lung compliance. Subsequent studies have demonstrated a reduced TLC in diabetic subjects whose respiratory muscle strength was normal [383]. There was also a reduced transfer factor [384–386] that was attributed to a reduced capillary blood volume, and there was an association with the presence of microangiopathy. These interpretations have been explored in further studies [e.g. 387].

In a large study that assessed 20% of type 2 diabetics amongst an urban population of 120,000 people there were 421 people in whom FVC and FEV_1 were reduced. The finding appeared to relate to the duration of diabetes and not to indices of glycaemic control [388]. However, type 2 diabetes is often associated with central obesity and this feature could have influenced the findings (cf. Section 25.5.1). A reduced FVC and FEV_1 in diabetes was also found in the Copenhagen City Heart Study but the rate of decline of lung function was unexceptional [389].

Sleep apnoea syndrome is a complication of obesity, including patients with type 2 diabetes. The syndrome was also observed amongst 5 out of 12 type 1 diabetes who were lean; sleep apnoea was related to the presence of neuropathy [390]. This finding has been confirmed in a study of 26 non-obese diabetic patients where obstructive sleep apnoea syndrome was found in 10 of the 18 patients with autonomic neuropathy but not in the 8 patients without autonomic neuropathy or in 10 matched controls [391]. No central apnoeas were found.

41.23.2 Amyloidosis

Amyloid can deposit in the lungs in the form of solitary or multiple nodules, bronchial amyloid plaques or diffuse reticulonodular interstitial lesions [392]. Nodules do not have any particular effect on lung function other than occupying space. Bronchial plaques can give rise to stenosis without or with atelectasis, whilst interstitial changes can be associated with a restrictive ventilatory defect and reduced gas transfer [393]. Case reports indicate pulmonary hypertension can occur due to diffuse vascular deposition of amyloid [394] and muscle involvement with amyloid can lead to a severe restrictive ventilatory defect, low maximal inspiratory pressures and ventilatory failure [395].

41.23.3 Gaucher disease and Niemann–Pick disease

In Gaucher disease (GD) there is a deficiency of acid β-glucosidase and in Niemann–Pick disease a deficiency of sphingomyelinase, with both leading to lysosymal accumulation of neutral glycosphingolipid in various tissues. A study of 95 patients with type 1 GD found pulmonary abnormalities in 68% with reduced FRC and gas transfer in just over 40% of subjects [396]. Airflow limitation was found in 33% and a high RV% in about 20%. A particular gene mutation may be responsible for susceptibility to pulmonary complications [397]. A subsequent study of 150 consecutive patients with type 1 GD only found pulmonary impairment in five of them (3%). The patients exhibited a restrictive defect, low gas transfer and pulmonary infiltrates on chest radiography [398]. Treatment had been with enzyme therapy that had not improved lung function or the concomitant pulmonary hypertension, despite reducing the visceral organomegaly [399].

A case study of Niemann–Pick disease with pulmonary involvement identified by basal infiltrates on chest radiograph found no evidence of airflow limitation but a profoundly low transfer factor [400]. Whole lung lavage in one case improved oxygenation [401].

41.23.4 Familial dysautonomia (Riley–Day syndrome)

This inherited condition affects the autonomic nervous system and can impair ventilatory control. A small study found some of these patients had elevated resting CO_2 levels despite an increased ventilatory response to CO_2 [402]. This indicated that chemosensitivity was still intact with a high gain that led to episodes of periodic breathing. In a more recent study of 26 cases the elevated end tidal CO_2 was confirmed, also the normal hyperoxic response to CO_2 [403]. However, the ventilatory response to hypoxia was severely blunted with central depression, bradypnoea and hypotension.

41.23.5 Obesity

Morbid obesity affects lung function due to changes in chest wall compliance and the presence of fat in and around the thorax, see Section 41.7.7.

41.24 Non-pulmonary infection

41.24.1 Septicaemia

Sepsis syndrome is a profound cause of acute lung injury. See Section 41.12.

41.24.2 Botulinism, Tetanus

These infections involve the lungs by interfering with neuromuscular transmission. In a study of 34 patients with botulism, pulmonary complications were found in over 85% of cases [404]. Hypoventilatory respiratory failure was present in a third of them whilst in 9 patients there was aspiration pneumonia. On long-term follow up, nearly half the cases remained dyspnoeic but with only minor pulmonary function changes. In another study of 13 patients who were assessed 2 years after botulism there was evidence of residual respiratory muscle weakness (low P_{I}max) in four of them [405]. In these post botulism patients the average maximal exercise workload and O_2 consumption were reduced compared to controls. The reasons included poor fitness and poor motivation.

41.25 Endocrine disease

41.25.1 Thyroid disease

Thyroid disease is the commonest cause for upper airway obstruction [2] (Section 41.2). In addition, both uncontrolled hyperthyroidism and myxoedma can cause heart failure and this can also affect lung function (Section 41.18). The deleterious effect of hyperthyroidism on patients with asthma has long been recognised and β-adrenergic responsiveness has been shown to be inversely related to the prevailing level of thyroid hormone [406]. However, artificially induced hyperthyroidism in normal subjects taking triiodothyronine did not affect bronchial responsiveness to methacholine [407].

In hyperthyroidism dyspnoea can be due to airflow obstruction, weakness of respiratory muscles, heart failure and other factors. One or other of these variables is likely to be the cause underlying a reduction in exercise capacity. In one study of 15 patients the maximal oxygen uptake was on average 53% (range 26–66) of predicted value with the majority stopping due to dyspnoea [408]. No increase in airway reactivity was found but respiratory muscle weakness was observed. This has been confirmed in subsequent studies [409, 410] which showed that weakness was the cause for reduced lung volumes (VC, IC, TLC). Diaphragm strength [411] and forced and static lung volumes improved after therapy [409–411].

In myxoedema body weight is increased and sleep apnoea is common. In a small series the apnoea was reduced on thyroxine treatment even in the absence of weight reduction [412].

41.25.2 Acromegaly

In acromegaly the lung size (FVC and TLC) is usually increased by about 15% above predicted value [413]. This increase is due to additional growth of the lungs rather than to hyperinflation [414] or increased inspiratory muscle strength [415]; indeed the strength tends to be reduced. One study found pulmonary distensibility to be normal despite large lungs [416]; the finding suggested that lung growth was achieved by an increased number of alveoli rather than an increase in alveolar size. Lung compliance tends to be increased with normal gas transfer after allowance has been made for lung size [417, 418]; a way for doing this is in Footnote 20.2, page 251.

Acromegalics can develop kyphosis and goitre, both of which independently affect lung function. Upper airway obstruction (UAO) was the most common abnormality found in a series of 35 subjects with acromegaly [419]. Obstruction was much more prevalent in men than women, a gender difference similar to that found for the effect of goitre on UAO [2].

41.25.3 Carcinoid syndrome

The condition arises from a carcinoid tumour of the bowel with liver metastases that secrete excessive amounts of pharmacologically active substances including serotonin, histamine and kinins. These agents enter the pulmonary circulation, adversely affect the right heart and can cause wheeze, flushing and gastrointestinal upset. The pulmonary aspects of this condition are usually only important in the context of anaesthetic practice if surgical procedures are to be undertaken [420].

41.25.4 Hypopituitarism

Hypopituitarism reduces the internal secretion of hormones, including growth hormone. In children this leads to impaired lung function with reductions in P_{I}max and P_{E}max that can persist into adult life [421]. In that study VC, FRC and TLC were reduced but RV, FEV_1% and gas transfer were normal. The reduction in lung volumes was not correlated to reduced muscle strength suggesting that reduced lung growth might be involved. An earlier study on children with hypopituitarism found that after treatment with growth hormone (GH) the lung function was appropriate for achieved height but not for age [422].

In adults who developed growth hormone deficiency only a small difference in FEV_1% was found [423] and when the GH was replaced there was no change in any aspect of lung function, including muscle strength, static and dynamic lung volumes and indices of tidal volume.

41.26 Toxicity from therapy

The lungs are affected by numerous pharmaceutical agents that can cause acute lung injury syndrome from liberation of free radicals (Section 41.12). The substances include: busulphan, bleomycin, amiodarone, methotrexate, nitrofurantoin, paraquat and radiotherapy (see Table 40.3, page 554). With a view to preventing damage to the lungs prophylactic monitoring of the lung function is sometimes carried out, but in two instances as least this appears not to have been cost effective.

41.26.1 Methotrexate

Methotrexate is used to suppress rheumatoid arthritis, psoriasis and related conditions. It may cause pneumonitis that is associated with cough, dyspnoea, fever, hypoxaemia and diffuse interstitial infiltrate on the chest radiograph [424]. In a prospective study of 124 patients 3% developed the complication. They experienced symptoms, a restrictive defect and reduced transfer factor. However, no test was found that predicted the onset of complications. Patients who received the drug but did not have symptoms only had minimal reductions ($<5\%$) in FVC, FEV_1 and transfer factor [425]. Thus, the case for prospective monitoring appears not to be strong. Cessation of methotrexate after the appearance of symptoms usually leads to improvement in lung function but further decline can occur and lung function does not necessarily return to normal [426].

41.26.2 Amiodarone

Amiodarone is used to control problematic cardiac dysrhythmias including atrial fibrillation and ventricular tachycardia. Pulmonary toxicity can occur in up to 10% of patients on high dosage (more than 400 mg day^{-1}) and 1.6% on conventional dosage [427]. The toxicity takes the form of hypersensitivity pneumonitis early in the course of therapy (Section 41.15.2) or interstitial fibrosis that starts later. Large prospective studies of lung function have not found any reliable predictor of toxicity [428, 429]. A reduction in transfer factor of 20% was a sensitive diagnostic criterion for toxicity but smaller reductions did not predict future toxicity. Thus, the best strategy is to measure the lung function at the onset of therapy, then repeat the tests if symptoms develop or the chest radiograph changes.

41.27 References

1. Miller D, Hyatt RE. Obstructing lesions of the larynx and trachea: clinical and physiological characteristics. *Mayo Clin Proc* 1969; **44**: 145–161.
2. Miller MR, Pincock AC, Oates GD et al. Upper airway obstruction due to goitre: detection, prevalence and results of surgical management. *Q J Med* 1990; **274**: 177–188.
3. Empey DW. Assessment of upper airways obstruction. *Br Med J* 1972; **3**: 503–505.
4. Bergeron D, Cormier Y, Desmeules M. Tracheobronchopathia osteochondroplastica. *Am Rev Respir Dis* 1976; **114**: 803–806.
5. Roberts HR, Wells AU, Milne DG et al. Airflow obstruction in bronchiectasis: correlation between computed tomography features and pulmonary function tests. *Thorax* 2000; **55**: 198–204.
6. Loubeyre P, Paret M, Revel D et al. Thin-section CT detection of emphysema associated with bronchiectasis and correlation with pulmonary function tests. *Chest* 1996; **109**: 360–365.
7. Koulouris NG, Retsou S, Kosmas E et al. Tidal expiratory flow limitation, dyspnoea and exercise capacity in patients with bilateral bronchiectasis. *Eur Respir J* 2003; **21**: 743–748.
8. Pang J, Chan HS, Sung JY. Prevalence of asthma, atopy, and bronchial hyperreactivity in bronchiectasis: a controlled study. *Thorax* 1989; **44**: 948–951.
9. Bahous J, Cartier A, Pineau L et al. Pulmonary function tests and airway responsiveness to methacholine in chronic bronchiectasis of the adult. *Bull Eur Physiopathol Respir* 1984; **20**: 375–380.
10. Ip M, Lam WK, So SY et al. Analysis of factors associated with bronchial hyperreactivity to methacholine in bronchiectasis. *Lung* 1991; **169**: 43–51.
11. Packe GE, Hodson ME. Changes in spirometry during consecutive admissions for infective pulmonary exacerbations in adolescent and adult cystic fibrosis. *Respir Med* 1992; **86**: 445–48.
12. Corey M, Edwards L, Levison H, Knowles M. Longitudinal analysis of pulmonary function decline in patients with cystic fibrosis. *J Pediatr* 1997; **131**: 809–814.
13. Moorcroft AJ, Dodd ME, Webb AK. Long-term changes in exercise capacity, body mass, and pulmonary function in adults with cystic fibrosis. *Chest* 1997; **111**: 338–343.
14. Wong EB, Regnis J, Shnier RC et al. The relationship between tests of lung function and three chest radiological scoring systems in patients with cystic fibrosis. *Australas Radiol* 1993; **37**: 265–269.
15. Rosenberg SM, Howatt WF, Grum CM. Spirometry and chest roentgenographic appearance in adults with cystic fibrosis. *Chest* 1992; **101**: 961–964.
16. Lebecque P, Stanescu D. Respiratory resistance by the forced oscillation technique in asthmatic children and cystic fibrosis patients. *Eur Respir J* 1997; **10**: 891–895.
17. Mellis CM, Levison H. Bronchial reactivity in cystic fibrosis. *Pediatrics* 1978; **61**: 446–450.
18. Van Haren EH, Lammers JW, Festen J et al. The effects of the inhaled corticosteroids budesonide on lung function and bronchial hyperresponsiveness in adult patients with cystic fibrosis. *Respir Med* 1995; **89**: 209–214.
19. Aurora P, Bush A, Gustafsson P et al. Multiple-breath washout as a marker of lung disease in preschool children with cystic fibrosis. *Am J Respir Crit Care Med* 2005; **171**: 249–256.
20. Kraemer R, Blum A, Schibler A et al. Ventilation inhomogeneities in relation to standard lung function in patients with cystic fibrosis. *Am J Respir Crit Care Med* 2005; **171**: 371–378.
21. Cotton DJ, Graham BL, Mink JT, Habbick BF. Reduction of the single breath CO diffusing capacity in cystic fibrosis. *Chest* 1985; **87**: 217–222.
22. Espiritu JD, Ruppel G, Shrestha Y, Kleinhenz ME. The diffusing capacity in adult cystic fibrosis. *Respir Med* 2003; **97**: 606–611.
23. Lebecque P, Lapierre JG, Lamarre A, Coates AL. Diffusion capacity and oxygen desaturation on exercise in patients with cystic fibrosis. *Chest* 1987; **91**: 693–697.
24. Cotton DJ, Graham BL, Mink JT. Pulmonary diffusing capacity in adult cystic fibrosis: reduced positional changes are partially reversed by hyperoxia. *Clin Invest Med* 1990; **13**: 82–91.
25. Leung AN, Fisher K, Valentine V et al. Bronchiolitis-obliterans after lung transplantation: detection using expiratory HRCT. *Chest* 1998; **113**: 365–370.
26. Schlesinger C, Veeraraghavan S, Koss MN. Constructive (obliterative) bronchiolitis. *Curr Opin Pulm Med* 1998; **4**: 288–293.
27. Arakawa H, Webb CR. Air trapping on expiratory high-resolution CT scans in the absence of inspiratory scan abnormalities: correlation with pulmonary function tests and differential diagnosis. *Am J Roentgenol* 1998; **170**: 1349–1353.
28. King TE, Mortenson RL. Cryptogenic organising pneumonitis. The North American experience. *Chest* 1992; **102**: Suppl 1: 8S–13S.
29. Epler GR. Bronchiolitis obliterans organising pneumonia. *Semin Respir Infect* 1995; **10**: 65–77.
30. Boots RJ, McEvoy JD, Mowat P, Le Fevre I. Bronchiolitis obliterans organising pneumonia: a clinical and radiological review. *Aust N Z J Med* 1995; **25**: 140–145.
31. Ezri T, Kunichezky S, Eliraz A et al. Bronchiolitis obliterans - current concepts. *Q J Med* 1994; **87**: 1–10.
32. Tobin MJ, Cook PJ, Hutchinson DC. Alpha$_1$ antitrypsin deficiency: the clinical and physiological features of pulmonary emphysema in subjects homozygous for Pi type Z. A survey by the British Thoracic Association. *Br J Dis Chest* 1983; **77**: 14–27.
33. Wilson JS, Galvin JR. Normal diffusing capacity in patients with PiZ alpha$_1$-antitrypsin deficiency, severe airflow obstruction, and significant radiographic emphysema. *Chest* 2000; **118**: 867–871.
34. Guest PJ, Hansell DM. High resolution computed tomography (HRCT) in emphysema associated with alpha$_1$-antitrypsin deficiency. *Clin Radiol* 1992; **45**: 260–266.
35. Parr DG, Stoel BC, Stolk J, Stockley RA. Pattern of emphysema distribution in α_1-antitrypsin deficiency influences lung function impairment. *Am J Resp Crit Care Med* 2004; **170**: 1172–1178.
36. Santolicandro A, Prediletto R, Fornai E et al. Mechanisms of hypoxemia and hypocapnia in pulmonary embolism. *Am J Respir Crit Care Med* 1995; **152**: 336–347.
37. Kline JA, Kubin AK, Patel MM et al. Alveolar dead space as a predictor of severity of pulmonary embolism. *Acad Emerg Med* 2000; **7**: 611–617.

38. Manier G, Castaing Y. Influence of cardiac output on oxygen exchange in acute pulmonary embolism. *Am Rev Respir Dis* 1992; **145**: 130–136.
39. Jones JS, Neff TL, Carlson SA. Use of alveolar-arterial oxygen gradient in the assessment of acute pulmonary embolism. *Am J Emerg Med* 1998; **16**: 333–337.
40. Stein PD, Goldhaber SZ, Henry JW. Alveolar-arterial oxygen gradient in the assessment of acute pulmonary embolism. *Chest* 1995; **107**: 139–143.
41. Riedel M, Stanek V, Widimsky J. Spirometry and gas exchange in chronic pulmonary thromboembolism. . *Bull Eur Physiopathol Respir* 1981; **17**: 209–221.
42. Riedel M, Stanek V, Widimsky J, Prerovsky I. Longterm follow-up of patients with pulmonary thromboembolism. *Chest* 1982; **81**: 151–158.
43. Roger N, Xaubet A, Agusti C et al. Role of bronchoalveolar lavage in the diagnosis of fat embolism syndrome. *Eur Respir J* 1995; **8**: 1275–1280.
44. Fabian TC, Hoots AV, Stanford DS, Patterson CR, Mangiante EC. Fat embolism syndrome: prospective evaluation in 92 fracture patients. *Crit Care Med* 1990; **18**: 42–46.
45. Chan KM, Tham KT, Chiu HS et al. Post-traumatic fat embolism: its clinical and subclinical presentations. *J Trauma* 1984; **24**: 45–49.
46. Williams AG, Mettler FA, Christie JH, Gordon RE. Fat embolism syndrome. *Clin Nucl Med* 1986; **11**: 495–497.
47. Gaine SP, Rubin LJ. Primary pulmonary hypertension. *Lancet* 1998; 352: 719-725. Erratum *Lancet* 1999; **353**: 74.
48. Riley MS, Porszasz J, Engelen MP et al. Gas exchange responses to continuous incremental cycle ergometry in primary pulmonary hypertension in humans. *Eur J Appl Physiol* 2000; **83**: 63–70.
49. Wensel R, Opitz CF, Ewert R et al. Effects of ileoprost inhalation on exercise capacity and ventilatory efficiency in patients with primary pulmonary hypertension. *Eur Respir J* 2003; **22** (Suppl 45): 88s.
50. Miyamoto S, Nagaya N, Satoh T et al. Clinical correlates and prognostic significance of six–minute walk test in patients with primary pulmonary hypertension. Comparison with cardiopulmonary exercise testing. *Am J Respir Crit Care Med* 2000; **161**: 487–492.
51. Sun XG, Hansen JE, Oudiz RJ, Wasserman K. Pulmonary function in primary pulmonary hypertension. *J Am Coll Cardiol* 2003; **41**: 1028–1035.
52. Meyer FJ, Ewert R, Hoeper MM et al. Peripheral airway obstruction in primary pulmonary hypertension. *Thorax* 2002; **57**: 473–476.
53. Mandel J, Mark EJ, Hales C. Pulmonary veno-occlusive disease. *Am J Respir Crit Care Med* 2001; **162**: 1964–1973.
54. Maltby JD, Gouverne ML. CT findings in pulmonary venooclusive disease. *J Comput Assist Tomogr* 1984; **8**: 758–761.
55. Elliott CG, Colby TV, Hill T, Crapo RO. Pulmonary veno-occlusive disease associated with severe reduction in single-breath carbon monoxide diffusion capacity. *Respiration* 1988; **53**: 262–266.
56. Scheibel R, Dedeker K, Gleason D et al. Radiographic and angiographic characteristics of pulmonary veno-occlusive disease. *Radiology* 1972; **103**: 47–51.
57. Bailey CL, Channick RN, Auger WR et al. High probability perfusion lung scans in pulmonary venoocclusive disease. *Am J Respir Crit Care Med* 2001; **162**: 1974–1978.
58. Pennington DW, Gold WM, Gordon RL et al. Treatment of pulmonary arteriovenous malformations by therapeutic embolization. Rest and exercise physiology in eight patients. *Am Rev Respir Dis* 1992; **145**: 1047–1051.
59. Sapru RP, Hutchinson DC, Hall JI. Pulmonary hypertension in patients with pulmonary arteriovenous fistulae. *Br Heart J* 1969; **31**: 559–569.
60. Trell E, Johansson BW, Linell F, Ripa J. Familial pulmonary hypertension and multiple abnormalities of large systemic arteries in Osler's disease. *Am J Med* 1972; **53**: 50–63.
61. Trembath RC, Thomson JR, Machado RD et al. Clinical and molecular genetic features of pulmonary hypertension in patients with hereditary hemorrhagic telangiectasia. *New Eng J Med* 2001; **345**: 325–334.
62. Marschke G, Haber L, Feinberg M. Pulmonary talc embolization. *Chest* 1975; **68**: 824–826.
63. Diaz-Ruiz ML, Gallardo X, Castaner E et al. Cellulose granulomatosis of the lungs. *Eur Radiol* 1999; **6**: 1203–1204.
64. Soin JS, Wagner HN, Thomashaw D, Brown TC. Increased sensitivity of regional measurements in early detection of narcotic lung disease. *Chest* 1975; **67**: 325–330.
65. Overland ES, Nolan AJ, Hopewell PC. Alteration of pulmonary function in intravenous drug abusers. Prevalence, severity, and characterization of gas exchange abnormalities. *Am J Med* 1980; **68**: 231–237.
66. Estenne M, Yernault JC, De Troyer A. Mechanism of relief of dyspnoea after thoracentesis in patients with large pleural effusions. *Am J Med* 1983; **74**: 813–819.
67. Zerahn B, Jensen BV, Olsen F et al. The effect of thoracentesis on lung function and transthoracic electrical bioimpedance. *Respir Med* 1999; **93**: 196–201.
68. Lardinois D, Krueger T, Dusmet M et al. Pulmonary function testing after operative stabilisation of the chest wall for flail chest. *Eur J Cardiothorac Surg* 2001; **20**: 496–501.
69. Morshuis W, Folgering H, Barentsz J et al. Pulmonary function before surgery for pectus excavatum and at long term follow-up. *Chest* 1994; **105**: 1646–1652.
70. Haller JA, Loughlin GM. Cardiorespiratory function is significantly improved following corrective surgery for severe pectus excavatum. Proposed treatment guidelines. *J Cardiovasc Surg* 2000; **41**: 125–130.
71. Koumbourlis AC, Stolar CJ. Lung growth and function in children and adolescents with idiopathic pectus excavatum. *Pediatr Pulmonol* 2004; **38**: 339–343.
72. Lisboa C, Moreno R, Fava M et al. Inspiratory muscle function in patients with severe kyphoscoliosis. *Am Rev Respir Dis* 1985; **132**: 48–52.
73. Iozzo A, Cosentino P, Ghai PC, Garbagni R. Alveolar-arterial gradients and small airways in kyphoscoliosis. *Respiration* 1983; **44**: 314–320.
74. Secker-Walker RH, Ho JE, Gill IS. Observations on regional ventilation and perfusion in kyphoscoliosis. *Respiration* 1979; **38**: 194–203.
75. Wong CA, Cole AA, Watson L et al. Pulmonary function before and after anterior spinal surgery in adult idiopathic scoliosis. *Thorax* 1996; **51**: 534–536.
76. Graham EJ, Lenke LG, Lowe TG et al. Prospective pulmonary function evaluation following open thoracotomy for anterior spinal fusion in adolescent idiopathic scoliosis. *Spine* 2000; **25**: 2319–2325.
77. Buyse B, Meersseman W, Demedts M. Treatment of chronic respiratory failure in kyphoscoliosis: oxygen or ventilation? *Eur Respir J* 2003; **22**: 525–528.

78. Phillips MS, Miller MR, Kinnear WJ et al. Importance of airflow obstruction after thoracoplasty. *Thorax* 1987; **42**: 348–352.
79. O'Connor TM, O'Riordan DM, Stack M, Bredin CP. Airways obstruction in survivors of thoracoplasty: reversibility is greater in non-smokers. *Respirology* 2004; **9**: 130–133.
80. Van Noord JA, Cauberghs M, Van de Woestijne KP, Demedts M. Total respiratory resistance and reactance in ankylosing spondylitis and kyphoscoliosis. *Eur Respir J* 1991; **4**: 945–951.
81. Baydur A, Swank SM, Stiles CM, Sassoon CS. Respiratory elastic load compensation in anesthetized patients with kyphoscoliosis. *J Appl Physiol* 1989; **67**: 1024–1031.
82. Vanderschueren D, Decramer M, Van den Daele P, Dequeker J. Pulmonary function and maximal transrespiratory pressures in ankylosing spondylitis. *Ann Rheum Dis* 1989; **48**: 632–635.
83. Sahin G, Calikoglu M, Ozge C et al. Respiratory muscle strength but not BASFI score relates to diminished chest expansion in ankylosing spondylitis. *Clin Rheumatol* 2004; **23**: 199–202.
84. van der Esch M, van 't Hul AJ, Heijmans M, Dekker J. Respiratory muscle performance as a possible determinant of exercise capacity in patients with ankylosing spondylitis. *Aust J Physiother* 2004; **50**: 41–45.
85. Romagnoli I, Gigliotti F, Galarducci A et al. Chest wall kinematics and respiratory muscle action in ankylosing spondylitis patients. *Eur Respir J* 2004; **24**: 453–460.
86. Kress JP, Pohlman AS, Alverdy J, Hall JB. The impact of morbid obesity on oxygen cost of breathing (Vo_{2RESP}) at rest. *Am J Respir Crit Care Med* 1999; **160**: 883–886.
87. Holley HS, Mili-Emili J, Becklake MR et al. Regional distribution of pulmonary ventilation and perfusion in obesity. *J Clin Invest* 1967; **46**: 475–481.
88. Li AM, Chan D, Wong E et al. The effects of obesity on pulmonary function. *Arch Dis Child* 2003; **88**: 361–363.
89. Guerra S, Wright AL, Morgan WJ et al. Persistence of asthma symptoms during adolescence: role of obesity and age at the onset of puberty. *Am J Respir Crit Care Med* 2004; **170**: 78–85.
90. Sin DD, Jones RL, Man SF. Obesity is a risk factor for dyspnea but not for airflow obstruction. *Arch Intern Med* 2002; **162**: 1477–1481.
91. De Bruin VS, Machado C, Howard RS et al. Nocturnal and respiratory disturbances in Steele—Richardson–Oslzewski syndrome. *Postgrad Med* 1996; **72**: 293–296.
92. Bach JR. Management of post-polio respiratory sequelae. *Ann N Y Acad Sci* 1995; **753**: 96–102.
93. Lechtzin N, Wiener CM, Shade DM et al. Spirometry in the supine position improves the detection of diaphragmatic weakness in patients with amyotrophic lateral sclerosis. *Chest* 2002; **121**: 436–442.
94. Howard RS, Wiles CM, Loh L. Respiratory complications and their management in motor neuron disease. *Brain* 1989; **112**: 1155–1170.
95. Pinto A, de Carvalho M, Evangelista T et al. Nocturnal pulse oximetry: a new approach to establish the appropriate time for non-invasive ventilation in ALS patients. *Amyotrop Lateral Scler Other Motor Neuron Disord* 2003; **4**: 31–35.
96. Morgan RK, McNally S, Alexander M et al. Use of sniff nasal-inspiratory force to predict survival in amyotrophic lateral sclerosis. *Am J Respir Crit Care Med* 2005; **171**: 269–274.
97. Wilson SR, Quantz MA, Strong MJ, Ahmad D. Increasing peak flow time in amyotrophic lateral sclerosis. *Chest* 2005; **127**: 156–160.
98. Suarez AA, Pessolano FA, Monteiro SG et al. Peak flow and peak cough flow in the evaluation of expiratory muscle weakness and bulbar impairment in patients with neuromuscular disease. *Am J Phys Med Rehabil* 2002; **81**: 506–511.
99. Ropper AH, Kehne SM. Guillain–Barre syndrome: management of respiratory failure. *Neurology* 1985; **35**: 1662–1665.
100. Sharshar T, Chevret S, Bourdain F, Raphael JC; French Cooperative Group on Plasma Exchange in Guillain-Barre Syndrome. Early predictors of mechanical ventilation in Guillain–Barre syndrome. *Crit Care Med* 2003; **31**: 278–283.
101. Zifko U, Chen R, Remtulla H et al. Respiratory electrophysiological studies in Guillain-Barre syndrome. *J Neurol Neurosurg Psychiatry* 1996; **60**: 191–194.
102. Keenan SP, Alexander D, Road JD et al. Ventilatory muscle strength and endurance in myasthenia gravis. *Eur Respir J* 1995; **8**: 1130–1135.
103. Mier-Jedrzejowicz AK, Brophy C, Green M. Respiratory muscle function in myasthenia gravis. *Am Rev Respir Dis* 1988; **138**: 867–873.
104. Teixeira A, Cherin P, Demoule A et al. Diaphragmatic dysfunction in patients with idiopathic inflammatory myopathies. *Neuromuscul Disord* 2005; **15**: 32–9.
105. Braun NM, Arora NS, Rochester DF. Respiratory muscle and pulmonary function in polymyositis and other proximal myopathies. *Thorax* 1983; **38**: 616–623.
106. Fathi M, Dastmalchi M, Rasmussen E et al. Interstitial lung disease, a common manifestation of newly diagnosed polymyositis and dermatomyositis. *Ann Rheum Dis.* 2004; **63**: 297–301.
107. Flaherty KR, Wald J, Weisman IM et al. Unexplained exertional limitation. Characterization of patients with mitochondrial myopathy. *Am J Respir Crit Care Med* 2001; **164**: 425–432.
108. Haller RG, Lewis SF, Estabrook RW et al. Exercise intolerance, lactic acidosis, and abnormal cardiopulmonary regulation in exercise associated with adult skeletal muscle cytochrome c oxidase deficiency. *J Clin Invest* 1989; **84**: 155–161.
109. Mohr CH, Hill NS. Long-term follow-up of nocturnal ventilatory assistance in patients with respiratory failure due to Duchenne-type muscular dystrophy. *Chest* 1990; **97**: 91–96.
110. Murdoch BE, Chenery HJ, Bowler S, Ingram JC. Respiratory function in Parkinson's subjects exhibiting a perceptible speech deficit: a kinematic and spirometric analysis. *J Speech Hear Disord* 1989; **54**: 610–626.
111. Solomon NP, Hixon TJ. Speech breathing in Parkinson's disease. *J Speech Hear Res* 1993; **36**: 294–310.
112. Sabate M, Rodriguez M, Mendez E et al. Obstructive and restrictive pulmonary dysfunction increases disability in Parkinson disease. *Arch Phys Med Rehabil* 1996; **77**: 29–34.
113. Maria B, Sophia S, Michalis M et al. Sleep breathing disorders in patients with idiopathic Parkinson's disease. *Respir Med* 2003; **97**: 1151–1157.
114. McElvaney NG, Wilcox PG, Churg A, Fleetham JA. Pleuropulmonary disease during bromocriptine treatment of Parkinson's disease. *Arch Int Med* 1988; **148**: 2231–2236.
115. Fugl-Meyer AR, Linderholm H, Wilson AF. Restrictive ventilatory dysfunction in stroke: its relation to locomotor function. *Scand J Rehabil Med* 1983; **9** Suppl: 118–124.
116. Annoni JM, Ackermann D, Kesselring J. Respiratory function in chronic hemiplegia. *Int Disabil Stud* 1990; **12**: 78–80.
117. Cohen E, Mier A, Heywood P et al. Diaphragm movement in hemiplegic patients measured by ultrasonography. *Thorax* 1994; **49**: 890–895.
118. Lanini B, Bianchi R, Romagnoli I et al. Chest wall kinematics in patients with hemiplegia. *Am J Respir Crit Care Med* 2003; **168**: 109–113.

119. Buyse B, Demedts M, Meekers J et al. Respiratory dysfunction in multiple sclerosis: a prospective analysis of 60 patients. *Eur Respir J* 1997; **10**: 139–145.
120. Blair HT, Greenberg SB, Stevens PM et al. Effects of rhinovirus infection on pulmonary function of healthy human volunteers. *Am Rev Respir Dis* 1976; **114**: 95–102.
121. Hall WJ, Douglas RG Jr, Hyde RW et al. Pulmonary mechanics after uncomplicated influenza A infection. *Am Rev Respir Dis* 1976; **113**:141–148.
122. Collier AM, Pimmel RL, Hasselblad V et al. Spirometric changes in normal children with upper respiratory infections. *Am Rev Respir Dis* 1978; **117**: 47–53.
123. Jenkins CR, Breslin AB. Upper respiratory tract infections and airway reactivity in normal and asthmatic subjects. *Am Rev Respir Dis* 1984; **130**: 879–883.
124. Empey DW, Laitinen LA, Jacobs L et al. Mechanisms of bronchial hypereactivity in normal subjects after upper respiratory tract infection. *Am Rev Respir Dis* 1976; **113**: 131–139.
125. Williamson HA Jr. Pulmonary function tests in acute bronchitis: evidence of reversible airway obstruction. *J Fam Pract* 1987; **25**: 251–256.
126. Huchon G, Woodhead M. European study on community-acquired pneumonia committee statement. Guidelines for management of adult community-acquired lower respiratory tract infections. *Eur Respir J* 1998; **11**: 986–991.
127. American Thoracic Society Statement. Guidelines for the initial management of adults with community-acquired pneumonia: diagnosis, assessment of severity, and initial antimicrobial therapy. *Am Rev Respir Dis* 1993; **148**: 1418–1426.
128. Kvale PA, Rosen MJ, Hopewell PC et al. A decline in pulmonary diffusing capacity does not indicate opportunistic lung disease in asymptomatic persons infected with the human immunodeficiency virus. *Am Rev Respir Dis* 1993; **148**: 390–395.
129. Mitchell DM, Fleming J, Harris JR, Shaw RJ. Serial pulmonary function tests in the diagnosis of P. carinii pneumonia. *Eur Respir J* 1993; **6**: 823–827.
130. Nelsing S, Jensen BN, Backer V. Persistent reduction in lung function after Pneumocystis carinii pneumonia in AIDS patients. *Scand J Infect Dis* 1995; **27**: 351–355.
131. Dreyer G, Burrel LST. The vital capacity constants applied to the study of pulmonary tuberculosis. *Lancet* 1920; **i**: 1212–1216; also *Lancet* 1922; **ii**: 374–376.
132. Hnizdo E, Singh T, Churchyard G. Chronic pulmonary function impairment caused by initial and recurrent pulmonary tuberculosis following treatment. *Thorax* 2000; **55**: 32–38.
133. Long R, Maycher B, Dhar A et al. Pulmonary tuberculosis treated with directly observed therapy: serial changes in lung structure and function. *Chest* 1998; **113**: 933–943.
134. Kimura H, Suda A, Sakuma T et al. Nocturnal oxyhemoglobin desaturation and prognosis in chronic obstructive pulmonary disease and late sequelae of pulmonary tuberculosis. *Intern Med* 1998; **37**: 354–359.
135. Brander PE, Salmi T, Partinen M, Sovijarvi AR. Nocturnal oxygen saturation and sleep quality in long-term survivors of thoracoplasty. *Respiration* 1993; **60**: 325–331.
136. Jackson M, Smith I, King M, Shneerson J. Long term non-invasive domiciliary assisted ventilation for respiratory failure following thoracoplasty. *Thorax* 1994; **49**: 915–919.
137. Alkrinawi S, Pianosi P. Pulmonary function following blastomycosis in childhood. *Clin Pediatr* 2000; **39**: 27–31.
138. Ploysongsang Y, Schonfeld SA. Pulmonary function studies in diffuse pulmonary North American blastomycosis. *Am Rev Respir Dis* 1983; **128**: 1095–1098.
139. Kritski AL, Lemle A, de Souza GR et al. Pulmonary function changes in the acute stage of histoplasmosis, with follow-up . An analysis of eight cases. *Chest* 1990; **97**: 1244–1245.
140. Lemle A, Wanke B, Miranda JL et al. Pulmonary function in paracoccidioidomycosis (South American blastomycosis). Analysis of the obstructive defect. *Chest* 1983; **83**: 827–828.
141. Larsen RA, Jacobson JA, Morris AH, Benowitz BA. Acute respiratory failure caused by primary pulmonary coccidioidomycosis. Two case reports and a review of the literature. *Am Rev Respir Dis* 1985; **131**: 797–799.
142. Meyer KC, McManus FJ, Maki DG. Overwhelming pulmonary blastomycosis associated with adult respiratory distress syndrome. *N Eng J Med* 1993; **329**: 1231–1236.
143. Ashbaugh DG, Bigelow DB, Petty TL, Levine BE. Acute respiratory distress in adults. *Lancet* 1967; **2**: 319–323.
144. Bernard GR, Artigas A, Brigham KL et al. The American-European consensus conference on ARDS: definitions, mechanisms, relevant outcomes, and clinical trial coordination. *Am J Respir Crit Care Med* 1994; **149**: 818–824.
145. Sartori C, Matthay MA. Alveolar epithelial fluid transport in acute lung injury: new insights. *Eur Respir J* 2002; **20**: 1299–1313.
146. Wiener-Kronish JP, Gropper MA, Matthay MA. The adult respiratory distress syndrome: definition and prognosis, pathogenesis and treatment. *Br J Anaesth* 1990; **65**: 107–129.
147. Nunes S, Uusaro A, Takala J. Pressure-volume relationships in acute lung injury: methodological and clinical implications. *Acta Anaesthesiol Scand* 2004; **48**: 278–286.
148. Dauber IM, Pluss WT, van Grondelle A et al. Specificity and sensitivity of non-invasive measurement of pulmonary protein leak. *J Appl Physiol* 1985; **59**: 564–574.
149. O'Brodovitch H, Coates G. Pulmonary clearance of ^{99m}Tc-DTPA: a non-invasive assessment of epithelial integrity. *Lung* 1987; **165**: 1–17.
150. Barrowcliffe MP, Zanelli GD, Jones JG. Pulmonary clearance of radiotracers after positive end-expiratory pressure or acute lung injury. *J Appl Physiol* 1989; **66**: 288–294.
151. Jones JG, Lawler JCW, Minty BD et al. Increased alveolar permeability in cigarette smokers. *Lancet* 1980; **i**: 66–68.
152. Schuster DP, Anderson C, Kozlowski J, Lange N. Regional pulmonary perfusion in patients with acute pulmonary edema. *J Nucl Med* 2002; **43**: 863–870.
153. Hert R, Albert RK. Sequelae of the adult respiratory distress syndrome. *Thorax* 1994; **49**: 8–13.
154. Elliott CG, Morris AH, Cengiz M. Pulmonary function and exercise gas exchange in survivors of the adult respiratory distress syndrome. *Am Rev Respir Dis* 1981; **123**: 492–495.
155. Weinart CR, Gross CR, Kangas JR et al. Health related quality of life after acute lung injury. *Am J Respir Crit Care Med* 1997; **156**: 1120–1128.
156. Ghio A, Elliott C, Crapo R et al. Impairment after adult respiratory distress syndrome. An evaluation based on American Thoracic Society recommendations. *Am Rev Respir Dis* 1989; **139**: 1158–1162.
157. Peters JI, Bell RC, Prihoda TJ et al. Clinical determinants of abnormalities in pulmonary functions in survivors of the adult respiratory distress syndrome. *Am Rev Respir Dis* 1989; **139**: 1163–1168.

158. McHugh LG, Milberg JA, Whitcomb ME et al. Recovery of function in survivors of acute respiratory distress syndrome. *Am J Respir Crit Care Med* 1994; **150**: 90–94.
159. Brooks SM, Weiss MA, Bernstein IL. Reactive airways dysfunction syndrome (RADS): persistent asthma syndrome after high level irritant exposures. *Chest* 1985; **88**: 376–384.
160. Fein A, Leff A, Hopewell PC. Pathophysiology and management of the complications resulting from fire and the inhaled products of combustion: review of the literature. *Crit Care Med* 1980; **8**: 94–98.
161. Kinsella J, Carter R, Reid WH et al Increased airways reactivity after smoke inhalation. *Lancet* 1991; **337**: 595–597.
162. Landa J, Avery WC, Sackner MA. Some physiologic observations in smoke inhalation. *Chest* 1972; **61**: 62–64.
163. Whitener DR, Whitener KM, Robertson KJ et al. Pulmonary function measurements in patients with thermal injury and smoke inhalation. *Am Rev Respir Dis* 1980; **122**: 731–739.
164. Kehrl HR, Vincent LW, Kowalsky RJ et al. Ozone exposure increases respiratory epithelial permeability in humans. *Am Rev Respir Dis* 1987; **135**: 1124–1128.
165. Hazucha MJ, Bates DV, Bromberg BA. Mechanism of action of ozone on the human lung. *J Appl Physiol* 1989; **67**: 1535–1541.
166. Horstman DH, Folinsbee LJ, Ives PJ et al. Ozone concentration and pulmonary response relationships for 6.6 hour exposures with 5 hours of moderate exercise to 0.08, 0.10, and 0.12 ppm. *Am Rev Respir Dis* 1990; **142**: 1158–1163.
167. Sandstrom T. Respiratory effects of air pollutants: experimental studies in humans. *Eur Respir J* 1995; **8**: 976–995.
168. Segev D, Szold O, Fireman E et al. Kerosene-induced severe acute respiratory failure in near drowning: reports on four cases and review of the literature. *Crit Care Med* 1999; **27**: 1437–1440.
169. Pujol JL, Barneon G, Bousquet J et al. Interstitial pulmonary disease induced by occupational exposure to paraffin. *Chest* 1990; **97**: 234–236.
170. Tashkin DP, Simmons MS, Sherrill DL, Coulson AH. Heavy habitual marijuana smoking does not cause an accelerated decline in FEV_1 with age. *Am J Respir Crit Care Med* 1997; **155**: 141–148.
171. Taylor DR, Fergusson DM, Milne BJ et al. A longitudinal study of the effects of tobacco and cannabis exposure on lung function in young adults. *Addiction* 2002; **97**: 1055–1061.
172. Tashkin DP, Coulson AH, Clark VA et al. Respiratory symptoms and lung function in habitual heavy smokers of marijuana alone, smokers of marijuana and tobacco, smokers of tobacco alone, and nonsmokers. *Am Rev Respir Dis* 1987; **135**: 209–216.
173. Renaud AM, Cormier Y. Acute effects of marihuana smoking on maximal exercise performance. *Med Sci Sports Exerc* 1986; **18**: 685–689.
174. Gil E, Chen B, Kleerup E et al. Acute and chronic effects of marijuana smoking on pulmonary alveolar permeability. *Life Sci* 1995; **56**: 2193–2199.
175. Tashkin DP, Simmons MS, Coulson AH et al. Respiratory effects of cocaine "freebasing" among habitual uses of marijuana with or without tobacco. *Chest* 1987; **92**: 638–644.
176. Tashkin DP, Khalsa ME, Gorelick D et al. Pulmonary status of habitual cocaine smokers. *Am Rev Respir Dis* 1992; **145**: 92–100.
177. Weiss RD, Tilles DS, Goldenheim PD, Mirin SM. Decreased single breath carbon monoxide diffusing capacity in cocaine freebase smokers. *Drug Alcohol Depend* 1987; **19**: 271–276.
178. Susskind H, Weber DA, Volkow ND, Hitzemann R. Increased lung permeability following long-term use of free-base cocaine (crack). *Chest* 1991; **100**: 903–909.
179. Kleerup EC, Koyal SN, Marques-Magallanes JA et al. Chronic and acute effects of "crack" cocaine on diffusing capacity, membrane diffusion, and pulmonary capillary blood volume in the lung. *Chest* 2002; **122**: 629–638.
180. Tashkin DP. Airway effects of marijuana, cocaine, and other inhaled illicit agents. *Curr Opin Pulm Med* 2001; **7**: 43–61.
181. Folgering H. The pathophysiology of hyperventilation syndrome. *Monaldi Arch Chest Dis* 1999; **54**: 365–372.
182. Hornsveld H, Garssen B, Dop MJ et al. Double-blind placebo-controlled study of the hyperventilation provocation test and the validity of the hyperventilation syndrome. *Lancet* 1996; **348**: 154–158.
183. Vansteenkiste J, Rochette F, Demedts M. Diagnostic tests of hyperventilation syndrome. *Eur Respir J* 1991; **4**: 393–399.
184. Saisch SG, Wessely S, Gardner WN. Patients with acute hyperventilation presenting to an inner-city emergency department. *Chest* 1996; **110**: 952–957.
185. Radwan L, Grebska E, Koziorowski A. Small airways function in pulmonary sarcoidosis. *Scan J Respir Dis* 1978; **59**: 37–43.
186. Argyropoulou PK, Patakas DA, Louridas GE. Airway function in stage I and stage II pulmonary sarcoidosis. *Respiration* 1984; **46**: 17–25.
187. Miller A, Chuang M, Teirstein AS, Siltzbach LE. Pulmonary function in stage I and II pulmonary sarcoidosis. *Ann N Y Acad Sci* 1976; **278**: 292–300.
188. Saumon G, Georges R, Loiseau A, Turiaf J. Membrane diffusing capacity and pulmonary capillary blood volume in pulmonary sarcoidosis. *Ann N Y Acad Sci* 1976; **278**: 284–291.
189. Magkanas E, Voloudaki A, Bouros D et al. Pulmonary sarcoidosis. Correlation of expiratory high-resolution CT findings with inspiratory patterns and pulmonary function tests. *Acta Radiol* 2001; **42**: 494–501.
190. Davies CW, Tasker AD, Padley SP et al. Air trapping in sarcoidosis on computer tomography: correlation with lung function. *Clin Radiol* 2000; **55**: 217–221.
191. Harrison BD, Shaylor JM, Stokers TC, Wilkes AR. Airflow limitation in sarcoidosis - a study of pulmonary function in 107 patients with newly diagnosed disease. *Respir Med* 1991; **85**: 59–64.
192. Stjernberg N, Thunell M. Pulmonary function in patients with endobronchial sarcoidosis. *Act Med Scand* 1984; **215**: 121–126.
193. Dines DE, Stubbs SE, McDougall JC. Obstructive disease of the airways associated with stage I sarcoidosis. *Mayo Clin Proc* 1978; **53**: 788–791.
194. Karetzky M, McDonaough M. Exercise and resting pulmonary function in sarcoidosis. *Sarcoidosis Vasc Diffuse Lung Dis* 1996; **13**: 43–49.
195. Baydur A, Alsalek M, Louie SG, Sharma OP. Respiratory muscle strength, lung function, and dyspnoea in patients with sarcoidosis. *Chest* 2001; **120**: 102–108.
196. Sovijarvi ARA, Kuusisto P, Muittari A, Kauppinen-Walin K. Trapped air in extrinsic allergic alveolitis. *Respiration* 1980; **40**: 57–64.
197. Remy-Jardin M, Remy J, Wallaert B, Muller NL. Subacute and chronic bird breeder hypersensitivity pneumonitis: sequential evaluation with CT and correlation with lung function tests and bronchoalveolar lavage. *Radiology* 1993; **189**: 111–118.

198. Sansores R, Perez-Padilla R, Pare PD, Selman M. Exponential analysis of the lung pressure-volume curve in patients with chronic pigeon-breeder's lung. *Chest* 1992; **101**: 1352–1356.
199. Bourke SJ, Carter R, Anderson K et al. Obstructive airways disease in non-smoking subjects with pigeon fanciers' lung. *Clin Exp Allergy* 1989; **19**: 629–632.
200. Schmidt CD, Jensen RL, Christensen LT et al. Longitudinal pulmonary function changes in pigeon breeders. *Chest* 1988; **93**: 359–363.
201. Ramirez-Venegas A, Sansores RH, Perez-Padilla R et al. Utility of a provocation test for diagnosis of chronic pigeon breeder's disease. *Am J Respir Crit Care Med* 1998; **158**: 862–869.
202. Geller DE, Kaplowitz H, Light MJ, Colin AA. Allergic bronchopulmonary aspergillosis in cystic fibrosis: reported prevalence, regional distribution, and patient characteristics. *Chest* 1999; **116**: 639–646.
203. Swyer PR, James GCW. Case of unilateral pulmonary emphysema. *Thorax* 1953; **8**: 133–136.
204. MacLeod VM. Abnormal transradiency of one lung. *Thorax* 1954; **9**: 147–153.
205. Moore AD, Godwin JD, Dietrich PA et al. Swyer-James syndrome: CT findings in eight patients. *Am J Roentgenol* 1992; **158**: 1211–1215.
206. Lucaya J, Gartner S, Garcia-Pena P et al. Spectrum of manifestations of Swyer-James-MacLeod syndrome. *J Comput Assist Tomogr* 1998; **22**: 592–597.
207. Avital A, Shulman DL, Bar-Yishay E et al. Differential lung function in an infant with Swyer-James syndrome. *Thorax* 1989; **44**: 298–302.
208. Ucan ES, Keyf AI, Aydilek R et al. Pulmonary alveolar microlithiasis: review of Turkish reports. *Thorax* 1993; **48**: 171–173.
209. Prakash UB, Barham SS, Rosenow EC et al. Pulmonary alveolar microlithiasis: a review including ultrastructural and pulmonary function studies. *Mayo Clin Proc* 1983; **58**: 290–300.
210. Freiberg DB, Young IH, Laks L et al. Improvement in gas exchange with nasal continual positive airways pressure in pulmonary alveolar microlithiasis. *Am Rev Respir Dis* 1992; **145**: 1215–1216.
211. Seymour JF, Presneill JJ. Pulmonary alveolar proteinosis. Progress in the first 44 years. *Am J Respir Crit Care Med* 2002; **166**: 215–235.
212. Goldstein LS, Kavaru MS, Curtis-McCarthy P et al. Pulmonary alveolar proteinosis: clinical features and outcomes. *Chest* 1998; **114**: 1357–1362.
213. Wang BM, Stern EJ, Schmidt RA, Pierson DJ. Diagnosing pulmonary alveolar proteinosis: a review and update *Chest* 1997; **111**: 460–466.
214. Murayama J, Fukuda K, Sato T et al. Pulmonary alveolar proteinosis. Xe-133 scintigraphic findings before and after bronchopulmonary lavage. *Clin Nucl Med* 1993; **18**: 123–125.
215. Delobbe A, Durieu J Dahamel A, Wallaert B. Determinants of survival in pulmonary Langerhans' cell granulomatosis. *Eur Respir J* 1996; **9**: 2002–2006.
216. Crausman RS, Jennings CA, Tuder RM et al. Pulmonary Histiocytosis X: pulmonary function and exercise pathophysiology. *Am J Respir Crit Care Med* 1996; **153**: 426–435.
217. Fartoukh M, Humbert M, Capron F et al. Severe pulmonary hypertension in Histiocytosis X. *Am J Respir Crit Care Med* 2000; **161**: 216–223.
218. Dawson J. Pulmonary tuberous sclerosis. *Q J Med* 1954; **23**: 113–145.
219. Carsillo T, Astrinidis A, Henske EP. Mutations in the tuberous sclerosis complex gene TSC2 are a cause of sporadic lymphangioleiomyomatosis. *Proc Natl Acad Sci USA* 2000; **97**: 6085–6090.
220. Lie JT, Miller RD, Williams DE. Cystic disease of the lungs in tuberous sclerosis: clinicopathologic correlation including body plethysmographic lung function tests. *Mayo Clin Proc* 1980; **55**: 547–553.
221. Castro M, Shepherd CW, Gomez MR et al. Pulmonary tuberous sclerosis. *Chest* 1995; **107**: 189–195.
222. Templeton PA, McLoud TC, Muller NL et al. Pulmonary lymphangioleiomyomatosis: CT and pathologic findings. *J Comput Assist Tomogr* 1989; **13**: 54–57.
223. Burger CD, Hyatt RE, Staats BA. Pulmonary mechanics in lymphangioleiomyomatosis. *Am Rev Respir Dis* 1991; **142**: 1030–1033.
224. Lazor R, Valeyre D, Lacronique J et al. Low initial KCO predicts rapid FEV_1 decline in pulmonary lymphangioleiomyomatosis. *Respir Med.* 2004; **98**: 536–541.
225. Taveira-DaSilva AM, Stylianou MP, Hedin CJ et al. Maximal oxygen uptake and severity of disease in lymphangioleiomyomatosis. *Am J Respir Crit Care Med.* 2003; **168**: 1427–1431.
226. Rosenberg DM, Weinberger SE, Fulmer JD et al. Functional correlates of lung involvement in Wegener's granulomatosis. Use of pulmonary function tests in staging and follow-up. *Am J Med* 1980; **69**: 387–394.
227. Daum TE, Specks U, Colby TV et al. Tracheobronchial involvement in Wegener's granulomatosis. *Am J Respir Crit Care Med* 1995; **151**: 522–526.
228. Bone RC, Vernon M, Sobonya RE, Rendon H. Lymphomatoid granulomatosis. Report of a case and review of the literature. *Am J Med* 1978; **65**: 709–716.
229. Pisani RJ, DeRemee RA. Clinical implications of the histopathologic diagnosis of pulmonary lymphomatoid granulomatosis. *Mayo Clin Proc* 1990; **65**: 151–163.
230. Ko GY, Byun JY, Choi BG, Cho SH. The vascular manifestations of Behçet's disease: angiographic and CT findings. *Br J Radiol* 2000; **73**: 1270–1274.
231. Basoglu T, Canbaz F, Bernay I, Danaci M. Bilateral pulmonary artery aneurysms in a patient with Behçet syndrome: evaluation with radionucleide angiography and V/Q lung scanning. *Clin Nucl Med* 1998; **23**: 735–738.
232. Ahonen AV, Stenius-Aarniala BS, Viljanen BC et al. Obstructive lung disease in Behçet's syndrome. *Scand J Respir Dis* 1978; **59**: 44–50.
233. Uysal H, Balevi S, Okudan N, Gokbel H. The relationship between HRCT and pulmonary function in Behcet's disease. *Lung* 2004; **182**: 9–14.
234. Wright PH, Buxton-Thomas M, Keeling PW, Kreel L. Adult idiopathic pulmonary haemosiderosis: a comparison of lung function changes and the distribution of pulmonary disease in patients with and without coeliac disease. *Br J Dis Chest* 1983; **77**: 282–292.
235. Wright PH, Menzies IS, Pounder RE, Keeling PW. Adult idiopathic pulmonary haemosiderosis and coeliac disease. *Q J Med* 1981; **50**: 95–102.
236. Beckerman RC, Taussig LM, Pinnas JL. Familial idiopathic pulmonary hemosiderosis. *Am J Dis Child* 1979; **133**: 609–611.
237. Allue X, Wise MB, Beaudry PH. Pulmonary function studies in idiopathic pulmonary haemosiderosis in children. *Am Rev Respir Dis* 1973; **107**: 410–415.

238. Frankel LR, Smith DW, Pearl RG, Lewiston NJ. Nitroglycerin-responsive pulmonary hypertension in idiopathic pulmonary hemosiderosis. *Am Rev Respir Dis* 1986; **133**: 170–172.
239. Cotes JE, Dabbs JM, Elwood PC et al. Iron-deficiency anaemia: its effect on transfer factor for the lung (diffusing capacity) and ventilation and cardiac frequency during sub-maximal exercise. *Clin Sci* 1972; **42**: 325–335.
240. Polange JA. Pulse oximetry: technical aspects of machine design. *Int Anesthesiol Clin* 1987; **25**: 137–175.
241. Park CM, Nagel RL. Sulfhemoglobinemia: clinical and molecular aspects. *N Eng J Med* 1984; **310**: 1579–1584.
242. Vichinsky EP, Neumayr LD, Earles AN et al. Causes and outcome of the acute chest syndrome in sickle cell disease. National Acute Chest Syndrome Study Group. *N Eng J Med* 2000; **342**: 1855–1865.
243. Aldrich TK, Dhuper SK, Patwa NS et al. Pulmonary entrapment of sickle cells: the role of regional hypoxia. *J Appl Physiol* 1996; **80**: 531–539.
244. Bellet PS, Kalinyak KA, Shukla R et al. Incentive spirometry to prevent acute pulmonary complications in sickle cell diseases. *N Eng J Med* 1995; **333**: 699–703.
245. Crawford MW, Speakman M, Carver ED, Kim PC. Acute chest syndrome shows a predilection for basal lung regions on the side of upper abdominal surgery. *Can J Anaesth* 2004; **51**: 707–711.
246. Emre U, Miller ST, Rao SP, Rao M. Alveolar-arterial oxygen gradient in acute chest syndrome of sickle cell disease. *J Pediatr* 1993; **123**: 272–275.
247. Bhalla M, Abboud MR, McLoud TC et al. Acute chest syndrome in sickle cell disease: CT evidence of microvascular occlusion. *Radiology* 1993; **187**: 45–49.
248. Santoli F, Zerah F, Vasile N et al. Pulmonary function in sickle cell disease with or without acute chest syndrome. *Eur Respir J* 1998; **12**: 1124–1129.
249. Koumbourlis AC, Hurlet-Jensen A, Bye MR. Lung function in infants with sickle cell disease. *Pediatr Pulmonol* 1997; **24**: 277–281.
250. Powars D, Weidman JA, Odom-Maryon T et al. Sickle cell chronic lung disease: prior morbidity and the risk of pulmonary failure. *Medicine* (Baltimore) 1988; **67**: 66–76.
251. Sylvester KP, Patey RA, Milligan P et al. Pulmonary function abnormalities in children with sickle cell disease. *Thorax* 2004; **59**: 67–70.
252. Kanj N, Shamseddine A, Gharzeddine W et al. Relation of ferritin levels to pulmonary function in patients with thalassaemia major and the acute effects of transfusion. *Eur J Haematol* 2000; **64**: 396–400.
253. Piatti G, Allegra L, Ambrosetti U et al. Beta-thalassaemia and pulmonary function. *Haematologica* 1999; **84**: 804–808.
254. Factor JM, Pottipati SR, Rappoport I et al. Pulmonary function abnormalities in thalassaemia major and the role of iron overload. *Am J Respir Crit Care Med* 1994; **149**: 1570–1574.
255. Luyt DK, Richards GA, Roode H et al. Thalassaemia: lung function with reference to iron studies and reactive oxidant status. *Pediatr Hematol Oncol* 1993; **10**: 13–23.
256. Isarangkura P, Chantarojanasiri T, Hathirat P et al. Pulmonary and platelet function in mild form Hb H disease. *Southeast Asian J Trop Med Public Health* 1993; **24**:(Suppl 1): 210–212.
257. Tai DY, Wang YT, Lou J et al. Lungs in thalassaemia major patients receiving regular transfusion. *Eur Respir J* 1996; **9**: 1389–1394.
258. Dimopoulou I, Kremastinos DT, Maris TG et al. Respiratory function in patients with thalassaemia and iron overload. *Eur Respir J* 1999; **13**: 602–605.
259. Freedman MH, Grisaru D, Olivieri N et al. Pulmonary syndrome in patients with thalassaemia major receiving intravenous deferoxamine infusions. *Am J Dis Child* 1990; **144**: 565–569.
260. Cooper DM, Mansell AL, Weiner MA et al. Low lung capacity and hypoxemia in children with thalassaemia major. *Am Rev Respir Dis* 1980; **121**: 639–646.
261. Andrews AT, Zmijewski CM, Bowman HS, Reihart JK. Transfusion reaction with pulmonary infiltration associated with HL-A-specific leukocyte antibodies. *Am J Clin Pathol* 1976; **66**: 483–487.
262. Gore EM, Lawton CA, Ash RC, Lipchik RJ. Pulmonary function changes in long-term survivors of bone marrow transplantation. *Int J Radiat Oncol Biol Pys* 1996; **36**: 67–75.
263. Fanfulla F, Locatelli F, Zoia MC et al. Pulmonary complications and respiratory function changes after bone marrow transplantation in children. *Eur Respir J* 1997; **10**: 2301–2306.
264. Curtis DJ, Smale A, Thien F et al. Chronic airflow obstruction in long-term survivors of allogeneic bone marrow transplantation. *Bone Marrow Transplant* 1995; **16**: 169–173.
265. Schultz KR, Green GJ, Wensley D et al. Obstructive lung disease in children after allogeneic bone marrow transplantation. *Blood* 1994; **84**: 3212–3220.
266. Schwarer AP, Hughes JM, Trotman-Dickenson B et al. A chronic pulmonary syndrome associated with graft-versus-host disease after allogeneic marrow transplantation. *Transplantation* 1992; **54**: 1002–1008.
267. Clark JG, Schwartz DA, Flournoy N et al. Risk factors for airflow obstruction in recipients of bone marrow transplants. *Ann Int Med* 1987; **107**: 648–656.
268. Chien JW, Martin PJ, Flowers ME et al. Implications of early airflow decline after myeloablative allogeneic stem cell transplantation. *Bone Marrow Transplant* 2004; **33**: 759–764.
269. Marras TK, Chan CK, Lipton JH et al. Long-term pulmonary function abnormalities and survival after allogeneic marrow transplantation. *Bone Marrow Transplant* 2004; **33**: 509–517.
270. Charoenratanakul S, Loasuthi K. Pseudohypoxaemia in a patient with leukaemia. *Thorax* 1997; **52**: 394–395.
271. Fox MJ, Brody JS, Weintraub LR. Leukocyte larceny: a cause of spurious hypoxaemia. *Am J Med* 1979; **67**: 742–746.
272. Bloom R, Taveira Da Silva AM, Bracey A. Reversible respiratory failure due to intravascular leukostasis in chronic myelogenous leukemia. Relationship of oxygen transfer to leukocyte count. *Am J Med* 1979; **67**: 679–683.
273. Jenney ME, Faragher EB, Jones PH, Woodcock A. Lung function and exercise capacity in survivors of childhood leukaemia. *Med Pediatr Oncol* 1995; **24**: 222–230.
274. Shaw NJ, Tweeddale PM, Eden OB. Pulmonary function in childhood leukaemia survivors. *Med Pediatr Oncol* 1989; **17**: 149–152.
275. Schunemann HJ, Dorn J, Grant BJ et al. Pulmonary function is a long-term predictor of mortality in the general population: 29-year follow up of the Buffalo Health Study. *Chest* 2000; **118**: 656–664.
276. Rhodes KM, Evemy K, Nariman S, Gibson GJ. Relation between severity of mitral valve disease and results of routine lung function tests in non-smokers. *Thorax* 1982; **37**: 751–755.
277. Dawson A, Rocamora JM, Morgan JR. Regional lung function in chronic pulmonary congestion with and without mitral stenosis. *Am Rev Respir Dis* 1976; **113**: 51–59.
278. Yernault J-C, De Troyer A. Mechanics of breathing in patients with aortic valve disease. *Bull Eur Physiopathol Respir* 1980; **16**: 491–499.

279. Ries AL, Gregoratos G, Friedman PJ, Clausen JL. Pulmonary function tests in the detection of left heart failure: correlation with pulmonary wedge pressure. *Respiration* 1986; **49**: 241–250.
280. Rolla G, Bucca C, Brussino L et al. Bronchodilating effect of ipratropium bromide in heart failure. *Eur Respir J* 1993; **6**: 1492–1495.
281. Yap JCH, Moore DM, Cleland JGF, Pride NB. Effect of supine posture on respiratory mechanics in chronic left heart failure. *Am J Respir Crit Care Med* 2000; **162**: 1285–1291.
282. Niset G, Ninane V, Antoine M, Yernault JC. Respiratory dysfunction in congestive heart failure: correction after heart transplantation. *Eur Respir J* 1993; **6**: 1197–1201.
283. Ravenscraft SA, Gross CR, Kubo SH et al. Pulmonary function after successful heart transplantation. One year follow-up. *Chest* 1993; **103**: 54–58.
284. Mustafa KY, Nour MM, Shuhaiber H, Yousof AM. Pulmonary function before and sequentially after valve replacement surgery with correlation to preoperative hemodynamic data. *Am Rev Respir Dis* 1984; **130**: 400–406.
285. Nishimura Y, Maeda H, Tanaka K et al. Respiratory muscle strength and hemodynamics in chronic heart failure. *Chest* 1994; **105**: 355–359.
286. Ambrosino N, Opasich C, Crotti P et al. Breathing pattern, ventilatory drive and respiratory muscle strength in patients with chronic heart failure. *Eur Respir J* 1994; **7**: 17–22.
287. Johnson BD, Beck KC, Olson LJ et al. Ventilatory constraints during exercise in patients with chronic heart failure. *Chest* 2000; **117**: 321–33.
288. McParland C, Krishnan B, Wang Y, Gallagher CG. Inspiratory muscle weakness and dyspnoea in chronic heart failure. *Am Rev Respir Dis* 1992; **146**: 467–472.
289. Sulc J, Samanek M, Zapletal A et al. Lung function in VSD patients after corrective heart surgery. *Pediatr Cardiol* 1996; **17**: 1–6.
290. Yau KI, Fang LJ, Wu MH. Lung mechanics in infants with left-to-right shunt congenital heart disease. *Pediatr Pulmonol* 1996; **21**: 42–47.
291. Hills EA, Geary M. Membrane diffusing capacity and pulmonary capillary volume in rheumatoid disease. *Thorax* 1980; **35**: 570–580.
292. Dawson JK, Fewins HE, Desmond J et al. Fibrosing alveolitis in patients with rheumatoid arthritis assessed by high resolution computed tomography, chest radiography, and pulmonary function tests. *Thorax* 2001; **56**: 622–627.
293. Perez T, Remy-Jardin M, Cortet B. Airways involvement in rheumatoid arthritis: clinical, functional, and HRTC findings. *Am J Respir Crit Care Med* 1998; **157**: 1658–1665.
294. Vergnenegre A, Pugnere N, Antonini MT et al. Airway obstruction and rheumatoid arthritis. *Eur Respir J* 1997; **10**: 1072–1078.
295. Begin R, Radoux V, Cantin A, Menard HA. Stiffness of the rib cage in a subset of rheumatoid patients. *Lung* 1988; **166**: 141–148.
296. Knook LM, de Kleer IM, van der Ent CK et al. Lung function and respiratory muscle weakness in children with juvenile chronic arthritis. *Eur Respir J* 1999; **14**: 529–533.
297. Gorini M, Ginanni R, Spinelli A et al. Inspiratory muscle strength and respiratory drive in patients with rheumatoid arthritis. *Am Rev Respir Dis* 1990; **142**: 289–294.
298. Chakravaty K, Webley M. A longitudinal study of pulmonary function in patients with rheumatoid arthritis treated with gold and D-penicillamine. *Br J Rheumatol* 1992; **31**: 829–833.
299. Geddes DM, Corrin B, Brewerton DA et al. Progressive airway obliteration in adults and its association with rheumatoid disease. *Q J Med* 1977; **46**: 427–444.
300. Turton CW, Williams G, Green M. Cryptogenic obliterative bronchiolitis in adults. *Thorax* 1981; **36**: 805–810.
301. Aquino SL, Webb CR, Golden J. Bronchiolitis obliterans associated with rheumatoid arthritis: findings on HRCT and dynamic expiratory CT. *J Comput Assist Tomogr* 1994; **18**: 555–558.
302. Warrington KJ, Moder KG, Brutinel WM. The shrinking lung syndrome in systemic lupus erythematosis. *Mayo Clin Proc* 2000; **75**: 467–472.
303. Hardy K, Herry I, Attali V et al. Bilateral phrenic paralysis in a patient with systemic lupus erythematosis. *Chest* 2001; **119**: 1274–1277.
304. Hawkins P, Davison AG, Dasgupta B, Moxham J. Diaphragm strength in acute systemic lupus erythematosis in a patient with paradoxical abdominal motion and reduced lung volumes. *Thorax* 2001; **56**: 329–330.
305. Forte S, Carlone S, Vaccaro F et al. Pulmonary gas exchange and exercise capacity in patients with systemic lupus erythematosis. *J Rheumatol* 1999; **26**: 2591–2594.
306. Scano G, Goti P, Duranti R et al. Control of breathing in a subset of patients with systemic lupus erythematosis. *Chest* 1995; **108**: 759–766.
307. Murin S, Wiedermann HP, Matthay RA. Pulmonary manifestations of systemic lupus erythematosis. *Clin Chest Med* 1998; **19**: 641–645.
308. Ooi GC, Ngan H, Peh WC et al. Systemic lupus erythematosis with respiratory symptoms: the value of HRCT. *Clin Radiol* 1997; **52**: 775–781.
309. Groen H, ter Borg EJ, Postma DS et al. Pulmonary function in systemic lupus erythematosis is related to distinct clinical, serologic, and nailfold capillary patterns. *Am J Med* 1992; **93**: 619–627.
310. Nakano M, Hasegawa H, Takada T et al. Pulmonary diffusion capacity in patients with systemic lupus erythematosus. *Respirology.* 2002; **7**: 45–49.
311. Pan TL, Thumboo J, Boey ML. Primary and secondary pulmonary hypertension in systemic lupus erythematosis. *Lupus* 2000; **9**: 338–342.
312. Papiris SA, Maniati M, Constantopoulos SH et al. Lung involvement in primary Sjogren's syndrome is mainly related to the small airway disease. *Ann Rheum Dis* 1999; **58**: 61–64.
313. Franquet T, Diaz C, Domingo P et al. Air trapping in primary Sjogren syndrome: correlation of expiratory CT with pulmonary function tests. *J Comput Assist Tomogr* 1999; **23**: 169–173.
314. La Corte R, Potena A, Bajocchi G et al. Increased bronchial responsiveness in primary Sjogren's syndrome. A sign of tracheobronchial involvement. *Clin Exp Rheumatol.* 1991; **9**: 125–130.
315. Gudbjornsson B, Hedenstrom H, Stalenheim G, Hallgren R. Bronchial hyperresponsiveness to methacholine in patients with primary Sjogren's syndrome. *Ann Rheum Dis* 1991; **50**: 36–40.
316. Lahdensuo A, Korpela M. Pulmonary findings in patients with primary Sjogren's syndrome. *Chest* 1995; **108**: 316–319.
317. Mialon P, Barthelemy L, Sebert P et al. A longitudinal study of lung impairment in patients with primary Sjogren's syndrome. *Clin Exp Rheumatol* 1997; **15**: 349–354.
318. Salaffi F, Manganelli P, Carotti M et al. A longitudinal study of pulmonary involvement in primary Sjogren's syndrome: relationship between alveolitis and subsequent lung changes on high-resolution computed tomography. *Br J Rheumatol* 1998; **37**: 263–269.
319. Spagnolatti L, Zoia MC, Volpini E et al. Pulmonary function in patients with systemic sclerosis. *Monaldi Arch Chest Dis* 1997; **52**: 4–8.

320. Kane GC, Varga J, Conant EF et al. Lung involvement in systemic sclerosis (scleroderma): relation to classification based on extent of skin involvement or autoantibody status. *Respir Med* 1996; **90**: 223–240.
321. Steen VD, Conte C, Owens GR, Medsger TA Jr. Severe restrictive lung disease in systemic sclerosis. *Arthritis Rheum* 1994; **37**: 1283–1289.
322. Kim EA, Johkoh T, Lee KS et al. Interstitial pneumonia in progressive systemic sclerosis: serial high-resolution CT findings with functional correlation. *J Comput Assist Tomogr* 2001; **25**: 757–763.
323. Marie I, Dominique S, Levesque H et al. Esophageal involvement and pulmonary manifestations in systemic sclerosis. *Arthritis Rheum* 2001; **45**: 346–354.
324. Schwaiblmair M, Behr J, Fruhmann G. Cardiorespiratory responses to incremental exercise in patients with systemic sclerosis. *Chest* 1996; **110**: 1520–1525.
325. Morelli S, Ferrante L, Sgreccia A et al. Pulmonary hypertension is associated with impaired exercise performance in patients with systemic sclerosis. *Scand J Rheumatol* 2000; **29**: 236–242.
326. Kon OM, Daniil Z, Black CM, du Bois RM. Clearance of inhaled technetium-99m-DTPA as a clinical index of pulmonary vascular disease in systemic sclerosis. *Eur Respir J* 1999; **13**: 133–136.
327. Konig P, Boxer R, Morrison J, Pletcher B. Bronchial hyperreactivity in children with Marfan syndrome. *Pediatr Pulmonol* 1991; **11**: 29–36.
328. Streeten EA, Murphy EA, Pyeritz RE. Pulmonary function in the Marfan syndrome. *Chest* 1987; **91**: 408–412.
329. Turner JA, Stanley NN. Fragile lung in the Marfan syndrome. *Thorax* 1976; **31**: 771–775.
330. Ayres JG, Pope FM, Reidy JF, Clark TJ. Abnormalities of the lungs and thoracic cage in the Ehlers-Danlos syndrome. *Thorax* 1985; **40**: 300–305.
331. Cavanaugh MJ, Cooper DM. Chronic pulmonary disease in a child with the Ehlers-Danlos syndrome. *Acta Paediatr Scand* 1976; **65**: 679–684.
332. Corbett E, Glaisyer H, Chan C et al. Congenital cutis laxa with a dominant inheritance and early onset emphysema. *Thorax* 1994; **49**: 836–837.
333. Mehregan AH, Lee SC, Nabai H. Cutis laxa (generalized elastolysis): a report of four cases with autopsy findings. *J Cutan Pathol* 1978; **5**: 116–126.
334. Rodriguez-Roisin R, Krowka MJ, Herve Ph et al. Pulmonary-hepatic vascular disorders (PHD). *Eur Respir J* 2004; **24**: 861–880.
335. Chao Y, Wang SS, Lee SD et al. Effect of large-volume paracentesis on pulmonary function in patients with cirrhosis and tense ascites. *J Hepatol* 1994; **20**: 101–105.
336. Angueira CE, Kadakia SC. Effects of large-volume paracentesis on pulmonary function in patients with tense ascites. *Hepatology* 1994; **20**: 825–828.
337. Berkowitz KA, Butensky MS, Smith RL. Pulmonary function changes after large volume paracentesis. *Am J Gastroenterol* 1993; **88**: 905–907.
338. Gupta D, Lalrothuama, Agrawal PN et al. Pulmonary function changes after large volume paracentesis. *Trop Gastroenterol* 2000; **21**: 68–70.
339. Chang SC, Chang HI, Chen FJ et al. Effects of ascites and body position on gas exchange in patients with cirrhosis. *Proc Natl Sci Counc Repub China B* 1995; **19**: 142–150.
340. Herve P, Lebrec D, Brenot F et al. Pulmonary vascular disorders in portal hypertension. *Eur Respir J* 1998; **11**: 1153–1166.
341. Castro M, Krowka MJ. Hepatopulmonary syndrome: a pulmonary vascular complication of liver disease. *Clin Chest Med* 1996; **17**: 35–48.
342. Rodriguez-Roisin R, Agusti AG, Roca J. The hepatopulmonary syndrome: new name, old complexities. *Thorax* 1992; **47**: 897–902.
343. Aller R, Moya JL, Avila S et al. Implications of estradiol and progesterone in pulmonary vasodilatation in cirrhotic patients. *J Endocrinol Invest* 2002; **25**: 4–10.
344. Gomez FP, Martinez-Palli G, Barbera JA et al. Gas exchange mechanism of orthodeoxia in hepatopulmonary syndrome. *Hepatology* 2004; **40**: 660–666.
345. Edell ES, Cortese DA, Krowka MJ, Rehder K. Severe hypoxaemia and liver disease. *Am Rev Respir Dis* 1989; **140**: 1631–1635.
346. Eriksson LS, Soderman C, Ericzon BG et al. Normalization of ventilation/perfusion relationships after liver transplantation in patients with decompensated cirrhosis: evidence for hepatopulmonary syndrome. *Hepatology* 1990; **12**: 1350–1357.
347. Ramsay MA, Simpson BR, Nguyen AT et al. Severe pulmonary hypertension in liver transplant candidates *Liver Transpl Surg* 1997; **3**: 494–500.
348. Kim WR, Krowka MJ, Plevak DJ et al. Accuracy of doppler echocardiography in the assessment of pulmonary hypertension in liver transplant candidates. *Liver Transpl* 2000; **6**: 453–458.
349. Wallace JG Jr, Tong MJ, Ueki BH, Quismorio FP. Pulmonary involvement in primary biliary cirrhosis. *J Clin Gastroenterol* 1987; **9**: 431–435.
350. Costa C, Sambataro A, Baldi S et al. Primary biliary cirrhosis: lung involvement. *Liver* 1995; **15**: 196–201.
351. Cazzato S, Bernardi F, Cinti C et al. Pulmonary function abnormalities in children with Henoch-Schonlein purpura. *Eur Respir J* 1999; **13**: 597–601.
352. Chaussain M, de Boissieu D, Kalifa G et al. Impairment of lung diffusing capacity in Schonlein-Henoch purpura. *J Pediatr* 1992; **121**: 12–16.
353. Greening AP, Hughes JM. Serial estimations of carbon monoxide diffusing capacity in intrapulmonary haemorrhage. *Clin Sci* 1981; **60**: 507–512.
354. Ferrer A, Roca J, Rodriguez-Roisin R et al. Bronchial reactivity in patients with chronic renal failure undergoing dialysis. *Eur Respir J* 1990; **3**: 387–391.
355. Metry G, Wegenius G, Wikstrom B et al. Lung density for assessment of hydration status in hemodialysis patients using the computed tomographic densitometry technique. *Kidney Int* 1997; **52**: 1635–1644.
356. Bazzi C, Amaducci S, Arrigo G et al. Bronchial responsiveness in patients on regular haemodialysis treatment of very long duration. *Am J Kidney Dis* 1994; **24**: 802–805.
357. Bush A, Gabriel R. Pulmonary function in chronic renal failure: effects of dialysis and transplantation. *Thorax* 1991; **46**: 424–428.
358. Herrero JA, Alvarez-Sala JL, Coronel F et al. Pulmonary diffusing capacity in chronic dialysis patients. *Respir Med* 2002; **96**: 487–492.
359. Beasley CR, Ripley JM, Smith DA, Ncalc TJ. Pulmonary function in chronic renal failure patients managed by continuous ambulatory peritoneal dialysis. *N Z Med J* 1986; **99**: 313–315.
360. Prezant DJ, Aldrich TK, Karpel JP, Lynn RI. Adaptations in the diaphragm's in vitro force-length relationship in patients on

continuous ambulatory peritoneal dialysis. *Am Rev Respir Dis* 1990; **141**: 1342–1349.

361. Pitcher WD, Diamond SM, Henrich WL. Pulmonary gas exchange during dialysis in patients with obstructive lung disease. *Chest* 1989; **96**: 1136–1141.
362. Fawcett S, Hoenich NA, Laker MF et al. Haemodialysis-induced respiratory changes. *Nephrol Dial Transplant* 1987; **2**: 161–168.
363. Mansfield LE, Stein MR. Gastro-oesophageal reflux and asthma: a possible reflex mechanism. *Ann Allergy* 1978; **41**: 224–226.
364. Andersen LI, Schmidt A, Bundagaard A. Pulmonary function and acid application in the oesophagus. *Chest* 1986; **90**: 358–363.
365. Wright RA, Millar SA, Corsello BF. Acid-induced oesophageal-bronchial-cardiac reflexes in humans. *Gastroenterol* 1990; **99**: 71–73.
366. Vincent D, Cohen-Jonathan AM, Leport J et al. Gastro-oesophageal reflux prevalence and relationship with bronchial reactivity in asthma. *Eur Respir J* 1997; **10**: 2255–2259.
367. Raiha IJ, Ivaska K, Sourander LB. Pulmonary function in gastro-oesophageal reflux disease of elderly people. *Age Aging* 1992; **21**: 368–373.
368. Swaminathan S, Quinn J, Stabile MW et al. Long-term pulmonary sequelae of meconium aspiration syndrome. *J Pediatr* 1989; **114**: 356–361.
369. Macfarlane PI, Heaf DP. Pulmonary function in children after neonatal meconium aspiration syndrome. *Arch Dis Child* 1988; **63**: 368–372.
370. Stevens JC, Eigen H, Wysomierski D. Absence of long term pulmonary sequelae after mild meconium aspiration syndrome. *Pediatr Pulmonol* 1988; **5**: 74–81.
371. Robertson DA, Traylor N, Sidhu H et al. Pulmonary permeability in coeliac disease and inflammatory bowel disease. *Digestion* 1989; **42**: 98–103.
372. Tarlo SM, Broder I, Prokipchuk EJ et al. Association between celiac disease and lung disease. *Chest* 1981; **80**: 715–718.
373. Douglas JG, McDonald CF, Leslie MJ et al. Respiratory impairment in inflammatory bowel disease: does it vary with disease activity? *Respir Med* 1989; **83**: 389–394.
374. Kuzela L, Vavrecka A, Prikazska M et al. Pulmonary complications in patients with inflammatory bowel disease. *Hepatogastroenterology* 1999; **46**: 1714–1719.
375. Tzanakis N, Bouros D, Samiou M et al. Lung function in patients with inflammatory bowel disease. *Respir Med* 1998; **92**: 516–522.
376. Marvisi M, Borrello PD, Brianti M et al. Changes in the carbon monoxide diffusing capacity of the lung in ulcerative colitis. *Eur Respir J* 2000; **16**: 965–968.
377. Herrlinger KR, Noftz MK, Dalhoff K et al. Alterations in pulmonary function in inflammatory bowel disease are frequent and persist during remission. *Am J Gastroenterol* 2002; **97**: 377–381.
378. Ussov WY, Peters AM, Savill J et al. Relationship between granulocyte activation, pulmonary granulocyte kinetics and alveolar permeability in extrapulmonary inflammatory disease. *Clin Sci* 1996; **91**: 329–335.
379. Murphy D, Pack AI, Imrie CW. The mechanism of arterial hypoxia occurring in acute pancreatits. *Q J Med* 1980; **49**: 151–163.
380. De Troyer A, Naeije R, Yernault JC, Englert M. Impairment of pulmonary function in actute pancreatits. *Chest* 1978; **73**: 360–363.
381. Basran GS, Ramasubramanian R, Verma R. Intrathoracic complications of acute pancreatitis. *Br J Dis Chest* 1987; **81**: 326–331.
382. Schnapf BM, Banks RA, Silverstein JH et al. Pulmonary function in insulin-dependent diabetes mellitus with limited joint mobility. *Am Rev Respir Dis* 1984; **130**: 930–932.
383. Cooper BG, Taylor R, Alberti K, Gibson GJ. Lung function in patients with diabetes mellitus. *Respir Med* 1990; **84**: 235–239.
384. Sandler M, Bunn AE, Stewart RI. Cross-section study of pulmonary function in patients with insulin-dependent diabetes mellitus. *Am Rev Respir Dis* 1987; **135**: 223–229.
385. Mori H, Okubo M, Okamura M et al. Abnormalities of pulmonary function in patients with non-insulin-dependent diabetes mellitus. *Intern Med* 1992; **31**: 189–193.
386. Marvisi M, Bartolini L, del Borrello P et al. Pulmonary function in non-insulin-dependent diabetes mellitus. *Respiration* 2001; **68**: 268–272.
387. Wanke T, Formanek D, Auinger M et al. Inspiratory muscle performance and pulmonary function changes in insulin-dependent diabetes mellitus. *Am Rev Respir Dis* 1991; **143**: 97–100.
388. Davis TM, Knuiman M, Kendall P et al. Reduced pulmonary function and its associations in type 2 diabetes: the Fremantle Diabetes Study. *Diabetes Res Clin Pract* 2000; **50**: 153–159.
389. Lange P, Parner J, Schnohr P, Jensen G. Copenhagen City Heart Study: longitudinal analysis of ventilatory capacity in diabetic and nondiabetic adults. *Eur Respir J* 2002; **20**: 1406–1412.
390. Mondini S, Guilleminault C. Abnormal breathing patterns during sleep in diabetes. *Ann Neurol* 1985; **17**: 391–395.
391. Bottini P, Dottorini ML, Cristina Cordoni M et al. Sleep-disordered breathing in nonobese diabetic subjects with autonomic neuropathy. *Eur Respir J* 2003; **22**: 654–660.
392. Cordier JF, Loire R, Brune J. Amyloidosis of the lower respiratory tract. Clinical and pathologic features in a series of 21 patients. *Chest* 1986; **90**: 827–831.
393. Sumiya M, Ohya N, Shinoura H et al. Diffuse interstitial pulmonary amyloidosis in rheumatoid arthritis. *J Rheumatol* 1996; **23**: 933–936.
394. Shiue ST, McNally DP. Pulmonary hypertension from prominent vascular involvement in diffuse amyloidosis. *Arch Intern Med* 1988; **148**: 687–689.
395. Santiago RM, Scharnhorst D, Ratkin G, Crouch EC. Respiratory muscle weakness and ventilatory failure in AL amyloidosis with muscular pseudohypertrophy. *Am J Med* 1987; **83**: 175–178.
396. Kerem E, Elstein D, Abrahamov A et al. Pulmonary function abnormalities in type 1 Gaucher disease. *Eur Respir J* 1996; **9**: 340–345.
397. Santamaria F, Parenti G, Guidi G et al. Pulmonary manifestations of Gaucher disease: an increased risk for L44P homozygotes? *Am J Respir Crit Care Med* 1998; **157**: 985–989.
398. Miller A, Brown LK, Pastores GM, Desnick RJ. Pulmonary involvement in type 1 Gaucher disease: functional and exercise findings in patients with and without clinical interstitial lung disease. *Clin Genet* 2003; **63**: 368–376.
399. Goitein O, Elstein D, Abrahamov A et al. Lung involvement and enzyme replacement therapy in Gaucher's disease. *Q J Med* 2001; **94**: 407–415.
400. Minai OA, Sullivan EJ, Stoller JK. Pulmonary involvement in Niemann-Pick disease: case report and literature review. *Respir Med* 2000; **94**: 1241–1251.
401. Nicholson AG, Wells AU, Hooper J et al. Successful treatment of endogenous lipoid pneumonia due to Niemann-Pick Type B disease with whole-lung lavage. *Am J Respir Crit Care Med* 2002; **165**: 128–131.

402. Maayan C, Carley DW, Axelrod FB et al. Respiratory system stability and abnormal carbon dioxide homeostatsis. *J Appl Physiol* 1992; **72**: 1186–1193.
403. Bernardi L, Hilz M, Stemper B et al. Respiratory and cerebrovascular responses to hypoxia and hypercapnia in familial dysautonomia. *Am J Respir Crit Care Med* 2003; **167**: 141–149.
404. Schmidt-Nowara WW, Samet JM, Rosario PA. Early and later complications of botulism. *Arch Intern Med* 1983; **143**: 451–456.
405. Wilcox P, Andolfatto G, Fairbarn MS, Pardy RL. Long-term follow-up of symptoms, pulmonary function, respiratory muscle strength, and exercise performance after botulism. *Am Rev Respir Dis* 1989; **139**: 157–163.
406. Harrison RN, Tattersfield AE. Airway response to inhaled salbutamol in hyperthyroid and hypothyroid patients before and after treatment. *Thorax* 1984; **39**: 34–39.
407. Irwin RS, Pratter MR, Stivers DH, Braverman LE. Airway reactivity and lung function in triiodothyronine-induced thyrotoxicosis. *J Appl Physiol* 1985; **58**: 1485–1488.
408. Kendrick AH, O'Reilly JF, Laszlo G. Lung function and exercise performance in hyperthyroidism before and after treatment. *Q J Med* 1988; **68**: 615–627.
409. McElvaney GN, Wilcox PG, Fairbarn MS et al. Respiratory muscle weakness and dyspnea in thyrotoxic patients. *Am Rev Respir Dis* 1990; **141**: 1221–1227.
410. Siafakas NM, Milona I, Salesiotou V et al. Respiratory muscle strength in hyperthyroidism before and after treatment. *Am Rev Respir Dis* 1992; **146**: 1025–1029.
411. Goswami R, Guleria R, Gupta AK et al. Prevalence of diaphragmatic muscle weakness and dyspnoea in Graves' disease and their reversibility with carbimazole therapy. *Eur J Endocrinol* 2002; **147**: 299–303.
412. Rajagopal KR, Abbrecht PH, Derderian SS et al. Obstructive sleep apnea in hypothyroidism. *Ann Intern Med* 1984; **101**: 491–494.
413. Harrison BDW, Millhouse KA, Harrington M, Nabarro JDN. Lung function in acromegaly. *Q J Med* 1978; **188**: 517–532.
414. Brody JS, Fisher AB, Gocmen A, Dubois AB. Acromegalic pneumomegaly: lung growth in the adult. *J Clin Invest* 1970; **49**: 1051–1060.
415. Iandelli I, Gorini M, Duranti R et al. Respiratory muscle function and control of breathing in patients with acromegaly. *Eur Respir J* 1997; **10**: 977–982.
416. Donnelly PM, Grunstein RR, Peat JK et al. Large lungs and growth hormone: an increased alveolar number? *Eur Respir J* 1995; **8**: 938–947.
417. Evans CC, Hipkin LJ, Murray GM. Pulmonary function in acromegaly. *Thorax* 1977; **32**: 322–327.
418. Garcia-Rio F, Pino JM, Diez JJ et al. Reduction in lung distensibility in acromegaly after suppression of growth hormone hypersecretion. *Am J Respir Crit Care Med* 2001; **164**: 852–857.
419. Trotman-Dickenson B, Weetman AP, Hughes JM. Upper airflow limitation and pulmonary function in acromegaly: relationship to disease activity. *Q J Med* 1991; **79**: 527–538.
420. Melnyk D. Update on carcinoid syndrome. *AANA J* 1997; **65**: 265–270.
421. Merola B, Sofia M, Longobardi S et al. Impairment of lung volumes and respiratory muscle strength in adult patients with growth hormone deficiency. *Eur J Endocrinol* 1995; **133**: 680–685.
422. Mansell AL, Levison H, Bailey JD. Maturation of lung function in children with hypopituitarism. *Am Rev Respir Dis* 1983; **127**: 166–170.
423. Meineri I, Andreani O, Sanna R et al. Effect of low-dosage recombinant human growth hormone therapy on pulmonary function in hypopituitary patients with adult onset growth hormone deficiency. *J Endocrinol Invest* 1998; **21**: 423–427.
424. Imokawa S, Colby TV, Leslie KO, Helmers RA. Methotrexate pneumonitis: review of the literature and histopathological findings in nine patients. *Eur Respir J* 2000; **15**: 373–381.
425. Cottin V, Tebib J, Massonnet B et al. Pulmonary function in patients receiving long-term low-dose methotrexate. *Chest* 1996; **109**: 933–938.
426. McKenna KE, Burrows D. Pulmonary toxicity in a patient with psoriasis receiving methotrexate therapy. *Clin Exp Dermatol* 2000; **25**: 24–27.
427. Sunderji R, Kanji Z, Gin K. Pulmonary effects of low dose amiodarone: a review of the risks and recommendations for surveillance. *Can J Cardiol* 2000; **16**: 1435–1440.
428. Ohar JA, Jackson F Jr, Redd RM et al. Usefulness of serial pulmonary function testing as an indicator of amiodarone toxicity. *Am J Cardiol* 1989; **64**: 1322–1326.
429. Gleadhill IC, Wise RA, Schonfeld SA et al. Serial lung function testing in patients treated with amiodarone: a prospective study. *Am J Med* 1989; **86**: 4–10.

Further reading

Enkhbaatar P, Traber DL. Pathophysiology of acute lung injury in combined burn and smoke inhalation injury. *Clin Sci (Lond)*. 2004; **107**: 137–143.

Mitzner W, Wagner EM. Vascular remodeling in the circulations of the lung. *J Appl Physiol* 2004; **97**: 1999–2004.

CHAPTER 42

Lung Function in Relation to General Anaesthesia and Artificial Ventilation

42.1 Introduction

General anaesthesia depresses the central mechanisms that control respiration. This affects the level and pattern of breathing and the special mechanisms that maintain the patency of the upper airways. There are also direct consequences for the airways, gas exchange and cardiac output (Table 42.1). These are aggravated by impaired lung function, that may itself contraindicate a particular procedure or influence the choice of anaesthetic technique or post-operative care.

This chapter reviews the consequences for lung function of general anaesthesia and indicates how ventilation can be maintained in a range of circumstances. The effects of regional and spinal anaesthesia are reviewed elsewhere [1].

42.2 Pre-operative assessment

All patients must be assessed prior to surgery with regard to possible risk of complications from the type of anaesthesia and surgical procedure that are envisaged. The assessment should be at its most rigorous when the lungs themselves are to be operated on (see Chapter 43). Procedures that entail upper abdominal incisions predispose to peri-operative complications, so also need special consideration [2]. Obesity (BMI > 25 kg m^{-2}) is another high- risk situation as it predisposes to upper airway occlusion during induction and post-operatively. It also increases the risk of atelectasis during anaesthesia. Patients who have required domiciliary oxygen therapy or previous mechanical ventilation for lung disease, those with myopathy or a history of previous problems in relation to general anaesthesia should also receive special consideration. The lung function assessment should start with questions about breathlessness, other respiratory symptoms and smoking habits (e.g. from Fig. 8.2, page 88) and form part of the pre-operative protocol. Spirometry should be performed routinely, but may be omitted if all the responses are normal. Conversely, dyspnoea on trivial exertion during daily living in a patient with lung disease indicates very poor respiratory reserve. Signs of cyanosis and right heart failure consequent from lung disease would also indicate high risk (Table 42.2).

42.2.1 Airway and thoracic anatomy

Abnormalities of the anatomy or configuration of the upper airway can indicate that intubation or protection of the airway will

Table 42.1 Effects of general anaesthesia on lung function.

Soft palate	Moves back, nasopharyngeal occlusion
Intercostal muscles	Diminished activity, reduced thoracic ventilatory movement
Diaphragm	Usually displaced towards the head
Rib cage volume	Decreased
Thoracic blood volume	May be increased
Functional residual capacity	Reduced in supine posture
Expiratory reserve volume	Reduced in supine posture
Regional ventilation	Superior to inferior ratio increased, alveolar dead space increased
Minute volume	Reduced
Tidal volume	Reduced
Respiratory frequency	Increased
Ventilatory response to $\uparrow P\text{CO}_2$ and $\downarrow P\text{O}_2$	Reduced
Airways resistance	Little change despite lower FRC. Most anaesthetic agents are bronchodilator
Lung compliance	Reduced, recoil pressure increased
Airway closure or atelectasis	Commonly occurs, thus anatomical shunt increased and compliance reduced
Alveolar blood shunting	Unchanged in normal subjects
Cardiac output	Reduced, so mixed venous $P\text{O}_2$ reduced
Pulmonary vasoconstrictor response to hypoxia	Reduced by inhalation anaesthetic agents
Arterial $P\text{O}_2$	Reduced
Arterial $P\text{CO}_2$	Increased

be difficult. Obesity, micrognathia, severe temporo-mandibular joint disease, neck abnormalities, such as fusion from ankylosing spondylitis or hypermobility with atlanto-axial subluxation due to rheumatoid disease, are all adverse features. Upper airway problems can also arise in patients with a goitre that encroaches on the thoracic inlet. A rigid thoracic cage, such as in ankylosing spondyolitis or kyphoscoliosis, is associated with reduced static lung volumes that may predispose to respiratory difficulties after induction of anaesthesia. With respect to lung function, a relatively low PEF (e.g. $\text{FEV}_1/\text{PEF}>10$, where FEV_1 is in ml and PEF in l min^{-1}) suggests upper airway obstruction; this should prompt a search for laryngeal or tracheal encroachment.

42.2.2 Spirometry and arterial gases

The lung function is of proven value for predicting the outcome of lung resections (Section 43.2.1, page 604). In other circumstances the information is largely unsatisfactory due to the studies being retrospective and inadequate allowances made for differences in anaesthetic technique, co-morbidities and surgical procedure. A recent prospective study of lung function pre- and post-cardiac surgery in 100 patients found no relationship between arterial saturation breathing air or spirometric values and either the time to extubation or radiological changes on CXR [3]. An earlier study of 106 subjects found those requiring 5 days or more on ICU had lower preoperative FEV_1 and FVC than those needing less than 5 days, but there was overlap between the groups so no cut off value could be defined that indicated increased operative risk [4]. However a raised $P\text{a,CO}_2$ was associated with a relatively increased mortality.

Table 42.2 Checklist of items to consider that may indicate potential problems for anaesthesia.

History	Cardiorespiratory or neuromyopathic symptoms, low exercise performance
Examination	Obesity, stridor, neck or jaw deformity, chest deformity, cyanosis, signs of heart failure
Investigation	Low PEF relative to FEV_1: upper airway obstruction
	Low PEF, low FEV_1, low FEV_1%: airflow limitation
	Raised arterial $P\text{CO}_2$: hypoventilation
	Low $P\text{O}_2$, anaemia: poor oxygen delivery

Severe airflow limitation is an independent risk factor for death after cardiac surgery with a mortality as high as 50% in those with FEV_1 less than half of their predicted value [5]. It is also a risk factor for post-operative complications requiring use of ICU facilities in patients with COPD, especially when the limitation is accompanied by hypercapnia (raised $P\text{a,CO}_2$) and other evidence for chronic respiratory failure. These features indicate a need for appropriate preoperative treatment that should be monitored by analysis of arterial blood. Simple oximetry preoperatively can provide warning of likely respiratory difficulties unless action is taken. Arterial saturation alone cannot predict outcome.

Unlike upper abdominal incisions, that predispose to respiratory complications [2], there is little risk associated with lower abdominal or other operations [6]. A review of five studies found no evidence that preoperative spirometry or arterial gases could accurately predict an individual's outcome or their chance of post-operative complications [7], indicating that some patients with poor pre-operative prognostic factors do well and conversely respiratory complications may arise in patients with normal lung function.

42.2.3 Muscle function

Anaesthetic agents and the incisions for either thoracic or upper abdominal surgery adversely affect diaphragm function. Accordingly, patients with disease affecting their respiratory muscles might be expected to be at risk of anaesthetic pulmonary complications. However, there are few data available to support this. One study of 13 patients with mytonic dystrophy found propofol anaesthesia to be safe with no change in post-operative arterial saturation and no respiratory complications despite a 42% reduction in mean VC immediately post-operatively [8]. Incentive spirometry has been found to leave post-operative diaphragm movement unimproved [9] but both incentive spirometry and physiotherapy have been shown to reduce post-operative complications [10] suggesting that improved muscle function is not the reason for the beneficial response.

42.2.4 Exercise capacity

There are data on the use of exercise testing for predicting operative risk with regard to lung resection (see Chapter 43), but not in relation to other forms of surgical intervention.

42.3 Physiological effects of anaesthesia

A wide variety of agents can be used to produce general anaesthesia and the pharmacological effects of these agents are diverse; this section provides a brief summary.

Pre-medication. Prior to induction, a benzodiazepine or other agent can be used to relieve anxiety. When given orally in pharmacological doses these drugs appear not to reduce respiratory drive but they may affect the muscles that determine the calibre of the upper airway (see below). The use of opiates and anticholinergic agents as pre-medication is no longer recommended since opiates depress ventilatory drive and can release histamine in asthmatic subjects.

Induction. Propofol and etomidate are two intravenous agents now commonly used for the induction of anaesthesia in preference to the barbiturates methohexitone and thiopentone. They cause dose dependent respiratory depression, which for propofol is at about three times the blood level required for anaesthesia. Maintenance of anaesthesia is usually with halogenated inhalational agents such as sevoflurane, enflurane, isoflurane or halothane. Total intravenous anaesthesia is sometimes employed using ketamine and/or propofol, together with other agents. Powerful and rapidly acting opiates are often used for intra-operative analgesia and these also depress respiration.

42.3.1 Upper airway

With the induction of general anaesthesia the upper airway tends to collapse and can occlude. This continues to be a risk post-operatively both when the patient is not fully conscious and during sleep for one or two nights subsequently. The problem is greatest in patients with obesity, micrognathia, or a short fat neck.

The upper airway collapse is probably due to the pharmacological agent altering the time of activation of the upper airway muscles during breathing. In awake subjects the muscles are phasically stimulated just prior to activation of the diaphragm [11]. During anaesthesia the activation of the upper airway muscles may be reduced and is then either synchronous with or may follow that of the diaphragm [12]. In this circumstance the descent of the diaphragm induces an intra-airway pressure that is negative relative to atmospheric pressure, hence the tendency for the upper airway to collapse is no longer resisted by the usual prior activation of the upper airway muscles. This effect is exacerbated by the prior use of benzodiazepines and by the usual supine posture of the patient during anaesthetic induction. If the head is elevated above the horizontal plane less neck extension is required to prevent upper airway occlusion [13]. The occlusion occurs at the level of the soft palate and not at the dorsum of the tongue or at the epiglottis [14]. This may explain why neck extension helps to relieve the obstruction but does not pull the tongue forward.

42.3.2 Ventilatory responses

General anaesthesia is often performed with the patient breathing spontaneously so preservation of ventilatory drive is important.

Inhalational anaesthetic agents depress the ventilatory response to CO_2; this is shown schematically in Fig. 42.1. The depression is also seen in sub-anaesthetic doses [15], indicating that a reduced ventilatory response to CO_2 may be present at the end of anaesthesia. Induction doses of barbiturates also depress the CO_2 response. In spontaneously breathing patients anaesthetists may on occasion allow a degree of hypercapnia during anaesthesia, arguing that this does not harm the patient and the P_{CO_2} returns to normal values in the post-operative period. The hypercapnoeic response is already reduced in patients with COPD [16] and in head injury or cerebral surgery a rise in P_{CO_2} can be dangerous on account of causing vasodilatation and hence a rise in intracranial pressure.

Most inhalational anaesthetic agents, and also nitrous oxide, depress the ventilatory response to hypoxia. Halothane in full anaesthetic concentration can abolish the response completely [17], whereas with isoflurane a blunted hypoxic response is found [18]. Sub-anaesthetic doses of isoflurane have little effect on the

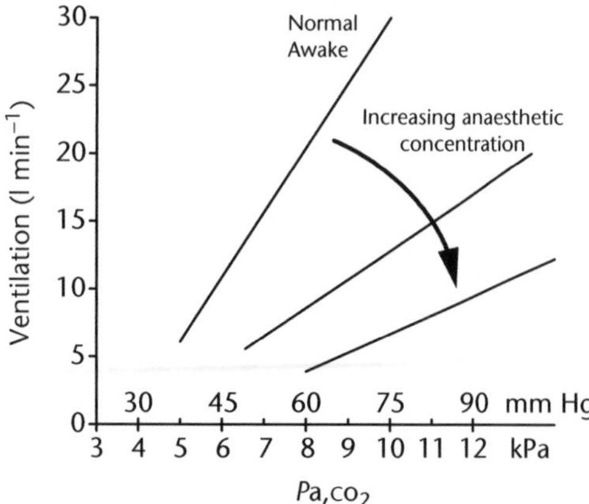

Fig. 42.1 Ventilatory responses to breathing carbon dioxide in normal awake subjects and after increasing concentrations of inhalational anaesthetic agent.

isocapnic hypoxic response [19], but sub-hypnotic doses of either propofol or halothane reduce the hypoxic response [20]. Post-operatively, healthy subjects will regain their usual CO_2 responsiveness and breathe normally despite any continued insensitivity to hypoxia. By contrast a patient with COPD, who ordinarily might be relatively insensitive to changes in CO_2, could be at risk of prolonged and dangerous apnoea if any insensitivity to hypoxia persists.

42.3.3 Muscle function

Diaphragm tone is reduced during anaesthesia leading to a higher (i.e. headwards) resting diaphragm position [21] with reduced movement of its dependent dorsal part [22]. This response is seen without the use of muscle relaxants; in adults these reduce the thoracic volume by an average of 500 ml [23].

In conscious subjects expiratory muscles are not activated during tidal breathing but they become phasically activate during anaesthesia [24]. On this account abdominal surgery is not possible without initiation of muscle paralysis to relax the abdominal muscles.

42.3.4 Lung volumes

The supine posture adopted for anaesthesia reduces FRC and the volume is reduced further (by about 20%) by the anaesthetised state [25]. The reduction in FRC develops within the first few minutes of supine anaesthesia and persists for some hours after recovery. It is not dependent on the use of paralysing agents, the use of oxygen or the use of artificial ventilation. Changes in diaphragm tone contribute to this [26]. As FRC is reduced the airway diameter in the dependent parts of the lungs becomes smaller and the local airway resistance higher. Thus, the upper parts of the lungs are preferentially ventilated and dependent atelectasis occurs (see Section 42.3.6).

42.3.5 Airway function

The suppression of upper airway reflexes is important for safe anaesthesia since reflex laryngospasm is extremely hazardous. Intravenous induction agents can cause irritability of the upper airway reflexes and one study has shown that cough or hiccup after induction occurred in about one third of patients receiving thiopentone, in one fifth of those receiving methohexitone and in none receiving propofol [27]. Volatile inhalational agents can give excitatory airway responses during induction, with isoflurane causing more problems than halothane [28]. Irritation of upper airway reflexes can induce bronchospasm through vagally mediated mechanisms.

Intravenous induction agents and muscle relaxants can on occasion cause histamine release and so increase airways resistance. By contrast, volatile inhalational anaesthetic agents cause bronchodilatation.

In supine anaesthetised patients the diminution in FRC has the consequence that the resting ventilatory position is relatively close to RV. This reduces airway calibre, causes airway closure and reduces lung compliance. The normal hyperbolic relationship between airway resistance and lung volume is enhanced in consequence [29]. It is also affected by obesity when FRC is often very close to RV and airway resistance is much higher than normal (see Fig. 42.2). Similar changes can occur in older persons as a result of loss of lung elasticity. Tidal volume may then encroach on closing volume and cause alveolar collapse hence increased shunting leading to impaired gas exchange.

42.3.6 Gas exchange

Gas exchange is impaired during anaesthesia leading to an increase in the A-a DO_2. This is partly caused by under-perfusion of ventilated alveoli in the most superior parts of the lungs. Hence, there is an increase in physiological deadspace that is due to an increase in alveolar deadspace [30]. However, the major reason for impaired gas exchange during anaesthesia is an increase in the

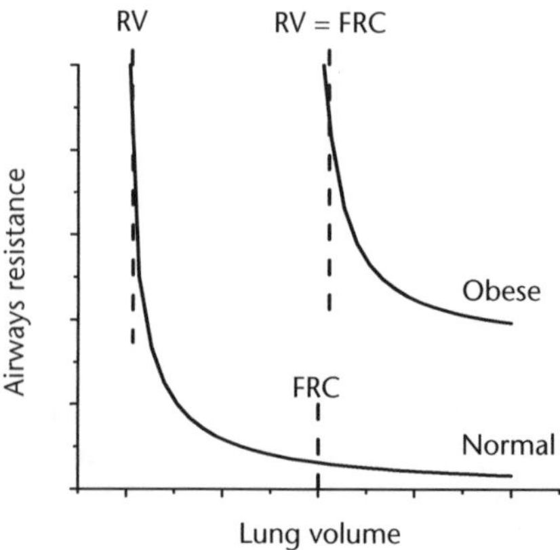

Fig. 42.2 Relationship of airway resistance to lung volume during anaesthesia for normal subjects and patients with obesity. Source [30]

proportion of low $\dot{V}/\dot{Q}$ areas [31, 32]. This may reflect impaired vaso-motor control.

An additional factor is a change in the function of the diaphragm consequent on its altered position in the thorax. This can lead to alveolar collapse in dorsal and dependent areas of the lungs. The positional factor alone appears not to explain the changes since, in an animal model, phrenic nerve stimulation was found to improve gas exchange to a greater extent than the application of positive end expiratory pressure. This suggested that it was the change in diaphragm position and recruitment rather than just lung volume *per se* that contributed to the impaired gas exchange [26]. This conclusion was born out by a study in humans in which CT measurement of lung collapse was combined with MIGET estimation of $\dot{V}_A/\dot{Q}$ relationships. There was a correlation between the increase in degree of shunt and the number of CT opacities. The number of opacities was reduced by PEEP but this did not improve gas exchange [33]. Atelectases during mechanical ventilation can be re-expanded by applying PEEP intermittently and maintaining for 8 s a vital capacity breath that is achieved using an airway pressure of 4 kPa (40 cm H_2O) [34].

Ventilating patients during anaesthesia with high inspired oxygen concentrations facilitates the development of atelectasis. The difficulty can be avoided by restricting the F_{I,O_2} to 0.4 (Section 35.7.2).

42.4 Physiological effects of intermittent positive pressure ventilation (IPPV)

For many operative procedures and for most patients on intensive care artificial ventilatory support is used. This section will describe the functional aspects of intermittent positive pressure ventilation (IPPV) on intubated subjects.

42.4.1 Phases of the respiratory cycle

During intermittent positive pressure ventilation (IPPV) the ventilator applies a positive pressure (i.e. pressure above atmospheric) to the airway and this inflates the lungs. The duration and speed of inflation and the prevailing resistance and compliance of the respiratory system all influence the outcome (see below). If the inflation is slow then the degree of lung inflation is largely determined by the compliance of the system. If the inflation is rapid then the regional airway resistance and local time constants of inflation determine which areas of the lungs are able to inflate in the time available. One of the adverse consequence of the method is that the raised pressure can diminish venous return and hence reduce cardiac output; the problem is greatest in patients who are hypovolaemic or vasodilated.

The expiratory phase of normal resting breathing is passive but control can be exercised by varying the calibre of the larynx [35] (hence laryngeal braking), and by activation of expiratory muscles [36]. When ventilation is by IPPV expiration can be either totally passive or retarded by maintenance of a positive expiratory pressure or application of an expiratory resistance.

In spontaneously breathing subjects the duration of inspiration (t_I) may be 1.5 s with expiration occupying about 2 s followed by an end expiratory pause. The total cycle will be about 5 s giving a frequency of 12 breaths per minute. Commonly the inspiratory cycle for IPPV is set, approximately, for between 1 and 1.5 s and expiration for about twice this amount, giving an inspiratory to expiratory ratio (t_I/t_E ratio) of 1: 2 and a breathing frequency of between 13 and 20 breaths per minute. If t_I falls below 1 s there is an increase in physiological deadspace [37, 38] (Section 18.4.1).

If the t_I/t_E ratio is changed so that inspiration is prolonged and expiration reduced, this may increase FRC and improve gas exchange. The improvement can be achieved by adopting a slowly progressive (ramp) flow on inspiration or introducing a post-inspiratory pause. This latter manoeuvre reduces the deadspace, improves gas mixing and provides more effective clearance of CO_2 for the level of alveolar ventilation [39]. By holding the lungs at end inspiration more airways are held open and so there are fewer lung regions with low $\dot{V}_A/\dot{Q}$ [40]. t_I/t_E ratios as high as 4: 1 have been used although 2:1 is more usual. The technique requires adequate time for expiration. This may not be available in the presence of airflow limitation when an unacceptable increase in FRC may occur.

42.4.2 Influence of airway pressure, resistance and lung compliance

The time course for lung inflation depends on the time constant for the lungs (i.e. the product of compliance and resistance) and the applied pressure (consult Section 16.1.9 for details). For a specified applied pressure of 1 kPa (10 cm H_2O) the consequences for ventilation of different values for compliance and resistance separately are illustrated in Figs 42.3 and 42.4. From Fig. 42.3 we can see that a lung of low compliance, as is caused by fibrosis or ARDS, has a small final inflation volume but it is achieved rapidly.

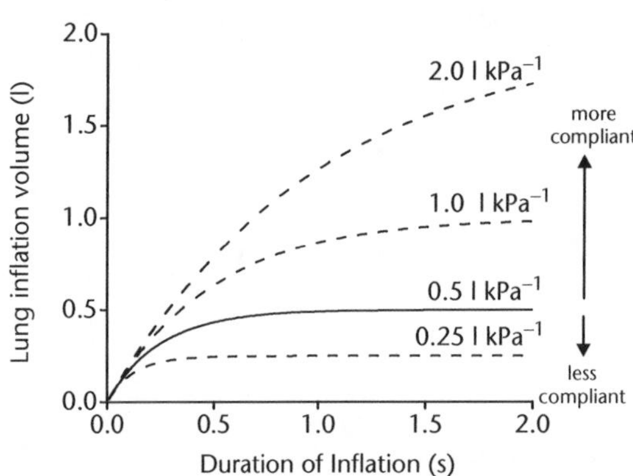

Fig. 42.3 Relationship of lung inflation volume to time for a constant inflation pressure of 1 kPa (10 cm H_2O). Solid line denotes normal position and dashed lines represent the effect of changing lung compliance.

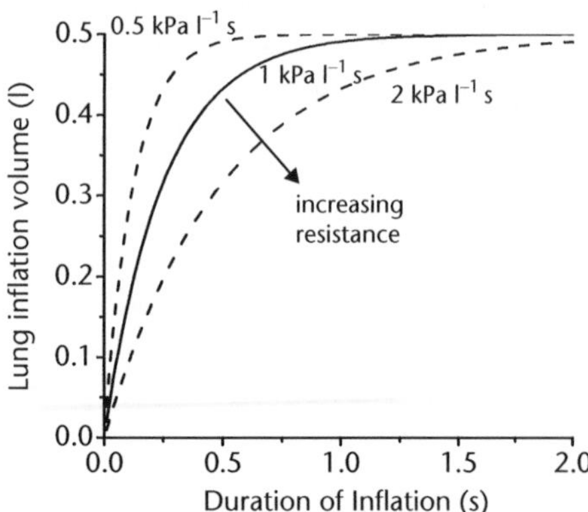

Fig. 42.4 Relationship of inflation volume to time for a constant inflation pressure of 1 kPa (10 cm H_2O). Solid line denotes normal position and dashed lines represent the effect of changing lung resistance.

If the lung is very compliant, as occurs with emphysema, the final inflation volume for a given inflation pressure is much increased, but the time required to achieve it is prolonged. If the time is short the volume is curtailed. However, with a set inspiratory time of 1 s the inflation volume would still be increased by about 70% for a doubling of compliance.

Isolated changes in airway resistance do not affect the volume change for a given applied pressure but greatly influence the time taken to achieve it (Fig. 42.4). Thus, for a t_I of 1 s a doubling of resistance reduces the inflation volume by 14%, whilst with a reduced resistance the inflation volume is achieved much faster. These effects are summarised in Table 42.3.

Ventilators are rarely set to produce a constant inflation pressure and the lungs are made up from a large number of units with differing resistance and compliance characteristics. Thus, how the system reacts in practice can only be assessed by trial and error.

Many ventilators produce a constant flow and will apply whatever pressure is required to deliver this against the given external impedance offered by the ventilator circuit and the patient's lungs, chest wall and abdomen. The operator can determine the magnitude of this flow ($\dot{v}$), the duration of inspiration (t_I) and duration of expiration (t_E). From these input values all appropriate variables can be calculated:

$$\text{Tidal volume}(V_t) = \dot{v} t_I$$
$$\text{Respiratory frequency}(f_R) = 60/(t_I + t_E)$$
$$\text{Minute ventilation} = V_t f_R$$
$$\text{I/E ratio} = t_I / t_E$$

Table 42.3 Effect of changes in lung compliance and resistance on lung inflation volume and inflation time when inflated with a constant inflation pressure.

		Condition	Inflation volume	Inflation time
Compliance	Increased	Emphysema	↑	↑
	Reduced	Fibrosis	↓	↓
Resistance	Increased	Asthma, COPD	↔	↑
	Reduced	Fibrosis	↔	↓

Inflation of the lungs by IPPV tends to distribute the ventilation predominantly to the non-dependent and under-perfused areas of the lungs, so the $\dot{V}_A/\dot{Q}$ balance is not as favourable as that during spontaneous ventilation. A common level of minute volume is approximately 10 ml kg^{-1} of body mass. In some lung conditions, because of the poor compliance of dependent areas, this level of ventilation can lead to over distension of the other areas of the lungs [41]. A recent study using low minute volumes of 5 ml kg^{-1} found a significant survival advantage in patients with adult respiratory distress syndrome [42].

42.4.3 Effects of IPPV on the circulation

During positive pressure ventilation the intrathoracic pressure (P_{ITP}) is raised compared with that during spontaneous breathing. This reduces the venous return to the heart and hence the filling and stroke volume of the right ventricle [43]. The effect is accentuated if the patient is already hypovolaemic. The changes percolate through the pulmonary circulation to affect the left ventricle where the preload and output are reduced a few beats later [44].

42.4.4 Positive end expiratory pressure

Application of a slightly raised (positive) pressure at end expiration (PEEP) is an established therapy for patients with acute lung injury. The positive pressure prevents airway collapse by increasing FRC above closing capacity. As a result the shunt fraction that would otherwise have arisen from perfusion of alveoli supplied by the collapsed airways is eliminated. In addition, the cardiac output is reduced and with it the blood flow to under ventilated areas [45]. The other effects are redistribution of extravascular lung water [46] and improved $\dot{V}_A/\dot{Q}$ matching. Thus, oxygenation is improved and a lower inspired fractional concentration of oxygen (F_{I,O_2}) can be used. In severely ill subjects this may allow an F_{I,O_2} of less than 0.6 to maintain adequate tissue oxygenation and so help minimise the lung toxicity that might otherwise result from using a high F_{I,O_2} (Section 35.7.2).

With progressive increases in PEEP the alveoli become stretched and FRC increases. The alveolar vessels then become compressed and pulmonary vascular resistance can increase [47]. The progressive reduction in blood flow can then affect perfusion of non-dependent areas of lung whilst increasing the flow in the lung periphery [48].These changes can impair gas exchange [49]. To achieve an optimal result it is common for PEEP to be titrated until the oxygen delivery (dependent on P_{I,O_2} and cardiac output) is optimal. Prolonged use of PEEP increases the risk of barotrauma where mediastinal emphysema and pneumothorax may develop [50], also Section 35.4.

42.4.5 Intrinsic positive end expiratory pressure

In the presence of airflow limitation the end expiratory lung volume (EELV) can exceed FRC. This is because the time required for passive exhalation is prolonged and either the patient or the ventilator may terminate expiration prematurely [51, 52]. The inspiratory muscles need to overcome this pressure, which is called auto positive end expiratory pressure or intrinsic PEEP (PEEPi), before gas flow can be reversed and inspiration can begin. The work of breathing is increased both on this account and because the inspiration is occurring at a raised lung volume so the energy cost is greater. When PEEPi is measured in spontaneously breathing subjects [53] an allowance should be made for overestimation due to expiratory muscle contraction [54].

In ventilated patients who are not in receipt of external PEEP or taking spontaneous breaths the *static* PEEPi can be measured, by occluding the airway at the end of expiration and recording the plateau pressure. This pressure will relate to airways resistance, tidal volume and expiratory time. PEEPi during the ventilation (*dynamic* PEEPi) can be estimated from the pressure in the airway at the time when inspiratory flow commences. By then any static PEEPi will have been overcome so the resulting pressure represents the lowest PEEPi within the lungs. Some areas may have a higher PEEPi but this is of no consequence as reversal of flow occurs when the lowest PEEPi in the lungs has been exceeded. In lungs with non-homogeneous ventilation the dynamic PEEPi may be considerably lower than static PEEPi.

When a patient with COPD is being ventilated the work of breathing can be reduced by the application of PEEP. Alternatively, if the patient is breathing spontaneously continuous positive airway pressure (CPAP) can be used instead [55, 56]. CPAP counterbalances the PEEPi and also enhances gas exchange by improving $\dot{V}_A/\dot{Q}$ distribution [57]. However, if the PEEP or CPAP exceeds 85% of PEEPi then hyperinflation tends to occur [58]. In patients with acute lung injury PEEPi can coexist with premature airway closure [59].

42.4.6 Weaning from artificial ventilation

In patients requiring prolonged artificial ventilation the respiratory muscles may become weak from disuse or a secondary metabolic disturbance. This can make the withdrawal of artificial ventilation very difficult. In this circumstance attention to nutrition and metabolic status can help to preserve muscle function. However, whilst diaphragm weakness can be very common the need to reinstitute artificial ventilation can precede the development of low frequency fatigue, thus failure to wean can have several causes [60]. Tracheotomy is often undertaken after a week of continuous artificial ventilation. Initially the aim was to prevent the long-term laryngeal damage caused by prolonged intubation. However, the beneficial effects also include reductions in the work of breathing, the deadspace and PEEPi [61].

Strategies to facilitate weaning include reducing the work associated with breathing and gradually increasing the amount of work the respiratory muscles are required to do. For example in patients with COPD requiring ventilation the careful matching of PEEP to PEEPi can reduce the respiratory workload [62]. Other strategies can also be used. A number of indices of function can help guide the clinician in these circumstances. Thus, in a study of over 200 patients with COPD, neurological diseases and acute respiratory failure, successful weaning was related to shorter duration of prior ventilation and could be predicted from the result of a 2-h trial of spontaneous ventilation through a T-piece. Favourable factors included (i) lower respiratory frequency to tidal volume ratio (f_R/V_T), (ii) higher MIP, (iii) higher airway occlusion pressure ($P_{0.1}$), (iv) higher MEP and (v) higher VC [63]. In a separate study of 163 patients after 1 h of spontaneous ventilation an $f_R/V_T > 100$ had a 33% sensitivity and 94% specificity for predicting weaning failure [64].

The ability to cough is a means of avoiding retention of pulmonary secretions and is a predictor of weaning success [65]. The measurement of cough peak flows during a trial of spontaneous breathing found that those with a cough PEF $\leq 60\ l\ min^{-1}$ were five times more likely to fail to wean and 19 times more likely to die than those with a cough PEF exceeding this limit [66].

No single index is a sufficient guide to the outcome of weaning and reliance is sometimes placed on a standard protocol [67]. However, a comparison between protocol driven weaning and usual care with regular physician rounds found no difference in outcome [68].

42.5 Modes of ventilation

A number of different ways of using artificial ventilation have been devised and these will be mentioned briefly. Most ventilators are set to deliver a given flow for a given time at a given frequency to achieve a specified minute volume, with the airway pressure determined by the impedance of the connecting tubing, airways, lungs, chest wall and abdomen.

42.5.1 Normal frequency ventilation

Controlled mandatory ventilation (CMV). This mode delivers a fixed number of breaths per minute at fixed time intervals irrespective of patient effort.

Intermittent mandatory ventilation (IMV). This mode allows the patient to take spontaneous breaths through a parallel inspiratory circuit, but if a predetermined level of minute ventilation is not met additional breaths are imposed by the ventilator. The imposed breaths are delivered without regard to the patient's own breathing pattern, so if the two are superimposed the lung may become excessively distended.

Synchronised intermittent mandatory ventilation (SIMV). This mode is the same as for IMV but the timing of the imposed breath from the ventilator is synchronised with the patient's own attempt at inspiration. This avoids 'stacking' of breaths through the imposition of a tidal volume on top of a patient's own inspiration.

Pressure support ventilation (PSV). In this mode the ventilator is triggered to give pressure support to a patient's inspiratory effort. The patient determines the inspiratory time and the respiratory rate, and the inspiratory flow is enhanced by the pressure support. The advantage of this mode is better patient acceptability but adequate ventilation is not assured by this mode alone.

Continuous positive airway pressure (CPAP). This mode of ventilation applies a continuous positive pressure during both inspiration and expiration in spontaneously breathing subjects. This is similar to the application of PEEP to patients being artificially ventilated where positive pressure is exerted but only during the expiratory phase.

Pressure control inverse ratio ventilation (PCIRV). This mode may be undertaken in an attempt to avoid very high inflation pressures when lung compliance is low ('stiff' lung). The level of pressure support, the respiratory frequency and t_I/t_E ratio are all predetermined (the later usually in the range 2:1–4:1). The required minute ventilation is achieved by adjusting the level of pressure support and the respiratory frequency. In ARDS the gas exchange may be improved by this technique through recruiting collapsed alveoli. The risk of barotrauma is low.

Airway pressure release ventilation (APRV). This is a modification of CPAP whereby the positive pressure is applied during the inspiratory phase to inflate the lungs and the pressure is either released to a lower level of pressure or to ambient pressure for expiration. The method may facilitate weaning.

Biphasic positive airway pressure (BiPAP). This mode is the application of two levels of CPAP whilst a patient is breathing spontaneously. The level of support is pressure controlled and time cycled. Two levels of pressure support are offered and the duration of each can be adjusted. P_{high} is applied during inspiration for duration t_{high}, and P_{low} is applied during expiration for duration t_{low}. This mode of pressure support can be combined with other modes of ventilation such as CMV or IMV. Patients can be changed from SIMV, which is a volume defined mode of ventilation, to BiPAP which is a pressure defined mode.

42.5.2 High frequency ventilation

High frequency ventilation provides a means for ventilating the lungs using relatively low peak airway pressures and with minimal disturbance to the cardiovascular system. The methods can be used when the lungs and/or chest wall are very stiff and so reduce the risks of barotrauma.

High frequency positive pressure ventilation (HFPPV). This mode uses a high-pressure source of gas that is delivered at a frequency of 60–120 Hz. The tidal volume can be as low as 3 to 5 ml kg^{-1}, which is not much more than the deadspace. Inspiratory time is about one third of the duty cycle and expiration is passive. Lower intratracheal and intrapleural pressures are found with HFPPV compared to IPPV despite comparable gas exchange [69].

High frequency jet ventilation (HFJV). This method of high frequency ventilation uses a jet injector of gas at high pressure at a frequency of 100–200 Hz. The tidal volume and duty cycle are as for HFPPV.

High frequency oscillation (HFO). This method has active inspiratory and expiratory phases. Any frequency in the range150–3000 Hz can be used together with relatively small tidal volumes (1–3 ml kg^{-1}).

42.6 Post-operative effects of anaesthesia on lung function

The effects of general anaesthesia can persist for hours to days after recovery. Failure to reverse neuromuscular blocking agents adequately can lead to type 2 respiratory failure (Section 38.5.2); this is mainly due to the muscle weakness, but the hypoventilation is aggravated by suppression of the hypoxic and hypercapnic drives to breathing during the recovery period. The hypoventilation can predispose to atelectasis. Thus, amongst 13 patients monitored using CT scans for up to 4 days after lower abdominal surgery six of them developed atelectasis during anaesthesia; these patients and also five of the remaining seven experienced atelectasis during the post-operative period [70]. Atelectasis was accompanied by hypoxaemia. Despite these findings lower abdominal surgery is usually free from serious post-operative complications [6].

The post-operative period is usually uneventful but diligent patient care is necessary if untoward events are to be avoided.

42.6.1 Post-operative monitoring

Adequate monitoring of patients after anaesthesia is essential with a view to avoiding critical respiratory deterioration and resulting demands on intensive care facilities.

Pulse oximetry is widely used to monitor oxy-haemoglobin saturation (Section 7.10.1). The measurement can be combined with varying the inspired oxygen concentration to construct a

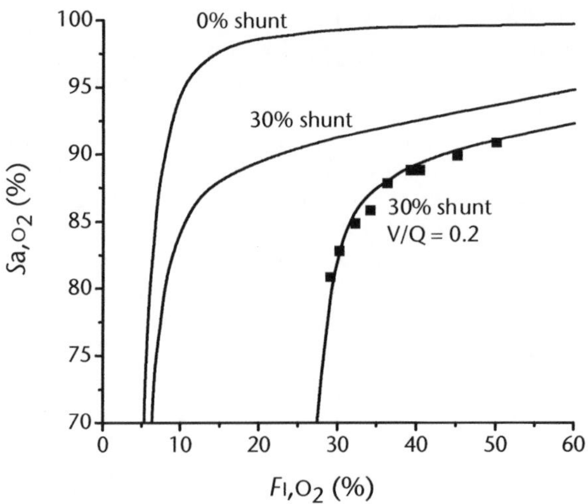

Fig. 42.5 Relaionship of Sa,O_2 to quantity of oxygen in inspired gas. Data points (black squares) are from a patient undergoing thoractomy with one lung ventilation whilst the collapsed lung was being operated on. The match with the isopleth for 30% shunt and $\dot{V}A/\dot{Q}$ ratio of 0.2 indicating that both shunt and $\dot{V}A/\dot{Q}$ imbalance were contributing to the poor gas exchange. Source: [71]

PI,O_2 versus SpO_2 diagram for assessing the degree of shunting and $\dot{V}A/\dot{Q}$ mismatch (see Section 21.6.3 and associated figures), also [71]. By this method a shunt depresses the PI,O_2 versus SpO_2 curve whilst $\dot{V}A/\dot{Q}$ inequality displaces the curve to the right. Figure 42.5 shows data from a patient undergoing single lung anaesthesia during an operation that entailed the collapse of the non-ventilated lung. In this circumstance there was $\dot{V}A/\dot{Q}$ mismatch due to increased dependent perfusion of poorly ventilated areas in the intact lung and a shunt that reflected continuing perfusion of the non-ventilated collapsed lung. The technique is a powerful tool for monitoring such patients.

Monitoring respiratory frequency. This can be undertaken by inductance plethysmography (also used in sleep studies and for studies in infants, Section 24.4.2), but non-invasive methods for accurately assessing tidal volumes are not yet available.

42.6.2 Epidural analgesia

Epidural analgesia is used in the post-operative period as a method for pain relief that, unlike opiates, does not suppress ventilatory drive. However, in a study of 10 subjects submitted to cervical epidural analgesia for upper limb surgery the epidural was found to carry a significant risk of reduced diaphragm excursion, reduced MIP (mean values 74 and 44 cm H_2O) and reduced FVC (mean values 3.8 and 2.8 l) [72] (cf. Section 9.5). A study comparing the effects of laparoscopic cholecystectomy (LPC), with and without thoracic epidural analgesia (TEA) versus subcostal incision found greatest reduction in FVC 24 h post-operatively with subcostal incision, less reduction with LPC, and least with LPC plus epidural analgesia [73]. An earlier randomised study of TEA, TEA and general anaesthesia (GA), and GA alone in 100 subjects found that FVC, FEV_1 and PEF measured within 24 h of operation were reduced by about 20% with TEA but by about 50% in patients receiving GA alone [74]. After the second post-operative day spirometric recovery was equivalent in all groups.

Thus, thoracic epidural anaesthesia is helpful in preserving respiratory function after surgery, but the cervical route for upper limb surgery is more hazardous on account of unintended involvement of the phrenic nerves.

42.6.3 Patient controlled analgesia

This technique is used for the management of post-operative pain. However the equipment needs to be robust and completely foolproof to avoid problems from overdosing leading to respiratory depression. Patients using patient controlled analgesia (PCA) must therefore be carefully trained and monitored. In elderly men post-operatively PCA has been shown to be superior to as-needed intramuscular injections of opiates, with a significant reduction in pulmonary complications [75]. Systematic review has confirmed this finding [76], but in chest trauma, epidural analgesia has been found to be superior to intravenous PCA [77].

42.7 References

1. von Ungern-Sternberg BS, Regli A, Bucher E et al. Impact of spinal anaesthesia and obesity on maternal respiratory function during elective Caesarian section. *Anaesthesia* 2004; **59**: 743–749.
2. Wightman JA. A prospective survey of the incidence of postoperative pulmonary complication. *Br J Surg* 1968; **55**: 85–91.
3. Macguire B, Royse C, Royse A et al. Lung function following cardiac surgery is not affected by postoperative ventilation time. *Ann Thorac Cardiovasc Surg* 2000; **6**: 13–18.
4. Carr HD, Stevens PM, Adamiya R. Preoperative pulmonary function and complications after cardiovascular surgery. *Chest* 1979; **76**: 130–135.
5. Kroenke K, Lawrence VA, Theroux JF et al. Operative risk in patients with severe obstructive pulmonary disease. *Arch Intern Med* 1992; **152**: 967–971.
6. Craig DB. Postoperative recovery of pulmonary function. *Anesth Analg* 1981; **60**: 46–52.
7. Zibrak JD, O'Donnell CR. Indications for preoperative pulmonary function testing. *Clin Chest Med* 1993; **14**: 227–236.
8. Bennun M, Goldstein B, Finkelstein Y, Jedeikin R. Continuous propofol anaesthesia for patients with myotonic dystrophy. *Br J Anaesth* 2000; **85**: 407–409.
9. Chuter TAM, Weissman C, Starker PM et al. Effect of incentive spirometry on diaphragmatic function after surgery. *Surgery* 1989; **105**: 488–493.
10. Hall JC, Tarala R, Harris J et al. Incentive spirometry versus routine chest physiotherapy for prevention of pulmonary complications after abdominal surgery. *Lancet* 1991; **337**: 953–956.
11. Strohl KP, Hensley MJ, Hallett M et al. Activation of upper airway muscles before onset of inspiration in normal humans. *J Appl Physiol* 1980; **49**: 638–642.

12. Rodenstein DO, Stanescu DC. The soft palate and breathing. *Am Rev Respir Dis* 1986; **134:** 311–325.
13. Boidin MP. Airway patency in the unconscious patient. *Br J Anaesth* 1985; **57**: 306–310.
14. Shorten GD, Opie NJ, Graziotti P et al. Assessment of upper airway anatomy in awake, sedated and anaesthetised patients using magnetic resonance imaging. *Anaesth Intensive Care* 1994; **22**: 165–169.
15. Dahan A, van den Elsen MJ, Berkenbosch A et al. Effects of subanesthetic halothane on the ventilatory responses to hypercapnia and acute hypoxia in healthy subjects. *Anesthesiology* 1994; **80**: 727–738.
16. Montes de oca M, Celli BR. Mouth occlusion pressure, CO_2 response and hypercapnia in severe chronic obstructive pulmonary disease. *Eur Respir J* 1998; **12**: 666–671.
17. Knill RL, Gelb AW. Ventilatory responses to hypoxia and hypercapnia during halothane sedation and anesthesia in man. *Anesthesiology* 1978; **49**: 244–251.
18. Sjogren D, Lindahl SG, Sollevi A. Ventilatory response to acute and sustained hypoxia during isoflurane anesthesia. *Anesth Analg* 1998; **86**: 403–409.
19. Van den Elsen MJ, Dahan A, Berkenbosch A et al. Does subanesthetic isoflurane affect the ventilatory response to acute isocapnic hypoxia in healthy volunteers? *Anesthesiology* 1994; **81**: 860–867.
20. Nagyova B, Dorrington KL, Gill EW, Robbins PA. Comparison of the effects of sub-hypnotic concentrations of propofol and halothane on the acute ventilatory response to hypoxia. *Br J Anaesth* 1995; **75**: 713–718.
21. Froese AB, Bryan CH. Effects of anaesthesia and paralysis on diaphragm mechanics in man. *Anaesthesiology* 1974; **41**: 242–255.
22. Muller N, Volgyesi G, Becker L et al. Diaphragmatic muscle tone. *J Appl Physiol* 1979; **47**: 279–284.
23. Hedenstierna G, Standberg E, Brismar B et al. Functional residual capacity, thoracoabdominal dimensions and central blood volume during general anaesthesia with muscle paralysis and mechanical ventilation. *Anaesthesiology* 1985; **62**: 247–254.
24. Kaul SU, Heath JR, Nunn JF. Factors influencing the development of expiratory muscle activity during anaesthesia. *Br J Anaesth* 1973; **45**: 1013–1018.
25. Bergman NA. Distribution of inspired gas during anaesthesia and artificial ventilation. *J Appl Physiol* 1963; **18**: 1085–1089.
26. Heneghan CPH, Jones JG. Pulmonary gas exchange and diaphragm position. *Br J Anaesth* 1985; **57**: 1161–1166.
27. Mackenzie N, Grant IS. Comparison of new emulsion formulation of propofol with methohexitone and thiopentone for induction of anaesthesia in day cases. *Br J Anaesth* 1985; **57**: 725–731.
28. Fisher DM, Robinsob S, Brett CM et al. Comparison of enflurane, halothane and isoflurane for diagnostic and therapeutic procedures in children with malignancies. *Anesthesiology* 1985; **63**: 647–650.
29. Jordan C, Lehane JR, Jones JG et al. Specific conductance using forced airflow oscillation in mechanically ventilated human subjects. *J Appl Physiol* 1981; **51**: 715–724.
30. Nunn JF, Hill DW. Respiratory dead space and arterial to end-tidal CO_2 tension difference in anesthetized man. *J Appl Physiol* 1960;**15**: 383–389.
31. Dueck R, Young I, Clausen J, Wagner PD. Altered distribution of pulmonary ventilation and blood flow following induction of inhalation anesthesia. *Anesthesiology* 1980; **52**: 113–125.
32. Bindslev L, Hedenstierna G, Santesson J et al. Ventilation-perfusion distribution during inhalation anaesthesia. Effects of spontaneous breathing, mechanical ventilation and positive end-expiratory pressure. *Acta Anaesth Scand* 1981; **25**: 360–371.
33. Tokics L, Hedenstierna G, Strandberg A et al. Lung collapse and gas exchange during general anaesthesia: effects of spontaneous breathing, muscle paralysis, and positive end-expiratory pressure. *Anesthesiology* 1987; **66**: 157–167.
34. Rothen HU, Neumann P, Berglund JE et al. Dynamics of re-expansion of atelectasis during general anaesthesia. *Br J Anaesth* 1999; **82**: 551–556.
35. Kuna ST, Insalaco G, Woodson GE. Thyroarytenoid muscle activity during wakefulness and sleep in normal adults. *J Appl Physiol* 1988; **65**: 1332–1339.
36. Abe T, Kusuhara N, Yoshimura N et al. Differential respiratory activity of four abdominal muscles in humans. *J Appl Physiol* 1996; **80**: 1379–1389.
37. Watson WE. Observations on physiological dead space during intermittent positive pressure respiration. *Br J Anaesth* 1962; **34**: 502–508.
38. Bergman NA. Effects of waveforms on gas exchange. *Anesthesiology* 1967; **28**: 390–395.
39. Fuleihan S, Wilson RS, Pontoppidan H. Effect of mechanical ventilation with end-inspiratory pause on blood-gas exchange. *Anesth Analg* 1976; **55**: 122–130.
40. Perez-Chada RD, Gardaz JP, Madgwick RG, Sykes MK. Cardiorespiratory effects of an inspiratory hold and continuous positive pressure ventilation in goats. *Intensive Care Med* 1983; **9**: 263–269.
41. Pelosi P, Crotti S, Brazzi L et al. Computed tomography in adult respiratory distress syndrome: what has it taught us? *Eur Respir J* 1996; **9**: 1055–1062.
42. The Acute Respiratory Distress Syndrome Network. Ventilation with lower tidal volumes as compared with traditional tidal volumes for acute lung injury and acute respiratory distress syndrome. *N Engl J Med* 2000; **342**: 1301–1308.
43. Scharf SM, Brown R, Saunders N et al. Hemodynamic effects of positive pressure inflation. *J Appl Physiol* 1980; **49**: 124–131.
44. Jardin FF, Farcot JC, Gueret P et al. Echocardiographic evaluation of ventricles during continuous positive pressure breathing. *J Appl Physiol* 1984; **56**: 619–627.
45. Stoller JK. Respiratory effects of positive end-expiratory pressure. *Respir Care* 1988; **33**: 454–463.
46. Pare PD, Warringer B, Baile EM et al. Redistribution of pulmonary extra-vascular water with positive end-expiratory pressure in canine pulmonary edema. *Am Rev Respir Dis* 1983; **127**: 590–593.
47. Baile EM, Albert RK, Kirk W et al. Positive end-expiratory pressure decreases bronchial blood flow in the dog. *J Appl Physiol* 1984; **56**: 1289–1293.
48. Hedenstierna G, White FC, Wagner PD. Spatial distribution of pulmonary blood flow in the dog with PEEP ventilation. *J Appl Physiol* 1979; **47**: 938–946.
49. Petty TL. Pulmonary perspectives. The use, abuse, and mystique of positive end-expiratory pressure. *Am Rev Respir Dis* 1988; **138**: 475–478.
50. Gammon RB, Shin MS, Buchalter SE. Pulmonary barotrauma in mechanical ventilation. *Chest* 1992; **102**: 568–572.
51. Kimball WR, Leith DE, Robins AG. Dynamic hyperinflation and ventilatory dependence in chronic obstructive pulmonary disease. *Am Rev Respir Dis* 1982; **126**: 991–995.

52. Pepe PE, Marini JJ. Occult positive end-expiratory pressure in mechanically ventilated patients with airflow obstruction. The auto-PEEP effect. *Am Rev Respir Dis* 1982; **126**: 166–170.
53. Zakynthinos SG, Vassilakopoulos T, Zakynthinos E et al. Contribution of expiratory muscle pressure to dynamic intrinsic positive end-expiratory pressure: validation using the Campbell diagram. *Am J Respir Crit Care Med* 2000; **162**: 1633–1640.
54. Gorini M, Misuri G, Duranti R et al. Abdominal muscle recruitment and PEEPi during bronchoconstriction in chronic obstructive pulmonary disease. *Thorax* 1997; **52**: 355–361.
55. Smith TC, Marini JJ. Impact of PEEP on lung mechanics and work of breathing in severe airflow obstruction. *J Appl Physiol* 1988; **65**: 1488–1499.
56. Petrof BJ, Legaré M, Goldberg P et al. Continuous positive airway pressure reduces work of breathing and dyspnea during weaning from mechanical ventilation in severe chronic obstructive pulmonary disease. *Am Rev Respir Dis* 1990; **141**: 281–289.
57. Rossi A, Santos C, Roca J et al. Effects of PEEP on VA/Q mismatching in ventilated patients with chronic airflow obstruction. *Am J Respir Crit Care Med* 1994; **149**: 1077–1084.
58. Ranieri VM, Giuliani R, Cinnella G et al. Physiologic effects of positive end-expiratory pressure in COPD patients during acute ventilatory failure and controlled mechanical ventilation. *Am Rev Respir Dis* 1993; **147**: 5–13.
59. Koutsoukou A, Armaganidis A, Stavrakaki-Kallergi C et al. Expiratory flow limitation and intrinsic positive end-expiratory pressure at zero positive end-expiratory pressure in patients with adult respiratory distress syndrome. *Am J Respir Crit Care Med* 2000; **161**: 1590–1596.
60. Laghi F, Cattapan SE, Jubran A et al. Is weaning failure caused by low-frequency fatigue of the diaphragm? *Am J Respir Crit Care Med* 2003; **167**: 120–127.
61. Diehl JL, El Atrous S, Touchard D et al. Changes in the work of breathing induced by tracheotomy in ventilator-dependent patients. *Am J Respir Crit Care Med* 1999; **159**: 383–388.
62. Guerin C, Milic-Emili J, Fournier G. Effect of PEEP on work of breathing in mechanically ventilated COPD patients. *Intensive Care Med* 2000; **26**: 1207–1214.
63. Vallerdu I, Calaf N, Subirana M et al. Clinical characteristics, respiratory functional parameters, and outcome of a two-hour T-piece trial in patients weaning from mechanical ventilation. *Am J Respir Crit Care Med* 1998; **158**: 1855–1862.
64. Leitch EA, Moran JL, Grealy B. Weaning and extubation in the intensive care unit. Clinical or index-driven approach? *Intensive Care Med* 1996; **22**: 752–759.
65. Khamiees M, Raju P, DeGirolamo A et al. Predictors of extubation outcome in patients who have successfully completed a spontaneous breathing trial. *Chest* 2001; **120**: 1262–1270.
66. Smina M, Salam A, Khamiees M et al. Cough peak flows and extubation outcomes. *Chest* 2003; **124**: 262–268.
67. Walsh TS, Dodds S, McArdle F. Evaluation of simple criteria to predict successful weaning from mechanical ventilation in intensive care patients. *Br J Anaesth* 2004; **92**: 793–799.
68. Krishnan JA, Moore D, Robeson C et al. A prospective, controlled trial of a protocol-based strategy to discontinue mechanical ventilation. *Am J Respir Crit Care Med* 2004; **169**: 673–678.
69. Malina JR, Nordstrom SG, Sjostrand UH, Wattwil LM. Clinical evaluation of high-frequency positive-pressure ventilation (HFPPV) in patients scheduled for open-chest surgery. *Anesth Analg* 1981; **60**: 324–330.
70. Lindberg P, Gunnarsson L, Tokics L et al. Atelectasis and lung function in the postoperative period. *Acta Anaesthesiol Scand* 1992; **36**: 546–553.
71. Jones JG, Jones SE. Discriminating between the effect of shunt and reduced VA/Q on arterial oxygen saturation is particularly useful in clinical practice. *J Clin Monit Comput* 2000; **16**: 337–350.
72. Capdevila X, Biboulet P, Rubenovitch J et al. The effects of cervical epidural anesthesia with bupivacaine on pulmonary function in conscious patients. *Anesth Analg* 1998; **86**: 1033–1038.
73. Rademaker BM, Ringers J, Odoom JA et al. Pulmonary function and stress response after laparascopic cholecystectomy: comparison with subcostal incision and influence of thoracic epidural analgesia. *Anesth Analg* 1992; **75**: 381–385.
74. Hendolin H, Lahtinen J, Lansimies E et al. The effect of thoracic epidural analgesia on respiratory function after cholecystectomy. *Acta Anaesthesiol Scand* 1987; **31**: 645–651.
75. Egbert AM, Parks LH, Short LM, Burnett ML. Randomized trial of postoperative patient-controlled analgesia vs. intramuscular narcotics in frail elderly men. *Arch Intern Med* 1990; **150**: 1897–1903.
76. Walder B, Schafer M, Henzi I, Tramer MR. Efficacy and safety of patient-controlled opioid analgesia for acute postoperative pain. A quantitative systematic review. *Acta Anaesthesiol Scand* 2001; **45**: 795–804.
77. Moon MR, Luchette FA, Gibson SW et al. Prospective, randomized comparison of epidural versus parenteral opioid analgesia in thoracic trauma. *Ann Surg* 1999; **229**: 684–691.

Further reading

Nunn's Applied Respiratory Physiology. Lumb AB. 5th ed. Butterworth–Heinemann & Co. 2000.

CHAPTER 43

Lung Function in relation to Surgery

43.1 Introduction

This chapter considers lung function in relation to thoracic surgery, including excisions, lung transplants and lung volume reduction surgery. It also revisits upper abdominal surgery where similar considerations apply.

43.2 Assessment for lung resection

An adult patient in whom FEV_1 is below 1.0 l usually has a greatly reduced exercise tolerance and is at increased risk of type 2 respiratory failure; the mortality approaches 10% per annum [1]. Many patients with lung tumours also have COPD where, if the FEV_1 is 0.75 l or less, the 5-year survival is about the same as in successfully resected stage 2 lung cancer [1, 2]. These figures indicate the approximate level of predicted post- operative FEV_1 at which thoracic surgery becomes inappropriate.

43.2.1 Resection for lung cancer

The likely post-operative FEV_1 is a major determinant of whether or not to operate. The estimate should take into account the probable extent of the excision, the quantity of functional lung tissue that will be removed and the condition of the lung tissue that will remain post-operatively. In some circumstances, e.g. where a lobe is collapsed due to bronchial occlusion, the post-operative function may not be changed by the operation. Thus, the algorithm for predicting post-operative FEV_1 should take into account whether the procedure is to be pneumonectomy, lobectomy or a lesser procedure.

Pneumonectomy

A patient whose pre-operative FEV_1 is greater than 2.0 l usually has enough ventilatory reserve to tolerate a pneumonectomy unless his or her ventilatory requirement is increased (Section 28.4.7). Such a patient is likely to experience undue dyspnoea on exertion. For lower levels of pre-operative FEV_1 the likely post-operative level should be adequate for a reasonable quality of life. The level will be less than the pre-operative FEV_1 by an amount that reflects the proportion of pulmonary vascular bed that is to be resected. This can be estimated from a perfusion scan [3]:

$$FEV_1\text{post-op (l)} = FEV_1\text{ pre-op} \times \text{proportion of perfusion going to the unresected lung} \quad \text{(RSD 0.19 l).}$$

In one study the relationship was found to account for over 80% of the variance in the post-operative FEV_1 [4]; the additional use of results from a ventilation scan did not improve the accuracy.

In the calculation, the left lung is taken as normally receiving 45% of total lung perfusion and the right lung 55%. Error in the prediction is greatest for central tumours (e.g. Fig. 43.1).

Lobectomy

For lobectomy, if the pre-operative FEV_1 is at least 1.5 l the patient is considered fit for surgery. Where pre-operative FEV_1 is less that 1.5 l the best predictor of FEV_1post-op is the proportion of lung segments that will remain (out of 19, Table 3.1, page 25):

$$FEV_1\text{post-op} = FEV_1\text{pre-op} \times \text{proportion of segments remaining.}$$

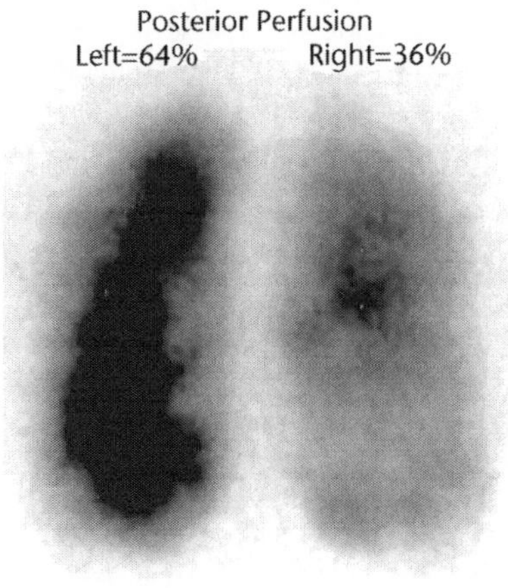

Posterior Perfusion
Left=64% Right=36%

Fig. 43.1 Posterior view of lung perfusion scan in a patient with a large right lung tumour. Pre-operative $FEV_1 = 1.65$ l, predicted post-operative $FEV_1 = 1.65 \times 0.64 = 1.06$ l.

The proportions of segments remaining after the different lobectomies are given in Table 43.1 (cf. Section 3.3.2). The use of data from ventilation and/or perfusion scans did not improve the predictions [4].

Lung function criteria of operability

A post-operative predicted $FEV_1 < 1.0$ l is taken by some as a relative contraindication to pneumonectomy and <0.8 l as an absolute contraindication. Some have argued that an absolute cut off level may disadvantage shorter, older or female patients who normally have a rather low absolute FEV_1. Thus, the use of per cent of predicted, with a cut off of 40% has been suggested instead [5], but this method introduces an age and height bias [6]. For patients with borderline lung function other tests can also be used. Pre-operative transfer factor can identify patients who have a high operative risk from lung resection (Fig. 43.2). Based on these data a threshold of <60% of the reference value for *Tl*,co has been proposed [7], alternatively a predicted post-operative level of <40% of the reference value might be used [5]. Other indices of transfer that have been proposed are the increase in transfer factor on exercise (cf. Section 29.2.2) and the method of measurement that makes separate estimates for

Table 43.1 Proportion of segments remaining after various lobectomy procedures for use in predicting post-operative FEV_1.

Lobectomy	Segments removed	Proportion remaining
Right upper	3	0.84
Right middle	2	0.89
Right middle and upper	5	0.74
Right lower	5	0.74
Left upper	5	0.74
Left lower	4	0.79

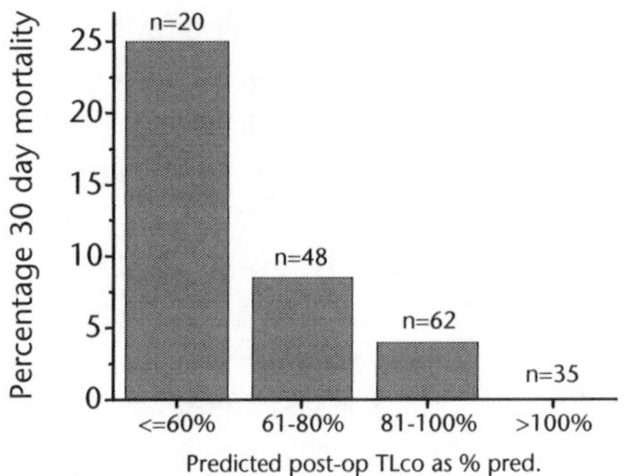

Fig. 43.2 Percentage of patients dying within 30 days following resection of lung carcinoma according to their preoperative *Tl*,co as per cent of predicted. Source: [7]

the inspiratory, breathhold, and expiratory part of the usual single breath CO transfer test (Section 20.4) [8].

Normally gas transfer increases on exercise due to recruitment of more pulmonary vasculature to accommodate the increased cardiac output. A study of cancer patients pre- and post-resection found that post-operative complications were likely if gas transfer did not rise by at least 10% on exercising up to 70% of exercise capacity [8]. This criterion had a 78% sensitivity in predicting post-operative complications.

In the past surgeons have felt that a patient who could not walk up a flight of stairs and conduct a conversation at the top was unsuitable for lung resection. This was confirmed in a study where the number of steps climbed was found to be an independent predictor of post-operative complications, whilst terms for pre-op FEV_1, predicted post-op FEV_1, age and coexisting cardiac disease were not significant [9]. Most (but not all) studies using conventional estimates of exercise performance have come to a similar conclusion. In one study a maximal oxygen uptake <50% predicted was associated with an increased mortality from post-operative complications [10]. In another study, patients tolerated resection well if their maximal oxygen uptake per kg body mass exceeded 15 ml kg^{-1} [11]. This work level corresponded to being able to complete 25 shuttles on a shuttle walk test [5], see (Section 29.9.3).

The difficulty with predictions is that the probability of post-operative survival has to be set against the probability of cure from the surgery. Here the perspective of the individual patient is all important. The role of the clinician is to present a fair and complete appraisal of the risks and benefits from the various treatment options so that an informed decision can be made.

43.2.2 Lung volume reduction surgery

An operative procedure to remove grossly damaged tissue from the lungs of emphysema patients was introduced in 1957 [12]. It was found to benefit some patients but was abandoned due to a high early mortality (approximately 16%). The rationale for this approach is as follows:

Patients with emphysema have hyperinflated lungs and airflow limitation. The hyperinflation can be seen as an adaptive mechanism to augment the lung elastic recoil and so reduce airway closure (Section 11.5.1). However, the higher FRC in these subjects has several detrimental effects:
(a) The chest wall operates over an adverse part of its volume–pressure relationship. So at end expiration the chest wall exerts a positive alveolar pressure that acts as an inspiratory load to be overcome at the beginning of inspiration, and total inspiratory work is increased [13, 14].
(b) The low, flat diaphragm position reduces the area of apposition between diaphragm and the thoraco-abdominal wall. This limits the ability of the diaphragm to lever the lower ribs outward and upward on inspiration [15].
(c) The low, flat resting position of the diaphragm sets the muscle fibres in the diaphragm at below their natural resting length so their ability to develop further tension is reduced. Their ability to increase thoracic volume by displacing abdominal contents downwards is diminished [16].

A successful operation will (i) reduce the level of hyperinflation so the respiratory pump can work at a position that is more advantageous, and (ii) increase the lung elastic recoil by removing some grossly emphysematous tissue. According to protocol the tissue to be removed is not contributing to gas exchange so the patient is better off without it. Thus, the criteria for successful LVRS [17, 18] include that the distribution of the emphysema, as assessed on CT scans, is heterogeneous. This enables the surgeon to select the worst affected areas for resection and leave the less damaged tissue to benefit from the reduced thoracic volume. In a study of unilateral lung volume reduction surgery in patients with asymmetric heterogenous emphysema there was sustained improvement over 3 years. At the end of this time FEV_1 was increased by an average 24% and RV was reduced by 12% [19].

The effectiveness of the operation was confirmed in one study where 80% of the patients experienced an increase in lung elastic recoil [20]. Unfortunately, few centres measure the recoil so other criteria are needed. Optimal benefit seems to be obtained in patients where the operation of LVRS reduces the RV more than the TLC, so the VC and FEV_1 are increased [21, 22]. Thus, if pre-operative assessment demonstrates severe airflow limitation, a very high RV as per cent of TLC and heterogeneous emphysema on CT scan, then the likelihood of benefit from LVRS is high.

The main concern from LVRS is the peri-operative mortality with the inter-quartile range across studies being 0–6% for 30 day mortality [23]. A mildly elevated Pa,CO_2 is not considered to be a problem despite early worries on this account [24, 25]. However, poor results have been obtained from patients with a low walking distance and high Pa,CO_2 [26], and in patients with a very low gas transfer (<20% of predicted value) the operative risks also outweigh the benefit [17].

A review of many studies [23] showed an expectation of an increase of 0.23–0.36 l in FEV_1 (inter-quartile range) from a baseline of 0.64–0.73 l, and an increase of 32–96 m on a baseline 6-min walking distance of 241–290 m. Individuals may respond differently to LVRS with some subjects experiencing increased exercise capacity of up to 40% [27] (correlated with increases in FEV_1), whereas in others an improvement in gas exchange was associated with reduction in pulmonary artery pressure that was unrelated to the FEV_1.

43.3 Lung transplantation

Lung function tests have an important role in lung transplant surgery. First, the decision to proceed to lung transplantation involves assessment as to whether transplantation is the best management plan for the patient. Then, there is a need to decide if the sizes of the donor lung and the recipient chest cavity are adequately matched. After transplantation early identification of rejection is the key to successful management.

43.3.1 Assessment for lung transplantation

Lung transplantation has now become an accepted method for treating a number of otherwise lethal pulmonary conditions. However, with an insufficient supply of lungs for transplantation, an inherently difficult procedure and an uncertain risk of some degree of rejection, the management of patients who are likely candidates for the procedure is extremely difficult. In addition, as the mortality and survival for lung transplantation improve so this risk assessment has to be modified.

Guidelines have been published for the selection of patients for lung transplantation [28]. Spirometry criteria have included, for COPD (FEV_1<25% predicted), for cystic fibrosis (CF) (FEV_1<30% predicted) and for pulmonary fibrosis (VC<60% predicted). Considerable difficulty surrounds predicting the optimal time for transplantation in CF and over reliance on the above data can distort the balance of risk involved [29]. The rapidity of decline is the most important consideration [30]. In one study of CF, amongst patients with a very low FEV_1 (<20% predicted) and hypercapnia, the risk of dying pre-transplant was increased by a factor of 1.43 for every increment in Pa,CO_2 of 1 kPa (7.5 mm Hg) above the normal level [31]. The inclusion of the 12-min walking distance improved the prediction, but there was no further improvement with the additional inclusion of FEV_1, arterial saturation, Pa,CO_2 or BMI [32]. The fact that from a group of 300 patients waiting for transplantation those with COPD/emphysema had the lowest death rate [33] may relate to the better ability to predict future decline in this condition.

Patients with idiopathic pulmonary fibrosis (IPF) are more likely to die whilst awaiting transplant than those with other diagnoses [34]. On this account patients under 65 years with IPF that has not responded to corticosteroids should be referred for transplant if either transfer factor or VC is less than 60% of predicted, or if there is resting hypoxia or pulmonary hypertension

[28]. A model including a CT score of fibrosis and transfer factor has shown that a gas transfer ≤39% predicted indicated worse survival awaiting transplant [35] so referral should not be left this late. Data from spirometry, static volumes, gas transfer and exercise tests such as 6-min walk tests or shuttle walk tests can all contribute to predicting how fast a subject's performance is declining.

43.3.2 Post-transplantation – rejection and infection

A rather small donor lung is usually able to expand to fill the recipient thorax with little functional effect whereas cramming too large a lung into a small thorax is less satisfactory. The final volume of the donor lung after double lung or heart and lung transplant is largely dictated by the recipient thorax and can increase for up to a year. If spirometry is to be useful in the early identification of rejection or infection the within subject variability needs to be known. For FEV_1 in single lung transplants a fall of 13% or more after 80 days post-transplant is likely to be significant and for double lung or heart–lung transplant a fall of 18% in the 1st year or 9% after the 1st year are likely to be significant [36].

Long-term survival for lung transplant recipients is best if the effects of rejection can be minimised through early detection and treatment. Any of several indices can be used of which spirometry is the simplest. In heart–lung transplants a significant change in FEV_1 has been found to have a 75% sensitivity in detecting either rejection or infection whereas chest radiograph only had 19% sensitivity for rejection and 58% sensitivity for infection [37]. For single lung transplants spirometry has been found useful in detecting rejection [38].

The onset of obliterative bronchiolitis (OB) following chronic rejection has a serious portent on graft survival. Attempts to detect specific physiologic change in OB using estimates of ventilation distribution from the alveolar slopes of He, N_2, and SF_6 have failed to show changes that distinguish this condition from acute infection or rejection [39].

43.4 Cardiothoracic surgery

Open-heart surgery for ischaemic heart disease is a common operation undertaken in some countries. The majority of the patients are smokers who, on this account, often have co-existing pulmonary disease and impaired lung function. However, the lung function does not predict the operative risk in this situation [40], whereas it does so for thoracic operations on the lungs (see above) and oesophagus [41].

Cardiac surgery can adversely affect lung function mechanically through the procedures of sternotomy or thoracotomy reducing the chest wall compliance [42] or damaging the muscles of respiration. The operation can also damage the phrenic nerve.

43.4.1 Effect of thoracotomy and sternotomy

Thoracotomy and median sternotomy can lead to the VC being reduced post-operatively, but sternotomy seems to cause less effect [43]. On discharge from hospital after open-heart surgery PEF has been found to be about 33% below pre-operative values [44] and lung volumes were reduced by between 20 and 33%. By 3 months these had largely recovered. Dissection for use of the internal mammary artery was associated with greater reductions. When compared with lateral thoracotomy, a sternotomy caused comparable changes in function that recovered more quickly [45]. Training the inspiratory muscles before the operation of coronary bypass surgery was found to reduce respiratory complications after the operation [46].

43.4.2 Effect on diaphragm function

The operation of open-heart surgery has been found to impair the function of the diaphragm in 10–85% of patients, depending on how the tests were carried out [47, 48]. A common cause is phrenic nerve dysfunction from direct damage during dissection, manipulation of the mediastinal structures or cold injury in circumstances when cold cardioplegia is employed [49]. Dissection of the left internal mammary artery is associated with left phrenic nerve dysfunction [50]. However, unilateral phrenic dysfunction is of little consequence in subjects with normal pre-operative lung function [51], whilst bilateral phrenic damage appears to be uncommon. In one series it was documented in 2% of cases [52].

43.5 General surgery

General surgery, as distinct from the general anaesthesia, only affects the lung function if the diaphragm and respiratory muscles are involved or the patient experiences a pulmonary embolus. Cerebral surgery can lead to oedema that is likely to affect the control of ventilation whilst head and neck surgery may compromise the upper airway. Abdominal surgery is worth more detailed consideration.

43.5.1 Abdominal incisions

For a hundred years the site of the abdominal incision has been known to influence the post-operative pulmonary complications [53]. Upper abdominal incisions cause respiratory muscle dysfunction in up to 40% of cases whereas with lower incisions this is seen in less than 5% of cases. MIP, MEP and transdiaphragmatic pressures are reduced after upper abdominal surgery [54] and this effect can last for up to 7 days [55]. There appears to be reflex reduction in diaphragm recruitment with increased use of intercostal muscles and rib cage movement [56]. Laparoscopic surgery also reduces MIP, but the effect is much less than that seen with open abdominal surgery [57]. Surgery involving dissection close to the diaphragm can also affect post-operative respiratory function. For example, the extensive dissection needed in orthoptic liver transplantation has been noted to cause right hemidiaphragm paralysis in about a third of patients [58].

A history of COPD increases the relative risk (RR) of post-operative pulmonary complications following abdominal surgery by a factor of between 2.7 and 4.7 [59]. The risk appears not to be related to the level of lung function as tested by spirometry and gas transfer, even with FEV_1 values as low as 0.45 l (i.e. RR = 1.0) [60]. However, where abnormalities were found on clinical examination of the patient's chest the RR was increased to 5.8 [61].

43.5.2 Laparoscopy

Artificial pneumoperitoneum is undertaken to allow access to the abdominal contents for video-assisted keyhole surgery in a number of general surgical and gynaecological conditions. The gas commonly used is carbon dioxide, of which some is absorbed raising the Pa,CO_2. The gas is quickly cleared through an increase in minute ventilation [62]. The pneumoperitoneum raises the abdominal pressure, hence raises the position of the diaphragm and reduces the respiratory compliance [63]. These effects are magnified in morbidly obese patients in whom the intraabdominal pressure can be elevated and there may be some pre-existing hypercapnia [64].

43.6 References

1. Diener CF, Burrows B. Further observations on the course and prognosis of chronic obstructive lung disease. *Am Rev Respir Dis* 1975; **111**: 719–724.
2. Mountain CF, Dresler CM. Regional lymph node classification for lung cancer staging. *Chest* 1997; **111**: 1718–1723.
3. Kristersson S, Lindell SE, Svanberg L. Prediction of pulmonary function loss due to pneumonectomy using ^{133}Xe-radiospirometry. *Chest* 1972; **60**: 694–698.
4. Wernly JA, DeMeester TR, Kirchner PT et al. Clinical value of quantitative ventilation-perfusion lung scans in the surgical management of bronchogenic carcinoma. *J Thorac Cardiovasc Surg* 1980; **80**: 535–543.
5. British Thoracic Society. Guidelines on the selection of patients with lung cancer for surgery. *Thorax* 2001; **56**: 89–108.
6. Miller MR, Pincock AC. Predicted values: how should we use them? *Thorax* 1988; **43**: 265–267.
7. Ferguson MK, Little L, Rizzo J et al. Diffusing capacity predicts morbidity and mortality after pulmonary resection. *J Thorac Cardiovasc Surg* 1988; **96**: 894–900.
8. Wang JS, Abboud RT, Evans KG et al. Role of CO diffusing capacity during exercise in the preoperative evaluation for lung resection. *Am J Respir Crit Care Med* 2000; **162**: 1435–1444.
9. Brunelli A, Al Refai M, Monteverde M et al. Stair climbing test predicts cardiopulmonary complications after lung resection. *Chest* 2002; **121**: 1106–1110.
10. Larsen KR, Svendsen UG, Milman N et al. Exercise testing in the preoperative evaluation of patients with bronchogenic carcinoma. *Eur Respir J* 1997; **10**: 1559–1565.
11. Beckles MA, Spiro SG, Colice GL, Rudd RM. The physiologic evaluation of patients with lung cancer being considered for resectional surgery. *Chest* 2003; **123**(Suppl 1): 105S–114S.
12. Brantigan O, Mueller E. Surgical treatment of pulmonary emphysema. *Am Surg* 1957; **23**: 789–804.
13. Pepe P, Marini J. Occult positive end-expiratory pressure in mechanically ventilated patients with airflow obstruction. *Am Rev Respir Dis* 1982; **126**: 166–170.
14. Rochester D, Braun N, Arora N. Respiratory muscle strength in chronic obstructive pulmonary disease. *Am Rev Respir Dis* 1979; **119**: 151–154.
15. Loring S, Mead J. Action of the diaphragm on the rib cage inferred from a force-balance analysis. *J Appl Physiol* 1982; **53**: 756–760.
16. Mead J. Functional significance of the area of apposition of diaphragm to rib cage. *Am Rev Respir Dis* 1979; **119**(Suppl): S31–S32.
17. Russi EW, Bloch KE, Weder W. Functional and morphological heterogeneity of emphysema and its implication for selection of patients for lung volume reduction surgery. *Eur Respir J* 1999; **14**: 230–236.
18. Yusen RD, Lefrak SS, Trulock EP. Evaluation and preoperative management of lung volume reduction surgery candidates. *Clinics Chest Med* 1997; **18**: 199–223.
19. Mineo TC, Pompeo E, Minoe D et al. Results of unilateral lung volume reduction surgery in patients with distinct heterogeneity of emphysema between lungs. *J Thorac Cardiovasc Surg* 2005; **129**: 73–79.
20. Sciurba FC, Rogers RM, Keenan RJ, et al. Improvement in pulmonary function and elastic recoil after lung reduction surgery for diffuse emphysema. *N Eng J Med* 1996; **334**: 1095–1099.
21. Cooper JD, Trulock EP, Triantafillou AN et al. Bilateral pneumectomy (volume reduction) for chronic obstructive pulmonary disease. *J Thorac Cardiovasc Surg* 1995; **109**: 106–119.
22. Brenner M, McKenna RJ Jr., Gelg AF et al. Objective predictors of response for staple versus laser emphysematous lung reduction. *Am J Respir Crit Care Med* 1997; **155**: 1295–1301.
23. Young J, Fry-Smith A, Hyde C. Lung volume reduction surgery (LVRS) for chronic obstructive pulmonary disease (COPD) with underlying severe emphysema. *Thorax* 1999; **54**: 779–789.
24. O'Brien GM, Furukawa S, Kuzma AM et al. Improvements in lung function, exercise, and quality of life in hypercapnic COPD patients after lung volume reduction surgery. *Chest* 1999; **115**: 75–84.
25. Eugene J, Dajee A, Kayaleh R et al. Reduction pneumoplasty for patients with a forced expiratory volume in 1 second of 500 ml or less. *Ann Thorac Surg* 1997; **63**: 186–190.
26. Szekely LA, Oelberg DA, Wright C et al. Preoperative predictors of operative morbidity and mortality in COPD patients undergoing bilateral lung volume reduction surgery. *Chest* 1997; **111**: 550–558.
27. Oswald-Mammosser M, Kessler R, Massared G et al. Effect of lung volume reduction on gas exchange and pulmonary hemodynamics at rest and during exercise. *Am J Respir Crit Care Med* 1998; **158**: 1020–1025.
28. American Thoracic Society Joint Statement. International guidelines for the selection of lung transplant candidates. *Am J Respir Crit Care Med* 1998; **158**: 335–339.
29. Doershuk CF, Stern RC. Timing of referral for lung transplantation for cystic fibrosis: overemphasis on FEV_1 may adversely affect overall survival. *Chest* 1999; **115**: 782–787.
30. Rosenbluth DB, Wilson K, Ferkol T, Schuster DP. Lung function decline in cystic fibrosis patients and timing for lung transplantation referral. *Chest* 2004; **126**: 412–419.

31. Sharples L, Hathaway T, Dennis C et al. Prognosis of patients with cystic fibrosis awaiting heart and lung transplantation. *J Heart Lung Transplant* 1993; **12**: 669–674.
32. Ruter K, Staab D, Magdorf K et al. The 12-min walk test as an assessment criterion for lung transplantation in subjects with cystic fibrosis. *J Cyst Fibros* 2003; **2**: 8–13.
33. Mannes GP, de Boer WJ, van der Bij W et al. Three hundred patients referred for lung transplantation. Experiences of the Dutch Lung Transplantation Program. *Chest* 1996; **109**: 408–413.
34. Hosenpud JD, Bennett LE, Keck BM et al. Effect of diagnosis on survival benefit of lung transplantation for end-stage lung disease. *Lancet* 1998; **351**: 24–27.
35. Mogulkoc N, Brutsche MH, Bishop PW et al. Pulmonary function in idiopathic pulmonary fibrosis and referral for lung transplantation. *Am J Respir Crit Care Med* 2001; **164**: 103–108.
36. Martinez JA, Paradis IL, Dauber JH et al. Spirometry values in stable lung transplant recipients. *Am J Respir Crit Care Med* 1997; **155**: 285–290.
37. Otulana BA, Higenbottam T, Scott J et al. Lung function associated with histologically diagnosed acute lung rejection and pulmonary infection in heart-lung transplant patients. *Am Rev Respir Dis* 1990; **142**: 329–332.
38. Becker FS, Martinez FJ, Brunsting LA et al. Limitations of spirometry in detecting rejection after single-lung transplantation. *Am J Respir Crit Care Med* 1994; **150**: 159–166.
39. Muylem AV, Antoine M, Yernault J-C et al. Inert gas single-breath washout after heart-lung transplantation. *Am J Respir Crit Care Med* 1995; **152**: 947–952.
40. Warner MA, Divertie MB, Tinker JH. Preoperative cessation of smoking and pulmonary complications in coronary artery bypass patients. *Anesthesiology* 1984; **60**: 380–383.
41. Law SYK, Fok M, Wong J. Risk analysis in resection of squamous cell carcinoma of the oesophagus. *World J Surg* 1994; **18**: 339–346.
42. Karlson KE, Seltzer B, Lee S et al. Influence of thoracotomy on pulmonary mechanics: association of increased work of breathing during anaesthesia and postoperative pulmonary complications. *Ann Surg* 1965; **162**: 973–980.
43. Peters RM, Wellons HA, Htwe TM. Total compliance and work of breathing after thoracotomy. *J Thorac Cardiovasc Surg* 1969; **57**: 348.
44. Shapira N, Zabatino SM, Ahmed S et al. Determinants of pulmonary function in patients undergoing coronary bypass operations. *Ann Thorac Surg* 1990; **50**: 268–273.
45. Cooper JD, Nelems JM, Pearson FG. Extended indications for median sternotomy in patients requiring pulmonary resection. *Ann Thorac Surg* 1978; **26**: 413–420.
46. Weinder P, Zeidan F, Zamir D, et al. Prophylactic inspiratory muscle training in patients undergoing coronary bypass graft. *World J Surg* 1998; **22**: 427–431.
47. Benjamin JJ, Cascade PN, Rubenfire M et al. Left lower lobe atelectasis and consolidation following cardiac surgery: effect of topical cooling on the phrenic nerve. *Radiology* 1982; **142**: 11–14.
48. Clergue F, Whitelaw WA, Charles JC et al. Inferences about respiratory muscle use after cardiac surgery from compartmental volume and pressure measurements. *Anesthesiology* 1995; **82**: 1318–1327.
49. Mills GH, Khan ZP, Moxham J et al. Effects of temperature on phrenic nerve and diaphragm function during cardiac surgery. *Br J Anaesth* 1997; **79**: 726–732.
50. O'Brien JW, Johnson SH, VanSteyn SJ et al. Effects of internal mammary artery dissection on phrenic nerve perfusion and function. *Ann Thorac Surg* 1991; **52**: 182–188.
51. Diehl JL, Lafaso F, Deleuze P et al. Clinically relevant diaphragmatic dysfunction after cardiac operations. *J Thorac Cardiovasc Surg* 1994; **107**: 487–498.
52. Dimopolou I, Daganou M, Dafani U et al. Phrenic nerve dysfunction after cardiac operations. Electrophysiologic evaluation of risk factors. *Chest* 1998; **113**: 8–14.
53. Pasteur W. Active lobar collapse of the lung after abdominal operations. *Lancet* 1910; **ii**: 1080–1083.
54. Ford GT, Whitelaw WA, Rosinal WT et al. Diaphragm function after abdominal surgery in humans. *Am Rev Respir Dis* 1983; **127**: 431–436.
55. Putensen-Himmer G, Putensen C, Lammer H et al. Comparison of postoperative respiratory function after laparoscopic or open laparotomy for cholecystectomy. *Anesthesiology* 1992; **77**: 675–680.
56. Ford GT, Rosenal TW, Clergue F et al. Respiratory physiology in upper abdominal surgery. *Clin Chest Med* 1993; **14**: 237–252.
57. Rovina N, Bouros D, Tzanakis N et al. Effects of laparascopic cholecystectomy on global respiratory muscle strength. *Am J Respir Crit Care Med* 1996; **153**: 458–461.
58. McAlister VC, Grant DR, Roy A et al. Right phrenic nerve injury in orthoptic liver transplantation. *Transplantation* 1993; **55**: 826–830.
59. Smetana GW. Preoperative pulmonary evaluation. *N Engl J Med* 1999; **340**: 937–944.
60. Jackson CV. Preoperative pulmonary evaluation. *Arch Intern Med* 1988; **148**: 2120–2127.
61. Lawrence VA, Dhandra R, Hilsenbeck SG, Page CD. Risk of pulmonary complications after elective abdominal surgery. *Chest* 1996; **110**: 744–750.
62. Tan PL, Lee TL, Tweed WA. Carbon dioxide absorption and gas exchange during pelvic laparoscopy. *Can J Anaesth* 1992; **39**: 677–681.
63. Rauh R, Hemmerling TM, Rist M, Jacobi KE. Influence of pneumoperitoneum and patient posture on respiratory system compliance. *J Clin Anaesth* 2001; **13**: 361–365.
64. Nguyen NT, Wolfe BM. The physiologic effects of pneumoperitoneum in the morbidly obese. *Ann Surg* 2005; **241**: 219–226.

Further reading

Zibrak JD, O'Donnell CR. Indications for preoperative pulmonary function testing. *Clinics Chest Med* 1993; **14**: 227–236.

CHAPTER 44

Pulmonary Rehabilitation

44.1 Introduction

Pulmonary rehabilitation programmes (PRP) are now widely promoted [1, 2]. Their aims are to ameliorate and control the patients' symptoms, minimise any complications from the illnesses and help the patients to live active lives with a minimum of restriction. The components of the programme may include education about the diseases, advice on smoking cessation, psychosocial support and guidance, optimisation of conventional medical therapies, nutritional advice and exercise conditioning. Several of the components require the active participation of the lung function laboratory. The outcome has been shown to be effective in a number of circumstances [3–5].

Most evidence is for patients with chronic obstructive pulmonary disease (COPD) and extrapolation to other diseases may not be justified. For COPD the beneficial effects can be long lasting. Thus, amongst more than 200 patients randomised to either a 6-week PRP (18 visits) or standard care with reassessment after a year the treated group had better walking ability and a record of fewer family practitioner visits and days in hospital. However, the number of hospital admissions was not reduced [6]. A similar randomised study with an 8-week PRP found better exercise tolerance at the end of a year [7] and a more complicated PRP confirmed this finding at 2 years [8], as well as the failure to reduce admissions despite reducing the number of exacerbations.

Exercise is a key part of PRP, so this chapter will review how exercise is limited in lung diseases and consider the place of lung function and exercise testing in rehabilitation programmes. Many of the topics are considered in greater detail in other chapters (see especially Section 28.12).

44.2 Limitation of exercise in lung disease

In patients with lung diseases the exercise limitation may be due to (1) ventilatory insufficiency and inability to achieve an adequate alveolar ventilation, (2) excessive energy cost of breathing such that an increase in ventilation mainly provides oxygen for the respiratory muscles, (3) impaired gas exchange in the lungs that increases the need for additional ventilation, (4) muscle deconditioning and dysfunction (skeletal and respiratory) that limits performance and (5) cardiac insufficiency that restricts the distribution of oxygen from the lungs to muscles and other tissues.

44.2.1 Ventilatory limitation

In respiratory patients activity during daily living is typically limited by breathlessness. This is a consequence of the damaged lungs not being able to satisfy the urge to breath because of constraints on ventilation (airflow limitation, restricted expansion etc). The balance between supply and demand is made worse by wasted ventilation for which there are three principal causes: (1) $\dot{V}\text{A}/\dot{Q}$ inequality enlarging the ventilation per minute of the alveolar deadspace, (2) shallow breathing wasting ventilation on the deadspace of the airways (high Vd/Vt) and (3) hypoxaemia causing additional chemoreceptor drive to respiration.

When ventilation is limited by narrowing of airways (airflow limitation) there is a compensatory increase in lung volume (hyperinflation). This increases the calibre of small airways by traction from the stroma of the lung (guy lines as in Section 11.2) but at the cost of reducing the inspiratory capacity [9]. During progressive exercise these changes occur dynamically at near to the breaking point; they include a rise in end- expiratory lung volume (EELV), shallow breathing (that adds to the deadspace ventilation as described above) and a change in shape of the Hey plot ($\dot{V}_E$ versus Vt) (Fig. 29.9, page 431)

The diminished ventilatory capacity is best described in terms of FEV_1 (e.g. Fig. 28.13, page 398) or by the flow–volume curve (Fig. 28.18, page 404). The increased ventilatory cost of exercise is measured during a progressive exercise test by comparing the observed ventilation with that expected for the patient's oxygen uptake, respiratory frequency and respiratory exchange ratio (Table 29.15, page 433). Examples are given in Tables 29.11 and 29.12 (pages 429 and 430).

The increase in EELV and consequent shallow breathing represent internal adaptations to narrowing of airways. In PRP (and also in the course of routine treatment) the need for these responses can be reduced or eliminated by energetic measures to expand and clear the airways (e.g. discontinuing smoking, bronchodilator and anti-inflammatory drug therapy, posture, physiotherapy, controlled coughing). These measures can increase the ventilatory capacity, reduce the hyperinflation and associated shallow breathing and exert a beneficial effect on the three causes of increased ventilatory cost of exercise. The case for their use is overwhelming. It would be satisfactory if the same held for an exercise training programme. However, in a recent study of patients with ventilatory limitation compared with others who had cardiovascular limitation (or non-cardiopulmonary limitation), the increase in exercise performance obtained from adding an exercise PRP to other components of the programme was much reduced in the ventilation limited group [10]. This indicated that the exercise programme *per se* did little to improve airflow limitation and its impact on performance in these patients. More effective help can often be given by prescription of portable oxygen equipment; this is beneficial when it reduces the ventilatory cost of exercise (Section 28. 8.1).

44.2.2 Energy cost of breathing

In conditions of low lung compliance (pulmonary fibrosis), of low chest wall compliance (obesity, ankylosing spondylitis) and with increased airway resistance (COPD, asthma, cystic fibrosis) the energy cost of breathing at rest is increased above normal by a factor of between 2 and 7 times [11–13]. Hence, the increased ventilation that accompanies exercise results in a disproportionate rise in the requirement for oxygen by the respiratory muscles. In the limiting situation, all the extra oxygen that is absorbed by the increased ventilation is used to power those muscles.

The energy expended on breathing can be reduced if circumstances are arranged so that the respiratory muscles perform less work. The work of overcoming airflow resistance can be reduced by breathing a helium–oxygen gas mixture instead of air. Part of the load borne by the respiratory muscles can be transferred to some form of assisted ventilation [14] and the total work can be reduced by lowering the ventilation through use of controlled oxygen therapy. There are disadvantages to all these remedies but at least they are available in an emergency situation.

44.2.3 Impaired gas exchange

In some patients hypoxaemia occurring during progressive exercise is due to defective gas transfer (e.g. if Tl,co is below 55% of the predicted value [15]). This mechanism can be the cause for exercise hypoxaemia in those patients with COPD in whom emphysema is the principal abnormality. However in most COPD patients the Pa,O_2 during exercise is relatively normal. Any small reduction is likely to be caused by uneven lung function ($\dot{V}_A/\dot{Q}$ inequality), as is also the case during near maximal exercise in a small proportion of healthy subjects (Section 28.8.2).

In patients with $\dot{V}_A/\dot{Q}$ inequality, taking exercise can affect the blood oxygen level by any of the three mechanisms: (1). The ventilation increases, including that to lung units which are relatively poorly ventilated; this can raise the Sa,O_2. (2) The blood flow through the lungs increases and its distribution tends to becomes more uniform; this can increase the flow through poorly ventilated lung units, hence reduce the Sa,O_2. (3) During exercise the saturation of mixed venous blood falls. This tends to promote desaturation, especially in patients with COPD where a significant proportion of lung units have a very low $\dot{V}_A/\dot{Q}$ ratio. The low saturation of the mixed venous blood then contributes to arterial desaturation [16, 17], with no evidence of change in the pattern of $\dot{V}_A/\dot{Q}$ inequality. The measured arterial desaturation can be wholly accounted for by this effect with no evidence of diffusion limitation.

In patients with interstitial fibrosis the situation is different. Diffusion limitation accounts for up to 14% of the A-aPO_2 at rest, as in normal subjects, but the proportion is increased to 50% or more when the patients exercise at sea level [18] (or are conveyed to altitude), cf. Fig. 21.2, (page 263), also Section 40.4.

44.2.4 Muscle dysfunction

Patients who are disabled with lung disease become inactive, their skeletal muscle loses its physical condition and exercise can then be limited by fatigue rather than breathlessness. Exercise training is then a therapeutic possibility. Where the deconditioning affects the respiratory muscles a programme of respiratory muscle training can also be considered (see below).

44.2.5 Cardiovascular dysfunction

Cardiac limitation of exercise occurs in diseases that affect the heart as a result of inactivity (deconditioning). The features include fatigue, lactacidaemia and the subject reaching his or her predicted maximal heart rate at a relatively low level of exercise. performance. Except when there is a heart failure, the condition usually responds to physical training, see Sections 28.12 and 44.4.1. By contrast, in severe respiratory conditions the cardiac output is usually relatively well preserved [19] and the features of limitation centre around breathlessness (Section 28.8).

44.3 Assessment for pulmonary rehabilitation programmes

44.3.1 Perspective

Advanced pulmonary disease limits a patient's ability to perform daily tasks. Initially the limitation applies to activities outside the house e.g. shopping and meeting with people. Later, even activities within the house (such as getting washed and dressed) lead to severe dyspnoea. The patient can then become depressed, isolated and lacking in motivation. It is often these factors as much as the actual reduction in lung function that determine whether a patient with an acute exacerbation of COPD can cope at home or requires admission to hospital.

In these circumstances conventional indices of lung function, such as FVC and FEV_1, may not correlate well with exercise limitation [20] and when exercise performance is improved by rehabilitation there may be little concomitant improvement in spirometry [21]. This suggests that the treatment should not be directed solely to therapies that improve the lung function but also to how the patient is affected by the disease. The relevant features then include psychological as well as physical support and attention to nutrition, body composition, muscle function, and cardiac performance. Physiotherapy and group therapy can make useful contributions.

The first stage in PRP is to measure the relevant characteristics of the disease from the patient's perspective. Without this it is not possible to evaluate the benefit and then assess whether the cost of the programme is justified.

44.3.2 Assessment of breathlessness

Relief of breathlessness on exertion is a principal objective of pulmonary rehabilitation. The symptom is not an 'on off' phenomenon but is experienced differently in the light of past, present and future experiences. For example the physical stress to a subject experiencing breathlessness at the end of sprinting in a 800-m race may be greater than that of a subject in a mild asthma attack but the breathlessness for the latter may be more distressing. The level of distress experienced by the runner may be different if the subject is about to win the race or is coming in last.

Breathlessness arises from many sensory inputs and is a concept made real by the language used to describe it. In order to measure breathlessness it is necessary to construct an agreed framework of language with an appropriate scale (Section 28.7).

In summary, the major methods for measurement of breathlessness are the Borg scale [22] (Table 29.9, page 426), visual analogue scales (VAS) [23] (Fig. 28.17, page 402) and a Medical Research Council (MRC) scale [24] (e.g. Table 44.1).

Table 44.1 Grades of abnormal breathlessness based on questions 8 of the MRC Questionnaire of respiratory symptoms (Fig. 8.2, page 88). The grades can also be defined in other ways (e.g. [24], also Table 38.3, page 532).

Grade	Description
3	The subject walks slower than a healthy person of the same age on the level because of breathlessness or has to stop for breath when walking at own pace on the level
4	Stops for breath after walking about 100 m or after a few minutes on the level
5	Too breathless to leave the house or breathless when dressing or undressing

A study comparing Borg score and VAS [25] indicated that there was large inter-individual variation in the relationship between ventilation during exercise ($\dot{V}_E$) and dyspnoea score, but the Borg score had a tighter relationship with $\dot{V}_E$ and was more repeatable, even up to 1 year [26].

In patients with obstructive lung disease the clinical scores of breathlessness have also been found to correlate with resting lung function in terms of FEV_1 or FVC [27]. Two separate aspects to the description of breathlessness, that is intensity and distress, have been explored [28]. Distress was highly correlated to $\dot{V}_E$ and on average was very repeatable and was scored lower than intensity. The relationship between intensity and distress differed between subjects. The distinction should probably be attempted more often than it is at present.

In the context of COPD the Borg scale or VAS score provide a better guide to general health status compared with conventional lung function tests [29]. However, multi-dimensional tests of respiratory symptoms and performance status (including the MRC grade of breathlessness) may be more effective at detecting improvements than these single scores on their own. The severity of dyspnoea in COPD patients has been found to be a better predictor of 5-year survival than an assessment of severity based on FEV_1 as per cent predicted (ATS) [30]. This indicates the importance of a simple but rigorous clinical evaluation of the patient.

44.3.3 Quality of life assessment

A number of generic Health Related Quality of Life questionnaires have been used in the assessment of patients with lung disease. These include the Quality of Well-Being scale (QWB) [31], the Sickness Impact Profile (SIP) [32], and the short form 36-item questionnaire (SF-36) [33]. Several questionnaires are specific for respiratory patients, including the Chronic Respiratory Questionnaire (CRQ) [34], Asthma Quality of Life (AQL) questionnaire [35], and the St George's Respiratory Questionnaire (SGRQ) [36]. See Table 44.2, also Section 8.2.6.

In COPD patients SGRQ score has been found to be related to Pa,O_2 whereas SIP score was not [38], and so in the context of

COPD and rehabilitation (where both SGRQ and CRQ are applicable and show improvement [1]), the disease specific questionnaires are likely to be more informative than generic ones [39]. It is possible to localise the benefit from a particular intervention by independently analysing the various domains within the questionnaires. For instance, when assessed with SGRQ, a long acting bronchodilator was found to have a significant effect on the psychosocial impact of disease whilst there was no effect on activity [40]. The SF-36 score was not as sensitive as SGRQ in detecting these changes, whilst the concomitant improvement in FEV_1 was small (120 ml) and only weakly correlated with the change in SGRQ score.

44.3.4 Functional assessment

Most PRP involve exercise, so patients for whom exercise might be dangerous should be closely monitored or excluded. Patients in this category include those with FEV_1 less than 20% of predicted, $Pa,o_2 < 7$ kPa, $Pa,co_2 > 7$ kPa (the equivalent in traditional units is 55 mm Hg), and myocardial infarction within 6 months. The hypoxaemia criterion should exclude patients with interstitial fibrosis who are at risk on account of pulmonary hypertension. Thus, initial assessment should include an adequate history and clinical procedures, simple spirometry, preferably also transfer factor (Tl,co), and arterial blood gases when breathing air. The latter tests provide a measure of internal consistency since FEV_1 or Tl,co probably has to fall to less than 50% of the predicted value before either attribute limits exercise performance (cf. Section 30.5.3). Patients whose exercise capacity is much below that expected for their lung function are particularly likely to be helped by PRP.

Functional assessment of ability to exercise must be undertaken. Preferably this should take the form of a progressive exercise test to identify the likely cause of exercise limitation, though there can be difficulty in distinguishing cardiac disease from deconditioning [41]. Where practicable a treadmill should be used as the limiting symptoms are then those likely to be experienced in life. This is not the case for cycle ergometry, except in cyclists (Section 29.4.1), though the numbers obtained using these two forms of ergometry are roughly equivalent [42, 43]. Exercise testing is covered in detail in Chapters 29 to 31.

Non-ergometric and field tests (Section 29.9) can be used to monitor the progress of PRP. They include the 6- and 12-min walk tests [44, 45] and the incremental and endurance shuttle walk tests [46, 47]. The former tests assess aspects of peak and endurance performance and motivation [48]. The results are not very reproducible [49], so their value for assessing improvements over time in a rehabilitation programme is limited. The incremental shuttle test (ISWT) has a high test–re-test correlation ($r \geq 0.98$), and after a single practice run the 95% confidence limits for subsequent test results are fairly tight (± 20 m). The test is more demanding than the self-paced 6-min walk test where the subjects can stop and pause as they wish. As a result with ISWT the final cardiac frequency is higher. The walking speed can be made equivalent to that normally adopted when crossing a road in an urban environment (80 m min^{-1}) [50], whilst the distance walked normally matches that estimated to be necessary to negotiate a community shopping environment [51]. However, these and other performance tests are not substitutes for physiologically orientated exercise testing which should be undertaken where possible.

44.4 Components of pulmonary rehabilitation programmes

Pulmonary rehabilitation is a multi-disciplinary approach to help patients with disabling chronic lung diseases to maximise their activities during daily living. The components of a full programme are given in Table 44.3; they require considerable resources in terms of staff, space, equipment, and time, but those who use the programmes consider them to be cost effective (Section 44.1). Guidelines on establishing such a programme have been written [1, 2, 52]. The lung function laboratory contributes mainly to the exercise conditioning and respiratory muscle training aspects of the programme, including monitoring the responses.

44.4.1 Exercise conditioning

The aim is to increase exercise endurance. This can be achieved for subjects in whom exercise is limited by circulatory factors,

Table 44.2 Summary details on five major quality of life questionnaires.

Name	Domains	No. of items	Administration	Duration
SIP	12	136	Self	15–25
SF-36	8	36	Self	5–10
CRQ	4	20	Interviewer	10–20
SGRQ	3	50	Self	10–15
AQL	4	32	Self	5–15

Source: [37].

Table 44.3 Topics that can be addressed in a pulmonary rehabilitation programme.

Patient education on their disease
Optimising conventional therapy
Smoking cessation*
Long term oxygen therapy*
Exercise conditioning
Respiratory muscle training
Respiratory physiotherapy
Nutritional support
Psychosocial support

* Items that have been shown to prolong life.

including the changes secondary to inactivity. The exercise is best undertaken three or more times per week at no less than 50% of maximum achievable work rate in sessions lasting 20 min or more and extending over 6 weeks (Section 28.12). This type of exercise can be either walking or cycling and lasting improvements in exercise performance can be obtained [53]. Recent evidence suggests this is a true training effect on muscle [54]. However, for the result to be beneficial to the patient the improvement should be demonstrable during walking or climbing stairs rather than during cycling.

Using the upper limbs reduces the stability of the upper thorax and so the inspiratory muscles including the diaphragm work at a disadvantage [55]. As a result upper limb exercise is often more potent at producing dyspnoea than equivalent amounts of leg exercise in patients with COPD. It seems that unsupported arm exercise as part of the programme helps patients with activities used in their daily living [56]. Pulmonary rehabilitation programmes for COPD need to include exercise training that is targeted at these muscles [57].

44.4.2 Respiratory muscle training

The role of respiratory muscle training in COPD rehabilitation is currently not clear [58]. Intuitively it would seem a good approach. Endurance training by low intensity, high frequency exercise can use flow resistive loading, threshold loading or voluntary isocapnic hyperpnoea. Resistive loading is achieved by breathing through a small orifice but the desired loading is only achieved if the tidal volume and inspiratory time are controlled. Threshold loading is achieved by requiring an increased inspiratory or expiratory pressure that is held constant irrespective of the flow achieved. Voluntary hyperpnoea with isocapnia for up to 15 min can also be used to train respiratory muscles. Recent evidence has suggested that respiratory muscle endurance training can increase inspiratory muscle endurance, MEP, 6-min walk distance, peak O_2 uptake, and physical aspects of HRQOL with no effect on dyspnoea, MIP or treadmill endurance [59]. The role of training schedules affecting expiratory as well as inspiratory muscles requires further exploration.

44.5 References

1. American Thoracic Society. Pulmonary rehabilitation – 1999. *Am J Respir Crit Care Med* 1999; **159**: 1666–1682.
2. BTS Standards of Care Subcommittee on Pulmonary Rehabilitation. Pulmonary rehabilitation. *Thorax* 2001; **56**: 827–834.
3. Goldstein RS, Gork EH, Stubbing D et al. Randomised controlled trial of respiratory rehabilitation. *Lancet* 1994; **344**: 1394–1397.
4. Cockroft AE, Saunders MJ, Berry G. Randomised controlled trial of rehabilitation in chronic respiratory disability. *Thorax* 1981; **26**: 200–203.
5. Lacasse Y, Wong E, Guyatt GH et al. Meta-analysis of respiratory rehabilitation in chronic obstructive pulmonary disease. *Lancet* 1996; **348**: 1115–1119.
6. Griffiths TL, Burr ML, Campbell IA et al. Results at 1 year of outpatient multidisciplinary pulmonary rehabilitation: a randomised controlled trial. *Lancet* 2000; **355**: 362–368.
7. Bestall JC, Paul EA, Garrod R et al. Longitudinal trends in exercise capacity and health status after pulmonary rehabilitation in patients with COPD. *Respir Med* 2003; **97**: 173–180.
8. Guell R, Casan P, Belda J et al. Long-term effects of outpatient rehabilitation of COPD: a randomized trial.*Chest* 2000; **117**: 976–983.
9. Regnis JA, Alison JA, Henke KG et al. Changes in end-expiratory lung volume during exercise in cystic fibrosis relate to severity of lung disease. *Am Rev Respir Dis* 1991; **144**: 507–512.
10. Plankeel JF, McMullen B, MacIntyre NR. Exercise outcomes after pulmonary rehabilitation depend on the initial mechanism of exercise limitation among non-oxygen-dependent COPD patients. *Chest* 2005; **127**: 110–116.
11. Bell SC, Saunders MJ, Elborn JS, Shale DJ. Resting energy expenditure and oxygen cost of breathing in patients with cystic fibrosis. *Thorax* 1996; **51**: 126–131.
12. Sridhar MK, Carter R, Lean ME, Banham SW. Resting energy expenditure and nutritional state of patients with increased oxygen cost of breathing due to emphysema, scoliosis and thoracoplasty. *Thorax* 1994; **49**: 781–785.
13. Mannix ET, Manfredi F, Farber MO. Elevated O_2 cost of ventilation contributes to tissue wasting in COPD. *Chest* 1999; **115**: 708–713.
14. Kramer NT, Meyer J, Meharg RD et al. Randomised prospective trial of non-invasive positive pressure ventilation in acute respiratory failure *Am J Respir Crit Care Med* 1995; **151**: 1799–1806.
15. Owens GR, Rogers RM, Pennock BE. The diffusing capacity as a predictor of arterial oxygen desaturation during exercise in patients with chronic obstructive pulmonary disease. *N Engl J Med* 1984; **310**: 1218–1221.
16. Dantzker DR, D'Alonzo GE. The effect of exercise on pulmonary gas exchange in patients with severe chronic obstructive pulmonary disease. *Am Rev Respir Dis* 1986; **134**: 1135–1139.
17. Wagner PD, Dantzker DR, Dueck R et al. Ventilation–perfusion inequality in chronic obstructive pulmonary disease. *J Clin Invest* 1977; **9**: 203–216.
18. Hughes JMB. Diffusive gas exchange. In: Whipp BJ, Wasserman K, eds. *Exercise: pulmonary physiology and pathophysiology.. Lung Biology in Health and Disease*, vol 52. New York: Marcel Dekker, 1991: 143–171.
19. Diaz O, Iglesia R, Ferrer M et al. Effects of non-invasive ventilation on pulmonary gas exchange and hemodynamics during acute hypercapnic exacerbations of chronic obstructive pulmonary disease. *Am J Respir Crit Care Med* 1997; **156**: 1840–1845.
20. Killian KJ, LeBlanc P, Martin DH et al. Exercise capacity and ventilatory, circulatory, and symptom limitation in patients with chronic airflow limitation. *Am Rev Respir Dis* 1992; **146**: 935–940.
21. Griffiths TL, Burr ML, Campbell IA et al. Results at 1 year of outpatient multidisciplinary pulmonary rehabilitation: a randomised controlled trial. *Lancet* 2000; **355**: 362–368.
22. Borg G. Psychophysical bases of perceived exertion. *Med Sci Sports Exerc* 1982; **14**: 377–381.
23. Aitken RCB. Measurement of feelings using visual analogue scales. *Proc R Soc Med* 1969; **62**: 989–993.
24. Altose MD. Assessment and management of breathlessness. *Chest* 1985; **88**(Suppl): 77–83.

25. Wilson RC, Jones PW. A comparison of the visual analogue scale and modified Borg scale for the measurement of dyspnoea during exercise. *Clin Sci* 1989; **76**: 277–282.
26. Wilson RC, Jones PW. Long-term reproducibility of Borg scale estimates of breathlessness during exercise. *Clin Sci* 1991; **80**: 309–312.
27. Mahler DA, Rosiello RA, Harver A et al. Comparison of clinical dyspnoea ratings and psychophysical measurements of respiratory sensation in obstructive airway disease. *Am Rev Respir Dis* 1987; **135**: 1229–1233.
28. Wilson RC, Jones PW. Differentiation between the intensity of breathlessness and the distress it evokes in normal subjects during exercise. *Clin Sci* 1991; **80**: 65–70.
29. Mahler DA, Harver A. A factor analysis of dyspnoea ratings, respiratory muscle strength, and lung function in patients with chronic obstructive pulmonary disease. *Am Rev Respir Dis* 1992; **145**: 467–470.
30. Nishimura K, Izumi T, Tsukino M, Oga T. Dyspnea is a better predictor of 5-year survival than airway obstruction in patients with COPD. *Chest* 2002; **121**: 1434–1440.
31. Kaplan RM, Atkins CJ, Timms R. Validity of a quality of well-being scale as an outcome measure in chronic obstructive pulmonary disease. *J Chronic Dis* 1984; **37**: 85–95.
32. Bergner M, Bobbitt RA, Carter WB et al. The Sickness Impact Profile: development and final revision of a health status measure. *Med Care* 1981; **19**: 787–805.
33. Ware JE Jnr, Sherbourne CD. The MOS 36-item short-form health survey (SF-36). 1. Conceptual framework and item selection. *Med Care* 1992; **30**: 473–483.
34. Guyatt GH, Berman LB, Townsend M et al. A measure of quality of life for clinical trials in chronic lung disease. Thorax 1987; **42**: 773–778.
35. Juniper EF, Guyatt GH. Evaluation of impairment of health related quality of life in asthma: development of a questionnaire for use in clinical trials. *Thorax* 1992; **47**: 76–83.
36. Jones PW, Quirk FH, Baveystock CM, Littlejohns P. A self-complete measure of health status for chronic airflow limitation. The St George's Respiratory Questionnaire. *Am Rev Respir Dis* 1992; **145**: 1321–1327.
37. Mahler DA, Jones PW. Measurement of dyspnoea and quality of life in advanced lung disease. *Clin Chest Med* 1997; **18**: 457–470.
38. Okubadejo AA, Jones PW, Wedzicha JA. Quality of life in patients with chronic obstructive pulmonary disease and severe hypoxaemia. *Thorax* 1996; **51**: 44–47.
39. Singh SJ, Sodergreen SC, Hyland ME et al. A comparison of three disease-specific and two generic health-status measures to evaluate the outcome of pulmonary rehabilitation. *Respir Med* 2001; **95**: 71–77.
40. Jones PW, Bosh TK. Quality of life changes in COPD patients treated with salmeterol. *Am J Respir Crit Care Med* 1997; **155**: 1283–1289.
41. Martinez FJ, Stanopoulos I, Acero R et al. Graded comprehensive cardiopulmonary exercise testing in the evaluation of dyspnoea unexplained by routine evaluation. *Chest* 1994; **105**: 168–174.
42. Mathur RS, Revill SM, Vara DD et al. Comparison of peak oxygen consumption during cycle and treadmill exercise in severe chronic obstructive pulmonary disease. *Thorax* 1995; **50**: 829–833.
43. Ries AL, Moser KM. Predicting treadmill-walking speed from the cycle ergometry exercise in chronic obstructive pulmonary disease. *Am Rev Respir Dis* 1982; **126**: 924–927.
44. Butland RJA, Pang J, Gross ER et al. Two-, six-, and 12-minute walking tests in respiratory disease. *Br Med J* 1982; **284**; 1607–1608.
45. McGavin CR, Gupta SP, McHardy GJR. Twelve-minute walking test for assessing disability in chronic bronchitis. *Br Med J* 1976; **1**: 822–823.
46. Singh SJ, Morgan MDL, Scott S et al. Development of a shuttle walking test of disability in patients with chronic airways obstruction. *Thorax* 1992; **47**: 1019–1024.
47. Revill SM, Morgan MDL, Singh SJ et al. The endurance shuttle walk test: a new field test for assessment of endurance capacity in chronic obstructive pulmonary disease. *Thorax* 1999; **54**: 213–222.
48. Guyatt GH, Pugsley SO, Sullivan MJ et al. Effect of encouragement on walking test performance. *Thorax* 1984; **39**: 818–822.
49. Knox AJ, Morrison JFJ, Muers MF. Reproducibility of walking test results in chronic obstructive airways disease. *Thorax* 1988; **43**: 388–392.
50. Fisher SV, Gullickson G. Energy cost of ambulation in health and disability: a literature review. *Arch Phys Med Rehabil* 1978; **59**: 124–133.
51. Lerner-Frankiel MB, Vargas S, Brown MB et al. Functional community ambulation: what are your criteria? *Clin Manag Phys Ther* 1986; **6**: 12–15.
52. Clark CJ. Setting up a pulmonary rehabilitation programme. *Thorax* 1994; **49**: 270–278.
53. Troosters T, Gosselink R, Decramer M. Short- and long-term effects of outpatient rehabilitation in patients with chronic obstructive pulmonary disease: a randomised trial. *Am J Med* 2000; **109**: 207–212.
54. Maltais F, Le Blanc P, Simard C et al. Skeletal muscle adaptation to endurance training in patients with chronic obstructive pulmonary disease. *Am J Respir Crit Care Med* 1996; **154**: 442–447.
55. Criner GJ, Celli BR. Effect of unsupported arm exercise on ventilatory muscle recruitment in patients with severe chronic airflow obstruction. *Am Rev Respir Dis* 1988; **138**: 856–861.
56. Martinez F, Montes de Oca M, Whyte R et al. Supported arm exercise vs. unsupported arm exercise in the rehabilitation of patients with severe chronic airflow obstruction. *Chest* 1993; **103**: 1397–1402.
57. Lacasse Y, Guyatt GH, Goldstein RS. The components of a respiratory rehabilitation program: a systematic overview. *Chest* 1997; **111**: 1077–1088.
58. Smith K, Cook D, Guyatt GH et al. Respiratory muscle training in chronic airflow limitation: a meta-analysis. *Am Rev Respir Dis* 1992; **145**: 533–539.
59. Scherer TA, Spengler CM, Owassapian D et al. Respiratory muscle endurance training in chronic obstructive pulmonary disease: impact on exercise capacity, dyspnoea, and quality of life. *Am J Respir Crit Care Med* 2000; **162**: 1709–1714.

Further reading

Adams L, Guz A, eds. *Respiratory sensation.* New York: Marcel Dekker . *Lung Biology in Health and Disease.* 1996; **90**.

Donner CF, Decramer M, eds. Pulmonary rehabilitation. *Eur Respir Mon* 2000; **13**: 1–200.

Whipp BJ, Wasserman K, eds. *Pulmonary physiology and pathophysiology.* New York: Marcel Dekker. *Lung Biology in Health and Disease.* 1991; **52**.

Index

Note: page numbers in *italics* refer to figures, those in **bold** refer to tables.

Printed and bound in the UK by
CPI Antony Rowe, Eastbourne